Head and Neck Pathology

HEAD AND NECK PATHOLOGY

With Clinical Correlations

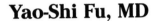

Yao-Shi Fu, MD
Senior Pathologist
Chief of Anatomic Pathology
Department of Pathology
Northridge Hospital Medical Center
Northridge, California

Bruce M. Wenig, MD
Professor of Pathology
Vice Chairman for Anatomic Pathology
Albert Einstein College of Medicine/
Montefiore Medical Center
Bronx, New York

Elliot Abemayor, MD, PhD
Professor and Vice Chief
Division of Head and Neck Surgery
University of California at Los Angeles
Los Angeles, California

Barry L. Wenig, MD, MPH
Professor of Otolaryngology–Head and Neck Surgery
Northwestern University Medical School
Director, Division of Head and Neck Surgery
Evanston Northwestern Hospital
Chicago, Illinois

Illustrator: Phillip Ashley Associates,
Philadelphia, Pennsylvania

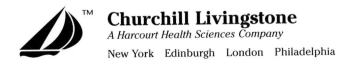

Churchill Livingstone
A Harcourt Health Sciences Company
New York   Edinburgh   London   Philadelphia

CHURCHILL LIVINGSTONE
A Harcourt Health Sciences Company

The Curtis Center
Independence Square West
Philadelphia, Pennsylvania 19106

Library of Congress Cataloging-in-Publication Data

Head and neck pathology with clinical correlations / [edited by] Yao-Shi Fu . . . [et al.].
        p. ; cm.
      Includes bibliographical references.
      ISBN 0-443-07558-1
      1. Head—Pathophysiology.   2. Neck—Pathophysiology.
      [DNLM: 1. Head—pathology.   2. Head and Neck Neoplasms—pathology.   3. Neck—
pathology.   WE 705 H4308 2001]   I. Fu, Yao S.
      RC936 .H4335   2001
      617.5'107—dc21

                                                                00–064377

Acquisitions Editor: Marc Strauss
Developmental Editor: Joanne Husovski

HEAD AND NECK PATHOLOGY WITH CLINICAL CORRELATIONS   ISBN 0–443–07558–1

Printed in the United States of America.

Last digit is the print number: 9   8   7   6   5   4   3   2   1

To my mentors Dr. Raffaele Lattes and Dr. Karl H. Perzin for their teaching and encouragement. To my family Anne, Karin, Victor, and Eva for their support. To all the contributors of this book for their great work!

Yao-Shi Fu, MD

To my family, my wife Ana and our children Sarah, Eli, and Jake, with love.

Bruce Wenig, MD

This book is dedicated to my past and present teachers. I am forever indebted to Paul H. Ward, MD, who gave me my roots and taught me the basics and subtleties of head and neck surgery. I am thankful to call Thomas C. Calcaterra, MD friend and colleague; he is a continuous and generous source of knowledge and innovation. And lastly, I thank all the members of my family, who continue to teach me the redemptive power of unconditional love.

Elliot Abemayor, MD, PhD

Although the production of a text involves countless individuals who labor and strive for excellence, it is an impossible task to adequately acknowledge all involved. For that I wish to apologize and offer collective thanks. I would like to single out, however, two groups of individuals who have had a direct bearing on my contribution to this text. For the past twenty years both my teachers and students have persistently and continuously challenged and educated me. Without their influence, my contribution to this work would not have been possible. I would also like to thank my family for just being themselves and for always being there even through the rough times. Words are inadequate to convey my feelings.

Barry Wenig, MD, MPH

To our parents, Sidonia and Louis Wenig for their love and support.

Bruce and Barry Wenig

Contributors

ELLIOT ABEMAYOR, MD, PhD
Professor and Vice Chief, Division of Head and Neck Surgery, University of California at Los Angeles School of Medicine, Los Angeles, California.

CAROL F. ADAIR, MD
Adjunct Clinical Professor, Department of Pathology, Uniformed Services University of Health Sciences, Bethesda, Maryland; Program Director, Pathology Residency Training Program, Walter Reed Army Medical Center, Washington, DC.

EDWARD L. APPLEBAUM, MD
Francis J. Lederer Professor, Chair, Department of Otolaryngology–Head and Neck Surgery, University of Illinois at Chicago School of Medicine, Chicago, Illinois.

B. HILL BRITTON, BA, MD
Professor Emeritus, Department of Otorhinolaryngology, Oklahoma University Health Sciences Center, Oklahoma City, Oklahoma.

JOHN F. CAREW, MD
Assistant Professor, Department of Otorhinolaryngology–Head and Neck Surgery, Cornell University Medical Center; New York Presbyterian Hospital, New York, New York.

THOMAS E. CAREY, PhD
Distinguished Research Scientist, Department of Otolaryngology–Head and Neck Surgery, University of Michigan Medical School, Ann Arbor, Michigan.

GEORGE D. CHONKICH, MD
Associate Professor of Surgery, Loma Linda University School of Medicine; Attending Physician, Loma Linda University Medical Center; Chief, Head and Neck Section, Department of Surgery, Loma Linda Veterans Administration Hospital, Loma Linda, California.

PETER D. COSTANTINO, MD
Co-Director, Cranial Base Surgery Center; Associate Professor, Department of Otolaryngology, Neurosurgery, and Oromaxillofacial Surgery, Mount Sinai School of Medicine, New York, New York.

PAUL DAGUM, MD, PhD
Cardiothoracic Research Fellow, Department of Cardiothoracic Surgery, Stanford University Hospital, Stanford, California.

KENNETH DEVANEY
Associate Professor, Department of Pathology, University of Michigan Medical Center, Ann Arbor, Michigan.

BRIAN E. DUFF, MD
Assistant Professor, Department of Otolaryngology, Tufts University School of Medicine, Boston, Massachusetts; Assistant Clinical Professor, Department of Surgery, Division of Otolaryngology, Brown University School of Medicine; Director of Otology, Neurotology, Skull Base Surgery, Rhode Island Hospital/Hasbro Children's Hospital, Providence, Rhode Island.

LEWIS EVERSOLE, DDS, MSD
Professor, Department of Pathology, University of the Pacific School of Dentistry, San Francisco, California.

WILLARD E. FEE, JR., MD
Edward and Amy Sewall Professor, Division of Otolaryngology–Head and Neck Surgery, Stanford University Medical Center, Stanford, California.

SARAH S. FRANKEL, MD
Staff Pathologist, Department of Infectious and Parasitic Disease Pathology, Armed Forces Institute of Pathology, Washington, DC; Pathologist, Division of Retrovirology, Walter Reed Army Institute of Research, Rockville, Maryland.

JAMES E. FREIJE, MD
Fayetteville, New York.

YAO-SHI FU, MD
Senior Pathologist, Chief, Anatomic Pathology, Department of Pathology, Northridge Hospital Medical Center, Northridge, California.

JOHN GOLDENBERG, MD
Otolaryngology Associates LLC; Clinical Assistant Professor of Otolaryngology–Head and Neck Surgery, Indiana University School of Medicine, Bloomington, Indiana.

GLEN D. HOUSTON, DDS, MSD
Professor and Chair, Department of Oromaxillofacial Pathology, Professor, Department of Pathology, Colleges of Dentistry and Medicine, University of Oklahoma Medical Center; Staff Pathologist, University Hospital; Veterans Affairs Medical Center; Children's Hospital of Oklahoma, Oklahoma City, Oklahoma.

GERNOT JUNDT, MD
Professor of Pathology, Institute of Pathology, Kantonsspital, University Clinics; Head, Bone Tumor Reference Center and Central Registry of DÖSAK, Basel, Switzerland.

MICHAEL KAPLAN, MD
University of California at San Francisco/Stanford Healthcare, Head and Neck Surgery, San Francisco, California.

ROBERT M. KELLMAN, MD
Professor and Chair, Department of Otolaryngology and Communication Sciences, State University New York, Upstate Medical University, Syracuse, New York.

DENNIS H. KRAUS, MD
Assistant Attending Surgeon, Head and Neck Service, Director, Speech, Hearing, and Rehabilitation Center, Department of Surgery, Memorial Sloan–Kettering Cancer Center, New York, New York.

LESTER J. LAYFIELD, MD
Professor, Department of Pathology, University of Utah School of Medicine, Salt Lake City, Utah.

VIRGINIA A. LIVOLSI, MD
Professor of Pathology, University of Pennsylvania; Surgical Pathology Section, Hospital of the University of Pennsylvania, Philadelphia, Pennsylvania.

JESUS E. MEDINA, MD
Paul and Ruth Jonas Professor and Chair, Department of Otolaryngology, Oklahoma University School of Medicine, Oklahoma City, Oklahoma.

KATHLEEN T. MONTONE, MD
Staff Pathologist, Department of Pathology, Abington Memorial Hospital, Abington, Pennsylvania.

SCOTT D. NELSON, MD
Associate Professor, Department of Pathology, University of California at Los Angeles School of Medicine, Los Angeles, California.

DAVID OSGUTHORPE, MD
Professor, Department of Otolaryngology, Medical University of South Carolina, Charleston, South Carolina.

KARL H. PERZIN, MD
Professor Emeritus of Clinical Surgical Pathology, College of Physicians and Surgeons of Columbia University; Attending Surgical Pathologist Emeritus, New York, New York.

GEORGE H. PETTI, JR., MD
Professor of Surgery, Division of Head and Neck Surgery, Loma Linda University Health Sciences Center; Attending Surgeon, Jerry Pettis Veterans Affairs Hospital, Loma Linda, California; Riverside Regional University Medical Center, Riverside, California.

SCOTT E. PHILLIPS, MD
Staff Otolaryngologist, Missouri Baptist Medical Center, St. Louis, Missouri.

LOUIS G. PORTUGAL, MD
Associate Professor, Department of Otolaryngology–Head and Neck Surgery, Director, Division of Head and Neck Surgery, University of Illinois at Chicago School of Medicine; Attending Physician, Veterans Administration Westside Medical Center, Chicago, Illinois.

JOACHIM PREIN, MD, DMD
Professor, Department of Maxillofacial Surgery, Head, Clinic for Reconstructive Surgery, University Hospital/Kantonsspital, Clinic for Reconstructive Surgery, Basel, Switzerland.

JAMES E. SAUNDERS, MD
Assistant Professor, Department of Otorhinolaryngology, University of Oklahoma Medical School, Health Sciences Center, Oklahoma City, Oklahoma.

STIMSON P. SCHANTZ, MD
Professor, Department of Otolaryngology, New York Medical College, Westchester, New York; Chief, Head and Neck Surgery, New York Eye and Ear Infirmary; Director, Head and Neck Laboratory, Strang Cancer Prevention Center, New York, New York.

RAINER SCHMELZEISEN, MD, DDS, PhD
Professor and Chair, Universitätsklinik für Zahn-, Mund-, und Kieferheilkunde, Abteilung Klinik und Poliklinik für Mund-, Kiefer-, und Gesichtschirurgie, Freiburg, Germany.

GLENN J. SCHWARTZ, MD
Attending Physician, Northwest Community Hospital, Arlington Heights, Illinois.

LEE J. SLATER, MS, DDS
Associate Professor, Department of Oral Pathology, School of Dental Medicine, University of Pittsburgh, Pittsburgh, Pennsylvania; Staff Pathologist, Department of Oral Pathology, Armed Forces Institute of Pathology, Washington, DC; Scripps Oral Pathology Service, San Diego, California.

LESTER D. R. THOMPSON, MD
Chief, Otorhinolaryngic–Head and Neck Pathology Division, Assistant Chair, Department of Scientific Laboratories, Armed Forces Institute of Pathology, Washington, DC.

MARILENE WANG, MD
Associate Professor, Division of Head and Neck Surgery, University of California at Los Angeles School of Medicine; Chief of Otolaryngology, VA Greater Los Angeles Healthcare System, Los Angeles, California.

PAUL H. WARD, MD
Professor and Chief Emeritus, Division of Head and Neck Surgery, University of California at Los Angeles School of Medicine, Los Angeles, California.

BARRY L. WENIG, MD, MPH
Director, Division of Head and Neck Surgery, Professor, Department of Otolaryngology–Head and Neck Surgery, Northwestern University Medical School, Chicago, Illinois.

BRUCE M. WENIG, MD
Professor, Department of Pathology, Vice Chair, Anatomic Pathology, Albert Einstein College of Medicine/Montefiore Medical Center, Bronx, New York.

JOHAN WENNERBERG, MD, PhD
Professor, Medical Faculty, University of Lund; Head, Clinical Department, Senior Surgeon, Department of Otorhinolaryngology–Head and Neck Surgery, University Hospital of Lund, Lund, Sweden.

PEAK WOO, MD
Associate Professor, Mount Sinai School of Medicine, Mount Sinai Medical Center, New York, New York.

SOOK-BIN WOO, MMSc, DMD
Assistant Professor, Department of Oral Medicine and Diagnostic Sciences, Harvard School of Dental Medicine; Attending Dentist, Division of Oral Medicine and Dentistry, Brigham and Women's Hospital, Boston, Massachusetts; Staff Pathologist, Pathology Services, Inc., Cambridge, Massachusetts.

GUOPEI YU, MD, MPH
Head, Epidemiology and Statistics Service, New York Eye and Ear Infirmary, New York, New York.

Preface

The initial concept and focus of this textbook were to produce a book that was primarily pathology driven. The approach was to include detailed discussions of the array of pathologic conditions that occur in the head and neck region. It became apparent to us early in the development of this textbook that complementary detailed discussions of the clinical parameters of each disease entity would be required to make this a valuable resource for health professionals interested in diseases of the head and neck. These considerations led us to entitle this textbook *Head and Neck Pathology with Clinical Correlations*.

The simplest way to accomplish the clinical correlation component of the book would have been to have pathologists fill in these clinical details. However, we felt that to produce the best textbook on head and neck diseases a collaborative effort between pathologists and clinical specialists was required. This approach would simulate the realities of daily clinical practice whereby the clinician and pathologist work as a team in the management of patients with head and neck diseases. To this end, the clinicians who have contributed to this text are renowned surgical specialists in the field of otorhinolaryngology. Similarly, the contributing pathologists are experts in head and neck pathology. This combined approach utilizing experts in clinical otolaryngology and experts in the pathology of head and neck diseases distinguishes this textbook from other textbooks on head and neck diseases that tend to be authored only by clinicians or only by pathologists. Our approach maximizes the usefulness of this textbook and makes it a valuable resource to a wide readership, including medical students, residents in pathology and otolaryngology, and practicing pathologists and otolaryngologists at all levels in their careers.

From a practical standpoint, this book is divided into the anatomic sites that make up the head and neck region. These sites include the sinonasal tract, oral cavity, pharynx, larynx, neck, thyroid gland, parathyroid gland, and the ear and temporal bone. The diseases of these anatomic sites are covered in depth, integrating the clinical parameters with the pathologic features. The clinical details include disease demographics, clinical presentation, epidemiology, treatment, and prognosis. The pathologic features include detailed descriptions of the gross pathology and histopathology, supplemented with appropriate ancillary studies such as histochemistry, immunohistochemistry, electron microscopy, and molecular biology evaluation. Dedicated chapters addressing the ethical considerations of the patient with head and neck disease, pathogenetic mechanisms of head and neck disease, fine-needle aspiration biopsy of head and neck lesions, and the head and neck manifestations of acquired immune deficiency syndrome are also included.

This textbook covers virtually every disease of the head and neck region. A notable exception is the exclusion of cervical lymph node hematolymphoid lesions, including lymphomas. Site specific (sinonasal, salivary gland, and so forth) hematolymphoid lesions are covered, but we felt that the topic of nodal-based hematolymphoid lesions was too expansive and would require an inordinate amount of textbook space to cover adequately. Further, a dedicated section on nodal-based hematolymphoid lesions would have precluded discussion of other head and neck diseases. For this reason, we decided not to address hematolymphoid lesions in this textbook; the reader is referred to "stand alone" texts on nodal hematolymphoid lesions for a detailed description of these diseases.

We wish to thank all the contributors who dedicated their time and effort in making this a valuable addition to medical literature. We would also like to thank our publisher Churchill Livingstone, specifically Marc Strauss and Joanne Husovski for their assistance and guidance throughout the entire development of this book.

Yao-Shi Fu, MD
Bruce M. Wenig, MD
Elliot Abemayor, MD, PhD
Barry L. Wenig, MD, MPH

Contents

HEAD AND NECK PATHOLOGY

PART I

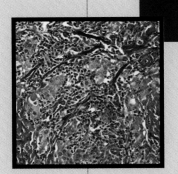

General Principles

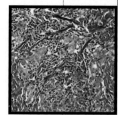

Cellular and Molecular Biology of the Cancer Cell

- THOMAS E. CAREY
- JOHAN WENNERBERG

OVERVIEW

This chapter is a summary of current views on molecular genetic changes in the cancer cell in general and in head and neck cancer in particular. Cancer of the head and neck comprises a wide variety of histologic types of tumors, but more than 80% are squamous cell carcinomas. Other head and neck tumors include thyroid and salivary gland carcinomas, adenocarcinomas of the sinonasal tract, esthesioneuroblastomas of the olfactory system, sarcomas of the facial bones, nasopharyngeal carcinomas, primary lymphomas in the tonsils and neck, malignant melanomas of the mucous membranes, as well as glomus tumors and acoustic neuromas arising in the inner ear. In addition, there are benign papillomas of the larynx, nose, and paranasal sinuses, as well as occasional squamous carcinomas arising from these benign precursors. Generally, this chapter discusses molecular mechanisms in head and neck squamous cell carcinomas (HNSCCs), but specific examples that have been worked out in other tumors may also be used for illustration.

Neoplasia and Tumor Progression

Neoplasia can be defined as all focal proliferative lesions, benign tumors, primary cancers, and metastases that may affect any given cell system.[1] Precursor states to invasive cancer are proliferative lesions and atypical cells confined to a single tissue compartment with a limited growth span and only rare examples of progression to cancer. Focal abnormal cell proliferation results in areas of increased cell number or areas of hyperplasia, whereas tissue hypertrophy is growth that causes an increase in cell mass within a tissue compartment. Hyperplasia may or may not involve atypia. Atypia describes individual cells with abnormal nuclear architecture. Dysplasia, on the other hand, refers to anomalous tissue organization. Dysplastic lesions are usually confined to a single tissue compartment and may progress to cancer, but do not always do so. Carcinomas in situ (CIS) or intraepithelial neoplasia are lesions that have the morphologic characteristics of cancer, including atypical cells and dysplastic tissue organization, but that, by definition, are confined to one tissue compartment and do not penetrate the basement membrane. In invasive cancer, the proliferating lesion is found growing in two or more tissue compartments; that is, it shows invasion through the basement membrane. These characteristic lesions have been well defined in the squamous epithelium of the uterine cervix, and similar lesions have been found in the upper aerodigestive tract (UADT) as well. Leukoplakia (leukoplasia) and erythroplasia are two types of premalignant lesions found in the UADT epithelium. Leukoplakia is a white, plaque-like lesion that can spread over wide areas, particularly in the oral cavity. This lesion, which may expand and contract over time, consists of mucosal cells that exhibit aberrant keratinization. Leukoplakias have a 1.5% to 6% annual rate of neoplastic progression and are frequently associated with smoking, oral tobacco or betel nut use, and diets lacking in vitamins of the carotenoid family.[2,3] Erythroplasia is a red lesion that can exhibit severe dysplasia. This type of lesion is less common than leukoplakias, but has a higher probability of progressing to invasive carcinoma. Although premalignant lesions do play a role in HNSCC development, most head and neck tumors appear to arise de novo, rather than from a recognizable premalignant lesion.

The ability to divide indefinitely, to overcome what is termed cellular or replicative senescence, is closely linked to tumor development, but is probably not a prerequisite for the early stages of carcinogenesis.[4] Most eukaryotic cells from higher organisms that can divide in vitro cannot do so indefinitely; they are said to have a finite replicative life span. This so-called in vitro senescence was first described for human fibroblasts in culture.[5] Because of the innate clock that limits the number of replications for a given cell, normal cells can be cultivated in vitro through only a limited number of passages unless they are transformed. Transformation involves immortalization and acquisition of a driving force to divide, characteristics which give cultivated cells the ability to achieve an unlimited number of passages in vitro. Immortalization is distinct from tumorigenicity, which is the ability to induce a tumor in vivo as, for example, when inoculated into immunodeficient animals, such as athymic mice and rats.

The development of neoplasia is a process of clonal expansion and clonal evolution. Initial events may affect the pathways that control the cell cycle. Later events appear to alter functions associated with tissue organization, cellular migration, and failure to respond to death signals. The clonal-evolution model of tumor progression, originally proposed by Nowell,[6] postulates that a transformed cell acquires successive genetic alterations and develops a proliferative advantage over other clones in a tumor. These acquired changes result in alterations in cellular behavior that are the hallmarks of malignant tumor cells, such as invasion, migration, angiogenesis, and the capacity for metastatic spread. Clonal expansion and clonal evolution are thought to be driven by genetic or epigenetic changes that affect expression of genes that regulate normal homeostasis. Chemical or physical mutagenesis and viral oncogenesis are thought to be the major pathways leading to neoplasia.

Carcinogenesis and Etiology of Head and Neck Cancer

CIGARETTES, ORAL TOBACCO, AND ETHANOL

For HNSCC, the links between carcinogen exposure and tumor development are well-established.[7] Cigarette smoking, in particular, is a common etiologic factor, and in many patients, this is accompanied by heavy ethanol consumption. The combined effects of smoking and alcohol appear to be more than additive.[8-10] This relationship is demonstrated in Figure 1-1.[11] In support of smoking and drinking as important etiologic factors is the fact that most patients with HNSCC are older men with long histories of heavy smoking and alcohol abuse. The number of women with HNSCC has increased in proportion to the increased incidence of smoking among women. Interestingly, the risk for cancer seems to be par-

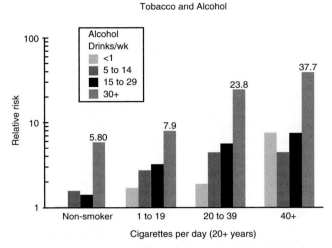

FIGURE 1-1 Combined effects of tobacco and alcohol on the risk of developing cancer. Adapted from Blot WJ, McLaughlin JK, Winn DM, et al. Smoking and drinking in relation to oral and pharyngeal cancer. *Cancer Res.* 1988; 48:3282–3287, with permission.

tially site-dependent within the oral cavity. For example, within the oral cavity, the percentage of cases of HNSCC in which smoking history is a factor ranges from 97% in cases of floor of the mouth (FOM) cancer to 64% in cases of cancer of the tongue, and only 50% of cases of gingival cancer.[12] The likelihood that smoking is a factor in FOM cancer is 32 times that for patients with gingival cancer. These figures suggest that there are other contributing etiologic factors involved in the genesis of head and neck cancers at different sites.

An increase in numerical and structural chromosomal rearrangements in the normal mucosa of smokers compared to nonsmokers has been reported.[13] This is consistent with the concept that carcinogens in tobacco smoke cause mutations that lead to aberrant cell growth. Tobacco smoke contains at least 40 known carcinogens. Carcinogens can bind to DNA, form adducts that interfere with DNA replication, and induce heritable errors in the DNA sequence. Carcinogens may also interfere with DNA repair. It has been shown that the frequency of p53 mutations in HNSCC is higher in tobacco users than in nonusers (33% vs. 17%) and even higher (58%) in smokers who also drink alcohol.[14] Because p53 is intimately involved in the cell cycle checkpoint required for DNA repair, mutations of this gene may increase the frequency of new mutations in subsequent cell divisions.

Although probably no one completely escapes morbidity from smoking, only about 10% of heavy smokers and drinkers develop HNSCC, suggesting that there may be a constitutional individual susceptibility to carcinogen-induced mutations. Many carcinogens require biotransformation to exert their activity. Thus, differences in carcinogen metabolism may affect individual susceptibility. In fact, there are large interindividual variations in the activity of a

number of enzymes implicated in carcinogen metabolism, such as arylhydrocarbon hydroxylase (AHH) and glutathione-S-transferase (GST). The ability to detoxify or to activate carcinogens effectively may be a result of the relative activity of these metabolizing enzymes. Patients in whom HNSCC develops may also have increased mutagen sensitivity as determined by bleomycin-induced chromatid breaks, when compared to individuals without cancer or patients with cancers not associated with carcinogens.[15] There is a dramatic increase in the odds ratios for head and neck cancer in mutagen-hypersensitive people who are also heavy smokers.[16] Further support for differences in susceptibility comes from lung cancer studies that indicate that, for a given level of smoking, blacks are at higher risk than whites, and women are at a higher risk than men.[17] Furthermore, among patients with lung cancer, the levels of aromatic/hydrophobic DNA adducts are higher in women than in men when adjusted for smoking dose.[18] This suggests the existence of important differences in the smoking-associated risk for lung cancer dependent upon sex and race. Whether this is also true for HNSCC has not yet been established.

The use of alcohol potentiates the carcinogenic effects of smoking. Possible mechanisms for alcohol-related carcinogenesis have been discussed by Kato and Nomura.[19] Ethanol per se is not mutagenic unless it is metabolized to acetaldehyde and superoxide. These metabolites are mutagenic and cytotoxic. Acetaldehyde is also carcinogenic. Alcohol can also promote carcinogenesis by solubilizing carcinogens from cigarette smoke, which may increase entry into cells, and by stimulating cell proliferation, which may facilitate mutagenic events. In addition, there are additives in many alcoholic drinks, such as the nitrosamines in beers made with open-fired hops, which may be mutagenic or carcinogenic.

In Asia, there is a high incidence of oral cancer related to the use of various forms of chewing tobacco and betel nut.[20] In the United States, chewing tobacco has been implicated as a major risk factor in oral cancer,[21] and the International Agency for Research on Cancer (IARC)[22] has concluded that oral tobacco is hazardous. Carcinogenic metabolites of tobacco-specific nitrosamines are found systemically in users of smokeless tobacco, which shows that these substances, which include specific metabolites linked to the development of leukoplakia, are absorbed and converted in the body, supporting the conclusion that smokeless tobacco products are dangerous.[23] Curiously, the risk of cancer from oral tobacco use has not been confirmed in Scandinavia where up to 15% of adult men use, or have used, moist oral snuff. A plausible explanation for the difference in cancer incidence in various geographic areas might be that Scandinavian oral snuff and chewing tobacco contain different amounts of carcinogenic agents owing to variations in added ingredients and in the production process. For example,

Scandinavian moist snuff is not fermented, but other types of snuff do go through a fermentation process. Fermentation of tobaccos can increase the amount of nitrosamines up to 10-fold.

VIRUSES

Epstein-Barr Virus

The Epstein-Barr virus (EBV) is an accepted etiologic factor in African Burkitt's lymphoma and in nasopharyngeal carcinoma in China. EBV infection is widespread in the world's population. On the basis of serologic studies, 80% to 90% of adults have been infected at some time with the virus. Presumably, EBV infects children early in life, as most individuals are seropositive for antibodies to EBV antigens by the time they are in their teens. Most people have no recognizable illness resulting from EBV infection, perhaps because infection may occur while the child is still protected by maternally transmitted EBV antibodies. Infectious mononucleosis (IM), a lingering but self-limiting disease characterized by swollen lymph nodes, sore throat, and unusual fatigue, is an exception. IM, also known as the kissing disease because it affects adolescents and college students, was linked to EBV infection by serologic studies performed on Yale University students. IM did not develop in students who were seropositive for EBV antibodies at entry into the study, but IM was frequently diagnosed among those in the seronegative group. Furthermore, those who developed IM became seropositive.[24]

It remains a mystery why, of the many people who are infected with EBV, only a few develop tumors related to this virus. The identification of EBV as a factor in Burkitt's lymphoma and nasopharyngeal carcinoma resulted from in vitro studies of cultured Burkitt's lymphoma cells and serologic studies of patients with both diseases. Denis Burkitt[25] postulated that the jaw lymphomas he described in central Africa were likely to have an infectious etiology because the cases tended to be clustered in time and space, with multiple cases occurring in the same village at the same time. Epstein and Barr[26] strengthened this hypothesis by placing Burkitt's lymphoma cells in culture and then demonstrating, by electron microscopic studies, that the cultured cells were producing a virus that belonged to the herpes virus family. Subsequent serologic studies showed that antigens induced by EBV are expressed in Burkitt's lymphoma cells, and that patients with Burkitt's lymphoma have elevated levels of antibodies to these antigens.[27] As a result of these findings, EBV is accepted to be the etiologic agent of this disease.

B lymphocytes express the receptor for the third component of complement (C3d), which also serves as a receptor for EBV, making these cells a natural target of EBV infection.[28] In vitro, EBV can infect and immortalize B lymphocytes, provided that the T lymphocytes in the cultures are suppressed by cy-closporin A.[29] EBV was linked to nasopharyngeal carcinoma (NPC) by serologic assays that revealed a high level of EBV antigens in NPC extracts and the presence of antibody to EBV antigens in sera from patients with NPC.[27,30] Burkitt's lymphomas and NPCs each express EBV-encoded antigens, such as Epstein-Barr virus nuclear antigen (EBNA) and latent membrane protein 1 (LMP1). NPCs are poorly differentiated epithelial tumors that arise from regions of the nasopharynx that are rich in lymphoid deposits (Waldeyer's ring). Presumably, these tissues harbor EBV, and the infected lymphoid cells provide a source of virus in this region. The actual mechanism by which EBV transforms epithelial cells is unknown. There are speculations that cell-to-cell fusion between an infected B lymphocyte and an overlying epithelial cell could lead to the development of the epithelial cancer cell. An alternative explanation is that some mucosal epithelial cells express receptors for the virus. As there is also a strong association of smoking with the development of NPC, a carcinogen-induced mutagenetic mechanism is also likely to be involved.

Human Papillomavirus

Infection with high-risk human papillomaviruses (HPVs) is strongly associated with risk for developing cervical carcinoma.[31] HPVs are highly polymorphic, with more than 70 known viral types. Some of these (HPV16, 18, 31, 52, etc.) are considered to be high-risk viruses, as infection with these virus types is much more likely to be associated with anogenital (cervix, penis, vulva, and anus) carcinoma. In contrast, low-risk types (HPV6, 11, etc.) are commonly associated with benign papillomas or condylomas, but usually not invasive cancers. In the head and neck region, HPV types 6 and 11 are the most common cause of laryngeal papillomatosis.[32,33] Laryngeal papillomas are benign tumors, but because of their location in the airway, they can be life-threatening. In children, laryngeal papillomatosis is thought to be the result of infection acquired during birth from mothers with active vaginal condylomas, most of which contain HPV6 or HPV11. Adults may also develop papillomatosis, although the incidence of adult-onset disease is thought to be lower than infantile infections, which number about 2000 cases per year in the United States. There have been only rare cases of laryngeal papillomas progressing to invasive cancer. Some such cases occurred after radiation treatment of the papilloma. Presumably, irradiation causes DNA breaks and facilitates viral insertion into the host cell genome. There are also rare reports of carcinomas arising from papillomas containing low-risk HPV types.[32] The mechanism of tumor formation in these cases is not understood, but may be the result of a mutation in the virus that increases its ability to transform an infected cell. Coinfection with low- and high-risk HPV has been associated with severe dysplasia.[34] Laryngeal verrucous carcinomas, which do not arise from papillomas but have a wart-like appearance, also may have an HPV16-related papillomavirus etiology.[35] Schneiderian or inverted papillomas of the nasal sinuses also seem to have an HPV etiology. HPV6 and HPV11, as well as types 16 and 18, have been found in inverted papillomas of the paranasal sinuses.[36–38] Beck et al[37] noted that 63% of inverted papillomas were HPV-positive, and that there was a greater likelihood of recurrent papilloma among these than among those that were HPV-negative. In a related study, the same group found that progression to dysplasia or to squamous cell carcinoma in inverting papilloma lesions was often associated with high-risk HPV types.[38] This finding suggests that the high-risk papillomaviruses may have a role in tumor development in the nasal epithelium.

HPV has also been detected in a variety of other HNSCC sites; however, the rate of HPV detection in HNSCC varies widely from one study to another.[39–44] Because polymerase chain reaction (PCR) is used to detect HPV, and because PCR contamination is difficult to rule out, the highest estimates are suspect. Most studies implicate HPV in 5% to 20% of HNSCC tumors. The highest rates of HPV DNA within head and neck tumors have been associated with tumors of the tonsillar pillar and tongue. The mechanism by which high-risk HPV viruses transform a cell is fairly well established. The E6 and E7 genes from high-risk viral types (HPV16 and 18) have transforming activity in vitro.[45] The E7 protein binds to the retinoblastoma protein, blocking the normal Rb sequestration of the transcription factor E2F. By inhibiting E2F binding, E7 frees E2F, which can then initiate transcription of genes that are involved in entry into the cell cycle and that are necessary for DNA replication.[46] Similarly, the viral E6 protein binds to p53, causing this protein to become ubiquinated, transported to the proteosome, and degraded.[47] As p53 regulates G1 arrest, DNA repair, and apoptosis, its degradation allows the cell to progress through the cell cycle checkpoint unimpeded. The expression of E6 and E7 is normally controlled by another early region gene in the HPV genome, E2. E2 is frequently disrupted by integration in cervical carcinoma cell lines, suggesting that loss of this regulatory gene product is responsible for overexpression of E6 and E7.[48] It is presumed that a similar transforming event occurs in HNSCC. Although HPV transcripts have been identified in head and neck tumors, interruption of E2 during integration has not been demonstrated in any HPV-positive head and neck tumors. Because only E6 and E7 from high-risk HPV types have been shown to have transforming activity, it remains to be determined what role the low-risk virus types have in tumors that harbor them. One possibility is that when there is both viral infection and exposure to carcinogens, the infected proliferating cells, as well as the viral genome they carry, are both susceptible to mutation and, therefore, at increased risk for transformation.

INDUSTRIAL EXPOSURES

Some industrial exposures are associated with an increased risk of head and neck cancers. Furniture workers have a higher-than-expected incidence of adenocarcinoma of the ethmoid sinuses, presumably due to the presence of carcinogenic compounds in hardwood dust, varnishes, and/or solvents.[49,50] Exposure to asbestos, a well-known risk factor for development of mesothelioma of the pleura, has also been discussed as a possible cause of laryngeal cancer. Some case-control studies have indicated an increased risk of up to 15-fold for laryngeal carcinoma;[51,52] however, these studies failed to include risks from alcohol and tobacco exposure. Other studies correcting for the effects of tobacco and alcohol could only find a small[9,53,54] or no[55–57] increased risk associated with exposure to asbestos. An increased risk for laryngeal cancer secondary to exposure to asbestos is thus not established, and is still being debated.[58–60]

Workers in the leather industry have a 3.5- to 8-fold increased risk for carcinoma of the larynx. Possible causes include exposure to chrome, a well-known carcinogen.[61] Other possible agents are aromatic amines, such as β-naphthylamine, and dyes based on benzidine, both of which are known to cause cancer of the urinary bladder. An increased risk for cancer of the pharynx and larynx (1.7- to 4.6-fold greater risk) has also been reported for workers in cement and concrete factories and for construction workers.[62,63] This increase in risk might also be attributable to the traces of chrome present in cement. Similarly, workers exposed to nickel have an increased risk for cancer of the nose and paranasal sinuses.[50,64] There are also reports of an increased risk for laryngeal cancer in those engaged in occupations in which there is exposure to tar and coal products, with the risk for supraglottic cancer of the larynx being estimated to increase sixfold.

INTERACTIONS OF SUSCEPTIBILITY FACTORS AND EXPOSURE

EBV is rarely found in NPCs that arise in individuals of northern European descent. Thus, it appears that there is a susceptibility factor, as well as a link to two etiologic factors. Susceptibility factors also may account for why some individuals do not develop cancers despite long-term exposure, whereas others develop head and neck cancer at an early age with much less exposure. This relationship between exposure and susceptibility factors is illustrated in Figure 1–2. Susceptibility factors can include immunologic factors that can alter susceptibility to viral infection or promote viral latency. Age at infection may also play a role. For example, neonates exposed to EBV may be protected by maternal antibodies and experience a very mild infection that produces immunity to subsequent infection. By contrast, seronegative young adults have a severe and protracted

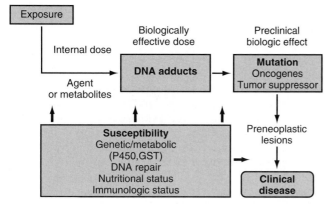

FIGURE 1-2 *Pathway of events in carcinogenesis illustrating the contributions to cancer risk from environmental and susceptibility factors. Individuals with increased susceptibility secondary to aberrant metabolizing pathways, depressed nutritional status, or depressed immunologic status may have a greater risk of developing cancer than someone without susceptibility but with equivalent environmental exposure. GST, glutathione-S-transferase. Courtesy of Dr. Andrew Olshan.*

illness when infected with EBV. In the case of African Burkitt's lymphoma, it has been postulated that coinfection with malaria stimulates B-cell proliferation and differentiation. Because B-cell differentiation involves rearrangement of the immunoglobulin genes, it is thought that the presence of EBV in the differentiating B cell increases the likelihood of the t(8;14) chromosome translocation that is characteristic of Burkitt's lymphoma.

Similarly, there are susceptibility factors for carcinogens. Genetic polymorphisms in metabolizing enzymes, such as the p450 system that can convert chemicals to active carcinogens, may predispose an individual to cancer development. By contrast, other systems, such as the GST and N-acetyltransferase enzymes, may exert a protective effect by rapidly converting potential carcinogens into water-soluble compounds that can be excreted easily. Thus, someone who has an increased sensitivity to viral infection and who also smokes may be at increased risk for virally induced cancer. Similarly, an individual with increased exposure to carcinogens and increased susceptibility for conversion of procarcinogens to proximal or active carcinogens may be at much greater risk than someone else who lacks either the exposures or the susceptibility factors.

Second Primary Cancers— Controversy and Current Findings

Second primary cancers are a leading cause of death among patients with early-stage head and neck cancers. In 1953, Slaughter et al[65] proposed the field cancerization hypothesis to explain the high incidence of multiple tumors involving the UADT. By examining tissue sections, these researchers observed areas of invasive tumor separated from areas of severe dysplasia or in situ carcinoma with apparently normal intervening mucosa. They postulated that multiple, independent, carcinogenic events were occurring in separate cells as a result of long-term exposure of the entire UADT to carcinogens in cigarette smoke (Fig. 1–3A). This hypothesis has dominated the way people view the problem of second primary cancers and has resulted in a wait-and-see approach to therapy. Thus, most physicians expect that about 15% to 25% of patients with early-stage head and neck tumors will develop a second primary cancer somewhere in the UADT within 5 years after the original diagnosis; however, an alternative hypothesis can be derived from the same observations.[66] If progeny of the initially transformed cell spread laterally from the primary site without disrupting the normal architecture of the adjacent epithelium, then secondary tumors from the same genetic legacy may arise at sites distant from the primary (Fig. 1–3B), just as Slaughter and colleagues observed.[65] These two alternative hypotheses to explain second primary cancers are illustrated in Figure 1–3. In fact, there is now mounting evidence that many second primary cancers are, in fact, progeny of the original cancer, and do not represent independent carcinogenic events. So-called second primary cancers also have been noted in other epithelia, such as the urinary bladder. In the bladder, it was presumed that the multiple tumors that arose over the surface of the bladder were attributable to field cancerization. However, Sidransky et al[67] examined X-chromosome inactivation in multiple bladder tumors from female patients and found that all of the tumors from each patient had the same inactive X chromosome. Furthermore, loss of heterozygosity (LOH) on 9p and 3p affected the same alleles in each of the tumors from the same patient. Worsham et al[68] studied synchronous head and neck tumors in a man with an FOM lesion and a pyriform sinus lesion. Using a combination of cultured cells, cytogenetics, and fluorescence in situ hybridization (FISH) on metaphase chromosomes and tissue sections, they showed that both tumors contained the same rearranged Y chromosome and the same numerical changes affecting multiple chromosomes. Thus, both tumors arose from the same original transformed cell. Bedi et al[69] applied the same techniques used previously on bladder carcinomas to examine multiple head and neck tumors from eight female patients. In four patients, both X chromosomes were present and the androgen receptor locus on X was heterozygous in normal cells. In all four cases, the same X was inactivated in each of the primary tumors. Similarly, analysis of LOH on 9p and 3p revealed the same break point in one set of primary tumors, loss of the same alleles in several tumors, and in one set, an identical microsatellite alteration in the two tumors, indicating that these were from the same clone. The probability that the second primary tumors were progeny of the same

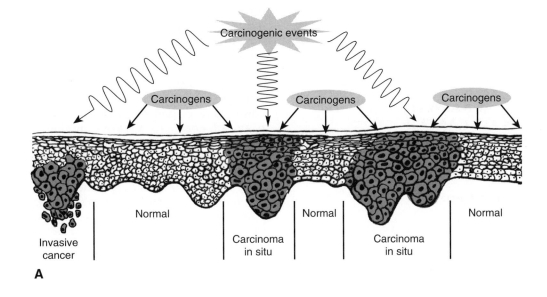

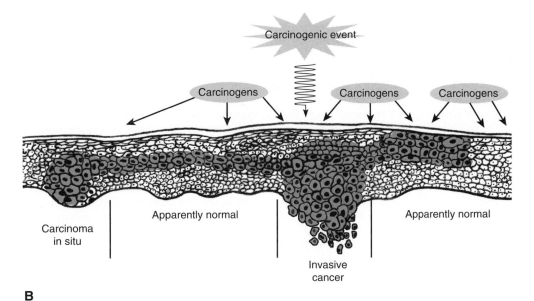

FIGURE 1–3 Alternative hypotheses to explain the origin of second primary cancers. *A*, Slaughter et al[65] proposed the "field cancerization" hypothesis in 1953 to explain the observation of multiple areas of carcinoma in situ or invasive carcinoma separated by normal tissue within an epithelium. These authors suggested that multiple carcinogenic events were occurring in widely separated cells, leading to the development of numerous independent cancerous foci. *B*, The alternative hypothesis, proposed by Carey and co-workers[66,68] and supported by other studies,[67,69,70] is that a single focus of tumor develops and spreads by arborization without disrupting the adjacent, apparently normal mucosa.

clone in most of these patients is very high, strongly supporting the idea that many second primary tumors actually represent extensions of the initial tumor clone. These observations are also consistent with the biologic behavior of head and neck tumors, which often exhibit local recurrence. Such behavior is to be expected in tumors that spread by local extension. In early-stage tumors, if the original transformed cells divide even slightly more often than their nontransformed neighbors, within a relatively short period of time, the transformed cells

will replace large segments of the normal epithelium, as indicated in the lower half of Figure 1–3. Califano et al[70] demonstrated that the apparently normal mucosa surrounding preinvasive and microinvasive HNSCCs shared common genetic aberrations with the tumor, supporting this concept. This type of arborization is also most likely responsible for the large patches of leukoplakias that spread over an area measuring many centimeters in the oral cavity of affected individuals. Supporting evidence that the cells in leukoplakias are the progeny of a single transformed cell comes from studies by Mao et al[71] in which the same genetic changes were identified in widely separated areas of such premalignant lesions.

GENETIC AND EPIGENETIC MECHANISMS OF CANCER DEVELOPMENT IN HEAD AND NECK SQUAMOUS CELL CARCINOMA

Genetic Basis for Cancer

Cancer is currently regarded as a genetic disease with mutations of genes essential for control of proliferation and maintenance of tissue organization. The role of genetic changes in neoplasia has been debated for more than a century. In 1890, von Hansemann[72] drew attention to the frequent occurrence of aberrant mitoses in cancer cells. The hypothesis of "somatic mutation" as the origin of cancer was formulated 25 years later by Boveri.[73,74]

Winge[75] first postulated the stemline concept in 1930. The mutation theory was further developed by the formulation of the clonal-evolution model.[6] The behavior of the malignant cell population was viewed as a microevolutionary process and described in Darwinian terms with genetic instability, variability through mutation, and subsequent selection. In 1982, it was demonstrated that carcinogenesis was a multistep, sequential process.[76] The concept of cancer genes or oncogenes was suggested by Huebner and Todaro[77] in 1969. The studies of Knudson[78] showed that an inherited defect in one allele of a protective gene can predispose an individual to cancer. Knudson postulated that such genetic changes affected so-called antioncogenes. Later, such genes were termed tumor suppressor genes.

The somatic mutation theory also has had its detractors, and epigenetic models of neoplasia that incorporate genetic events have been proposed.[1,79,80] The term epigenetic refers to the acquisition of heritable characteristics without a change in the primary sequence of genes.[81]

A single mutation is not enough to cause cancer. During the course of a lifetime, approximately 10^{16} cell divisions take place in the human body. It is estimated that, in a mutagen-free environment, mutations will occur spontaneously at a rate of about 10^{-6}; thus, in a lifetime, every single gene is likely to have undergone mutation on about 10^{10} separate occasions in any individual human being. One could expect many of these mutations to engage genes involved in the intricate control of cell division. The problem of cancer could thus be formulated not as a question of why cancer occurs, but rather why its development is so infrequent.

The concept of multiple mutations as a requisite for cancer development stems from the observation that the incidence of cancer rises steeply as a function of age.[82,83] If only one mutation is needed to initiate the process of carcinogenesis, the incidence would not be age-dependent. The idea of multiple genetic changes has been strongly supported by the example of colorectal malignant disease with its accumulation of genetic alterations during progression from adenoma to invasive malignant tumor.[84] A similar model has been proposed for HNSCC,[70] but in the absence of a clear, stepwise, adenoma-to-invasive-cancer model like that in the colon, it has not yet gained widespread acceptance. However, despite the massive amount of accumulated data on chromosomal and molecular rearrangements in human cancer,[85] the basic question—How many mutations are required for the pathogenesis of a specific malignant tumor?—has not yet been answered.

A variety of mathematical models of human carcinogenesis have been presented. Early multistage models did not make any assumptions about the number of genetic changes.[82,83] Later models have been developed to calculate the number of genetic changes needed for development of manifest cancer. Renan[86] estimated the number of mutations necessary for cancer development using the following assumptions: (1) malignant tumors are caused by the accumulation of genetic changes in a single cell; (2) the number of mutations in a specific tumor is independent of the dose of exogenous carcinogens; (3) the cell proliferation rate of a particular tissue remains constant throughout life; (4) only mutations after birth are considered; and (5) mortality rates provide an indication of the incidence rates of tumor types. He plotted the log of the age-specific mortality rate against the log of age (in years) for 28 different malignant diseases and then used the slope of the line to derive estimates of the number of mutations needed for tumor development. He found that some commonly occurring solid tumors, including those of the lip and skin, needed seven to eight mutations for an overt cancer to appear. A second set of tumors, which included tumors of the esophagus and larynx, required nine or more genetic events. A third group, including thyroid tumors, required five or fewer genetic mutations. Data on tumors of the nasal cavities and salivary glands have indicated two distinct subpopulations: those individuals who develop such tumors at relatively young ages (<40 yr) and those who develop them later. The suggested number of mutations for late-onset salivary gland tumors is seven, for tumors of the nose and nasal cavities, it is six. The corresponding number for early-onset tumors is two or three, implying the existence of up to three mutations at birth in individuals developing these early tumors (Fig. 1–4). Carey et al[87,88] compared chromosomal abnormalities in cell cultures from primary and metastatic tumors of two patients with HNSCC. In both cases, the primary and metastatic tumors each

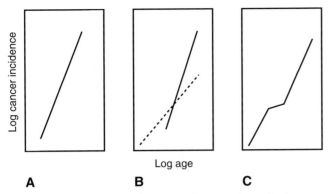

FIGURE 1-4   Cancer incidence as a function of age for three different populations. *A*, The incidence of cancer is shown to increase linearly by age. The linear regression coefficient of this plot varies from 5 to 7, indicating that six to eight independent events are necessary before cancer appears as a clinical entity. *B*, When plots of cancer incidence versus age yield a line with these characteristics, it indicates there are two subpopulations, one developing cancer at an early age and a second at a later age. *C*, Incidence plots with this shape and approximately the same slope indicate a bimodal age distribution, suggesting the presence of a subpopulation with inherited susceptibility who develop cancer at an earlier age than the sporadic group, who develop a tumor later in life. Adapted from Renan MJ. How many mutations are required for tumorigenesis? Implications from human cancer data. *Mol Carcinogen.* 1993; 7:139–146, with permission of Wiley-Liss, Inc., a subsidiary of John Wiley & Sons, Inc.

had numerous different chromosomal abnormalities, but also in each case, the primary and metastatic tumors shared five common chromosomal rearrangements, which is consistent with Renan's predictions.[86] However, Worsham et al[89,90] found two examples of head and neck tumor cell lines in which only two or three initial chromosomal changes were visible. Of course, visible cytogenetic changes can easily underestimate the changes that have occurred at the individual base pair level. Nevertheless, it is interesting that these gross changes correlate rather well with Renan's[86] statistical predictions, supporting the concept that several pathways must be inactivated in the genesis of solid tumors.

Oncogenes and Tumor Suppressor Genes (Knudson's Hypothesis)

All methods of analysis have indicated that, although squamous cell carcinomas have very complex karyotypes, these karyotypes also indicate many regions of consistent loss and several regions of consistent gain. This suggests that both loss of tumor suppressor genes and amplification of dominantly acting, growth regulatory genes are likely involved in the progression of solid tumors. The significance of this balance has been expressed colorfully by Jean Marx: "If you're tooling along the interstate in your aging Austin-Healey 3000, brake failure can

be every bit as catastrophic as a stuck accelerator."[91] The authors, each of whom has had experience with aging British sports cars and genetic changes in squamous carcinoma, found this comment, paraphrasing Bert Vogelstein's brake and accelerator analogy, to be highly appropriate. It highlights the intricate interaction between inactivated tumor suppressor genes (the failed brakes) (e.g., p53 and cyclin-dependent kinase inhibitors) and amplified genes that stimulate cell division (the stuck accelerator) (e.g., the cyclins and their kinases). Loss of suppressor function and unscheduled activation of cell cycle regulatory genes in combination can be disastrous for regulation of cell proliferation.

Activated oncogenes have been linked to chromosomal changes in multiple tumor types. The Philadelphia chromosome in chronic myelogenous leukemia is a t(9;22) that results in a fusion protein *BCR/ABL* that activates the *C-ABL* proto-oncogene by converting the protein to a constitutively active protein kinase. Similarly, the t(8;14) translocation in Burkitt's lymphoma activates C-MYC oncogene expression by bringing this gene into proximity with the immunoglobulin promoters, resulting in C-MYC overexpression. Homogeneously staining regions and double minute chromosomes have been linked to gene amplification of *N-MYC* in neuroblastoma and the dihydrofolate reductase gene in cells resistant to methotrexate. Retinoblastoma (*RB*), the prototypical tumor suppressor gene, was discovered after consistent deletions affecting chromosome 13q14 were discovered in both the inherited and sporadic form of retinoblastoma, suggesting that the deleted region contained a gene involved in the pathogenesis of this tumor. Knudson[78] had analyzed the age at diagnosis for both congenital cases of retinoblastoma and for sporadic cases. He demonstrated that the former followed first-order kinetics, whereas the latter followed second-order kinetics. From this, he postulated that two events were required for tumor development, and that in the inherited form of the disease, affected children were born with the first event and thus developed retinoblastoma at an early age. In contrast, children with sporadic disease had a delayed onset, consistent with the longer time required for two events to develop. From this, Knudson[78] postulated that both copies of an antioncogene must be inactivated. When the *RB* gene was identified and cloned, it became clear that Knudson's hypothesis was correct. In tumors, one copy of the *RB* gene is typically inactivated, and the other is lost by chromosomal deletion. Similar findings were subsequently identified for the *TP53* (*p53*) gene, in which mutation and loss of heterozygosity are typically observed. As a result of these discoveries, consistent rearrangements and regions of gain and regions of loss are considered to be markers that predict the loci of gene amplification and the loss of tumor suppressor genes, respectively. As discussed in the following section, several regions of consistent gain and loss have already led to the identification of genes that are involved in HNSCC.

Epigenetic Mechanisms of Gene Inactivation

In some cases, genes located at regions of consistent loss are not inactivated by mutation, yet the gene product is not expressed. This factor was puzzling until the genomic DNA for the remaining gene copy was analyzed in multiple tumors. In such cases, multiple methylated bases were found. Methylation blocks the RNA polymerase complex from being activated, and methylated genes are thus not expressed. This mechanism has been implicated in HNSCC for inactivation of the *p16* gene on 9p21.[92] Consistent LOH on 9p in multiple tumor types led to the discovery of the *p16* locus and its gene product. This gene, initially called *MTS1* for multiple tumor suppressor gene-1 because it was implicated in several tumor types, was later shown to be an inhibitor of cyclin-dependent kinase (*p16INK4a*).[93] In HNSCC, there is a high rate of LOH affecting 9p21,[94] but an initial investigation of *p16* showed a relatively low rate of mutation,[95] raising questions about whether this gene is the important 9p gene in this tumor type. However, a subsequent study revealed that *p16* was frequently inactivated by epigenetic mechanisms, such as hypermethylation.[92] Presumably, this type of mechanism serves to silence other tumor suppressor genes as well.

Genomic Instability and DNA Repair

The DNA of normal and tumor cells is continuously exposed to damage. The frequency of error in DNA replication has been calculated to be 1 per 10^9 base pairs and cell generation. A gene coding for a medium-sized protein with about 10^3 coding base pairs will mutate only once in every 10^6 cell generations. In humans, this corresponds to an amino acid change about once every 200,000 years.[96] In resting cells, the DNA is subject to continuous exogenous breakdown. It is estimated that about 5000 purine bases per cell are lost daily owing to cleavage of the N-glycosyl bond to deoxyribose. The fact that only a few stable mutations accumulate is explained by very efficient DNA repair mechanisms.

Throughout evolution, there has been a process favoring a phenotype with enzymes that recognize and repair DNA lesions to ensure gene stability and provide a high fidelity in DNA replication. Because the possibility for DNA damage is so vast, the successful organism or cell has become equipped with a battery of repair enzymes specialized to cope with different DNA lesions. As there is an overlap between the different DNA repair pathways, alternate repair pathways can repair most DNA lesions. Most repair mechanisms rely on the existence of the com-

plementary information in the two-stranded DNA helix; if the sequence in one of the strands is distorted, the sequence of nucleotides of the complementary strand can be used to restore the damaged strand. The two major pathways are *base excision repair* and *nucleotide excision repair*. The former repairs small lesions, whereas the latter repairs bulky, helix-distorting lesions. In nucleotide excision repair, DNA damage is identified and removed by a protein complex as a part of an oligonucleotide fragment and is then replaced by a newly synthesized DNA using the intact DNA strand as a template. It has been estimated that more than 50 genes code for proteins involved in DNA repair, demonstrating the importance of this system. Furthermore the repair system focuses on maintaining fidelity of the genome that are in use in a cell, as opposed to regions between genes and regions that are not expressed. Thus, cells preferentially repair DNA sequences that are frequently transcribed and there is a preference for repair of the DNA strand used as a template for transcription, rather than the noncoding strand.[97-99]

The base and the nucleotide excision repair systems are important to correct mistakes in DNA strand replication during the S-phase. However, the cell also has an emergency DNA repair process to handle severe DNA damage, termed the *SOS-repair response*. Severe DNA damage triggers an arrest in DNA replication and induces transcription of genes of the salvage pathway that allows a cell to survive the otherwise potentially lethal effects of large-scale DNA damage. The cost of this emergency response seems to be an increased mutation rate owing to an increasing number of errors in copying DNA sequences.[96]

Mismatch repair genes have been found in a variety of species. In the absence of an intact mismatch repair system, cells accumulate mutations at a rate that may be 1000 times faster than that in normal cells. When frequent examples of microsatellite instability were found in hereditary nonpolyposis colorectal cancer (HNPCC), it was suggested that there might be a defect in the mismatch repair system. Subsequent experiments have demonstrated that the human homologues of the bacterial DNA repair genes *mutL* and *mutS* are not functional in certain tumors, suggesting that failure to repair mutations might have a role in tumor development in these patients. Further evidence that the strand-specific repair pathways function in mutation avoidance has been derived from studies showing that a hypermutable, cultured cell line is defective in mismatch repair. This finding was later clinically paralleled when it was shown that certain sporadic cancers and practically all tumors associated with HNPCC are highly prone to mutation. Furthermore, cell lines derived from such cancers were found to accrue mutations at a rate of more than a 100 times that of normal human cells.[100] The majority of cases of HNPCC are attributable to a defect in one of four repair genes: *hMSH2*, *hMLH1*, *hPMS1*, and *hPMS2*.

HNPCC is inherited in an autosomal pattern. One of the alleles is mutated in the germline, and in tumor cells, the wild-type allele is lost through somatic mutation.

In contrast to HNPCC cell lines, in vitro cultivated cell lines established from HNSCC are usually genetically stable and do not exhibit a mutator phenotype. Similarly, microsatellite instability is relatively uncommon in head and neck tumors, although occasional examples are reported.[69,101] It remains to be determined if one of the DNA repair genes is inactivated in these unusual cases. HNSCC tumor cell lines tend to be stable in in vitro culture. Tumor lines that have been karyotyped over a span of 100 in vitro passages have shown essentially no new chromosomal changes.[87] However, there appears to be significant pressure for tumors to evolve in vivo, as cells removed from primary and metastatic tumors in the same individual often differ by up to 20 chromosomal changes.[88] In these cases, there are typically four to six consistent genetic changes that are identical in the primary tumor and the metastatic lesion.[88] Xenografted tumors generally exhibit constant growth rates and a stable histopathologic appearance during long-term serial passages, but there are reports of changes in growth rate, differentiation, and chemosensitivity, indicating the presence of increased in vivo genetic instability.[102]

It is not necessary to presume a mutator phenotype in order to explain most cancer in epithelial cells. Estimation of the frequency of microsatellite alterations and mutation of the hypoxanthine phosphoribosyltransferase (HPRT) gene in epithelial cells indicate a mutation frequency of around 10^{-5} per cell for a marker gene such as HPRT, a frequency that increases with age in an exponential way. This rate of mutation is adequate to account for the incidence of cancer that exists,[103] and is compatible with the exponential nature of increased cancer incidence with age.[82,83,86]

Mutagen sensitivity in patients who develop HNSCC has been studied using bleomycin-induced chromosomal breakage in lymphocytes. This end point represents only a fraction of the total mutations, but has the advantage of identifying individuals with a deficiency in the DNA maintenance pathways. In a normal population, there is a wide gaussian-distributed variation in mutagen sensitivity.[104] If the cutoff value is set at 1.0 break per cell (which equals the mean value for control individuals + one SD), then 16% of the population is hypersensitive to bleomycin. The authors found that patients with cancers originating from tissues exposed to environmental carcinogens, such as HNSCC and lung cancer, preferentially exhibited increased bleomycin sensitivity, indicating that both a mutator phenotype and exposure to carcinogens are important for the development of this type of cancer. In contrast, individuals with breast cancer, which is not linked to carcinogen exposure, showed no elevation over that in the normal population with respect to mutagen sensitivity. It has since been shown that young adults with HNSCC exhibit an increased mutagen sensitivity compared to that in elderly men without tumors but with an extensive history of tobacco and alcohol exposure, the latter of whom were predominantly insensitive.[105] It also seems as if mutagen-sensitive patients with HNSCC have an increased risk for development of second primary tumors, compared to nonsensitive individuals.[15,106,107] It was later confirmed that constitutional mutagen sensitivity is associated with a dose-dependent increase in risk for HNSCC after exposure to carcinogenic compounds. There is a dramatic increase in odds ratios from 10.6 to 45.1 for head and neck cancer in mutagen-hypersensitive individuals who are also heavy smokers; however, a hypersensitive phenotype does not appear to result in an increased cancer risk in nonsmokers. The use of alcohol further potentiates the effect of smoking in hypersensitive persons.[16]

The spontaneous mutation rate is crucial, both for evolution and for maintenance of the intact organism. No species can allow mutations to accumulate at a high rate in germ cells; on the other hand, variation is necessary for natural selection. A low mutation rate does not allow adaptation to environmental alterations, but a high mutation rate leads to instability of the organism. The mutation rate also limits the complexity of the organism. The observed mutation rate allows encoding for 60,000 proteins; a 10-fold higher mutation rate would limit this to about 6000 proteins, which is inconsistent with an organism more complex than a fruit fly.[96] Thus, it may be that the risk of developing cancer with increasing age in some individuals is the price a population of complex organisms has to pay to allow for evolution.

CONSISTENT CHROMOSOMAL GAINS AND LOSSES IN TUMORS OF THE HEAD AND NECK

Nonrandom patterns of chromosomal aberrations have been detected in all tumor types investigated. In leukemias and lymphomas, which constitute 75% of the more than 27,000 aberrant cases reported in the literature, karyotypic findings have been shown to correlate with clinical findings and outcome. Although carcinomas are much more common, there is much less information available about the genetic changes because these tumors are more difficult to culture and have far more complex karyotypes. In contrast to leukemias and lymphomas, which commonly have balanced structural aberrations, carcinomas exhibit combinations of unbalanced translocations, deletions, and segmental amplifications that affect multiple chromosomal segments.

Chromosomal rearrangements are usually studied in short-term cultures of malignant cells that are terminated after 5 to 10 days through colchicine treatment, which arrests the cells in metaphase and allows the karyotype to be studied. The field of cancer cytogenetics experienced its first striking success in 1960 when Nowell and Hungerford[108] discovered the Philadelphia (Ph) chromosome in chronic myeloid leukemia. A major improvement in the cytogenetic procedure was the chromosome banding technique, introduced by Caspersson and colleagues in 1970, which allowed each chromosome to be identified on the basis of its particular banding pattern. This made the characterization of chromosome rearrangements more precise and stringent.

Up to June of 1996, a total of 26,523 recurrent chromosomal aberrations in hematologic malignant diseases and solid tumors had been reported in the literature,[85] most of which (more than 70%) were hematologic malignant lesions or lymphomas. In this compilation, all numerical anomalies were excluded, as were aberrations involving unidentified chromosomes or regions. Anomalies with uncertain breakpoints were also excluded. Using these restrictions, a total of 215 balanced and 1588 unbalanced recurrent aberrations were identified. When the cytogenetic and diagnostic information from the 75 different tumor types were compared, it became evident that the balanced structural chromosomal rearrangements (mostly translocations, but also some inversions) were decidedly more disease-specific than the unbalanced changes. Squamous carcinomas have complex abnormalities with frequent unbalanced chromosomal rearrangements (Table 1–1).

Thyroid and Parathyroid Tumors

In thyroid adenomas, gains of chromosomes 5, 7, and 12, as well as structural changes of 19q, have been reported. Papillary carcinomas of the thyroid characteristically have an inv(10)(q11q21), which is associated with the fusion gene RET/PTC.[110] Interestingly, an inherited activating mutation of the RET oncogene, a protein tyrosine kinase, is also implicated in multiple endocrine neoplasia, a syndrome in which individuals are predisposed to develop endocrine gland tumors, including thyroid carcinoma. In addition, RET oncogene rearrangements have been noted in papillary thyroid carcinomas arising in children exposed to radiation following the Chernobyl nuclear accident in Soviet Union.[111] Parathyroid adenomas often have a pericentric inversion of chromosome 11 that brings the active parathyroid hormone (PTH) locus at 11p15 into close proximity with the BCL-1 locus mapped to 11q13. Analysis of this breakpoint resulted in the discovery and cloning of parathyroid adenoma gene 1 (PRAD1),[112] which was later found to be the mammalian equivalent of the invertebrate cyclin genes, resulting in the renaming of this gene as cyclin D1.[113] Chromosome 11q13 abnormalities and cyclin D1 also play a prominent role in squamous cell carcinomas, as discussed in the following text.

Pleomorphic Adenoma of the Salivary Gland

Pleomorphic adenomas are the most common types of salivary gland tumor. Although these are benign tumors, a subset contains recurrent chromosomal rearrangements with breakpoints affecting 3p21, 8p12, and 12q13-15. A consistent t(3;8)(p21;q12) translocation results in promoter swapping between PLAG1, a zinc finger protein, and β-catenin. It appears that the constitutively active promoter of the catenin gene results in unregulated expression of PLAG1, and this protein contributes to salivary gland adenoma tumorigenesis.[114]

TABLE 1–1	SUMMARY OF HEAD AND NECK NEOPLASMS WITH RECURRENT ABNORMALITIES		
TYPE OF NEOPLASIA	NO. OF CASES	NO. OF BALANCED ABNORMALITIES[a]	NO. OF UNBALANCED ABNORMALITIES[a]
Thyroid	71	2 (2)	0
Mucoepidermoid carcinoma of the salivary gland	19	1 (1)	0
Squamous cell carcinoma	197	3	52 (4)
Tongue	39	1 (0)	19 (1)
Oral cavity, other sites	50	0	15 (0)
Oropharynx	28	1 (0)	8 (0)
Nasal cavity	5	0	1 (0)
Nasopharynx	25	0	4 (1)
Larynx	50	1 (0)	5 (2)

[a] Number of cytogenetically different abnormalities detected in each tumor group. The number of aberrations reported as sole anomalies are given in parentheses.
Modified from Mitelman F, Mertens F, Johansson B. A breakpoint map of recurrent chromosomal rearrangements in human neoplasia. *Nature Genet.* 1997; 15:417–474.

Squamous Cell Carcinomas

CYTOGENETIC ANALYSIS

Cytogenetic information from 206 short-term cultures of HNSCC published by Mertens et al[115] and 29 HNSCC cell lines published by Van Dyke et al[116] are illustrated in Table 1–2. In both short-term cultures of primary tumors[115] and in established cell cultures,[116] losses are more common than gains, and unbalanced aberrations are far more common than balanced ones. Similar results reported by others[87,117–122] have supported these consistent regions of genetic changes and the premise that losses are the most common type of event. Analysis of cell lines (see left side of Table 1–2) reveals more regions of consistent loss and gain than does study of primary tumors. There are several reasons for this. In primary tumors, there are only a limited number of metaphases that can be analyzed. This reduces the possibility of confirming consistent changes. Also, cell lines are likely to include more representations of advanced tumors as many come from recurrent or metastatic tumors. Thus, such cell lines contain changes associated with tumor progression, as in, for example, loss of 18q, which Frank et al[101] have shown occurs with progression and is a marker of poor prognosis.[123] Similarly, gain of 11q13-q24 is also more commonly found in cell lines (see Table 1–2), and Åkervall et al[124] have shown

rearrangement at this locus to be a poor prognostic indicator in patients with HNSCC. One could argue that these changes are best represented in cell lines because the cell lines do not accurately represent the in vivo situation. However, that would be an incorrect assumption as analysis of tumors and cell lines from the same individuals by Jones et al[125] and by Frank et al[101] have shown that the tumors and cell lines have identical allelic losses and even identical microsatellite instabilities. In fact, the data suggest that cell lines are a snapshot of the status of the tumor at the time of its removal, and that the tumor cell lines are very stable in vitro, showing few, if any, in vitro chromosomal changes.[68,87] The significance of these chromosomal aberrations will be discussed further after a discussion of the other methods that have been used to characterize the consistent genetic changes in HNSCC.

MOLECULAR ANALYSIS OF LOSS OF HETEROZYGOSITY AND ALLELIC IMBALANCE

As noted previously, gains and losses are the common chromosomal aberrations in many carcinomas, and allelotyping has been used extensively to examine chromosomes from nonviable (i.e., fixed or frozen) tumor tissue for evidence of LOH or allelic imbalance. LOH is evident when a genetic locus that is heterozygous in normal somatic cells has only one

TABLE 1 – 2	CHROMOSOMAL IMBALANCES IN HEAD AND NECK SQUAMOUS CELL CARCINOMA (HNSCC)		
VAN DYKE ET AL[116]		MERTENS ET AL[115]	
Gain[a] (28%–38% of tumors)	Loss[a] (30%–60% of tumors)	Gain[b] (at least 15% of tumors)	Loss[b] (at least 15% of tumors)
	Y (70%)		Y
	Inactive X (70%)		
3q21-qter	3p13-p24 (60%)		3p11-26
	4p12-p16		4p15-16
5p	5q12-q23 (40%)		
7p		7p22-q21	
8p	8q (40%)		8p11-23
	9p21-p24 (40%)		
	10p13-pter		
11q13-q23			
	13q13-14		13p11-13
			14p11-13
			15p11-13
	16		
	17p		
	18q22-q23 (50–55%)		
	19q		
			21p13-q10
	21q11.1-q21 (55%)		21q22

[a] Modified from Van Dyke DL, Worsham MJ, Benninger MS, et al. Recurrent cytogentic abnormalities in squamous cell carcinomas of the head and neck region. *Genes Chromosomes Cancer*. 1994; 9:192–206, with permission. These authors examined 29 HNSCC cell lines established from 19 males and 10 females.

[b] Modified from Mertens F, Johansson B, Höglund M, Mitelman F. Chromosomal imbalance maps of malignant solid tumors: A cytogenetic survey of 3185 neoplasms. *Cancer Res*. 1997; 57:2765–2780.

allele in the tumor. Allelic imbalance—that is, a strong signal from one allele and a weak signal from the other—is observed when there are more copies of one allele than of the other allele in tumor tissue. Allelic imbalance can result from either amplification or duplication of a gene or chromosomal segment, or from a gain of one homologue in the tumor (e.g., three copies of a chromosome in which one homologue is represented twice and the other only once). This happens frequently after tetraploidization and subsequent loss of supernumerary chromosomes.[90] Allelic imbalance also occurs when there is loss of a chromosomal segment or a whole homologue in the tumor, but normal cells contaminate the DNA preparation. In this case, the contaminating normal tissue contributes a weak signal from both chromosomes that is proportional in strength to the amount of normal cells contaminating the tumor sample. By contrast, the chromosome that is present in only one copy in the tumor, together with the signal from the same chromosome in the normal cells, generates a strong signal.

Allelotyping relies on polymorphic markers that differ on the maternal and paternal chromosomes in an individual. Initially, this type of analysis used polymorphic restriction enzyme sites. However, the discovery of the much more frequent and more highly polymorphic dinucleotide, trinucleotide, and tetranucleotide repeat sequences (such as the dinucleotide $CACACA_n$) that differ in the number of repeats on individual chromosomes has made the former type of study almost obsolete.[126] Allelotyping analysis involves the study of normal DNA, derived, for example, from lymph nodes, blood, or other normal tissue from the patient, and tumor DNA, isolated from regions of the tumor specimen that contain at least 70% tumor nuclei. Primer sets that flank the nucleotide repeats, or microsatellite repeat polymorphisms, as they are also called, are used to amplify the maternal and paternal sequences using polymerase chain reaction (PCR) amplification with a labeled nucleotide or a labeled primer in the reaction mixture. The amplified sequences, which typically differ in size because of the difference in the number of repeat subunits on the maternal and paternal chromosomes, are then separated by size by polyacrylamide gel electrophoresis (PAGE) under denaturing conditions. The alleles are detected by autoradiography or fluorescence, depending on the type of label used to tag the PCR products. If there are two alleles in the normal DNA and only one in the tumor, then the tumor is judged to have LOH at that allele. When one allele is 50% more intense than the other, the sample is judged to have allelic imbalance. This may be attributable either to LOH and contamination of the tumor DNA with normal DNA, or the presence of more copies of one chromosome than the other.

Allelotyping analysis has been applied to HNSCC by a number of researchers,[127–129] and results generally similar to those obtained by karyotyping and comparative genomic hybridization (CGH) analysis have been obtained. Examples from the three studies cited here are shown in Table 1–3. Several points can be appreciated from this comparison. First, detection of LOH is dependent on the number of marker alleles studied. A typical allelogram includes at least two markers on every chromosome arm. However, as more markers are used, the likelihood of finding regions of loss increases. Furthermore, if the markers used by different investigators are not located in the same region of the chromosome arm, then different results may be obtained. Nawroz et al[127] used a marker within 9p21 and found a high frequency of 9p LOH. Ah-See et al[128] did not report the same frequency of loss on this arm, presumably because they selected a different marker. All three groups found LOH on 17p. This was not observed as frequently in cytogenetic analysis because the p arm is small. In contrast to cytogenetic studies, which revealed frequent gain of 11q (see Table 1–2), investigators using allelotyping reported LOH on 11q. It may be that, in allelotyping, the additional copies of one homologue in tumors with chromosome gain appears as allelic imbalance, so that the allelic gain is scored as a loss. However, it is also possible that a marker located near a breakpoint could be lost, although there is amplification of adjacent chromosome segments.

TABLE 1–3 REGIONS OF LOSS DETECTED BY ALLELOTYPE ANALYSIS IN HEAD AND NECK SQUAMOUS CELL CARCINOMAS

NAWROZ ET AL[127]	AH-SEE ET AL[128]	LI ET AL[129]
3 (50%)	3p	3p
4 (35%)		
	5q	
6p (35%)		
8 (35%)		8p
9 (72%)	9q	
11q (50%)	11q	
13q (50%)		13q
14q (35%)		
17p (50%)	17p	17p
19q (35%)		

Data from Nawroz H, van der Riet P, Hruban RH. Allelotype of squamous cell carcinoma. *Cancer Res.* 1994; 54:1152–1155; Ah-See KW, Cooke TG, Pichford IR, Soutar D, Balmain A. An allelotype of squamous carcinoma of the head and neck using microsatillite markers. *Cancer Res.* 1994; 54:1617–1621; and Li X, Lee NK, Ye Y-W, et al. Allelic loss at chromosomes 3p, 8p, 13q, and 17p associated with poor prognosis in head and neck cancer. *J Natl Cancer Inst.* 1994; 86:1524–1529.

COMPARATIVE GENOMIC HYBRIDIZATION

Comparative genomic hybridization (CGH) is a technique used to visualize losses and gains of chromosomal segments using DNA extracted from tumor tissue.[130] Its ability to interrogate the entire genome is comparable to karyotyping, and it has the advantage of being applicable even in the absence of viable tissue. Tumor DNA is extracted from frozen or fixed tissue samples and labeled by nick translation with biotin–d-uridine triphosphate (dUTP). Normal control DNA is isolated from lymphocytes or other normal tissue of a donor of the same sex as the tumor patient and labeled with digoxigenin-dUTP. In contrast to loss of heterozygosity studies, in which specific alleles in normal and tumor tissue are compared, in CGH there is no requirement that the normal DNA come from the same individual as the tumor. The labeled tumor and normal DNA samples are mixed in equimolar amounts and hybridized to normal chromosomes on a slide containing well-spread metaphase chromosomes. The hybridization signal from tumor DNA is detected by staining the chromosomes with fluorescein-avidin, which binds to the biotinylated UTP. Similarly, the signal from the normal DNA is detected by simultaneously staining with antidigoxigenin-rhodamine. The metaphase chromosomes are counterstained with 4'-6-diamidino-2-phenyl-indole (DAPI). Three separate fluorescence images per metaphase can be recorded, and by superimposing the digitized images, imbalances between tumor and normal DNA can be visualized as green staining of chromosomal segments where there is amplification in the tumor and red staining where there are losses in the tumor[131] (Fig. 1–5).

CGH is a powerful tool for screening tumors for genetic changes as it only requires a reasonably pure source of tumor DNA from the patient. It can detect three- to five-fold gains, relative to the normal copy number, down to a size of 2 Mb and deletions of 10 to 20 Mb. False-positive findings are rare. However, centromeres and heterochromatin regions cannot be analyzed, nor can balanced translocations or aneuploidy be detected. There is good concordance (89% to 95%) with conventional cytogenetic techniques, as well as with LOH studies.

Thus far, CGH has been applied to only a limited number of HNSCCs. As in conventional cytogenetic analysis, there is a complex picture with multiple segmental gains and losses of chromosomes. In a mixed series of 30 HNSCCs (of which 13 were laryngeal), deletions were found in more than 50% of cases on chromosomes 1p, 3p, 4, 5q, 6q, 8p, 9p, 11q, 13q, 18q, and 21q.[132] Note the strong correlation with the changes detected by conventional cytogenetic analysis (see Table 1–1). Furthermore, by this method, accurate assessment of both gains and losses are obtained. Deletions are very frequent in chromosome 3p, whereas increases are frequently seen in all or part of chromosome 3q (3q24 and 3q27-qter). Increases were also documented in 11q13, 8q, 19q, 19p and 17q. These findings are consistent with two smaller series that also reported a high level of amplification of the regions 3q26-qter and 11q13 and copy number decreases at 3p and 5q.[133,134]

MICROARRAYS

Microarrays represent an area of new technology that is revolutionizing the ability to detect genetic changes and to identify alterations in gene expression in tissues or cells. Microarrays use hybridization of DNA, RNA, or cDNA to various targets that represent either chromosome fragments such as those already cloned into bacterial artificial chromosomes or cDNA sequences that represent 600, 1000, and eventually 30,000 or more expressed genes.

Genomic DNA Arrays

The chromosome segment approach is based on CGH and instead of using a spread of metaphase chromosomes as the target DNA, an array of small segments that represents the entire genome is used. The location of each chromosome segment placed on the array is known and then normal and tumor DNA labeled with different fluorochromes are mixed in equal amounts and hybridized to the array. A fluorescent reader determines the color of each spot and if the segment or gene is lost in the tumor then the spot will hybridize predominantly with the normal DNA and be stained red. If the gene is amplified in the tumor then the spot will hybridize predominantly with the tumor DNA and will be stained green.

Expression Arrays

Similar arrays are being developed to represent cDNA for all human genes as well as for other species. Currently filter arrays containing from 600 to 1000 expressed genes and microarrays spotted on special microscope slides are in wide use. Development of microchip arrays is in progress and prototypes are being tested at the Human Genome Center of NIH and in private technology firms. Some arrays are selected gene expression sets, such as genes known to be involved in the cell cycle. Others represent specific areas of interest. For example there are several cancer gene arrays that include genes known to be aberrently expressed in various tumors. For the expression arrays, total RNA is collected from a test and normal sample and the expression of genes in the normal is compared to the test system. If one wishes to detect changes in gene expression associated with a tumor development then RNA would be collected from fresh tumor and from the corresponding normal tissue. If the RNA is relatively abundent it can be converted directly to cDNA using reverse transcription and the cDNA samples can be used to probe the array. If the RNA is limiting then a variety of startegies are employed to amplify the signal. Currently most investigators use linear amplification to avoid errors induced by PCR approaches that might change the relative abundance of transcripts. As with the genomic arrays, the test cDNA is labeled with a green fluorochrome and the control

Comparative genomic hybridization

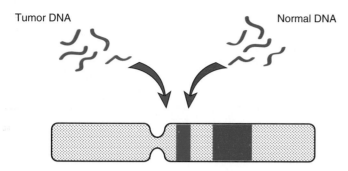

Tumor DNA   Normal DNA

Hybridization to metaphase chromosome spread

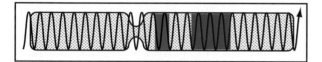

Digitalized image analysis

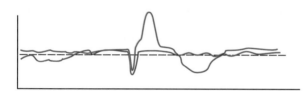

Superimposed curves

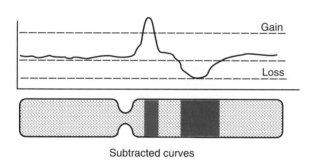

Gain

Loss

A   Subtracted curves

FIGURE 1–5 Diagram illustrating the principle of comparative genomic hybridization (CGH). *A*, DNA samples isolated from tumor cells and from normal cells (of a sex-matched donor) are labeled with different fluorescent markers, green for tumor and red for normal DNA. The DNA samples are mixed in equal amounts and hybridized to normal chromosome spreads. The images from the normal chromosomes are examined and digitized, and areas with different intensities of red or green fluorescence are plotted against the length of each chromosome. Where the color intensities are equal, the contribution of red and green signal is the same. Where there is more red signal, it indicates that there was loss of this region in the tumor; when there is more green signal, it indicates that there is a gain of genetic material in the tumor. *B*, An example of CGH in a tumor showing both amplification and loss of chromosome segments in the tumor DNA. Note that the amplification of 8p in the tumor results in increased green staining, whereas the loss of the midsection of 15q, combined with gain of the distal region of 15q, results in both red staining and green staining of the indicator chromosome. Redrawn from van Dekken H, Geeten E, Dinjens WJM, et al. Comparative genomic hybridization of cancer of the gastroesophageal junction: Deletion of 14q 31–32.1 discriminates between esophageal (Barrett's) and gastric cardia adenocarcinomas. *Cancer Res.* 1999; 59:748–752, with permission.

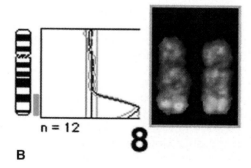

n = 12

8

B

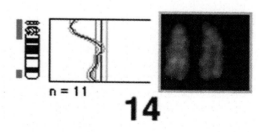

n = 11

14

sample is labeled with a red flurochrome. Genes that are upregulated in the test tissue (tumor) will appear as predominantly green whereas those that have been shut off in the test sample will appear as predominantly red. Microarray technology is very powerful and is being used for a myriad of applications.

Bioinformatics

Microarray experiments result in huge amounts of data. This has necessitated the development of a specialized field of data management that is termed bioinformatics. To evaluate the information for whole classes of genes that are regulated by complex biological phenomena requires specialized algorithms for data storage and analysis. Automated readers collect the data, the fluorescence intensity and relative color is recorded and hundreds to hundreds of thousands of data points are recorded. The algorithms then manipulate and evaluate the results of the experiments. As with most technological advances, the quality of the samples and the design of the experiment, as well as the sophistication of the technological devices are equally important factors in gaining accurate new information.

CANDIDATE GENES ASSOCIATED WITH REGIONS OF CONSISTENT GAIN OR LOSS

In general, the cytogenetic aberrations seen in HNSCC are very complex. Despite this complexity, specific gene abnormalities are being associated with consistent chromosomal rearrangements, indicating that the complexity is not just the result of random, widespread, genomic damage. Possible tumor suppressor genes on 3p, a common site of loss, include the *FHIT* (fragile histidine triad) gene located within 3p14.2 and the *VHL* (von Hippel-Lindau disease) tumor suppressor gene on 3p25-p26. There is no evidence that VHL is involved in a significant number of tumors other than renal cell carcinoma.[135] However, *FHIT*, a human homologue of a yeast adenosine triphosphate–adenosine monophosphate (ATP-AMP) hydrolase, shows frequent abnormalities in many tumor types with LOH at 3p14. In head and neck tumors, LOH, homozygous deletions of one or more exons, and aberrant transcripts have been documented, suggesting that FHIT may have tumor suppressor properties in this tumor type.[136,137] Candidate genes for 3q26-qter amplifications are *LAZ3*, a zinc finger protein mapping to 3q27 and *BLC-6*, also a zinc finger protein that maps to 3q27. BCL-6 is a gene that often shows rearrangements in diffuse, large cell lymphomas.

Consistent gains of 7p may be related to the frequent overexpression and activation of the epidermal growth factor receptor (EGFR). Activation of this pathway may be an early event in HNSCC carcinogenesis.[138] The prime candidates for the very frequent (up to 70% of HNSCC) deletion on 9p are the

p16 gene and its homologue *p15,* as well as *p14^ARF,* which are overlapping genes located within 9p21. The *p16* gene is frequently inactivated in HNSCC by mutation and deletion and by methylation and deletion.[92] The p16 is also known as *p16^INK4a*, and as *CDKN2* (cyclin-dependent kinase inhibitor 2), as well as *CKI2*. CDKN2 protein antagonizes the function of CDK4 (cyclin-dependent kinase 4) and CDK6 (cyclin-dependent kinase 6), which are activated by binding cyclin D1. This complex then activates transcription of genes required for transit through the cell cycle. There are families of cyclins and of cyclin-dependent kinase inhibitors (CKIs) that are regulated in part by ubiquitin-mediated proteosome degradation (see Fig. 1–6A). Interestingly, the *CCND1* gene, which encodes cyclin D1, is located within the 11q13 region that is frequently amplified in HNSCC. Although seen in only about 15% of newly diagnosed cases of HNSCC[124] and about 30% of HNSCC cell lines,[116,119] rearrangements of 11q13 seem to be associated with cyclin D1 overexpression and poor prognosis.[124,139] Furthermore, studies of cyclin-D1 messenger RNA and protein expression also correlate with rearrangement and/or gain of 11q13,[139] suggesting that cyclin D1 overexpression is itself associated with aggressive malignant behavior. A combination of loss of the *p16* gene and amplification of the cyclin D1 oncogene could abrogate the cell cycle regulatory pathway at the G1 restriction point and enhance tumor progression.

Although it is difficult to detect loss of the short arms of acrocentric chromosomes, 17p loss was found by cytogenetic analysis in roughly 30% of cell lines.[116] Consistent with this finding, LOH on 17p has been detected in roughly 50% of HNSCCs by microsatellite analysis.[127–129] This loss correlates with mutation of the *p53* gene in roughly 40% of tumors and cell lines.

Losses on other chromosomal segments suggest the presence of tumor suppressor genes at these loci as well. Loss of 18q appears to be a late event, possibly associated with tumor progression.[101] On 18q, there are three candidate tumor suppressor genes: *DCC*, *DPC4*, and *Smad2*. It is not yet known whether these genes, whose products appear to be involved in cell adhesion (*DCC*) and TGFβ signaling (*DPC4* and *Smad2*), respectively, have a role in HNSCC.

CELL CYCLE REGULATION AND APOPTOSIS

Two critical areas of imbalance in cellular behavior in tumors are aberrant regulation of the cell cycle and aberrant regulation of programmed cell death. These processes are tightly regulated in normal cells to maintain homeostasis. Typically, cancer cells lose the ability to regulate these processes and may even gain mechanisms that drive cells through the cell cycle, or gain methods to avoid cell death. In some cases, knowledge of these abnormal mechanisms has been gained by studies of other tumor types, but as more is learned about tumors in general, researchers have found that head and neck tumors also have genetic or epigenetic changes that alter these pathways. Therefore, the next two sections present overviews of cell cycle regulation and programmed cell death, with specific reference to changes acquired by tumor cells to overcome the normal regulation of these processes.

Cell Cycle and Tumor Doubling Time

The cell cycle is the process by which DNA is faithfully replicated and by which it is ensured that identical chromosomal copies are equally distributed to the two daughter cells. Early light microscopic studies showed that cell division was preceded by mitosis (the M phase), during which the cells condensed their chromosomes and segregated sister chromatids to opposite poles of the cell. The cell cycle was divided into two fundamental parts: interphase, which occupies the majority of the cell cycle, and M-phase or mitosis, which normally lasts about 30 minutes and which terminates with the division of the cell. Interphase, or the period between two mitoses, was obscure until 1951 when Howard and Pelc used the incorporation of radioactive phosphorus into the DNA of bean roots (*Vica faba*) to divide interphase into four phases: G1, S, G2, and M.[140,141] G1 and G2 were defined as gap phases, separating the DNA synthesis (S) and mitosis (M) phases. In S-phase, the DNA content is duplicated, whereas in M-phase, the cell divides. During G1, the cell prepares to replicate the DNA, whereas during G2, the cell prepares for mitosis. The cell cycle of growing eukaryotic cells lasts from 90 minutes to more than 24 hours, and can be as short as 10 minutes in embryonic cells. In rapidly dividing human cells, the cell cycle normally lasts about 24 hours. The duration of the cell cycle shows considerable variation within a population of cells.

In normal proliferating tissues, such as epidermis and oral/oropharyngeal and intestinal mucosa, the gain in cell number by the proliferative activity in the basal cell layers is balanced by cell loss through differentiation and desquamation; the net volume is unaltered although the proliferative activity is high. The cell cycle time in normal tissue is usually shorter than in malignant cells[142–144] (Table 1–4). Cell cycle time calculations are difficult because there is usually a complex mixture of growing and dying cells, as well as quiescent cells, within tumors. Perfusion and competition for nutrients also affect the behavior of individual cells within a tumor. Not surprisingly, there is a striking discrepancy between cell cycle time and tumor volume doubling time (Table 1–5).[142,143] Tumor volume growth, measured

TABLE 1–4	CELL CYCLE TIMES OF NORMAL AND MALIGNANT CELLS
CELL TYPE	CELL CYCLE TIME (hr)
Embryonic cells	0.15
Colon epithelial cells	25
Rectum epithelial cells	48
Stomach epithelial cells	24
Bone marrow cells	18
Basal cell carcinoma	67
Acute myeloblastic leukemia	49
Acute lymphoblastic leukemia	35
Epidermoid carcinoma	24–90

Modified from Gussack GS, Brantley BA, Former JC Jr. Biology of tumors and head and neck cancer chemotherapy. *Laryngoscope.* 1984; 94: 1181–1187.

as tumor volume doubling time (T_D) is also highly variable within tumor types, and it can (e.g., in epidermoid carcinoma of the lung) span between 20 and 300 days.[144] In HNSCC, it varies from 12 to more than 107 days (Table 1–6).[143]

The balance between cell production and cell loss determines T_D. Cell production is influenced by the balance between several factors, such as the growth fraction, the cell cycle time, and cell loss. The compartment model proposed by Mendelsohn and Dethlefsen[145] suggests that the actual tumor volume is the consequence of the flow of cells between the proliferating (P), quiescent (Q) lethal (L) compartments. The growth fraction is the relation between proliferating and quiescent cells. Cells are lost from the tumor through shedding, necrosis, apoptosis, and differentiation. Stromal cells (vessels, connective tissue) and inflammatory cells also contribute to the

TABLE 1–5	DOUBLING TIMES (MEAN) OF TUMORS
TYPE OF TUMOR	MEAN DOUBLING TIME (days)
Squamous cell carcinoma of the lung	84
Breast carcinoma	96
Adenocarcinoma of colon	632
Hodgkin's disease	49
Ewing's sarcoma	17
Malignant melanoma	53
Osteosarcoma	30
Head and neck squamous cell carcinoma	12–>107

Modified from Gussack GS, Brantley BA, Former JC Jr. Biology of tumors and head and neck cancer chemotherapy. *Laryngoscope.* 1984; 94: 1181–1187 and Bresciani F, Paoluzi R, Benassi M, et al. Cell kinetics and growth of squamous cell carcinoma in man. *Cancer Res.* 1974; 34: 2405–2415.

TABLE 1–6	GROWTH OF SQUAMOUS CELL CARCINOMAS OF THE HEAD AND NECK IN HUMANS					
				RATE IN CELLS/hr/10^4		
TUMOR	CELL CYCLE (hr)	DOUBLING TIME (hr)	GROWTH FRACTION (%)	*Cell Birth*	*Cell Loss*	*Tumor Growth*
1	62	312	62	100	78	22
2	62	600	39	61	50	11
3	88	1362	41	47	43	4

Modified from Bresciani F, Paoluzi R, Benassi M, et al. Cell kinetics and growth of squamous cell carcinoma in man. *Cancer Res.* 1974; 34:2405–2415 and Gussack GS, Brantley BA, Former JC Jr. Biology of tumors and head and neck cancer chemotherapy. *Laryngoscope.* 1984; 94:1181–1187.

volume of the tumor. Rapidly growing tumors may be more susceptible to chemotherapy or radiation therapy; therefore, T_D may be useful in guiding the selection of patients for therapy.

Clinically, cell proliferation in tissues can be estimated by several means. By simple counting of mitoses with light microscopy, the fraction of cells in mitosis, known as the *mitotic index,* can be calculated. However, the M-phase is short and constitutes only a small fraction of the cell cycle, thus, the mitotic index will be low in slowly proliferating tissue/tumors. Therefore, the method has limited clinical value. Many nuclear proteins vary in their concentration during the cell cycle. They can be detected and quantified through immunohistochemical procedures, some of which can also be applied to archival paraffin-embedded material. The Ki-67 antibody recognizes a 345- and 395-kd antigen encoded by a single gene on chromosome 10. The antigen is expressed in proliferating cells, but not in G0 cells. It has been used to calculate the growth fraction of tumors, but has the limitation of only being applicable on cryostat sections. Recently, MIB1, a monoclonal antibody, has become available. This antibody can be used on paraffin-embedded material after antigen retrieval by microwave heating. Proliferating cell nuclear antigen (PCNA) is a 36-kd nuclear protein. It has been identified as an auxiliary protein of DNA polymerase δ, which is necessary for adequate strand synthesis during DNA replication. It is used to estimate the S-phase fraction (SPF). However, because it also is expressed during DNA repair (unscheduled DNA synthesis) in nonproliferating cells in association with neoplasia, and because it has a relatively long half-life (20 hours), it can give a falsely high impression of the SPF.

The fraction of cells in S-phase in a sample can be measured easily using flow cytometry. In nondiploid tumors, in which the malignant G1/G0 cells can be distinguished from the benign, stromal G0 cells of the tumor, the denominator for calculating the proportion of cells in S-phase can be calculated rather accurately. In diploid tumors, however, the malignant G1/G0 cells and the benign G0 cells cannot be differentiated; therefore, the denominator will include benign cells of the diploid G1/G0 peak, and

the SPF will be falsely low. In static cytometry, the malignant cells can be identified visually, but the number of cells that can be calculated in this way is considerably lower (2 to 300 compared to 10,000 to 20,000 in flow cytometry), and the SPF estimation is less accurate. Using in vivo pulse labeling or in vitro incubation techniques with either radiolabeled thymidine or 5-bromodeoxyuridine (BrdU) incorporation, the labeled S-phase can be identified by radiography or immunohistochemical techniques. These procedures are the common reference in cell kinetic studies and can be regarded as the "gold standards."

By combining in vivo pulse labeling and repeated tumor sampling through two cell cycles, a percent-labeled mitoses (PLM) curve can be constructed, and the various cell kinetic parameters can be calculated. However, this technique is not feasible for clinical use. When cell production is exactly balanced by cell loss, there is no net increase in tumor volume and so the T_D becomes infinitely long. The more cell production exceeds cell loss, the faster the tumor will grow. The theoretically maximum growth rate would occur when there is no cell loss, and this is usually expressed as the potential doubling time (T_{pot}).[146] Using BrdU in vivo pulse labeling and flow cytometric analysis of a tumor biopsy sampled 4 to 8 hours later, the T_{pot} can be calculated.[147]

Regulation of the Cell Cycle

ENTRY INTO THE CELL CYCLE AND CELL CYCLE CHECKPOINTS

Cells are in the resting phase of the cell cycle G0, most of the time. Tissue stem cells are triggered by growth factors to leave G0 and enter the cell cycle to undergo growth, DNA synthesis, and cell division. Several of the dominantly acting oncogenes, including activated growth factor receptors (*EGFR, Her2/Neu*), growth factors (transforming growth factor alpha [TGF-α], platelet-derived growth factor [PDGF]), and signaling molecules (*MYC, RAS*), affect this aspect of cell growth regulation by stimulating cells to enter the cell cycle. Once cells embark upon entry into the cell cycle, there is a series of phases that the cells go through, and there are checkpoints that regulate progress through the cycle to ensure that each of the new cells has an accurate copy of the genome.

To ensure high fidelity in DNA replication and mitosis, the cell cycle is subject to controls that regulate the cell cycle phases. The surveillance mechanisms is often referred to as a series of checkpoints because the cells can arrest at the checkpoints if necessary. The checkpoints are positions in the cell cycle at which processes being monitored are completed or in which transitions are blocked. Originally, checkpoints meant surveillance mechanisms, but they have since been redefined as any control that ensures the order of cell cycle events.[148,149] The protein p53 is often referred to as the guardian of the genome because it plays a critical role in regulating the cell cycle and in causing cell cycle arrest at either the G1 or G2 checkpoints. Growth factors can trigger the resting G0 cell or the G1 cell (cells in G1 and G0 cannot be easily distinguished) into the cell cycle. During the G1 phase, the cells respond to extracellular signals. However, once the cell has passed the restriction point (R-point), it becomes refractory to growth factor–induced signals. Instead, it will rely on an intrinsic clock that regulates the progression through the cell cycle and mitosis.

CYCLINS, CYCLIN-DEPENDENT KINASES, AND CYCLIN-DEPENDENT KINASE INHIBITORS

Central to the regulation of progression through the cell cycle is a highly conserved family of protein kinases, the CDKs and their activating partners, the cyclins.[150] These proteins regulate transition through the cell cycle and ensure that G2 nuclei do not re-replicate until they pass through mitosis. Cyclins were originally defined as proteins that were specifically degraded at every mitosis, but once several cyclin cDNAs had been cloned and sequenced, the definition changed to that of a protein containing a 100-amino-acid region of sequence homologous to the consensus "cyclin box." Today, more than 10 animal cell cyclins have been described.[150] The activity of the cyclin-CDK complex is regulated by phosphorylation, by the binding of specific inhibitor proteins, or by changes in the level of the cyclin itself (Fig. 1–6 A and B).

Cyclins D and E function during G1, cyclins E and A during S-phase, and cyclins A and B during mitosis. Cyclins D, E, and A and their CDKs sequentially regulate passage through the R-point and entry into the S-phase. There are three D-type cyclins (D1, D2, and D3). D-type cyclins are sensitive to growth factors, which stimulate cyclin synthesis, leading to assembly with their corresponding CDKs (CDK4 and CDK6). The D-cyclins can be regarded as growth factor sensors, induced as part of the delayed early response to growth factor stimulation and important for the transition from a quiescent

(G0) state to G1 status. The D cyclins are unstable, and are rapidly degraded by the ubiquitin-proteasome proteolytic pathway. Several different ubiquitin-conjugating enzymes are known, and these may recognize particular motifs. One candidate motif is a "destruction box" shared by mitotic cyclins.[151] The degradation of the D-cyclins is a mechanism that helps to restrict cells from unscheduled cell replication. As noted previously, cyclin D1 is encoded by the CCND1 gene on the chromosome 11q13 and is frequently overexpressed in HNSCC. Both cyclin D1 (originally designated PRAD1) overexpression[112,113] and chromosome 11q13 aberrations are signs of poor prognosis in patients with HNSCC.[124,139] This finding is consistent with the requirement for cyclin D1 to drive the G0 to G1 transition. Cells with constitutive overexpression of cyclin D1 are continuously ready to progress into the cell cycle. Cyclin D2 is encoded by the CCND2 gene on chromosome 12p13. So far, no rearrangements have been found in CCND2. CCND3 on the 6p21 locus has not yet been identified as a proto-oncogene.[152]

The CDKs consist of a catalytic subunit, usually of 34 kd, which requires formation of a complex with the corresponding cyclin component to become catalytically active. The catalytic activity can be regulated at three levels (see Fig. 1–6). First, the CDKs are regulated by association with a cyclin that is necessary to activate the protein kinase activity of the CDK. Therefore, these enzymes are inactive in the absence of the cyclin partner. Furthermore, an active CDK can be made inactive by degradation of the cyclin. Second, protein phosphorylation of a tyrosine in the active site of the enzyme inhibits its activity, and a tyrosine phosphatase can reactivate the enzyme by dephosphorylation of the active site. Third, the CDKs are regulated via specific CKIs.[153] CKIs include p16 (also called MTS1/INK4/CDKN2),[93] which, as described previously, is frequently inactivated in HNSCC. In carcinogenesis, the regulation of the cell cycle checkpoints, like the START checkpoint in the G1-S-phase transition, is disturbed, often because of deregulation of the cyclin-CDK complexes and their inhibitors. The first CKI cloned was the WAF1/Cip1 gene (independently cloned by two research teams) coding for the p21 protein. p53 promotes the expression of p21, and the G1 arrest seen after induction of p53 in response to DNA damage is mediated via p21 inhibition of cyclin D1-CDK4/6 activity. There are other specific polypeptide inhibitors of CDK4 and CDK6—the so-called INK4 proteins—that can directly block cyclin D–dependent kinase activity and cause G1 phase arrest. The four known 15- to 19-kd INK4 proteins (p16^{INK4a}, p15^{INK4b}, p18^{INK4c}, and p19^{INK4d}) bind and inhibit CDK4 and CDK6, but not other CDKs.[154] Mutations of the INK4a gene (also called CDKN2 or MTS1, on chromosome 9p21) are associated with familial malignant melanoma. Homozygous deletions of the INK4a locus have also been found in two of five NPCs.

The critical target of the cyclin D1-p34 CDK com-

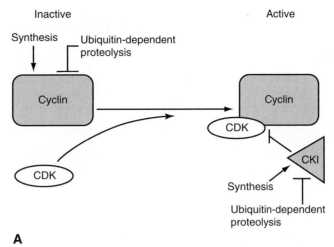

A

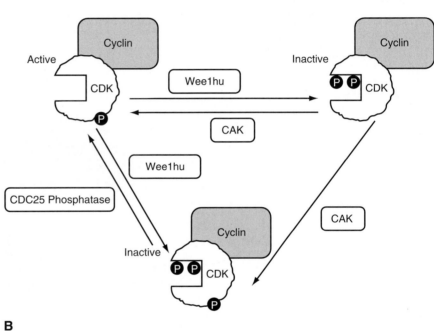

B

FIGURE 1–6 Interactions between cyclins, cyclin-dependent kinases (CDKs) and cyclin-dependent kinase inhibitors (CKIs). *A,* The CDK is inactive until it forms a complex with its cyclin partner. The CDK-cyclin complexes can be inactivated by CKIs. Both cyclins and CKIs can be removed by ubiquitin-dependent proteolysis. As noted in the text, CKIs such as *p16 (p16^INK4A, CDKN2, CKI2*), and *p21 (WAF1/cip1*) are important regulators of cell cycle progression. *B,* CDKs are further regulated by phosphorylation status. Dephosphorylation within the active site by CDC25 phosphate and phosphorylation by a CDK-activating kinase (CAK) (cyclin H/CDK7) activate the cyclin-bound CDK. Phosphorylation of the active site by human homologues (Wee1hu) (phosphorylates CDC2 and CDK2 on tyrosine 15) of the yeast Wee1 gene product can inactivate the kinase. Much of what has been learned about cell cycle control has come from the study of yeast cell division incompetent mutants such as Wee1. It is clear that there are multiple mechanisms that control cell cycle progression and ensure that each step is successfully completed and properly scheduled.

plex is the retinoblastoma protein, or Rb. Rb is encoded by the *RB* gene on chromosome 13q14 and is inactivated by mutation of one copy and loss of the remaining copy in the juvenile ocular tumor of the same name. Rb is the main gatekeeper for the transition from G0 to G1. There are several Rb family members (e.g., p107, p130). Presumably, these work similarly to the 107-kd Rb protein in regulating transcription of other key proteins required for DNA replication and cell division. Rb has a binding pocket that binds to and sequesters E2F, a DNA-binding protein that is essential for formation of the transcriptional complex.[155] When Rb is in its unphosphorylated form, E2F is bound and unavailable for binding to DNA transcription sites, and so the cell remains in G0. Phosphorylation of Rb by the cyclin-D/CDK4 complex releases E2F, which binds to DNA sites and initiates transcription and expres-

sion of genes required for DNA synthesis and chromosome replication. The interrelationship between Rb, E2F, cyclin D1, CDK4/CDK6, and CKIs is shown in Figure 1–7. Rb is nearly always wild-type and expressed in HNSCC; however, as noted before, this pathway is often inactivated by loss of expression of the CKI p16 and/or by overexpression of cyclin D1. The simian virus 40 (SV40) and HPV viral oncoproteins, large T antigen, and E7, respectively, can also inactivate Rb function by displacing E2F.[46,156] Thus, this critical regulatory process can be affected by several mechanisms.

p53 EXPRESSION AND MUTATION

In the search for clues to carcinogenesis, much attention has focused on the dominantly acting oncogenes, such as *c-erbB1* (epidermal growth factor recep-

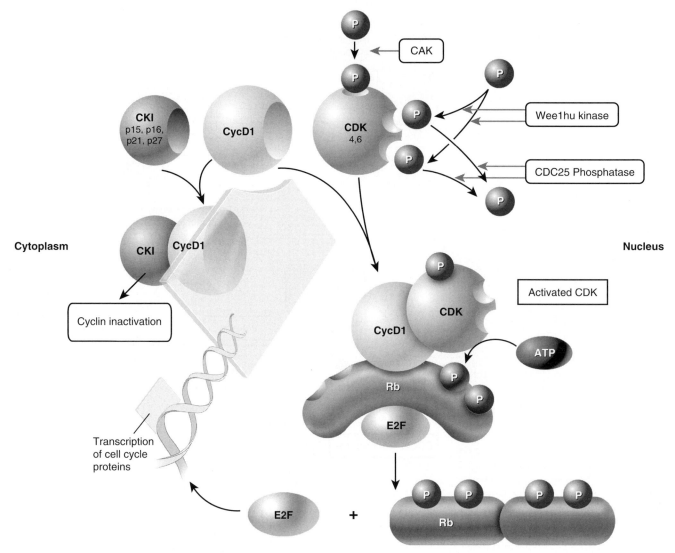

FIGURE 1–7 Cyclin D1/CDK4 or CDK6 complexes lead to phosphorylation of Rb and release of E2F1. This schematic diagram illustrates the protein-protein interactions regulating RB-mediated entry into the cell cycle. CAK, CDK-activating kinase; CDK, cyclin-dependent kinase; ATP, adenosine triphosphate.

tor gene), *CCND1* (the cyclin D1 gene) and *C-YMC*, which function through activation. They exercise their function in the carcinogenic process by abnormal expression (inappropriate overexpression, expression at the wrong time in the cell cycle, or expression in the wrong cell). In contrast to the oncogenes, the activity of a tumor suppressor gene has to be lost to facilitate tumorigenesis. The retinoblastoma gene, *p53*, and the CKIs are all examples of tumor suppressor genes, the products of which act as brakes to proliferation. The loss of both copies of such a gene by allelic loss, by methylation, by inactivation through mutation, or by inhibition of function of the normal protein all can cause an increase in proliferation by removing important regulatory mechanisms. The central role played by *p53* is one

of the reasons why this is one of the most frequently mutated genes in human cancers.

The p53 protein was identified in 1979 independently by two groups as a cellular protein that interacts with the large T antigen of the SV40 virus.[157,158] Initially, p53 was considered to be an oncogene because it was often overexpressed in tumor cells. When p53 was sequenced from a normal cell, it became evident that the p53 protein expressed in most tumors was mutant p53, and that the mutations were loss-of-function mutations, suggesting that p53 was a tumor suppressor gene, like Rb.

A 53-kd protein of 393 amino acids, p53 is encoded by a gene located on chromosome 17p. Mutation in the *p53* tumor suppressor gene is the most frequently reported genetic aberration in human cancer.[159] The normal p53 protein functions as a cell cycle checkpoint and sensor of DNA damage in the cell, and modulates such events as G1-arrest, DNA repair, and apoptosis.[159,160] Cells with mutated *p53* are predisposed to further genetic alterations because of inadequate DNA repair, escape from apoptosis, and manifestation of additional DNA damage in subsequent cell cycles. The gene consists of 11 exons, and more than 80% of the mutations are reported to be in exons 5-8, a region highly conserved through evolution. In HNSCC, mutations outside exons 5-8 are even less frequent.[161] Other mechanisms of p53 inactivation include binding to DNA tumor virus proteins, such as the papillomavirus E6 protein, or to overexpressed cellular genes, such as the *MDM2* oncogene.[162] Germline mutations of *p53* are the basis for the Li-Fraumeni familial cancer syndrome. The mutation is not lethal, and transgenic mice without a functioning *p53* gene develop normally, but develop tumors within a few months. Because the protein functions as a homo-tetramer, mutation of one allele leads to partial functional inactivation of p53 activity in a dominant-negative manner. The wild type p53 protein has a short half-life and normally cannot be detected by immunohistochemical techniques. However, mutation usually leads to a stabilization of the protein, with subsequent accumulation in the cell that can be detected by immunohistochemistry, except in the case of mutations resulting in a stop codon or mutant protein without increased stability. By using PCR and single-strand conformational polymorphism (PCR-SSCP) analysis, mutant forms can be detected. However, it is necessary to sequence the mutant forms, as some silent mutations can result in a codon coding for the same amino acid as the nonmutated gene. In head and neck cancer, there is an association between carcinogenic factors, such as alcohol or tobacco use, and p53 overexpression or *p53* mutation in head and neck carcinogenesis.[14,163,164]

Immunohistochemical studies have shown *p53* overexpression to be an early event in HNSCC carcinogenesis, being found in dysplastic lesions and CIS before the development of invasive carcinoma. It is not known if this event reflects p53 protein accumulation due to gene mutation or merely a normal p53 response to DNA damage and the activity of a carcinogen.[165–170] Generally, an association between mutation and overexpression is assumed. However, in HNSCC, there is emerging evidence of a discrepancy between the results achieved with molecular analysis and those obtained by immunohistochemical methods.[171,172] False-negative findings (mutation without overexpression) can be attributed to p53 mutations at splice sites, frame shifts, or nonsense mutations that would be predicted to encode for a truncated p53 protein undetectable by immunohistochemistry. Furthermore, Boyle et al[165] showed that mutation of p53 increases with tumor progression, suggesting that the overexpression of wild-type p53

seen in preinvasive lesions or the mucosa of smokers might be a normal p53 response to DNA damage caused by carcinogens in smoke.

Recently, the crystal structure of the p53 tumor suppressor–DNA complex was elucidated, and it was made clear how p53 mutations inactivate the protein.[173,174] p53 contains three functional domains: an amino-terminal transcriptional activation domain; a central, sequence-specific, DNA-binding domain; and a carboxy-terminal oligomerization domain. Most p53 point mutations affect the residues within the core domain. These class 1 mutations inactivate the protein's function by abolishing its sequence-specific, DNA-binding capacity and its ability to regulate gene transcription. Class 2 mutations involve residues that are important in folding of the core domain, leading to abnormal conformation of the protein and loss of function either by loss of specific DNA-binding capacity or loss of one or more of its many protein-protein interactions. Therefore, the discrepancy between the PCR-SSCP and the immunohistochemical results may depend on the site of p53 mutation or the anti-p53 antibody employed, which vary in sensitivity and specificity for different types of p53 alterations. Overexpression is not only seen in gene mutation, but also in cases with retention of the target protein detectable by the p53 antibody in the tumor cell. Both mutational stabilization of the p53 protein and elevated levels of wild-type p53 protein allow detection by immunohistochemistry. Thus, if the secondary stabilization of p53 occurs by some mechanism(s) other than gene mutation, overexpression can be demonstrated. Accumulation of wild-type p53 protein has been found in inherited cancer[175] and in cancers treated with chemotherapeutic drugs or radiation.[176,177] The mechanism for such nonmutational stabilization of the p53 protein is unknown, but is most likely the result of interruption of the normal degradative pathway of p53. Other proteins, such as the products of cellular oncogene *mdm-2*,[178,179] have p53 binding sites, as do the protein products of several DNA viruses, including SV40 large T antigen, E1b of adenovirus,[180,181] and E6 of HPV.[47,182] These viral proteins can bind to the *p53* gene and inactivate its ability to act as a negative regulator of DNA synthesis via its function as a transcription factor for other regulatory proteins, such as p21 (Waf1/Cip1/CKI).

Studies have implicated p53 protein expression as an independent prognostic factor in carcinomas of the breast, stomach, colon/rectum, bladder, and in non–small cell lung cancer (NSCLC).[183,184] The clinical relevance of p53 overexpression in HNSCC has been subject to debate. There are studies indicating a correlation between p53 overexpression and survival, with some reporting improved survival in patients with p53 overexpression.[185] Overexpression has also been strongly associated with a histologic malignancy grading scale with prognostic capability.[186] However, the lack of correlation between p53 expression and clinicopathologic parameters or survival, originally reported by Field et al,[163] has subsequently been substantiated by many reports.[187]

Studies on the relationship between p53 mutation in HNSCC and clinicopathologic parameters or survival are sparse. Brennan et al[188] found an association with recurrence, but not survival. Ahomadegbe et al[189] could not find any correlation between mutation and clinical stage or 5-year survival. They reported a high frequency of mutations (69%), as well as a good correlation between mutation and overexpression. Nylander et al[172] in a study of 80 HNSCCs of the oral cavity using archival specimens, could not find any relation between p53 mutation and survival. Their research revealed a high frequency of a novel nonrandom 14 bp deletion in exon 8.[190] Bradford et al[191] did find an association between p53 mutation and poor prognosis in patients with advanced laryngeal carcinoma.

p53 SENSES DNA DAMAGE, REGULATES CELL CYCLE ARREST, AND INDUCES APOPTOSIS

DNA damage (e.g., that induced by ionizing radiation) induces an arrest of cells in G1 phase. This arrest is mediated by and requires a functional p53 protein. Loss of expression of wt-p53 or overexpression of a mutant p53 protein results in lack of G1 arrest following DNA damage. DNA strand breaks are believed to be the primary signal leading to induction of p53 expression, and this, in turn, activates the expression of several genes, including GADD45 (growth arrest and DNA damage-inducible), p21 (WAF-1/cip1) and MDM2 (Fig. 1–8). Overexpression of GADD45 results in the inhibition of progression of cells into S-phase, and recent studies have suggested an association of GADD45 with proliferating cell nuclear antigen (PCNA), whereby GADD45 facilitates the interaction between PCNA, a component of DNA polymerase delta, and DNA repair complexes.[192]

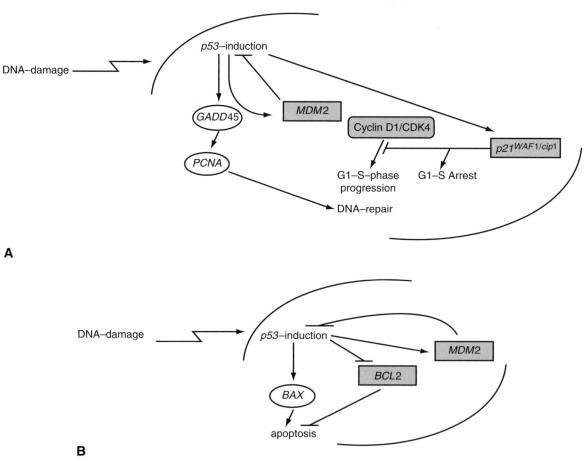

FIGURE 1–8   Cell cycle progression, DNA repair, and apoptosis are regulated by p53. A, DNA damage induces p53 expression, which in turn affects DNA repair processes and inhibits cell cycle progression. B, DNA damage, if extensive, can also trigger programmed cell death via up-regulated p53, which in turn leads to increased expression of BAX, a proapoptotic member of the BCL-2 family. This is accompanied by down-regulation of BCL-2, an antiapoptotic protein that favors cell survival. In both cases, MDM2 acts as a regulator of p53 expression and function. PCNA, proliferating cell nuclear antigen.

Up-regulation of p21 inhibits the cyclin D/CDK2 complex and the associated phosphorylation of several proteins, including the Rb protein, a phosphorylation necessary for G1 to S-phase progression. The concomitant induction of the *MDM2* gene, a down-regulator of p53, serves as a negative feedback loop limiting the extent of G1 arrest after DNA damage. These relationships are illustrated in Figure 1–8B. When a cell arrests in G1 as a result of DNA damage, it either repairs the damage or the cell is directed to undergo programmed cell death, or apoptosis. Apoptosis is a distinct mode of cell death, morphologically different from necrotic cell death and responsible for deletion of cells in normal tissues. It also occurs in neoplasia. It is characterized by chromatin condensation to the nuclear membrane, which occurs before any loss of plasma membrane integrity, and is followed by shrinkage of the cells and modification of the cytoskeleton, leading to plasma membrane blebbing. The whole nucleus collapses at the time other organelles are still relatively unchanged, and the cell excludes vital dyes. Associated with these morphologic changes is DNA degradation into oligonucleosomal fragments. These oligonucleosomal fragments appear as a ladder pattern of DNA bands upon electrophoretic separation of isolated DNA and serve as one assay for detection of apoptotic cells. Formation of nuclear fragments and protuberances follows condensation of the cytoplasm and convolution of nuclear and cell outlines on the cell surface, resulting in the production of apoptotic bodies. These are phagocytosed by nearby cells and degraded within lysosomes. There is no associated inflammation.

Most, or maybe even all, cells in an organism have the ability to undergo programmed cell death. This process removes redundant as well as damaged cells and is a central mechanism in embryologic development for removing unneeded cells, such as those between the fingers and toes, or for selecting out unwanted, autoreactive T cells in the developing thymus. In proliferating tissues, such as epithelium, programmed cell death contributes to the physiologic control of cell number. As in DNA-damage–induced growth arrest and repair, p53 plays a critical role in the induction of apoptosis following DNA damage, and it has been suggested that the cellular decision of growth arrest versus apoptosis is dependent upon cell type or "cellular context."[192] The process of apoptosis is controlled by an increasing number of evolutionarily conserved genes, with some gene products being activators and others being inhibitors of apoptosis.

BCL-2 AND *BAX*: SURVIVAL VERSUS DEATH

The apoptosis-promoting gene *BAX* seems to be the only member of a family of apoptosis-regulating genes that is up-regulated by p53 in response to DNA damage. The *BAX* gene was originally identified as a *BCL*-2–associated protein. The *BCL*-2 gene, in turn, was initially discovered by chromosome analysis of the most common t(14;18) translocation in human B-cell follicular lymphoma. The BCL-2 protein is localized on the mitochondrial and nuclear membranes and the endoplasmic reticulum. It is widely expressed during embryonic development but is restricted to immature and stem cell populations in adult tissues. Unlike other oncogenes, *BCL*-2 has the unusual property to extend cell survival rather than to excite cell proliferation.[193] *Bcl*-2 knockout mice are surprisingly normal at birth, but manifest a catastrophic, postnatal, immune function failure due to loss of mature B and T cells through apoptosis. Overexpression, on the other hand, is associated with human B-cell lymphoma and has also been described in a wide variety of human solid cancers, including HNSCC. The mechanism by which the BCL-2 protein exerts its action is unknown. It has been suggested that BCL-2 acts by blocking the generation of reactive oxygen species caused by activation of cytochrome p450 in the mitochondria. No longer considered a single entity, *BCL*-2 is one member of a growing multigene family (for review, see White[193]). The *BCL-X* gene has homology to *BCL*-2 and also regulates cell death, but in contrast to *bcl*-2, *bcl*-*x* knockout mice have an embryonic lethal phenotype. *BAK*, a pro-apoptotic member of the *BCL*-2 family, also has a sequence homology to *BCL*-2. Similar to *BAX*, *BAK* can form complexes with pro-apoptotic family members and can accelerate cell death. There are also viral counterpoints to *BCL*-2, the best characterized being the adenovirus E1B 19-kd protein. It is required to block apoptosis during adenovirus infection. *BAX* can suppress the capacity of *BCL*-2 to block apoptosis. These proteins can form heterodimers and it is thought that the ratio of BCL-2 to BAX protein determines cell survival or death following a stimulus capable of inducing apoptosis. Interactions between *p53* and the *BAX*–*BCL*-2 family are presented schematically in Figure 1–8B. Figure 1–9 summarizes the interrelationships between growth inhibiting signals such as TGFβ, mitogenic signals mediated by growth factors and their receptors, and signals generated by DNA damage on the cell cycle regulatory machinery of the mammalian cell.

IMMORTALITY: CANCER CELLS EXPRESS TELOMERASE

Senescence

Most eukaryotic cells are capable of only a limited number of cell divisions; thus, they are said to have a finite replicative life span. As mentioned earlier, this was described 30 years ago by Hayflick,[5] who

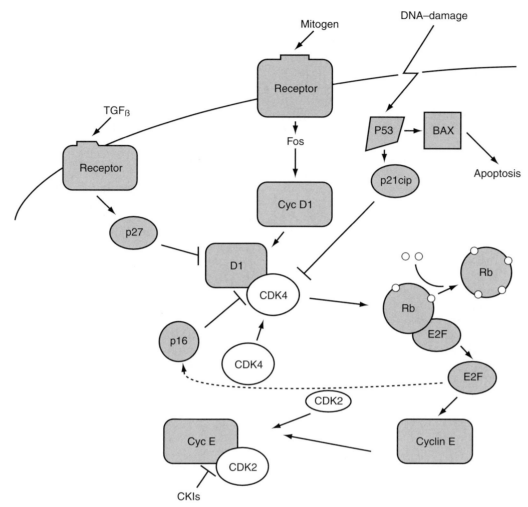

FIGURE 1-9 This schematic diagram illustrates the interactions between growth stimulatory and cell cycle regulatory mechanisms in a normal cell. Many of the players in this carefully orchestrated mechanism are targets of mutation, amplification, or inactivation in cancer, leading to unregulated cell cycle progression, increased genetic instability, and loss of growth control. In the simplest paradigm, a normal cell receives growth stimulatory signals through its membrane receptor, leading to cyclin D expression, activation of CDK4, phosphorylation of Rb, and release of E2F, which then leads to expression of other cell cycle proteins. Note that multiple inhibitory pathways limit the ability of cells to progress through the cell cycle. Of particular importance is the ability to arrest for DNA repair via the p21^{CIPI} CKI. TGFβ, transforming growth factor beta.

noted that in vitro cultivated fibroblasts could be passed through only a limited number of passages, with a mean of many tens of population doublings ending in a state of proliferative quiescence. Since then, it has been shown that many animal cell types have finite replicative life spans when cultivated in vitro. Studies in vivo are sparse, but support replicative senescence.[194] Apart from terminally differentiated cells, most proliferation-competent mammalian cells senesce, but there are a few exceptions. Germ cells are capable of continuous replication. The senescent phenotype is acquired during embryonic development; however, stem cells, even in the adult organism, can divide infinitely. Many malignant tumors seem to circumvent replicative senescence.

Telomere Shortening Limits Life Span

The mechanism by which cells sense the number of divisions they have completed appears to depend, at least in part, on the length of their telomeres. It appears that telomere shortening is a cell division counting mechanism. A telomere is the DNA at the chromosome end. The lagging strand of DNA molecules (the 5' end of double-stranded DNA) is incompletely replicated by conventional DNA polymerases owing to the polarity of the normal replication machinery. A DNA end cannot be fully replicated.[195] Therefore, unless other mechanisms intercede, the telomere will shorten by 30 to 150 bp per cell division. Telomeres consist of repetitive DNA sequences specific for telomeres and serve different functions. They are important in the pairing of homologous chromosomes in meiotic nuclear division, in the movement of chromosomes during division, and in the protection of chromosome termini.

The Telomerase Complex

Telomerase is a special DNA polymerase used by most eukaryotic cells to solve the problem of the telomere end replication. It has an essential RNA component, implicating a primordial origin, and unusual polymerization properties.[196] Telomerase adds repeated telomere sequences to the chromosome ends. Telomerase activity is generally absent in normal somatic tissues, but can be detected in adult testes (germ cells) and activated lymphocytes. Lower levels are expressed in proliferative cells of renewal tissues, such as the basal layer of the human epidermis. Telomerase activity has also been detected in 85% to 90% of all human cancers,[197] including 89% to 100% of HNSCCs.[198,199] There are two targets for detecting telomerase expression that are currently in use: the biochemical activity of telomerase (the TRAP assay); and the RNA component of telomerase.[200] Recent investigations have shown that there are multiple components to the telomerase complex. There are two noncatalytic proteins that are homologous to the tetrahymena p80 and p95 telomerase–associated proteins. The absence of catalytic units in these proteins led to the search for the enzymatic unit. It is of interest that a telomerase catalytic protein with homology to the retroviral reverse transcriptases has been cloned and shown to be the telomerase enzyme. This protein is highly expressed in immortalized cells, but is absent from mortal cells, giving greater tumor specificity than the other telomerase subunits.[201] There is much excitement for developing tumor-specific therapies based on inhibition of telomerase function.

The Dominance of Senscence over Immortality

In normal senescence, the proliferatively inactive cells retain viability and biochemical activity. Cell fusion experiments have shown that replicative senescence is a dominant phenotype. Hybrids between cells with an infinite replicative life span and normal cells senesce, which implies that immortal cells have lost, mutated, or inactivated genes required for the senescent phenotype. One explanation for the restoration of senescence in cell fusion experiments is that one or more of the introduced genes suppresses telomerase activity. The senescence program can probably activated via multiple pathways with multiple steps. For human fibroblasts, for example, the most likely number of pathways is three, one in-

volving pRb, one involving p53, and one involving an unknown gene, possibly on chromosome 6. It has been shown that, in some, but not all cell lines, introduction of chromosome 3 induces senescence and represses telomerase activity.[202]

IMMORTALITY WITH E6, E7, AND *hTERT* AND NEOPLASIA WITH *hTERT, H-RAS*, AND SV40 T ANTIGEN

The catalytic subunit of human telomerase, *hTERT*, when ectopically expressed, extends the life span of normal fibroblasts and, when combined with other changes in gene expression, can allow indefinite replication of differentiated cells. This is a crucial observation because previous attempts to immortalize cells have also disrupted the differentiation program. It has also been particularly difficult to immortalize normal human cells in vitro until the discovery by Kiyono et al[203] that *hTERT* can prevent senescence and immortalize primary normal human keratinocytes, provided that the Rb/p16INK4 signaling pathway is also inactivated. This discovery was quickly followed by a demonstration by Hahn et al[204] that primary human epithelial cells and fibroblasts could be made not only immortal, but also tumorigenic, by expression of the telomerase catalytic subunit in combination with expression of activated *H-RAS* and the simian virus large T antigen. SV40 T antigen, like the HPV E6 and E7 proteins, targets both p53 and Rb, the gatekeepers of the cell cycle, whereas *H-RAS* can bypass the need for external stimulation by growth factors that signal through *RAS*. That only these three pathways are sufficient for tumorigenesis may be an instrumental factor in the development of new therapeutic strategies. On the other hand, there may be other factors induced by T antigen that have been previously unrecognized. In any case, knowledge of the minimal requirements for converting normal human epithelial cells into tumor cells is important in understanding the development and progression of squamous cell carcinoma.

ANGIOGENESIS AND TUMOR SPREAD

Angiogenesis

Angiogenesis or neovascularization is the process by which new blood vessels are produced. New vessels are generated as capillaries by sprouting from existing small vessels. The cells bud from an existing capillary or small venule and form a solid cord, which then hollows out to form a tube. The process continues until the new vessel encounters and connects to another capillary. This is a normal process in wound healing, in which there is a phase of rapid neovascularization associated with cell proliferation and tissue repair. In tumorigenesis, neovascularization is a rate-limiting step in most instances. Malignant cells cannot grow beyond the limits of oxygenation permitted by diffusion without induction of new blood vessels. As early as the 1950s, Thomlinson and Gray[205] demonstrated, in a study of squamous cell carcinoma of the lung, that consumption of oxygen causes a falling gradient from the vessels throughout the tumor cell mass. Furthermore, they showed that tumor necrosis developed in tumor cords with a central vessel and a radius exceeding 160 μm.

The concept of tumors being angiogenesis-dependent diseases means that angiogenesis is necessary for primary tumor growth, progression, and metastasis, and that inhibition leads to cessation of growth or tumor remission. The hypothesis that tumor growth is largely dependent on the induction of neovascularization was originally proposed by Folkman[206] more than 2 decades ago. It is now well established that the progression of tumor growth beyond the limit of 3 to 5 mm^3 requires the recruitment of new blood vessels. Angiogenesis, as part of the normal wound healing process with the formation and maturation of granulation tissue, is, unlike tumor neovascularization, a time-limited and self-regulating process. Tumors are often likened to wounds that do not heal, indicating neovascularization as a possible target for systemic antitumor therapy.[207] Support for the hypothesis that tumors are angiogenesis-dependent has been derived from experimental observations. For example, it has been noted that experimental tumors in either the liver or the anterior chamber of the eye fail to grow larger than 1 mm^3 unless there is vessel proliferation into the tumor. Similarly, neutralizing antibodies to the angiogenic factor bFGF (basic fibroblast growth factor) can inhibit tumor cell growth.[208]

The formation of new blood vessels involves interactions between endothelial cells and the extracellular matrix. The neovascularization is triggered by the release of polypeptide growth factors and cytokines[207-209] (Table 1–7) by the tumor cells and the cells of the host response to the tumor. The ability to bind to heparin is a common characteristic associated with many of these factors. The angiogenic molecules function as autocrine and paracrine growth signals between the tumor cells and surrounding stroma. During the past several years, at least 14 different proteins that can trigger blood vessel growth have been identified, along with several others than can halt it. Recent discoveries indicate that there is a balance between substances inhibiting and stimulating angiogenesis in tumors, and that this balance is crucial in determining whether angiogenesis will proceed or not. Using three different transgenic mouse models (pancreatic islet B-cell tumor, dermal fibrosarcoma, and HPV 16–expressing epidermal squamous cell carcinoma), Hanahan and co-workers[210] found that discrete stages of premalig-

TABLE 1 – 7	GROWTH FACTORS PROMOTING ANGIOGENESIS

GROWTH FACTOR	DESCRIPTION/CHARACTERISTICS
Angiogenein	14 kd-polypeptide; stimulates angiogenesis, but is neither mitogenic nor chemotactic
Angiotropin	4.5-kd polypeptide; angiogenic and mitogenic for endothelial cells
bFGF	Basic fibroblast growth factor, an 18-kd polypeptide; both chemotactic and mitogenic for endothelial cells and fibroblasts
EGF	Epidermal growth factor
Fibrin	
HGF	Hepatocyte growth factor
HIV-1-Tat	Transactivator of HIV-1 genes
IL-8	Interleukin 8
Nicotinamide	
NO	Nitric oxide
PAF	Platelet-activating factor
PD-ECGF	Platelet-derived endothelial cell growth factor, a 45-kd protein; endothelial cell mitogen
PDGF	Platelet-derived growth factor
PGF	Placental growth factor
TGF-α	Transforming growth factor α, a 5.5-kd polypeptide
TGF-β	Transforming growth factor β, a 25-kd polypeptide; neither chemotactic nor mitogenic for endothelial cells, but stimulates endothelial cell differentiation and ECM production
TNF-α	Tumor necrosis factor α, a 17-kd polypeptide; promotes endothelial cell differentiation and extracellular matrix organization
VEGF	Vascular endothelial growth factor, a 23-kd dimer composed of two identical subunits; angiogenic and mitogenic for endothelial cells

Compiled from Gasparini G. Angiogenesis research up to 1996. A commentary on the state of art and suggestions for future studies. *Eur J Cancer.* 1996; 32A:2379–2395; Petruzzili GJ. Tumor angiogenesis. *Head Neck.* 1996; 18:283–291; and Ellis LM, Fidler IJ. Angiogenesis and metastasis. *Eur J Cancer.* 1996; 32A:2451–2460.

nant progression were evident. They found a hyperplastic phase that was followed by a stochastic angiogenic stage, and they determined that neovascularization developed well before the emergence of an invasive malignant lesion. They suggested the hypothesis that the induction of neovascularization during the multistage carcinogenic process is coordinated by a discrete event, an angiogenic switch. During the development of squamous cell carcinoma, the lesion progresses from hyperplasia through increasing degrees of dysplasia to carcinoma in situ. In the transgenic mouse model with the HPV 16 oncogenes controlled by the keratin 14 regulatory region, there was a striking increase both in the number and distribution of dermal capillaries in the early and advanced dysplastic lesions, with numerous vessels lying in close apposition to the basement membrane. The pattern of development was indicative of an angiogenic switch from vascular quiescence to an initial condition of modest neovascularization, followed by a second, striking, upregulation of angiogenesis in high-grade neoplasias, as well as in invasive cancers. Similar patterns of activation of neovascularization are evident in human premalignant lesions, such as dysplastic nevi, mammary ductal carcinoma in situ, and dysplasias of the uterine cervix.

ANGIOSTATIN AND ENDOSTATIN

In normal tissue, the antiangiogenic pathway is likely to predominate. There are several naturally occurring antiangiogenic substances. For more than 50 years, it has been recognized clinically and experimentally that metastases do not grow independent of the primary tumor, and that removal of the primary tumor can result in enhanced growth of the metastases. Whether these interactions were due to immunologic phenomena, hormonal interactions, or metabolic changes was unclear, however. A few years ago, it was demonstrated that the total tumor burden could affect angiogenesis in remote metastases. The primary tumor can suppress angiogenesis, a process mediated by an endogenous angiogenesis inhibitor—angiostatin—produced by the primary tumor.[211] Angiostatin is a 38-kd protein with homology to the first four kringle structures of plasminogen, and it is a specific inhibitor of endothelial cell proliferation. Angiostatin can block development of metastases after resection of large tumors in mice, and it can suppress tumor growth by inducing involution of vessels.[211] Although this molecule does not appear to have a direct effect on tumor cells, the residual tumor cells exhibit increased apoptosis during angiostatin treatment.[212] Endostatin is an angiogenesis inhibitor, produced by hemangioendothelioma, that is a 20-kd C-terminal fragment of collagen XVIII. Endostatin inhibits endothelial cell growth and induces regression of established tumors.[212] Reports in the popular press state that the combination of angiostatin and endostatin results in complete elimination of murine tumors, raising high hopes for these noncytotoxic drugs as therapeutic agents in humans.[213]

THROMBOSPONDIN-1

Thrombospondin-1 (TSP-1) is produced by fibroblasts, activated macrophages, and platelets. TSP-1 is of interest because it is in the antiangiogenic pathway[214] and is influenced by the tumor suppressor gene p53.[215] Furthermore, loss of heterozygosity for p53 has been shown to result in loss of TSP-1 expression, as well as loss of the antiangiogenic phenotype with increased vessel density.[215]

INTEGRINS

Angiogenesis is a cascade of events. The formation of new blood vessels involves the extracellular matrix (ECM) and its adhesive and proteolytic enzymes. Quiescent endothelial cells, activated by angiogenic factors, react with cellular proliferation, migration, and invasion. They exhibit elevated expression of adhesion molecules and induction of proteolytic enzymes. Vascular cells must have the capacity to sense and respond to changes occurring in the structure and composition of the surrounding ECM. A group of molecules engaged in this part of the complex signaling system of the angiogenesis cascade is the integrin class of transmembrane cell adhesion receptors. Integrins are a family of cell adhesion molecules composed of associated α and β chains. To date, there are at least 15 α and 8 β chains identified, allowing a wide variety of heterodimers with different ligand specificities. These ECM receptors can bind to ECM components, such as fibronectin, laminin, collagen, and fibrinogen, and thus correspond to the composition of the matrix surrounding the vessels. Integrins have been shown to regulate different cellular responses, such as proliferation, migration, adhesion, invasion, and also apoptosis.[216] In angiogenesis, both $\beta1$ and $\alpha v\beta3$ seem to be implicated. Recent experiments suggest that ligation of $\alpha v\beta3$ with proteolyzed or denatured collagen suppresses p53 activity, blocks expression of the p53-inducible cell cycle inhibitor p21$^{WAF1/CIP1}$, and increases the BCL-2/BAX ratio, thus providing a critical survival signal necessary for growth and maturation of blood vessels during the angiogenic process.[217]

MICROVESSEL DENSITY AND PROGNOSIS

Benign, nonmetastasizing tumors are usually, but not always, sparsely vascularized, whereas most malignant solid tumors are well vascularized. A rich vasculature is likely to enhance the possibility that tumor cells will enter the circulation. An association between the intratumor microvessel density, the number of intravascular tumor cells, and the occurrence of pulmonary metastasis was demonstrated by Liotta et al[218] using an animal tumor model more than 20 years ago. An association between the clinical course of a tumor and its angiogenic capacity was first supported by studies of cutaneous melanomas.[219] A few years later, using immunohistochemical staining of breast cancer sections with antibodies to factor VIII, which is expressed on the surface of endothelial cells, Weidner and co-workers[220] demonstrated that the density of microvessels correlated directly with metastasis and inversely with survival. This relationship has been found in other types of tumors, non–small cell lung cancer, testicular cancer, cancer of the prostate, and cancer of the head and neck. In squamous cell carcinoma of the uterine cervix,[221] as well as in squamous cell carcinoma of the head and neck,[222] a high tumor vessel density also corresponds to response to radiotherapy. This finding is probably attributable to the fact that adequately oxygenated tissues respond better to radiotherapy than anoxic cells. In contrast, tumor vascularity in HNSCC does not seem to be predictive of the response to chemoradiotherapy.[223] This seems conflicting, but probably depends upon the sequence of the therapy and could reflect effects of chemotherapy on the microvasculature of the tumor. Antiangiogenic agents show promise of potentiating the effects of ionizing radiation[224,225] and may soon find clinical application.

METASTASIS AND EARLY RELAPSE

Metastasis, the spread of cancer from the primary tumor to distant sites in the body, is one of the characteristics of malignancy and is, in fact, what makes cancer so lethal in most tumor types. In head and neck cancer, distant spread beyond the locoregional area is equivalent to incurable disease. The metastatic process is complex, with many steps. To successfully metastasize, the cancer cell has to acquire several new properties[226] (Fig. 1–10). The metastatic process is rather inefficient. The detachment of cells from a clinically manifest tumor has been estimated to occur at a rate of 10^6 to 10^8 cells per 24 hours, and probably fewer than 10^{-4} of the cells that reach the circulation survive to establish a new tumor at a distant site. In 1889, the clinical observation that metastases from different tumor

types had preferences for different organs stimulated Paget[227] to formulate the "seed and soil" hypothesis.[227] Such specificity has been verified; however, the general rule is that the first organ of metastasis tends to be the first capillary bed that the detached cells encounter. For tumors draining to the vena cava system, this organ is the lungs. For tumors draining to the portal system, it is the liver. From those primary metastases, there is then spread (metastasis from metastasis) to tumor-specific organs.

CONCLUSION

Clearly, the work of the future is to achieve a better understanding of the mechanisms responsible for the behavior of tumor cells at each stage of the tumor progression pathway, and to search for novel strategies to overcome these mechanisms. As can be gleaned from this short review, there are many new targets developing. Of special interest are those genetic markers that predict response to therapy so that the current armamentarium can be used with greater effectiveness. For example, tumors that overexpress cyclin D1 respond better to chemotherapy with cisplatinum and 5-fluorouracil. This knowledge allows the physician to turn a bad prognostic sign into improved outcome. Likewise, the exciting developments with respect to angiogenesis inhibitors suggest that knowledge of the biology of tumor growth can lead to new targets for treatment and may provide a means to eradicate or control many types of tumors.

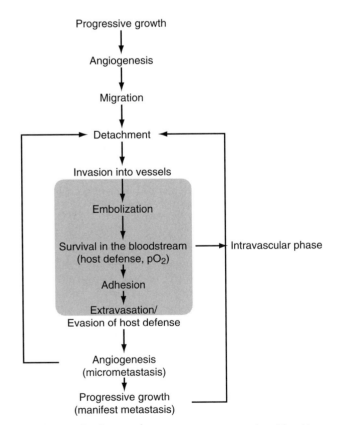

FIGURE 1–10 Steps in the metastatic process. Adapted from Hart IA, Saini A. Biology of tumor metastasis. *Lancet.* 1992; 339:1453–1457, with permission.

REFERENCES

1. Clark, WH. The nature of cancer: Morphogenesis and progressive (self)-disorganization in neoplastic development and progression. *Acta Oncol.* 1995; 34:3–21.
2. Harinder GS, Schantz S. Emerging role of beta carotene and antioxidant nutrients in prevention of oral cancer. *Arch Otolaryngol/Head Neck Surg.* 1995; 121:141–144.
3. Silverman S, Shillitoe EJ. Etiology and predisposing factor in oral cancer. In: Silverman S, ed. *Oral Cancer.* 3rd ed. New York: American Cancer Society; 1990:7–39.
4. Campesi J. The biology of replicative senescence. *Eur J Cancer.* 1977; 33:703–709.
5. Hayflick L. The limited in vitro lifetime of human diploid cell strains. *Exp Cell Res.* 1965; 37:614–636.
6. Nowell P. The clonal evolution of tumor cell populations. *Science.* 1976; 194:23–28.
7. Wynder EL, Bross IJ, Feldman BA. A study of the etiological factors in cancer of the mouth. *Cancer.* 1957; 10:1300–1323.
8. Rothman K, Keller A. The effect of joint exposure to alcohol and tobacco on risk of cancer of the mouth and pharynx. *J Chron Dis.* 1972; 25:711–716.
9. Blot WJ, Morris LE, Stroube R, Tagnon I, Fraumeni JF Jr. Lung and laryngeal cancer in relation to shipyard employment in Coastal Virginia. *JNCI.* 1980; 65:571–575.
10. Franceschi S, Bidoli E, Negri E, Barbone F, La Vecchia C. Alcohol and cancers of the upper aerodigestive tract in men and women. *Cancer Epidemiol Biomarkers Prev.* 1994; 3:299–304.

11. Blot WJ, McLaughlin JK, Winn DM, et al. Smoking and drinking in relation to oral and pharyngeal cancer. *Cancer Res.* 1988; 48:3282–3287.

12. Barasch A, Morse DE, Krutchoff DJ, Eisenberg E. Smoking, gender, and age as risk factors for site-specific intraoral squamous cell carcinoma. *Cancer.* 1993; 73:509–513.

13. Jin C, Jin Y, Wennerberg J, et al. Clonal chromosome aberrations accumulate with age in upper aerodigestive tract mucosa. *Mutat Res.* 1997; 374:63–72.

14. Brennan JA, Boyle JO, Koch WM, et al. Association between cigarette smoking and mutation of the p53 gene in squamous-cell carcinoma of the head and neck. *N Engl J Med.* 1995; 332:712–717.

15. Cloos J, Braakhuis BJM, Steen I, et al. Increased mutagen sensitivity in head and neck squamous cell carcinoma patients, particularly those with multiple primary tumors. *Int J Cancer.* 1994; 56:816–819.

16. Cloos J, Spitz MR, Schantz SP, et al. Genetic susceptibility to head and neck squamous cell carcinoma. *J Natl Cancer Inst.* 1996; 88:530–535.

17. Harris RE, Zang EA, Anderson JI, Wynder EL. Race and sex differences in lung cancer risk associated with cigarette smoking. *Int J Epidemiol.* 1993; 22:592–599.

18. Ryberg D, Hewer A, Phillips DH, Haugen A. Different susceptibility to smoking-induced DNA damage among male and female lung cancer patients. *Cancer Res.* 1994; 54:5801–5803.

19. Kato I, Nomura AMY. Alcohol in the aetiology of upper aerodigestive tract cancer. *Eur J Cancer Oral Oncol.* 1994; 75–81.

20. Ranasinghe A, Macgeoch C, Dyer S, Spurr N, Johnson WN. Some oral carcinomas from Sri Lankan betel/tobacco chewers overexpress p53 oncoprotein but lack mutations in exon 5–9. *Anticancer Res.* 1993; 13:2065–2068.

21. Winn DM, Blot WJ, Shy CM, et al. Snuff dipping and oral cancer among women in the southern United States. *N Engl J Med.* 1981; 304:745–749.

22. International Agency for Research on Cancer (IARC). Betel-quid and areca-nut chewing; and some related nitrosamines. *Monogr Eval Carcinog Risk Chem Hum.* 1985; 37: 137–202.

23. Kresty LA, Carmella SG, Borukhova A, et al. Metabolites of a tobacco-specific nitrosamine, 4-(methylnitrosamino)-1-(3-pyridyl)-1-butanone (NNK), in the urine of smokeless tobacco users: Relationship between urinary biomarkers and oral leukoplakia. *Cancer Epidemiol Biomarkers Prev.* 1996; 5: 521–525.

24. Sawyer RN, Evans AS, Neiderman JC, McCollum RW. Prospective studies of a group of Yale University freshman. I. Occurrence of infectious mononucleosis. *J Infect Dis.* 1971; 123:263–270.

25. Burkitt D, Wright D. Geographical and tribal distribution of the African lymphoma in Uganda. *Br Med J.* 1966; 5487:569–573.

26. Epstein MA, Achong BG, Barr YM. Virus particles in cultured lymphoblasts from Burkitt's lymphoma. *Lancet.* 1964; I: 702–703.

27. Klein G, Geering G, Old LJ, et al. Comparison of the anti-EBV titer and the EBV-associated membrane reactive and precipitating antibody levels in the sera of Burkitt lymphoma and nasopharyngeal carcinoma patients and controls. *Int J Cancer.* 1970; 5:185–194.

28. Frade R, Barel M, Ehlin-Hendriksson B, Klein G. gp 140, the C3d receptor of human B lymphocytes, is also the Epstein-Barr virus receptor. *Proc Natl Acad Sci USA.* 1985; 82:1490–1493.

29. Bejarano MT, Masucci MG, Ernberg I, Klein E, Klein G. Effect of cyclosporin-A (CsA) on the ability of T-lymphocyte subsets to inhibit the proliferation of autologous EBV-transformed B cells. *Int J Cancer.* 1985; 35:327–333.

30. Kline G. The Epstein-Barr virus and neoplasia. *N Engl J Med.* 1975; 293:1353–1357.

31. zur Hausen H. Human papillomavirus in the pathogenesis of anogenital cancer. *Virology.* 1991; 184:9–13.

32. Corbitt G, Zarod AP, Arrand JR, Longson M, Farrington WT. Human papillomavirus (HPV) genotypes associated with laryngeal papilloma. *J Clin Pathol.* 1988; 41:284–288.

33. Rihkanen H, Aaltonen LM, Syrjanen SM. Human papillomavirus in laryngeal papillomas and in adjacent normal epithelium. *Clin Otolaryngol.* 1993; 18:470–474.

34. Lin KY, Westra WH, Kashima HK, Mounts P, Wu TC. Coinfection of HPV-11 and HPV-16 in a case of laryngeal squamous papillomas with severe dysplasia. *Laryngoscope.* 1997; 107:942–947.

35. Brandsma JL, Steinberg BM, Abramson AL, Winkler B. Presence of human papillomavirus type 16 related sequences in verrucous carcinoma of the larynx. *Cancer Res.* 1986; 46:2185–2188.

36. Brandwein M, Steinberg B, Thung S, et al. Human papillomavirus 6/11 and 16/18 in Schneiderian inverted papillomas. In situ hybridization with human papillomavirus RNA probes. *Cancer.* 1989; 63:1708–1713.

37. Beck JC, McClatchey KD, Lesperance MM, et al. Presence of human papillomavirus predicts recurrence of inverted papilloma. *Otolaryngol Head Neck Surg.* 1995; 113:49–55.

38. Beck JC, McClatchey KD, Lesperance MM, et al. Human papillomavirus types important in progression of inverted papilloma. *Otolaryngol Head Neck Surg.* 1995; 113:558–563.

39. Lindeberg H, Fey SJ, Ottosen PD, Larsen MP. Human papillomavirus (HPV) and carcinomas of the head and neck. *Clin Otolaryngol.* 1988; 13:447–454.

40. DeVilliers EM, Weidauer H, Otto H, zur Hausen H. Papillomavirus DNA in human tongue carcinomas. *Int J Cancer.* 1985; 36:575–588.

41. Bradford CR, Zacks SE, Androphy EJ, et al. Human papillomavirus DNA sequences in cell lines derived from head and neck squamous cell carcinomas. *Otolaryngol Head Neck Surg.* 1991; 104:303–310.

42. Snijders P, Cromme F, van den Brule A, et al. Prevalence and expression of human papillomavirus in tonsillar carcinomas, indicating a possible viral etiology. *Int J Cancer.* 1992; 51:845–850.

43. Snijders P, Meijer C, van den Brule A, et al. Human papillomavirus (HPV) type 16 and 33 E6/E7 region transcripts in tonsillar carcinomas can originate from integrated and episomal HPV DNA. *J Gen Virol.* 1992; 73:2059–2066.

44. Clayman GL, Stewart MG, Weber RS, El-Naggar AK, Grimm EA. Human papillomavirus in laryngeal and hypopharyngeal carcinomas. *Arch Otolaryngol Head Neck Surg.* 1994; 120: 743–748.

45. Munger K, Phelp WC, Bubb V, Howley PM, Schlegel R. (1989) The E6 and E7 genes of the human papillomavirus type 16 together are necessary and sufficient for transformation of primary human keratinocytes. *J Virol.* 1989; 63:4417–4421.

46. Munger K, Werness BA, Dyson N, et al. Complex formation of human papillomavirus E7 proteins with the retinoblastoma suppressor gene product. *EMBO J* 1989; 8:4099–4105.

47. Werness BA, Levine AJ, Howley PM. Association of human papillomavirus types 16 and 18 E6 proteins with p53. *Science* 1990; 248:76–79.

48. Baker CC, Phelps WC, Lindgren V, et al. Structural and transcriptional analysis of human papillomavirus type 16 sequences in cervical carcinoma cell lines. *J Virol* 1987; 61:962–971.

49. Acheson ED, Cowdell H, Hadfield E, Macbeth RG. Nasal cancer in woodworkers in the furniture industry. *Br Med J.* 1970; 2:587–596.

50. Hernberg S, Westerholm P, Schultz-Larsen K, et al. Nasal and sinonasal cancer. Connection with occupational exposures in Denmark, Finland and Sweden. *Scand J Work Environ Health.* 1983; 9:315–326.

51. Morgan RW, Shettigara PT. Occupational asbestos exposure, smoking and laryngeal carcinoma. *Ann NY Acad Sci.* 1976; 271:308–310.

52. Stell PM, McGill T. Exposure to asbestos and laryngeal carcinoma. *J Laryngol Otol.* 1975; 89:513–517.

53. Burch JD, Howe GR, Miller AB, Semenciw R. Tobacco, alco-

hol, asbestos, and nickel in the etiology of cancer of the larynx: A case-control study. *JNCI*. 1981; 67:1219–1224.

54. Olsen J, Sabroe S. Occupational causes of laryngeal cancer. *J Epidemiol Commun Health*. 1984; 38:117–121.

55. Hinds MW, Thomas DB, O'Reilly HP. Asbestos, dental x-rays, tobacco and alcohol in the epidemiology of laryngeal cancers. *Cancer*. 1979; 44:1114–1120.

56. Elwood JM, Pearson JCG, Skippen DH, Jackson SM. Alcohol, smoking, social and occupational factors in the aetiology of cancer of the oral cavity, pharynx and cancer of the larynx. *Int J Cancer*. 1984; 34:603–612.

57. Finkelstein MM. Mortality rates among employees potentially exposed to chrysotile asbestos at two automobile parts factories. *Can Med Assoc J*. 1989; 141:125–130.

58. Chan CK, Gee JBL. Asbestos exposure and laryngeal cancer: An analysis of the epidemiologic evidence. *J Occup Med*. 1988; 30:23–27.

59. Edelman DA. Laryngeal cancer and occupational exposure to asbestos (review). *Int Arch Occup Environ Health*. 1989; 61: 223–227.

60. Smith AH, Handley MA, Wood R. Epidemiological evidence indicates asbestos causes laryngeal cancer. *J Occup Med*. 1990; 32:499–507.

61. World Health Organization–International Agency for Research on Cancer (WHO-IARC). *Biennial Report 1986–1987*. Lyon, France: WHO-IARC; 1987.

62. Olsen J, Sabroe S, Lajer M. Welding and cancer of the larynx: A case-control study. *Eur J Cancer Clin Oncol* 1984; 20: 639–643.

63. Haugenoer JM, Cordier S, Mortel C, Lefebvre JL, Hermon D. Occupational risk factors for upper respiratory tract and upper digestive tract cancers. *Br J Ind Med*. 1990; 47:380–383.

64. Doll R. Cancer of the lung and nose of nickel workers. *Br J Med*. 1958; 15:217–223.

65. Slaughter DP, Southwick HW, Smejkal W. "Field cancerization" in oral stratified squamous epithelium: Clinical implications of multicentric origin. *Cancer*. 1953; 6:963–968.

66. Carey TE. Field cancerization: Are multiple primary cancers monoclonal or polyclonal? *Ann Med*. 1996; 28:183–188.

67. Sidransky D, Frost P, von Eschenbach A, et al. Clonal origin of bladder cancer. *N Engl J Med*. 1992; 326:737–740.

68. Worsham MJ, Wolman SR, Carey TE, et al. Common clonal origin of synchronous primary head and neck squamous cell carcinomas: Analysis by tumor karyotypes and fluorescence in situ hybridization. *Hum Pathol*. 1995; 26:251–261.

69. Bedi GC, Westra WH, Gabrielson E, Koch W, Sidransky D. Multiple head and neck tumors: Evidence for common clonal origin. *Cancer Res*. 1996; 56:2484–2487.

70. Califano J, van der Riet P, Westra W, et al. Genetic progression model for head and neck cancer: Implications for field cancerization. *Cancer Res*. 1996; 56:2488–2492.

71. Mao L, Lee JS, Fan YH, et al. Frequent microsatellite alterations at chromosomes 9p21 and 3p14 in oral premalignant lesions and their value in cancer risk assessment. *Nature Med*. 1996; 2:682–685.

72. von Hansemann D. Über asymmetrische zellteilung in epitelkrebsen und deren biologische bedeutung. *Virchows Arch [A]*. 1890; 119:299–326.

73. Boveri T. *Zur Frage der Entstehung maligne tumoren*. Jena: Verlag von Gustav Fisher; 1914.

74. Boveri T. *The Origin of Malignant Tumors*. Baltimore: Williams & Wilkins; 1929.

75. Winge O. Zytologische unterschungunden ueber di natur maligner tumoren. II. Teerkarzinomen bei maeusen. *Z Zellforsch Mikrosk Anat*. 1930; 10:683–735.

76. Berenblum I. Sequential aspects of chemical carcinogenesis. In: Becker F, ed. *Cancer: A Comprehensive Treatise*. Vol. 1. New York: Plenum Press; 1982:451.

77. Huebner RJ, Todaro GJ. Oncogenes of RNA tumor viruses as determinants of cancer. *Proc Natl Acad Sci USA*. 1969; 77: 1087–1094.

78. Knudson AG. Genetics of human cancer. *Ann Rev Genet*. 1986; 20:231–251.

79. Rubin H. Cancer development: The rise of epigenetics. *Eur J Cancer*. 1992; 28:1–2.

80. Strohman R. Epigenesis: The missing beat in technology. *Biotechnology*. 1994; 12:156–164.

81. Rubin H. On the nature of enduring modifications in cells and organisms. *Am J Physiol*. 1990; 258 (Lung Cell Molec Physiol 2): L19–L24.

82. Nordling CO. A new theory on the cancer-inducing mechanism. *Br J Cancer*. 1953; 7:68–72.

83. Armitage P, Doll R. The age distribution of cancer and a multi-stage theory of carcinogenesis. *Br J Cancer* 1954; 8:1–12.

84. Fearon ER, Vogelstein B. A genetic model for colorectal tumorigenesis. *Cell*. 1990; 61:759–767.

85. Mitelman F, Mertens F, Johansson B. A breakpoint map of recurrent chromosomal rearrangements in human neoplasia. *Nature Genet*. 1997; 15:417–474.

86. Renan MJ. How many mutations are required for tumorigenesis? Implications from human cancer data. *Mol Carcinogen*. 1993; 7:139–146.

87. Carey TE, Van Dyke DL, Worsham MJ, et al. Characterization of human laryngeal primary and metastatic squamous cell carcinoma cell lines UM-SCC-17A and UM-SCC-17B. *Cancer Res*. 1989; 49:6098–6107.

88. Carey TE, Worsham MJ, Van Dyke DL. Chromosomal biomarkers in the clonal evolution of head and neck squamous neoplasia. *J Cell Biochem [Suppl]*. 1993; 17F:213–222.

89. Worsham MJ, Benninger MJ, Zarbo RJ, Carey TE, Van Dyke DL. Deletion 9p22-pter and loss of Y as primary chromosome abnormalities in a squamous cell carcinoma of the vocal cord. *Genes Chromosomes Cancer*. 1993; 6:58–60.

90. Worsham MJ, Carey TE, Benninger MS, et al. Clonal cytogenetic evolution in a squamous cell carcinoma of the skin from a xeroderma pigmentosum patient, HFH-SCC-XP-1. *Genes Chromosomes Cancer* 1993; 7:158–164.

91. Marx J. New tumor suppressor may rival p53. *Science*. 1994; 264:344–345.

92. Reed AL, Califano J, Cairns P, et al. High frequency of *p16* (*CDKN2/MTS-1/INK4A*) inactivation in head and neck squamous cell carcinoma. *Cancer Res*. 1996; 56:3630–3633.

93. Serrano M, Hannon GJ, Beach D. A new regulatory motif in cell-cycle control causing specific inhibition of cyclinD/CDK4. *Nature*. 1993; 366:704–707.

94. van der Riet P, Nawroz H, Hruban RH, et al. Frequent loss of chromosome 9p21–22 early in head and neck cancer progression. *Cancer Res*. 1994; 54:1156–1158.

95. Cairns P, Mao L, Merlo A, et al. Rates of p16 (*MTS1*) mutations in primary tumors with 9p loss. *Science*. 1994; 265:415–416.

96. Alberts B, Bray D, Lewis J, et al. *Molecular Biology of the Cell*. New York: Garland Publishing, Inc; 1994.

97. Bohr VA, Smidt CL, Okumoto DS, Hanawalt PC. DNA repair in an active gene: Removal of pyridine dimers from the DHRF gene of CHO cells is much more efficient than in the genome overall. *Cell*. 1985; 40:359–369.

98. Mellon I, Spivak G, Hanawalt PC. Preferential DNA repair of an active gene in human cells. *Proc Natl Acad Sci USA*. 1986; 83:8878–8882.

99. Mellon I, Spivak G, Hanawalt PC. Selective removal of transcription-blocking DNA damage from the transcribed strand of mammalian DHFR gene. *Cell*. 1987; 51:241–249.

100. Modrich P. Mismatch repair, genetic stability and cancer. *Science*. 1994; 266:1959–1960.

101. Frank CJ, McClatchey KD, Devaney KO, Carey TE. Evidence that loss of chromosome 18q is associated with tumor progression. *Cancer Res*. 1997; 57:824–827.

102. Rydell R, Lybak S, Wennerberg J, Willén R. Increased response to cisplatin after long-term serial passage of a squamous cell carcinoma xenograft. *In Vivo*. 1991; 5:23–28.

103. Simpson AJG. The natural somatic mutation frequency and human carcinogenesis. In: *Advances in Cancer Research*. Vol. 71. Orlando, FL: Academic Press; 1997:209–240.

104. Hsu TC, Johnston DA, Cherry LM, et al. Sensitivity to geno-

toxic effects of belomycin in humans: Possible relationship to environmental carcinogenesis. *Int J Cancer.* 1989; 43:403–409.

105. Schantz SP, Hsu TC, Ainslie N, Moser RP. Young adults with head and neck cancer express increased susceptibility to mutagen-induced chromosome damage. *JAMA.* 1989; 262: 3313–3315.

106. Schantz SP, Spitz MR, Hsu TC. Mutagen sensitivity in patients with head and neck cancers: A biological marker for risk of multiple primary malignancies. *J Natl Cancer Inst.* 1990; 82:1773–1775.

107. Spitz MR, Hoque A, Trizna Z, et al. Mutagen sensitivity as a risk factor for second malignant tumors following malignancies of the upper aerodigestive tract. *J Natl Cancer Inst.* 1994; 86:1681–1684.

108. Nowell PC, Hungerford DA. A minute chromosome in human chronic granulocytic leukemia. *Science.* 1960; 132:1497.

109. Caspersson T, Zech L, Johansson C. Differential binding of alkylating fluorochromes in human chromosomes. *Exp Cell Res.* 1970; 60:315–319.

110. Santoro M, Dathan NA, Berlingieri MT, et al. Molecular characterization of RET/PTC3: A novel rearranged version of the RET proto-oncogene in a human thyroid papillary carcinoma. *Oncogene* 1994; 9:509–516.

111. Nikiforov Y, Rowland JM, Bove KE, Monteforte-Munoz H, Fagin JA. Distinct pattern of ret oncogen rearrangements in morphological variants of radiation-induced and sporadic thyroid papillary thyroid carcinomas in children. *Cancer Res.* 1997; 57:1690–1694.

112. Motokura T, Bloom T, Kim HG, et al. A novel cyclin encoded by a *bcl1*-linked candidate oncogene. *Nature.* 1991; 350: 412–515.

113. Motokura T, Arnold A. PRAD1/cyclin D1 proto-oncogene: genomic organization, 5′ DNA sequence, and sequence of a tumor-specific rearrangement breakpoint. *Genes Chromosomes Cancer.* 1993; 7:89–95.

114. Kas K, Voz ML, Roijer E, et al. Promoter swapping between the genes for a novel zinc finger protein and beta-catenin in pleomorphic adenoms with t(3;8)(p21;q12) translocations. *Nature Genet.* 1997; 15:170–174.

115. Mertens F, Johansson B, Höglund M, Mitelman F. Chromosomal imbalance maps of malignant solid tumors: A cytogenetic survey of 3185 neoplasms. *Cancer Res.* 1997; 57:2765–2780.

116. Van Dyke DL, Worsham MJ, Benninger MS, et al. Recurrent cytogenetic abnormalities in squamous cell carcinomas of the head and neck region. *Genes Chromosomes Cancer.* 1994; 9: 192–206.

117. Heo DS, Snyderman C, Gollin SM, et al. Biology, cytogenetics, and sensitivity to immunological effector cells of new head and neck squamous cell carcinoma cell lines. *Cancer Res.* 1989; 49:5119–5123.

118. Bradford CR, Kimmel KA, Van Dyke DL, et al. Chromosome 11p deletions and breakpoints in squamous cell carcinoma: Association with altered reactivity with the UM-E7 antibody. *Genes Chromosomes Cancer.* 1991; 3:272–282.

119. Cowan JM, Beckett MA, Ahmed-Swam S, Weichselbaum RR. Cytogenetic evidence of the multistep origin of head and neck squamous cell carcinomas. *J Natl Cancer Inst.* 1992; 84: 793–797.

120. Sreekantiah C, Rao PH, Xu L, et al. Consistent chromosome losses in head and neck squamous cell carcinoma cell lines. *Genes Chromosome Cancer.* 1994; 11:29–39.

121. Jin Y, Mertens F, Mandahl N, et al. Chromosome abnormalities in eighty-three head and neck squamous cell carcinomas: Influence of culture conditions on karyotypic pattern. *Cancer Res.* 1993; 53:2140–2146.

122. Jin Y, Mertens F, Jin F, et al. Nonrandom chromosome abnormalities in short-term cultured primary squamous cell carcinomas of the head and neck. *Cancer Res.* 1995; 55:3204–3210.

123. Pearlstein RP, Benninger MS, Carey TE, et al. Loss of 18q predicts poor survival in patients with squamous cell carci-

noma of the head and neck. *Genes Chromosomes Cancer.* 1998; 21:333–339.

124. Åkervall JA, Jin Y, Wennerberg J, et al. Chromosomal abnormalities involving 11q13 are associated with poor prognosis in patients with squamous cell carcinoma of the head and neck. *Cancer.* 1995; 76:853–859.

125. Jones JW, Raval JR, Beals TF, et al. Frequent loss of heterozygosity on chromosome arm 18q in squamous cell carcinomas: Identification of two regions of loss-18q11.1-q12.3 and 18q21.1-q23. *Arch Otolaryngol Head Neck Surg.* 1997; 123:610–614.

126. Weber JL, May PE. Abundant class of human DNA polymorphisms which can be typed using the polymerase chain reaction. *Am J Hum Genet.* 1989; 44:388–396.

127. Nawroz H, van der Riet P, Hruban RH, et al. Allelotype of squamous cell carcinoma. *Cancer Res.* 1994; 54:1152–1155.

128. Ah-See KW, Cooke TG, Pickford IR, Soutar D, Balmain A. An allelotype of squamous carcinoma of the head and neck using microsatellite markers. *Cancer Res.* 1994; 54:1617–1621.

129. Li X, Lee NK, Ye Y-W, et al. Allelic loss at chromosomes 3p, 8p, 13q, and 17p associated with poor prognosis in head and neck cancer. *J Natl Cancer Inst.* 1994; 86:1524–1529.

130. Kallioniemi A, Kallioniemi OP, Sudar D, et al. Comparative genomic hybridization for molecular cytogenetic analysis of solid tumors. *Science.* 1992; 258:818–821.

131. van Dekken H, Geelen E, Dinjens WNM, et al. Comparative genomic hybridization of cancer of the gastroesophageal junction: Deletion of 14q31-32.1 discriminates between esophageal (Barrett's) and gastric cardia adenocarcinomas. *Cancer Res.* 1999; 59:748–752.

132. Bockmuhl U, Schwendel A, Dietel M, Petersen I. Distinct patterns of chromosomal alterations in high- and low-grade head and neck squamous cell carcinomas. *Cancer Res.* 1996; 56:5325–5329.

133. Speicher MR, Howe C, Crotty P, et al. Comparative genomic hybridization detects novel deletions and amplifications in head and neck squamous cell carcinomas. *Cancer Res.* 1995; 55:1010–1013.

134. Brzoska PM, Levin NA, Fu KK, et al. Frequent novel DNA copy number increase in squamous cell head and neck tumors. *Cancer Res.* 1995; 55:3055–3059.

135. Gnarra JR, Tory K, Weng Y, et al. Mutations of the *VHL* tumour suppressor gene in renal carcinoma. *Nature Genet* 1994; 7:85–90.

136. Mao L, Fan Y-H, Lotan R, Hong WK. Frequent abnormalities of *FHIT*, a candidate tumor suppressor gene, in head and neck cancer cell lines. *Cancer Res.* 1996; 56:5128–5131.

137. Virgilio L, Shuster M, Gollin SM, et al. FHIT gene alterations in head and neck squamous cell carcinomas. *Proc Natl Acad Sci USA.* 1996; 93:9770–9775.

138. Grandis JR, Tweardy DJ. Elevated levels of transforming growth factor alpha and epidermal growth factor receptor messenger RNA are early markers of carcinogenesis in head and neck cancer. *Cancer Res.* 1993; 53:3579–3584.

139. Åkervall JA, Michalides RJAM, Mineta H, et al. Amplification of cyclin D1 in squamous cell carcinoma of the head and neck and the prognostic value of chromosomal abnormalities and cyclin D1 overexpression. *Cancer.* 1997; 79:380–389.

140. Howard A, Pelc SR. Nuclear incorporation of P32 as demonstrated by autoradiographs. *Exp Cell Res.* 1951; 2:178–187.

141. Howard A, Pelc SR. Synthesis of nucleoprotein in bean root cells. *Nature.* 1951; 167:599–600.

142. Gussack GS, Brantley BA, Farmer JC Jr. Biology of tumors and head and neck cancer chemotherapy. *Laryngoscope.* 1984; 94:1181–1187.

143. Bresciani F, Paoluzi R, Benassi M, et al. Cell kinetics and growth of squamous cell carcinoma in man. *Cancer Res.* 1974; 34:2405–2415.

144. Shackney SE, McCormack GW, Cuchural GJ. Growth rate patterns of solid tumors and their relation to responsiveness to therapy. *Ann Int Med.* 1978; 89:107–121.

145. Mendelsohn ML, Dethlefsen LA. Cell kinetics of breast cancer: The turnover of nonproliferating cells. *Recent Results Cancer Res.* 1973; 42:73–86.

146. Steel GG. *Growth Kinetics of Tumours.* Oxford, England: Clarendon Press; 1977.

147. Begg AC, McNally NJ, Shrieve DC, Kärcher H. A method to measure the duration of DNA synthesis and the potential doubling time from a single sample. *Cytometry.* 1985; 6:620–626.

148. Hartwell LH, Weinert T. Checkpoints: Controls that ensure the order of cell cycle events. *Science.* 1989; 246:629–634.

149. Nasmyth K. Viewpoint: Putting the cell cycle in order. *Science.* 1996; 274:1643–1645.

150. Pines J. Cyclins and cyclin dependent kinases: A biochemical view. *Biochem J.* 1995; 308:697–711.

151. Hochstrasser M. Ubiquitin, proteasomes, and the regulation of intracellular protein degradation. *Curr Opin Cell Biol.* 1995; 7:215–223.

152. Hunter T, Pines J. Cyclins and cancer II: Cyclins D and CDK inhibitors come of age. *Cell.* 1994; 79:573–582.

153. Nurse P. Regulation of the eukaryotic cell cycle. *Eur J Cancer.* 1997; 33:1002–1004.

154. Sherr CJ. Cancer cell cycles. *Science.* 1996; 274:1672–1677.

155. Martelli F, Livingston DM. Regulation of endogenous E2F1 stability by the retinoblastoma protein. *Proc Natl Acad Sci USA.* 1999; 96:2858–2863.

156. Livingston DM. Functional analysis of the retinoblastoma gene product and RB-SV40 T antigen complexes. *Cancer Surv.* 1992; 12:153–160.

157. Lane DP, Crawford LV. T-antigen is bound to a host protein in SV40 transformed cells. *Nature.* 1979; 278:261–263.

158. Linzer DI, Levine AJ. Characterization of a 54k Dalton cellular SV40 tumour antigen present in SV40 transformed cells and uninfected embryonal carcinoma cells. *Cell.* 1979; 17:43–52.

159. Harris CC, Hollstein M. Clinical implications of the p53 tumor-suppressor gene. *N Engl J Med.* 1993; 329:1318–1327.

160. Levine AJ, Momand J, Finlay CA. The p53 tumour suppressor gene. *Nature (Lond).* 1991; 351:453–456.

161. Greenblatt MS, Bennett WP, Hollstein M, Harris CC. Mutations in the p53 tumour suppressor gene: Clues to cancer etiology and molecular pathogenesis. *Cancer Res.* 1994; 54:4855–4878.

162. Levine AJ, Perry ME, Chang A, et al. The 1993 Walter Hubert Lecture: The role of the p53 tumour-suppressor gene in tumorigenesis. *Br J Cancer.* 1994; 69:409–416.

163. Field JK, Spandidos DA, Malliri A, et al. Elevated p53 expression correlates with a history of heavy smoking in squamous cell carcinoma of the head and neck. *Br J Cancer.* 1991; 64:573–577.

164. Field JK, Spandidos DA, Stell PM. Over-expression of p53 gene in head and neck cancer, linked with heavy smoking and drinking. *Lancet.* 1992; 339:502–503.

165. Boyle J, Hakim J, Koch W, et al. The incidence of p53 mutations increases with progression of head and neck cancer. *Cancer Res.* 1993; 53, 4477–4480.

166. Nees M, Homann N, Discher H, et al. Expression of mutated p53 occurs in tumor-distant epithelia of head and neck cancer patients: A possible molecular basis for the development of multiple tumors. *Cancer Res.* 1993; 53:4189–4196.

167. Pavelic ZP, Li YQ, Stambrook PJ, et al. Overexpression of p53 protein is common in premalignant head and neck lesions. *Anticancer Res.* 1994; 14:2259–2266.

168. Shin DM, Kim J, Ro JY, et al. Activation of p53 gene expression in premalignant lesions during head and neck tumorigenesis. *Cancer Res.* 1994; 54:321–326.

169. Wang LD, Shi ST, Zhou Q, et al. Changes in p53 and cyclin D1 protein levels and cell proliferation in different stages of human oesophageal and gastric-cardia carcinogenesis. *Int J Cancer.* 1994; 59:514–519.

170. el-Naggar AK, Lai S, Luna MA, et al. Sequential p53 mutation analysis of pre-invasive and invasive head and neck squamous carcinoma. *Int J Cancer.* 1995; 64:196–201.

171. Mineta H, Borg Å, Dictor M, Wahlberg P, Wennerberg J. Discordance between p53 protein expression and suppressor gene mutation in H&N squamous cell carcinoma. *Eur J Cancer.* 1995; 31(suppl A):5, 92.

172. Nylander K, Nilsson P, Mehle C, Roos G. p53 mutations, protein expression and cell proliferation in squamous cell carcinomas of the head and neck. *Br J Cancer.* 1995; 71:826–830.

173. Cho Y, Gorina S, Jeffrey PD, Pavletich NP. Crystal structure of a p53 tumor suppressor-DNA complex: Understanding tumorigenic mutations. *Science.* 1994; 265:346–355.

174. Milner J. DNA damage, p53 and anticancer therapies. *Nature Med.* 1995; 1:879–880.

175. Barnes DM, Hanby AM, Gillett CE, et al. Abnormal expression of wild type p53 protein in normal cells of a cancer family patient. *Lancet.* 1992; 340:259–263.

176. Kastan MB, Onyekwere O, Sidransky D, Vogelstein B, Craig RW. Participation of p53 protein in the cellular response to DNA damage. *Cancer Res.* 1991; 51:6304–6311.

177. Vogelstein N, Kinzler KW. p53 function and dysfunction. *Cell.* 1992; 70:523–526.

178. Monaud J, Zambetti GP, Olson DC, George D, Levine AJ. The mdm-2 oncogene product forms a complex with the p53 protein and inhibits p53-mediated transactivation. *Cell.* 1992; 69:1237–1245.

179. Meltzer PS. MDM2 and p53: A question of balance. *J Natl Cancer Inst.* 1994; 86:1265–1266.

180. Gannon JV, Greaves R, Iggo R, Lane DP. Activating mutations in p53 produce a common conformational effect. A monoclonal antibody specific for the mutant form. *EMBO J.* 1990; 9:1595–1602.

181. Cesarman E, Inghirami G, Chadburn A, Knowles DM. High level of p53 protein expression do not correlate with p53 gene mutations in anaplastic large cell lymphoma. *Am J Pathol.* 1993; 143:845–856.

182. Scheffner M, Werness BA, Hibregtse JM, Levine AJ, Howley PM. The E6 oncoprotein encoded by human papillomavirus types 16 and 18 promotes the degradation of p53. *Cell.* 1990; 63:1129–1136.

183. Dowell SP, Hall PA. The clinical relevance of the p53 tumour suppressor gene. *Cytopathology.* 1994; 5:133–145.

184. Chang F, Syrjänen S, Syrjänen K. Implications of the p53 tumor-suppressor gene in clinical oncology. *J Clin Oncol.* 1995; 13:1009–1022.

185. Sauter ER, Ridge JA, Gordon J, Eisenberg BL. p53 overexpression correlates with increased survival in patients with squamous carcinoma of the tongue base. *Am J Surg.* 1992; 164:651–653.

186. Watling DL, Gown AM, Coltrera MD. Overexpression of p53 in head and neck cancer. *Head Neck.* 1992; 14:437–44.

187. Field JK, Pavelic ZP, Spandidos DA, et al. The role of the p53 tumor suppressor gene in squamous cell carcinoma of the head and neck. *Arch Otolaryngol Head Neck Surg.* 1993; 119:1118–1122.

188. Brennan JA, Boyle JO, Koch WM, et al. Effect of p53 mutations on survival in head and neck squamous carcinoma. *Head Neck* 1994; 16:510–514.

189. Ahomadegbe JC, Barrois M, Fogel S, et al. High incidence of p53 alterations (mutation, deletion, overexpression) in head and neck primary tumors and metastases: Absence of correlation with clinical outcome. Frequent protein overexpression in normal epithelium and in early non-invasive lesions. *Oncogene* 1995; 10:1217–1227.

190. Nylander K, Schildt EB, Eriksson M, et al. A nonrandom deletion in the p53 gene in oral squamous cell carcinoma. *Br J Cancer.* 1996; 73:1381–1386.

191. Bradford CR, Zhu S, Poore J, et al., for the Department of Veterans Affairs Laryngeal Cancer Cooperative Group. P53 mutation as a prognostic marker in advanced laryngeal carcinoma. *Arch Otolaryngol Head Neck Surg.* 1997; 123:605–609.

192. Morgan SE, Kastan MB. p53 and ATM: Cell cycle, cell death, and cancer. In: *Advances in Cancer Research.* Vol. 71. Orlando, FL: Academic Press; 1997:1–21.

193. White E. Life, death, and the pursuit of apoptosis. *Genes Devel.* 1997; 10:1–15.

194. Campesi J. Replicative senescence: An old lives tale? *Cell.* 1996; 84:497–500.

195. Watson JD. Origin of concatemeric DNA. *Nature.* 1972; 239: 197–201.

196. Morin GB. The implications of telomerase biochemistry for human disease. *Eur J Cancer.* 1997; 33:750–760.

197. Shay JW, Wright WE. Telomerase activity in human cancer. *Curr Opin Oncol.* 1996; 8:66–71.

198. Mao L, El-Naggar AK, Fan Y-H, et al. Telomerase activity in head and neck squamous cell carcinoma and adjacent tissues. *Cancer Res.* 1996; 56:5600–5604.

199. Hohaus S, Cavallo S, Bellacosa A, et al. Telomerase activity in human laryngeal squamous cell carcinomas. *Clin Cancer Res.* 1996; 2:1895–1900.

200. Kim NW. Clinical implications of telomerase in cancer. *Eur J Cancer.* 1997; 33:781–786.

201. Nakamura TU, Morin GB, Chapman KB, et al. Telomerase catalytic subunit homologs from fission yeast and human. *Science.* 1997; 277:955–959.

202. Oshimura M, Barrett JC. Multiple pathways to cellular senescence: Role of telomerase repressors. *Eur J Cancer.* 1997; 33: 710–715.

203. Kiyono T, Koop SA, Jenn I, et al. Both Rb/p16^{INK4a} inactivation and telomerase activity are required to immortalize human epithelial cells. *Nature.* 1998; 396:84–88.

204. Hahn WC, Counter CM, Lundberg AS, et al. Creation of human tumour cells with defined genetic elements. *Nature.* 1999; 400:401–402.

205. Thomlinson RH, Gray LH. The histological structure of some human lung cancers and the possible implications for radiotherapy. *Br J Cancer.* 1955; 9:539–549.

206. Folkman J. Tumor angiogenesis: Therapeutic implications. *N Engl J Med.* 1971; 285:1182–1186.

207. Gasparini G. Angiogenesis research up to 1996. A commentary on the state of art and suggestions for future studies. *Eur J Cancer.* 1996; 32A:2379–2385.

208. Petruzzelli GJ. Tumor angiogenesis. *Head Neck.* 1996; 18:283–291.

209. Ellis LM, Fidler IJ. Angiogenesis and metastasis. *Eur J Cancer.* 1996; 32A:2451–2460.

210. Hanahan D, Christofori G, Naik P, Arbeit J. Transgenic mouse models of tumour angiogenesis: The angiogenic switch, its molecular controls, and prospects for preclinical therapeutic studies. *Eur J Cancer.* 1996; 32A:2386–2393.

211. O'Reilly M, Holmgren M, Shing Y, et al. Angiostatin: A novel angiogenesis inhibitor that mediates the suppression of metastases by a Lewis lung carcinoma. *Cell.* 1994; 79:315–328.

212. Cao Y, O-Reilly MS, Marshall B, et al. Expression of angiostatin cDNA in a murine fibrosarcoma suppresses primary tumor growth and produces long term dormancy of metastases. *J Clin Invest.* 1998; 101:1055–1063.

213. Kolata G. A cautious awe greets drugs that eradicate tumors in mice. *NY Times.* 1998; 148:1, 20.

214. Castle VP, Dixit VM, Polverini PJ. Thrombospondin 1 suppresses tumorigenesis and angiogenesis in serum- and anchorage-independent NIH3T3 cells. *Lab Invest.* 1997; 77:51–61.

215. Grossfeld GD, Ginsberg DA, Stein JP, et al. Thrombospondin-1 expression in bladder cancer: Association with p53 alterations, tumor angiogenesis and tumor progression. *JNCI.* 1997; 89:219–227.

216. Lester BR, McCarthy JB. Tumor cell adhesion to the extracellular matrix and signal transduction mechanisms implicated in tumor cell mobility, invasion and metastasis. *Cancer Metastasis Rev.* 1992; 11:31–44.

217. Brooks PC. Role of integrins in angiogenesis. *Eur J Cancer.* 1996; 32A:2423–2429.

218. Liotta LA, Kleinerman J, Saidel GM. Quantitative relationship of intravascular tumor cells, tumor vessels, and pulmonary metastases following tumor implantation. *Cancer Res.* 1974; 34:997–1004.

219. Srivastava A, Laidler P, Davies R, Horgan K, Huges L. The prognostic significance of tumor vascularity in intermediate-thickness (0.76-4.0 mm thick) skin melanoma: A quantitative histologic study. *Am J Pathol.* 1988; 133:419–423.

220. Weidner N, Folkman J, Pozza F, et al. Tumor angiogenesis: A new significant and independent prognostic indicator in early-stage breast carcinoma. *J Natl Cancer Inst.* 1992; 84: 1875–1887.

221. Kolstad P. Vascularization, oxygen tension and radiocurability in cancer of the cervix. Oslo: University of Oslo, Norway; 1964.

222. Zätterstroöm UK, Brun E, Willen R, Kjellen E, Wennerberg J. Tumor angiogenesis and prognosis in squamous cell carcinoma of the head and neck. *Head Neck.* 1995; 17:312–318.

223. Gasparini G, Weidner N, Maluta S, et al. Intratumoral microvessel density and the p53 protein: Correlation with metastasis in head and neck squamous cell carcinoma. *Int J Cancer.* 1993; 55:739–744.

224. Gorski DH, Mauceri HJ, Salloum RM, et al. Potentiation of the antitumor effect of ionizing radiation by brief concomitant exposures to angiostatin. *Cancer Res.* 1998; 58: 5686–5689.

225. Gorski DH, Beckett MA, Jaskowiak NT, et al. Blockade of the vascular endothelial growth factor stress response increases the antitumor effects of ionizing radiation. *Cancer Res.* 1999; 59:3374–3378.

226. Hart IA, Saini A. Biology of tumor metastasis. *Lancet.* 1992; 339:1453–1457.

227. Paget F. The distribution of secondary growth in cancer of the breast. *Lancet.* 1889; 1:571–573.

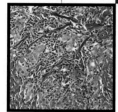

Epidemiology

■ STIMSON P. SCHANTZ

■ GUOPEI YU

Head and neck cancer is a paradigm for understanding the causes and prevention of environmentally induced disease. The preponderance of information suggests that tobacco is a significant etiologic determinant. Yet, despite this well-known association, efforts to curb tobacco use, thereby controlling disease, have met with limited success. Indeed, recent data suggest that head and neck cancer is actually increasing within certain segments of the U.S. population. A better understanding of the determinants of host-environmental interactions is needed so that treatment can be applied accordingly. This chapter presents current knowledge of the epidemiology of squamous cell carcinoma of the oral cavity, pharynx, and larynx, that is, head and neck cancer. Although the epidemiology of the disease worldwide is discussed, most of this chapter focuses on head and neck cancer within the United States. Information that points to the etiologic role of tobacco is summarized. Likewise, the confounding factors that promote disease are reviewed. It is hoped that such information will set the stage for future cancer preventive strategies.

INCIDENCE AND MORTALITY FROM HEAD AND NECK CANCER

It is estimated that 41,000 new cases of head and neck cancer will occur annually and that 13,000 of those affected will subsequently die of disease.[1] Overall rates have remained relatively constant over the last 20 years.[1,2] Although head and neck cancer within the United States represents less than 5% of neoplasias, worldwide, it is one of the most frequently identified cancers, with the highest incidence of disease being reported in southeastern and south-central Asia (Tables 2–1 and 2–2).[3] Factors that account for differences in head and neck cancer incidence are detailed in the sections that follow.

Within the United States, the 1992 incidence of oral cavity/pharynx cancer and larynx cancer was reported to be 10.3 and 4.4 per 100,000, respectively.[1] Mortality rates in 1992 for oral cavity/pharynx cancer and larynx cancer were 2.8 and 1.4 per 100,000, respectively. Rates are higher for male pa-

TABLE 2-1	THE MOST FREQUENT CANCERS WORLDWIDE, 1985 (ESTIMATED NUMBERS AND PERCENT TOTAL)								

MALES			FEMALES			ALL CASES		
Site	Number (thousands)	Percent	Site	Number (thousands)	Percent	Site	Number (thousands)	Percent
1. Lung	667	18	1. Breast	719	19	1. Lung	896	12
2. Stomach	473	12	2. Cervix	437	12	2. Stomach	755	10
3. Colon/rectum	331	9	3. Colon/rectum	346	9	3. Breast	720	9
4. Prostate	291	8	4. Stomach	282	8	4. Colon/rectum	678	9
5. Mouth/pharynx	270	7	5. Lung	219	6	5. Cervix	437	6
6. Liver	214	6	6. Ovary	162	4	6. Mouth/pharynx	412	5
7. Esophagus	196	5	7. Mouth/pharynx	143	4	7. Lymphoma	316	4

Adapted from Parkin DM, Pisani P, Ferlay J. Estimates of the worldwide incidence of eighteen major cancers in 1985. *Int J Cancer.* 1993; 54:594–606.

tients than for female patients. Black males, in particular, have the greatest risk for either oral cavity/pharyngeal or laryngeal disease, and they are at greatest risk of dying of this disease. Table 2–3 reveals the rank order of head and neck cancer mortality by state within the United States. A significantly increased incidence of disease is found within the District of Columbia, South Carolina, Florida, and Louisiana. The determinants of this differential increase in head and neck cancer are discussed later in this chapter.

Changing Incidence Rates

Within the last 20 years, there have been several significant trends in head and neck cancer incidence and mortality rates. Overall incidence and mortality from oral cavity and pharyngeal cancer have decreased significantly.[1] No significant change has been noted in laryngeal cancer rates. Changes in oral cavity/pharyngeal cancer incidence, however, must take into account specific sites. The observed decrease in oral cavity cancer is primarily a reflection of decreasing lip cancer.[3] Other sites within the oral cavity and pharynx have not shown similar trends. Indeed, the incidence rates of tongue cancer have actually increased significantly over this period.[2]

It is not only the current head and neck cancer incidence and mortality rates that are of concern, but also the changing patterns of the disease. Indeed, in certain populations within the United States, the problem is increasing, as detailed in the following sections.

DISEASE IN WOMEN

Chen et al[4] utilized the Connecticut tumor registry to determine male:female ratio for oral cavity cancer. Prior to 1940, this ratio was approximately 10:1. Between 1980 and 1985, the ratio decreased to 3:1 as a result of the increase in head and neck cancer among women. Birth cohort analysis revealed that

TABLE 2-2	THE ESTIMATED NUMBER OF NEW CANCER CASES (THOUSANDS) BY SITE, SEX, AND GEOGRAPHIC AREA, 1985			

GEOGRAPHIC AREA	ORAL CAVITY/ PHARYNX		LARYNX	
	Males	Females	Males	Females
Western Africa	1.5	1.4	0.5	0.1
South America (Tropical)	12.9	3.7	7.3	0.9
North America	21.4	9.4	11.5	2.4
Eastern Asia (China)	37.9	26.7	11.6	4.8
Southern Asia (including India)	90.5	52.4	26.7	4.5
Western Europe	16.1	4.3	8.5	0.8
Australia/New Zealand	1.6	0.6	0.6	0.1

Adapted from Parkin DM, Pisani P, Ferlay J. Estimates of the worldwide incidence of eighteen major cancers in 1985. *Int J Cancer.* 1993; 54:594–606.

TABLE 2 – 3	MORTALITY RATES IN SPECIFIC STATES: RANK ORDER OF THE 10 STATES WITH HIGHEST RATES

ORAL CAVITY/PHARYNX			LARYNX		
Rank	State	Mortality[a]	Rank	State	Mortality[a]
1.	District of Columbia	7.3[b]	1.	District of Columbia	1.3
2.	Delaware	4.5	2.	Montana	0.8
3.	South Carolina	3.9[b]	3.	Kentucky	0.7
4.	Alaska	3.7	4.	Nevada	0.7
5.	Louisiana	3.7[b]	5.	New York	0.7
6.	Florida	3.5[b]	6.	Massachusetts	0.7
7.	Maryland	4.5	7.	Delaware	0.6
8.	Mississippi	3.5	8.	Georgia	0.6
9.	Maine	3.5	9.	Louisiana	0.6
10.	Hawaii	3.4	10.	Virginia	0.5

[a] Mortality rates are from the National Center Health Service public use tapes.[1]
Rates are per 100,000 population and are age-adjusted to the 1920 U.S. standard.
[b] $P < 0.05$ as compared to the total U.S. mortality rate.

the greatest risk among women occurred in those born between 1900 and 1920. The determinants of this process undoubtedly relate to the increased prevalence of tobacco use among women that occurred during the early decades of the century.[5] This assumption would be predicated on a median time from initial exposure to cancer development of approximately 40 years.[6] Data from the Surveillance, Epidemiology, and End Results (SEER) program suggest that differences in the incidence of head and neck cancer between men and women have not changed appreciably since 1973, with the incidence for men being approximately 17 per 100,000 and for women, approximately 6.5 per 100,000 for the entire time period from 1973 to 1987.[2]

In addition to incidence rates, mortality rates may also be informative. Indeed, mortality rates are more widely collected and less subject to population selection bias and, thus, may be more reflective of real trends than incidence rates. Mortality rates are also not distorted by the efficiency of a particular cancer registry. Overall, from 1973 to 1987, a significant decrease in oral cavity and pharyngeal cancer mortality was noted.[2] The estimated annual decrease, however, was greater for men than for women (1.7% per year versus 0.7% per year, respectively). The authors conclude that the problem of head and neck cancer in women has changed appreciably since the beginning of the century, possibly reflecting changes in tobacco use habits. These habits among men and women have mostly stabilized, so further alterations in male : female incidence ratio are likely to be of decreased magnitude.

DISEASE IN AFRICAN-AMERICANS

The most significant increase in head and neck cancer over the last 20 years has been within the Afri-

can-American population.[1,2] In 1973, the combined oral cavity/pharyngeal cancer incidence was approximately 11 per 100,000 individuals for blacks and whites, an incidence that has remained relatively constant over time for whites. However, for African-Americans, the incidence increased dramatically to 14.7 between 1983 and 1987. The greatest change in the incidence of head and neck cancer involves black men, and the site of disease in which this change is most apparent is within the pharynx.

Multiple factors undoubtedly account for this increasing disease incidence among African-Americans. However, Day et al[7] have shown that combined tobacco and alcohol exposure may represent the greatest determinants. These authors performed a population-based case-control study that utilized the cancer registries of four communities. Over 1000 cases and 1000 controls were studied. Potential determinants assessed in this study included diet, occupation, family history, and socioeconomic status. When all factors were considered, the most explanatory variable was alcohol consumption. A greater proportion of black men, as compared to either whites or black females, were heavy alcohol users; however, it is also important to note that levels of consumption cannot be considered to be the sole explanatory variable. For instance, a differential risk ratio for a given level of alcohol exposure was noted. Greater than 30 drinks per week resulted in a 17-fold increase in risk among African-Americans, as compared to a 9-fold increase among whites. Other determinants, discussed later in this chapter, include diet, innate susceptibility factors, and factors related to socioeconomic status.

In addition to a growing disparity in head and neck cancer incidence between blacks and whites, there appear to be differences in the disease process between the two groups.[2,7–14] Blacks develop disease at an earlier age than do whites. Likewise, the disease is more advanced in blacks at the time of diagnosis, and mortality rates on a stage-by-stage basis are uniformly higher in the black population.

DISEASE IN YOUNG ADULTS

By examining the incidence and mortality rates, one can conclude that head and neck cancer is a disease of aging. The disease typically occurs in the fifth and sixth decade of life. Within affected individuals, a number of comorbid conditions often exist, such as coronary artery disease, hypertension, and stroke, all of which are diseases that could also be considered to be reflective of the aging process For those who treat this illness, such considerations only make the problem of head and neck cancer in young adults even more perplexing; they also make the frequently noted increasing incidence of head and neck cancer in this population a major concern.[15-19] Shemen et al[15] were the first to raise this issue, citing the hospital registry of Memorial Sloan-Kettering Cancer Center, as well as data from the SEER registry. Similar observations regarding an increase in the disease among young adults were subsequently reported by MD Anderson Cancer Center.[17] Using death certificate rates from the National Center for Health Statistics, Depue[16] showed an increase in head and neck cancer mortality among young adults under the age of 30 years. The increase was reported to have begun in the mid-1970s. Such increases are not exclusively limited to young adults within the United States. Franchesci et al[19] examined mortality trends in 24 European countries based on death certificates recorded from 1955 to 1989. In 10 countries, the incidence of head and neck cancer among men younger than 44 years of age increased by more than twofold; three countries showed a similar increase for women. The countries in which such an increase was reported were principally central European countries, including Austria, Germany, Hungary, Poland, and Bulgaria. Fortunately, head and neck cancer among individuals younger than 40 years of age is still considered a relatively rare event in the United States.

Factors that may account for disease development in young adults have not been defined. Suggested causative agents include smokeless tobacco, various forms of drug abuse, and viruses, as well as host susceptibility factors.[16,19-22] However, there remains no clear evidence to support the significance of any single determinant. In light of the importance placed on smokeless tobacco, the tobacco habits of young adult patients with head and neck cancer at MD Anderson Cancer Center from 1947 to 1987 were reviewed.[17] Although the number of young adults affected by the disease increased over this period, no evidence for a causative association with smokeless tobacco use could be identified. Indeed, the authors noted that the number of young adults who used tobacco in any form represented a minority,

leading them to conclude that causes other than tobacco must be considered. Undoubtedly, no single factor will explain disease in these individuals.

A major consideration is also whether or not the mortality rate associated with the disease in this population is greater than that typically observed in the older population. Although considerable controversy persists, there is no clear evidence that the disease carries an increased mortality rate in the young adult population.[23-25]

TOBACCO USE

Analytic epidemiology has provided considerable insight into factors that contribute to the development of head and neck cancer. In order to judge the significance of these factors, a framework based on a modification of Koch's postulates has been provided by Wynder and Day.[26,27] These postulates include the following:

1. The factor has to increase the risk of cancer.
2. Global distribution should be consistent with the rate of cancer.
3. After its removal or reduction in a given population, the rate of cancer should decline after a suitable latent period.

Perhaps the first report demonstrating a causal relationship between tobacco and head and neck cancer was published by Wynder et al[28] in 1956. These authors compared 1444 patients with larynx cancer to 1339 age- and sex-matched controls and noted that the odds-ratio of developing head and neck cancer increased 10-fold among smokers. Furthermore, a dose-response relationship was observed; those individuals who smoked the heaviest were at greatest risk. After adjusting for alcohol and other factors, the greatest risk was noted to be 6.0 higher as a result of tobacco use. Most research articles cite risk-ratios of disease ranging from 5-fold to 25-fold, depending on the duration and intensity of tobacco consumption (reviewed in references 29 to 31). The odds-ratio, however, is influenced by the overall proportion of individuals among the controls who smoke. It is, therefore, relevant that the prevalence of tobacco use among patients with head and neck cancer is approximately 80% to 90%.[29-31]

Epidemiologic data also suggest that the type of tobacco habit influences the site of disease development within the upper aerodigestive tract. Wynder et al,[28] for instance, has noted that cigar and pipe smokers are at increased risk for developing cancers of the oral cavity, pharynx, and extrinsic larynx. The risk of development of intrinsic laryngeal cancer did not seem to be influenced, however. The use of smokeless tobacco is known to induce disease within the oral cavity, but not the lung.[32,33] Furthermore, one must distinguish between dark and light (flu-cured) tobacco in epidemiologic studies,[34–39] as the former contains increased levels of carcinogens and larger particulate matter.[37] Particles are more frequently trapped in the proximal aerodigestive tract, leading to genetic damage in these locations. Thus, cancers of the oral cavity and larynx are more commonly seen in users of black tobacco, as compared to lung cancer in the users of flu-cured tobacco.[40,41]

Consistent with one of the postulates noted earlier—i.e., that after the removal of a suspected causative agent, the risk of cancer should decline—Franco et al[34] demonstrated that the risk of head and neck cancer among smokers approximated that of nonsmokers following 10 years of smoking cessation. Similar reports of decreasing risk with smoking cessation have been noted by others. [32,39,42,43]

Smokeless Tobacco and Oral Cavity Cancer

The relationship between oral cancer and smokeless tobacco has been well established, principally through epidemiologic investigations in developing countries. Indeed, the world's highest incidence of cancer occurs within regions where the chewing of pan (a mixture of various regional ingredients including areca nut, slaked lime, and tobacco) represents a traditional custom.[40,44] Within the United States, smokeless tobacco use has been associated with an increased risk of oral cancer, primarily among older women in the southeastern region of the country.[45] However, several other studies within the United States have yielded inconclusive data (reviewed in references 46 and 47). The study by Blot et al,[42] which involved more than 1000 cases and controls from several counties within the United States, found similar numbers of individuals in both groups who used smokeless tobacco. Other studies have been limited by the low prevalence of cases and controls associated with the use of smokeless tobacco.[48] Moreover, smokeless tobacco is rarely

used as the sole source of tobacco, and is most often consumed with smoked products.[48] Additionally, case-control studies have demonstrated little relationship to cancer development outside of the oral cavity.[46] The exception may relate to a potential increase in salivary gland tumors among smokeless tobacco users.[49]

The current increase in smokeless tobacco use among young adults has raised concern over a potential epidemic of oral cancer. To date, there is no evidence to support that claim. However, several studies have shown a high incidence of oral leukoplakia lesions in groups that frequently use smokeless tobacco.[50] Given the high level of tobacco-specific carcinogens found in these products, as well as the demonstration of snuff-induced cancers within animal models, there is cause for concern that these cancers will become manifest as the young adult population ages over the ensuing years.

ALCOHOL

Just as the evidence to support the causative role of tobacco is extensive, so is the evidence for the cancer-causative role of alcohol. A plethora of studies have demonstrated that the odds-ratio of head and neck cancer, after adjusting for tobacco use, increases from 3- to 15-fold in individuals who consume alcohol[51–55] Furthermore, a multiplicative effect is observed when interactions between tobacco and alcohol are considered.[51–53] The greater the use of each agent when used in combination, the more likely an individual is to develop disease. Perhaps the most representative study of alcohol effect was performed by Blot et al.[51] In this study, the risk of disease increased to greater than 30-fold in heavy smokers who consumed more than 30 drinks per week (Table 2–4).

Epidemiologic studies demonstrate that the effect of alcohol on cancer risk must also take into account the location of the cancer within the upper aerodi-

T A B L E 2 - 4	**ODDS-RATIOS OF ORAL CAVITY AND PHARYNGEAL CANCER IN MALES ACCORDING TO TOBACCO SMOKING AND ALCOHOL CONSUMPTION**				
SMOKING STATUS (cigarettes/day)	**NO. OF ALCOHOLIC DRINKS (per week)**				
	<1	**1–4**	**5–14**	**15–29**	**30+**
None	1.0	1.3	1.6	1.4	5.8
<20	1.7	1.5	2.7	5.4	7.9
20–39	1.9	2.4	4.4	7.2	23.8
≥40	7.4	0.7	4.4	20.2	37.7

Adapted from Blot WJ, McLaughlin JK, Winn DM, et al. Smoking and drinking in relation to oral and pharyngeal cancer. *Cancer Res.* 1988; 48:3282–3287.

gestive tract (Table 2–5).[31,56–59] The oral cavity and pharynx appear to be more adversely influenced than the larynx. Within the larynx, the extrinsic mucosa appears to be at greater risk than the intrinsic mucosa. Such information provides clues as to the mechanism by which alcohol promotes cancer risk. It would suggest that the greatest effect is through a topical, rather than a systemic, influence. The intrinsic larynx is spared direct contact through normal protective mechanisms provided by movement of the epiglottis, as well as through sensory responses induced by the contact of fluids upon intrinsic laryngeal mucosa. Although not as extensively studied as differences related to subsites within the larynx, relative risks within the oral cavity would support the same conclusion regarding alcohol's topical influence. In the study by Jovanic et al,[59] alcohol was associated with a greater risk of disease within the floor of mouth as compared to the tongue, perhaps because the floor of the mouth represents a reservoir for oral secretions and is a site of prolonged contact.

A fundamental question in head and neck carcinogenesis is whether or not alcohol alone represents a carcinogenic influence. Recalling Wynder's modification of Koch's postulates, described earlier in this chapter, the evidence for alcohol as a cancer-producing substance is not as strong as that for tobacco. For instance, no reproducible animal studies exist in which the direct, topical application of alcohol alone induces cancer (reviewed in reference 51). Likewise, the influence of alcohol cessation on reducing cancer risk has not been clearly established. The only study to address this latter point showed that risks approached that of the normal controls in those individuals who had achieved alcohol abstinence for 10 years.[60] These latter results were not, however, adjusted for tobacco use. Likewise, it is difficult to sort out the relative impact of tobacco consumption on alcohol-related risks, as most individuals who consume alcohol also smoke. A study by Blot et al,[42] however, had the advantages of a large case size and control size, and was able to establish the impact of alcohol alone in those individuals who did not use tobacco in any form. Risks in nonsmokers ranged from 1.6 in moderate drinkers to 5.8 in those who consumed more than 30 drinks per week. Similar observations were reported by Elmwood et al.[55]

Several studies have addressed the influence of various types of alcohol on cancer risk. Blot et al[42] and others[57,61,62] have noted similar risks of oral and pharyngeal cancer associated with beer and hard liquor intake. Risks were greater than those associated with wine. Most studies, however, simply demonstrate the dose-response relationship between alcohol exposure with disease, without addressing the type of alcohol consumed. Day et al[7] have suggested that a distinction needs to be made between dark alcohol, such as bourbon and scotch, and light alcohols, such as gin and vodka. In a case-control study, these authors noted that alcohol remained the single greatest risk factor to which the increased incidence of head and neck cancers among African-American men could be attributed. These researchers further found that there were differences in alcohol consumption patterns in this ethnic group. Specifically, black men were found to drink a greater proportion of dark alcohol than light alcohol. Dark alcohol represents a far more complex mixture of substances than light alcohol and thus may provide greater carcinogenic exposure.[63]

Various types of alcohol are known to contain various congeners that may have a carcinogenic effect (reviewed in reference 51). For instance, beer may contain increased levels of N-nitroso compounds.[64] Other carcinogenic substances that can be found in particular liquors include mycotoxins, tannins, aldehydes, and pesticides.[51] These impurities tend to increase in certain regions of the world in which the beverage is indigenous and locally made.

The mechanism by which alcohol may function as a causative agent is multifactorial. Blot,[51] Schottenfeld,[31] and others[65,66] have provided excellent reviews of this role. The effects may be through direct mucosal contact as well as through systemic influences. However, most experimental studies have

			SITE (RR)						
			Oral Cavity				Larynx		
AUTHOR	YEAR	NO. OF CASES	Tongue	FOM	NOS	Pharynx	Intrinsic	Extrinsic	NOS
Elmwood et al[55a]	1984	374	—	—	1–5	1–12	1–2	1–6	—
Brugere et al[56a]	1988	3465	—	—	3–70	3–62	1–6	3–21	—
Tuyns et al[57a]	1988	1147	—	—	—	2–13	1–3	1–11	—
Baron et al[58]	1993	532	—	—	4–350	4–305	—	—	1–21
Jovanic[59]	1993	740	1	2–3	—	—	—	—	—

TABLE 2–5 THE RISK OF HEAD AND NECK CANCER ATTRIBUTABLE TO ALCOHOL USE: DIFFERENCES BASED ON ANATOMIC SUBSITE

[a] Adjusted for tobacco exposure.
RR, relative risk range; FOM, floor of mouth; NOS, site not otherwise specified.

ruled out a direct carcinogenic effect upon cellular DNA. Alcohol, by itself, does not have a detectable clastogenic influence. Likewise, no animal study to date has directly linked alcohol exposure to cancer initiation.[51] However, as mentioned earlier in this section, identifiable contaminants may be found within alcohol that could exert a direct carcinogenic influence.[63,64] Likewise, intermediate metabolites of alcohol may be related to cancer risk. Acetaldehyde, a metabolic product of alcohol generated by enzymes within the aerodigestive mucosa, may induce mutational events as well as inhibit critical DNA repair mechanisms.[66,67]

The direct effect of alcohol on cancer development may be through mechanisms independent of initiation. Such mechanisms reflect so-called promotional effects and include the production of prostaglandins, lipid peroxidation, and the generation of free radical oxygen, all of which enhance cell turnover and cell growth.[65,68] Alcohol may also modulate carcinogen effect by enhancing membrane permeability.[59] Furthermore, the influence of carcinogens may be enhanced by the toxic effect of alcohol on mucosa.

There are other cancer-causing effects associated with alcohol that may not be strictly categorized as either tumor-initiating or promotional. As an example, tobacco may induce specific DNA mutations that are normally repaired. In the presence of alcohol, such damage-control mechanisms may be retarded, thereby allowing mutations to persist and to eventuate in the cancer-initiated state.[69-71] Other means by which alcohol may increase the risk of cancer may be through its influence on the xenobiotic enzyme systems (i.e., enzymes that metabolize foreign compounds). For instance, alcohol may retard enzymes that normally protect the host from carcinogen-DNA interactions.[72,73] Conversely, host enzymes that activate carcinogens to their more DNA damaging intermediates may be induced by alcohol.[74] Alcohol may lead to a depressed immunologic state.[75-77] Identifiable alterations include decreased T-lymphocyte activation, mitogen responsiveness, cytokine production, and cell-mediated cytotoxicity. Likewise, alcohol may influence cancer risk through systemic effects, principally by means of its toxic effect on the liver. The liver is critical to the detoxification of numerous carcinogenic compounds, such as tobacco-specific nitrosamines. As a result of alcohol-induced liver dysfunction, these substances may be free to circulate, leading to enhanced tissue damage. The liver is also critical to the generation of various circulating hormones which, in the diseased state, may lead to tumor initiation. Estrogen levels, for instance, are elevated in individuals with alcoholic liver disease, and estrogens have been demonstrated to have a promotional effect on head and neck cancer.[78] Finally, alcohol may directly or indirectly influence host nutritional status, thereby contributing to disease. The impact of nutritional deficiencies on head and neck cancer risk is discussed later in this chapter.

SOCIOECONOMIC DETERMINANTS OF HEAD AND NECK CANCER PROGRESSION

It has been generally accepted that the problem of head and neck cancer reflects a lifestyle disease that is most prevalent among individuals of certain socioeconomic strata.[7,55,79-82] A critical question remains the relevance of socioeconomic correlates after adjusting for known risk factors, such as alcohol and/or tobacco. Ernster et al provided evidence for the significance of socioeconomic status within the United States population through the use of the Third National Cancer Survey, conducted in the United States from 1969 to 1971.[79] Each cancer patient was assigned to one of three income levels based on the median income of his or her census tract of residence in nine survey areas. Denominator data for the population came from the 1970 tapes of the U.S. Bureau of the Census. Table 2–6 shows that, for every age group and sex, low annual income was associated with an increased risk of head and neck cancer. This risk was most significant when comparing low-income male subjects to high-income male subjects in the group that was 55 to 64 years of age.

In a more recent study, Elmwood et al[55] performed a case-control study in Vancouver, British Columbia using more than 300 patients treated at a major referral center. Controls were derived from the patient population admitted to the same center with cancer diagnoses other than aerodigestive tumors, and were matched for age and sex. Results demonstrated that unskilled workers showed a crude relative risk of 2.2 compared to skilled workers and professionals. The risk remained significant after adjustment for alcohol, smoking, and marital status. Similar results were noted by Day et al,[7] who also showed that low employment levels were independently associated with increased oral cancer risks among both African-Americans and whites.

Two additional factors were noted to be significant in the study by Elmwood et al,[55] namely, marital status and regular dental care. The observation regarding marital status may reflect the significance of social support systems as a factor in head and neck carcinogenesis. Unmarried persons can be characterized as having both fewer social support systems and a more deficient health status.[7,81] A similar significance had been ascribed to marital status in a report by Day et al,[7] although the data to support that observation were not included. In a report by Greenberg et al,[82] lack of social support systems, as reflected in a lower percentage of potential working life spent in employment and being unmarried, was a stronger correlate of oral cancer risk than socioeconomic status per se.

The preceding evidence suggests that socioeconomic factors and, perhaps more specifically, social

TABLE 2 – 6	INCIDENCE RATES PER 100,000 POPULATION FOR HEAD AND NECK CANCER ACCORDING TO INCOME LEVEL				
		SITE			
		Oral Cavity		Larynx	
AGE (years)	INCOME LEVEL	Males	Females	Males	Females
35–44	Low	1.7	2.7	3.1	1.5
	Intermediate	1.4	0.7	2.6	0.0
	High	1.0	0.7	1.9	0.8
45–54	Low	11.2	4.1	17.6	4.8
	Intermediate	5.4	4.1	14.3	2.6
	High	3.7	2.6	9.2	1.7
55–64	Low	18.8	8.0	41.6	4.9
	Intermediate	16.8	6.3	29.5	4.0
	High	11.6	5.2	22.6	4.0

Adapted from Ernster VL, Selvin S, Sacks ST, Merrill DW, Holly EA. Major histologic types of cancers of the gum and mouth, esophagus, larynx, and lung by sex and income level. *JNCI*. 1982; 69:773–776.

stability factors are independent risk factors for the development of head and neck cancer. These findings have a profound implication in terms of the way this disease is viewed. What are the true determinants of disease related to social status? That is, are individuals from these groups more likely to have poor nutritional habits? Are they more likely to have associated risk factors, such as poor dentition or infectious diseases? The potential significance of social stability factors for head and neck cancer risk should be regarded seriously in light of the rising incidence and mortality rates among African-American males.

NUTRITION

Certain dietary factors appear to exert a protective effect on the risk of head and neck cancer. Data from case-control studies, in many circumstances, are confounded by the lack of control for other variables, such as tobacco and alcohol (reviewed in references 83 and 84). Many of the studies assessing nutrition are limited by sample size. Likewise, case-control studies have their own inherent limitations, such as ascertainment bias, that may lead to overestimates of nutrient effects. Thus, evidence must also be drawn from additional methodologies, such as ecologic studies that examine for risk factors among groups rather than individuals. Cohort studies, which make risk assessments within individuals who are then followed over time for the development of disease, are also valuable. Unfortunately, a paucity of head and neck cancer studies has been performed using these latter techniques. Thus, the overall role of diet in modifying risk is not entirely clear.

Tables 2–7 and 2–8 present the results of several case-control studies organized by site of disease within the upper aerodigestive tract.[85–94] As summarized by Steinmetz and Potter,[84] the beneficial effect depends on the type of food and the site of index cancer within the upper aerodigestive tract. For

TABLE 2 – 7	SELECTED EPIDEMIOLOGIC STUDIES, NUTRITION, AND LARYNGEAL CANCER				
AUTHOR	YEAR	NO. OF PATIENTS	FOOD/NUTRIENT INTAKE	OR (95% CI)	SIGNIFICANCE
Graham et al[85a]	1981	374	Low in vitamin A	3.1 (not stated)	<0.01
			Low in vitamin C	2.5 (not stated)	<0.05
DeStefani et al[86]	1987	170	Low in fruit	2.7 (1.3–5.4)	<0.05
			Low in vegetables	— (—)	NS
Notani and Jayant[87a]	1987	80	Low in fruit	2.0 (1.0–4.1)	NS
			Low in vegetables	2.7 (1.4–5.3)	<0.05

[a] Adjusted for tobacco and alcohol use.
OR, odds-ratios; CI, confidence interval; NS, not significant.

TABLE 2-8	SELECTED EPIDEMIOLOGIC STUDIES, NUTRITION, AND ORAL/PHARYNGEAL CANCER				
AUTHOR	YEAR	NO. OF PATIENTS	FOOD/NUTRIENT INTAKE	OR (95% CI)	SIGNIFICANCE
Winn et al[91a]	1984	227	High in fruit	0.6 (0.4–0.08)	<0.001
			High in green, leafy vegetables	0.7 (0.5–1.1)	NS
			High in dairy products	1.0 (not stated)	NS
McLaughlin et al[88a]	1988	871	High in retinol	1.6 (not stated)	<0.01
			High in carotene	0.8 (not stated)	0.11
			Vitamin C	0.6 (not stated)	<0.001
Franco et al[89a]	1989	235	High in carotene vegetables	0.4 (0.2–1.0)	NS
			High in citric fruits	0.5 (0.3–0.9)	<0.05
			High in green vegetables	0.7 (0.4–1.4)	NS

[a] Adjusted for tobacco and alcohol use.
OR, odds-ratios; CI, confidence interval; NS, not significant.

instance, fruit intake appears to be more beneficial against oral cavity cancer than the level of vegetable intake. Risk reduction estimates related to fruit vary twofold to fourfold in those with the highest intake versus those with the lowest intake. Within the larynx, neither fruit nor vegetable intake conveys a readily apparent benefit. In the studies reviewed by Steinmetz and Potter,[84] the beneficial effect of vegetable intake, for instance, was described as significant in only one case-control study involving laryngeal disease. Whether or not diet is significant after adjusting for tobacco exposure has not been well established, but it does appear to be the case.[88,90] More studies are required in order to obtain definitive answers.

Some have speculated that diet may not play as significant a role as one might expect, as demonstrated by Graham et al.[93] In this study, which involved more than 550 cases, no significant influence of diet could be identified. In the authors' case-control study, a multivariate analysis of various risk factors was performed for more than 150 cases and 150 controls.[95] Factors analyzed in multivariate analysis included dietary intake and tobacco and alcohol use, as well as the genetic susceptibility marker, mutagen sensitivity. Those factors found to be significant were tobacco, alcohol, and mutagen sensitivity. Various nutrient intakes were not found to contribute to risk estimates after accounting for the aforementioned measures. One cannot exclude a potential influence of dietary factors on overall mutagen-sensitivity measures that may obscure results.

Several studies have evaluated head and neck cancer risk as a function of specific nutrient intake, including nutrient supplements, rather than by food groups (reviewed in reference 83). The nutrients most suggestive of a protective benefit included vitamins C and E. The benefit of vitamin A has not been substantiated. Most information related to beta-carotene intake has shown no relationship between beta-carotene intake and head and neck cancer risk.

Most studies that attempt to establish risk estimates based on nutrient intake do so through recall questionnaires. The value of such methodology has not been universally accepted and has been associated with several deficiencies, including adequacy of recall, especially among older patients. Furthermore, food intake does not necessarily reflect bioavailability of a particular nutrient. As previously alluded to in the section on alcohol, heavy alcohol intake may lower vitamin A reserves through mechanisms independent of consumption levels.[96] This has led to a growing interest in the establishment of tissue and serum nutrient levels as markers of risk. In one of the few studies involving head and neck cancer, Zheng et al[97] reported an inverse relationship between serum vitamin levels—principally, beta-carotene and α-tocopherol—and head and neck cancer risk. This study involved 25,802 individuals in Maryland beginning in 1974. Twenty-eight individuals went on to develop oral or pharyngeal cancer. Interestingly, increased levels of both serum retinol and serum selenium were associated with an increased risk of cancer.

Perhaps the longest standing association between dietary deficiencies and head and neck cancer risk relates to the iron deficiency syndromes, specifically, the Plummer-Vinson syndrome. This syndrome is characterized by glossitis, esophageal webs, and iron deficiency anemia. Wynder et al[98] were the first to draw attention to the high incidence of head and neck cancers in individuals with this syndrome. The disease has mostly disappeared in previously endemic areas as a result of iron supplementation.

Multiple mechanisms may be involved in the host protection provided by various nutrients. Probably the best understood effect may be the ability of various nutrients to function as free radical scavengers. The interaction between dietary factors and carcinogens, such as tobacco, that produce free radical oxygen would then be reflected in risk estimates. In support of this biologic premise, Winn et al[83] noted that the adverse effect of low fruit and vegetable intake was most apparent in smokers. In addition to free radical scavenging, other factors must also be considered, such as the ability of nutrients to control cellular differentiation. This latter effect has most often been ascribed to vitamin A and its retinol derivatives.[99] Certain foodstuffs may influence DNA repair capacities, carcinogen metabolizing systems, as well as various signal transduction pathways that influence DNA synthesis.[99]

Although many studies have suggested that specific fruits and vegetables are beneficial in terms of head and neck cancer risk, only a few have identified types of foods associated with an increased risk. Notani et al[87] provided evidence that the risk of head and neck cancer increases in individuals with a high intake of red chili peppers. These authors found that a compound—capsaicin—within red peppers had both a mutagenic and a tumor-promoting effect in laboratory model systems. In a study from India, the risk of oral cancer among pan chewers was increased significantly in individuals who consumed high levels of the cereal raji.[100] Franchesci et al[101] reported that maize intake enhanced oral cancer risk. The mechanisms underlying these authors' observations are not clear, but may relate to an associated nutritional deficiency in those who consume these staples as a principal food source.[102] Likewise, the manner in which a food is prepared, such as overcooking vegetables, grilling foods, or cooking over a woodstove, may enhance cancer risk.[89]

OCCUPATION

The lack of well-established occupational risk factors for head and neck cancer may be as informative as their existence. Conceivably, this suggests the requirement of more chronic exposures as a determinant of disease. As mentioned earlier, the median duration of tobacco use among head and neck cancer patients is 40 years. Employment at any particular trade rarely extends over such a prolonged interval. Likewise, one would also have to take into account other confounding factors, such as additional lifestyle habits as well as host susceptibility factors. Given all these covariates, few studies have identified enough cases to achieve statistical significance (reviewed in references 29 and 103). It is also relevant that no reported occupational exposure has been related to disease of any site within the head and neck (i.e., oral cavity, pharynx, and larynx). Rather, analytical epidemiologic studies that demonstrate enhanced risks associated with a specific occupation are usually restricted to a particular region within the upper aerodigestive tract.[104–120] Among those occupations that have been attributed to an enhanced risk of oral cancer, the most extensively studied has been textile working within Europe and

printing occupations within the United States.[106–110] Several occupational exposures have been related to laryngeal carcinoma, including exposure to asbestos, nickel, sulfuric acid, and mustard gas.[111,112,114–117] Of all these factors, exposure to asbestos has been the most extensively investigated.[111,114]

GENETIC SUSCEPTIBILITY

In recent years, analytical epidemiology has focused on the role of heritable susceptibility factors as a determinant of head and neck cancer. Such investigations are intended to provide insight as to why only a small proportion of the 25 million individuals who use tobacco develop head and neck cancer annually. Factors other than tobacco, acting either in concert with tobacco or alone, may contribute to cancer development. Potential host susceptibility factors can be assigned to various categories to allow a better understanding (Table 2–9). These may include host factors that control the metabolism of carcinogens (i.e., the so-called xenobiotic enzyme system), traits related to gender and race, genetic determinants found in individuals with various cancer family syndromes, as well as syndromes associated with DNA repair deficiency.

Carcinogen Metabolizing Systems

Most carcinogenic compounds within tobacco will not act directly upon host DNA. Rather, these compounds must be metabolized to electrophilic inter-

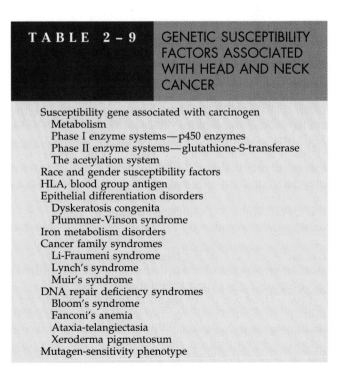

T A B L E 2 - 9	GENETIC SUSCEPTIBILITY FACTORS ASSOCIATED WITH HEAD AND NECK CANCER

Susceptibility gene associated with carcinogen
  Metabolism
    Phase I enzyme systems—p450 enzymes
    Phase II enzyme systems—glutathione-S-transferase
    The acetylation system
Race and gender susceptibility factors
  HLA, blood group antigen
Epithelial differentiation disorders
  Dyskeratosis congenita
  Plummner-Vinson syndrome
Iron metabolism disorders
Cancer family syndromes
  Li-Fraumeni syndrome
  Lynch's syndrome
  Muir's syndrome
DNA repair deficiency syndromes
  Bloom's syndrome
  Fanconi's anemia
  Ataxia-telangiectasia
  Xeroderma pigmentosum
Mutagen-sensitivity phenotype

mediates. The latter intermediates are termed ultimate carcinogens; their production is governed by a family of enzymes that acts either to enhance or diminish their intracellular levels. The enzymes that control these metabolic states are termed xenobiotic enzymes. It has been recognized for many years that innate differences exist within individuals in their capacity to express such enzyme activity.[121–124] Furthermore, the relative functional capacity of these enzymes within an individual may determine the degree to which that individual is at risk.

The most extensively studied xenobiotic enzyme superfamily is the p450 system, one of the so-called phase I enzymes.[125,126] Phase I enzymes are involved principally in carcinogen activation, that is, the generation of more genotoxic intermediates. There are more than 20 families that are further composed of more than 150 gene products. It has also been well established that various tissues express differing types of p450 enzymes, and that this may be a factor as to why certain tissues, and not others, may be at risk. Typically, various p450 enzymes are classified by the prefix CYP, indicating cytochrome, followed by a combination of two separate numbers and a letter. The first arabic number represents the respective family. Following the respective family symbol is a letter and a final number representing the subfamily and gene, respectively. Thus, CYP 1A1, which exists at high levels within the laryngeal mucosa and is involved in the metabolism of tobacco-related carcinogens, represents family 1, subfamily A, and gene 1 of the p450 enzyme superfamily. It is also important to understand that each enzyme has substrate specificity. Thus, p450 1A1 will act upon polycyclic aromatic hydrocarbons, but will not interact with other substances, such as tobacco-specific nitrosamines. Conversely, enzymes 2D6 and 2E1 interact principally with the latter.

The significance of p450 enzymes in tobacco carcinogenesis stems from the study of multiple cancers, including cancers of the head and neck, lung, and bladder. The first study to draw attention to this host susceptibility factor was performed by Kellerman et al[127] in 1973. These researchers utilized the arylhydrocarbon hydroxylase assay to assess CYP 1A1 function, rather than looking at specific genotypes. They noted that the risk of lung cancer was increased more than 30-fold in those who expressed elevated function. Several years later, these authors and others reported on the role of this enzyme in the epidemiology of laryngeal cancer, again documenting increased risk in those who had elevated function.[128–130] However, few studies using other measures of host p450 status have yielded results of similar significance.[124] Most, however, have utilized genotyping rather than functional assays.

Phase II enzymes, in contrast to the p450 enzyme family, are involved in carcinogen detoxification, and thus serve to protect the host. The most well-known enzyme within the phase II system is glutathione-S-transferase (GST). It would be logical to assume that individuals with innately more active phase II systems would be at decreased risk. Indeed, this has been substantiated by the few studies that have investigated the relationship. However, risk estimates have been relatively modest, rarely exceeding a threefold difference, and in several instances, the results have not been significant.[131–133] In the authors' own preliminary study involving patients with head and neck cancer treated at Memorial Sloan-Kettering Cancer Center, GST as a single risk factor could not be associated with a readily apparent increased risk.[133] Additional investigations in this potentially meaningful field are warranted.

The relatively modest risks associated with heritable xenobiotic enzyme status are not entirely unexpected. Head and neck cancer is undoubtedly governed by multiple factors, including polygenic susceptibility traits. The use of these enzyme measures would, consequently, be more relevant when used in combination than when used individually. In one of the few reports that investigated both p450 enzyme and GST enzyme activity within the same individual, Hayashi et al[134] noted that the combination of measures yielded greater estimates of risk for lung cancer than either alone. Similar studies relating to head and neck carcinogenesis remain to be investigated. Additional enzymes that have been reportedly involved with head and neck cancer risk include the acetylation pathways in which active levels of this enzyme serve to detoxify carcinogens and, thus, reduce risk.[135]

Gender

As stated earlier in this chapter, data from the Connecticut Cancer Registry indicate that the incidence of head and neck cancer has increased among women.[4] Such trends have been attributed to increasing tobacco use. However, the question remains as to whether other influences may account for these trends. Indeed, although tobacco is a determinant in most circumstances, elderly women, as well as many young adult females who present with the disease, frequently deny ever using tobacco. Furthermore, one must also consider that women may be inherently more susceptible to tobacco-induced carcinogenesis. In this regard, several studies have shown higher cancer risks for women as compared with men for any given level of tobacco exposure.[48,136]

Clues from molecular epidemiologic studies, as detailed later in this chapter, may provide some answers. Molecular studies of DNA adduct formation show that the ratio of exposure to genetic damage may not be equivalent between genders.[137] DNA adduct formation represents the covalent binding of chemical carcinogens with the host genome. Such binding sets the stage for subsequent genetic damage, including DNA breaks as well as abnormal repair. It has also been shown that the greater the exposure to a particular carcinogen, the more likely one is able to identify such adducts (reviewed in reference 138). Likewise, epidemiologic studies involving one particular adduct—i.e., those generated by polycyclic aromatic hydrocarbons (PAH)—have shown that cancer patients with a history of tobacco exposure are more likely to express such adducts than healthy, nonsmoking controls.[138] Ryberg et al[137] have investigated the relative quantity of PAH related adducts among male and female smokers. In their study, DNA was isolated from 63 patients with lung cancer. For both men and women, the amount of tobacco use governed the total quantity of DNA adducts formed. Individuals who used tobacco were more likely to express an increased level of adducts; however, a great deal of variability was noted. Most significantly, for any given level of tobacco consumption, women had higher levels of adducts than men. These data raise the possibilities that women may be more sensitive to tobacco damage than men, and that factors that promote carcinogen metabolism and the binding of those carcinogens to DNA may be influenced by gender. Alternatively, the DNA adducts measured may not necessarily be specific to tobacco. Randerath et al[139] have demonstrated that bulky adducts, not unlike the ones discussed in Ryberg et al, may be formed as a consequence of normal metabolic activites. Furthermore, the greater the metabolic activity, the more likely these so-called indigenous adducts will be generated. The specificity of any adduct is, thus, questionable. Its measurement may reflect disparate exposures, as well as metabolic activities. The adducts described by Ryberg et al[137] are potentially generated from multiple sources, which may be influencing an increased cancer risk among women.

Studies of estrogen receptors within aerodigestive mucosa raise the question of the role of hormonal influences in cancer risk among men and women. Aerodigestive mucosa has been shown to contain high levels of hormonal receptors, including both estrogen and androgen types.[78] The role of these receptors and their corresponding ligands is uncertain. Laboratory studies have suggested that such receptors may control cellular proliferation.[140] The greater the binding of estrogen, for instance, the more likely that increased cellular turnover will occur. Estrogen may also promote the metabolism of carcinogens to more toxic intermediate stages.[141]

Race

Just as gender-related factors may be relevant to cancer risk, so may influences attributable to race and ethnicity. As previously reviewed in this chapter, head and neck cancer is a much greater problem among African-American males within the United States than for any other group. The factors that account for this increased incidence are multiple. Head and neck cancer is a disease of misfortune; that is, individuals at risk are characterized by an increased prevalence of unemployment, diminished education, disrupted family units, alcohol abuse, and poor nutrition. These same factors are typically expressed to a higher degree in certain minority populations within the United States, including African-Americans. Moreover, as compared to whites, blacks present with head and neck cancer at an earlier age, present with more advanced disease, and have worse prospects for survival on a stage-by-stage basis.

As mentioned previously in this chapter, an important process in tobacco carcinogenesis is the conversion of tobacco-containing compounds into active carcinogens, a process that, in many circumstances, requires active metabolism by host enzyme systems. Hecht et al[142] have focused on one such metabolic system; namely, the enzymes involved in the metabolism of tobacco-specific nitrosamines. They studied the degree to which 4-(methylnitrosamino)-1-(3-pyridyl)-1-butanone (NNK) is converted to the metabolite 4-(methylnitrosamino)-1-(3-pyridyl)-1-butanol (NNAL), and the extent to which the latter metabolite is conjugated to NNAL-glucuronide. They found that the greater the glucuronidation, the more likely the DNA would be protected from carcinogen exposure. Hecht et al[142] noted that blacks had much lower levels of glucuronidation than did whites. This, in turn, results in a higher NNAL/NNAL-glucuronide ratio in blacks than whites, thereby suggesting that, for a given level of exposure, blacks are at increased risk. Additional studies are needed.

Other genetic markers of carcinogen metabolism are, likewise, not equally distributed among racial groups. For instance, studies involving the p450 enzyme system have shown a higher frequency of the "risk" alleles for lung cancer among blacks as compared to whites.[143,144] However, no association with lung cancer in African-Americans has been identified with these markers. In addition, Wagenknecht et al[145] have shown that blacks metabolize nicotine differently than whites. For any given level of nicotene exposure, blacks have higher levels of circulating cotinine, a metabolite of nicotene. Such differences in metabolic activity may contribute to an increased level of nicotene dependence and an associated increased risk of cancer.

Although not specifically related to head and neck cancer, additional studies have focused on racial differences involving polymorphisms of genes that are associated with the development and progression of diseases considered to be tobacco-related. Evaluated genetic loci include the polymorphic p53 gene, as well as L-MYC loci.[146–148] In each of these studies, African-Americans were found to express the allelotype associated with more aggressive disease.

Day et al[7] have observed two factors that are relevant to an understanding of genetic susceptibility. In their extensive case-control study involving more than 1000 head and neck cancer cases, the authors examined for explanatory variables that might account for the increasing incidence of cancer among

African-Americans. They noted that the single most explanatory variable was alcohol. Using population-attributable risk estimates and disregarding alcohol use, the risk of disease for blacks or whites was essentially similar. Furthermore, when examining for risks attributable to tobacco, similar odds-ratios were identified for both races after adjusting for alcohol use. These data minimize the role of heritable factors attributable to race in head and neck cancer development. The authors do emphasize, however, that the risk of disease when high levels of both alcohol and tobacco or alcohol alone are consumed appeared to be greater for blacks than whites. Furthermore, the incidence of cancer among siblings was higher for African-American patients than for white patients. The significance of genetic factors that could account for racial differences in disease risk remains to be defined.

Cancer Family Syndromes

Within the past 20 years, the heritable nature of cancer has been more clearly elucidated through the study of so-called cancer family syndromes. These sydromes are characterized by both a high incidence of cancer, as well as specific types of cancer within a family unit. There are several cancer family syndromes recently described which may be relevant to our understanding of the etiology of head and neck cancer. These include the Li-Fraumeni syndrome and the Lynch syndrome, the latter of which is more commonly referred to today as hereditary nonpolyposis colorectal cancer (HNPCC).

LI-FRAUMENI SYNDROME

The Li-Fraumeni syndrome was first recognized in 1969 by Li and Fraumeni,[149] who noted that afflicted family members had a dramatically increased history of cancer. The types of cancer occurring within these families are listed in Table 2–10. Soft tissue sarcomas and breast cancer are the predominant cancer types. An individual with laryngeal carcinoma could also be identified. Recent years have established the existence of more than 20 families with this syndrome.[150–152] The molecular basis of this process has been determined and includes a mutation in the p53 gene.[153,154]

It should be emphasized that a single incidence of laryngeal cancer does not establish a causal relationship between disease susceptibility and a particular genetic trait. In the authors' review of the literature, only three additional cases of head and neck cancer were identified. Thus, it cannot be concluded that the problem of head and neck cancer is increased in this disease entity, nor is there sufficient information regarding the interaction between heritable traits and environmental exposures as a determinant of the disease.

HEREDITARY NONPOLYPOSIS COLORECTAL CANCER

As was true for the lack of association between Li-Fraumeni syndrome and head and neck cancer, similar observations have been made for HNPCC. The HNPCC syndrome was first described by Henry Lynch[155,156] and was based on the assessment of an extended family in which a high degree of cancer prevalence was noted in family members. Table 2–11 lists the types of cancer typically associated with this syndrome. Again, as was the case for the Li-Fraumeni syndrome, a case of laryngeal cancer was identified.[157]

The molecular basis of HNPCC has, likewise, been extensively investigated. Through linkage analysis, susceptibility traits have been mapped to chromosome 2 and chromosome 3p21.[154,156,158] The responsible genes are currently considered to be involved in "genetic housekeeping", that is, the maintenance of normal genetic structure and sequence. Mutations in

TABLE 2–10	FREQUENTLY IDENTIFIED CANCERS IN PATIENTS AND THEIR FAMILIES WITH CANCER-PRONE SYNDROMES	
LI-FRAUMENI SYNDROME	HEREDITARY NONPOLYPOSIS COLON CANCER	CHROMOSOME FRAGILITY SYNDROMES[a,b]
Sarcoma, soft tissue	Colorectal	Leukemia
Sarcoma, bone	Breast	Lymphoma
Breast	Stomach	Lymphosarcoma
Brain	Ovary	Liver
Leukemia	Small intestine	Head and neck
Lung	Kidney	Stomach
Adrenocortical		

[a] Includes xeroderma pigmentosum, Fanconi's anemia, Bloom's syndrome, and ataxia-telangiectasia.
[b] Excludes skin cancers in patients with xeroderma pigmentosum.

TABLE 2–11	SELECTED CANCER RISK IN MEMBERS OF FAMILIES WITH HEREDITY NONPOLYPOSIS COLORECTAL CANCER

CANCER SITE	OBSERVED	EXPECTED	OR	SIGNIFICANCE
Stomach	17	4.1	4.1	<0.001
Small intestine	10	0.4	25.0	<0.001
Kidney	10	3.1	3.2	<0.01
Ovary	13	3.6	3.5	<0.001
Lung	5	12.0	0.4	<0.05
Larynx	1	2.2	0.4	NS
Breast	19	22.0	0.9	NS

OR, odds-ratio; NS, not significant.
Adapted from Watron P, Lynch HT. Extracolonic cancer in hereditary nonpolyposis colorectal cancer. *Cancer.* 1993; 71:677–685.

these genes are responsible for the so-called mismatch repair process and are characterized by microsatellite instability. Such deficiencies in gene housekeeping, particularly in DNA repair, set the stage for subsequent mutational events.

Watson and Lynch[159] have recently reviewed the patterns of cancer within the individuals diagnosed with HNPCC syndrome. Table 2–11 presents the relative risks of selected cancers of the total cancers reported by Watson and Lynch.[159] Interestingly, although the original family described by Lynch had a laryngeal cancer, only sporadic cases of head and neck cancer have been identified. Indeed, it is most relevant that the number of head and neck cancers, as well as the number of lung cancer cases, is actually lower than that of the general population,[159] and is actually significantly lower in the case of the number of lung cancers. Such rates are not attributable to tobacco consumption characteristics, and they suggest the involvement of genetic influences which may be protective.

DNA Repair Syndromes

The most compelling evidence for the heritable nature of head and neck cancer may be derived from the assessment of the so-called chromosome fragility syndromes, syndromes that can be characterized principally by deficiencies in DNA repair. These syndromes include xeroderma pigmentosum, Bloom's syndrome, Fanconi's anemia, and ataxia-telangiectasia. For a more comprehensive review of these syndromes, the reader is referred to *Chromosome Mutation and Neoplasia*, edited by James German.[160] This excellent review provides a clear description of the various abnormalities associated with each of the syndromes. To review the genetic basis of each syndrome is beyond the scope of this chapter. However, there have been several genetic defects that have been described. Xeroderma pigmentosum, for instance, has been related to a deficit

in DNA polymerase activity.[161] Defects in such activity result in the inbility of cells to repair gaps in DNA structure induced by excised abnormal nucleotides. Bloom's syndrome has been related to a defect in ligase function, a process that rejoins reconstructed DNA sequences to originally damaged genes.[162] Recently, the gene responsible for ataxia-telangiectasia has been isolated and cloned.[163]

Table 2–10 summarizes the various types of malignant disease associated with these syndromes. There are several important differences, as well as similarities. Leukemia and lymphoma are the predominant cancers identified within these syndromes. Although not the predominant cancer type, each of these syndromes has also been associated with head and neck cancer. Most of these latter cancers have been reported to occur prior to the age of 30 years, and without a history of prolonged environmental exposures. Likewise, each of these syndromes is associated with cancers that are limited to specific sites within the upper aerodigestive tract.[95] Patients with xeroderma pigmentosum, for instance, develop disease within the oral cavity, but not the larynx or pharynx. Conversely, patients with Bloom's syndrome only develop head and neck cancer outside the oral cavity. The basis for the differential expression of head and neck cancer within the upper aerodigestive tract is not well understood. A better understanding of this process may provide insight into not only head and neck carcinogenesis, but other environmentally induced cancers as well.

Mutagen Sensitivity

It can be presumed that chromosome fragility, as expressed in the chromosome fragility syndromes, is not an all-or-none phenomenon. Rather, a gradient exists within the general population whereby some individuals have greater DNA repair capacity than others. It is those individuals with the least capacity to repair DNA damage who are most likely to develop disease. This general perception has stimulated many investigators to explore the role of DNA damage and repair in patients with tobacco-induced disease.[164] Perhaps the most extensive investigations of DNA repair in the head and neck cancer population were performed using the chromosomal fragility assay.[165] This assay makes use of chromosomal preparations from peripheral blood lymphocytes. Briefly, lymphocytes are harvested from the peripheral blood and cultured for a short period in vitro. They are then exposed to the clastogen bleomycin, which is capable of inducing chromatid breaks through its generation of free-radical oxygen.[166] Metaphase spreads are then created following bleomycin exposure, and the number of chromatid breaks per cell are quantitated. The number of breaks are then compared between individuals. It is the inability to repair free-radical damage among individuals prone to head and neck cancer that may contribute to the disease state.

In initial studies of patients with head and neck cancer, it was noted that affected individuals were highly sensitive to bleomycin.[165] The number of chromatid breaks induced in lymphocyte preparations from such individuals was much greater than in healthy volunteers. Similar results have been seen in subsequent multiple case-control studies.[167-170] Interactions between chromosomal sensitivity and tobacco exposure, suggestive of a multiplicative effect, were also noted to exist.[167-170] The odds-ratio for the disease was greatly enhanced in those individuals who both expressed bleomycin sensitivity and smoked, as compared to either marker alone. The strength of this marker in defining the risk of disease is limited by the small number of studies performed.

The significance of the bleomycin assay is also noted in its relationship to other known risk factors for head and neck cancer. Spitz et al[167] have pointed to the significant interaction between bleomycin sensitivity and alcohol consumption. In a case-control study involving more than 100 cases of head and neck cancer, the odds-ratio for head and neck cancer increased 45-fold in mutagen-sensitive users of alcohol as compared to nondrinking, mutagen-resistant individuals. Several investigators have subsequently performed in vitro analyses in order to explain this phenomenon.[171,172] These researchers noted that alcohol had a profound ability to inhibit the repair of bleomycin-induced damage.

Bleomycin-induced damage has also been noted to be influenced by the presence of free-radical scavengers, such as are found in many nutrients. Trizna et al[173] noted that bleomycin-induced damage in vitro is inhibited by the presence of vitamins A, C, and E. The authors have previously performed a case-control study involving patients with head and neck cancer in whom these in vitro observations were extended.[95] The odds-ratio for head and neck cancer was increased in those individuals who demonstrated both mutagen-sensitivity and low levels of vitamins C and E intake. This interaction, however, was not as great as that observed between mutagen sensitivity with either tobacco or alcohol.

Mutagen sensitivity as a measure of risk for head and neck cancer has been extended in other studies as well. For instance, a study of young adults with head and neck cancer has shown that this cancer population is more sensitive to free-radical damage than either age-matched controls or young adult patients with cancers other than squamous cell cancer,[27] including those with sarcomas and central nervous system tumors. Mutagen sensitivity also has provided information about the risk of second primary tumors.[174] Those individuals who expressed the greatest sensitivity were the individuals who were most likely to develop additional cancers within the aerodigestive tract.

Additional measures of DNA repair relevant to tobacco carcinogenesis have been developed, but have not yet been applied to head and neck cancer. These assays include benzo[a]pyrene (BP) sensitivity assays, assays of sensitivity to irradiation, as well as assays that explore the capacity to repair specific DNA adducts, that is, the 0-methylguanine repair assay.[175–177]

THE ROLE OF VIRUSES

The modifications of Koch's postulates, as described earlier in this chapter, provide a framework for judging the significance of viral agents as an etiologic factor in head and neck carcinogenesis. Certain viruses are more frequently found in patients with head and neck cancer than in the general population; the wordwide distribution of these viruses is consistent with the relative frequency of head and neck cancer; and the experimental data supporting the role of viruses in carcinogenesis have been extensive. Review the discussion in Chapter 1 of Epstein-Barr virus (EBV) and its role in head and neck neoplasia and non-neoplastic lesions. Yet, questions as to the true role of various viruses still remain. The one postulate that would provide conclusive evidence is still lacking; that is, that the removal of the agent from individuals at risk would result in a deceased incidence of disease. This section discusses epidemiologic studies that have focused on the two principal viruses linked to upper aerodigestive tract cancer; the human papilloma virus (HPV) and the herpes simplex virus (HSV).

Human Papillomavirus

The epidemiology, as well as the molecular biology, of HPV-related carcinogenesis has been detailed in numerous reviews.[178–181] The number of known HPV types is increasing on a regular basis. To date, there are approximately 70 known types, of which 41 can be considered relevant to upper aerodigestive mucosa. Within the latter 41 types, certain of the HPV types are considered to be of low malignant potential, such as types 6, 11, and 13. Others, such as types 16 and 18, are considered to be carcinogenic. However, clear distinctions have not been found. For instance, Balarum et al[182] found a high incidence of polyclonal infections within oral cavity lesions containing both the low-risk and high-risk HPV groups. Likewise, the carcinogenic potential of any single virus type must be considered in light of exposure to other carcinogens. It is relevant that, within most epidemiologic and laboratory-based studies, HPV infection alone has not been sufficient to induce malignant transformation.[182–184] Likewise, when compared to other HPV-related malignant diseases (most notably, cervical cancer), HPV copies exist at low levels.

Franchesci et al[179] have performed the most recent review of the epidemiologic data relating to HPV and upper aerodigestive tract cancers. The wide variance in HPV prevalence described by the various studies is notable. The percentage of tumors that are identified as containing HPV varies from 14% to 79%. Such variance may reflect several factors, including investigator bias, geographic location of the population studied, number of cases, and the methods employed to detect the viral genome. It can also be concluded that certain sites within the upper aerodigestive tract may be at greater risk than others, with the highest risks being identified within the oral cavity and pharynx and the lowest risks being identified within the larynx. A critical determinant may be the type of mucosal epithelium. For instance, the most frequent site of HPV infection and malignant transformation within the cervix is the transitional epithelium. A similar transition zone does not exist in the head and neck. Rather, sites at risk may be in areas where mucosa changes from keratinizing to nonkeratinizing epithelium.

One of the most thorough assessments of HPV status and head and neck cancers was performed by Balarum et al.[182] These researchers were able to identify HPV types in nearly 74% of the lesions. The frequency of identified genotypes, in increasing order, were HPV 6 (13% of the cancers), HPV 11 (20%), HPV 16 (42%), and HPV 18 (47%). Significantly, 41% of the lesions were noted to have multiple HPV infections. This study is meaningful for several reasons. First, it is one of the largest studies, as more than 90 patients with cancer were analyzed. Second, both the type of cancer (oral cavity) and the patient population (Indian betel nut chewers) were relatively homogeneous. Finally, the method of analysis was relatively rigorous, utilizing both consensus and specific primers, and then HPV sequencing, in order to establish the presence of and to identity the specific virus. The authors noted that the strongest correlate for the presence of the virus was the extent of concomitant exposures to tobacco. Those individuals who were the heaviest users of tobacco were at the greatest risk. An increased prevalence of virus was also identified in younger patients and those

patients with poorly differentiated disease. Gillison et al[184A] reported evidence for a causal association between HPV and subsets oropharyngeal squamous cell carcinoma. These authors found that high-risk tumorigenic type HPV 16 was present in 90% of the HPV-positive tumors and that poor tumor grade and oropharyngeal site independently increased the probability of HPV presence.

The mechanisms by which HPV induces cellular transformation have been made evident.[178] The principal incriminating factor is the production of the transforming proteins E6 and E7. These proteins may disrupt normal host cellular mechanisms by binding to critical nuclear proteins that control progression through the cell cycle, that is, the p53 and the pRb proteins. Binding has been associated with an increased degradation rate of these cell cycle regulators. This association has been most evident when assessing genital cancers. The significance of the mutated p53 gene in carcinogenesis has been well known. Within cervical cancers, the gene itself is rarely mutated. However, the presence of HPV is identified in the vast majority of lesions, suggesting an alternative pathway to p53 disregulation. The role of HPV in upper aerodigestive tract cancers is not as apparent. The mutation of the p53 gene can be directly correlated with extent of tobacco exposure. Correlative analyses have shown that various HPV types can be found even in the presence of such mutations. Thus, whether or not HPV disregulation of known cell-cycle regulators is the underlying mechanism in head and neck carcinogenesis is not certain. Furthermore, studies have shown that more individuals will express HPV than actually develop cancer, suggesting that HPV infection alone is an insufficient determinant.[179]

Within the laboratory setting, however, it has been determined that HPV integration into the oral epithelial cell leads to cellular immortilization and sets the stage for enhancing carinogenic potential of relevant chemical compounds.[183] HPV integration may act as a means to enhance genetic instability in such instances, and may promote the loss of critical tumor suppressor genes.

Herpes Simplex Virus

The evidence for the causative role of HSV, specifically HSV-1, in cancer is not as clear as for the papillomaviruses. To the authors' knowledge, no one has yet isolated HSV DNA from head and neck tumors. Nonetheless, an incriminating role for the virus has been investigated,[185–188] principally through serologic studies.[185,186] Levels of anti-HSV antibodies have been noted to be higher in patients with head and neck cancer as compared to healthy controls. Those who point to the relevance of HSV as a carcinogenic factor reconcile the absence of an HSV genome within cancers as a function of a particular property of the virus. Namely, HSV can function as a "hit-and-run" agent. The virus can induce genetic damage without the requirement of host genomic integration. It is then free to leave the cell, leaving no evidence of infection.

MOLECULAR EPIDEMIOLOGY

Molecular epidemiology refers to the use of molecular analyses to define the relationship of disease to various exposures, host susceptibility, and cellular damage.[189,190] The authors have reviewed many of the molecular epidemiology studies that relate to host susceptibility, such as the genetic polymorphisms that may control carcinogen metabolism. This section briefly reviews the current understanding of molecular markers of carcinogen exposures. The authors then discuss how these exposures may lead to genetic mutational events that contribute to head and neck carcinogenesis.

Molecular measures of exposure have revolved around the quantitation of carcinogen adducts. Adducts represent the covalent binding of xenobiotic or indigenous chemicals with macromolecules, such as DNA and/or protein.[191,192] Means to measure these adducts vary, and each has its own limitations and qualities.[138] Most studies have focused on adduct measurements that are presumably related to tobacco exposure. In one of the initial investigations, Perera and colleagues[193] demonstrated that cancer patients in Eastern Europe expressed polycyclic aromatic hydrocarbon DNA adducts significantly more frequently than did healthy controls, and that levels of adducts within blood cells corresponded to those found in lung tissue. Related studies have, likewise, demonstrated that activated enzyme systems may account for the increased adduct levels in such patients.[194] However, only a few studies of DNA adduct formation relevant to head and neck cancer development have been performed.[195-199] In a field study conducted within southern and central Asia, Dunn et al[195] identified elevated adducts within the exfoliated mucosal cells of tobacco users. Adduct formation was greater in the smoking population than in nonsmokers. Furthermore, the types of adducts could be distinguished by the mode of tobacco use (i.e., tobacco chewers vs. reverse smokers). Randerath et al[196] measured bulky, nonpolar, aromatic hydrocarbon DNA adducts in laryngeal and lung mucosa and noted an increase in adduct formation with increasing tobacco consumption. Adducts were noted to diminish with smoking cessation.

The ability to quantitate adducts raises questions regarding head and neck carcinogenesis that might not otherwise have been asked. For instance, whether or not one can ascribe an increased risk of head and neck cancer based on qualititive and quantitative assessment of these compounds remains to be determined. In one of the only studies to address this issue, Foiles et al[198] prospectively followed a group of veterans in whom DNA adducts had been measured. Contrary to the expectations raised in the latter study, elevated adduct levels were more commonly seen in those who remained cancer-free.

It is also clear that many of the measureable adducts, although capable of being generated by tobacco, may originate from other sources. BP is an important example. Although found in high levels within tobacco combustion products, BP is found both within polluted air and food products, such as barbecued foods.[200] Nearly all BP exposure comes from the food chain, with only a small proportion generated from ambient air exposure. Although increased levels of BP adducts may be measured in an individual smoker with cancer, and although that adduct may be responsible for subsequent DNA damage, the source of the adduct may have been generated by means other than tobacco consumption alone. Furthermore, current limitations include the degree to which an adduct is specific for a single exposure. Presumed BP adducts may represent other chemical compounds, some of which may have been generated from endogenous metabolism in the course of aging.[201] Additional research is required in this field to investigate the determinants of differential levels within various tissues, the identification of specific regions within the genome that are more susceptible to adduct formation, and the mechanisms that control the progression of adducts to specific mutational events.

Recent advances in molecular biology have allowed for explorations into the relationship between environmental exposures and specific mutational events within head and neck cancers. Certain genetic regions may be more susceptible to environmental damage than others, and this may govern the pathway of disease progression. It is the *p53* gene that has served as a paradigm for this process. Numerous studies of patients with head and neck cancer have demonstrated that the type and quantity of a particular carcinogenic exposure will relate to the probability and characteristics of *p53* mutation.[202-205]

LESSONS TO BE LEARNED FROM MULTIPLE PRIMARY MALIGNANCIES

The problem of head and neck cancer could be considered a sign of an underlying disease process, rather than a single disease entity by itself. The basis of the problem, in most circumstances, is chronic, uncontrolled, carcinogen exposure leading to cellular and multiorgan genetic damage. Certain "signs" would reflect any manifestation of that underlying disease process and would involve multiple organ systems, such as atherothrombotic disease involving the heart and brain, chronic pulmonary disease, and severe liver abnormalities. Indeed, long-term follow-up studies of patients with head and neck cancer have shown that 30% of patients die within 5 years of causes other than the index cancer.[206] Perhaps the best illustration of distinguishing "signs" of the disease process versus the root problem is the well-known tendency of patients with head and neck cancer to develop multiple primary malignant lesions.[207–210] Such malignant tumors typically occur within the tissues exposed to tobacco carcinogens, such as the lung and esophagus. The incidence of second primary malignant tumors varies considerably between reports, ranging between 6% and 20% depending on the extent of underlying exposures to tobacco and alcohol, as well as the length of the follow-up period.[207–210] Perhaps the most representative estimate has been developed by Tepperman and Fitzpatrick.[211] In this study from Canada, 377 individuals with oral cancer underwent longitudinal follow-up study for a median of 58 months. The rate of second primary malignant tumors within the upper alimentary and respiratory tract was approximately 4% per year. Similar results were demonstrated by Day et al,[207] who utilized a combination of population-based registries within the United States involving more than 1000 patients with head and neck cancer. At Memorial Sloan-Kettering Cancer Center, investigators have reported that the average annual incidence for second primary carcinomas of the respiratory and upper digestive systems was 18.2 per 1000 in men and 15.4 per 1000 in women.[206]

The wide variance in rates of second primary malignant carcinomas suggests multiple factors as determinants, including site of disease, extent of carcinogenic exposures, and diligence in follow-up strategies. The results of a meta-analysis of second primary cancer risk performed by Haughey et al,[212] for instance, suggest that the rate of second primary cancers may differ among various countries, with the lowest rates being reported in Japan and Israel. The representative Israeli study, however, evaluated only individuals with an index laryngeal cancer which, as is emphasized in the following section, may be associated with a lower second primary cancer rate as compared to other sites within the upper aerodigestive tract.[213]

Based on the authors' overall review and that of others, it can be concluded that one of the major determinants of risk for a second primary cancer relates to the degree of carcinogenic exposure. For instance, the population-based study by Day et al[207] examined the relationship between intensity and duration of tobacco exposure and showed that the risk of metachronous malignant carcinomas was enhanced nearly fivefold in those individuals who smoked cigarettes for more than 40 years as compared to those who had smoked for less than 20 years. Likewise, the intensity of smoking was also significant. Individuals who smoked more than 40 cigarettes per day were 3.6 times more likely to develop a second cancer as compared to those who smoked less than 20 cigarettes per day. Likewise, studies from Memorial Sloan-Kettering Cancer Center have attempted to quantitate alcohol exposure and assess for the risk of second primary malignant lesions.[214] Results have demonstrated that 37% of the male patients with a second primary cancer, as compared to 9% of the male patients with a single primary cancer could be characterized as heavy drinkers. These results would suggest that alcohol exposure is a cofactor in multiple primary cancer risk. Schottenfeld et al,[206] in a prospective study from the same institution, identified the extent of alcohol consumption as the single most distinguishing characteristic between individuals who developed multiple cancers and those who had only a single cancer. The risk of second primary malignant carcinoma was approximately fourfold higher in those identified as heavy alcohol and tobacco users compared to individuals with low combined exposures. In contrast, the significance of alcohol in the study by Day et al[207] was not as readily apparent. After controlling for degree of tobacco use, alcohol as a single factor could not be identified as a significant variable. However, Day and colleagues[207] did note a multiplicative effect between tobacco and alcohol as a risk factor for second primary disease.

Additional clues as to the relevance of exposure histories as determinants of second primary cancers can be derived from studies of smoking and alcohol cessation. Moore[215] was the first to draw attention to this phenomenon by demonstrating that individuals who stopped smoking were more likely to have fewer second primary malignant carcinomas. However, Moore selected only individuals who had been free of disease for at least 3 years. Similar benefits were reported by Stevens et al[216] and Silverman and associates.[217] Others, however, have not been able to confirm the protective effect of smoking cessation.[218] Day et al[207] suggest that the risk of second cancers is principally determined by the length of follow-up after achieving smoking cessation, with risk reduction becoming significant in those individuals who abstain from such exposures for 5 years or longer. These findings suggest the need for more intensive intervention in the initial years following smoking cessation, such as with chemoprevention or intensive screening.

The risk of second primary malignant carcinoma may depend not only upon the degree of exposure to tobacco and alcohol, but also on the site of the index cancer. In one of the most comprehensive reports on this subject, Haughey et al[212] noted that the prevalence of second cancers was 23% in patients with a primary cancer within the oral cavity and 11% for those with an index cancer of the larynx. Likewise, the site of the second cancer may differ depending on the index disease. Patients with laryngeal cancer most often have second cancers in the lung. Patients with index cancers of the oral cavity and pharynx most often develop a second cancer within the upper aerodigestive tract. Haughey et al[212] also noted similar site-dependent rates in their meta-analysis involving 25 studies and more than 38,000 patients.

The influence of radiation therapy on the risk of second primary malignant lesions has not been extensively studied, but should be considered. In an early investigation, Wynder et al[214] reported an increased risk in those individuals who had previously received radiation therapy as part of their initial treatment. Conversely, subsequent studies by others have found no increased incidence in those treated by surgery alone versus those receiving radiation therapy, either within the head and neck region or more inclusive aerodigestive sites.[211,219,220] We have recently evaluated the incidence of second primary cancers using the SEER data in approximately 52,000 individuals with index cancers within the upper aerodigestive tract, including the esophagus. Patients who received radiation therapy as part of the treatment for their index head and neck cancer had elevated rates of second primary cancers within the lung and esophagus.[221] There exist numerous confounding factors that were not controlled for in this study. The relationship is emphasized here only to suggest that more comprehensive studies are needed. Should there exist such a relationship, therapeutic decision processes would need to be adjusted accordingly.

Several studies suggest that the risk of second cancers may differ between men and women. Tepperman and Fitzpatrick[211] noted that the risk of an additional cancer was 13-fold higher in men than in the general population, and was a dramatic 82-fold higher in women. In the report of the SEER data, Begg et al[221] found similar increased risks in women. Although no gender-related differences in overall second primary malignant carcinomas could be identified in the study by Schottenfeld et al,[206] this group pointed to two observations that may be relevant to an understanding of the risk of second primary malignant lesions in men and women. First, women with multiple primary tumors were more likely to be nonsmokers than similarly affected men (29% versus 3%, respectively). This factor led researchers to examine the role of determinants other than tobacco that may be gender related. Second, Schottenfeld et al[206] noted differences in alcohol consumption patterns between men and women. Men were more likely than women to stop heavy alcohol consumption following the diagnosis of the index cancer; thus, differences in the risk of second primary malignant carcinoma may be the result of multiple factors, including both gender-specific and lifestyle determinants.

One of the difficulties in assessing the true incidence of multiple primary malignant lesions in the population with head and neck cancer is discriminating between disease recurrence and a new primary lesion. This is particularly a problem for local disease when the cancer occurs in the same anatomic location, as is the case in multiple cancers occurring on the hard palate or floor of the mouth. Likewise, a major question as it relates to disease within the lung is whether or not the second cancer represents metastasis or a primary cancer. It is noteworthy that one of the original criteria for defining a second cancer, as reported by Warren and Gates,[222] was simply that the "probability of one['s] being a metastasis of the other be excluded." Within the lung, this may be difficult, given that both cancers may be of a similar histologic type.

A general rule is that the definition of a true second primary within the lung must be characterized histologically by a transition from normal mucosa to in situ disease to invasive cancer, a strict criterion that may lead to an underestimation of the true second primary incidence. Furthermore, definitive tissue sampling in order to satisfy these criteria may not have occurred for a variety of reasons. Molecular advances that allow for analysis at a subcellular level may help to clarify this issue further. Such techniques can prove the existence of separate primary disease through the identification of tumor clones with disparate genetic mutational events. Furthermore, distinct clones can be identified with only a few cells, obviating the need for more invasive procedures simply to establish a tissue diagnosis. Chung et al[223] examined patients with head and neck and lung cancers for the p53 mutational profile, demonstrating the utility of this method by identifying discordant mutations in the separately isolated tumors.

Molecular epidemiology may also play a role in the understanding of risk of multiple primary disease. The authors have already discussed the relationship between environmental exposures and the predisposition to specific mutational events. For instance, it has been frequently reported that the risk of p53 mutations within head and neck cancers can be related to the degree of tobacco exposure, with prolonged exposures leading to increased mutations. Given that prolonged exposure in a patient with head and neck cancer is also associated with a greater risk of a second malignant primary cancer, it would stand to reason that the expression of p53 mutations within an index tumor would, likewise, identify individuals who are more likely to develop additional cancers. In one of the only studies to explore this relationship, Shin et al[224] noted that patients whose index tumor overexpressed p53 protein by immunohistochemical staining with the DO7 anti-p53 antibody were greater than three times more likely to develop second primary malignancies than patients with p53-negative tumors. This may represent a critical area of research in the coming years.

Host susceptibility factors may also play a role in identifying risk of second primary disease, although to date, only a few studies have addressed this issue. The authors recently reported that the risk of second primary cancers was fourfold higher in patients who express sensitivity to mutagens (bleomycin) as compared to those patients with head and neck cancer who were more mutagen-resistant.[174] Mutagen sensitivity was presumed to be innate and not influenced by the extent of carcinogenic exposures or dietary intake. These findings have been supported by independent analyses by Cloos et al.[169] Other heritable risk factors that have been identified relate to patients' human leukocyte antigen (HLA) types and immunoglobulin allotypes.[225] The potential significance of heritable host susceptibility factors as determinants of second primary cancer risk was further supported by the work of Bongers et al.[226] These authors assessed for the risk of upper aerodigestive tumors in family members of patients with head and neck cancer and either a single or multiple primary malignant carcinomas. Significantly, those patients with multiple primary malignant lesions were more likely to have a positive family history for respiratory and upper digestive tract cancers. The results appeared to be unrelated to the smoking history of either the proband or the family members, although all the probands were smokers, which limited analysis.

REFERENCES

1. *SEER Cancer Statistics Review, 1973–1992.* Bethesda, MD: U.S. Department of Health and Human Services; 1996. NIH Publication No. 96-2789.
2. Centers for Disease Control, National Institute of Dental Research. *Cancers of the Oral Cavity and Pharynx: A Statistics Review Monograph, 1973–1987.* Bethesda, MD: National Institutes of Health; 1991.
3. Parkin DM, Pisani P, Ferlay X. Estimates of the worldwide incidence of eighteen major cancers in 1985. *Int J Cancer.* 1993; 54:594–606.
4. Chen J, Katz RV, Krutchkoff DJ. Intraoral squamous cell carcinoma: Epidemiologic patterns in Connecticut from 1935 to 1985. *Cancer.* 1990; 66:1288–1296.
5. Harris JE. Cigarette smoking among successive birth cohorts of men and women in the United States during 1900–1980. *JNCI.* 1983; 71:473–479.
6. Ostroff JS, Jacobsen PB, Moadel AB, et al. Prevalence and predictors of continued tobacco use following diagnosis of head and neck cancer. *Cancer.* 1995; 75:569–576.
7. Day GL, Blot WJ, Austin DF, et al. Racial differences in risk of oral and pharyngeal cancer: Alcohol, tobacco, and other determinants. *JNCI.* 1993; 85:465–473.
8. Devesa SS, Blot WJ, Fraumeni JF Jr. Cohort trends in mortality for oral, pharyngeal, and laryngeal cancers in the United States. *Epidemiology.* 1990; 1:116–121.
9. Slotman GJ, Swaminathan AP, Rush BF Jr. Head and neck cancer in a young age group: High incidence in black patients. *Head Neck Surg.* 1983; 5:293–298.
10. Wasfie T, Newman R. Laryngeal carcinoma in black patients. *Cancer.* 1988; 61:167–172.
11. Bang KM, White JE, Gause BL, Leffall LD Jr. Evaluation of recent trends in cancer mortality and incidence among blacks. *Cancer.* 1988; 61:1255–1261.
12. Boring CC, Squires TS, Heath CW Jr. Cancer statistics for black Americans. *CA.* 1992; 42:7–17.
13. Fiore MC, Novotny TE, Pierce JP, et al. Trends in cigarette smoking in the United States. *JAMA.* 1989; 261:49–55.
14. Kabat GC, Morabia A, Wynder EL. Comparison of smoking habits of blacks and whites in a case-control study. *Am J Publ Health.* 1991; 81:1483–1486.
15. Shemen LJ, Klotz J, Schottenfeld D, Strong E. Increase of tongue cancer in young men. *JAMA* 1984; 252:1857.
16. Depue RH. Rising mortality from cancer of the tongue in young white males. *N Engl J Med.* 1986; 315:647.
17. Schantz SP, Byers RM, Goepfert H. Tobacco and cancer of the tongue in young adults. *JAMA.* 1988; 259:1943–1944.
18. Davis S, Severson RK. Increasing incidence of cancer of the

19. Franchesci S, Levi F, Lucchini F, et al. Trends in cancer mortality in young adults in Europe, 1955–1989. *Eur J Cancer.* 1994; 30A:2096–2118.
20. Endicott JN, Skipper P, Hernandez L. Marijuana and head and neck cancer. *Adv Exp Med Biol.* 1994; 335:107–113.
21. Das C, Schantz SP, Shillitoe EJ. Antibody to a mutagenic peptide of herpes simplex virus in young adult patients with cancer of the head and neck. *Oral Surg.* 1993; 75:610–614.
22. Schantz SP, Hsu TC, Ainslie N, Moser RP. Young adults with head and neck cancer express increased susceptibility to mutagen-induced chromosomal damage. *JAMA.* 1989; 262: 3313–3315.
23. Byers RM. Squamous cell carcinoma of the oral tongue in patients less than 30 years of age. *Am J Surg.* 1975; 30:475–478.
24. Carniol PJ, Fried MP. Head and neck carcinoma in patients under 40 years of age. *Ann Otol Rhinol Laryngol* 1982; 91:152–155.
25. Schantz SP, Byers RM, Goepfert H, Shallenberger RS, Beddingfield N. The implication of tobacco use in the young adult with head and neck cancer. *Cancer.* 1988; 62:1374–1380.
26. Wynder EL, Day E. Some thoughts on the causation of chronic disease. *JAMA.* 1961; 175:997–999.
27. Wynder EL. Listen to nature. The challenge of lifestyle medicine. *Soz Praventivmed.* 1991; 36:137–146.
28. Wynder EL, Bross IJ, Day E. A study of environmental factors in cancer of the larynx. *Cancer.* 1956; 9:86–110.
29. Spitz MR. Epidemiology and risk factors for head and neck cancer. *Semin Oncol.* 1994; 21:281–288.
30. Rothman KJ, Cann CI, Flanders D, et al. Epidemiology of laryngeal cancer. *Epidemiol Rev.* 1980; 2:195–209.
31. Schottenfeld D. The etiology and prevention of aerodigestive tract cancers. *Adv Exp Med Biol.* 1992; 320:1–21.
32. Wynder EL, Stellman SD. Comparative epidemiology of tobacco-related cancers. *Cancer Res.* 1977; 37:4608–4622.
33. Wynder EL, Bross IJ, Feldman RM. A study of the etiological factors in cancer of the mouth. *Cancer.* 1957; 6:1300–1322.
34. Franco EL, Kowalski LP, Oliviera BV, et al. Risk factors for oral cancer in Brazil: A case-control study. *Int J Cancer.* 1989; 43:992–1000.
35. DeMarini DM. Genotoxicity of tobacco smoke and tobacco smoke condensate. *Mutat Res.* 1983; 114:59–83.
36. Ruhl C, Adams JD, Hoffman D. Comparative assessment of volatile and tobacco-specific N-nitrosamines in the smoke of selected cigarettes from United States, West Germany and France. *J Anal Toxicol.* 1980; 4:255–259.
37. Parsa I, Foye CA, Cleary CM, Hoffman D. Differences in metabolism and biological effects of NNK in human target cells. *Banbury Rep.* 1986; 23:133–146.
38. Hecht SS, Hoffmann D. The relevance of tobacco-specific nitrosamines to human cancer. *Cancer Surv.* 1989; 8:273–294.
39. Wynder EL, Covey LS, Mabuchi K, et al. Environmental factors in cancer of the larynx: A second look. *Cancer.* 1976; 38:1591–1601.
40. Gupta PC, Bhonsle RB, Mehta FS, Pindborg JJ. Mortality experience in relation to tobacco smoking and chewing habits from a 10-year follow-up study in Ernakulam district, Kerala. *Int J Epidemiol.* 1984; 13:184–187.
41. DeStefani E, Correa P, Oreggia F, et al. Risk factors for laryngeal cancer. *Cancer.* 1987; 60:3087–3091.
42. Blot WJ, McLaughlin JK, Winn DM, et al. Smoking and drinking in relation to oral and pharyngeal cancer. *Cancer Res.* 1989; 48:3282–3287.
43. Freedman DA, Navidi WC. Ex-smokers and multistage model of lung cancer. *Epidemiology.* 1990; 1:21–29.
44. Thomas SJ, MacClennan R. Slaked lime and betel nut cancer in Papua, New Guinea. *Lancet.* 1992; 340:577–578.
45. Winn DM, Blot WJ, Shy CM, et al. Snuff dipping and oral cancer among women in the southern United States. *N Engl J Med.* 1981; 304:745–749.
46. Winn DM. Smokeless tobacco and aerodigestive tract cancers: Recent research directions. In: Newell GR, Hong WK,

eds. *The Biology and Prevention of Aerodigestive Cancers.* New York: Plenum; 1992:39–46.

47. Winn DM. Smokeless tobacco in the USA: Usage patterns, health effects, and extent of morbidity and mortality. In: Gupta PC, Hamner JE III, Murti PR, eds. *Control of Tobacco-Related Cancers and Other Diseases.* Bombay: Oxford Press; 1992.

48. Spitz MR, Fueger JJ, Goepfert H, Hong WK, Newell GR. Squamous cell carcinoma of the upper aerodigestive tract: A case-control analysis. *Cancer.* 1988; 61:203–208.

49. Stockwell HG, Lyman GH. Impact of smoking and smokeless tobacco on the risk of cancer of the head and neck. *Head Neck Surg.* 1986; 9:104–110.

50. Ernster VL, Grady DG, Greene JC, et al. Smokeless tobacco use and health effects among baseball players. *JAMA* 1990; 264:218–224.

51. Blot WJ. Alcohol and cancer. *Cancer Res.* 1992; 52:2119s–2123s.

52. Rothman K, Kellar AZ. The effect of joint exposure to alcohol and tobacco on risk of cancer of the mouth and pharynx. *J Chronic Dis.* 1972; 25:711–716.

53. Flanders WD, Rothman KJ. Interaction of alcohol and tobacco in laryngeal cancer. *Am J Epidemiol.* 1982; 115:371–379.

54. Kato I, et al. Alcohol in the etiology of upper aerodigestive tact cancer. *Eur J Cancer B Oral Oncol.* 1994; 30B:75–81.

55. Elmwood JM, Pearson JCG, Skipper DH, Jackson SM. Alcohol, smoking, social and occupational factors in the aetiology of cancer of the oral cavity, pharynx, and larynx. *Int J Cancer.* 1984; 34:603–612.

56. Brugere J, Grenel P, LeClerc A, Rodriguez J. Differential effects of tobacco and alcohol in cancer of the larynx, pharynx, and mouth. *Cancer.* 1986; 57:391–395.

57. Tuyns AJ, Esteve J, Raymond L, et al. Cancer of the larynx/hypopharynx, tobacco, and alcohol. *Int J Cancer.* 1988; 41:483–491.

58. Baron AE, Franchesci S, Barra S, Talamani R, LaVecchia C. A comparison of the joint effects of alcohol and smoking on the risk of cancer across sites in the upper aerodigestive tract. *Cancer Epidemiol Biomed Prev.* 1993; 2:519–523.

59. Jovanic A. Tobacco and alcohol related to the anatomical site of oral squamous cell cancer. *J Oral Pathol Med.* 1993; 22:459–462.

60. Martinez I. Factors associated with cancer of the esophagus, mouth, and pharynx in Puerto Rico. *JNCI.* 1969; 42:1069–1094.

61. Kabat GC, Wynder EL. Type of alcoholic beverage and oral cancer. *Int J Cancer.* 1989; 43:190–196.

62. Rothman KJ, Cann CI, Fried MP. Carcinogenicity of dark liquor. *Am J Public Health.* 1989; 79:1516–1520.

63. International Agency for Research on Cancer (IARC). *Alcohol Drinking.* Lyon, France: IARC; 1988. IARC Monographs on the Evaluation of the Carcinogenic Risk to humans, vol. 44.

64. Walker EA, Castegnaro M, Garren L, Toussant G, Kowalski B. Intake of volatile nitrosamines from consumption of alcohols. *JNCI.* 1979; 69:947–951.

65. Mufti SI. Alcohol acts to promote the incidence of tumors. *Cancer Detect Prev.* 1992; 16:157–162.

66. Smith M. Genetics of human alcohol and aldehyde dehydrogenases. *Adv Hum Genet.* 1986; 15:249–290.

67. Obe G, Ristow H. Acetaldehyde but not alcohol induces sister chromatid exchanges in Chinese hamster cell in vitro. *Mutat Res.* 1977; 56:211–213.

68. Mufti SI, Eskelson CD, Odeleye OE, Nachiappan V. Alcohol associated generation of oxygen free radicals and tumor promotion. *Alcohol Alcohol.* 1993; 28:621–628.

69. Popp W, Wolf R, Vahrenholz C, et al. Sister chromatid exchange frequencies in lymphocytes of oral cancer patients seem to be influenced by drinking habits. *Carcinogenesis.* 1994; 15:1603–1607.

70. Hsu TC, Furlong C. The role of ethanol in oncogenesis of the upper aerodigestive tract: Inhibition of DNA repair. *Anticancer Res.* 1991; 11:1995–1998.

71. Kumano A, Kajii T. Synergistic effect of aphidocolin and ethanol on the induction of common fragile sites. *Hum Genet.* 1987; 75:74–78.

72. Shaw S, Rubin KP, Lieber CS. Depressed hepatic glutathione and increased diene conjugates in alcoholic liver disease: Evidence of lipid peroxidation. *Dig Dis Sci.* 1983; 28:585–589.

73. Murphy SE, Hecht SS. Effects of chronic ethanol consumption on benzo[a]pyrene metabolism and glutathione-S- transferase activities in Syrian golden hamster cheek pouch and liver. *Cancer Res.* 1986; 46:141–146.

74. Park SS, Ko I, Patten C, Yang CS, Gelboin HV. Monoclonal antibodies to ethanol induce cytochrome P450 that inhibit aniline and nitrosamine metabolism. *Biochem Pharmacol.* 1986; 35:2855–2858.

75. Palmer DL. Alcohol consumption and cellular immunocompetence. *Laryngoscope.* 1978; 88:13–17.

76. Brodie JC, Domenio J, Gelfand EW. Ethanol inhibits early events in T-lymphocyte activation. *Clin Immunol Immunopathol.* 1994; 70:129–136.

77. Spitzer JJ, Bautista AP. Alcohol, cytokines, and immunodeficiency. *Adv Exp Med Biol.* 1994; 335:159–164.

78. Reiner Z, Cvrtila D, Petric V. Cytoplasmic steroid receptors in cancer of the larynx. *Arch Otorhinolaryngol.* 1988; 245:47–49.

79. Ernster VL, Selvin S, Sacks ST, Merrill DW, Holly EA. Major histologic types of cancers of the gum and mouth, esophagus, larynx, and lung by sex and income level. *JNCI.* 1982; 69:773–776.

80. Williams RR, Horn JW. Association of cancer sites with tobacco and alcohol consumption and socioeconomic status of patients. Interview study from the Third National Cancer Survey. *JNCI.* 1977; 5:301–306.

81. Polednak AP. *Racial and Ethnic Differences in Disease.* New York: Oxford University Press, 1989.

82. Greenberg RS, Haber MJ, Clark WS, et al. The relation of socioeconomic status to oral and pharyngeal cancer. *Epidemiology.* 1991; 2:194–200.

83. Winn DM. Diet and nutrition in the etiology of oral cancer. *Am J Clin Nutr.* 1995; 61:437S–445S.

84. Steinmetz KA, Potter JD. Vegetables, fruit, and cancer. I. Epidemiology. *Cancer Causes Control.* 1991; 2:325–357.

85. Graham S, Mettlin C, Marshall J, et al. Dietary factors in the epidemiology of cancer of the larynx. *Am J Epidemiol.* 1981; 113:675–680.

86. DeStefani C, Correa P, Oreggia F, et al. Risk factors for laryngeal cancer. *Cancer.* 1987; 60:3087–3091.

87. Notani PN, Jayant K. Role of diet in upper aerodigestive tract cancers. *Nutr Cancer.* 1987; 10:103–113.

88. McLaughlin JK, Gridley G, Block G, et al. Dietary factors in oral and pharyngeal cancer. *JNCI.* 1988; 80:1237–1243.

89. Franco EL, Kowalski LP, Oliveira BV, et al. Risk factors for oral cancer in Brazil. *Int J Cancer.* 1989; 43:992–1000.

90. La Vecchia C, Negri E, D'Avanzo B, Boyle P, Franceschi S. Dietary indicators of oral and pharyngeal cancer. *Int J Epidemiol.* 1991; 20:39–44.

91. Winn DM, Ziegler RG, Pickle LW, Gridley G, et al. Diet in the etiology of oral and pharyngeal cancer among women from the southern United States. *Cancer Res.* 1984; 44:1216–1222.

92. Marshall J, Graham S, Mettlin C, et al. Diet in the epidemiology of oral cancer. *Nutr Cancer.* 1982; 3:145–149.

93. Graham S, Dayal H, Rorher T. Dentition, diet, tobacco, and alcohol in the epidemiology of oral cancer. *JNCI.* 1977; 59:1611–1688.

94. Rogers MAM, Thomas DB, Davis S, Vaughan TL, Nevissi AE. A case-control study of element levels and cancer of the upper aerodigestive tract. *Cancer Epidemiol Biomarkers Prev.* 1993; 2:305–312.

95. Schantz SP, Zhang ZF, Spitz MR, Hsu TC. Genetic susceptibility to head and neck cancer: Interactions between mutagen sensitivity and nutrition. *Laryngoscope.* 1997; 107:765–781.

96. Salaspuro M. Nutrient intake and nutritional status in alcoholics. *Alcohol Alcohol.* 1993; 28:85–88.

97. Zheng W, Blot WJ, Diamond EL, et al. Serum micronutrients

and the subsequent risk of oral and pharyngeal cancer. *Cancer Res.* 1993; 53:795–798.

98. Wynder EL, Hultberg S, Jacobsson F, et al. Environmental factors in cancer of the upper alimentary tract. A Swedish study with special reference to Plummer-Vinson syndrome. *Cancer.* 1952; 10:470–487.

99. Berger MR, Berger I, Schmahl D. Vitamins and cancer. In: Rowland IR, ed. *Nutrition, Toxicity, and Cancer.* Ann Arbor MI: CRC Press; 1991:517–548.

100. Nandakumar A, Thimmasetty KT, Sreeramareddy NM, et al. A population-based case-control investigation on cancers of the oral cavity in Bangalore, India. *Br J Cancer.* 1990; 62:845–851.

101. Franceschi S, Bidoli E, Baon AE, La Vecchia C. Maize and risk of cancers of the oral cavity, pharynx, and esophagus in Northeastern Italy. *JNCI.* 1990; 82:1407–1411.

102. Herbert JR, Landon J, Miller DR: Consumption of meat and fruit in relation to oral cancer and esophageal cancer: a cross sectional study. *Nutr Cancer.* 1993; 19:169–179.

103. Boyle P, Macfarlane GJ, McGinn R, Zheng T, LaVecchia C: International epidemiology of head and neck cancer. In: deVries N, Gluckman JL, ed. *Multiple Primary Tumors in the Head and Neck.* New York: Thieme; 1990:80–139.

104. Vogler WR, Lloyd JW, Millmore BK. A retrospective study of etiological factors in cancer of the mouth, pharynx, and larynx. *Cancer.* 1962; 15:246–248.

105. Binnie WH, Cawson RA, Hill GB, Soaper AE. *Oral Cancer in England and Wales: A National Study of Morbidity, Mortality, Curability and Related Factors.* London: HMSO; 1972. OPCS Studies on Medical and Population Subjects, 23.

106. Moss E, Lee WR. Occurrence of oral and pharyngeal cancers in textile workers. *Br J Ind Med.* 1974; 31:224–232.

107. Moulin JJ, Mur JM, Perreaux JP, Pham QT. Oral cavity and laryngeal cancers among man-made mineral fibre production workers. *Scand J Work Environ Health.* 1986; 12:27–31.

108. Nicholson WJ, Seidman H, Selikoff JJ. *The Mortality Experience of New York City Newspaper Pressmen, 1950–1976.* New York: Environmental Sciences Laboratory, Mount Sinai School of Medicine, University of New York; 1981.

109. Lloyd JW, Decoufle P, Salvin LG. Unusual mortality experience in printing press men. *J Occup Med.* 1977; 19:543–550.

110. Paganini-Hill A, Glazer E, Henderson BE, Ross RK. Cause-specific mortality among newspaper web pressman. *J Occup Med.* 1980; 22:542–544.

111. Newhouse ML, Berry G. Asbestos and laryngeal carcinoma. *Lancet.* 1973; 2:615.

112. Olsen J, Sabroe S. Occupational causes of laryngeal cancer. *J Epidemiol Community Health.* 1984; 38:117–121.

113. Maier H, Dietz A, Gewelke V, et al. Occupational exposure to hazardous substances and risk of cancer in the area of the mouth cavity, oropharynx, hypopharynx, and larynx. A case-control study. *Laryngol Rhinol Otol.* 1991; 70:93–98.

114. Burch JD, Howe GR, Miller AB, et al. Tobacco, alcohol, asbestos, and nickel in the etiology of cancer of the larynx. A case-control study. *JNCI.* 1981; 67:1219–1224.

115. Zagraniski RT, Kelsey JL, Walter SD. Occupational risk factors for laryngeal carcinoma: Connecticut, 1975–1980. *Am J Epidemiol.* 1986; 124:67–76.

116. Wada S, Nishimoto Y, Miyanishi M, et al. Mustard gas as a cause of respiratory neoplasia in man. *Lancet.* 1968; 1:1161–1163.

117. Soskolne CI, Zeighami EA, Hanis NM, et al. Laryngeal cancer and occupational exposure to sulfuric acid. *Am J Epidemiol.* 1984; 120:358–369.

118. Young TB, Ford CN, Brandenburg JH. An epidemiologic study of oral cancer in a statewide network. *Am J Otolaryngol.* 1986; 7:200–208.

119. Flanders WD, Cann CI, Rothman KJ, Fried MP. Work-related risk factors for laryngeal cancer. *Am J Epidemiol.* 1984; 119:23–32.

120. Huebner WW, Schoenberg JB, Kelsey JL, et al. Oral and pharyngeal cancer and occupation: A case-control study. *Epidemiology.* 1992; 3:300–309.

121. Nebert DW. Role of genetics and drug metabolism in human cancer risk. *Mutat Res.* 1991; 247:267–281.

122. Idle JR. Is environmental carcinogenesis modulated by host polymorphism? *Mutat Res.* 1991; 247:259–266.

123. Harris CC. Interindividual variation among humans in carcinogen metabolism, DNA adduct formation, and DNA repair. *Carcinogenesis.* 1989; 10:1563–1566.

124. Shields PG, Harris CC. Molecular epidemiology and the genetics of environmental cancer. *JAMA.* 1991; 266:681–687.

125. Nebert DW, Nelson DR, Coon M, et al. The p450 superfamily: Update on new sequences, gene mapping, and recommended nomenclature. *DNA Cell Biol.* 1991; 10:1–14.

126. Guengerich FP, Shimada T. Oxidation of toxic and carcinogenic chemicals by human cytochrome p450 enzymes. *Chem Res Toxicol.* 1991; 4:391–407.

127. Kellermann G, Shaw CR, Luyten-Kellermann M. Aryl hydrocarbon hydroxylase inducibility and bronchogenic carcinoma. *N Engl J Med.* 1973; 298:934–937.

128. Brandenberg JH, Kellerman G. Aryl hydrocarbon hydroxylase inducibility in laryngeal carcinoma. *Arch Otolaryngol.* 1978; 104:151–152.

129. Andreasson L, Bjorlin G, Hocherman M, et al. Laryngeal cancer, aryl hydrocarbon hydroxylase inducibility and smoking. A follow-up study. *ORL J Otorhinolaryngol Relat Spec.* 1987; 49:187–192.

130. Trell E, Korsgaard R, Hood B, et al. Aryl hydrocarbon hydroxylase inducibility and laryngeal carcinomas. *Lancet* 1976; 2: 140–144.

131. LaFuente A, Pujol F, Carretero P, Perez-Villa J, Cuchi H. Human glutathione *S*-transferase m (GSTm) deficiency as a marker of susceptibility to bladder and larynx cancer among smokers. *Cancer Lett.* 1993; 68:49–54.

132. Trizna Z, Clayman GL, Spitz MR, Briggs KL, Goepfert H. Glutathione-s-transferase genotypes as risk factors for head and neck cancer. *Am J Surg.* 1995; 170:499–501.

133. Lazarus P, Ren Q, Strudwick S, et al. GSTM1 and CYP 1A1 polymorphisms and oral cavity cancer risk. *Proc Am Assoc Cancer Res.* 1996; 37:107.

134. Hayashi S, Watanabe J, Kawajiri K. High susceptibility to lung cancer analyzed in terms of combined genotypes of the p450 1A1 and mu-class glutathione-s-transferase genes. *Jpn J Cancer* 1992; 83:866–870.

135. Drozdz M, Gierek T, Jendryczko A. N-acetyltransferase phenotype of patients with cancer of the larynx. *Neoplasma.* 1987; 34:481–486.

136. Wynder EL, Stellman SD. Impact of long-term filter cigarette usage on lung and larynx cancer risk: A case-control study. *JNCI.* 1979; 62:471–477.

137. Ryberg D, Hewer A, Phillips DH, Hangen A. Different susceptibility to smoking-induced DNA damage among male and female lung cancer patients. *Cancer Res.* 1994; 54:5801–5803.

138. Beach AC, Gupta RC. Human monitoring and the ^{32}P-postlabeling assay. *Carcinogenesis.* 1992; 13:1053–1074.

139. Randerath K, Li D, Randerath E. Age-related DNA modifications (I-compounds): Modulation by physiological and pathological processes. *Mutat Res.* 1990; 238:245–253.

140. Grenman R, Virolainen, E, Shapira A, et al. In vitro effects of Tamoxifen on UM-SCC head and neck cancer cell lines: Correlation with the estrogen and progesterone receptor content. *Int J Cancer.* 1987; 39:77–81.

141. Roy D, Floyd RA, Liehr JG. Elevated 8-hydroxydeoxyguanosine levels in DNA of diethylstilbestrol-treated Syrian hamsters: Covalent DNA damage by free radicals generated by redox cycling of diethylstilbestrol. *Cancer Res.* 1991; 51:3882–3885.

142. Hecht SS, Carmella SG, Akerkar S, Ritchie JP Jr. 4-(Methylnitrosamino)-1-(3-pyridyl)-1-butanol (NNAL) and its glucuronide metabolites of a tobacco specific carcinogen in the urine of black and white smokers. *Proc Am Assoc Cancer Res.* 1994; 35:286.

143. Shields PG, Caparoso NE, Falk RT, et al. Lung cancer, race, and a CYP1A1 genetic polymorphism. *Cancer Epidemiol Biomarkers Prev.* 1993; 2:481–485.

144. Relling MV, Cherrie J, Schell MJ, et al. Lower prevalence of the debrisoquine oxidative poor metabolizer phenotype in American black versus white subjects. *Clin Pharmacol Ther.* 1991; 50:308–313.

145. Wagenknecht LE, Cutter G, Haley NJ, et al. Racial differences in serum cotinine levels among smokers in the coronary artery risk development in adults study. *Am J Public Health.* 1990; 80:1053–1056.

146. Weston A, Pervin LS, Forrester K, et al. Allelic frequency of a p53 polymorphism in human lung cancer. *Cancer Epidemiol Biomarkers Prev.* 1993; 2:481–483.

147. Tamai S, Sugimuru H, Caporaso NE, et al. Restriction fragment length polymorphism analysis of the L-*myc* gene locus in a case-control study of lung cancer. *Int J Cancer.* 1990; 46:411–415.

148. Lun D, Cherney BW, Lalande M, et al. A duplicated region is responsible for the poly(ADP-Ribose) polymerase polymorphism on chromosome 13, associated with a predisposition for cancer. *Am J Hum Genet.* 1993; 52:124–134.

149. Li FP, Fraumeni JF Jr. Soft-tissue sarcomas, breast cancers, and other neoplasms: A familial syndrome? *Ann Intern Med.* 1969; 7:747–752.

150. Li FP, Fraumeni FF, Mulvihill JJ, et al. A cancer family syndrome in twenty-four kindreds. *Cancer Res* 1988; 48:5358–5362.

151. Duncan MH, Miller RW. Another family with the Li-Fraumeni cancer syndrome. *JAMA.* 1983; 249:195.

152. Williams WR, Strong LC. Genetic epidemiology of soft tissue sarcomas in children. In: Muller HR, Weber W, eds. *Familial Cancer, First International Research Conference.* Basel: S Karger AG; 1985:151–153.

153. Malkin D, Li FP, Strong LC, et al. Germ line p53 mutations in a familial syndrome of breast cancer, sarcomas, and other neoplasms. *Science.* 1990; 250:1233–1238.

154. White R. Inherited cancer genes. *Curr Opin Genet Dev.* 1992; 2:53–57.

155. Lynch HT, Mutcahy GM, Harris RE, Gurgis HA, Lynch JF. Genetic and pathologic findings in a kindred with hereditary sarcoma, brain cancer, brain tumors, leukemia, lung, laryngeal, and adrenal cortical carcinoma. *Cancer.* 1978; 41:2055–2064.

156. Lynch HT. The Lynch syndromes. *Curr Opin Oncol.* 1993; 5:687–696.

157. Lynch HT, Kriegler M, Christiansen TA, et al. Laryngeal carcinoma in a Lynch syndrome II kindred. *Cancer.* 1998; 62:1007–1013.

158. Papadopoulos N, Nicolaides NC, Wei YF, et al. Mutation of a mutL homolog in hereditary colon cancer. *Science.* 1994; 263:1625–1629.

159. Watson P, Lynch HT. Extracolonic cancer in hereditary non-polyposis colorectal cancer. *Cancer.* 1993; 71:677–685.

160. German J. Patterns of neoplasia associated with the chromosome breakage syndromes. In: German J, ed. *Chromosome Mutation and Neoplasia.* New York: Alan R. Liss, Inc.; 1983: 97–134.

161. Kraemer KH, Lee MM, Scotto J. DNA repair protects against cutaneous and internal neoplasia: Evidence from xeroderma pigmentosum. *Carcinogenesis.* 1994; 5:511–514.

162. Tomkinson AE, Lasko DD, Lindahl T, et al. Biochemical properties of mammalian DNA ligase I and the molecular defect in Bloom's syndrome. *Prog Clin Biol Res.* 1990; 340A(2):283–294.

163. McConville CM, Byrd PJ, Ambrose HJ, Taylor AM. Genetic and physical mapping of the ataxia-telangiectasia locus on chromosome 11q22–23. *Int J Radiat Biol.* 1994; 66:545–556.

164. Hsu TC. Genetic instability in the human population: A working hypothesis. *Hereditas.* 1983; 98:1–11.

165. Schantz SP, Hsu TC. Mutagen-induced chromosome fragility within peripheral blood lymphocytes of head and neck cancer patients. *Head Neck.* 1989; 11:337–342.

166. Povirk LF, Austin MJ. Genotoxicity of bleomycin. *Mutat Res.* 1991; 257:127–143.

167. Spitz MR, Fueger JJ, Beddingfield NA, et al. Chromosome sensitivity to bleomycin-induced mutagenesis in patients with upper aerodigestive cancers: A case-control analysis. *Cancer Res.* 1989; 49:4626–4638.

168. Spitz MR, Fueger JJ, Halabi S, et al. Mutagen-sensitivity in upper aerodigestive tract cancer. *Cancer Epidemiol Biomarkers Prev.* 1993; 2:329–333.

169. Cloos J, Braakhuis BJ, Steen I, et al. Increased mutagen sensitivity in head and neck squamous cell carcinoma patients, particularly those with multiple primary tumors. *Int J Cancer.* 1994; 56:816–819.

170. Cloos J, Spitz MR, Schantz SP, et al. Genetic susceptibility to upper aerodigestive tract cancers. *JNCI.* 1996; 88:530–535.

171. Hsu TC, Furlong C, Spitz M. Ethyl alcohol as a carcinogen with special reference to the aerodigestive tract: A cytogenetic study. *Anticancer Res.* 1991; 11:1097–1102.

172. Li AT, Wang TD, Yang RT. Pingyangomycin-induced chromosome damage in lymphocytes of laryngeal cancer patients and healthy control subjects. *Head Neck.* 1994; 16:510.

173. Trizna Z, Schantz SP, Lee JJ, et al. In-vitro protective effects of chemopreventive agents against bleomycin-induced genotoxicity in lymphoblastoid cell lines and peripheral blood lymphocytes of head and neck cancer patients. *Cancer Detect Prevent.* 1993; 17:575–583.

174. Schantz SP, Spitz MR, Hsu TC. Mutagen sensitivity in patients with head and neck cancers: A biologic marker for risk of multiple primary malignancies. *JNCI.* 1990; 82:1773–1775.

175. Wei Q, Spitz MR, Gu J, et al. DNA repair correlates with mutagen sensitivity in lymphoblastoid cell lines. *Cancer Epidemiol Biomarkers Prev.* 1996; 5:199–204.

176. Sanford KK, Parshad R, Gantt RR, Tarone RE. A deficiency in chromatin repair, genetic instability, and predisposition to cancer. *Crit Rev Oncol.* 1989; 1:323–341.

177. Rudiger HW, Schwartz U, Serrand E, et al. Reduced 0⁶-methylguanine repair in fibroblast cultures from patients with lung cancer. *Cancer Res.* 1989; 49:5623–5626.

178. ZurHausen H. Viruses in human cancers. *Science.* 1991; 254:1167–1173.

179. Franceschi S, Munoz N, Bosch XF, Snijders PJF, Walboomers JMM. Human papillomavirus and cancers of the upper aerodigestive tract: A review of the epidemiological and experimental evidence. *Cancer Epidemiol Biol Biomarkers Prev.* 1996; 5:567–575.

180. Scully C, Prime S, Maitland N. Papillomaviruses: Their possible role in oral disease. *Oral Surg.* 1985; 60:166–174.

181. Madan C, Beckman AM, Thomas DB, et al. Human papillomaviruses, herpes simplex viruses, and the risk of oral cancer in men. *Am J Epidemiol.* 1992; 135:1093–1102.

182. Balarum P, Nalinakumad KR, Abraham E, et al. Human papillomaviruses in 91 oral cancers from Indian betel quid chewers: High prevalence and multiplicity of infections. *Int J Cancer* 1995; 61:450–454.

183. Li SL, Kim MS, Cherrick HM, Doniger JP, Park NH. Sequential combined tumorigenic effects of HPV 16 and chemical carcinogens. *Carcinogenesis.* 1992; 13:1981–1987.

184. Steenbergen RDM, Hemsen MAJA, Walboomers JMM, et al. Integrated human papillomavirus type 16 and loss of heterozygosity at 11q22 and 18q21 in an oral carcinoma and its derivative cell line. *Cancer Res.* 1995; 55:5465–5471.

184A. Gillison ML, Koch WM, Capone RB, et al. Evidence for a causal association between human papillomavirus and a subset of head and neck cancers (see comments). *J Natl Cancer Inst.* 2000; 92(9):675–677, 709–720.

185. Larsson PA, Edstrom S, Westin T, et al. Reactivity against herpes simplex virus in patients with head and neck cancer. *Int J Cancer.* 1991; 49:14–18.

186. Shillitoe EJ, Greenspan D, Greenspan JS, et al. Antibody to early and late antigens of herpes simplex virus type 1 in patients with oral cancer. *Cancer.* 1986; 54:266–273.

187. Kassim KH, Daley TD. Herpes simplex virus type proteins in human oral squamous cell carcinoma. *Oral Surg.* 1988; 65:445–448.

188. Schantz SP, Shillitoe EJ, Brown B, Campbell. Natural killer

cell activity and head and neck cancer: A clinical assessment. *JNCI.* 1986; 77:869–875.

189. Perera FP, Weinstein IB. Molecular epidemiology and carcinogen-DNA adduct detection: New approaches to studies of human cancer causation. *J Chronic Dis.* 1982; 35:581–600.

190. McMichael AJ. Molecular epidemiology: New pathway or new travelling companion. *Am J Epidemiol.* 1994; 140:1–11.

191. Turtletaub KW, Frantz CE, Creek MR, et al. DNA adducts in model systems and humans. *J Cell Biochem (Suppl)* 1993; 17F: 2–17.

192. Hemminki K. DNA adducts, mutations, and cancer. *Carcinogenesis.* 1993; 14:2007–2012.

193. Perera FP, Hemminki K, Gryzybowska E, et al. Molecular and genetic damage from environmental pollution in Poland. *Nature.* 1992; 360:256–258.

194. Bartsch H, Petruzzeli S, De Flora S, et al. Carcinogen metabolism and DNA adducts in human lung tissues as affected by tobacco smoking or metabolic phenotype: A case-control study on lung cancer patients. *Mutat Res.* 1991; 250: 103–114.

195. Dunn BP, Stich HF. ^{32}P-postlabeling analysis of aromatic DNA adducts in human oral mucosal cells. *Carcinogenesis.* 1986; 7:1115–1120.

196. Randerath E, Miller RH, Mittal D, et al. Covalent DNA damage in tissues of cigarette smokers as determined by ^{32}P-postlabeling assay. *JNCI.* 1989; 81:341–347.

197. Chacko M, Gupta RC. Evaluation of DNA damage in the oral mucosa of tobacco users and non-users by ^{32}P-adduct assay. *Carcinogenesis.* 1988; 9:2309–2313.

198. Foiles PG, Miglietta LM, Quart AM, et al. Evaluation of ^{32}P-postlabeling analysis of DNA from exfoliated oral mucosa cells as a means of monitoring exposure of the oral cavity to genotoxic agents. *Carcinogenesis.* 1989; 10:1429–1434.

199. Stern SJ, Degawa M, Martin MV, et al. Metabolic activation, DNA adducts, and H-*ras* mutations in human neoplastic and non-neoplastic larygeal tissue. *J Cell Biochem (Suppl).* 1993; 17F:129–138.

200. Hattemer-Frey HA, Travis CC. Benzo-*a*-pyrene. Environmental partitioning and human exposure. *Toxicol Ind Health.* 1991; 7:141–157.

201. Marnett LJ, Burcham PC. Endogenous DNA adducts. Potential and paradox. *Chem Res Toxicol.* 1993; 6:771–785.

202. Harris CC. At the crossroads of molecular carcinogenesis and risk assessment. *Science.* 1993; 262:1980–1981.

203. Field JK, Spandidos DA, Malliri A, et al. Elevated p53 expression correlates with a history of heavy smoking in squamous cell carcinoma of the head and neck. *Br J Cancer.* 1991; 64:573–577.

204. Somers KD, Merrick MA, Lopez ME, et al. Frequent p53 mutations in head and neck cancer. *Cancer Res.* 1992; 52: 5997–6000.

205. Lazarus P, Steen J, Zweibel N, et al. Relationship between p53 mutation incidence in oral cavity squamous cell carcinomas and patient tobacco use. *Carcinogenesis.* 1996; 17:733–739.

206. Shottenfeld D, Gantt RC, Wynder EL. The role of alcohol and tobacco in multiple primary cancers of the upper digestive system, larynx, and lung: A prospective study. *Prev Med.* 1974; 3:277–293.

207. Day GL, Blot WJ. Second primary tumors in patients with oral cancer. *Cancer.* 1992; 70:14–19.

209. Cooper JS, Pajak TF, Rubin P, et al. Second malignancies in patients who have head and neck cancers: Incidence, effect on survival and implications for chemoprevention based on the RTOG experience. *Int J Radiat Oncol Biol Phys.* 1989; 17: 449–456.

210. Lippman SM, Hong WK. Second malignant tumors in head and neck squamous cell carcinoma: The overshadowing threat for patients with early-stage disease. *Int J Radiat Oncol Biol Phys.* 1989; 17:691–694.

211. Tepperman BS, Fitzpatrick PJ. Second respiratory and upper aerodigestive tract cancers after oral cancer. *Lancet.* 1981; 2: 547–549.

212. Haughey BH, Gates GA, Arfken CL, Harvey J: Meta-analysis of second malignant tumors in head and neck cancer: The case for an endoscopic screening protocol. *Ann Otol Laryngol.* 1992; 101:105–112.

213. Deviri E, Bartal A, Goldsher M, et al. Occurrence of additional primary neoplasms in patients with laryngeal carcinoma in Israel (1960–1976). *Ann Otol Rhinol Laryngol.* 1982; 91:261–265.

214. Wynder EL, Dodo H, Bloch DA, Gantt RC, Moore OS. Epidemiologic investigation of multiple primary cancer of the upper alimentary and respiratory tracts. 1. A retrospective study. *Cancer.* 1969; 24:730–739.

215. Moore C. Cigarette smoking and cancer of the mouth, pharynx, and larynx. *JAMA.* 1971; 218: 553–558.

216. Stevens MH, Gardner JW, Parkin JL, et al. Head and neck cancer survivial and lifestyle change. *Arch Otolaryngol.* 1983; 109:746–749.

217. Silverman S Jr, Gorsky M, Greenspan D. Tobacco usage in patients with head and neck carcinomas: A follow-up study on habit changes and second primary oral/orpharyngeal cancers. *J Am Dent Assoc.* 1983; 106:33–35.

218. Castigliano SG. Influence of continued smoking on the incidence of second primary cancers involving mouth, pharynx, and larynx. *J Am Dent Assoc.* 1968; 77:580–585.

219. Seydel HG. The risk of tumor induction following medical irradiation for malignant neoplasms. *Cancer.* 1975; 35:1641–1645.

220. Parker RG, Enstrom SE. Second primary cancers of the head and neck following treatment of initial primary head and neck cancers. *Int J Radiat Oncol Biol Phys.* 1988; 14:501–564.

221. Begg CB, Zhang ZF, Sun M, Herr HW, Schantz SP. Methodology for evaluating incidence of second primary cancers with application to smoking-related cancers from SEER. *Am J Epidemiol.* 1995; 142:653–655.

222. Warren S, Gates O. Multiple primary malignant tumors: A survey of the literature and a statistical study. *Am J Cancer.* 1932; 16:1358–1414.

223. Chung KY, Mukhopadhyay T, Kim J, et al. Discordant p53 gene mutations in primary head and neck cancers and corresponding second primary cancers of the upper aerodigestive tract. *Cancer Res.* 1993; 53:1676–1683.

224. Shin DM, Lee JS, Lippman SM, et al. p53 expression: Predicting recurrence and second primary tumors in head and neck squamous cell carcinoma. *JNCI.* 1996; 88:519–529.

225. DeVries N, Drexhage HA, DeWaal L, DeLange G, Snow G. Human leukocyte antigens and immunoglobulin allotypes in head and neck cancer patients with and without multiple primary cancers. *Cancer.* 1987; 60:957–961.

226. Bongers V, Braakhuis BJM, Tobi H, Lubsen H, Snow G. The relation between cancer incidence among relatives and the occurrence of multiple primary carcinomas following head and neck cancer. *Cancer Epidemiol Biomarkers Prev.* 1996; 5: 595–598.

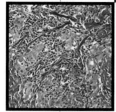

CHAPTER 3

Ethical Considerations

■ PAUL H. WARD

■ ELLIOT ABEMAYOR

This text deals with the pathology and treatment of head and neck disease. By contrast, this chapter is concerned with the patient receiving treatment. In the words of the essayist E. B. White, this is "one man's meat." This chapter presents, in an abbreviated fashion, a philosophical approach to the treatment of patients with head and neck tumors. These heartfelt views are derived from three decades of extensive clinical practice, observation, and teaching of residents in several university hospitals. There is no attempt toward political correctness or statistical validation.

In addition to the ethical challenges facing all contemporary physicians, the head and neck oncologist (surgeon, radiotherapist, or chemotherapist) is presented with certain unique dilemmas. These include, but certainly are not limited to, respecting patient autonomy, as well as properly allocating limited health care resources. When confronted with such divergent demands, what moral compass should guide a physician's decisions? For almost 2000 years, the answer has been relatively clear. The ethical principles of physician-patient relationships originate in the Hippocratic Oath, which a physician takes upon assuming the mantle of healer, one who possesses skills and knowledge acquired to benefit others.[1] At the core of the Oath is pursuit of what is "good" for the whole patient, not just a body part. The "good" can be in the form of beneficence, an active promotion of welfare (as in sustaining life and relieving pain) or nonmalfeasance (doing no harm or not causing pain or disability).[1] In any case, the Oath emphasizes active participation by the physician in his patients' welfare, rather than passive attendance to his fate. While the Oath has undergone several cosmetic changes since its inception in ancient Greece, its underlying emphasis is unwavering. Ethical dilemmas are bound to result if these principles are ignored or forgotten.

The Oath has been condemned for purported paternalism, elitism, and a subsequent deprivation of patient autonomy. On the contrary, the Oath is a vibrant affirmation of patient advocacy, not a neutral string of philosophical platitudes. It recognizes the singular, unique nature of each individual. Hippocratic physicians cannot passively stand by while their patient is suffering, nor do they take it upon themselves to decide their patient's fate. The Oath and its philosophical underpinnings are what separate true physicians from practicing hucksters, degreed technicians, or mere "health care providers."

Medicine today is under siege. A curtailment of resources has been foisted on physicians by the proliferation of managed care organizations with a subsequent cutback in health benefits. Physicians are enjoined to spend less time and money in caring for their patients. In turn, these forces have adversely affected the physician-patient relationship, often shaping it into an adversarial one. In so doing, ethical dilemmas have taken more of a prominent position in the national health care debate. However, for the thoughtful physician, a difficult ethical problem is best resolved by keeping the patient's welfare uppermost, an increasingly formidable task. Two prominent dilemmas include: how much information can, or should, a physician provide a patient on disease treatment options and probable outcome, and what does one do for a patient who insists on being helped to die because of a terminal cancer? If the principles of Hippocratic medicine are forgotten or ignored, a physician is likely to be lost down dark alleys of ethical ambiguity. The physician-patient relationship is based on trust and hope. It is an obligation that all physicians accept when they first take the Hippocratic Oath. For the head and neck oncologist, this is especially true, from beginning to end.

FIRST RIGHTS

Once diagnosed with disease, a patient will likely seek treatment. As discussed earlier, by virtue of experience and education, the physician as healer is empowered to assist the patient in choosing what is "good" for them. This, in turn, requires effective and forthright communication; the courts have assisted us in this task. In 1914, *Schloedoerf vs. Society of NY Hospital* asserted that a surgeon who performs an operation without the patient's consent commits an assault.[2] Approximately 40 years later, in 1957, the courts ruled that "consent" needs to be coupled with factual information. *Salgo vs. Leland Stanford University Board of Trustees* affirmed that a full disclosure of facts is necessary in order for a patient to form an informed consent to a procedure.[3] Interestingly, as pointed out by Katz,[4] the judge's written decision was, in great part, derived from a legal brief submitted by the American College of Surgeons. The courts dictated, but it was a society of surgeons who ultimately helped foster the modern concept of informed consent. These and other decisions emphasize an important point: it is the patient who controls his body, and it is he who has the right to say "yes" or "no" to treatment. Further, these cases rightfully recognize that the physician-patient relationship is trust-based (fiduciary) and not merely contractual or business-based. The image of a paternalistic, godly, physician who chooses what is "right" for the patient is supplanted by one of a partnership forged between an informed patient and an informative physician. These laws underscore patient self-determination and compel the physician to provide maximum information regarding the disease process, treatment options, and expected outcome. Whereas many physicians resent the intrusion of legal "technicalities" in patient interactions, informed consent, as articulated in these laws, enhances patient-physician relations by reinforcing the concept of patient autonomy. They encourage increased dialogue with patients and alleviate some of the physician's moral burden, as it is the patient who must ultimately decide which plan of treatment to undertake. Until society at large takes it upon itself to ration care, it is the legal and ethical obligation of a head and neck oncologist to discuss fully treatment options and probable disease outcome, no matter what the "organization" to which the physician belongs dictates.[5,6]

Nonetheless, even after having spent long hours with patients, physicians realize that despite their best efforts, true, educated, informed consents are rare. More than words are needed to convey certain vital concepts. Patients often cease to listen after certain words, such as "cancer," "operation," or "deformity," have been voiced. In order to assist these patients, it may be helpful to encourage patients to contact individuals who have been successfully treated (e.g., a laryngectomy patient with good esophageal speech), or a maxillofacial prosthodontist in order to better come to grips with the rehabilitation as well as potential treatment outcome. This approach can often make otherwise unbearable news somewhat palatable.

Just as oncologists are obligated to outline all available options in order to facilitate true informed consent, they also have the duty to know when not to treat. In surgery, resectability is not always commensurate with curability. An extensive head and neck tumor may pose an "interesting" technical challenge to the surgeon; however, the result of its attempted removal can be devastating to the patient. Heroic surgery may shorten or prematurely terminate a patient's existence. Moreover, what quality of life can be afforded if the patient's last days are spent recovering in a hospital bed? It is not an easy decision for either physician or patient to make, but in the presence of incurable disease, "no treatment" should still be an option. Palliative therapy is important, but it should alleviate, not accelerate suffering. Patients with inoperable, incurable disease or those who are curable but opt for no treatment are the ones who present the greatest challenge. This is the situation for which the most compassion is needed.

LAST RIGHTS

The "right to die" is the focus of a great deal of debate in the United States. Since 1976, when the New Jersey Supreme Court ruled in the Quinlan case, it has been estimated that more than 200 judgments have been handed down pertaining to the role of medical decisions in the dying process.[7] In 1996, the Second and Ninth Circuit Courts of Appeals handed down decisions upholding a constitutional right to physician-assisted suicide. This ruling was reversed in 1997 when the Supreme Court unanimously held that physician-assisted suicide was not a fundamental liberty protected by the 14th Amendment of the Constitution (reviewed in ref. 7). Nonetheless, in their concurring opinions, several justices wisely noted that no legal barriers should exist between qualified physicians and patients in requiring aggressive palliation of pain, even to the point of ". . . causing unconsciousness and hastening death."[7] This legal decision revealed what many already knew: patients go to their physicians in search of relief from pain and suffering, even to the point of promoting death. Given this premise, physicians should be appropriately responsive to their patients' requests. In that regard, the results of a study by Meier et al[8] are interesting. They found that up to 18% of physicians had received a request from a patient for assistance with suicide, 11% would be willing to hasten a patient's death under current legal constraints, and 6% had complied with such a request at least once. Legal decisions also reflect another point: difficult issues of life and death need to be evaluated within the context of an individual case; they should not be dictated by case law. For example, in order to arrive at a common constitutional formula,[9] the three courts lumped together different groups of terminally ill patients. Yet, as clinicians know, not all terminal patients can or should be grouped together. Moreover, whereas the Supreme Court looks to the defense of fundamental societal liberties, the physician's duty is to care for the individual patient. Society's welfare cannot be ignored, but it seldom takes precedence in the pursuit of what is right for the individual seeking care.

As long ago as the 18th century, the British novelist Fielding noted that ". . . it is not death, but dying which is terrible." What can we do to ameliorate this process? As physicians we tend to underutilize the large arsenal of available pain-relieving medications. Addiction is not an issue in a terminal patient. Patients should be given the option of increasing the potency of pain medications as needed. Patients and their families need to be absolved of their learned societal reluctance to use potent and effective narcotic balms. Such medication is given on a fixed schedule, not on an "as needed" basis. In this way, pain is not allowed to crescendo to the point of requiring relief, which may take some time to achieve. If oral feeding is difficult, rather than placing an uncomfortable nasogastric feeding tube, early placement of a percutaneous gastrostomy tube under local anesthesia can be recommended. Hospice care is provided if the patient or family feels overwhelmed. If a patient is clearly terminal, realistic advice should be given about getting his or her affairs in order, drawing up a living will, and determining the circumstances under which they wish to be rescucitated. As noted by Gostin,[7] it would be difficult to prosecute a case if a patient's death were due to aggressive pain control and palliative care. Such legal protection, in turn, helps preserve the dignity and autonomy of the patient.

Physicians are privileged to be healers, not just health care providers. They take an oath to do what is right for the patient and to alleviate suffering. They may be enjoined by society to participate in onerous decisions requiring the allocation of health care, but they must never forget their commitment to "cure sometimes, relieve often, and comfort always."

REFERENCES

1. Pellegrino E, Thomasma DC. *For the Patient's Good. The Restoration of Beneficence in Health Care.* New York: Oxford University Press; 1988:26, 32.
2. *Schloendorff v The Society of New York Hospital,* 211, NY, 125, 105 NE 92 (1914).
3. *Salgo v Leland Stanford Jr. University Board of Trustees,* 154, Cal. App 2d, 560, 317 p.2d 170 (1957).
4. Katz J. Reflections on informed consent. 40 years after its birth. *J Am Coll Surg.* 1998; 186:466–474.
5. English DC. Surgeon's role in ethical decisions. *Am Surg.* 1985; 51:423–425.
6. Ward PH. Informed consent in the patient with advanced cancer of the aerodigestive tract. In: Kagan AR, Miles J, eds. *Head and Neck Oncology: Clinical Management.* New York: Pergammon Press; 1989:12–15.
7. Gostin LD. Deciding life and death in the court room. *JAMA* 1997; 278:1523–1528.
8. Meier DE, Emmons C-A, Wallenstein S, et al. A national survey of physician-assisted suicide and euthanasia in the United States. *N Engl J Med.* 1998; 338:1193–1201.
9. Alpers A, Lo B. Does it make clinical sense to equate terminally ill patients who require life-sustaining interventions with those who do not? *JAMA* 1997; 277:1705–1708.

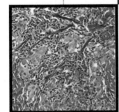

CHAPTER 4

Human Immunodeficiency Virus and Acquired Immunodeficiency Syndrome

■ SARAH S. FRANKEL

■ BRUCE M. WENIG

Acquired immunodeficiency syndrome (AIDS) was first recognized in 1981.[1] The clinical syndrome was characterized by opportunistic infection(s) and/or neoplasia with associated immunodeficiency. AIDS-related pathology may be seen in every organ system as a result of infection by the human immunodeficiency virus type 1 (HIV-1), the causative agent for AIDS.[1] The head and neck represents a microcosm of the entire body with respect to the manifestations of AIDS. Virtually every conceivable pathologic process associated with HIV infection and AIDS can be found within the head and neck, including a wide variety of opportunistic infections, reactive lymphoproliferative processes, and hematolymphoid and nonlymphoid neoplasms. These pathologic changes may be the initial manifestations of HIV infection or AIDS, or they may represent a component of systemic disease. Regardless of the context or site of occurrence, clinicians and pathologists must be aware of the pathologic manifestations of AIDS. Once the diagnosis is established, therapy can then be initiated that may potentially enhance the quality of life of the infected individual.

This chapter briefly discusses the pathogenetic mechanisms of HIV infection and immunodeficiency and various HIV- and AIDS-related pathologic lesions of the head and neck region.

PATHOGENESIS

Overview

Infection with HIV-1 initiates a series of events within the host immune system that ultimately lead to the destruction of cellular immunity. This results in immunosuppression, which renders the host susceptible to the opportunistic infections and tumors that are the hallmark of AIDS.

HIV-1 is a human retrovirus of the lentivirus genus. The virus is a membrane-bound, double-stranded RNA that is characterized by the presence of a unique enzyme—reverse transcriptase—at its core. This enzyme allows the viral RNA to be transcribed "backward" into DNA and then inserted into the host genome.[2] The virus preferentially infects CD4+ (helper) T-cell lymphocytes and other cells of the immune system that bear both the CD4 receptor and one of two chemokine receptors (CCR-5 and CXCR-4) on their surface.[2] These cells include CD4+ lymphocytes, dendritic cells, and macrophages.[3] Worldwide, more than 30 million persons are infected with HIV-1. World Health Organization (WHO) estimates that, worldwide, there are 16,000 new infections every day; 44,000 new cases of HIV-1 infection are predicted in the United States in 1998.[4]

Transmission of HIV occurs through blood, sexual (body fluids), and maternofetal routes. The overwhelming majority of early cases of HIV infection and AIDS in the United States and Europe were reported in men who had sexual relations with men. Although this remains the major risk group (53%), intravenous drug users (36%) and women (18%) are the two groups that have experienced the greatest increase in incidence rates of AIDS in the United

States and Europe. Most cases in Africa and Asia are heterosexually transmitted. Because infected females are usually at peak reproductive ages, the incidence of vertical transmission is also high. The recipients of contaminated blood and blood products (e.g., hemophiliacs) were at much greater risk of acquiring the infection prior to the routine screening of blood products for HIV that was begun in 1984. This mode of transmission continues to be a threat in areas of the world where the blood supply is not screened.

Spectrum of Disease

HIV-1 causes a spectrum of disease. With initial infection, a constellation of findings are reported that are caused directly by infection with HIV-1 and the patient's immune response. The transient, symptomatic illness is associated with high-titer viremia and a vigorous response to the invading virus. In the United States, 40% to 90% of infected patients will manifest this syndrome. The clinical manifestations of the primary infection are quite nonspecific and include a flu-like viral syndrome characterized by fever, fatigue, pharyngitis, lymphadenopathy (including tonsillar and adenoidal enlargement), and a maculopapular rash. The diagnosis of this syndrome has become much more critical because there is now effective antiretroviral therapy that may, if administered in the earliest phase of infection, have a major positive impact on prognosis and long-term survival. Owing to the abundance of lymphoid tissue in the head and neck, including lymph nodes and extranodal lymphoid tissues (e.g., Waldeyer's tonsillar ring and parotid gland), this anatomic region is especially likely to manifest these findings. During primary HIV infection, a peak in viral load occurs which then decreases and levels out at what is known as the set-point. This viral set-point is prognostically significant. Those individuals with a low viral set-point are much more likely to progress slowly (>10 years) to AIDS, whereas those with a

T A B L E 4 – 1 CDC CLASSIFICATION SYSTEM FOR HIV INFECTION			
	CLINICAL CATEGORIES		
CD4+ T-CELL CATEGORIES	A (Asymptomatic, Acute, or PGL)	B (Symptomatic, B-Conditions)	C (AIDS Indicator Conditions)
1 = >500 cells/mm³ or CD4 percentage ≥29%	A1	B1	C1[a]
2 = 200–500 cells/mm³ or CD4 percentage 14%–28%	A2	B2	C2[a]
3 = <200 cells/mm³ or CD4 percentage <14% Immunologic AIDS	A3[a]	B3[a]	C3[a]

[a] Persons in subcategories A3, B3, C1, C2, and C3 are reportable as AIDS cases in the United States and its territories (effective January 1, 1993).
   Data from Centers for Disease Control and Prevention (CDC). 1993 revised classification system and expanded surveillance case definition for AIDS among adolescents and adults. *MMWR* 1992;41(No. RR-17):1–19.

high viral set-point are likely to progress rapidly to AIDS (<5 years).[4]

During primary infection the immune system responds vigorously to the virus. The patient is not immunodeficient. The patient is HIV-1 infected but does not have AIDS. As the disease proceeds, especially if left untreated, the virus begins to destroy the cellular arm of the patient's immune system. As the CD4+ cells of the immune system are destroyed, the patient loses the ability to fight off

T A B L E 4 – 2	INDICATORS OF HIV DISEASE AND AIDS

Category A

Asymptomatic HIV infection
Persistent generalized lymphadenopathy
Acute (primary) HIV infection with accompanying illness or history of acute HIV infection

Category B

Candidiasis of the oropharynx (thrush)
Candidiasis of the vulva and vagina that is persistent, frequent, or poorly responsive to therapy
Cervical dysplasia, moderate to severe, or cervical carcinoma in situ
Constitutional symptoms, such as fever (38.5° C) or diarrhea lasting more than 1 month
Herpes zoster (shingles), involving at least two distinct episodes or more than one dermatome
Idiopathic thrombocytopenic purpura
Listeriosis
Oral hairy leukoplakia
Pelvic inflammatory disease complicated by tubo-ovarian abscess
Peripheral neuropathy
Bartonellosis (Rochalimiasis) (bacillary angiomatosis/cat-scratch disease complex)

Category C

Candidiasis of bronchi, trachea, lungs, or esophagus
Cervical cancer, invasive
Coccidioidomycosis, disseminated or extrapulmonary
Cryptococcosis, extrapulmonary
Cryptosporidiosis, intestinal, chronic (>1 month's duration)
Cytomegaloviral disease, including retinitis with loss of vision (other than liver, spleen, or nodes)
HIV-related encephalopathy (>1 month's duration)
Herpes simplex (chronic ulcer[s] >1 month's duration; or bronchitis, pneumonitis, or esophagitis)
Histoplasmosis, disseminated or extrapulmonary
Isosporiasis, intestinal, chronic (>1 month's duration)
Kaposi's sarcoma
Lymphoma, Burkitt's or immunoblastic (or equivalent terms)
Lymphoma of brain, primary
Mycobacteriosis (*M. avium* complex disease, *M. kansasii*), disseminated or extrapulmonary
Mycobacteriosis (*M. tuberculosis*), pulmonary or extrapulmonary
Pneumocystosis, any site (i.e., *P. carinii* pneumonia)
Recurrent pneumonia
Progressive multifocal leukoencephalopathy
Salmonella species septicemia, recurrent
Toxoplasmosis of brain
Wasting syndrome secondary to HIV

the myriad pathogens that are ubiquitous in our world. AIDS is the disease that results from HIV-1 infection. Infections seen in AIDS include pathogenic organisms, as well as opportunistic infections. The diagnosis of HIV-1 infection is conceptually simple; like most infections, it begins when the pathogen invades the host. The diagnosis of AIDS is much less clear-cut. AIDS is a diagnosis based on criteria. In the United States, the diagnosis is established by fulfilling criteria developed by the Centers for Disease Control (CDC). Elsewhere in the world, WHO criteria are applied. The CDC classification system (Tables 4–1 and 4–2) is based on three clinical categories (A, B, and C) and three CD4-T-cell count categories (1, 2, and 3). HIV-1 viral load, which has become a critical tool in diagnosing and managing patients with HIV-1 infection, is not included in the CDC criteria at this time.

HIV- AND AIDS-RELATED DISEASES OF THE HEAD AND NECK

INFECTIONS

As a result of the immunodeficiency produced by HIV, HIV-infected patients and those with AIDS are susceptible to a variety of infectious agents, including protozoa, viruses, bacteria, and fungi. Any one of these organisms can produce disease in the head and neck region. Only the more common infectious diseases of the head and neck associated with HIV infection are discussed here. For a more complete overview of HIV- and AIDS-related infectious diseases, the reader is referred to a more detailed text on this subject.[5]

Protozoa

Pneumocystis carinii is an opportunistic organism that is usually associated with pneumonia in the immunosuppressed host, and it is one of the most common life-threatening infections in patients with AIDS.[6] It is unusual for Pneumocystis to cause clinical manifestations outside of the pulmonary system;[7] however, infections caused by *P. carinii* have been identified in many organ systems. In the head and neck, Pneumocystis infection has been reported to involve the external auditory canal[8] and the middle ear.[9] The clinical manifestations, which differ according to the site of infection, may include ear pain, hypomobility of the tympanic membrane, and otitis media, as well as conductive and sensorineural hearing losses. The pathologic findings are similar to

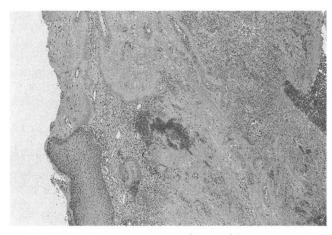

FIGURE 4-1 *Pneumocystis carinii* infection of the ear canal. Focally ulcerated squamous epithelium is evident, with identification of a foamy eosinophilic infiltrate in the submucosa.

those seen in the lung and include a foamy exudate within which the organism can be identified (Figs. 4–1 and 4–2). The presumed mode of dissemination to the ear from the lung is via vascular channels.[8] Typically, the pulmonary manifestations of Pneumocystis infection precede those of extrapulmonary involvement; however, occasionally, the initial diagnosis of AIDS is made following identification of its associated pathology in extrapulmonary locations.[8]

Viruses

The specific morphologic alterations related to HIV infection are discussed in the section on lymphoid lesions. Other than HIV, viral infection of head and neck sites in HIV-positive patients is common. Included in the spectrum of virus-associated infections are cytomegalovirus (CMV), herpes virus (simplex and zoster), Epstein-Barr virus (EBV), and human papillomavirus (HPV).

CYTOMEGALOVIRUS
Gross Pathology

When it occurs in the head and neck, CMV infection is seen as an ulcerative mucocutaneous lesion (Fig. 4–3).

Microscopic Pathology

The histologic appearance includes ulceration, necrosis, and cytomegaly with characteristic intranuclear and/or intracytoplasmic inclusions (Fig. 4–4).

Special Techniques

CMV infection can be confirmed on the basis of positive anti-CMV immunoreactivity (see Fig. 4–4).

Clinicopathologic Correlation

CMV is the most common opportunistic pathogen recognized at autopsy in patients with AIDS.[5] In general, CMV infection involving the head and neck is not common.

HERPES
Gross Pathology

Herpes simplex virus (HSV) is a cause of mucocutaneous disease in HIV-positive patients. Head and neck manifestations include an ulcerated lesion with involvement of intraoral, nasal cavity, lip, and external ear sites. Nasal cavity involvement may include septal perforation.

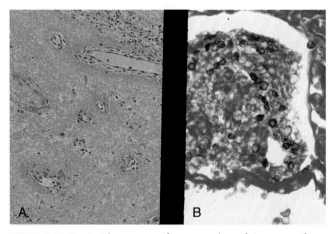

FIGURE 4-2 *A,* Characteristic foamy exudate of *P. carinii* infection in the submucosa of the ear, including perivascular localization. *B,* Gomori methenamine silver stain is used to delineate *P. carinii* organisms within the foamy exudate.

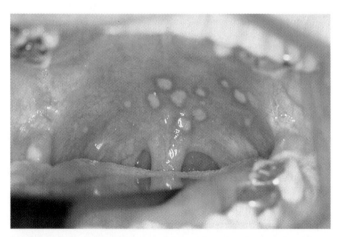

FIGURE 4-3 CMV infection of the oral cavity characterized by well-demarcated, round to oval lesions.

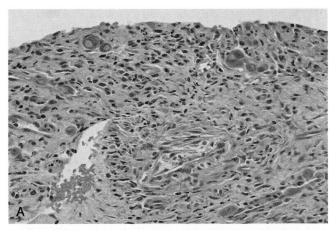

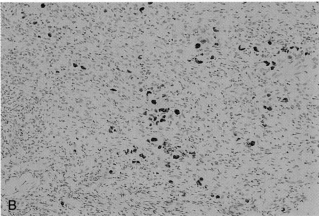

FIGURE 4-4 CMV pharyngitis. *A,* Ulcerated lesion with markedly enlarged cells having intranuclear and intracytoplasmic inclusions. *B,* Positive anti-CMV immunoreactivity confirms the diagnosis.

Microscopic Pathology

The histopathologic appearance is that of an intraepidermal vesicle marked by acantholysis and balloon degeneration of epithelial cells. Intranuclear inclusions may be identified within the degenerating epithelial cells (Fig. 4–5), and multinucleated giant cells may be numerous.

Special Techniques

As with CMV infection, herpetic infections can be identified by their positive anti-HSV immunoreactivity (see Fig. 4–5).

Clinicopathologic Correlation

Herpes zoster may occur as varicella (chickenpox) or as dermatomal zoster (shingles). The latter, although not specific for HIV infection, appears to be related to HIV infection and may represent an early marker for the immunosuppression associated with HIV infection.[10,11] Herpes zoster can localize to any dermatome and cause unremitting pain. The head and

neck manifestations include involvement of the eighth nerve or geniculate ganglion (Ramsay Hunt syndrome), producing severe ear pain, hearing loss, vertigo, and facial nerve paralysis. Intranuclear inclusions that are indistinguishable from those seen in herpes simplex are identified.

EPSTEIN-BARR VIRUS

Gross Pathology

EBV has been associated with oral hairy leukoplakia,[12] which is an asymptomatic, white thickening of the mucosa of the oral cavity (lateral tongue) and oropharynx.

Microscopic Pathology

On histologic examination, oral hairy leukoplakia is characterized by hyperkeratosis, parakeratosis, acanthosis, submucosal chronic inflammation, and fungal overgrowth (Candida species).

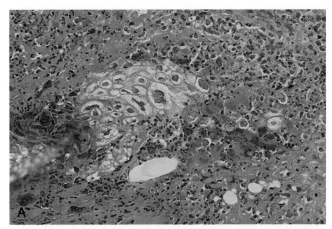

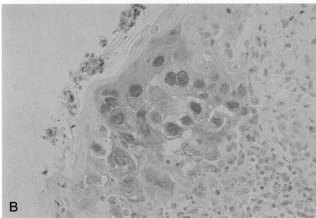

FIGURE 4-5 HSV infection. *A,* Ulcerated cutaneous lesion with clustering of enlarged, atypical epithelial cells in the ulcer bed showing intranuclear inclusions. *B,* Confirmation of HSV infection as demonstrated by positive anti-HSV immunoreactivity.

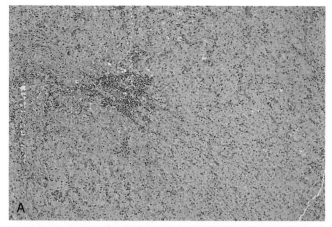

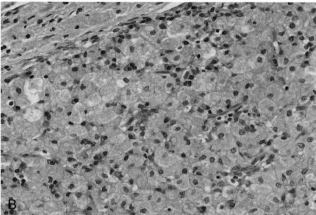

FIGURE 4-6 Atypical mycobacterial infection. A, Cervical lymph node showing effacement of the normal architecture by a diffuse cellular proliferation. B, Higher magnification shows that this cellular infiltrate is composed of histiocytes.

Clinicopathologic Correlation

EBV is a pathogen that is frequently identified in association with infections and neoplasms of the head and neck. EBV infection may cause fever, fatigue, and lympadenopathy. More often than not, this association involves patients who are not infected with HIV. However, EBV-related disease can be seen in HIV-positive patients, and virtually all patients with AIDS demonstrate serologic evidence of EBV infection. The role of EBV in causing disease in patients with AIDS remains uncertain.

Aside from its mucocutaneous (infectious) manifestations, EBV-associated pathology in HIV-infected patients may include malignant lymphoproliferative neoplasms (non-Hodgkin's and Hodgkin's lymphomas). EBV infection has also been linked to epithelial malignant neoplasms, specifically nasopharyngeal carcinoma, but there is no known similar association occuring in patients with HIV or AIDS.

HUMAN PAPILLOMAVIRUS

HPV has been implicated in several head and neck pathologic processes occurring in patients with AIDS. These include condyloma acuminata and epithelial hyperplasia of the oral cavity.[10]

Bacteria

MYCOBACTERIAL INFECTION

Gross Pathology

Typically, mycobacterial infection in the head and neck is found in cervical lymph nodes and presents as lymphadenopathy.

Microscopic Pathology

The histologic appearance is that of an architecturally effaced lymph node replaced by confluent, caseating granulomas. Within the areas of necrosis, giant cells and/or epithelioid histiocytes are seen. The presence of giant cells and epithelioid histiocytes is indicative of a hyperergic reaction, which typically is devoid of mycobacterial organisms. Patients with more advanced disease (i.e., those who are more immunocompromised) may not be able to mount a granulomatous reaction to the mycobacteria. In these patients, a diffuse proliferation of histiocytes may be seen without a granulomatous inflammatory response (Fig. 4-6).

Special Techniques

Special stains, such as acid-fast bacilli (AFB) or Ziehl-Neelsen stain may be helpful in the identification of mycobacterial organism. When identified, the organisms are curved and beaded, and they are seen within giant cells or histiocytes (Fig. 4-7).

Clinicopathologic Correlation

Mycobacterial infections have been identified with frequency among HIV-infected patients and are usu-

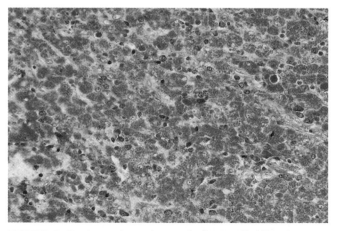

FIGURE 4-7 Atypical mycobacterial infection. Ziehl-Neelsen staining reveals the presence of innumerable mycobacteria within the cytoplasm of the histiocytes.

ally related to the *Mycobacterium tuberculosis* and the *M. avium-intracellulare* species. Localized and disseminated mycobacterial infection occurs in HIV-infected patients and those with AIDS. Spindle cell lesions or pseudotumors caused by nontuberculous mycobacteria (*M. avium-intracellulare*) may occur in patients with AIDS.[13-16] These spindle cell lesions occur in lymph nodes or cutaneous sites and are characterized by the presence of spindle cells with a storiform or fascicular growth. In lymph nodes, the spindle cells efface the normal nodal architecture, whereas in the skin, these lesions tend to be located in subepidermal areas. A variable chronic inflammatory cell infiltrate may be present, as may a variable number of dense bands of collagen. The spindle-shaped cells are phagocytic cells containing numerous mycobateria. These may be confirmed by histochemical stains (AFB). Immunohistochemical studies of the spindle cell lesions indicate that they are of monocytic/macrophage origin.[13,14] Umlas et al[14] have reported desmin immunoreactivity in these mycobacterial spindle cell lesions. Ultrastructural studies have shown differentiation along fibroblastic (presence of abundant intracytoplasmic rough endoplasmic reticulum and investment of collagen) and phagocytic cell lines with numerous intracytoplasmic microorganisms.[13]

OTHER BACTERIA

Other bacterial infections seen in the head and neck in association with HIV infection include *Staphylococcus aureus*, *Streptococcus pneumoniae*, and *Hemophilus influenza*. These organisms have been implicated in causing upper respiratory infections. It is not entirely clear whether these infections occur more frequently in patients with AIDS than in the general population. With the advent of the AIDS era, a rise in the incidence of syphilis has also been noted.[17,18] A number of reports have suggested a different natural history of syphilis in HIV-infected patients compared to syphilis in other patients.[19,20] These findings suggest that syphilis occurring in HIV-infected individuals has an atypical or uncommon presentation, a shorter incubation period for development of central nervous system involvement (neurosyphilis), and an altered serologic response, and it may not respond to standard therapy. Head and neck involvement by syphilis may manifest as an otologic problem, presenting with sensorineural hearing loss.[21] Diagnosis is confirmed by serologic testing.

Fungi

Many fungi occur in association with HIV infection or AIDS. However, the Candida species is the single most important fungal pathogen in the head and neck.

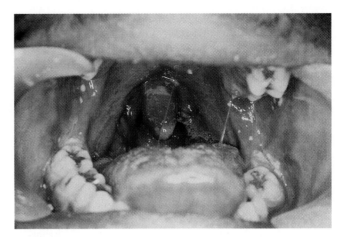

FIGURE 4–8 Oral candidiasis (thrush), which manifests as a cheesy or creamy appearing mucosal plaque.

Gross Pathology

The most common form of oral candidiasis (thrush) appears as a cheesy or creamy mucosal plaque (Fig. 4–8).

Microscopic Pathology

Histologically, budding yeasts and pseudohyphae typical of *C. albicans* are identified.

Special Techniques

Special stains for fungi, including Gomori methenamine silver (GMS) and periodic acid–Schiff (PAS), are used to highlight the fungal forms (Fig. 4–9).

Clinicopathologic Correlation

Oral candidiasis frequently occurs in patients with AIDS, and its presence is a strong indication for the

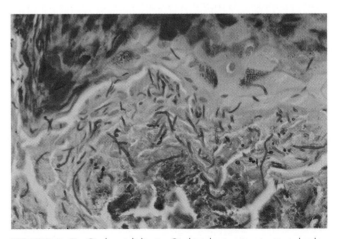

FIGURE 4–9 Oral candidiasis. On histologic examination, budding yeasts and pseudohyphae typical of *C. albicans* are identified by PAS staining.

subsequent development of AIDS.[22] As previously detailed, Candida is seen in association with oral hairy leukoplakia, where it is identified on the surface of the lesion.

BENIGN LESIONS

Benign Reactive Lymphoproliferative Lesions

Patients with AIDS are at risk for the development of a lymphoproliferative disorder.[23] The pathology of lymph node involvement includes both reactive and neoplastic diseases. Although the head and neck is an anatomically small area, it is a region that is rich in lymphoid tissues and, therefore, prone to development of an HIV- or AIDS-related lymphoproliferative lesion. The lymphoproliferative lesion may represent the initial manifestation of HIV infection or may be part of a smoldering, progressive process.

Lymphadenopathy is an early and prominent feature of HIV-infected patients and can be considered to be a sign suggestive of HIV infection in the appropriate patient population.[24] Sites of involvement include regional lymph nodes, as well as extranodal lymphoid tissues, such as Waldeyer's tonsillar tissue ring (palatine tonsils, adenoids, and base of tongue) and the salivary glands.

There is a wide spectrum of clinical manifestations in patients infected with HIV. With regard to lymph node involvement, this spectrum ranges from persistent generalized lymphadenopathy (PGL) (also referred to as lymphadenopathy syndrome [LAS]), which is commonly found in patients with early HIV infection, to generalized lymphadenopathy, which is found in patients with AIDS-related complex (ARC) and those with frank AIDS. PGL is a CDC category A indicator condition of HIV infection. Palpable lymphadenopathy with lymph nodes measuring greater than 1 cm in more than two extrainguinal sites for a duration of more than 3 months is the clinical definition of persistent generalized lymphadenopathy.

Lymphadenopathy

Microscopic Pathology

The histologic findings in patients with HIV infection or AIDS and PGL can be divided into three distinct patterns, including follicular hyperplasia, follicular involution, and lymphocyte depletion.[25,26] In follicular hyperplasia, there are enlarged germinal centers present in cortical regions, as well as in deeper locations. The germinal center enlargement may be so pronounced as to suggest confluence with other germinal centers. In addition, there is follicle lysis, paracortical hyperplasia, and focal hemorrhage, and the germinal centers are mitotically active and demonstrate prominent tingible body macrophages. Monocytoid B-lymphocyte hyperplasia and Warthin-Finkeldey–like multinucleated giant cells may be present.

During follicular involution, there is diffuse lymphoid hyperplasia with effacement of the lymph node architecture. Germinal centers are atrophic or completely absent, and mantle zones are thin. Intrafollicular plasmacytosis and erythrophagocytosis can be seen. A prominent vascular proliferation is present, suggesting Castleman's disease or Kaposi's sarcoma. Fibrosis of the capsule or subcapsular sinus begins during this stage.

In the lymphocyte depletion stage, lymphoid nodes are atrophic, almost invariably lack germinal centers, and show marked depletion of lymphocytes. Fibrosis is increasingly evident. Sinus histiocytosis is present, often with erythrophagocytosis. This latter finding is identified in all three patterns, but is most frequently observed in the stage of lymphocyte depletion. Although there is a marked reduction of lymphocytes, plasma cells may be numerous.

Extranodal Lymphoid Tissues of the Head and Neck

The HIV-associated morphologic changes are not restricted to nodal lymphoid tissues, but also affect extranodal lymphoid tissues, such as in Waldeyer's tonsillar tissues.[27–31] HIV-1 infection is a fatal retroviral infection that may first present clinically as enlargement of the lymphoid tissues of Waldeyer's ring. These tissues are a major site of viral replication.

Microscopic Pathology

The presence of the virus in Waldeyer's tissues causes a unique constellation of diagnostic histopathologic features, including florid follicular hyperplasia, follicle lysis, and HIV-1–infected multinucleated giant cells of probable dendritic cell origin. The histomorphologic changes in HIV-induced tonsillar and adenoidal enlargement vary with the progression of disease. In the early stages of infection, the histomorphology may include florid follicular hyperplasia (Fig. 4–10), with or without follicular fragmentation, and follicle lysis with areas of follicular involution (Fig. 4–11). Additional findings include the presence of monocytoid B-cell hyperplasia, paracortical and interfollicular zone expansion with immunoblasts and plasma cells, interfollicular clusters of high endothelial venules, intrafollicular hemor-

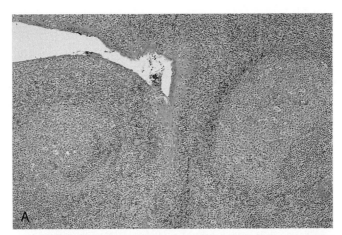

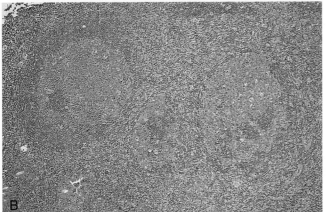

FIGURE 4-10 *A,* Early histologic manifestations of HIV infection include the presence of florid follicular hyperplasia characterized by enlarged and irregularly shaped germinal centers, some of which approximate the surface epithelium. *B,* Three follicles in varying stages. The two larger ones show attenuated to partially absent mantle cell lymphocytes; the smaller germinal center (*center*) is infiltrated by small lymphocytes (follicle lysis).

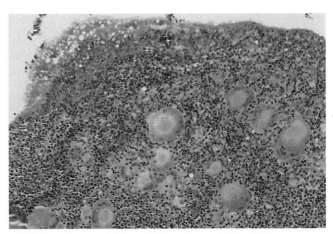

FIGURE 4-12 Multinucleated giant cells in HIV infection. The giant cells are characteristically localized to the surface (as seen here) or crypt epithelium (not shown).

rhage, and the presence of multinucleated giant cells. The giant cells characteristically cluster adjacent to or within the adenoidal surface epithelium or the tonsillar crypt epithelium (Fig. 4–12).

The histologic features in patients with more advanced stages of disease contrast with those just described and correlate with the lymphoid obliteration seen in the terminal stages of HIV infection or AIDS. In these cases, effacement of nodal architecture, loss of the normal lymphoid cell population with subsequent replacement by a benign plasma cell infiltrate, and the presence of increased vascularity are noted (Fig. 4–13). The multinucleated giant cells characteristically seen in the early and chronic stages of disease are not identified in the more advanced stages of HIV infection.

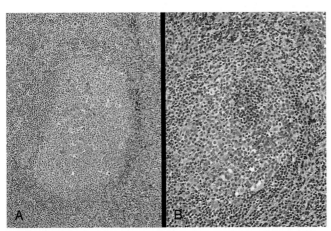

FIGURE 4-11 Histologic changes suggesting early HIV infection. *A,* Follicular hyperplasia with absent mantle cell lymphocytes. *B,* Follicle lysis characterized by "infiltrating" small lymphocytes and an absence of clearly defined mantle zones.

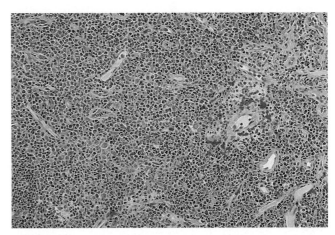

FIGURE 4-13 The histologic features in patients with more advanced stages of AIDS or HIV infection include the effacement of lymphoid tissue architecture, loss of the normal lymphoid cell population with replacement by a benign plasma cell infiltrate, and the presence of increased vascularity.

Special Techniques

Special stains for microorganisms other than HIV yield negative results.[30] Reactivity for the HIV core antigen p24 (GAG protein), an indicator of active HIV infection,[30,31] is consistently identified in the early and chronic stages of disease.[30] Anti-HIV p24 reactivity is seen within the follicular dendritic cell network of the germinal centers, in scattered interfollicular lymphocytes, in the multinucleated giant cells, and within intraepithelial cells of the crypt epithelium (Figs. 4–14 and 4–15).[30] The HIV p24–positive intraepithelial cells are positive for S-100 protein (a dendritic cell marker), and their morphologic appearance correlates with the appearance of dendritic cells.[30,32] Reactivity with both B-cell (CD20) and T-cell markers or subsets (CD45RO, CD3, OPD4) is seen within the germinal centers and in the interfollicular regions, as well as in scattered intraepithelial cells.

Patients with more advanced disease, characterized by loss of germinal centers and the presence of

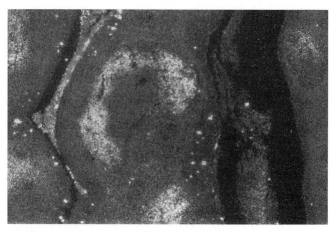

FIGURE 4–15 In situ hybridization for HIV-1 RNA, using antisense riboprobe, darkfield microscopy, shows signal in enlarged and irregularly shaped germinal centers, as well as in scattered interfollicular cells and multinucleated giant cells, with the latter approximating the epithelial layer.

a predominant plasma cell infiltrate, show a relative absence of lymphoid cell markers (CD45RB, CD3, or OPD4). In these cases, the plasma cell infiltrate shows reactivity with κ and λ light chains, indicative of a benign proliferation. Surface and crypt epithelia are cytokeratin-reactive. Immunoreactivity with EBV-latent membrane protein (EBV-LMP), HSV, or CMV is not present.[30]

Evidence of HIV RNA by in situ hybridization is seen in the follicular dendritic cell network, in the multinucleated giant cells, and in mature lymphocytes localized to the germinal centers, interfollicular zones, and within the surface and/or crypt epithelia (Fig. 4–15).[30] The strongest signal is present in the multinucleated giant cells.

Clinicopathologic Correlation

The morphologic changes seen in affected lymph nodes and peripheral lymphoid tissues represent a continuum that varies according to the duration and progression of disease.[33] The clinical spectrum of HIV infection includes three phases: early or acute, chronic, and crisis or final.[34] The morphologic changes parallel the course of HIV infection. In the early stages of disease, the florid follicular hyperplasia of lymphoid tissues results in enlargement of the affected sites. This not only causes lymphadenopathy but also results in enlarged adenoids and/or tonsils. This enlargement may, in turn, cause airway obstruction or otitis media, or both, and raises clinical concern for neoplastic involvement of these sites.[28,30] Similar to the lymphoid tissue changes that occur with progression of the disease, the identification of HIV also changes over time. In nodal tissues, the follicular dendritic cells of the germinal centers have been shown to be reservoirs of HIV RNA.[35–37]

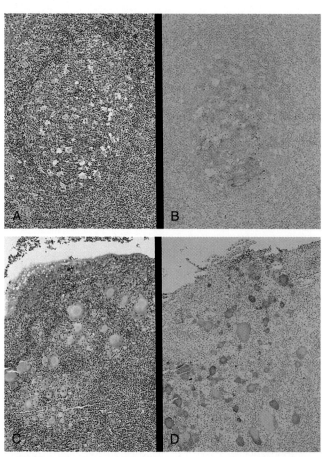

FIGURE 4–14 Confirmation of HIV infection by immunohistochemical reactivity with HIV p24 core antigen. A and B, HIV-infected tonsillar tissue shows alterations of the germinal center demonstrating HIV p24 immunoreactivity within follicular dendritic cells. C and D, HIV-infected tonsillar tissue shows characteristic multinucleated giant cells that also demonstrated HIV p24 immunoreactivity.

The follicular dendritic cells entrap but do not actively produce HIV, allowing for presentation of the virus to competent immune cells of B-cell lineage.[34] With progression of disease and continued immunosuppression, the germinal centers involute and then disappear. Serologic evaluation is confirmatory of HIV infection. With the recent advances in antiretroviral chemotherapy, the early institution of which may significantly prolong life and disease-free interval, the recognition of the clinical and pathologic parameters of HIV-related enlargement of Waldeyer's ring tissues is essential.

The clinical features of tonsillar and adenoidal disease in patients with HIV have been extensively detailed elsewhere.[27–30] In brief, HIV-induced tonsillar and adenoidal enlargement is more common in men than women, and occurs most frequently in the third to fifth decades of life (median age, fourth decade). The clinical presentation varies and may include nasal congestion, airway obstruction, sore throat (pharyngitis), otitis media that is unresponsive to antibiotic therapy, otalgia, facial weakness, fever, and a nasopharyngeal or tonsillar mass. Clinically, the tonsils and adenoids are enlarged, usually bilaterally; however, unilateral enlargement may also occur. The enlargement of the tonsils or adenoids may raise the concern of a hematolymphoid or epithelial neoplasm, prompting surgical removal of the enlarged organ. Concurrent (unilateral) cervical adenopathy may be present.[28,30] Large ulcers leading to complete destruction of the tonsil have also been reported, but no causative agents could be identified by histopathologic, microbiologic, and laboratory tests.[38] It is difficult to determine whether these lesions are a type of giant aphthous ulcer or a malady unique to tonsils in patients with AIDS. Wenig et al[30] report that, of their entire group of 12 patients, 4 were known or suspected at the time of presentation to be infected with HIV or suffering from AIDS, or both. The four patients known or suspected to be HIV-positive were seropositive for HIV but were without evidence of opportunistic infections. The remaining eight patients were not known to be HIV-infected and were not known to be in any of the risk groups associated with HIV infection. Other than enlarged tonsils or adenoids, these patients presented without any of the clinical stigmata of HIV infection. The risk factors for the patients who were known or suspected to be HIV-positive included homosexuality, blood transfusions, and intravenous drug abuse.

HIV-Related Salivary Gland Disease

Gross Pathology

HIV-related salivary gland disease (SGD) is manifested by cystic lesions. These may be single or multiple, unilateral or bilateral (Fig. 4–16).

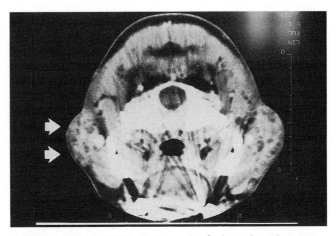

FIGURE 4–16 HIV-SGD. Radiographic findings show the presence of bilateral parotid gland cysts (*arrows*).

Microscopic Pathology

On histologic examination, lymphoepithelial cysts are evident. The cysts are lined by an epithelium that may vary from cuboidal to squamous. The epithelium is surrounded by a lymphoid tissue, including mature lymphocytes with or without germinal centers (Fig. 4–17). The lymphoid infiltrate may be so extensive as to obscure the lining epithelium. Lymphoid changes vary and may include florid follicular hyperplasia, follicle lysis, and attenuated or absent mantle zone. Multinucleated giant cells may be present. These giant cells can be found in interfollicular or intrafollicular sites, or they may tend to localize adjacent to or within the lining epithelium (Fig. 4–18). Adjacent salivary gland tissue is infiltrated by the lymphoid cells with destruction of the salivary gland parenchyma and formation of epimyoepithelial islands (Fig. 4–19).

Special Techniques

The lymphoid cell infiltrate is polyclonal. HIV-1 p24 immunoreactivity may be associated with follicular dendritic cells and the multinucleated giant cells.

Clinicopathologic Correlation

HIV-SGD includes those HIV-infected individuals with xerostomia, enlargement of one or more major salivary glands, or both of the above.[39] Patients may also complain of dry eyes or arthralgia. HIV-SGD may represent the initial manifestations of HIV infection. HIV-SGD typically affects adults between the ages of 20 and 60 years, with more than 90% of cases occuring in men. HIV-SGD may occur in children born of HIV-infected mothers. Under these circumstances, there is no gender predilection. HIV-SGD primarily involves the parotid gland; the

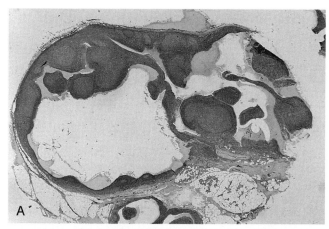

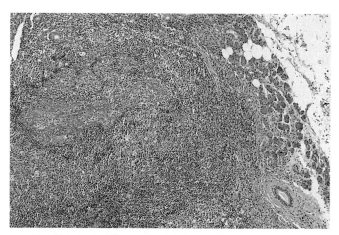

FIGURE 4-19 HIV-SGD. The adjacent salivary gland tissue is infiltrated by lymphoid cells, with destruction of the salivary gland parenchyma and formation of epimyoepithelial islands (*left of center*).

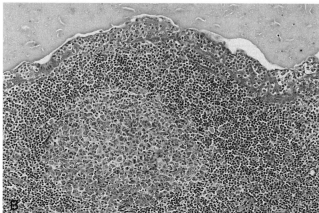

FIGURE 4-17 HIV-SGD. *A,* This parotid gland shows the presence of multiple cysts surrounded by a lymphoid cell infiltrate and numerous germinal centers. *B,* At higher magnification, the cystic structures appear to be lined by a disrupted squamous epithelium. The cyst wall includes a benign lymphoid infiltrate and a germinal center that lacks mantle cell lymphocytes.

submandibular gland is involved in a small percentage of cases. Bilateral gland involvement occurs in up to 60% of cases. Computed tomography (CT) and magnetic resonance imaging (MRI) studies show unilateral or bilateral multicentric cysts of varying sizes. Serologic markers confirm HIV positivity. Treatment for HIV-SGD is surgical resection. HIV-SGD is benign, but malignant lymphoma may occur in a small percentage of cases, especially in patients with low CD4 counts.[40]

The origin of these cysts appears to be the salivary gland (parotid) epithelial structures arising in intraparotid or periparotid lymph nodes accounting for the lymphoid component. Similar cysts can be found in HIV-negative patients.[41] The presence of HIV-1 suggests that the pathogenesis of the salivary gland lymphoepithelial lesions is primarily attributable to this virus.[42] Sjögren's syndrome–like illness has also been identified in patients with AIDS representing additional evidence of the severely damaged immune system in these patients.[43]

Bacillary Angiomatosis

Gross Pathology

The gross appearance of bacillary angiomatosis (BA) varies widely from cutaneous erythematous papules to mushroom-shaped papules and nodules, to deep-seated, rounded lesions without a change in skin color.[44] Uncommonly, BA may appear as a mucosa-based, erythematous, nodular proliferation.

Microscopic Pathology

Regardless of its clinical presentation, the histologic features of BA are the same and include a well-circumscribed, lobular, capillary proliferation. The

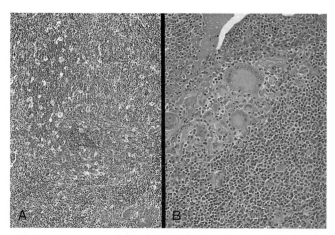

FIGURE 4-18 HIV-SGD. Similar to the changes in HIV-infected lymph nodes and tonsillar tissues, early histologic features suggestive of HIV infection include follicular hyperplasia (*A*) and multinucleated giant cells (*B*).

overall features are similar to those seen in lobular capillary hemangioma. Small capillaries are arranged around ectatic vessels, which are lined by prominent-appearing epithelioid endothelial cells (Fig. 4–20). In general, cytologic atypia, mitotic figures, and necrosis are not usually present, but they may occasionally be seen. Solid areas may be present and may obscure the vascular proliferation. A variable edematous, mucinous, or fibrotic stroma is seen separating the lobular proliferation. An important histologic feature in BA is the presence of neutrophils and neutrophilic debris adjacent to the capillary proliferation. Associated with the neutrophils are granular clumps that represent aggregated bacilli (Fig. 4–21). BA typically lacks spindled cells, interconnecting vascular channels, and hyaline globules, features seen in Kaposi's sarcoma.

The overlying epithelium may be ulcerated or thinned, or it may show pseudoepitheliomatous hyperplasia.

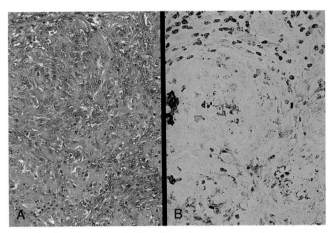

FIGURE 4–21 Bacillary angiomatosis. *A,* Vascular proliferation with prominent epithelioid endothelial cells and scattered neutrophils are associated with granular-appearing areas. *B,* Warthin-Starry staining reveals bacteria in the granular material. The bacteria are interstitially located.

Special Techniques

Warthin-Starry staining reveals bacteria in the aforementioned granular material. These bacteria are interstitially located.

Differential Diagnosis

The histologic differential diagnosis includes lobular capillary hemangioma, epithelioid hemangioma, angiosarcoma, and Kaposi's sarcoma. The presence of granular material, neutrophils, and neutrophilic debris, as well as the absence of cytologic atypia, ramifying and interconnecting vascular channels, necrosis, mitotic activity, and hyaline globules, assists in differentiating BA from these other vascular lesions.

Clinicopathologic Correlation

BA is a pseudoneoplastic capillary proliferative lesion that occurs as a complication of HIV infection and usually presents as a cutaneous vascular lesion.[44] The causative opportunistic infection involves a bacteria of the Rochalimaea species (*R. henselae*).[45] The treatment for BA is directed at the causative microorganism. Full-dose erythromycin is effective, often resulting in the resolution of the lesions.[45] However, if left untreated, BA is progressive and potentially life-threatening.[45,46]

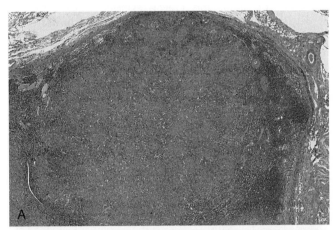

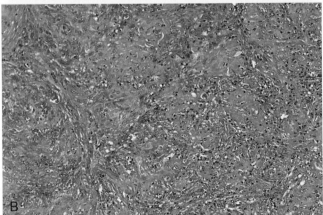

FIGURE 4–20 Bacillary angiomatosis. *A,* The architecture of this cervical lymph node is effaced by a circumscribed lobular capillary proliferation. *B,* Small capillaries are arranged around ectatic vessels, which are lined by prominent-appearing endothelial cells. A fibrotic stroma is seen separating the lobular proliferation. Scattered neutrophils and neutrophilic debris can be seen adjacent to the capillary proliferation.

MALIGNANT LESIONS

Hematolymphoid Neoplasms

In 1985, the CDC expanded the case definition criteria for AIDS to include individuals with high-grade lymphomas with positive serology for HIV.[47] Malignant lymphoma is the second most common malignant disease in HIV-infected patients.[48] In contrast to the general population, most patients with HIV infection or AIDS who have malignant lymphomas tend to have extranodal disease, most likely involving mucosa-associated lymphoid tissues, the central nervous system, and body cavities.[48] Most of the malignant lymphomas in such patients are high-grade B-cell tumors. CD30 (Ki-1)–positive, large-cell, anaplastic lymphomas have also been reported.[40] Up to 50% of patients with AIDS and malignant lymphoma have elevated EBV titers, and immunoreactivity for EBV-LMP can be identified in the malignant cells. Despite the predominance of the high-grade type of non-Hodgkin's lymphoma, both low-grade and intermediate-grade malignant lymphomas have been identified in patients with AIDS.

Hodgkin's disease is rather uncommon in patients with HIV infection or AIDS, accounting for approximately 1% of the malignant lesions in this patient population. As such, Hodgkin's disease is not considered by the CDC to be an indicator condition. Compared to non-HIV patients, HIV-infected patients and those with AIDS who have Hodgkin's disease tend to have more clinically aggressive tumors, and they present with a more advanced stage of disease with extranodal involvement. Further, these patients have lower survival rates and increased incidence of secondary malignant lymphomas and opportunistic infections.

Nonhematolymphoid Malignant Neoplasms

Various solid tumors have been seen in the HIV-infected and AIDS populations, including lung carcinoma, cervical carcinoma, and gastrointestinal (anal) carcinoma.[40] Although there is no known direct association with HIV infection or AIDS, oropharyngeal squamous cell carcinoma and cutaneous basal cell carcinoma have been identified in affected patients.[11,18,34] The most common malignant disease in patients with HIV infection or AIDS is Kaposi's sarcoma.

Kaposi's Sarcoma

Gross Pathology

Kaposi's sarcoma may involve almost every head and neck site, including the skin, oral cavity, and pharynx (oropharynx and hypopharynx). Involvement of the salivary glands, as well as of the sinonasal and nasopharyngeal regions, is uncommon and, when present, is usually seen in patients with AIDS.[49] Kaposi's sarcoma in patients with AIDS appears as a blue-red or violaceous mucosal papule or nodule (Fig. 4–22).

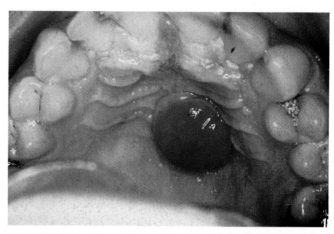

FIGURE 4–22 Kaposi's sarcoma of the palate appearing as a delineated, raised, round to oval, red nodule.

Microscopic Pathology

In mucosal sites, the characteristic histopathologic findings vary according to the stage of the disease. In the early patch stage, there is a slight increase in vascular spaces. In the more advanced nodular stage, Kaposi's sarcoma is unencapsulated and infiltrative and is composed of spindle cells in a fascicular growth. The spindle cells are elongated and rather uniform, with scant cytoplasm and indistinct cell borders (Fig. 4–23). Scattered mitotic figures can be identified. Separating the spindle cell proliferations are slit-like spaces containing erythrocytes that commonly extravasate into the spindle cell component. Intracellular and extracellular, diastase-resistant, PAS-positive, hyaline globules can be seen. Lymph node involvement by Kaposi's sarcoma is

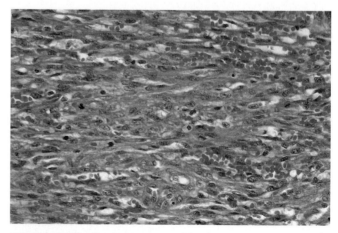

FIGURE 4–23 Kaposi's sarcoma. Histologic examination reveals this tumor to be composed of elongated spindle cells with scant cytoplasm and indistinct cell borders. Separating the spindle cell proliferations are slit-like spaces containing erythrocytes that extravasate into the spindle cell component. Intracellular and extracellular hyaline globules can be seen, as can scattered mitotic figures.

characterized by multiple tumor foci located in the capsular and sinusoid regions of the lymph nodes.

Special Techniques

Intracellular and extracellular, diastase-resistant, PAS-positive, hyaline globules can be seen. Immunoreactivity is often absent with endothelial cell markers (Factor VIII–related antigen, CD31, CD34). There is an association between Kaposi's sarcoma and herpes hominis virus-8 (HHV-8). Nucleic acid sequences specific to HHV-8 are found in tissue samples from various forms of Kaposi's sarcoma. Hexagonal nucleocapsids and mature envelope virions typical for herpesvirus have been found by electron microsopy in Kaposi's sarcoma.[50]

Clinicopathologic Correlation

Kaposi's sarcoma is a malignant vascular neoplasm that occurs in three forms: classic, epidemic or AIDS-related, and transplantation-associated. Other than for diagnostic purposes, surgery is not utilized in treatment. Patients with AIDS and Kaposi's sarcoma have a more aggressive disease course marked by increased mortality rates as a result of the constellation of problems in this group, including opportunistic infections and visceral Kaposi's sarcoma. The presence of HHV-8 in Kaposi's sarcoma suggests that this organism may be the cause for this neoplasm. Further, the identification of HHV-8 may be of diagnostic utility for Kapsosi's sarcoma.

With the relatively recent recognition of AIDS has come the recognition of its association with a unique form of Kaposi's sarcoma. In contrast to the classic Kaposi's sarcoma, AIDS-associated Kaposi's sarcoma, referred to as epidemic Kaposi's sarcoma, is more aggressive and is characteristically progressive and rapidly fatal.[51] In the head and neck, epidemic Kaposi's sarcoma may manifest as a cutaneous, mucosal, or lymph node lesion with symptoms related to the site of origin.[52]

REFERENCES

1. Essex M. Origin of AIDS. In: DeVita VT, Hellman S, Rosenberg SA, eds. *Acquired Immunodeficiency Syndrome—Etiology, Diagnosis, Treatment, and Prevention.* 4th ed. Philadelphia: Lippincott-Raven; 1997:3–14.
2. Hirsch M, Curran J. Human immunodeficicency viruses. In: Fields B, Knipe D, Howley P, eds. *Fields Virology.* Vol 2. Philadelphia: Lippincott-Raven Press; 1996:1953–1969.
3. Banchereau J, Steinman RM. Dendritic cells and control of immunity. *Nature.* 1998; 392:245–252.
4. Kahn J, Walker B. Acute human immunodeficiency virus type 1 infection. *N Engl J M.* 1998; 339:33–39.
5. DeVita VT, Helman S, Rosenberg SA. Clinical manifestations. In: DeVita VT, Hellman S, Rosenberg SA, eds. *Acquired Immunodeficiency Syndrome—Etiology, Diagnosis, Treatment, and Prevention.* 4th ed. Philadelphia: Lippincott-Raven; 1997:203–443.
6. Masur H, Michelis MA, Greene JB, et al. An outbreak of community-acquired *Pneumocystis carinii* pneumonia: Initial manifestation of cellular immune dysfunction. *N Engl J Med.* 1981; 305:1431–1438.
7. Coulman CU, Greene I, Archibald RWR. Cutaneous pneumocystosis. *Ann Intern Med.* 1987; 106:396–398.
8. Sandler ED, Leboit PE, Wenig BM, et al. *Pneumocystis carinii* otitis media in AIDS: A case report and review of the literature regarding extrapulmonary pneumocystosis. *Otolaryngol Head Neck Surg.* 1990; 103:817–821.
9. Gherman CR, Ward RR, Bassis ML. *Pneumocystis carinii* otitis media and mastoiditis as the initial manifestation of the acquired immunodeficiency syndrome. *Am J Med.* 1988; 85:250–252.
10. Friedman-Kien AE, Lafleur FL, Gendler E, et al. Herpes zoster: A possible early clinical sign for the development of acquired immunodeficiency syndrome in high-risk individuals. *J Am Acad Dermatol.* 1986; 14:1023–1028.
11. Melbye M, Grossman RJ, Goedert JJ, et al. Risk of AIDS after herpes zoster. *Lancet.* 1987; 1:728–730.
12. Silverman S, Migliorati CA, Lozada-Nur F, et al. Oral findings in people with or at high risk for AIDS: A study of 375 homosexual males. *J Am Dent Assoc.* 1986; 112:187–192.
13. Brandwein M, Choi HSH, Strauchen J, Stoler M, Jagirdar J. Spindle cell reaction to nontuberculous mycobacteriosis in AIDS mimicking a spindle cell neoplasm. Evidence for dual histiocytic and fibroblast-like charcteristics of spindle cells. *Virch Arch [A].* 1990; 416:281–286.
14. Umlas J, Federman M, Crawford C, et al. Spindle cell pseudotumor due to mycobacterium avium-intracellulare in patients with acquired immunodeficiency syndrome (AIDS). Positive staining for cytoskeleton filaments. *Am J Surg Pathol.* 1991; 15:1181–1187.
15. Chen KT. Mycobacterial spindle cell pseudotumor of lymph nodes. *Am J Surg Pathol.* 1992; 16:276–281.
16. Wolf DA, Wu CD, Medeiros LJ. Mycobacterial pseudotumors of lymph node. A report of two cases diagnosed at the time of intraoperative consultation using touch imprint preparations. *Arch Pathol Lab Med.* 1995; 119:811–814.
17. Spence MR, Abrutyn E. Syphilis and infection with the human immunodeficiency virus. *Ann Intern Med.* 1987; 107:587.
18. Tramont EC. Syphilis in the AIDS era. *N Engl J Med.* 1987; 316:1600–1601.
19. Johns DR, Tierney M, Felsenstein D. Alteration in the natural history of neurosyphilis by concurrent infection with the human immunodeficiency virus. *N Engl J Med.* 1987; 316:1569–1572.
20. Berry CD, Hooten TM, Collier AC, et al. Neurologic relapse after benzathine penicillin therapy for secondary syphilis in a patient with HIV infection. *N Engl J Med.* 1987; 316:1587–1589.
21. Smith ME, Canalis RF. Otologic manifestations of AIDS: The otosyphilis connection. *Laryngoscope.* 1989; 99:365–372.
22. Klein RS, Harris CA, Small CB, et al. Oral candidiasis in high-risk patients as the initial manifestation of the acquired immune deficiency syndrome. *N Engl J Med.* 1984; 311:354–358.
23. Lang W, Anderson RE, Perkins H, et al. Clinical, immunologic, and serologic findings in men at risk for acquired immunodeficiency syndrome. *JAMA.* 1987; 257:326–330.
24. Pantaleo G, Cohen O, Graziosi C, et al. Immunopathogenesis of human immunodeficiency virus infection. In: DeVita VT, Hellman S, Rosenberg SA, eds. *Acquired Immunodeficiency Syndrome—Etiology, Diagnosis, Treatment, and Prevention.* Philadelphia: Lippincott-Raven; 1997:75–88.
25. Ewing EP, Chandler FW, Spira TJ, et al. Primary lymph node pathology in AIDS and AIDS-related lymphadenopathy. *Arch Pathol Lab Med.* 1985; 109:977–981.
26. Öst Å, Baroni CD, Biberfeld P, et al. Lymphadenopathy in HIV infection: Histological classification and staging. *Acta Pathol Microbiol Immunol Scand.* 1989; 8(suppl):7–15.
27. Barzan L, Carbone A, Tirelli U, et al. Nasopharyngeal lymphatic tissue in patients infected with human immunodeficiency virus: A prospective clinicopathologic study. *Arch Otolaryngol Head Neck Surg.* 1990; 116:928–931.
28. Shahab I, Osborne BM, Butler JJ. Nasopharyngeal lymphoid tissue masses in patients with human immunodeficiency virus-1: Histologic findings and clinical correlation. *Cancer.* 1994; 74:3083–3088.

29. Stern JC, Lin PT, Lucente FE. Benign nasopharyngeal masses and human immunodeficiency virus infection. *Arch Otolaryngol Head Neck Surg.* 1990; 116:206–208.

30. Wenig BM, Thompson LDR, Frankel SS, et al. Lymphoid changes of the nasopharynx and tonsils that are indicative of human immunodeficiency virus infection: A clinicopathologic study of 12 cases. *Am J Surg Pathol.* 1996; 20:572–587.

31. Burke AP, Benson W, Ribas JL, et al. Postmortem localization of HIV-1 RNA by in situ hybridization in lymphoid tissues of intravenous drug addicts who died unexpectedly. *Am J Pathol.* 1993; 142:1701–1713.

32. Frankel SS, Wenig BM, Burke AP, et al. Active HIV-1 replication in dendritic cells and syncytia at the mucosal surface of the pharyngeal tonsil (adenoids). *Science.* 1996; 272:115–117.

33. Wood GS. The immunohistology of lymph nodes in HIV infection: A review. In: Rotterdam H, ed. *Progress in AIDS Pathology.* Philadelphia: Field and Wood; 1990:25–32.

34. Pantaleo G, Graziosi C, Fauci AS. The immunopathogenesis of human immunodeficiency virus infection. *N Engl J Med.* 1993; 328:327–335.

35. Biberfeld P, Chayt KJ, Marselle LM, et al. HTLV-III expression in infected lymph nodes and relevance to pathogenesis of lymphadenopathy. *Am J Pathol.* 1986; 125:436–442.

36. Fox CH, Tenner-Rácz K, Rácz P, et al. Lymphoid germinal centers are reservoirs of human immunodeficiency virus type 1 RNA. *J Infect Dis.* 1991; 164:1051–1057.

37. Racz P, Tenner-Racz K, Schmidt H. Follicular dendritic cells in HIV-induced lymphadenopathy and AIDS. *Acta Pathol Microbiol Immunol Scand.* 1989; 8(suppl):16–23.

38. Chaudhry R, Akhtar S, Lucente FE, Kim DS. Large oral ulcers leading to destruction of the tonsils in patients with AIDS. *Otolaryngol Head Neck Surg.* 1996; 114:474–478.

39. Auclair P, Ellis G. HIV-associated salivary gland disease (multiple lymphoepithelial cysts of the parotid gland). In: Rosai J, Sobin LH, eds. *Atlas of Tumor Pathology/Tumors of the Salivary Glands.* Fascicle 17; third series. Washington, DC: Armed Forces Institute of Pathology; 1996:430–433.

40. Klassen MK, Lewin-Smith M, Frankel SS, Nelson AM. Pathology of human immunodeficiency virus infection: Noninfectious conditions. *Ann Diagn Pathol.* 1997; 1:57–64.

41. Bernier JL, Bhaskar SN. Lymphoepithelial lesions of salivary glands: Histogenesis and classification based on 168 cases. *Cancer.* 1958; 11:1156–1179.

42. Labouyrie E, Merlio JP, Beylot-Barry M, et al. Human immunodeficiency virus type 1 replication within cystic lymphoepithelial lesion of the salivary gland *Am J Clin Pathol.* 1993; 100: 41–46.

43. Ulirsh RC, Jaffe ES. Sjögren's syndrome–like illness associated with the acquired immunodeficiency syndrome-related complex. *Hum Pathol.* 1987; 18:1063–1068.

44. LeBoit PE, Berger TG, Egbert BM, et al. Bacillary angiomatosis. The histopathology and differential diagnosis of a pseudoneoplastic infection in patients with human immunodeficiency virus infection. *Am J Surg Pathol.* 1989; 13:909–920.

45. Batsakis JG, Ro JY, Frauenhoffer EE. Bacillary angiomatosis. *Ann Otol Rhinol Laryngol.* 1995; 104:668–672.

46. Cockerell CJ, Webster GF, Whitlow MA, Friedman-Kien AE. Epithelioid angiomatosis: A distinct vascular disorder in patients with the acquired immunodeficiency syndrome or AIDS-related complex. *Lancet.* 1987; 2:654–656.

47. Centers for Disease Control. Revision of the case definition of acquired immunodeficiency syndrome for national reporting—United States. *Ann Intern Med.* 1985; 103:402–403.

48. Kaplan LD. HIV-associated lymphoma. *AIDS Clin Rev.* 1997–1998; 349–373.

49. Goldberg AN: Kaposis's sarcoma of the head and neck in acquired immunodeficiency syndrome. *Am J Otolaryngol.* 1993; 14:5–14.

50. Orenstein JM, Alkan S, Blauvelt A, et al. Visualization of human herpesvirus type 8 in Kaposi's sarcoma by light and transmission electron microscopy. *AIDS.* 1997; 11:F35–F45.

51. Gottlieb GJ, Ackerman AB. Kaposi's sarcoma: An extensively disseminated form in young homosexual men. *Hum Pathol.* 1982; 13:882–892.

52. Stafford ND, Herdman RCD, Forster S, et al. Kaposi's sarcoma of the head and neck in patients with AIDS. *J Laryngol Otol* 1989; 103:379–382.

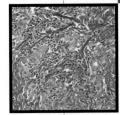

Fine-Needle Aspiration Biopsy

■ L E S T E R J . L A Y F I E L D

Fine-needle aspiration (FNA) biopsy has become an accepted method for the work-up of many palpable and radiographically demonstrable lesions within the head and neck. FNA biopsy is the preferred technique for the evaluation of cervical lymphadenopathy in patients with known or suspected head and neck squamous carcinoma primary tumors. In this clinical setting, the purpose of FNA cytology is to exclude or establish the diagnosis of metastatic squamous cell carcinoma. Under these circumstances, contraindications are few, and diagnostic accuracy is high. The finding of a positive aspirate is of great clinical importance in determining prognosis and the direction of future therapy. FNA biopsy can also be used for the work-up of cervical lymphadenopathy in young patients. Here, the diagnos-

tic aim is to confirm the clinical suspicion of reactive lymphadenopathy and to support the clinician's decision to follow such patients expectantly for resolution of the lymphadenopathy.

The second major use of needle aspiration cytology in the head and neck area is for the evaluation of thyroid nodules. In this case, FNA is used to increase the percentage of surgically removed nodules that contain carcinoma, rather than hyperplastic or degenerative conditions (multinodular goiter). FNA is the most reliable technique currently available for the nonoperative distinction of benign from malignant thyroid nodules. Judicious use of needle aspiration of thyroid nodules can significantly reduce the number of operative procedures involving the thyroid.

FNA has been utilized for the investigation of other lesions arising within the head and neck. In some cases, these lesions are aspirated inadvertently because of their misidentification as cervical lymphadenopathy. A variety of lesions occurring within the lateral neck can be confused clinically with cervical lymph nodes. Schwannomas, carotid body tumors, branchial cleft cysts, and other less common neoplasms have all been aspirated because of a clinical desire to exclude metastatic squamous cell carcinoma. Hence, familiarity with the cytologic appearance of these lesions is important for anyone interpreting FNA smears derived from the head and neck.

Because a wide variety of reactive and reparative processes, cysts, and neoplasms occurs within the head and neck, diagnosis by FNA biopsy is best accomplished when the differential diagnosis is narrowed by establishing sets of differential diagnoses based on the anatomic site of aspiration. In this manner, site-specific, reasonably limited differential diagnoses can be used when evaluating smears. Such anatomically based divisions include the (1) lateral neck, including the cervical lymph node chain; (2) thyroid; (3) salivary glands; (4) nasopharynx; (5) oral cavity; (6) nose and paranasal sinuses; (7) skin; and (8) orbit. In the following sections, the cytopathology of the most common or diagnostically important lesions in the first six of these categories are discussed.

TECHNIQUE

Although the technique of FNA is theoretically simple, it requires practice to develop and maintain the necessary expertise for consistency in cellular sampling and yield. Several modifications of the technique have been developed over the years, but the basic approach has remained the same. Only two significant variations in the technique are widely used. In one, FNA is performed without vacuum aspiration. In the second, more traditional methodology, a syringe is used to apply a small vacuum when extracting the tissue fragments. Both techniques utilize 22- to 25-gauge needles as the basic biopsy instrument. When using the traditional method, a syringe holder greatly facilitates the application of suction. A variety of these are commercially available.

Traditional Approach

In the traditional technique, the nodule of interest is palpated prior to the area being cleaned with 95% ethanol–soaked pads. Following this aseptic precaution, the nodule is fixed between the index and middle fingers of one hand (Fig. 5–1). The skin is drawn tensely over the nodule for the purpose of fixation. The needle is rapidly introduced through

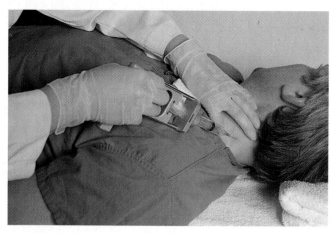

FIGURE 5–1 The lesion is fixed with the index and middle fingers. Sample cells are loosened by back-and-forth strokes of the needle and aspirated into the needle hub with negative pressure.

the skin and into the nodule, at which point 10 to 20 rapid back-and-forth strokes are made within the lesion. During this time, 2 to 3 cc of negative pressure is applied via the syringe to optimize extraction of tissue. After about 10 seconds of manipulation, or when material appears within the needle hub, the aspiration is stopped, the vacuum is released, and the needle is quickly withdrawn from the patient. Hemostasis is achieved with gauze and local pressure. At this point, the needle is removed from the syringe, air is drawn into the syringe, the needle is reattached, and the material is expressed onto a clean glass slide. A second slide is gently placed over the top of the first slide, compressing the sample (Fig. 5–2). The second slide is gently and rapidly brought down to the end of the first slide in a single stoke, producing a uniform smear (Fig. 5–3). If the material is to be stained by the Papanicolaou technique, the slide is immediately placed in 95% ethanol. If the material is to be stained by a Romanovsky technique, it is allowed to air-dry.

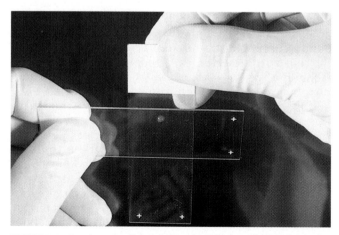

FIGURE 5–2 Aspirated material is placed on a glass slide and a second slide is laid on top.

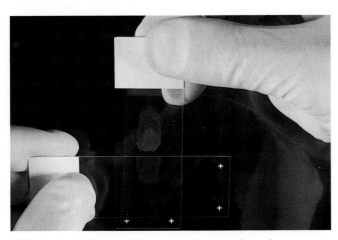

FIGURE 5–3 The two slides are gently pressed together using a smooth, downward, smearing stroke.

Modified Approach

In the modified technique, no syringe is used for obtaining a sample. Only a 22- or 25-gauge needle is utilized, which is placed into the nodule. Rapid excursions are made, as described earlier, and the needle is withdrawn. Material is then expelled onto the glass slide using a syringe, as described for the traditional technique. Smears are prepared in the same manner as described before.

Much controversy exists concerning the optimal staining method for fine-needle aspirates. Both the Papanicolaou technique and the Romanovsky technique have their ardent supporters, and each has significant advantages. The Papanicolaou technique optimizes the cytopathologist's ability to examine the nuclei, whereas the Romanovsky technique optimizes the study of intracellular and extracellular substances. The air-dried Romanovsky method appears to be superior for the investigation of lymphoid lesions and lesions of the salivary gland. The Papanicolaou technique is probably superior for the investigation of squamous lesions. FNA diagnosis can be optimized by using both the Papanicolaou and Romanovsky staining methods. By obtaining two to three aspirates per visit, sufficient material for both techniques can usually be obtained.

DIAGNOSTIC ACCURACY

The diagnostic accuracy of FNA cytology is site-specific and varies considerably with the location and type of lesion being investigated. The diagnostic accuracy of FNA biopsy for the study of cervical lymphadenopathy and thyroid and salivary gland nodules has been most widely studied and reported in the literature.[1] Needle aspiration of cervical lymphadenopathy appears to be highly accurate, with false-negative rates reported to be between 3.4% and 5%, and false-positive rates between 0% and 0.9%.[2–4]

In a study by Steel et al,[2] diagnosis of lymphoma by FNA biopsy was the most difficult, accounting for 15 (65%) of the 23 false-negative diagnoses in that series. The needle aspiration diagnosis of metastatic squamous carcinoma demonstrated a considerably higher degree of accuracy.

FNA biopsy has been shown to be more accurate than physical or radiographic examination in the diagnosis of salivary gland nodules,[5,6] and appears to be at least as accurate as frozen section for the diagnosis of salivary gland neoplasms.[5,7,8] In experienced hands, FNA biopsy of salivary gland nodules has a sensitivity of 90% or greater and a specificity of approximately 95.[5,7,9–13] Sampling error appears to be the most significant cause of false-negative diagnosis.[11,14] Because of sampling errors, negative results from FNA biopsy of suspicious masses should result in reaspiration or surgical biopsy. Certain lesions of the salivary gland, including mucoepidermoid carcinoma, chronic sialadenitis, and malignant lymphoma, are associated with an increased rate of inaccuracy.[5,7]

Needle aspiration cytology has been widely accepted as the preferred diagnostic technique for investigation of thyroid nodules. The false-negative rate for FNA biopsy of the thyroid has been reported to be between 5% and 10%.[15–18] The false-positive rate varies from 0.5% to 1%.[15] Approximately 10% of FNA specimens are unsatisfactory for diagnosis.[15,19]

Needle aspiration cytology of head and neck lesions is a safe procedure, with few complications being reported. Localized hemorrhage and infection do occur infrequently, but these appear to be of limited clinical importance. Rarely, the extent of bleeding has compromised vital structures, but in more than 3000 aspirates of the head and neck, the author has not personally experienced this complication. Aspiration of a carotid body tumor appears to be the most hazardous needle aspiration procedure in the head and neck. Complications following FNA biopsy of the carotid body include local hematoma, resulting in compression of vascular structures and a potential for carotid artery emboli.[20] In cases of suspected carotid body tumor, angiography should be performed in an attempt to document the classic vascular pattern. FNA should be carried out only when a neoplasm is suspected and angiographic findings are not diagnostic.

CYTOMORPHOLOGY OF SELECTED LESIONS OF THE LATERAL NECK

Branchial Cleft Cysts

Branchial cleft cysts are benign cystic lesions that represent malformations of the branchial cleft apparatus. They are relatively common, with most occurring in the lateral neck along the anterior portion of the sternocleidomastoid muscle. However, they may also be found around the external ear, auditory canal, and in the area of the parotid gland. Their importance to the aspiration cytologist is predominantly in the requirement that they be distinguished from well-differentiated cystic squamous cell carcinomas with which they may be confused both clinically and cytologically.

Upon aspiration, branchial cleft cysts yield 1 mL or more of turbid or cloudy, straw-colored to brown fluid. Golden yellow discoloration secondary to cholesterol crystals is seen in some cases. Secondary hemorrhage with bloody discoloration of the cyst fluid occurs following traumatic aspiration.

In most cases, the smears obtained are hypocellular and contain a mixture of anucleate and keratotic superficial cells, occasional parakeratotic squamous cells, and a small number of foamy or pigment-laden histiocytes (Fig. 5–4).[21–23] The squamous component is usually sparse but may be cellular. The anucleate squamous cells will have a glassy "robin's egg" blue cytoplasm (on Giemsa staining) and, frequently, ghost-like outlines of nuclei. The parakeratotic cells have small, hyperchromatic nuclei with smooth nuclear membranes (Fig. 5–5). In general, nuclear atypia is absent. With Papanicolaou staining, the keratotic cells demonstrate cytoplasmic orangeophilia, but the cytoplasmic staining of these cells is often less intense than that seen in cervical/vaginal preparations. The parakeratotic cell nuclei stain deeply with the Papanicolaou method, demonstrating a dense, hyperchromatic chromatin and smooth nuclear membranes. Mitotic activity is not seen in the squamous component.

The smears usually contain a small number of histiocytes with a round or polygonal shape and moderately abundant cytoplasm. The nuclei are bland and reniform or oval in shape. Nucleoli may be seen in these cells. The cytoplasm may contain

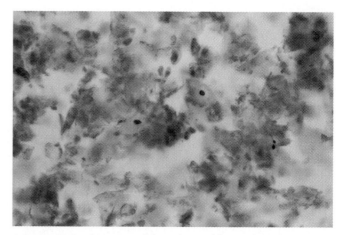

FIGURE 5–5 Squamous debris obtained from a branchial cleft cyst. Numerous anucleate keratinizing squamous cells are present, along with several parakeratotic cells with small hyperchromatic nuclei (Papanicolaou, × 132).

abundant granular material which, on Papanicolaou staining, has a golden appearance that is consistent with hemosiderin. This pigment stains deep blue with Romanovsky-based stains. Occasionally, lymphoid cells are admixed with the squamous cells and histiocytes. This component is usually not prominent and is composed of small mature lymphocytes.

Occasionally, branchial cleft cysts will show inflammatory or degenerative changes with atypia in the squamous lining (Fig. 5–6); in these cases, significant nuclear atypia may be seen in the parakeratotic element. In general, these smears are dominated by anucleate squamous cells, but atypical cells, including metaplastic elements, may closely resemble the cells of well-differentiated cystic squamous cell carcinomas.

Branchial cleft cysts and epidermal inclusion cysts may overlap cytologically.[21–23] Although differentia-

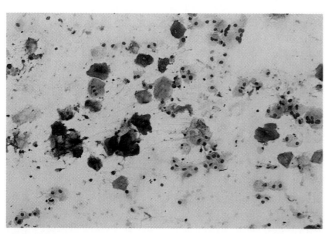

FIGURE 5–4 Aspirated material from a branchial cleft cyst shows numerous pigment-laden and foamy histiocytes (Diff-Quik, × 33).

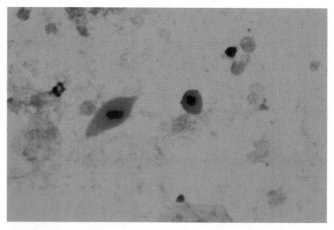

FIGURE 5–6 Keratinizing squamous cells obtained from a branchial cleft cyst. These cells show slightly enlarged, hyperchromatic nuclei representing reactive atypia (Diff-Quik, × 198).

tion is not clinically important, it can be achieved by recognizing the looser, more watery appearance of the branchial cleft cyst or by noting the presence of foamy or pigmented histiocytes in material obtained from branchial cleft cysts. The material in epidermal inclusion cysts is usually of greater cellularity, with abundant, superficial, anucleated squamous cells showing marked overlapping. The clinical findings also differ, in that branchial cleft cysts lie deeper within the neck than do epidermal inclusion cysts. The latter occur within the skin and subcutaneous fat.

Pilomatricomas (calcifying epithelioma of Malherbe) that are sampled by FNA biopsy can be misinterpreted as malignant neoplasms. Pilomatricomas display sheets of small, round, basaloid cells with hyperchromatic nuclei, scant cytoplasm, and high nucleocytoplasmic ratios. In the background, keratin debris and granular material often simulate tumor necrosis. Atypical squamous cells, foreign body giant cells, inflammatory cells, calcium deposits, and ghost cells occur in varying numbers. The presence of basaloid cells and ghost cells in an FNA specimen obtained from a young patient should raise the possibility of pilomatricoma.

The most important distinction to be made in this differential diagnosis is between branchial cleft cysts and well-differentiated cystic squamous cell carcinomas.[24] Well-differentiated squamous cell carcinomas arising within Waldeyer's ring may metastasize to the neck, where they form cystic deposits. These may be difficult to distinguish from branchial cleft cysts by cytologic examination. Differentiation is generally facilitated by recognition of the greater degrees of nuclear atypia seen in the carcinomas. Although the parakeratotic and metaplastic cells of branchial cleft cysts may have nuclear hyperchromasia, these cells are generally small. The nuclei, although hyperchromatic, have smooth nuclear membranes and the nuclear/cytoplasmic ratio is within the normal range. Cells from squamous cell carcinomas show increased degrees of nuclear atypia, with at least some cells demonstrating clearly malignant features, including significantly increased nuclear/cytoplasmic ratios, nuclear membrane irregularities, and marked degrees of hyperchromasia (Fig. 5–7). In branchial cleft cysts, the atypical elements are usually few in number and represent only a small proportion of the total cellularity. The atypical elements in squamous cell carcinomas are more numerous. A distinction between the two is also aided by a careful search for the more immature and atypical elements present in most squamous cell carcinomas. These latter cells do not demonstrate keratinization and have a considerably higher nuclear/cytoplasmic ratio than do branchial cleft cysts. The higher cellularity of squamous cell carcinomas, the overall increased degree of nuclear atypia, the presence of necrotic debris, and the occurrence of rare, immature, atypical nonkeratinized cells all favor the diagnosis of squamous cell carcinoma over that of branchial cleft cyst.

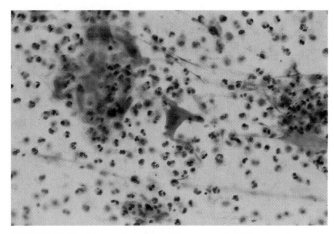

FIGURE 5–7 Material aspirated from a well-differentiated squamous cell carcinoma. The cells show individual cell keratinization with hyperchromatic, somewhat irregular nuclei. Numerous neutrophils are present in the backgound (Papanicolaou, × 132).

Cervical Lymph Nodes

In most cases, FNA biopsy of the cervical lymph nodes is performed to establish or exclude the diagnosis of metastatic carcinoma. Most metastases originate from squamous primary lesions within the head and neck. The pattern of metastatic spread is somewhat predictive of the site of origin. Establishment of metastatic disease within the cervical lymph node chain by FNA biopsy has significant prognostic value, as well as therapeutic implications, so careful study of all enlarged cervical lymph nodes for metastatic deposits is warranted.

The cytologic features of lymph nodes containing metastatic squamous cell carcinoma vary with the degree of differentiation[24] present in the carcinomas, as well as the percentage of nodal replacement. Although most metastases associated with cervical lymphadenopathy replace the bulk of the lymph node, some lymph nodes will be seen, on FNA biopsy, to contain microscopic metastases. Smears from these nodes are dominated by a mixed lymphoid infiltrate or acute inflammation in which are scattered rare to modest numbers of clusters and individual squamous cells (see Fig. 5–7). A thorough search at low, medium, and high power is necessary to detect these deposits. Metastatic malignant melanoma may also result in cervical adenopathy that is detectable by FNA biopsy.

Lymph node aspirates that are obtained to exclude metastatic squamous cell carcinoma should be scanned at low power for cohesive groups of cells. Such groups generally represent metastatic carcinoma, but at times, may correspond to follicular center fragments or aggregates of histiocytes. Medium- and high-power microscopic study will confirm or disprove the epithelial nature of these cells. Low-power study of Papanicolaou-stained material is helpful in identifying rare individual dyskeratotic

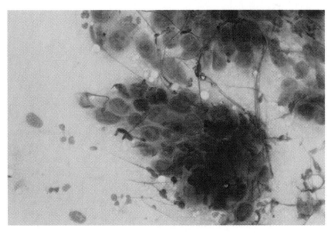

FIGURE 5–8 Clusters and small sheets of atypical squamous cells obtained from a poorly differentiated squamous cell carcinoma. Note the tight nuclear overlapping and marked nuclear hyperchromasia and atypia (Diff-Quik, × 198).

cells. These cells are best appreciated with the Papanicolaou staining technique because they have a bright orange color, which contrasts with the background green-blue lymphoid cells. Most metastatic squamous cell carcinomas arising within the head and neck display a keratinizing morphology (see Fig. 5–7), facilitating their distinction from other metastatic malignant lesions and lymphoma. Differentiation of well-differentiated squamous cell carcinomas from branchial cleft cysts may be difficult, but the presence of true nuclear anaplasia and less differentiated epithelial cells in the carcinomas should allow the distinction to be made.

Some metastatic squamous cell carcinomas will be poorly differentiated and may appear as sheets or loose groupings of cells with occasional solitary neoplastic cells (Fig. 5–8). Nuclear crowding is usually prominent. The cells are more irregular than those seen in well-differentiated squamous cell carcinoma, and have a higher nuclear/cytoplasmic ratio and large, pleomorphic nuclei containing granular chromatin and large nucleoli. These lesions may be difficult to distinguish from metastatic adenocarcinoma, but the cells of squamous carcinoma usually have a more irregular shape than those of adenocarcinoma. In addition, the cytoplasm of squamous cell carcinomas has a rigid metaplastic appearance. Despite these differences, it may be impossible to distinguish some poorly differentiated adenocarcinomas from poorly differentiated squamous cell carcinomas.

Deposits of malignant melanoma may occur within lymph nodes of the cervical chain. The cytologic findings in metastatic malignant melanoma vary widely and have been discussed in several publications.[25–27] In general, metastases from malignant melanoma appear in aspiration smears as isolated or loosely cohesive cells displaying marked nuclear pleomorphism. The cells often have a plasmacytoid configuration (Fig. 5–9) with huge eccentric nuclei and moderate to abundant amounts of cytoplasm. These cells are most frequently noncohesive and may be difficult to distinguish from surrounding lymphoid elements. Marked variation in cell size and a high degree of nuclear anaplasia are clues to the nature of these cells. Melanoma may assume one of several other morphologic characteristics in lymph node deposits, including a spindle cell, small cell (lymphocyte-like), epithelioid or giant cell pleomorphic appearance. When such shapes are present, immunohistochemistry performed on Cytospin or cell block material to demonstrate the presence or absence of S-100 protein and melanoma-associated antigens using antibody HMB-45 can be immensely helpful in establishing a specific diagnosis.

Other neoplasms occasionally metastasize to the cervical chain, including prostatic and mammary adenocarcinomas. Prostatic adenocarcinoma appears cytologically as sheets of rather bland epithelial cells which may form gland-like groupings. The cytoplasm is generally modest in amount and surrounds round nuclei with small but distinctive nucleoli. Mitotic activity is low. Immunocytochemical demonstration of prostatic-specific antigen or prostatic acid phosphatase is helpful in confirming the diagnosis. Metastatic adenocarcinoma of the breast is more difficult to diagnose definitively. The cells of adenocarcinoma of the breast are round to slightly ovoid with scanty to modest amounts of cytoplasm and large hyperchromatic nuclei, often with distinct nucleoli. Magenta bodies are highly suggestive of a mammary origin and can be demonstrated with the May-Grünwald-Giemsa stain. The cytoplasmic inclusions probably represent a form of mucin.

LYMPHADENOPATHY SECONDARY TO PRIMARY LYMPHOPROLIFERATIVE PROCESSES

Cytologic diagnosis of lymphoproliferative lesions is more difficult than the diagnosis of metastatic carci-

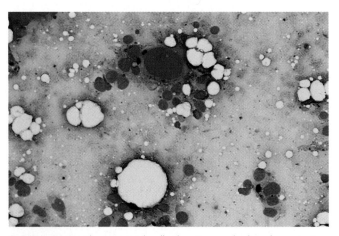

FIGURE 5–9 Plasmacytoid cells showing marked nuclear atypia, including rare giant cell forms. Occasional cells contain intracytoplasmic pigment. Such cells are common in melanomas (Diff-Quik, × 66).

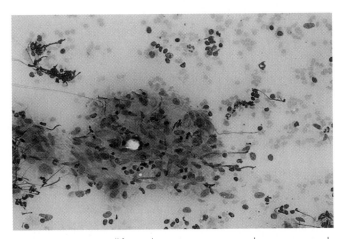

FIGURE 5–10 Well-formed, noncaseating granuloma composed of elongated epithelioid histiocytes with pale to granular cytoplasm. Scattered lymphocytes are present in the backgound (Diff-Quik, × 66).

noma.[2] Hence, a careful and systematic approach is necessary for accurate interpretation of lymphoid proliferations. Cytologic assessment of primary lymphadenopathies must take into consideration not only the cytology of the individual cells, but the mixture of cell types present, including the presence or absence of an orderly maturational sequence and architectural clues (cell aggregates) present in the smear.[28–30] Aspirates from lymph nodes should be studied at low, medium, and high power. Low-power examination is performed to assess the overall cellularity of the smear and the pattern of cell arrangement. Recognition of an isolated or aggregated cell pattern is important in distinguishing purely lymphoid reactions from either metastatic disease or granulomatous inflammation (Fig. 5–10). Medium-power examination is performed to evaluate the polymorphous or monomorphous nature of the cell population, to identify the presence or absence of occasional pleomorphic cells (Reed-Sternberg cells, giant cells of melanoma, or anaplastic carcinoma), to recognize the presence of certain cell types (eosinophils, neutrophils, and plasma cells), and finally, to confirm the presence or absence of necrosis or granulomata. In addition, medium-power examination is used to divide the lymphoid population into one of four categories represented by: (1) predominantly small cell population; (2) mixed cell population with an ordered sequence of maturation; (3) mixed cell population lacking a sequence of maturation; and (4) lymphoid population composed of predominantly or exclusively large cells. High-power examination is performed to confirm the morphologic categorization of the individual cells and to more closely assess their nuclear characteristics. Under × 40 magnification or oil immersion, hematoxylin-eosin-stained or Papanicolaou-stained preparations should be studied for the presence of nuclear convolutions or cleaves within the lymphoid cell nuclei. The chromatin distribution and the presence of nucleoli should also be assessed. High-

power examination can document the presence of differentiation within nonlymphoid cell types, particularly the presence of melanin pigment in examples of melanoma, keratinization or the presence of intracytoplasmic mucin in metastatic carcinomas.

While a complete discussion of the cytologic appearances of various benign and malignant lymphoproliferative processes is beyond the scope of this chapter, the most common entities are described. Preliminary studies have found good correlations between the cytologic and histologic features based on the Revised European–American Classification of Lymphoid Neoplasms (REAL). However, more studies are needed.

REACTIVE LYMPHOID HYPERPLASIA

Aspirates from benign hyperplastic lymph nodes vary in cellularity.[28–30] The smear cellularity depends on the degree of hyperplasia present. The more florid the hyperplasia, the higher the cellularity of the smears obtained. Aspirates from lymph nodes showing mild reactive hyperplasia are usually of low to moderate cellularity. Most of the cells are small to medium-sized lymphocytes; less than 5% of cells are of large cell morphology. Tingible body macrophages are present in small numbers. Follicular center fragments are often present, as are plasma cells and plasmacytoid lymphocytes. The constellation of a mixed lymphoid infiltrate dominated by small mature lymphocytes, occasional tingible body macrophages, and follicular center fragments is characteristic of mild hyperplasia (Fig. 5–11). As the hyperplasia increases in degree, overall cellularity and the percentage of large cells increase. In moderate hyperplasia, the smears are generally highly cellular, with between 5% and 20% of the component lymphocytes being of a large cell morphology (Figs. 5–12 and 5–13). Despite this relative prominence of large cells, the lymphoid population shows an orderly maturation from small mature lymphocytes

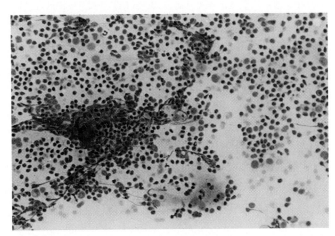

FIGURE 5–11 Mixed lymphoid infiltrate demonstrating an orderly maturational sequence in cell sizes, along with occasional tingible body macrophages (Diff-Quik, × 66).

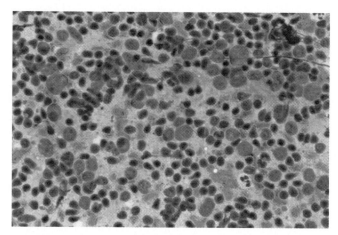

FIGURE 5–12   Material aspirated from a lymph node showing moderate hyperplasia. The lymphocytes show an orderly maturation, with cells ranging from small, mature lymphocytes to immunoblasts (Diff-Quik, × 132).

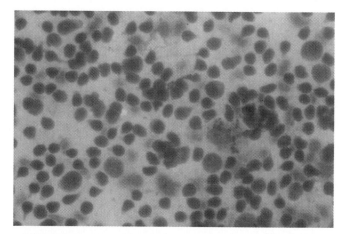

FIGURE 5–14   Mixed lymphoid population surrounding a tingible body macrophage. The tingible body macrophage has abundant pale cytoplasm in which are dispersed dark nuclear fragments (Diff-Quik, × 198).

through immunoblasts to plasma cells (see Figs. 5–12 and 5–13). Tingible body macrophages are common (Fig. 5–14) and follicular center fragments (Fig. 5–15) are present. In marked hyperplasia, cellularity is universally high with a predominance of large cells, generally representing more than 25% of the lymphoid population. The population is polymorphous with an orderly maturational sequence. Tingible body macrophages are plentiful. There is a range of plasmacytoid cells, including mature plasma cells, and follicular center fragments are present in significant numbers although they may be hard to resolve owing to the heavy surrounding cellularity. At times, the cellularity may be so high that cells overlap or closely abut each other, making evaluation of cytoplasmic features difficult.

Cytologic findings in tuberculosis and many fungal infections are similar. In general, both necrosis and fragments of granulomata are seen. At times, only necrosis may be apparent, and a careful search may be necessary before fragments of granulomata or individual histiocytes are seen. The epithelioid histiocytes of the granulomata appear as elongated, spindle-shaped cells with bland nuclei. These cells frequently overlap and form tight clusters (see Fig. 5–10). In tuberculosis and many fungal infections, multinucleated histiocytic giant cells are seen and may be found engulfing organisms. Culture of aspirated material, as well as special staining techniques, may be helpful in establishing a specific diagnosis. Gupta et al[31] have demonstrated a relationship between the presence of necrosis, epithelioid histiocytes, and inflammation and the likelihood of obtaining positive cultures and the presence of clinically documentable tuberculosis.

Sarcoidosis can be recognized by FNA biopsy.[32] In

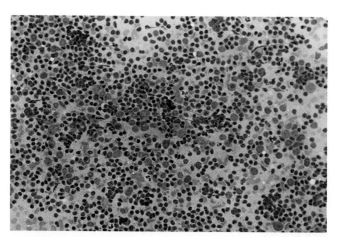

FIGURE 5–13   Lower-power view of moderate hyperplasia showing a mixed lymphoid infiltrate along with aggregates of histiocytes and follicular center fragments (Diff-Quik, × 66).

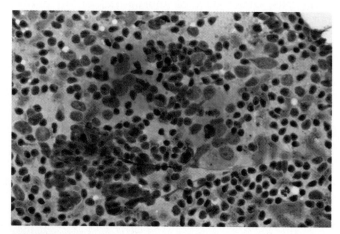

FIGURE 5–15   Follicular center cell fragment in an aspirate obtained from a patient with follicular hyperplasia involving the lymph nodes. Note the mixture of lymphocytes and histiocytes (Diff-Quik, × 132).

most cases, many tightly cohesive granulomata will be seen in the aspirated material. These are made up of spindle-shaped, epithelioid histiocytes with pale cytoplasm and moderately dark, elongated nuclei. These epithelioid histiocytes are tightly clustered and lie in a background of mature lymphocytes and plasma cells. Necrosis is usually absent in smears obtained from cases of sarcoidosis.

Material aspirated from lymph nodes affected by cat-scratch disease has a variable appearance depending on the stage of the disease. In the early phase, only a marked follicular hyperplasia is seen, similar to that described for reactive lymph nodes. As the disease progresses, granulomatous elements appear, with aggregates of epithelioid histocytes being characteristic. In later stages, the smears contain prominent areas of necrosis along with clusters of epithelioid histiocytes and, often, aggregates of neutrophils.

The differential diagnosis of reactive lymphadenopathy includes lymph nodes partially replaced by metastatic carcinoma, metastatic melanoma (particularly of the small-cell type) and lymphomas of both Hodgkin's and non-Hodgkin's type. Careful low- and medium-power evaluation, by identifying aggregates of cohesive atypical cells, is most helpful in establishing the presence of metastatic disease. Confirmation of the epithelial nature of these cells is then made at medium or high power. Care must be exercised in distinguishing follicular center fragments and granulomata from true epithelial cell aggregates. Although most malignant melanomas metastatic to the lymph nodes are characterized by highly pleomorphic, polygonal or spindle-shaped cells and anaplastic giant cells, occasionally, they present a more uniform population of plasmacytoid cells. These may closely resemble lymphocytes. The identification of melanin pigment and rare bizarre cells, as well as the immunohistochemical demonstration of melanoma specific antigen or S-100 protein, is helpful in the cytologic diagnosis of metastatic melanoma. Reactive lymph nodes are best distinguished cytologically from non-Hodgkin's lymphomas by recognizing the mixed cell population with a directed maturational sequence in the former, which differs from the monomorphous or abnormally stratified lymphoid population in the latter. In addition, follicular center fragments and tingible body macrophages in the setting of a mixed lymphoid population support the diagnosis of reactive hyperplasia. The differentiation of Hodgkin's disease from reactive lymphoid hyperplasia can be extremely difficult or impossible. Careful study at low and medium power to identify bizarre cells (Reed-Sternberg cells and their variants) is critical. Other clues that are helpful in distinguishing Hodgkin's disease from reactive adenopathy include the absence of tingible body macrophages in most cases of Hodgkin's disease and the prominence of eosinophils and plasma cells in many cases of Hodgkin's disease. When doubt exists as to the nature of a lymphoid proliferation, excisional biopsy is mandatory.

WELL-DIFFERENTIATED LYMPHOCYTIC LYMPHOMA

Aspirates obtained from well-differentiated lymphocytic lymphoma are usually of high cellularity with monomorphous populations of small, round lymphocytes. The lymphoid cells are slightly larger than mature lymphocytes and have a coarsely clumped nuclear chromatin. The chromatin may show beading along the nuclear membrane when studied under oil immersion after staining with hematoxylin-eosin or Papanicolaou stain. When proliferation centers are not present, the hallmark of this lymphoma is monotony of the cell population (Fig. 5–16). When growth centers are present, a restricted range of cell sizes is seen. Most of the cells are small lymphocytes, but there is a continuum of cells, with some larger forms being present. These larger cells have a finer, less deeply staining chromatin and may contain conspicuous nucleoli. An important finding in these cases is the absence of follicular center fragments and tingible body macrophages.

Well-differentiated lymphocytic lymphomas are difficult to distinguish from mild forms of hyperplasia, small cleaved cell lymphomas, and lymphocyte-predominant Hodgkin's disease. In general, examples of mild hyperplasia will have a greater range of cell sizes, tingible body macrophages, and follicular center fragments. Distinction from small cleaved cell lymphocytic lymphoma is less important clinically, but lymphomas of the small cleaved type will have a biphasic pattern and a more irregular chromatin distribution. Examination of aspirate under oil immersion after hematoxylin-eosin or Papanicolaou staining reveals the presence of cleaved cells in the smears from most of these lymphomas.

Lymphocyte-predominant Hodgkin's disease shows a greater range of cell types, including histio-

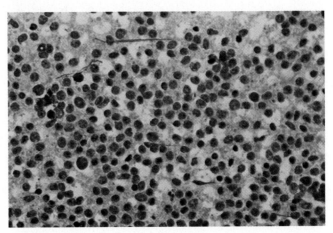

FIGURE 5-16 Monomorphous population of small, round lymphocytes obtained from a small cell lymphoma (Diff-Quik, × 132).

cytes and occasional Reed-Sternberg cell variants. When these latter cells are not seen, lymphocyte-predominant Hodgkin's disease may be very difficult, if not impossible, to distinguish from either mild hyperplasia or well-differentiated lymphocytic lymphoma. In such cases, flow cytometry or immunohistochemistry, performed to document lymphocyte cell type and clonality, may be helpful for diagnosis.

POORLY DIFFERENTIATED LYMPHOCYTIC LYMPHOMA

Poorly differentiated lymphocytic lymphomas (lymphoma, small cleaved type) are characterized, on FNA smears, by a moderate to high degree of cellularity. Most of the cells are small lymphocytes that are about 1.5 times the size of a mature lymphocyte. There is a bimorphic cell distribution within the lymphoid population of small, darkly staining cells and a lesser number of larger cells, which are approximately twice the size of a mature lymphocyte. Occasionally, the small cell component will form tight, grape-like clusters. Examination of material under oil immersion after Papanicolaou or hematoxylin-eosin staining will reveal some cells to have distinct nuclear folds or cleaves (Fig. 5–17). Low- and medium-power examination discloses an absence of tingible body macrophages and follicular center fragments.

Poorly differentiated lymphocytic lymphoma must be distinguished from mild hyperplasia, well-differentiated lymphocytic lymphoma, and lymphoblastic lymphoma. Poorly differentiated lymphocytic lymphoma may be distinguished from mild hyperplasia by recognition of tingible body macrophages, follicular center fragments, and a maturational sequence in the latter. Well-differentiated lymphocytic lymphoma has a more monotonous cell population

and a more regular chromatin distribution than that seen in poorly differentiated lymphocytic lymphoma. Lymphoblastic lymphoma has a finer, more evenly distributed chromatin pattern than that seen in poorly differentiated lymphocytic lymphoma.

MIXED FOLLICULAR CENTER CELL LYMPHOMA

Mixed small and large cell follicular center cell lymphomas yield aspirates of high cellularity characterized by a mixture of large and small lymphoid cells. In general, the small cells predominate, whereas the large cell component forms a distinct and prominent subpopulation. The two populations may be discrete, without transitional forms, or intermediate forms may be present. Tingible body macrophages are generally absent. When aspirates stained with hematoxylin-eosin or Papanicolaou preparations are examined under oil immersion, the cells are found to have an irregular chromatin distribution, and many nuclei have irregular contours. Flow cytometric examination is helpful in that these lesions are of B-cell origin and demonstrate monoclonality for κ or λ light chains. In addition, these lymphomas are positive for CD19, CD20, or CD22.

Mixed large and small cell lymphomas must be distinguished from moderate or severe hyperplasia. These lymphomas lack the ordered maturational sequence seen in hyperplasia and also usually lack the tingible body macrophages and follicular center fragments that are characteristic of hyperplasia. The mixture of large and small lymphoid cells distinguishes these lymphomas from other common lymphomas, including well-differentiated lymphocytic lymphoma, poorly differentiated lymphocytic lymphoma, lymphoblastic lymphoma, and small non–cleaved cell lymphomas. Hodgkin's disease of mixed cellularity is distinguished from mixed large and small cell lymphoma by recognition of Reed-Sternberg cells and their variants in the former. In most cases, aspirates of mixed cellularity Hodgkin's disease will contain larger numbers of eosinophils and plasma cells than are seen in non-Hodgkin's lymphomas.

LARGE CELL LYMPHOMA

Cytologic material aspirated from large cell lymphomas is of variable, but generally abundant, cellularity. The cells are usually uniform in size but may show some variability. Lymphoglandular bodies (small cytoplasmic fragments) are prominent in the background. Most cells are noncohesive, but they may occasionally form small, loose aggregates. Moderate to abundant cytoplasm is present. The neoplastic cells are several times the size of a mature lymphocyte and have nuclei that often contain prominent nucleoli (Fig. 5–18).

Differentiation of large cell lymphomas from marked reactive hyperplasia is generally straightforward. Examples of florid hyperplasia display a

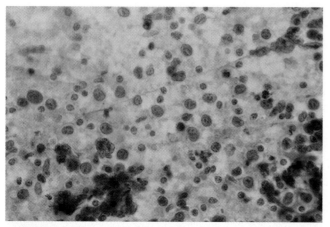

FIGURE 5–17 A relatively monomorphous population of slightly enlarged lymphoid cells. Some lymphoid cells have nuclear folds or clefts that are consistent with a small cleaved cell lymphoma (H&E, × 198).

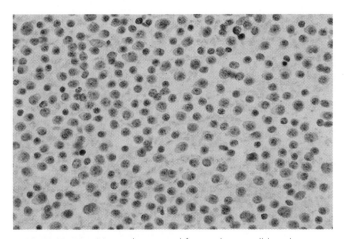

FIGURE 5-18 Material aspirated from a large cell lymphoma showing a rather uniform population of large, atypical lymphoid cells (Papanicolaou, × 132).

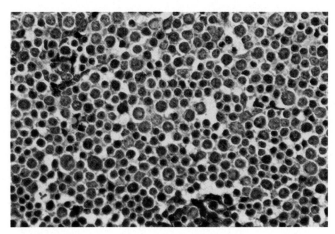

FIGURE 5-19 Monomorphous population of lymphoid cells obtained from a patient with Burkitt's lymphoma. Scattered throughout the smear of lymphocytes are tingible body macrophages (Diff-Quik, × 132).

range of cells with an orderly maturational sequence that is not seen in large cell lymphomas. In addition, florid hyperplasia has a smaller percentage of large cells than is seen in large cell lymphoma. Distinguishing large cell lymphoma from poorly differentiated carcinoma and melanoma is possible with the aid of immunohistochemistry and flow cytometry. FNA specimens of undifferentiated carcinomas usually contain cohesive malignant cells that mark with antibodies directed against low-molecular-weight keratins, whereas melanoma cells are mostly isolated and decorate with antibodies directed against melanoma specific antigen or S-100 protein. The presence of lymphoglandular bodies in the smear background strongly supports the diagnosis of lymphoma. Almost all lymphomas display a pattern of loose, single, noncohesive cells.

SMALL NON–CLEAVED CELL LYMPHOMA

Small non–cleaved cell lymphomas (Burkitt's and non-Burkitt's subtypes) are associated with aspirate smears of high cellularity. The lymphoid population is monotonous, with little variability in nuclear size or shape. Individual cells are approximately 2 to 2.5 times the size of a mature lymphocyte (Fig. 5–19). In general, the individual cells have a narrow rim of blue cytoplasm that may contain clear vacuoles that are best demonstrated on Diff-Quik or Giemsa staining. Examples of Burkitt's lymphoma frequently display multiple nucleoli associated with a clumped chromatin pattern that is best appreciated by oil immersion examination of specimens prepared with hematoxylin-eosin or Papanicolaou stain. Mitotic figures are numerous, and tingible body macrophages are abundant. Necrotic debris is commonly present in the backgound.

Because of their monotony of cell type, these lesions are easily distinguishable from reactive hyperplasias. Cell size and nuclear features aid in the

differentiation of Burkitt's and non-Burkitt's lymphoma from other lymphomas. Burkitt's lymphoma may be difficult to distinguish from nonlymphoid small round cell malignant tumors of childhood, particularly neuroblastoma and, less commonly, Ewing's sarcoma. Immunohistochemical staining for neuroendocrine markers and the protein product of the MIC2 oncogene aid in the diagnosis of neuroblastoma and Ewing's sarcoma, respectively.

LYMPHOBLASTIC LYMPHOMA

Examples of lymphoblastic lymphoma reveal a monomorphic population of lymphoid cells ranging in size from 1.5 to 2.5 times the size of a mature lymphocyte (Fig. 5–20). Occasionally, smaller cell forms are seen. The cells are round and frequently have convoluted nuclei. The nuclear convolutions are seen almost exclusively in Papanicolaou- or hematoxylin-eosin–stained material. Cytoplasm is scant. The nu-

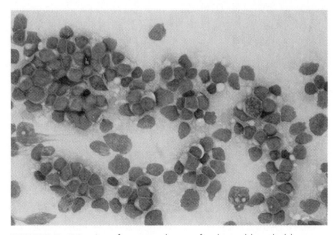

FIGURE 5-20 A uniform population of enlarged lymphoblastic cells characteristic of lymphoblastic lymphoma (Diff-Quik, × 132).

clear chromatin is powdery and nucleoli are absent or inconspicuous. Mitotic figures are numerous. Tingible body macrophages may be present.

Diagnosis of lymphoblastic lymphoma is greatly aided by either flow cytometric or immunocytochemical analysis. Most lymphoblastic lymphomas are of T-cell type, demonstrate TDT positivity, and may be positive for CD1A, CD3, CD5, CD7, and CD8.

The powdery appearance of the chromatin, the nuclear size, and the T-cell phenotype help distinguish this lymphoma from the other lymphoid proliferations. Lymphoblastic lymphoma may be differentiated from nonlymphoid small round cell neoplasms of childhood by using the markers discussed for Burkitt's lymphoma.

HODGKIN'S DISEASE

Diagnosis of Hodgkin's disease is achievable by FNA cytology, but subcategorization is relatively inaccurate.[33-36] In general, aspirates obtained from lymph nodes affected by Hodgkin's disease are of moderate or high cellularity. Most of the cells present are mature lymphocytes, although a maturational range of cell sizes is seen. Admixed with the lymphoid elements are lesser numbers of eosinophils and plasma cells. Rarely, epithelioid granulomata are identified. The diagnostic cell type is the Reed-Sternberg cell or one of its variants. Cytologic diagnosis of Hodgkin's disease depends on the recognition of this cell type in the appropriate background.

The classic Reed-Sternberg cell (Fig. 5–21) is binucleate with an "owl's eye" appearance. Each nucleus contains a large, often eosinophilic nucleolus which is approximately the size of a mature lymphocyte nucleus. The amount of cytoplasm is variable but generally moderate in amount. Reed-Sternberg cell variants are mononuclear with similar nuclear cytology; alternatively, the nuclei may be multilobulated (Fig. 5–22).

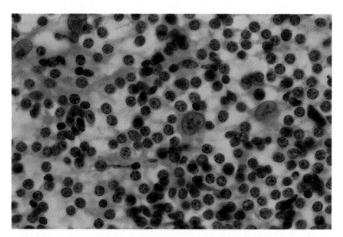

FIGURE 5-22   Material obtained from a lymph node involved by Hodgkin's disease. Two Reed-Sternberg cell variants are present; these are surrounded by a mixed population of predominantly mature lymphocytes (H&E, × 198).

In general, the number of Reed-Sternberg cells and their variants is lowest in lymphocyte-predominant Hodgkin's disease, whereas bizarre forms are most frequent in the lymphocyte-depleted type. Reed-Sternberg cells and their variant forms can be identified by screening the smears at medium power. High-power examination confirms the diagnostic impression. CD15 staining by immunohistochemistry supports a diagnosis of Hodgkin's disease, but some T-cell lymphomas will also react positively with antibodies directed against CD15.

Schwannoma (Neurilemmoma)

The cytologic findings in schwannomas are reasonably specific and, when combined with clinical findings, a cytologic diagnosis of schwannoma can be made with a high level of confidence.[37-40] Schwannomas are characterized by the finding of a lateral neck nodule that can be moved from side to side but not in the inferosuperior direction along the course of a nerve. In addition, penetration of the nodule by a needle frequently results in significant pain or a tingling sensation. Cytologically, the smears are of low to modest cellularity with cells lying singly and in small clusters. The predominant cell type is an elongated spindle cell with bipolar cytoplasmic processes (Fig. 5–23). The cytoplasm has a wispy appearance and surrounds a fusiform nucleus that often displays bends or creases within the nuclear membrane. The chromatin is fine. The nuclei show little atypia although occasionally, there are rare cells that exhibit significant nuclear enlargement and hyperchromasia. Intranuclear cytoplasmic invaginations may be seen in a small number of

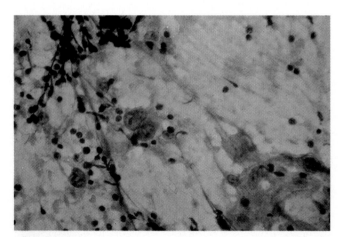

FIGURE 5-21   Material aspirated from a lymph node involved by Hodgkin's disease. Note the large, binucleated, Reed-Sternberg cell (Papanicolaou, × 198).

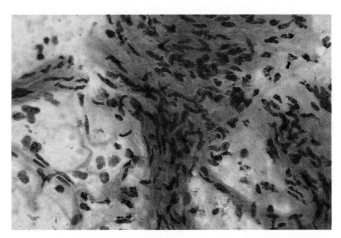

FIGURE 5-23 A population of elongated spindle cells with wavy nuclei characteristic of a low-grade nerve sheath tumor (schwannoma). No mitotic activity is seen, and most of the nuclei are bland and either arranged in bundles or in the form of palisades (Diff-Quik, × 132).

cells. Mitotic activity is absent. The cytoplasm is fragile, and scattered naked nuclei are seen in the background. The background may be clean, myxoid, or contaminated with a small number of red blood cells. Mast cells may be scattered within the background. Within the tissue fragments, the nuclei run in bundles with a palisading pattern. The tissue fragments often have a fibrillary stroma between cells.

Carotid Body Tumor

Carotid body tumors or cervical paragangliomas are infrequently aspirated. The cellularity of the resultant smears varies markedly.[20,41,42] Many smears are dominated by blood, with only a few spindle or polygonal cells. Others are highly cellular with cells lying both individually and in clusters (Fig. 5-24). The cells may have an epithelioid or spindle-shaped morphology.

Within each distinct cell population, the cells may be of a uniform appearance (Fig. 5-25) or show marked pleomorphism. Frequently, the polygonal cells form rosettes that closely resemble microacinar structures (see Fig. 5-25). Cases with a prominent number of rosettes may be confused with adenocarcinoma, particularly one arising in the thyroid. Other, more solid aggregates representing "Zellballen" are also seen. The nuclei of the individual cells vary from round to ovoid or fusiform. The chromatin has a salt-and-pepper appearance, and intranuclear cytoplasmic pseudoinclusions are common.[41] Individual cells have abundant, finely granular cytoplasm which, when present in the cells forming the clusters, can result in a lattice-like appearance. Cytoplasmic granules are seen with Giemsa-based stains and are mauve or reddish-purple. These granules are not seen with Papanicolaou or hematoxylin-eosin staining. Distinguishing carotid body tumors from thyroid carcinoma, either follicular or medullary in type, can be difficult. The mixture of cell types (polygonal and spindle-shaped) aids in the exclusion of these follicular neoplasms of the thyroid. Although the presence of microacinar structures can cause confusion with follicular neoplasms of the thyroid, the presence of a significant component of spindle cells intimately admixed with the microfollicular structures should suggest the appropriate diagnosis. Similarly, the neuroendocrine appearance of material obtained from paragangliomas can result in confusion of these neoplasms with medullary carcinoma of the thyroid. Immunocytochemistry for calcitonin can be helpful in differentiating between these two neoplasms. The more lateral position of carotid body tumors in the neck also aids in this distinction. When doubt persists, computed tomography (CT)

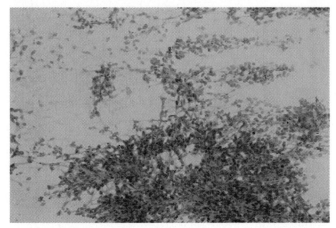

FIGURE 5-24 A cellular smear aspirated from a carotid body tumor containing both single cells and clusters of oval shaped cells (H&E, × 33).

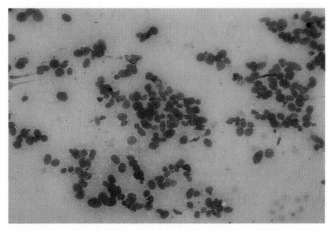

FIGURE 5-25 A population of relatively uniform and bland oval cells lying in small clusters. Occasional gland-like formations are seen (Diff-Quik, × 66).

and angiographic studies can generally distinguish cartoid body tumors from neoplasms of the thyroid. Mitotic activity is a poor indicator of clinical aggressiveness for cervical paragangliomas.

SALIVARY GLAND

The salivary gland is the site of origin for a wide variety of neoplastic and inflammatory conditions. Fortunately, most nodules undergoing FNA biopsy represent pleomorphic adenomas, Warthin's tumors, or examples of sclerosing chronic sialadenitis. These are usually easily recognized by cytologic study. Adenoid cystic carcinoma and mucoepidermoid carcinoma are the only other conditions seen with any significant frequency. Diagnostic difficulty may be encountered in the recognition of mucoepidermoid carcinoma and in distinguishing adenoid cystic carcinoma from some forms of monomorphic adenoma. The remaining lesions occurring within the salivary gland are most easily diagnosed by using the following differential diagnostic categories: (1) squamous-containing lesions; (2) lymphocyte-rich lesions; (3) clear cell–containing lesions; and (4) neoplasms containing cords and cores of stroma. Once the most common lesions have been excluded, these categories are helpful in establishing the nature of the lesion. Table 5–1 lists the most common lesions within each diagnostic category.

Material obtained by aspiration from pleomorphic adenomas is usually abundant and is composed of fragments of myxoid-chondroid stroma, epithelial cells, and myoepithelial cells (Fig. 5–26).[43] This appearance on low-power magnification of air-dried Giemsa-stained specimens is diagnostic for pleomorphic adenoma. The myxoid-chondroid stroma is usually abundant and entraps and partially obscures the epithelial and myoepithelial components (see Fig. 5–26). The myxoid-chondroid stroma stains mauve or magenta on Romanovsky preparations and has a vaguely fibrillary appearance. The epithelial and myoepithelial cells have a round, spindle-shaped, or plasmacytoid morphology. The nuclei are round to ovoid, small in size, and possess a dark, uniform chromatin. Mitotic activity is not seen. In many cases, the nuclear features are obscured by the myxoid-chondroid ground substance. With Papanicolaou staining, the myxoid-chondroid material stains green and has a waxy appearance. The nuclear features of the cells are best demonstrated with Papanicolaou staining, which shows a bland uniform morphology with finely granular chromatin. Nucleoli are absent.

In some examples of pleomorphic adenoma, the cellular component dominates, and little myxoid-chondroid substance is present. In these cases, most of the cells have a plasmacytoid or oval shape with moderate amounts of cytoplasm. The nuclei are bland, uniform in size and shape, and have a fine but dark chromatin pattern. Nucleoli are not seen. The small amount of myxoid-chondroid material

TABLE 5–1	DIAGNOSTIC CATEGORIES FOR SALIVARY GLAND LESIONS

Cystic Lesions

Benign lymphoepithelial cyst
Retention cyst
Warthin's tumor
Cystic pleomorphic adenoma
Mucoepidermoid carcinoma

Squamous Cell Containing Lesions

Chronic sialadenitis
Warthin's tumor
Pleomorphic adenoma (infarcted)
Mucoepidermoid carcinoma
Squamous cell carcinoma

Clear Cell Containing Lesions

Clear cell oncocytoma
Acinic cell carcinoma
Mucoepidermoid carcinoma
Epithelial myoepithelial carcinoma
Clear cell adenocarcinoma
Metastatic renal cell carcinoma

Lymphocyte-Rich Lesions

Intraparotid lymph nodes
Chronic sialadenitis
Benign lymphoepithelial cyst
Benign lymphoepithelial lesion
Warthin's tumor
Primary salivary gland lymphoma

Stroma-Rich Lesions

Pleomorphic adenoma
Monomorphic adenoma
Adenoid cystic carcinoma

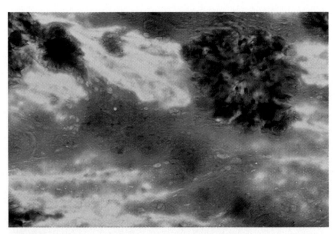

FIGURE 5–26 Myxoid-chondroid and epithelial elements obtained from a pleomorphic adenoma. Note the distortion and masking of nuclear detail by the abundant myxoid-chondroid stroma (Diff-Quik, × 33).

present surrounds individual cells, as well as small groups of cells, and has a finely fibrillar character.

Differentiation of pleomorphic adenoma from monomorphic adenoma and adenoid cystic carcinoma represents the major diagnostic concern. The clinical importance of distinguishing pleomorphic adenoma from monomorphic adenoma is trivial, but the distinction between pleomorphic adenoma and adenoid cystic carcinoma has significant clinical consequences. In general, the stromal element in adenoid cystic carcinoma forms well-defined cords and cores with more distinct outlines than seen in pleomorphic adenoma. The core material seen in adenoid cystic carcinomas is denser and lacks the fibrillary character seen in the stroma of most adenomas. Also, the nuclei of adenoid cystic carcinoma are slightly larger than those of adenomas and possess nucleoli. In practice, differentiation between adenoid cystic carcinoma and pleomorphic adenoma by nuclear size is difficult and imprecise. In these cases, clinical findings (presence of pain or nerve function loss in adenoid cystic carcinoma but an absence of these signs in pleomorphic adenoma) helps to distinguish the two lesions. When doubt exists, histologic examination is necessary.

Chronic Sialadenitis

In the author's initial series of 171 cases, chronic sialadenitis was the second most frequent lesion involving the salivary gland for which needle aspiration biopsy was performed. In most cases, aspirates were obtained to exclude recurrent squamous cell carcinoma as a diagnosis. The submandibular gland frequently undergoes a sclerosing and inflammatory process following surgery or irradiation directed at squamous primary lesions involving the floor of the mouth. This therapeutic regimen frequently causes enlargement and hardening of the submandibular gland, raising clinical suspicion for carcinoma. Aspirates from such lesions are of low cellularity but contain small fragments of atypical epithelium (Fig. 5-27).[44] The tissue fragments are composed of enlarged epithelial cells with hyperchromatic nuclei and an increased nuclear/cytoplasmic ratio. The tissue fragments are tight clusters of cells with sharp borders and prominent overlapping of nuclei (Fig. 5-28). The background is either bloody or proteinaceous, but necrosis is absent. Only occasionally are single cells scattered in the smear, and these are frequently represented by naked nuclei. The nuclei can be hyperchromatic but do not show true anaplasia. Occasionally, mature lymphocytes will be present.

Smears from cases of chronic sialadenitis may be overdiagnosed as either mucoepidermoid carcinoma or metastatic squamous cell carcinoma.[7] The nuclear crowding, metaplastic change, nuclear enlargement, and hyperchromasia can lead to misdiagnosis; however, the overall low level of cellularity, as well as

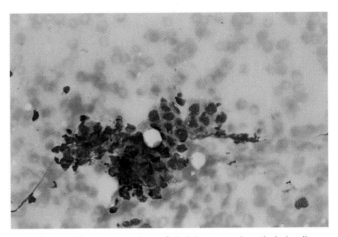

FIGURE 5-27 A tight cluster of slightly atypical epithelial cells characteristic of chronic sialadenitis. Note that the background is clean except for scattered red blood cells. Few individual cells have exfoliated from the cell clusters (Diff-Quik, × 132).

the low-power appearance of tightly clustered tissue fragments with sharp borders and tubular shape, should allow the correct diagnosis of chronic sialadenitis to be made. The absence of mucin-producing cells and intermediate cells excludes the diagnosis of mucoepidermoid carcinoma.

Benign Oncocytic Proliferations, Including Warthin's Tumor

A variety of oncocytic lesions occur within the salivary glands. Most are found in the parotid gland. Oncocytosis, oncocytic nodule, oncocytoma, and Warthin's tumor are the most important of these lesions. Oncocytosis and oncocytic nodule probably represent metaplastic changes and rarely are subject to needle aspiration. The oncocytic appearance is at-

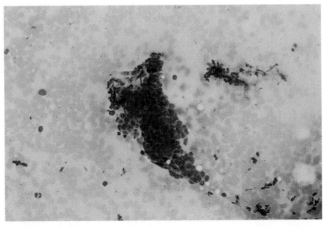

FIGURE 5-28 A tight, tube-like aggregate of cells is characteristic of chronic sialadenitis (Diff-Quik, × 66).

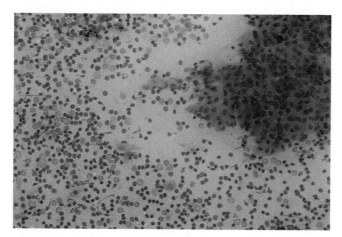

FIGURE 5-29 Material aspirated from a Warthin's tumor. Sheets of oncocytic cells lie in a dirty proteinaceous background with a large population of predominantly mature lymphocytes (Diff-Quik, × 66).

tributable to a component of the salivary gland epithelium that accumulates mitochondria, resulting in an abundant granular cytoplasm. The precise relationship of these metaplastic changes to the more circumscribed neoplasms of Warthin's tumor and oncocytoma is unclear. The cytologic features of the individual cells in oncocytosis, oncocytic nodule, oncocytoma, and Warthin's tumor are identical.[45] In each case, the epithelial component is characterized by large polygonal cells with abundant granular cytoplasm surrounding a round or oval nucleus with a bland chromatin. The nuclei may contain distinct nucleoli. Nuclear size frequently varies, but nuclear membrane irregularities and irregularities of the chromatin pattern are absent.

In both oncocytoma and Warthin's tumor, the epithelial component is exclusively or nearly exclusively oncocytic. Oncocytomas are characterized by a pure population of oncocytic cells lying in a clean or bloody background. Warthin's tumor is characterized by a triad of a dirty proteinaceous background, a variable number of mature lymphocytes, and scattered aggregates of oncocytic epithelium (Fig. 5-29).

These oncocytic epithelial cells are identical to those seen in oncocytosis and oncocytoma. Differentiating Warthin's tumor from the aforementioned lesions depends on the finding of the classic triad. Rarely, Warthin's tumor can undergo infarction with atypical squamous metaplasia, in which case it must be distinguished from squamous cell carcinoma.[7,46] The metaplastic squamous epithelium seen in Warthin's tumor is generally scant and has a degenerative metaplastic appearance. The background may reveal necrosis, and careful scrutiny of the aspirated material will usually show classic Warthin's tumor in other areas. True squamous cell carcinomas yield more abundant squamous epithelium with nuclear atypia occurring in well-preserved cells lacking a degenerative appearance. The scanty nature of the

epidermoid component, along with its degenerative appearance, should alert the cytologist to the presence of squamous metaplasia in a Warthin's tumor and aid in the exclusion of squamous cell carcinoma. The absence of intermediate cells and mucin-containing cells facilitates differentiation between Warthin's tumor and mucoepidermoid carcinoma.

Mucoepidermoid Carcinoma

Mucoepidermoid carcinomas account for approximately one third of all salivary gland malignant neoplasms. They are responsible for a disproportionately high number of diagnostic errors. This is, in part, due to their wide morphologic spectrum and mixture of cell types, including mucinous, epidermoid, and intermediate cells.[47,48] Cytologically, mucoepidermoid carcinomas are classified as high grade or low grade based on the relative numbers of mucin-producing and epidermoid cells present.

Low-grade mucoepidermoid carcinomas are frequently cystic, and aspirates contain a prominent amount of extracellular mucin in which is dispersed a variable number of histiocytes, mucin-containing epithelial cells, and intermediate cells (Fig. 5-30).[44,45] In these carcinomas, the epidermoid component is either scanty or absent. The predominant epithelial cell is columnar and mucin-containing, with a bland, round or oval nucleus. The cytoplasm is abundant and is largely composed of intracellular mucin (see Fig. 5-30). Mucin stains are strongly positive. The nuclei are displaced toward one end of the cell and are best seen with Papanicolaou staining. The chromatin is bland and condensed within a small nucleus. The mucin-containing cells lie individually or form small clusters and strips. Intermediate cells are almost always present and have bland nuclear features with modest amounts of cytoplasm (Fig. 5-31; see also Fig. 5-30).

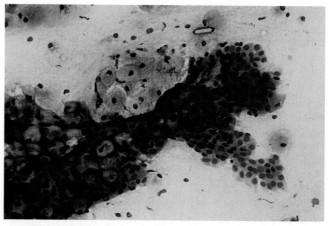

FIGURE 5-30 Clusters of cells obtained from a low-grade mucoepidermoid carcinoma. Note the mixture of rather small intermediate cells and larger clear or foamy cells. The larger cells with abundant cytoplasm are mucin-positive (Diff-Quik, × 66).

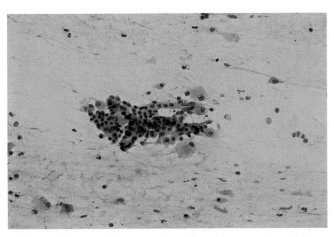

FIGURE 5–31 Cell cluster aspirated from a mucoepidermoid carcinoma. The cell cluster contains both intermediate cells and larger, pale orange–staining, mucin-rich cells. These latter cells have bland nuclei and abundant granular or clear cytoplasm. The background contains mucoid debris, as well as individual intermediate cells and mucin-rich cells (Papanicolaou, × 33).

High-grade mucoepidermoid carcinomas contain fewer mucin-producing cells, an increased number of intermediate cells, and a marked number of epidermoid cells (Fig. 5–32). The epidermoid cells have the appearance of metaplastic squamous cells. True keratinization is almost never seen. In addition to the significant number of epidermoid cells, high-grade mucoepidermoid carcinomas display increased degrees of nuclear atypia, significant chromatinic hyperchromasia, clumped chromatin, and distinct nucleoli. Mitotic figures may be seen. Although mucin-producing cells are not prominent, mucin staining will disclose occasional cells with intracytoplasmic mucin. This mucin positivity, along with the presence of intermediate and epidemioid cells, confirms the diagnosis of mucoepidermoid carcinoma.

Mucoepidermoid carcinomas must be distinguished from several lesions.[48] Low-grade mucoepidermoid carcinomas need to be distinguished from mucoceles. High-grade mucoepidermoid carcinoma must be distinguished from squamous cell carcinoma and chronic sialadenitis with marked nuclear atypia. Low-grade mucoepidermoid carcinomas can be very difficult to distinguish from mucoceles and mucus-retention cysts. In general, the amount of epithelium is greater in mucoepidermoid carcinomas than in benign cysts, but the overlap in cellularity is significant. The finding of intermediate cells and occasional cells with a metaplastic squamous appearance is most helpful in establishing the diagnosis of low-grade mucoepidermoid carcinoma.

High-grade mucoepidermoid carcinoma may be difficult to distinguish from some cases of chronic sialadenitis. The tissue fragments from chronic sialadenitis are smaller, tubular, and more sharply delineated than those seen in mucoepidermoid carci-

noma. In addition, specimens of mucoepidermoid carcinoma will contain some cells with intracytoplasmic mucin demonstrable by mucin staining. This is not generally seen in cases of chronic sialadenitis. Mucoepidermoid carcinoma must be distinguished from squamous cell carcinoma. Mucoepidermoid carcinomas almost never show true keratinization, a phenomenon that is very common in metastatic squamous cell carcinoma. The demonstration of intracytoplasmic mucin establishes the diagnosis of mucoepidermoid carcinoma and excludes squamous cell carcinoma.

Adenoid Cystic Carcinoma

Adenoid cystic carcinomas represent approximately 10% of all salivary gland neoplasms. The neoplasms are divided into three types histologically, but only two are distinguishable by cytologic review. The cylindromatous and tubular patterns of adenoid cystic carcinoma are essentially indistinguishable by cytologic examination, whereas the solid form can often be identified. The classic appearance of adenoid cystic carcinoma with the cylindromatous and/or tubular patterns is that of oval or cuboidal cells forming ring-like configurations.[49] These rings surround dense hyalin stromal cores that stain magenta or red on Romanovsky preparations (Fig. 5–33). Individual epithelial cells have bland nuclei containing small, often distinctive nucleoli. The nuclei are slightly larger than those seen in pleomorphic and monomorphic adenomas. Mitotic activity is not present. At times, the stromal material will be distributed in cords rather than cores, making differentiation from monomorphic adenomas more difficult. In most cases, the well-formed, ring-like appearance dominates specimens of adenoid cystic carcinoma. The stromal material that is characteristic of adenoid

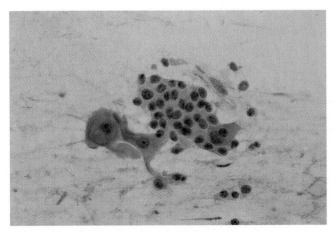

FIGURE 5–32 Material obtained from a high-grade mucoepidermoid carcinoma contains both intermediate cells and epidermoid cells. Some of the epidermoid cells have cytoplasmic tails and extensions (Papanicolaou, × 132).

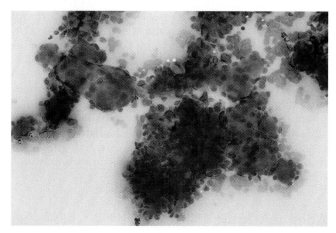

FIGURE 5-33 Cellular material obtained from an adenoid cystic carcinoma demonstrates relatively small, bland, round cells associated with cores of magenta-colored stroma (Diff-Quik, × 66).

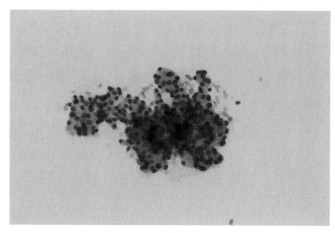

FIGURE 5-35 A cluster of bland epithelial cells with small, round or oval nuclei associated with a granular or finely foamy cytoplasm. These findings are characteristic of acinic cell carcinoma (Diff-Quik, × 33).

cystic carcinoma is more homogeneous and less fibrillar than that seen in adenomas. The background of the smears is either clean or bloody, and the overall smear cellularity is moderate. Necrosis is absent.

The solid form of adenoid cystic carcinoma is difficult to distinguish cytologically from basal cell adenoma.[50] Smears of solid adenoid cystic carcinomas are moderately cellular, with most cells lying in small, tight clusters and occasional sheets (Fig. 5-34). The clusters are composed of relatively small but hyperchromatic cells with a high nuclear/cytoplasmic ratio. Nucleoli may be seen. The nuclei tend to overlap and may have slightly irregular nuclear membranes. Although this appearance closely resembles that of monomorphic adenoma, the nuclei of solid adenoid cystic carcinomas are more atypical and larger. These differences are modest, though, and differentiation is subjective.[50] In many cases,

histologic study is necessary to establish the correct diagnosis.

Acinic Cell Carcinoma

Aspirates obtained from acinic cell carcinomas are usually of moderate or high cellularity.[51] Most of the cells lie in small sheets, papillary formations, or clusters (Fig. 5-35). Occasionally, gland-like arrangements may be seen. The backgound is clean except for red blood cells and a small number of scattered acinar cell nuclei. These are randomly distributed or aggregated around intact epithelial clusters. The individual cells are polygonal with abundant, finely granular or vacuolated cytoplasm (Fig. 5-36). Occasionally, clear cells are noted upon staining by the Papanicolaou or the hematoxylin-eosin

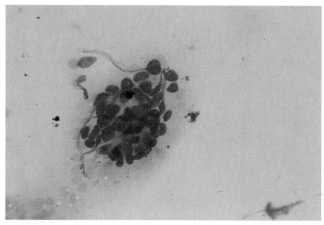

FIGURE 5-34 Solid ball of relatively bland basaloid cells. These cells have little cytoplasm, and the nuclei are modestly enlarged and deeply hyperchromatic. This appearance is characteristic of the solid form of adenoid cystic carcinoma (Diff-Quik, × 132).

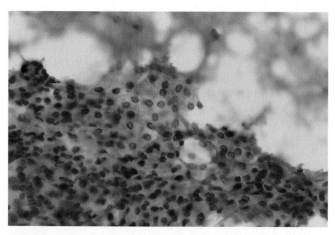

FIGURE 5-36 Smeared material from an acinic cell carcinoma is characterized by a large sheet of bland cells with abundant granular or finely vacuolated cytoplasm. Nuclear atypia is minimal, and mitotic activity is not seen (H&E, × 132).

method. The nuclei are uniformly bland in character with dark chromatin. The nuclear outline is round. Small nucleoli may be seen. In a minority of cases, Giemsa-stained preparations disclose dense metachromatic granules. These granules are found within the cytoplasm but may spill into the background. When found in a salivary gland neoplasm, they are nearly pathognomonic of acinic cell carcinoma. Similar granules can be found in medullary carcinoma of the thyroid and carotid body tumors.

Less Common Salivary Gland Neoplasms and Proliferations

SQUAMOUS CELL CONTAINING LESIONS

Table 5–1 lists proliferations arising within the salivary gland that may have a prominent or predominant squamous cell component. The most commonly occurring is Warthin's tumor with squamous metaplasia, as described earlier.[52] The other lesions are relatively uncommon.

Rarely, pleomorphic adenomas undergo spontaneous infarction and contain areas of squamous metaplasia. Aspirates from infarcted pleomorphic adenomas show extensive necrosis and small fragments of atypical, metaplastic, squamous epithelium. Rare individual cells show keratinization and degenerative changes within the nuclei. As with infarcted Warthin's tumor, the squamous epithelium is usually a minor component within the smear, and the associated nuclei are frequently smudged, and have a degenerative appearance. Squamous metaplasia sometimes occurs after FNA and is evident in the excised specimens.

Squamous epithelium can be seen in benign lymphoepithelial cysts occurring in immunocompromised patients. The background is watery and predominantly lymphoid in character, but rare squamous cells are mixed with the lymphocytes. The watery background is associated with a mixed but predominantly mature lymphoid population. Squamous, ciliated, or nonciliated columnar epithelial cells help to establish the diagnosis of benign lymphoepithelial cyst.

Primary squamous carcinomas of the salivary gland are rare. Most squamous carcinomas found within the parotid gland represent metastases to intraparotid lymph nodes. The cytologic features of these neoplasms are identical to those of metastatic squamous cell carcinomas occurring elsewhere. The abundant cellularity of the neoplastic component, along with the clear-cut nuclear atypia in at least a component of the cells, should distinguish these neoplasms from other squamous-containing lesions occurring within the parotid. In addition, squamous cell carcinomas frequently display distinct keratinization, allowing them to be distinguished from mucoepidermoid carcinoma.

SALIVARY GLAND LESIONS CONTAINING A PROMINENT OR PREDOMINANT POPULATION OF LYMPHOCYTES

Table 5–1 lists the lymphoid-containing lesions occurring within the salivary glands, of which Warthin's tumor is the most common. The lymphoid component of Warthin's tumor is an intrinsic component of the neoplasm, but other primary salivary gland neoplasms also have an associated lymphoid infiltrate. Most are malignant, but occasionally, benign lesions, including oncocytomas, may be associated with a lymphoid component.

Intraparotid lymph nodes may become enlarged, presenting as palpable nodules. Aspirates of these lymph nodes are highly cellular and contain a mixed population of lymphoid cells showing an ordered maturational sequence. Tingible body macrophages and follicular center fragments are present. With the exception of contaminating acinar tissue, aspirates of reactive intraparotid lymph nodes will not contain an epithelial component. The absence of epithelial cells aids in the differentiation of reactive lymph nodes from other lesions with a prominent lymphoid component (see Table 5–1).

Benign lymphoepithelial cysts contain a prominent lymphoid population similar to that seen in reactive lymph nodes. However, the lymphoid population in these cysts is diluted by a watery proteinaceous fluid and the overall cellularity is lower. Rare squamous or columnar epithelial cells are present in the cysts.

The benign lymphoepithelial lesion of Sjögren's syndrome rarely is sampled by needle aspiration, but when it presents as a dominant unilateral nodule, needle aspiration cytology may be performed. The resultant smears are highly cellular with a mixed population of lymphocytes showing a normal maturational sequence (Fig. 5–37). Tingible body

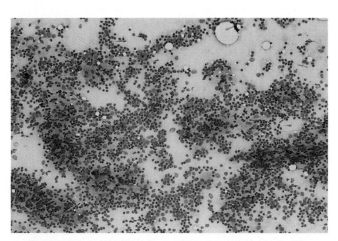

FIGURE 5–37 Mixed lymphoid infiltrate associated with aggregates of histiocytes and rare epimyoepithelial islands. These findings are characteristic of benign lymphoepithelial lesions (Sjögren's syndrome) (Diff-Quik, × 33).

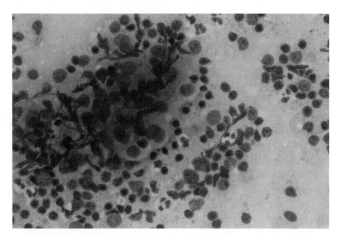

FIGURE 5-38 Epimyoepithelial aggregate composed of large cells with abundant pale cytoplasm. These cells are surrounded by a mixed lymphoid population (Diff-Quik, × 198).

macrophages and follicular center fragments are present. The morphologic feature with the greatest diagnostic utility is the epimyoepithelial island (Fig. 5-38). Cytologically, these structures appear as clusters of relatively large, pale cells containing ill-defined, abundant, and pale-staining cytoplasm. The nuclei are relatively large, often ovoid, and contain distinct nucleoli. The epimyoepithelial islands are infiltrated by small, round, mature lymphocytes.

Lymphomas may develop in the setting of Sjögren's syndrome. Because the neoplastic cells are often admixed with residual non-neoplastic lymphocytes, these lymphomas may be difficult, if not impossible, to diagnose by cytologic analysis. When the lymphoma largely or completely replaces a salivary gland, diagnosis by FNA biopsy is possible with the aid of flow cytometric analysis. In cases of primary salivary gland lymphomas, the smears are highly cellular and contain a monomorphic population of enlarged, atypical lymphocytes. The finding of a monomorphous population of large and atypical lymphocytes should raise suspicion for lymphoma and prompt either open biopsy or repeat FNA to obtain specimens for flow cytometry or immunohistochemical analysis for lymphoid markers.

CLEAR CELL CONTAINING LESIONS

Table 5-1 lists the clear cell containing lesions occurring within the salivary gland. Among these, mucoepidermoid carcinoma, epithelial myoepithelial carcinoma, clear cell adenocarcinoma, and metastatic renal cell carcinoma are the most frequent.[53] Mucoepidermoid carcinomas with a prominent mucinous component contain many large globular cells with abundant clear cytoplasm. This appearance is best appreciated with hematoxylin-eosin or Papanicolaou staining, whereby cytoplasmic clarity represents intracytoplasmic mucin or glycogen. The recognition

of intermediate cells and staining for mucin will establish the correct diagnosis.

Epithelial myoepithelial carcinomas contain a component of clear cells seen both in alcohol-fixed and air-dried Giemsa-stained material. These neoplasms have a rather characteristic FNA appearance. Most of the cells form grape-like clusters composed of well-formed cell balls (Fig. 5-39). The balls are composed of a ring of small dark cells surrounding central larger cells with pale or clear cytoplasm. The background contains naked nuclei derived from myoepithelial cells and some small epithelial cells. This architectural pattern is nearly pathognomonic for epithelial myoepithelial carcinoma. The nuclei of the myoepithelial cells are larger than those seen in pleomorphic adenoma and show greater degrees of hyperchromasia. Mitotic activity is generally not seen. Cytologic features of clear cell adenocarcinoma have not been clearly defined.

Many neoplasms can metastasize to intraparotid lymph nodes. Squamous cell carcinomas arising in the head and neck are the most frequent examples, followed by metastases from the lung, breast, and kidney. When examining hematoxylin-eosin– or Papanicolaou-stained material, the presence of large atypical cells with a clear to slightly granular cytoplasm should raise the possibility of metastatic renal cell carcinoma. Although nuclear atypia can be variable in renal cell carcinomas, the nuclei are almost always larger than those seen in acinic cell carcinoma, epithelial myoepithelial carcinoma, and well-differentiated mucoepidermoid carcinoma. The presence of clear cells with significant nuclear atypia should prompt the cytopathologist to seek additional clinical history or imaging studies to establish or exclude the diagnosis of metastatic renal cell carcinoma.

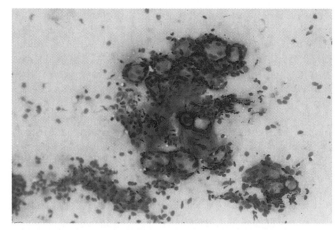

FIGURE 5-39 Grape-like clusters, composed of balls of epithelial and myoepithelial cells, are characteristic of epithelial myoepithelial carcinoma. These balls have an inner core of pale-appearing cells surrounded by a ring of darker, smaller, epithelial cells (Diff-Quik, × 66).

NEOPLASMS WITH CORES OR CORDS OF STROMA

Pleomorphic adenoma and adenoid cystic carcinoma represent the most important and most frequent neoplasms containing significant amounts of extracellular stroma.[54] Generally, these two lesions are easily distinguishable because the myxoid-chondroid stroma of pleomorphic adenomas is usually abundant, has a feathery or filamentous appearance, and surrounds the cellular elements. By contrast, the stromal material of adenoid cystic carcinoma forms round or oval cores and elongated cords. This material is more waxy appearing and is surrounded by cells. Difficulties in diagnosis occur because of rare monomorphic adenomas that contain significant amounts of stromal material. Dermal anlage tumor and trabecular adenoma can contain round cords or cores of stroma similar to those seen in adenoid cystic carcinoma. Points of distinction are subjective. Adenoid cystic carcinomas are said to have larger and more hyperchromatic nuclei than the bland nuclei seen in monomorphic adenomas (Fig. 5–40). In addition, the stromal material is often more prominent in monomorphic adenomas and more frequently forms long, cord-like structures. Differentiation is extremely difficult, and some authorities recommend that a definitive diagnosis of adenoid cystic carcinoma only be made when clinical findings (pain or nerve dysfunction) support such an interpretation.[55]

Basaloid squamous cell carcinoma may contain hyaline extracellular stroma. The cell population in this variant of squamous cell carcinoma is markedly pleomorphic and heterogeneous, a feature not seen in adenoid cystic carcinoma.

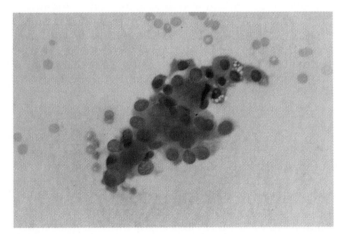

FIGURE 5–40 A smear from a monomorphic adenoma contains an aggregate of small bland cells with scanty to modest amounts of pale cytoplasm. The individual nuclei are bland and round (Diff-Quik, × 132).

THYROID GLAND

Palpable, solitary, nonfunctioning thyroid nodules are relatively common and raise a suspicion for carcinoma. When examined histologically, most of these nodules represent hyperplastic or degenerative processes. Because of the low rate of neoplastic disease in patients who undergo surgical exploration of thyroid nodules, protocols have been developed for preoperative differentiation of neoplastic and non-neoplastic nodules. Ultrasonographic and radionucleotide uptake studies have been used to increase the percentage of patients with carcinoma among individuals undergoing operative investigation. Although these techniques have been moderately successful, the introduction of FNA biopsy has greatly improved the overall yield of carcinomas in nodules undergoing resection. Needle aspiration cytology has been shown to be the most cost-effective technique for the investigation of palpable thyroid nodules.[56]

FNA biopsy has a sensitivity of approximately 92% and a specificity of 95% for detection of carcinoma of the thyroid. Accuracy is highest when aspiration cytology is performed and interpreted by individuals trained in the technique and practicing it on a frequent basis. Specimen adequacy is an important issue, and precise criteria exist to define an adequate smear. Most authorities agree that two slides, each containing at least 6 groups of at least 10 well-preserved, well-visualized cells is a reliable criterion for specimen adequacy.[57]

Smears of hyperplastic or colloid nodules are dominated by colloid with scattered clusters and sheets of follicular epithelium.[58] The colloid stains blue on air-dried Diff-Quik material, and it stains green or orange with the Papanicolaou method. Depending on the consistency and amount of colloid present, it may appear thin and watery, or thick. Frequently, the colloid has a "cracked plate glass" pattern that is best appreciated on Papanicolaou staining. The thyroid epithelium usually forms sheets of well-defined, uniform epithelial cells arranged in an even "honeycomb" pattern (Fig. 5–41). The individual epithelial cells have well-defined cytoplasmic borders, moderate amounts of cytoplasm, and uniform round or ovoid nuclei. In some cases of marked hyperplasia, the nuclei vary considerably in size but maintain a bland chromatin pattern and smooth nuclear membrane. In addition to sheets of cells, individual follicular epithelial cells and macrofollicles are found. The macrofollicles have a sphere-like three-dimensional appearance. Macrofollicles are more than 10 cells (frequently 30 or more) in circumference. Microfollicles are 10 or fewer cells in circumference. Individual follicular epithelial cells are often present and may be represented by naked nuclei.

Because goiters often contain foci undergoing cys-

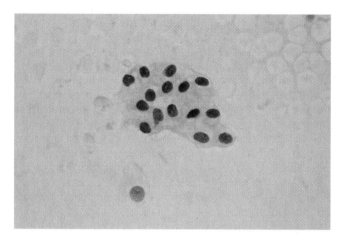

FIGURE 5–41 A honeycomb cluster of bland follicular cells is present in this smear obtained from a patient with goiter. These cells have moderately abundant, granular to pale cytoplasm surrounding a small, dark nucleus. Abundant colloid is present in the background (Papanicolaou, × 198).

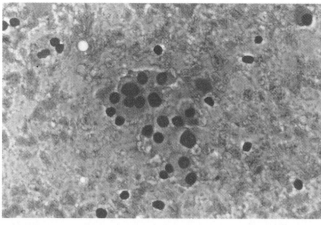

FIGURE 5–42 Smear material obtained from a patient with Graves' disease. The background is bloody and contains relatively little colloid. The cells are enlarged and have somewhat reactive or atypical nuclei. The cytoplasm is moderately abundant and may have a "fire flare" appearance around its periphery (Diff-Quik, × 198).

tic degeneration, aspirated material usually contains histiocytes as well as small clusters of epithelial cells showing the morphologic features of repair. The histiocytes have a foamy or pigment-laden cytoplasm. The histiocyte nuclei are shaped like coffee beans and are larger than those of the thyroid epithelial cells. Epithelial cells showing repair have enlarged, somewhat atypical nuclei, and cytoplasm is present in amounts greater than that seen in normal follicular epithelial cells. The cytoplasm of cells demonstrating repair has a spreading appearance, often with pseudopodia-like extensions. The atypia seen in these cells may suggest neoplastic change, but the cytoplasmic characteristics (similar to those seen in cervical repair) should help to establish the correct diagnosis.

Hyperthyroid states may be associated with a diffuse or nodular pattern of follicular cell proliferation. Associated with the clinical findings of Graves' disease is a characteristic FNA smear appearance.[59] The smears are bloody and contain, at most, scanty amounts of background colloid. Most of the epithelial cells lie in clusters and have a syncytial appearance. Monolayered sheets and macrofollicular structures are uncommon findings in patients with Graves' disease. The individual cells have a delicate cytoplasm that may be highly vacuolated. The vacuoles vary in size from minuscule to larger than the cell nucleus. The "fire flare" cell is a characteristic finding in Graves' disease (Fig. 5–42). These cells have peripheral globules of metachromatic pink material (Romanovsky technique). This pink material is not apparent in Papanicolaou-stained preparations where a marginal vacuole appearance is more characteristic. The fire flare cells, with their "marginal vacuoles," are characteristic of the hyperplastic state,

but may also be found in follicular and papillary carcinomas.

Acute thyroiditis is a rare condition and is infrequently the reason for FNA. Needle aspiration specimens may contain frankly purulent material associated with large numbers of bacteria or fungal organisms. Atypical reparative cells, similar to those seen in goiters, are frequently present. Care must be taken to exclude high-grade carcinoma whenever a background of necrotic debris is seen.

Chronic Lymphocytic Thyroiditis

Patients with chronic lymphocytic thyroiditis may present with clinically palpable nodules. Aspirated material contains a prominent population of small, mature to intermediate-sized lymphocytes and clusters of thyroid epithelial cells.[60] When the thyroid epithelium shows oncocytic change (Hürthle cells), a diagnosis of Hashimoto's thyroiditis should be made (Fig. 5–43).[60]

The benign oncocytes have large round bland nuclei with prominent nucleoli. Benign oncocytes can vary tremendously in size. When a Hürthle cell component is not identified, a diagnosis of chronic lymphocytic thyroiditis is made. In both chronic lymphocytic and Hashimoto's thyroiditis, the lymphoplasmacytic infiltrate has a mixed appearance and frequently contains germinal center fragments, tingible body macrophages, and multinucleated histiocytic giant cells. It is important to distinguish small mature lymphocytes from stripped nuclei derived from follicular epithelial cells. Small mature lymphocytes retain a rim of intact cytoplasm.

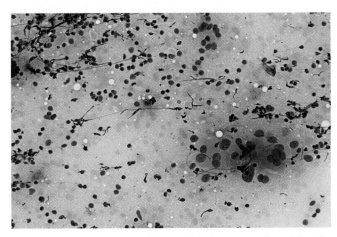

FIGURE 5-43 A mixture of benign lymphocytes and Hürthle cell epithelium is characteristic of Hashimoto's thyroiditis (Diff-Quik, × 66).

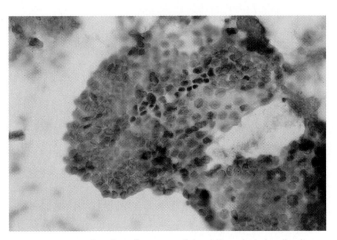

FIGURE 5-45 Papillary fragment of thyroid epithelial cells obtained from a papillary carcinoma. Some nuclei contain nuclear grooves (Papanicolaou, × 132).

Subacute Thyroiditis

Because of the characteristic clinical presentation of subacute thyroiditis, FNA biopsy is performed only rarely. Aspirated examples have contained lymphocytes, plasma cells, foreign body giant cells and Langerhans' type giant cells. The thyroid epithelium may show atypia secondary to inflammatory change and repair. Multinucleated giant cells frequently surround and engulf fragments of colloid. In most cases of subacute thyroiditis, the follicular epithelial component is sparse. Subacute or granulomatous thyroiditis must be differentiated, from sarcoid, tuberculosis, and fungal infections. Special stains for microorganisms are helpful. Caseous necrosis suggests tuberculosis.

Papillary Carcinoma

Papillary carcinoma is the most frequent malignant tumor involving the thyroid gland, and its cytologic appearance is characteristic. Diagnostic accuracy of FNA biopsy for papillary carcinoma is high. Key features for the diagnosis of papillary carcinoma include: (1) intranuclear cytoplasmic pseudoinclusions; (2) metaplastic (squamoid) cytoplasm; (3) papillary structures without internal vessels; (4) nuclear grooving; and (5) enlargement of the nuclei with clearing of the chromatin (Figs. 5–44 through 5–46).[61–63] Psammoma bodies are almost pathognomonic of papillary carcinoma, but they are rarely identified (Fig. 5–47). Occasionally, giant cells of epithelial or histiocytic origin are seen in some papil-

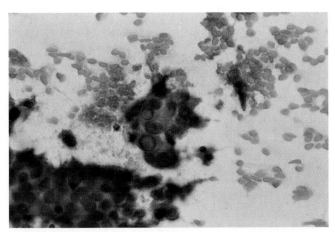

FIGURE 5-44 Clusters of thyroid epithelial cells in a bloody background. The thyroid epithelial cells have enlarged hyperchromatic nuclei, and some nuclei (center fragment) have intranuclear cytoplasmic pseudoinclusions (Papanicolaou, × 132).

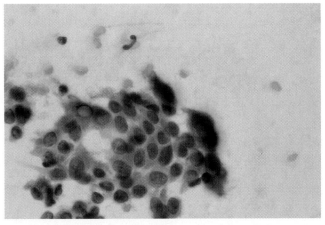

FIGURE 5-46 Material obtained from a papillary carcinoma of the thyroid. Occasional cells contain intranuclear cytoplasmic pseudoinclusions. These inclusions have a pale center with a rim of condensed chromatin (Papanicolaou, × 198).

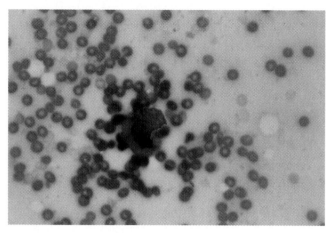

FIGURE 5-47 A psammoma body, which is characteristic of papillary carcinoma of the thyroid (Diff-Quik, × 132).

other criteria should be sought to support the diagnosis. When papillary clusters, bubble gum–like colloid, or psammoma bodies are found in association with the aforementioned nuclear features, a definitive diagnosis of papillary carcinoma can be made. The "Orphan Annie" eye nucleus seen in Papanicolaou-stained material also supports the diagnosis of papillary carcinoma.

Occasionally, papillary carcinomas may be cystic, and careful study is required to establish the diagnosis. The finding of cells with fine cytoplasmic vacuoles and fragments of thick bubble gum–like colloid in cyst contents should alert the pathologist to the possibility of papillary carcinoma.

Follicular Neoplasms

The most diagnostically challenging area in FNA biopsy of the thyroid is the differentiation between hyperplastic nodules and follicular adenomas and follicular carcinomas. Because the architectural features of capsular or vascular invasion are not identifiable in cytologic material, other, less specific criteria are used. Lesions that are cytologically identified as follicular neoplasms should undergo open biopsy or diagnostic suppressive therapy. When surgically excised, 15% of such nodules reveal carcinoma, 15% represent hyperplastic nodules, and the remainder are follicular adenomas. In needle aspiration smears, follicular neoplasms are characterized by a minimal amount of extracellular colloid and cellular smears with microfollicles and syncytial clusters of follicular cells (Figs. 5–49 and 5–50).[65] The syncytial clusters have irregular edges and poorly defined cytoplasmic membranes.[65] The microfollicles have a circumference of between five and nine cells. (see Fig. 5–49). The nuclei of follicular neoplasms are slightly larger than those found in hyperplastic nodules. Follicular carcinomas have nuclei larger than follicular adeno-

lary carcinomas, especially those with cystic change. Thick bubble gum–like colloid has been reported as a marker of papillary carcinoma. The cytoplasm of cells characteristic of papillary carcinoma is well defined and may be columnar in shape. Epithelial fragments obtained from papillary carcinomas show nuclear crowding, often with overlapping of cells (Fig. 5–48). The cytoplasm of these cells may show fine vacuolization that is best identified with Romanovsky staining.

No single feature is absolutely diagnostic of papillary carcinoma, so multiple features should be sought. Intranuclear cytoplasmic pseudoinclusions and nuclear grooves are particularly helpful in establishing the diagnosis of papillary carcinoma.[64] Both of these features have been described in other lesions, including goiters and medullary carcinoma. Therefore, before a definitive diagnosis of papillary carcinoma is made on the basis of nuclear features,

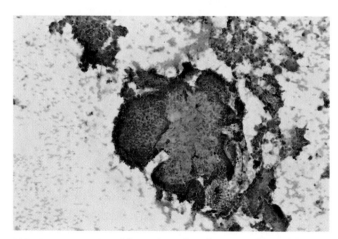

FIGURE 5-48 A well-formed papillary fragment obtained from a papillary carcinoma of the thyroid. Note the marked nuclear overlapping and crowding (H&E, × 33).

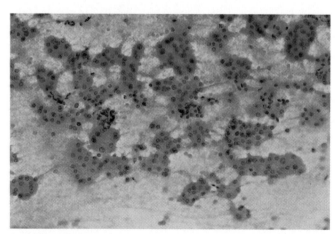

FIGURE 5-49 Abundant material obtained from a follicular neoplasm. Note the absence of colloid in the background and the overall high cellularity of the smear. Several microfollicles are also evident. (H&E, × 66).

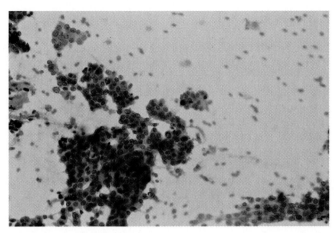

FIGURE 5-50 Syncytial clusters composed of thyroid epithelial cells obtained from a follicular neoplasm. Note the virtual absence of colloid in the background (H&E, × 66).

mas. Kini et al[65] have published specific criteria for distinguishing follicular carcinoma from follicular adenoma. She believes that marked nuclear crowding, overlapping of nuclei, enlarged nuclear size, and prominent nucleoli are characteristic of follicular carcinoma. Coarsely granular chromatin favors follicular carcinoma. Other authorities have had less success in distinguishing follicular carcinoma from follicular adenoma. Because diagnostic accuracy in the diffentiation of follicular adenoma from follicular carcinoma has been imperfect, the use of the term follicular neoplasm is recommended by many authors. The diagnosis of follicular neoplasm should be made whenever there are numerous microfollicles, along with syncytial aggregates of follicular epithelium that are dispersed in a background containing only scant colloid.

Hürthle Cell Neoplasms

Hürthle cell neoplasms are not easily subdivided into benign and malignant forms by aspiration cytology. Hürthle cell tumors are characterized cytologically by a nearly uniform population of oncocytic cells with abundant granular cytoplasm surrounding enlarged nuclei with prominent nucleoli (Fig. 5–51).[66] With Papanicolaou staining, the presence of large, cherry-red nucleoli in oncocytic cells supports the diagnosis of Hürthle cell neoplasm. The background of smears from Hürthle cell neoplasms contains little colloid and few or no lymphocytes. Nuclear atypia is variable and may at times be marked. Given this variability, it is not a useful criterion for differentiating between benign and malignant Hürthle cell neoplasms. Hürthle cell neoplasms must be distinguished from Hashimoto's thyroiditis and focal oncocytic metaplasia in goiters. Hashimoto's thyroiditis will invariably have a prominent mature lymphoid population. Multinodular

goiters showing focal Hürthle cell metaplasia yield smears with abundant colloid and a prominent follicular epithelial cell population.

Anaplastic Carcinoma

Anaplastic carcinomas are easily diagnosed as malignant tumors by FNA cytology. Differentiating them from a metastatic malignant lesion may be difficult, but the characteristic clinical findings are helpful in this regard. Smears contain a variable number of epithelioid or spindle-shaped cells with marked nuclear anaplasia. Intranuclear cytoplasmic pseudoinclusions may be present. Because these carcinomas may be densely fibrotic, smear cellularity can be low. At other times, smears are highly cellular. The individual epithelial cells vary considerably in size and shape, with bizarre forms frequently dominating the smears. Many of the epithelioid cells are multinucleated with bizarre, irregular nuclei. Mitotic activity is prominent. The background often contains necrotic debris. Colloid is absent in most cases.

Medullary Carcinoma

Medullary carcinomas can be diagnosed definitively by needle aspiration cytology.[67] Smears from medullary carcinomas have a bloody background and contain scant colloid. Smear cellularity is high. Although colloid is absent, the background may contain aggregates of amyloid.

Amyloid is difficult to identify with Papanicolaou staining, but appears bright pink in Giemsa-stained specimens. Characteristically, medullary carcinomas contain both polygonal or plasmacytoid cells and

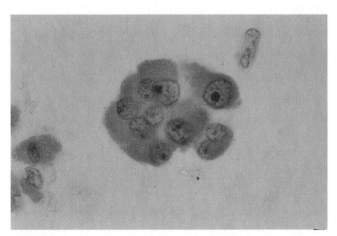

FIGURE 5-51 A cluster of cells obtained from a Hürthle cell neoplasm. Note the abundant granular cytoplasm and the enlarged nuclei. Prominent cherry-red nucleoli are present (Papanicolaou, × 250).

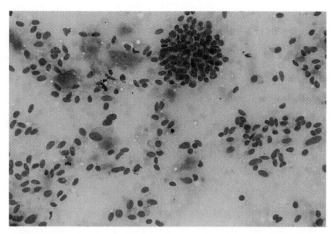

FIGURE 5-52 A mixture of spindle-shaped and polygonal cells obtained from a medullary carcinoma. Within the background are fragments of somewhat amorphous to waxy material characteristic of amyloid (Diff-Quik, × 66).

spindle cells (Fig. 5–52). This bimorphic appearance is helpful in differentiating medullary carcinoma from Hürthle cell neoplasms. For definitive diagnosis of medullary carcinoma, both the spindle and polygonal cell elements must be present. In a minority of cases, small, pink, intracytoplasmic granules will be demonstrable in Giemsa-stained material (Fig. 5–53). These granules are highly suggestive of medullary carcinoma, but can be found in carotid body tumors and acinic cell carcinomas of the salivary gland, as well. The granules are not seen with Papanicolaou staining. Both the spindle cells and epithelioid cells have enlarged nuclei with a salt-and-pepper chromatin pattern. Multinucleated cells and intranuclear inclusions are commonly seen.

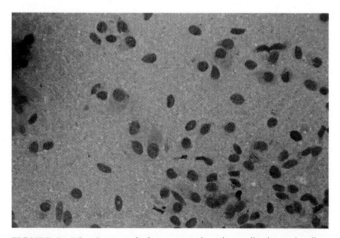

FIGURE 5-53 Scattered plasmacytoid and spindle-shaped cells with enlarged, somewhat hyperchromatic nuclei. Several cells in the central portion of the photomicrograph have granular cytoplasm. These granules stain magenta and are characteristic of medullary carcinoma of the thyroid (Diff-Quik, × 132).

Lymphoma

The thyroid may be a primary site of involvement by malignant lymphoma. Such lesions can be recognized by needle aspiration cytology using the criteria described for lymphoma involving cervical lymph nodes. In general, these lymphomas are of the B-cell type, and smears contain large numbers of atypical lymphoid elements lying in a background containing cytoplasmic fragments (lymphoglandular bodies). The use of flow cytometry or immunohistochemistry for the analysis of lymphoid markers is helpful in confirming the diagnosis.

Metastatic Lesions of the Thyroid

The thyroid can play host to a variety of metastatic carcinomas.[68] Renal cell carcinoma and carcinoma of the lung are most frequent and should be kept in mind whenever a population of markedly atypical cells is obtained by FNA biopsy of the thyroid. Clinical history and immunohistochemistry are usually helpful in establishing the correct diagnosis.

ORAL CAVITY AND OTHERS

Because most neoplasms arising within the oral cavity are squamous cell carcinomas arising from the surface epithelium, they are investigated by punch-grasp or excisional biopsy. However, occasionally, lesions are more deeply seated, in which case needle aspiration biopsy may be warranted. Such lesions include granular cell tumor of the tongue and tonsillar carcinoma. On morphologic examination, squamous cell carcinomas arising within the oral cavity resemble metastases to the cervical lymph nodes. A discussion of squamous cell carcinoma can be found in the earlier section dealing with cervical lymph node metastases.

Granular Cell Tumor

Granular cell tumors are found within the tongue. Aspirates are generally highly cellular, with both single and syncytial clusters of large granular cells (Fig. 5–54).[69] The individual cells contain abundant granular cytoplasm with indistinct cell borders. Single cells often present as stripped nuclei lying in a dirty, somewhat granular background. Within the syncytial clusters, the nuclei may be arranged in a vaguely acinar pattern. The nuclei are small and round. Small nucleoli are generally present. Occasionally, the nuclei of the granular cells vary markedly in size. Nonetheless, the chromatin pattern remains bland and the nucleoli are small. The granules react with the periodic acid–Schiff (PAS)

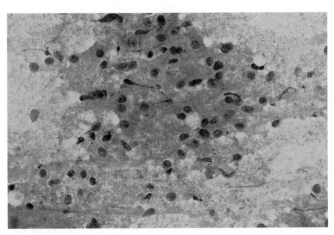

FIGURE 5–54 This syncytial aggregate of enlarged cells contains abundant granular cytoplasm and bland but enlarged nuclei. The background contains abundant granular material. This cytologic appearance is characteristic of granular cell tumor (Papanicolaou, × 132).

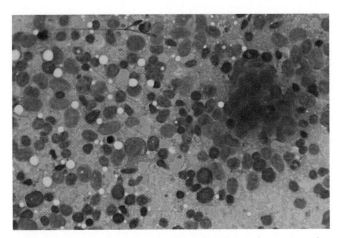

FIGURE 5–55 Enlarged cells with atypical hyperchromatic nuclei surrounded by scanty cytoplasm. The background has abundant granular debris and contains a mixed population of lymphocytes. These findings are typical of lymphoepithelioma (Diff-Quik, × 132).

stain, test positive for S-100 protein, and are variably reactive to carcinoembryonic antigen (CEA) when stained by the immunoperoxidase technique.

Malignant Lesions of the Tonsil

The tonsils can give rise to primary squamous cell carcinomas, as well as lymphomas. The histologic and cytologic characteristics of these neoplasms are similar to those previously described for the same lesions occurring at other sites.

Nasopharyngeal Carcinomas

Nasopharyngeal carcinomas are divided into three types depending on the degree of differentiation. Types I and II comprise keratinizing and nonkeratinizing squamous cells, respectively. Type II is subclassified into (A) differentiated and (B) undifferentiated. The latter includes the classic lymphoepithelioma, which is associated with a heavy lymphoid infiltrate.

Cytologically, types I and IIA are usually easily diagnosed and are similar in morphology to squamous cell carcinomas arising elsewhere. Type IIB, undifferentiated carcinoma, is more difficult to diagnose because of the large number of benign lymphocytes present. Cytologic study shows variable proportions of undifferentiated carcinoma cells and lymphocytes (Fig. 5–55).[70] The lymphocytes are predominately small and mature, but intermediate forms may be found. The epithelial cells occur individually or in loosely cohesive clusters. In general, the cytoplasm is ill defined and scanty or modest in amount. The nuclei are round or oval, possess a finely granular chromatin, and have small but distinct nucleoli on air-dried preparations. With hematoxylin-eosin or Papanicolaou staining, the nuclei appear large and vesicular, with chromatin clearing and large, distinct, central nucleoli. Immunoperoxidase staining for cytokeratin may be helpful in identifying the epithelial component within cell block preparations. At times, distinction from lymphoma is difficult, and ancillary studies are helpful.

Olfactory Neuroblastoma

Olfactory neuroblastomas (esthesioneuroblastomas) are uncommon malignant lesions arising within the olfactory epithelium of the superior portion of the nasal cavity. The patients may be of any age, but the median age of occurrence is 49 years. Histologically, these neoplasms are composed of nests of small, round, tumor cells, often lying in an edematous fibrous stroma. Neoplastic cells may grow in a diffuse fashion or form rosettes. The individual neoplastic cells will decorate with antibodies directed against neuroendocrine markers and S-100 protein. On cytologic examination, the smears are cellular and are composed of both individual cells and aggregates of cohesive cells.[71] The neoplastic cells have scanty, ill-defined cytoplasm, round nuclei, and distinct nucleoli (Fig. 5–56). At times, nuclear smearing artifact is prominent (Fig. 5–57). Some authors have described an intercellular fibrillary background that they believe is diagnostic of olfactory neuroblastoma. Occasionally, binucleate cells may be seen, and although exceedingly rare, rosette-like structures may be identified. In some cases, a marked smearing artifact of the nuclei is observed, particularly in air-dried material.

A variety of other lesions occur within the head and neck. These include angiofibroma, synovial sar-

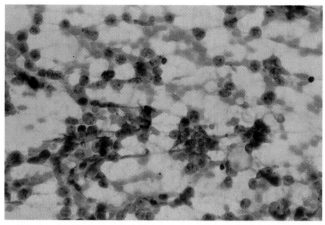

FIGURE 5–56 Individual and small clusters of hyperchromatic, small, round cells obtained from a patient with esthesioneuroblastoma. The individual cells often show significant smearing artifact of the nuclei. The nuclei have a blotchy or somewhat granular chromatin pattern. Pyknotic cells are present (H&E, × 132).

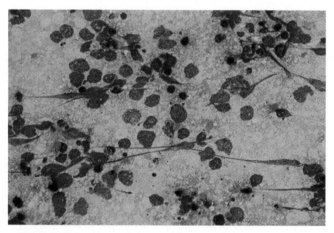

FIGURE 5–57 Material obtained from an esthesioneuroblastoma. The background has a dirty granular appearance. The individual cells have enlarged hyperchromatic nuclei. Many nuclei show extensive smearing artifact, which characterizes olfactory neuroblastoma (Diff-Quik, × 132).

coma, rhabdomyosarcoma, chordoma, extraskeletal Ewing's sarcoma, myxoma, fibromatosis, nodular fasciitis, and a variety of skin tumors. Readers are referred to several specialty texts for the cytologic findings that characterize these lesions.[72–74]

REFERENCES

1. Chen VSM, Qizilbash A, Young JEM. *Guides to Clinical Aspiration Biopsy: Head and Neck*. New York: Igaku-Shoin; 1996:1.
2. Steel BL, Schwartz MR, Ramzy I. Fine needle aspiration biopsy in the diagnosis of lymphadenopathy in 1,103 patients. Role, limitations and analysis of diagnostic pitfalls. *Acta Cytol*. 1995; 39:76.
3. Betsill WL, Hajdu SI. Percutaneous aspiration biopsy of lymph nodes. *Am J Clin Pathol*. 1980; 73:471.
4. Frable WJ. Thin needle aspiration biopsy—A personal experience with 469 cases. *Am J Clin Pathol*. 1976; 65:168.
5. Cohen MB, Reznicek MJ, Miller TR. Fine-needle aspiration biopsy of the salivary glands. *Pathol Annu*. 1992; 27:213.
6. Owen ERTC, Banerjee AK, Prichard AJN, et al. Role of fine needle aspiration cytology and computed tomography in the diagnosis of parotid swellings. *Br J Surg*. 1989; 76:1273.
7. Layfield LJ, Tan P, Glasgow BJ. Fine needle aspiration of salivary gland lesions: Comparison with frozen sections and histologic findings. *Arch Pathol Lab Med*. 1987; 111:346.
8. Gansler TS, Morris RC. Fine needle aspiration and frozen section of salivary gland lesions. *South Med J*. 1990; 83:283.
9. Candel A, Gattuso P, Reddy V, et al. Is fine needle aspiration biopsy of salivary gland masses really necessary? *Ear Nose Throat J* 1993; 72:485.
10. Eneroth C-M, Franzen S, Zajicek J. Cytologic diagnosis on aspirate from 1000 salivary gland tumours. *Acta Otolaryngol*. 1967; 224(suppl):168.
11. Frable MAS, Frable WJ. Fine needle aspiration biopsy of salivary glands. *Laryngoscope*. 1991; 101:245.
12. Roland NJ, Caslin AW, Smith PA, et al. Fine needle aspiration cytology of salivary gland lesions reported immediately in a head and neck clinic. *J Laryngol Otol*. 1993; 107:1025.
13. Young JA, Smallman LA, Thompson H, et al. Fine needle aspiration cytology of salivary gland lesions. *Cytopathology*. 1990; 1:25.
14. MacLeod CB, Frable WJ. Fine needle aspiration biopsy of the salivary gland: Problem cases. *Diagn Cytopathol*. 1993; 9:216.
15. Ashcraft MW, Van Herle AJ. Management of thyroid nodules. II: Scanning techniques, thyroid suppressive therapy, and fine needle aspiration. *Head Neck Surg*. 1981; 3:297.
16. Caruso D, Mazzaferi EL. Fine needle aspiration biopsy in the management of thyroid nodules. *Endocrinologist*. 1991; 1:194.
17. Frable WJ. The treatment of thyroid cancer: The role of fine-needle aspiration cytology. *Arch Otolaryngol Head Neck Surg*. 1986; 112:1200.
18. Mazzaferri EL. Thyroid cancer in thyroid nodules: Finding a needle in a haystack. *Am J Med*. 1992; 93:359.
19. Gharib H, Goellner JR, Johnson DA. Fine needle aspiration cytology of the thyroid: A 12 year experience with 11,000 biopsies. *Clin Lab Med*. 1993; 13:699.
20. Engzell U, Franzén S, Zajicek J. Aspiration biopsy of tumors of the neck. II. Cytologic findings in 13 cases of carotid body tumor. *Acta Cytol*. 1971; 15:25.
21. Engzell U, Zajicek J. Aspiration biopsy of tumors of the neck. I. Aspiration biopsy and cytologic findings in 100 cases of congenital cysts. *Acta Cytol*. 1970; 14:51.
22. Ramzy I, Rone R, Schantz HD. Squamous cells in needle aspirates of subcutaneous lesions: A diagnostic problem. *Am J Clin Pathol*. 1986; 85:319.
23. Dejmek A, Lindholm K. Fine needle aspiration biopsy of cystic lesions of the head and neck, excluding thyroid. *Acta Cytol*. 1990; 34:443.
24. Burgess KL, Hartwick RWJ, Bedard YC. Metastatic squamous carcinomas presenting as a neck cyst. Differential diagnosis from inflamed branchial cleft cyst in fine needle aspirates. *Acta Cytol*. 1993; 37:494.
25. Kapila K, Kharbanda K, Verma K. Cytomorphology of metastatic melanoma—Use of S-100 protein in the diagnosis of amelanotic melanoma. *Cytopathology*. 1991; 2:229.
26. Layfield LJ, Ostrzega N. Fine needle aspirate smear morphology in metastatic melanoma. *Acta Cytol*. 1989; 33:606.
27. Perry NM, Seigler HF, Johnston WW. Diagnosis of metastatic malignant melanoma by fine needle aspiration biopsy. A clinical and pathologic correlation of 298 cases. *JNCI*. 1986; 77: 1013.
28. Frable WJ, Kardos TF. Fine needle aspiration biopsy: Applications in the diagnosis of lymphoproliferative diseases. *Am J Surg Pathol*. 1988; 12(suppl):62.
29. Daskalopoulou D, Harhalakis N, Maouni N, Markidou SG. Fine needle aspiration cytology of non-Hodgkin's lymphomas: A morphologic and immunophenotypic study. *Acta Cytol*. 1995; 39:180.
30. Kardos TF, Maygarden SJ, Blumberg AK, et al. Fine needle

aspiration biopsy in the management of children and young adults with peripheral lymphadenopathy. *Cancer.* 1989; 63:703.

31. Gupta AK, Nayar M, Chandra M. Critical appraisal of fine needle aspiration cytology in tuberculous lymphadenitis. *Acta Cytol.* 1992; 36:391.

32. Frable MA, Frable WJ. Fine needle aspiration biopsy in the diagnosis of sarcoid of the head and neck. *Acta Cytol.* 1984; 28:175.

33. Kardos TF, Vinson JH, Behm FG, et al. Hodgkin's disease: Diagnosis by fine needle aspiration biopsy. *Am J Clin Pathol.* 1986; 86:286.

34. Dmitrovsky E, Martin SE, Krudy AG, et al. Lymph node aspiration in the management of Hodgkin's disease. *J Clin Oncol.* 1986; 4:306.

35. Friedman M, Kim U, Shimaoka K, et al. Appraisal of aspiration cytology in management of Hodgkin's disease. *Cancer.* 1980; 45:1653.

36. Das DK, Gupta SK Datta BN, et al. Fine needle aspiration cytodiagnosis of Hodgkin's disease and its subtypes: I. Scope and limitations. *Acta Cytol.* 1990; 34:329.

37. Ramzy I. Benign schwannoma: Demonstration of Verocay bodies using fine needle aspiration. *Acta Cytol.* 1977; 21:316.

38. Navas-Palacios JJ, de Agustin PP, Alvaroz de los Hevos F, et al. Ultrastructural diagnosis of facial nerve schwannoma using fine needle aspiration. *Acta Cytol.* 1983; 27:441.

39. Hood IC, Qizilbash AH, Young JEM, Archibald SD. Needle aspiration cytology of a benign and a malignant schwannoma. *Acta Cytol.* 1984; 28:157.

40. Stastny JF, Frable WJ. Diagnosis of primary nerve sheath tumor of the sphenoid sinus by fine needle aspiration biopsy. A case report. *Acta Cytol.* 1993; 37:242.

41. Jacobs DM, Waisman J. Cervical paraganglioma with intranuclear vacuoles in a fine needle aspirate. *Acta Cytol.* 1987; 31:29.

42. Fleming MV, Oertel YC, Rodriguez ER, Fidler WJ. Fine needle aspiration of six carotid body paragangliomas. *Diagn Cytopathol.* 1993; 9:510.

43. Eneroth CM, Zajicek J. Aspiration biopsy of salivary gland tumors. III. Morphologic studies on smears and histologic sections from 368 mixed tumors. *Acta Cytol.* 1966; 10:440.

44. Droese M. Cytological diagnosis of sialadenosis, sialadenitis and parotid cysts by fine needle aspiration biospy. *Adv Otol Rhinol Laryngol* 1981; 26:89.

45. Eneroth CM, Zajicek J. Aspiration biopsy of salivary gland tumors: II. Morphologic studies on smears and histologic sections from oncocytic tumors (45 cases of papillary cystadenoma lymphomatosum and 4 cases of oncocytoma). *Acta Cytol.* 1965; 9:355.

46. Van den Brekel MWM, Risse EKJ, Tiwari RM, Stel HV. False-positive fine needle aspiration cytologic diagnosis of a Warthin's tumor with squamous metaplasia as a squamous cell carcinoma. *Acta Cytol.* 1991; 35:477.

47. Zajicek J, Eneroth CM, Jakobsson P. Aspiration biopsy of salivary gland tumors. VI. Morphologic studies on smears and histologic sections from mucoepidermoid carcinoma. *Acta Cytol.* 1976; 20:35.

48. Cohen MB, Fisher PE, Holly EA, et al. Fine needle aspiration biopsy diagnosis of mucoepidermoid carcinoma. Statistical analysis. *Acta Cytol.* 1990; 34:43.

49. Eneroth CM, Zajicek J. Aspiration biopsy of salivary gland tumors. IV. Morphologic studies on smears and histologic sections from 45 cases of adenoid cystic carcinoma. *Acta Cytol.* 1969; 13:59.

50. Orell SR, Nettle WJS. Fine needle aspiration biopsy of salivary gland tumours: Problems and pitfalls. *Pathology.* 1988; 20:332.

51. Eneroth CM, Jakobsson P, Zajicek J. Aspiration biopsy of salivary gland tumors. V. Morphologic investigations on smears and histologic sections of acinic cell carcinoma. *Acta Radiol.* 1971; 310(suppl):85.

52. Mooney EE, Dodd LG, Layfield LJ. Squamous cells in fine needle aspiration biopsies of salivary gland lesions: Potential pitfalls in cytologic diagnosis. *Diagn Cytopathol.* 1996; 15:47.

53. Layfield LJ, Glasgow BJ. Aspiration cytology of clear cell lesions of the parotid gland: Morphologic features and differential diagnosis. *Diagn Cytopathol.* 1993; 9:705.

54. Wax T, Layfield LJ. Epithelial-myoepithelial cell carcinoma. A case report and comparison of cytologic features with other stromal, epithelial and myoepithelial cell containing lesions of the salivary gland. *Diagn Cytopathol.* 1996; 14:298.

55. Löwhagen T, Tani EM, Skoog L. Salivary gland and rare head and neck lesions. In: Bibbo M, ed. *Comprehensive Cytopathology.* Philadelphia; WB Saunders; 1991: 634.

56. Van Herle AJ, Rich P, Ljung B-ME, et al. The thyroid nodule. *Ann Intern Med.* 1982; 96:221.

57. Kini SR, Miller JM, Hamburger JI. Cytopathology of thyroid nodules. *Henry Ford Hosp Med J.* 1982; 30:17.

58. Frable WJ, Frable MA. Fine needle aspiration biopsy of the thyroid: Histopathologic and clinical correlations. *Prog Surg Pathol.* 1980; 1:105.

59. Jayaram G, Singh B, Marwaha RK. Graves' disease: Appearance in cytologic smears from fine needle aspirates of the thyroid gland. *Acta Cytol.* 1989; 33:36.

60. Guarda LA, Baskin HJ. Inflammatory and lymphoid lesions of the thyroid gland: Cytopathology by fine needle aspiration. *Am J Clin Pathol.* 1987; 87:14.

61. Francis IM, Das DK, Sheikh AZ, et al. Role of nuclear grooves in the diagnosis of papillary thyroid carcinoma. *Acta Cytol.* 1995; 39:409.

62. Kini SR, Miller JM, Hamburger JI, et al. Cytopathology of papillary carcinoma of the thyroid by fine needle aspiration. *Acta Cytol.* 1980; 24:511.

63. Leung C-S, Hartwick RWJ, Bedard YC. Correlation of cytologic and histologic features in variants of papillary carcinoma of the thyroid. *Acta Cytol.* 1993; 37:645.

64. Akhtar M, Ali MA, Huq M, et al. Fine needle aspiration biopsy of papillary thyroid carcinoma: Cytologic, histologic and ultrastructural correlations. *Diagn Cytopathol.* 1991; 7:373.

65. Kini SR, Miller JM, Hamburger JI, et al. Cytopathology of follicular lesions of the thyroid gland. *Diagn Cytopathol.* 1981; 1:123.

66. Kini SR, Miller JM, Hamburger JI. Cytopathology of Hûrthle cell lesions of the thyroid gland by fine needle aspiration. *Acta Cytol.* 1981; 25:647.

67. Kini SR, Miller JM, Hamburger JI. Cytopathologic features of medullary carcinoma of the thyroid. *Arch Pathol Lab Med.* 1984; 108:156.

68. Kini SR, Smith MJ, Miller JM, et al. Fine needle aspiration cytology of tumors metastatic to the thyroid gland. *Acta Cytol.* 1982; 26:743.

69. Franzen S, Stenkvist B. Diagnosis of granular cell myoblastoma by fine-needle aspiration biopsy. *Acta Pathol Microbiol Scand.* 1968; 72:391.

70. Chan MKM, McGuire LJ, Lee JCK. Fine-needle aspiration cytodiagnosis of nasopharyngeal carcinoma in cervical lymph nodes. A study of 40 cases. *Acta Cytol.* 1989; 33:344.

71. Fagan MF, Rone R. Esthesioneuroblastoma: Cytologic features with differential diagnostic considerations. *Diagn Cytopathol.* 1989; 1:322.

72. Chen VSM, Qizilbash A, Young JEM. *Guides to Clinical Aspiration Biopsy. Head and Neck.* New York: Igaku-Shoin; 1996:273.

73. DeMay RM. *The Art and Science of Cytopathology.* Chicago: ASCP Press; 1996:560.

74. Orell SR, Sterrett GF, Walters MNI, Whitaker D. *Manual and Atlas of Fine Needle Aspiration Cytology.* 3rd ed. London: Churchill Livingstone; 1999:372.

PART II

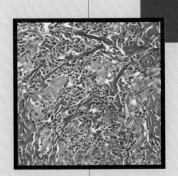

Diseases by Anatomic Site

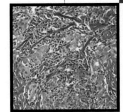

CHAPTER 6

Nasal Cavity and Paranasal Sinuses

I. CLINICAL CONSIDERATIONS FOR THE DISEASES OF THE NASAL CAVITY AND PARANASAL SINUSES

■ MARILENE WANG

■ DAVID OSGUTHORPE

■ ELLIOT ABEMAYOR

Inflammatory and benign disorders of the nasal cavity and paranasal sinuses are common. Early diagnosis and successful treatment of neoplasms in this region are often difficult, despite their common occurrence, because of the relative rarity of some of the pathologic entities encountered, as well as unfamiliarity with the tortuous regional anatomy. To further compound the issue, clinical signs and symptoms of aggressive disease may mimic benign processes.

This chapter reviews common, uncommon, benign and malignant diseases of the nasal cavity, nasopharynx, and paranasal sinuses. As with other regions of the head and neck, a close collaboration and careful communication is mandatory among pathologists and clinicians if rational diagnosis and treatment plans are to be formulated.

EMBRYOLOGY

The maxilla, nose, and paranasal sinuses are derivatives of the first pharyngeal (branchial) arch, which splits into a caudad-mandibular section and cepha-

113

lad/lateral maxillary swellings.[1,2] Between the maxillary swellings and frontal prominence, nasal placodes develop on either side of the midline at about 4.5 weeks of life. The lateral portions of the placodes form the nasal alae, and the medial portions of the placodes and the maxillary swellings form the upper lip. These merge over the stomodeum to create the primary palate (i.e., premaxilla). By the sixth week of life, the medial aspects of the maxillary processes bud palatal shelves, initially separated by the tongue. As the tongue descends to the floor of the oral cavity by the 15th week of life, the shelves fuse in the midline to separate the nasal from the oral cavities, creating a posterior choana at the junction of the posterior nasal cavity and the nasopharynx. During the palatal fusion process, a vertical outcropping of the primitive nasal roof (i.e., precursor to the nasal septum) extends ventrally in the midline to partition two separate nasal cavities from the common cavity formed shortly after invagination of the nasal pits.

The paranasal sinuses develop as diverticula from the lateral nasal walls, with their first appearance in the 6th fetal week when maxilloturbinal swellings (precursors of inferior turbinates and uncinates) appear on anterolateral nasal walls. One week later, ethmoturbinals appear at the junctions of the nasal roof and lateral walls. The space between these two swellings becomes the middle meatus. By 9 weeks a pouch precursor of the maxillary sinus buds from the middle meatus, and by 15 to 17 weeks the frontal recess and anterior ethmoid precursors appear. Shortly thereafter the superior meatal structures evolve. By the end of the 4th fetal month, all the structures of the adult paranasal region can be identified, although the sinuses do not reach adult dimensions until around age 16. Aeration of the sinuses and the development of the maxillary teeth substantially affect the dimensions and shape of the adult face. The embryonal arterial supply to the first pharyngeal arch becomes the terminal branches of the external carotid artery, principally the internal maxillary artery. The nerve to the first arch is the trigeminal, with the maxillary and—to a lesser extent—ophthalmic divisions innervating the sinuses and midface.

SURGICAL ANATOMY

The nasal cavities extend from the anterior choana at the limen nasi (level of the junction of the upper and lower lateral nasal cartilages, and the transition from facial skin to nasal mucosal lining) to the posterior choana that lie directly above the posterior end of the hard palate.[2–4] The floor of the nasal cavity is formed by the maxillary and palatine bones, the roof by the cribriform plate, the lateral walls by the turbinates and the medial walls of the maxillary and the ethmoid sinuses. The nasal cavi-

ties are bisected by a septum that anteriorly is composed of septal cartilage, posterosuperiorly the bony perpendicular plate of the ethmoid and posteroinferiorly the vomer extending from the anterior face of the sphenoid. Only the thick, bony floor of the nasal cavity presents a significant barrier to the egress of malignancy from the nasal cavities. The lateral nasal walls are thin, and each cribriform plate is not only thin but penetrated by 15 to 25 terminal branches of the olfactory nerve (Fig. 6–1).

The maxillary sinus is a blunt-edged triangle in shape, with its base being the lateral wall of the nasal cavity and its apex a depression in the undersurface of the malar bone and zygomatic process of the maxilla. The floor of the maxillary sinus dips inferiorly into the alveolar arch and is commonly 5 to 10 mm caudad to the floor of the nasal cavity. The roots of the molar teeth may penetrate into the floor of the antrum. The medial antral wall contains a small ostium that communicates with the nasal cavity through the middle meatus, below which is attached the inferior turbinate. The posterolateral wall of the maxillary sinus separates it from the pterygoid muscles laterally and the contents of the infratemporal fossa posteriorly, including branches of the second division of the fifth cranial nerve and the inferior maxillary artery (which enters the nasal cavity through the sphenopalatine foramen just behind the posterosuperior wall of the maxillary sinus). The thin roof of the maxillary sinus is also the floor of orbit, through which courses the infraorbital branch of the maxillary nerve.

With respect to midline, the ethmoid sinuses are a symmetrical labyrinth of air cells, immediately medial to the orbits and lateral to the middle turbinates. They fuse in the midline to form the perpendicular plate of the septum (see Fig. 6–1). The bony

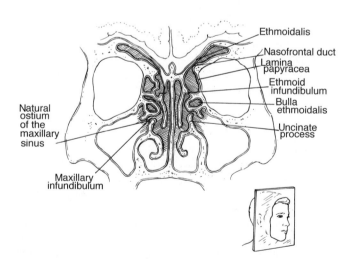

FIGURE 6–1 Anatomy of the paranasal sinuses, fully developed, in a coronal view. Note the relationship between the ethmoid sinuses and the orbits (laterally) as well as the floor of the cranial fossa (superiorly). From Wang MB and Berke GS. Paranasal sinus endoscopy. In: King WA, Frazee JG, De Salles AAF, eds. *Endoscopy of the Central and Peripheral Nervous System.* New York: Thieme; 1998, with permission.

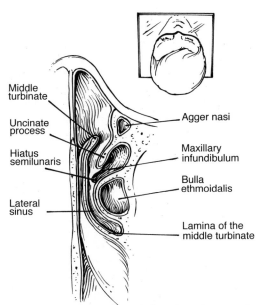

FIGURE 6–2 Axial section through the ethmoid sinuses illustrating the relationship of the sinuses to the turbinates and septum (medially) and the orbit (laterally). From Wang MB, Berke GS. Paranasal sinus endoscopy. In: King WA, Frazee JG, De Salles AAF, eds. *Endoscopy of the Central and Peripheral Nervous System.* New York: Thieme; 1998, with permission.

Middle turbinate

Uncinate process

Hiatus semilunaris

Lateral sinus

Agger nasi

Maxillary infundibulum

Bulla ethmoidalis

Lamina of the middle turbinate

septa between the ethmoid cells are thin and do not impede tumor spread. The thin lateral wall of the ethmoid sinus, the lamina papyracea, is penetrated by the anterior and posterior ethmoidal neurovascular bundles, and so afford direct access of tumor to the orbits. The ethmoid sinuses are separated from the maxillary sinuses by a thin shelf of bone located on the superomedial corner of the maxillary sinus, the antroethmoidal septum. It is common for antral malignancies to invade the inferior ethmoids and adjacent orbit through this route.

The frontal sinuses are aerated cells between the anterior and posterior tables of the frontal bones, with both tables being fairly thick, but the intersinus septum is thin and offers little resistance to tumors. The floor of the frontal sinuses, which enters the middle meatus through the frontonasal recesses or anterior ethmoid cells, is thin and represents the pathway of least resistance for expansion of a frontal malignancy. The size and aeration of the frontal sinuses vary considerably among individuals, and may be asymmetrical within the individual.

The sphenoid sinuses also exhibit varying degrees of aeration and are bounded laterally by the cavernous sinuses, superomedially by the optic nerves, posterosuperiorly by the sella, inferiorly by the clivus, anteroinferiorly by the nasopharynx and anterosuperiorly by the posterior choana. As with the frontal sinuses, the thin intersinus septum separating the two sides offers little resistance to the spread of malignancy. Indeed, the sphenoid sinuses are surrounded by thin bone on all but their inferior margins (the clivus).

The orbits are bounded inferiorly by the maxillary sinuses, medially by the ethmoid labyrinths, anterosuperiorly by the frontal sinuses and posterolaterally by the sphenoid sinuses (Fig. 6–2). Spread of tumors from any sinus through these thin, bony orbital walls occurs readily, with the periorbita being the final plane of resistance before the orbital soft tissues are invaded (and, hence, exenteration common with tumor extirpations).

Invasion of the infratemporal fossa, pterygoid muscles, or oral cavity is most frequent with maxillary malignancies, as the antrum is not only the most likely location for sinus malignancies but also shares a common wall with the aforementioned regions. The central nervous system is most commonly invaded through the cribriform plate or roof of an ethmoid sinus, although the frontal and sphenoid sinuses also share walls with the anterior fossa.

PHYSIOLOGY

The sinus epithelium forms a mucociliary system that supplies the nose with a mucous covering to warm and humidify inspired air. Both parasympathetic and sympathetic nerves supply this mucous blanket, which is renewed every 10 to 15 minutes.[5] The cilia beat 10 to 15 times per second and move the mucous blanket toward the natural ostia of the sinuses. Environmental factors influence ciliary function: humidity increases the activity, while dehydration and cold temperatures decrease flow.[6] Bacterial and vital proliferation may increase when there is dysfunction of the cilia and relative stasis of the mucous blanket.

In addition to mucociliary dysfunction, any condition that obstructs the drainage of the sinuses (i.e., polyps or inflammation and edema of the nasal mucosa) will lead to sinusitis. Benign and malignant tumors of the nasal cavity, paranasal sinuses, and skull base can also lead to a post-obstructive sinusitis of one or more of the paranasal sinuses.

CONGENITAL ANOMALIES

Congenital masses of the nose and parasinus region usually occur at or near an embryonic midline fusion and primarily consist of dermoids, gliomas, and encephaloceles.[2,7] Nasal dermoids usually present on the upper nasal dorsum, heralded by a small cutaneous pit with an extruding hair, although their location can vary from the columella to the sphenoid sinus. Unlike teratomas, which contain all three embryonal germ layers, dermoids only contain ectodermal and mesodermal elements, usually in the form of hair follicles, sweat or sebaceous glands, and the like. One theory on the origin of nasal dermoids is a failure of the neuropore to close, with dermal elements invaginating into the open prenasal space (primarily into the frontonasal suture in the late second to third month of fetal life.)[7] Dermoids can be solid or have a cystic component but in either case usually present as a firm and poorly compressible mass. Intracranial connections are unusual, although substantial effacement of the anterior cribriform bony barrier by a large dermoid can occur. Therefore, a presurgical imaging study should be obtained. Management consists of excision, taking a cuff of skin around the cutaneous pore; such surgery can be delayed until the age of 4 to 5 years if the dermoid growth is not causing progressive deformity of the nasal bones or interfering with vision or nasal respiration.

Gliomas and encephaloceles share an embryonic origin: faulty closure of the foramen caecum in the third week of fetal life with incomplete separation of epithelial from brain elements.[2,7] Since brain tissue remains in contact with the skin, a bony defect occurs between the glabella and the anterior fossa. Since all but 15% of the gliomas have lost their neural connection with the central nervous system, the connection is merely a fibrous stalk in the remainder. Approximately 60% of the gliomas are extranasal (i.e., outside the nasal cavity, usually paramedian along the nasal dorsum), with the remainder having an intranasal or a combined intra/extranasal presentation. They appear as polypoid masses beneath the nasal mucosa or skin. Encephaloceles are divided into "sincipital" if the transcranial bony dehiscence is anterior to the crista galli (through the frontal or ethmoid bones) and "basal" if presenting as an intranasal mass along an axis from the cribriform plate to a posterior clinoid. Basal encephaloceles tend to be compressible and bluish in color underneath the mucosa and to exhibit Furstenburg's sign (i.e., mass expansion when the jugular veins are compressed). As encephaloceles contain both neural tissue and a subarachnoid space containing cerebrospinal fluid, an intracranial/extracranial approach for closure of the dural defect is mandatory. Because of the risk of meningitis from a secondary infected encephalocele during an upper respiratory infection, surgical correction in the first 6 months of life is advisable.

INFLAMMATORY CONDITIONS

Acute and Chronic Rhinosinusitis

Acute rhinosinusitis is one of the most common health care problems afflicting the population and is increasing in both incidence and prevalence.[8] Costs associated with this disease are enormous and include significant loss of productivity at work and school.[9,10] Acute rhinitis is often found in conjunction with a viral upper respiratory infection and generally lasts 4 weeks or less.[11] Edema and inflammation of the nasal mucosa, including the turbinates, result in symptoms of nasal congestion, rhinorrhea, post-nasal drip, and fever. Inflammation can extend to involve the mucosa of the paranasal sinuses. Edema and mucus production within the sinuses lead to partial or complete blockage of the natural ostia. This, in turn, can result in further fluid accumulation, causing pain and pressure of the involved sinus. Without treatment, the sinusitis may progress to a cellulitis and/or abscess of the orbit and eventually a cavernous sinus thrombosis.[12]

Bacterial etiologies of acute rhinitis and sinusitis include the common upper respiratory pathogens: streptococcus, staphylococcus aureus, haemophilus influenza, and many others.[13-15] Fungal sinusitis is less common and may be classified as invasive or allergic. Invasive fungal sinusitis usually afflicts patients with diabetes and other immunocompromised hosts. Mucormycosis is a life-threatening invasive fungal sinusitis with a propensity for spreading to the central nervous system via blood vessels.[16] Thrombosis of the blood vessels results in a necrotic-appearing black nasal mucosa. A patient suspected of having mucormycosis requires immediate biopsy of the nasal tissue and crusts. Emergency surgical debridement is mandatory once the diagnosis of mucormycosis is obtained. Aggressive resection of all affected tissue may require radical maxillectomy, orbital exenteration, or even craniotomy. Aspergillus and other fungi are less commonly involved in invasive sinusitis.

Allergic fungal sinusitis usually affects a younger population of patients. These patients often have concurrent asthma and nasal polyps and do not respond to repeated courses of antibiotics. They often have elevated IgE levels and are atopic to both fungal and nonfungal antigens.[17,18] Their sinuses are filled with thick mucoid secretions that contain eosinophils and fungal elements.[19,20] In contrast to the fungal sinusitis of immunocompromised patients, these fungal elements are not angioinvasive, and radical surgical intervention is not required.

No specific treatment is necessary for uncomplicated acute rhinitis associated with an upper respiratory infection. Symptomatic relief may be obtained with antihistamines, decongestants, and nonsteroidal anti-inflammatory agents. Acute sinusitis is initially treated with oral antibiotics. Refractory sinusitis may require intravenous antibiotics. Surgical drainage is necessary for sinusitis that fails to respond to medical therapy or if there is concomitant orbital or brain involvement, or invasive fungal sinusitis. Endoscopic drainage is appropriate for most cases of sinusitis, except when debridement of tissue is necessary as in mucormycosis.

Chronic rhinosinusitis is most often allergic in etiology and lasts longer than 12 weeks. Symptoms are similar to acute rhinosinusitis and include nasal congestion, rhinorrhea, facial pressure and pain, postnasal drip, halitosis, hyposmia, and headache. Nasal polyps may be present as well. Other concurrent conditions should be sought, including cystic fibrosis, aspirin sensitivity, and asthma. A CT scan in chronic rhinosinusitis will reveal mucoperiosteal thickening or complete opacification of one or more sinuses.

Medical treatment for chronic rhinosinusitis includes antibiotics, antihistamines, nasal steroid sprays, and short courses of oral steroids.[21] In addition, the underlying allergies should be addressed, and immunotherapy may be of benefit. Surgery is indicated when medical treatment has not resulted in satisfactory improvement of symptoms. Patients with recurrent episodes of acute rhinosinusitis may also be candidates for surgery.

A variety of destructive granulomatous conditions can involve the nose. Numerous terms have been applied to these disease processes, including Wegener's granulomatosis and polymorphic reticulosis, to name a few. For the latter two, immunohistochemical and molecular genetic studies have determined that the majority of these are lymphomas of the sinonasal tract.[22]

Wegener's Granulomatosis

Wegener's granulomatosis is a systemic necrotizing vasculitis that involves the upper and lower respiratory tracts and the kidneys. It was first described in 1939 as a necrotizing granuloma.[23] The etiology of this condition is unknown, but it is thought to be a hypersensitivity reaction to unknown inhaled antigens. Symptoms of Wegener's granulomatosis include purulent nasal discharge, septal perforation, mucosal ulcerations, and sinusitis. There is usually a slowly progressive destruction and ulceration of the nose and paranasal sinuses with eventual saddle nose deformity. Pulmonary granulomas and vasculitis ensue, as well as focal and crescentic glomerulonephritis and progressive renal failure.

The majority of patients also have ocular involvement, including conjunctivitis, scleritis, uveitis, optic nerve vasculitis, and blindness. The larynx and trachea may be involved as well, causing hoarseness, stridor, and odynophagia. Otologic disease may also be present in the form of an otitis media, tympanic membrane perforation, and sensorineural hearing loss.[24]

Diagnosis is made on the basis of disease involvement in two of the three systems—upper respiratory tract, lung, or kidneys—with tissue biopsy to confirm the diagnosis. Antineutrophil cytoplasmic antibodies (ANCA) titers have been described as a sensitive and specific marker for Wegener's granulomatosis.[25] Other nonspecific laboratory abnormalities may be present, including an elevated erythrocyte sedimentation rate, positive rheumatoid factor, and anemia. The differential diagnosis includes other midline destructive processes of the respiratory tract such as nasal lymphomas, sarcoidosis, and tuberculosis.

In the past, untreated patients with Wegener's granulomatosis had a 93% mortality rate at 2 years.[26] Currently, patients can be treated with a combination of cyclophosphamide and corticosteroids. More than 90% of patients undergo remission on this regimen. Oral trimethoprim-sulfamethoxizole and plasmapharesis have also been tried in cases that are resistant to cyclophosphamide and steroids. Serum ANCA levels can be used to monitor treatment.

The nose and sinuses may be involved in tuberculosis, leprosy, syphilis, and rhinoscleroma. These infections are endemic in parts of the world and should be suspected in immigrants and patients with a history of world travel. Diagnosis is made on the basis of tissue histology and specific stains.

BENIGN NEOPLASMS

The epithelial elements of the nose and sinuses may give rise to benign neoplasms, including papillomas, dermoids, and adenomas. Benign mesenchymal tumors may arise as well, including hemangiomas, osteomas, chondromas, and neurofibromas.

Other tumors, while not histologically malignant, behave more aggressively and tend to recur if incompletely removed. They include angiofibromas, inverted papillomas, fibrous dysplasia, and giant cell tumors.

Nasosinus Papillomas

Nasosinus papillomas have been classified into three major types: fungiform, inverted, and cylindrical.[27,28] The fungiform type usually arises from the anterior portion of the nasal septum, while inverted and cylindrical types arise from the lateral nasal wall. Fungiform papillomas are not considered premalignant, and complete surgical excision is the treatment of choice. There is a relatively low incidence of associated invasive squamous cell carcinoma with fungiform papillomas.

Inverted papillomas occur in an older population than do fungiform. They most commonly originate from the lateral nasal wall in the region of the middle turbinate. The maxillary antrum is often involved and, less commonly, the ethmoids. Though inverted papilloma is considered a benign neoplasm, it can be locally aggressive and invade other sinuses and the orbit. There is a significant incidence of coexisting in situ or invasive squamous cell carcinoma within an inverted papilloma (10% to 20%). Complete surgical extirpation of the disease is the treatment of choice. The lateral rhinotomy approach and medial maxillectomy have achieved the lowest rates of recurrence in this disease,[29,30] although selected cases of smaller lesions limited to the lateral nasal wall may be completely removed endoscopically.[31,32]

Cylindrical cell papilloma is very rare and usually originates on the lateral nasal wall and maxillary sinus in a similar fashion as inverted papilloma.[28]

Angiofibromas

Nasal angiofibromas are commonly called juvenile nasal angiofibromas (JNA) because of the almost exclusive occurrence in prepubescent males. JNA originates in the nasopharynx and is histologically benign, although it is sometimes clinically aggressive. There are many theories as to the cell of origin of this tumor. Schiff[33] proposed that vascular tissue similar to that found in the turbinates may migrate to the nasopharynx during embryonic development. The site of origin of JNA on the posterolateral wall of the roof of the nose represents the approximate location of the attachment of the buccopharyngeal membrane between the stomadeal ectoderm and the foregut ectoderm.[34] There may be wide variations in the caliber of vessels in the tumor and in the cellularity of the surrounding stroma.[35] Taxy[36] described the ultrastructural appearance of stromal cells as having characteristics of both fibroblasts and smooth muscle cells. The vessel walls in JNA lack the contractile components important in vessel constriction following trauma, thus explaining the tendency of these tumors to bleed profusely during surgery.

The tumor may be sessile or pedunculated and is usually attached laterally in the nasopharynx. It may grow to fill the nasal cavity and is a polypoid, reddish, ulcerated mass. Early symptoms, which are often unilateral, include intermittent epistaxis and nasal congestion. Later symptoms include conductive hearing loss from obstruction of the eustachian tube, disturbance of speech, swelling of the cheek and eye, and visual changes.

CT and MRI are used to delineate tumor boundaries, including intracranial extension (Fig. 6–3A). Angiography, essential in the workup of JNA, is characterized by an appearance of multiple tortuous vessels with a dense blush during the capillary phase (Fig. 6–3B). Large venous channels are present, and there is rapid circulation through the tumor. In tumors with intracranial extension, the internal carotid artery involvement must be evaluated to determine feasibility of surgical resection.

In the past, JNA has been unsuccessfully treated with sclerotherapy, hormones, cryotherapy, and embolization. The current preferred methods of treatment for JNA are surgery and radiation therapy, with both modalities achieving high levels of local control. In a large series of patients with JNA from the UCLA Medical Center, local control was achieved in more than 92% of patients treated with primary surgical resection.[37] Radiation therapy was

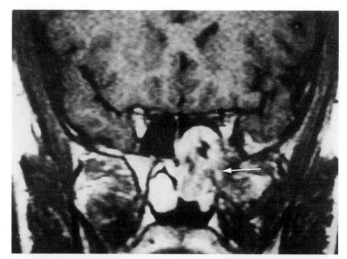

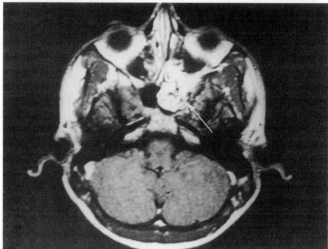

A

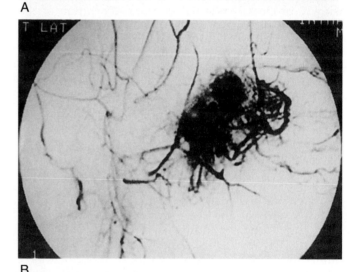

B

FIGURE 6–3 *A,* MRI of a teenaged boy with juvenile nasal angiofibroma involving the left nasopharynx and paranasal sinuses (*arrows*): Coronal view (*upper*) and axial view (*lower*). *B,* Angiogram of patient in part *A* demonstrating multiple feeding vessels and intense blush during the capillary phase. From Myers EN, Suen JY. *Cancer of the Head and Neck,* 3rd ed. Churchill-Livingstone; 1996:650: Fig. 31–4 A and B, Fig. 31–5, with permission.

reserved for patients who had intracranial disease or tumors fed by parasellar feeding vessels.

Surgical resection of most tumors can be done via a transpalatal approach, avoiding an external facial scar.[37] There is adequate exposure of the nasopharynx, pterygopalatine fossa, and nasal cavity for tumors up to about 6 cm in diameter. A lateral rhinotomy approach may be necessary for larger tumors. The most important consideration during an operation for JNA is complete extirpation of the tumor. Prior to packing and closure, the cavity should be carefully inspected for residual disease.

Preoperative embolization should be done within 48 hours of surgery and can significantly decrease the operative blood loss.[38] External carotid artery ligation may be required when facilities for embolization are not available.

Patients with tumors that have intracranial extension or intracranial feeding vessels should receive primary radiation therapy.[37] A significant proportion of these patients respond to one course of radiation therapy (3600 cGy), while some require a second course. An important consideration in this group of young patients is the delayed effect of radiation therapy on facial bone growth and maturation. In addition, there may be predisposition to the later development of malignancy.

Other Benign Neoplasms

Most hemangiomas are of the capillary type and are found in the nasal septum.[39] Cavernous hemangiomas and other vascular malformations are rare. Clinically, these vascular lesions can cause symptoms of bleeding and nasal obstruction.

Fibrous and fibro-osseous tumors include fibrous dysplasia, and ossifying fibroma.[40–42] These must be distinguished from low-grade fibrosarcoma on the basis of mitotic activity and nuclear atypia. Treatment for these benign fibrous lesions is complete excision with clear surgical margins.

MALIGNANT NEOPLASMS

Incidence and Epidemiology

Tumors of the nasal cavity and sinuses comprise 0.2% to 0.8% of all neoplasms and 3% of those of the upper aerodigestive tract. In the United States they occur with a frequency of 0.1 to 0.3 per 100,000 in the first decade of life, gradually escalating to 7 per 100,000 by the eighth decade.[3,43–45] Approximately 40% to 50% can be ascribed to a particular environmental origin, ranging from tobacco smoke to salted or smoked foods to (most commonly) occupational exposures. Heavy metal particles or their (heated) fumes such as occur in nickel or chromium mining, smelting, or welding increase the incidence of paranasal carcinomas in workers at least 10-fold. This to a lesser extent in the refining/processing of volatile hydrocarbons or isopropyl oils.[3,44,46] Inhaled organic fibers in leather and textile industries raise the incidence of paranasal malignancies three- to fivefold above the general population. In the woodworking industries, from milling to furniture, the incidence is up to 540-fold (especially if coupled with hydrocarbon adjuncts such as formaldehyde or similarly based glues in particleboard and the like).[3,46,47] With organic product exposures, adenocarcinomas are more frequent than carcinomas (22:1 ratio). There is a 2:1 male-to-female predominance in paranasal malignancies, possibly due to a predominance of male workers in the aforementioned industries. Human papillomavirus has been cited as a cofactor, particularly subtypes 6 and 12, in up to 24% of inverting papillomas.[3,48] Chronic irritation of the nose and sinuses from chronic sinusitis and/or inhalant allergies has been designated as a risk factor for nasal neoplasia in some series, but not in others.

Approximately 50% of paranasal neoplasms are malignant, with squamous cell carcinomas comprising 50% to 80%. Minor salivary gland carcinomas and olfactory neuroblastomas form the majority of remaining tumors. The other half of paranasal neoplasms are benign, most commonly inverted and other squamous papillomas. The sites of origin of paranasal tumors are the maxillary sinuses in 55% to 63%, the nasal walls in 27% to 35%, the ethmoid sinuses in 9% to 10%, and the frontal and sphenoid sinuses in 1% to 2% each.[3,43–45]

Staging Classifications

There are a number of classification schemes for tumors of the nose and paranasal sinuses, but the one endorsed by the American Joint Committee on Cancer (AJCC) is only for maxillary sinus tumors (Table 6–1).[49,50] The AJCC system—at least the first two stages thereof—is based on Ohngren's line, a theoretical plane oriented between the medial canthus of the eye and the angle of the mandible, dividing the antrum into an "infrastructure" (anteroinferior antrum) and a "suprastructure" (posterosuperior antrum). The basis for this distinction is that anteroinferior tumors initially spread into the adjacent cheek or hard palate, areas easier to extirpate en bloc than those adjacent to the posterosuperior walls—that is, the orbital and pterygopalatine regions.

Many use the University of Florida staging system for tumors of the nasal cavity and of the ethmoid, sphenoid, and frontal sinuses.[4] Some also apply it to maxillary sinus tumors.[3] This system, which was developed by radiation oncologists, was designed so that Stage I malignancies could be treated with equal effectiveness by irradiation or surgery, Stage II malignancies optimally by combined therapy, and

TABLE 6 – 1	STAGING SYSTEM OF PARANASAL SINUS TUMORS

AJCC:[5]

T0:	No primary tumor
T1:	Tumor confined to mucosa of antral infrastructure without bony erosion or destruction
T2:	Tumor confined to mucosal suprastructure without bony destruction, or, to infrastructure with only medial or inferior bony destruction
T3:	More extensive tumor invading cheek skin, orbit, anterior ethmoid sinuses, or pterygoid muscles
T4:	Massive tumor with invasion of cribriform plate, posterior ethmoids, sphenoid, nasopharynx, or skull bone

UNIVERSITY OF FLORIDA:[4]

Stage I:	Limited to site of origin
Stage II:	Extension to adjacent sites (e.g., orbit, nasopharynx, paranasal sinuses, skin)
Stage III:	Base of skull or pterygoid plate destruction, intracranial extension

Stage III malignancies by either combined therapy or palliative modalities, depending on involvement of the brain, carotid artery, and the like. The University of Florida system correctly places malignancies with the poorest prognoses—that is, those with intracranial extension or base of skull—into Stage III.

Anteriorly in the nasal cavity, tumors of the nasal vestibule, columella, and adjacent anterior septum can be classified according to the AJCC system for skin cancers.[4,50] In general, the prognosis for tumors of similar histologies diminishes as one progresses from anterior to posterior in the paranasal region, and such must be kept in mind when evaluating the case mix of any particular series report.

Clinical Presentation

It has been stated that the best strategy for diminishing mortality from a paranasal malignancy is education of the primary-care physician and patients, particularly in occupationally exposed populations.[3,4,43] The median delay between the first symptoms of paranasal neoplasm and the diagnosis is 6–8 months. By then most tumors have reached an advanced stage. Initial symptoms may include unilateral nasal airway compromise, increased mucoid or purulent discharge from local obstruction, or decreased olfaction. For all nasal cavity lesions and sinus neoplasms eroding into the nasal cavities, epistaxis is common. Tumors involving the ethmoid, maxillary, or frontal sinuses can cause proptosis, restriction of eye motility, diplopia or loss of vision, and epiphora from lacrimal sac or duct invasion. Either direct invasion at the tumor site or perineural spread can compromise the functions of cranial nerves 1 through 6. Anterior tumor extension from the maxillary sinus can cause facial swelling as well as cheek paresthesias from infraorbital nerve involvement. Inferior extension can loosen teeth and cause bleeding and pain. Posterior extension can cause trismus from pterygoid muscle invasion. In addition to orbital manifestations, frontal, ethmoid, and sphenoid tumors will cause dull headaches as the cranial vault is eroded and the dura invaded. Metastatic parotid or cervical adenopathy occurs in 9% to 19% of patients.

Given that most tumors have reached an advanced stage by the time of clinical presentation, the histologic diagnosis is usually obtainable transnasally should tumor involvement be confined to a sinus. Endoscopically guided biopsy is possible via a gingivobuccal approach.

Diagnostic Imaging

Computer tomography (CT) and magnetic resonance imaging (MRI) are the principal imaging modalities for paranasal malignancies. Arteriography is reserved for highly vascular tumors (e.g., hemangiopericytomas, some sarcomas) in which preoperative embolization is desired and for tumors that abut the carotid artery. Such delineation of artery/tumor interface and a perioperative trial balloon occlusion is desirable in order to establish whether that vessel can be temporarily or permanently occluded during extirpative surgery.[3,4,51,52]

Computed tomography is the initial test applied to most paranasal processes, whether inflammatory or neoplastic. In general, malignant tumors destroy bone, particularly the squamous cell carcinomas that comprise up to 80% of paranasal malignancies. Some malignancies, principally sarcomas and minor salivary gland carcinomas, may incite a thickening or remodeling of adjacent bone, findings more characteristic of benign neoplasms or chronic inflammatory processes such as fungal sinusitis.[51] Inflammatory pseudotumors may cause frank bony destruction and mimic a malignancy.[53] The reaction to an expanding neoplasm differs between the skull and the facial bones. In the former, there tends to be an impaired remodeling ability with a more likely appearance of erosion from benign lesions. The facial bones remodel around benign processes or demonstrate increased bony density as is common in chronic inflammations.[51] Computed tomography is superior to MRI in bony delineation when bone reconstruction algorithms are utilized, and thin (3 mm) slices are taken. Coronally oriented scans are particularly useful for planning the surgical approach and for evaluating the anterior skull base, orbital, ethmoid, and lateral sphenoid walls. Axial scans are preferred for evaluating the soft tissues in the orbital apex and face, the pterygopalatine fossa, and the anterior and posterior walls of the maxillary, frontal, and sphenoid sinuses. Sagittal recon-

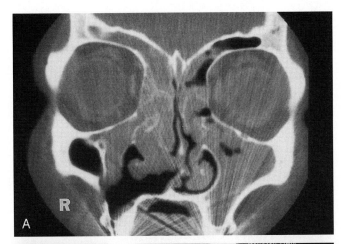

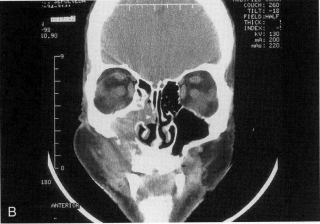

FIGURE 6–4 *A,* Coronal CT scan of the paranasal sinuses showing bilateral opacification with probable inflammatory mucosa. *B,* Coronal CT scan demonstrating unilateral maxillary sinus opacification with local destruction of bone and soft tissue invasion. This is typical for carcinoma (as opposed to bilateral opacification with inflammatory disease).

inspissated secretions, with a high water content, have high signal intensity on T2-weighted images. In contrast, cellular paranasal neoplasms have lesser amounts of water and demonstrate intermediate signal intensities on T2-weighted images (Fig. 6–5). Those few paranasal tumors that have a high signal intensity on T2-weighted images include minor salivary gland carcinomas and hemangiomas. Tumor enhancement with intravenous gadolinium is best demonstrated on T1-weighted images; most sinus neoplasms enhance to an intermediate degree and are homogeneous in character. Tumor enhancement makes detection of spread to or through dural or periorbital margin easier to discern. As inflammatory processes also demonstrate enhancement, non-contrasted T1- and T2-weighted studies should be completed before the injection of gadolinium.[51,52]

Salient questions to be answered by the radiographic imaging include the tumor soft tissue margins, particularly the periorbital and dural planes, and the relationship of tumor to the internal carotid artery and cavernous sinus. Most CT or MRI studies for paranasal malignancies extend to the level of the hyoid bone, thereby affording detection of metastatic adenopathy, particularly the retropharyngeal nodes, which are not accessible to physical examination. Extension of imaging to the hyoid should be specified, if not routine, with any paranasal malignancy that extends into the soft tissues of the face, oral cavity, or infratemporal fossa, as these regions are rich in lymphatics and hence are associated with a higher rate of metastatic adenopathy.

Certain malignancies, particularly adenoid cystic carcinomas, have a predilection for perineural spread. Such is best detected by a gadolinium contrasted MRI and T1-weighted images with fat suppression. Evidence of perineural spread must be sought in any patient with a disturbance of extraocular mobility, facial paresthesia, or weakness of the muscles of mastication. Typically denervated muscle

structions are commonly eschewed, but can be valuable in detailing some walls of the frontal and sphenoid sinuses, the cribriform plate, and the floor of the anterior fossa. Tumors usually exhibit a soft tissue density on CT scans, whereas normal or inflamed mucosa and most secretions have a lower, or water, density. Differentiation of tumor margins from areas of inflamed mucosa and the like are best addressed when the CT is obtained with an iodinated intravenous contrast, an approach that also makes it easy to detect tumor involvement of the dura or periorbita with both enhancing when invaded by tumor (Fig. 6–4).

Magnetic resonance imaging offers superior delineation of the soft tissue margins of a tumor, particularly when there is adjacent inflammation. The addition of intravenous gadolinium for magnetic resonance angiography (MRA) details tumor vascularity and its afferent blood supply; such studies can render diagnostic arteriography superfluous in some cases.[3,4,51,52] Inflamed mucosa, polyps, and non-

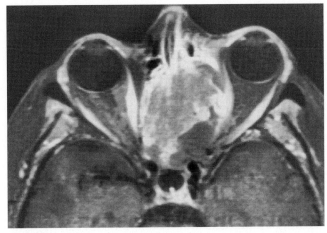

FIGURE 6–5 Axial MRI scan showing tumor invasion at the left orbital apex with surrounding inflammatory reaction.

exhibits a fatty infiltration that is easily detected by MRI.

The first post-therapy imaging is obtained 3 to 4 months after the treatment. Most prefer an MRI with gadolinium, as it is more sensitive to the early soft tissue changes of an early recurrence. The initial post-treatment images act as the new "baseline" for the patient, and a change from that baseline is commonly the earliest sign of tumor persistence. Positron emission tomography (PET), with tagged fluorodeoxyglucose, can in some cases distinguish surgical, radiation, or inflammatory changes from a recurrent tumor. The availability of that modality, however, is limited at present, and the study should be reserved for equivocal MRI findings in an area difficult to access for biopsy.

Patterns of Tumor Spread

Regional metastases from paranasal malignancies are uncommon, occurring in 9% to 14% of squamous cell carcinomas and 10% to 19% of most of the remaining malignancies. Lymphomas, plasmacytomas, melanomas, and some sarcomas have, as elsewhere in the body, a high propensity for distant spread.[3,4,43,44,54] The lymphatics of the nasal vestibule and anterior septum drain into the submandibular nodes, with the first echelon being the perivascular nodes along the facial vein as it crosses the mandible. The lymphatics of the posterior nasal cavity and the sphenoid connect to the deep parotid and retropharyngeal nodes of Rouviere that are located medial to the internal carotid arteries below the skull base; both of the aforementioned drain into the jugulodigastric nodes. In general, neoplasms confined within intact sinus walls rarely metastasize, either regionally or to a distant site. Only with erosion into the lymphatics of the soft tissues outside the sinuses does the incidence of metastases increase. Frontal malignancies that erode to the forehead skin eventually appear in the parotid nodes, as do malignancies of the maxillary sinus that spread to the pterygoid muscles. Maxillary carcinomas eroding inferiorly into the soft palate present in the jugulodigastric nodes; those spreading into the cheek skin present in the submandibular nodes. Since the ethmoid sinuses are bordered on two sides by the orbit and brain (neither with a defined lymphatic drainage pattern), access to lymphatics requires posterior invasion into the nasopharynx (retropharyngeal nodes) or anterior invasion into the medial canthal region (submandibular or parotid nodes). Distant metastases from paranasal malignancies are far less common than regional metastases, and usually only manifest in advanced disease states, frequently with regional metastases already present.[3,4,43,44,54] Adenoid cystic carcinoma tends to spread, in order of frequency, by perineural invasion, bloodborne metastases (primarily to the lung), and regional lymphatics. An assessment of the functions of cranial nerves traversing the paranasal sinus region is therefore important at the initial examination of patients with adenoid cystic carcinoma, and an enhanced MRI is obtained if nerve compromise is detected.

Given the relatively low incidence of regional and distant spreads of common paranasal malignancies, an extensive metastatic work-up is unwarranted in the pre-treatment evaluation of most of these tumors. A chest X-ray and liver function tests suffice in most patients unless specific evidence of distant organ dysfunction is gleaned from the patient history, or adenopathy is detected during the physical examination.

Perioperative Considerations

For most congenital malformations or benign tumors (excepting large clival chordomas and the like) no special preoperative preparation is needed aside from those associated with the patient's general physical condition. For malignancies, particularly when an intracranial portion of an extirpation is anticipated, careful attention must be directed to positioning the endotracheal tube and the head. For extracranial procedures, prophylactic antibiotics are started just prior to the operation and are continued for the duration of nasal packing, with CSF-penetrating characteristics being favored if an intracranial portion of the procedure is anticipated.

Intraoperative considerations include controlled hypotension for vascular tumors or those abutting vascular structures such as the internal carotid artery. Intravenous steroids and controlled hyperventilation to lower arterial pCO_2 are appropriate during intracranial portions of a procedure, with an osmotic diuretic such as mannitol administered when needed.[55-58] A lumbar subarachnoid drain is sometimes placed to drain cerebrospinal fluid during the procedure, thereby easing brain retraction, and left in place for 3 to 5 days postoperatively if a dural repair is required at the extirpation site. Hemostasis is desirable at the end of any operative procedure, but the limited ability to access all the arteries feeding the paranasal region—most of which enter through a bony foramen (e.g., sphenopalatine for the internal maxillary artery)—favors the placement of an antibiotic ointment–coated nasal and sinus pack for 3 to 5 days. Hemorrhage is the most common perioperative complication, occurring in up to 20% of patients, albeit minor in most.

Cerebrospinal fluid leak occurs in up to 14% of those in whom dura is exposed.[57-60] A watertight closure around any dural defect is mandatory. When the dura has not been violated, full thickness mucosal or skin grafts applied to any exposed dura, and supported by a nasal pack, are the simplest method for defect resurfacing. With intracranial intervention, a pericranial flap pedicled on the supraorbital vascular bundles is raised separately from the bicoronal forehead flap and utilized to resurface the floor of the anterior fossa. When the pericranium has been compromised by prior operations, temporalis muscle flaps may be sufficient if they can reach across the midline of the anterior fossa and be sutured to each other in a "pants over vest" fashion. Prior operations, especially if irradiation has been utilized, compromise vascularity in the surgical field, and consideration to repairing dural defects with a vascularized free flap is appropriate; a radial forearm free flap is commonly selected.[58–63]

Epiphora is frequent after paranasal tumor operations. If the distal nasolacrimal duct has been interrupted by the resection (e.g., midfacial degloving), a silastic stent threaded through the canaliculi into the nasal cavity and left for 6 to 8 weeks assures patency. If the proximal nasolacrimal duct has been divided at its junction with the lacrimal sac (e.g., lateral rhinotomy), a dacryocystorhinostomy is performed. Even without an anatomic disruption, edema in the anterior nasal/orbital region from a tumor extirpation is frequently sufficient for epiphora to last up to 1 to 2 months postoperatively. If it continues thereafter, the patency of the nasolacrimal drainage system is evaluated by probing or dacryocystography, and addressed by dacryocystorhinostomy (DCR) if ductal obstruction is verified.[3,57,60]

Enophthalmos and/or diplopia occur most frequently after orbital floor resections, such as after maxillectomy, and can be addressed by temporalis muscle slings placed under the orbital soft tissues at the time of operation. A split-thickness skin graft over exposed periorbita is a satisfactory alternative, as postoperative graft contracture usually provides sufficient orbital support within a few months. Irradiation substantially increases postoperative orbital complications and should be kept in mind when making a decision to spare an orbit during resection of a malignancy.[3,4,43,57,60,64]

Osteomyelitis after sinus tumor surgery is infrequent, even after irradiation, unless an intracranial procedure is required. In such a case, the bifrontal bone flap, which becomes a free bone flap when replaced at the end of a procedure, may become infected or necrose. Reconstruction at a later date can range from an acrylic plate or hydroxyapatite paste to a fine mesh metal sheet.[58–63]

Surgical Approaches

The surgical approach to a paranasal neoplasm is based on such factors as the size and location of the tumor, its histology, and its relationship to the skull base, orbits, and the cavernous sinuses. Regardless of the approach, incisions are placed along the junctions of the anatomic units to minimize visible scarring (e.g., lateral rhinotomy incision positioned at junction of the nose and cheek). Aesthetic units are mobilized en bloc where necessary (e.g., nasal bones and caudal septum mobilized in one piece for an extended lateral rhinotomy), and most dissection is

accomplished in subperiosteal or subfascial planes to preserve blood supply and minimize damage to innervation.[58,59,63–67] The basic surgical approaches can be divided into extracranial and intracranial ones, and they will be discussed separately.

EXTRACRANIAL

The simplest extracranial approach is via the transnasal cavity. Whether performed with endoscopes, magnification loupes, or a microscope, the process involves access through the nostrils to neoplasms confined to the lateral nasal walls or floor, the septum, the ethmoids (if no orbital, sphenoid, or frontal sinus involvement), or the turbinates.[3,67] Septal mobilization, such as with a submucosal "septoplasty," affords wide access to the nasal cavity by displacing the septum into the contralateral nasal cavity. Inverted papillomas and the other squamous papillomas of the nasal walls can be easily extirpated by such an intranasal approach. Tumor extension into the floor of the frontal sinus, to the lamina papyracea, laterally in the maxillary sinus or substantially into the sphenoid sinus are usually contraindications to an endonasal en bloc resection of benign or malignant neoplasms.

For neoplasms that extend to the aforementioned regions, a lateral rhinotomy (most commonly in conjunction with a "medial maxillectomy") is commonly undertaken (Fig. 6–6 A and B).[3,43,54,68–70] This affords access to the medial orbit, the nasal roof, and the frontal, ethmoid, and sphenoid sinuses. For malignancies that penetrate the periorbita, as verified by frozen section, unilateral orbital exenteration can be accomplished by extending the lateral rhinotomy approach to an adjacent orbitotomy. This approach can also serve as the transfacial portion of a combined intracranial/extracranial procedure—for example, for an olfactory neuroblastoma that has eroded the cribriform plate.[71–76] An "extended" lateral rhinotomy incision can also cross the nasion for full bony nasal pyramid and caudal septum mobilizations, with a vascular supply based on the contralateral cheek. Such affords access from the lateral wall of one orbit to the medial wall of the contralateral orbit, encompassing the entire nasal cavity, including the medial walls of the maxillary sinuses, the frontal sinuses, and the sphenoid sinuses.

An alternative to a lateral rhinotomy is a midfacial degloving that passes through the upper gingivobuccal and gingivolabial sulci and upwardly mobilizes the soft tissues of the cheeks and lower nose from the maxilla and caudal septum, thereby providing access to the paranasal region below the inferior orbital rims.[77,78] This approach avoids an external incision but is limited by the infraorbital nerves. Moreover, the most anterior ethmoid cells and the frontal sinuses are not well visualized, and managing any orbital or anterior fossa disease extension may be challenging unless combined with an intracranial access. Benign or early-stage maxillary malig-

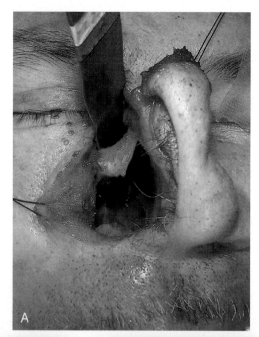

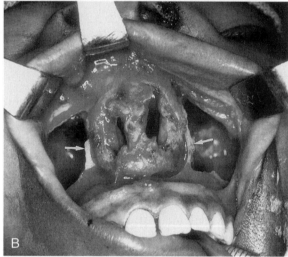

FIGURE 6-6 *A*, Medial maxillectomy of the paranasal sinus via a lateral rhinotomy approach. *B*, Bilateral medial maxillectomies via a midfacial degloving approach. Intact pyriform aperture bony struts are demonstrated (*arrows*).

nancies can be removed via a degloving approach, since this allows access to all walls of the maxillary sinus. If the infraorbital rim and the pyriform aperture bony strut are retained, cosmetic deformity is minimal (see Fig. 6–6B).

Radical maxillectomy that encompasses the orbital contents, the walls of the maxillary sinus, and most of the ethmoid labyrinth can usually be performed through a degloving approach plus medial and lateral canthotomies. However, such an extirpation is usually approached through an extended lateral rhinotomy with a lip split and lateral rotation of the soft tissues of the cheek from the maxilla and or-

bit.[3,43,49] With either approach, the defect is lined with a split-thickness skin graft. It is prudent in any procedure where tumor abuts periorbita, and when exenteration is being considered, to explore that periorbita early during the procedure and to obtain frozen section studies. In this way, a decision to save or sacrifice the orbit can be made and en bloc tumor resection planned accordingly.

Tumors of the posterior nasal cavity, the sphenoid sinuses, and the most posterior ethmoid sinuses can be accessed by midfacial approaches, but lateral extensions of tumor, particularly into the pterygomaxillary region, the orbital apex, and/or the anterior fossa usually demand a combination of surgical approaches.[3,56,58,61,66,70–73,79–82] With lateral tumor extension, carotid artery abutment can frequently be assessed by preoperative diagnostic imaging. In such an instance, it is prudent to expose the internal carotid artery in the neck, then trace it through the skull base as needed. For maxillary tumors that extend through the pterygoid plates, a lower lip split and stairstep paramedian mandibular osteotomy, along with a superior exposure involving a lateral rhinotomy and lip split, allow exposure of the carotid artery from the bifurcation in the neck to the skull base, with the ability to control the internal maxillary and other arteries that may supply the tumor region.[58,80]

For the most posterior ethmoid and sphenoid tumors, a lateral facial split may be necessary. This involves an ipsilateral parotidectomy-type preauricular incision that extends to the submandibular region, frequently a direct extension of a bicoronal incision.[56,58,66] After identifying and tagging (for later reanatomosis) the upper and lower trunks of the facial nerve in the parotid, mobilization of the lateral facial structures such as the zygomatic arch, temporalis muscle, mandible, and parotid in an anterior and lateral direction allows access to the internal carotid artery, the pterygoid plates and parapharyngeal space, the inferior orbital fissure, and—with neurosurgical assistance—the cavernous sinus and optic nerve.

INTRACRANIAL

Intracranial access to the paranasal region is more straightforward than the plethora of extracranial choices and usually involves some modification of a bifrontal craniotomy for paramedian tumors or a frontotemporal (so-called "pteryonal") approach for lateral tumors that can be combined with zygomatic arch and temporal muscle transpositions as needed.[58,66,71,72,82] The intracranial portion of a planned "craniofacial disassembly" is performed first, to assess dural, cavernous sinus, carotid artery, and orbital involvements with the tumor. This approach allows protection of these vital structures during the extracranial procedure. The anterior osteotomy of a bifrontal craniotomy was traditionally placed a few centimeters above the supraorbital rims. However, a "sub-basal" approach that mobilizes the supraorbital rims between the zygomaticofrontal sutures en bloc with the lower half of the frontal bones is now often preferred. This intracranial/extracranial access with one bony excision allows the necessary inferior traction on the orbits to be split with superior retraction on the frontal lobes, hence diminishing the pressure on both during subsequent tumor resection.[58,82]

Radiation Therapy

A minority of sinus neoplasms such as lymphomas and plasmacytomas are highly sensitive to irradiation alone. For other early paranasal malignancies, both surgery and primary irradiation result in 5-year survival rates in the 40% to 75% range. A higher end of that range is seen with olfactory neuroblastomas and squamous cell carcinomas, the middle of the range with salivary gland carcinomas, and the low end of the range for sarcoma and melanomas.[3,4,43,45,68,76,83–90] As with surgery, the tumor histology, the site of origin, and the stage at diagnosis determine the prognosis. In general, the prognosis is best for malignancies confined to the walls of the nasal cavities followed, in order, by ethmoid, antral, frontal, and sphenoid malignancies. Advanced malignancies (T3 and early T4 per AJCC[50] and Stage II per University of Florida system[4,52]) have 5-year survival rates from 10% to 66%, depending on the aforementioned factors. These malignancies are commonly subjected to planned combined therapy, with most favoring postoperative irradiation, although there is no statistical difference in survival rates between preoperative and postoperative irradiation protocols.[3,4,43] Preoperative irradiation is preferred in some centers, especially with relatively radiosensitive tumors such as olfactory neuroblastomas, when there is an indication of tumor abutment to the periorbita or dura. The goal of preoperative irradiation is to "sterilize" tumor in those regions and to avoid exenteration or allow preservation of a preponderance of dura.[64] In all other situations, postoperative irradiation is favored, as this lowers the incidence of postoperative complications such as CSF leaks, suture line healing, and osteomyelitis. Additionally, unirradiated tumor margins are more easily discerned intraoperatively by the surgeon.[3,57,60,68] Preoperative irradiation is commonly given to the 50 Gy range, many favoring a 1.1 to 1.2 Gy twice-a-day dosing protocol, and postoperative irradiation to 60 Gy utilizing the same delivery technique for cure of advanced malignancies.[83,88] High-dose irradiation alone, in the 74–79 Gy range, was favored by some groups until late onset unilateral blindness in approximately 19% of patients; bilateral blindness in 5.6% from optic neuropathy was reported.[88] Such therapy has fallen out of favor for all but "unresectable" tumors. The latter are defined by tumor extension into the brain, bone marrow of the skull base,

through a lateral or posterior wall of a sphenoid sinus, or into the internal carotid artery. Although all of the aforementioned may be technically resectable, morbidity is high and cure low.[55,58,74,83,88,90–92] High-dose irradiation for "unresectable" malignancies can be associated with 5-year survival rates of up to 10%; in such circumstances radiation retinopathy is an acceptable risk.[88] Prophylactic lymphadenectomy is not a part of most surgical treatments of paranasal malignancy. Similarly, elective neck irradiation is avoided unless the neoplasm is poorly differentiated, or there is an extensive recurrence that has extended into areas outside the paranasal region affording tumor access to abundant lymphatics, (e.g., the pterygoid muscles, soft palate, cheek, or the nasopharynx).

Combination therapy for advanced sinus malignancies is superior to either surgery or irradiation alone. External beam irradiation can be supplemented by brachytherapy administered via implants or removable dental-type prostheses as appropriate. Cure following en bloc resection of a paranasal malignancy with "clear" margins is reported to be increased an average of 11% to 15% with the addition of irradiation.[3,83,88] It should be kept in mind that surgical margins in the paranasal region are usually much less than the 2 or more centimeters traditionally obtained in the oral cavity and pharynx. Since the paranasal region is an anatomically complex region, a truly "wide" margin of resection would entail disabling morbidity. For most paranasal malignancies regional and distant metastatic rates combined are less than 25%, thus the increased cure rate from preoperative or postoperative irradiation is mainly attributable to increased local control.[83,88,91,92]

There are some reports on the use of stereotactic radiosurgery, with the "gamma knife" or 3D oriented high-energy external beam therapy in treating paranasal sinus tumors. This allows the delivery of curative doses while minimizing the potential for damage to the retina or major cranial nerves. However, these techniques are too new to fully evaluate their efficacy. Similarly, intraoperative irradiation can increase the cure rates for locally extensive disease with inadequate surgical margins, but insufficient long-term follow-up and the potential for late complications limit this form of treatment to a small number of institutions.[3,88,92]

Chemotherapy

Chemotherapy for paranasal malignancies has usually been reserved for the palliative treatment of advanced or recurrent tumors. Cisplatin-base protocols are favored for squamous cell carcinomas and doxorubicin or fluorouracil regimens for tumors of salivary gland origin.[3,43] Intravenous induction chemotherapy combined with irradiation doses below those causing optic nerve or retinal damage has been the subject of encouraging reports, but data is insufficient.

Non–Squamous Cell Malignant Neoplasms

GLANDULAR NEOPLASMS

Most nonsquamous carcinomas of the paranasal sinuses arise from either the salivary glands or respiratory epithelium of the mucosa.[93] The most common nonsquamous carcinomas are adenocarcinoma, adenoid cystic carcinoma, and mucoepidermoid carcinoma.[94]

Adenocarcinomas have a predilection for the ethmoid sinuses. There is an association between wood and furniture work and development of this carcinoma. Nearly 90% of cases are in males, with a peak age incidence of 50 to 60 years.

Adenocarcinomas can be classified as high- or low-grade based on the histologic features. There are three basic growth forms—papillary, sessile, and alveolar-mucoid—but tumors may possess combinations of patterns.[95] The papillary type has a fibrovascular core and arises from the surface epithelium. The sessile type resembles adenocarcinoma of the gastrointestinal tract. The alveolar-mucoid type is characterized by multiple goblet cells and nests of tumor cells within a mucinous background. Tumors with a predominance of the papillary type may have a better prognosis.

Adenoid cystic carcinoma is the predominant tumor type arising from minor salivary glands and represents 5% to 15% of malignant tumors arising in the paranasal sinuses. These tumors occur in equal numbers in males and females and occur most frequently in the fourth to sixth decades. The most common site is the maxilla, followed by the nasal cavity, ethmoids, nasopharynx, and other sinuses.[28]

Although adenoid cystic carcinoma is characterized by slow growth, it is locally aggressive with perineural spread and skull base invasion. Because recurrences can occur 10 to 20 years after treatment, short-term survival rates must be interpreted with extreme caution.[95] Because of the propensity for perineural spread to the cranial cavity and central nervous system, adenoid cystic tumors of the paranasal sinuses have the worst prognosis of all head and neck adenoid cystic carcinomas.[96]

Lymphatic spread is unusual in adenoid cystic carcinoma, while distant metastases are more common, occurring in approximately 40% of cases.[97] The most frequent sites of metastases are to lung and bone. Systemic metastases usually occur with failure to control disease at the primary site, thus mandating aggressive efforts for local control. Although distant metastases are usually associated with poor prognosis, the 5-year survival rate of patients with metastatic adenoid cystic carcinoma is more than 20%.

The treatment of choice for adenoid cystic carcinoma is complete tumor extirpation. The tumor is considered radiosensitive but not radiocurable. The propensity for perineural spread makes obtaining clear margins difficult. Postoperative radiation has been used to improve local control, especially in cases with microscopic residual disease or close margins.[98] Aggressive local therapy is warranted even in patients with distant metastases, since a significant number of patients will live for many years with their disease.

Other malignant neoplasms of the minor salivary glands can occur in the nasal cavity and paranasal sinuses, including mucoepidermoid carcinomas, malignant mixed tumors, and acinic cell carcinomas. These types are found much less frequently than adenoid cystic carcinomas. Benign salivary gland neoplasms, such as pleomorphic adenomas, are likewise rarely found in the nasal cavity and paranasal sinuses and have histologic and clinical features similar to those found in the major salivary glands.

MALIGNANT MELANOMA

Melanomas of the sinonasal tract are rare. In the nasal cavity the most frequently involved site is the anterior septum. In the sinuses, the maxillary antrum is more frequently involved than the ethmoids.[99,100] Examination usually reveals a pigmented mass; however, some melanomas lack the typical pigment and may appear pink-tan. Metastastic melanomas to the nasal cavity and paranasal sinuses have been described.[101]

Prognosis for sinonasal melanomas is poor. Wide local excision is the treatment of choice. Only 10% to 20% of patients have cervical metastases, and a therapeutic neck dissection is indicated in these patients. In one series, the 5-year survival rate was 11% and the 20-year survival rate was 0.5%.[102] In another series only patients with mucosal melanomas measuring less than 8 mm in thickness survived.[103] Death usually results from disseminated metastases.

OLFACTORY NEUROBLASTOMA

Olfactory neuroblastoma, or esthesioneuroblastoma, is believed to originate from neural crest cells that are found in the upper part of the nasal cavity.[104–106] These are specialized olfactory epithelial cells that can also give rise to neuroendocrine tumors within the nasal cavity. Olfactory neuroblastomas usually occur after age 40 and produce symptoms of nasal obstruction, facial swelling, epistaxis, and—at late stages—cranial nerve deficits.

Histologically the tumor is composed of small round cells, larger than lymphocytes, with dense nuclei. In well-differentiated tumors, the cells are arranged in rosettes and pseudorosettes, while poorly differentiated tumors contain solid sheets of anaplastic cells.

A clinical staging system was proposed by Kadish[107] in 1976, based on a series of 17 patients treated over 30 years:

Group A: Tumor confined to nasal cavity

Group B: Tumor extending into paranasal sinuses

Group C: Tumor spread beyond nasal cavity and paranasal cavity

Dulguerov and Calcaterra[108] proposed a new staging system using CT and MRI scanning to ascertain disease extent. Patients treated by radiation or surgery can be staged. A better correlation with outcome was found utilizing the following system:

T1: Tumor involving the paranasal cavity and/or paranasal sinuses (excluding sphenoid), sparing the most superior ethmoid cells

T2: Tumor involving the nasal cavity and/or paranasal sinuses (including the sphenoid) with extension to or erosion of the cribriform plate

T3: Tumor extending into the orbit or protruding into the anterior cranial fossa

T4: Tumor involving the brain

Complete surgical resection is the treatment of choice for these tumors. Because of tumor location at the cribriform plate, a combined craniofacial resection is required to obtain clear surgical margins. Postoperative radiation is usually given with excellent local control rates.[108]

OTHER NONEPITHELIAL TUMORS

Malignant fibrous tumors encompass a range of lesions from low-grade fibromatosis to fibrosarcoma.[42] Wide local excision is the treatment of choice for low-grade lesions. Postoperative radiation therapy is utilized for recurrent tumors or positive margins.

Rhabdomyosarcoma involves the nose and paranasal sinuses in about 3% to 4% of cases.[28] In this region, it is classified as a nonorbital parameningeal site and tends to have a more aggressive behavior than tumors from other sites.[109] The Intergroup Rhabdomyosarcoma Study reports an improved prognosis for patients when intensive chemotherapy and radiation therapy are used in nonorbital parameningeal tumors in the pediatric population.[110] However, most adult rhabdomyosarcomas are treated with wide surgical resection and postoperative radiation. Chemotherapy and/or radiation therapy is used to manage recurrences or unresectable tumors.

Osteogenic and chondrosarcomas are uncommon in the maxilla. These lesions are best treated aggressively with wide surgical resection, radiation therapy, and chemotherapy.[111] Prognosis is poor because of the aggressive behavior of high-grade tumors. Five-year survival rates approximate 10% to 20%. Some promising results have been obtained with neutron beam therapy in these patients.[112]

Treatment for sinonasal lymphomas consists of primary radiation therapy when the disease is confined to one site. Chemotherapy is reserved for patients with systemic disease. In one large series of 18 patients with polymorphic reticulosis at the Mayo Clinic, the Kaplan-Meier estimate of survival was 63% at 5 years and 50% at 15 years.[113]

CONCLUSION

For effective diagnosis and treatment, it is necessary to have a thorough understanding of the anatomy and disease processes of the complex region surveyed in this chapter. Clinicians should be aware of the difficulties a pathologist may have in rendering a definitive diagnosis, and pathologists should be familiar with the clinical ramifications of their decisions.

REFERENCES

1. Langman J. Head and neck. In: *Medical Embryology*. 6th ed. Baltimore: Williams & Wilkins; 1990:280.
2. Anon JB, Rontal M, Zinreich SJ. Embryology and anatomy of the paranasal sinuses. In: Bluestone C, Stool S, Kenna M, eds. *Pediatric Otolaryngology*. 3rd ed. Philadelphia: W.B. Saunders; 1966:719.
3. Osguthorpe JD. Sinus neoplasia. *Arch Otolaryngol Head Neck Surg*. 1994; 120:19.
4. Parsons JT, Stringer SP, Mancuso AA, Million RR. Nasal vestibule, nasal cavity, and paranasal sinuses. In: Million RR, Cassisi NJ, eds. *Management of Head and Neck Cancer: A Multidisciplinary Approach*. 2nd ed. Philadelphia: J.B. Lippincott; 1994:551.
5. Hilding AC. The role of the respiratory mucosa in health and disease. *Minn Med*. 1967; 50:915.
6. Grossman M. The saccharin test of nasal mucociliary function. *ENT*. 1975; 54:415.
7. Hengerer AS, Yanofsky SD. Congenital malformations of the nose and paranasal sinuses. In: Bluestone C, Stool S, Kenna M, eds. *Pediatric Otolaryngology*. 3rd ed. Philadelphia: W.B. Saunders; 1996:831.
8. Benson V, Marano MA. Current estimates from the 1993 National Health Interview Survey. National Center for Health Statistics. *Vital Health Stat 10*. 1994; 190.
9. Collins JG. Prevalence of selected chronic conditions: United States, 1986–1988. National Center for Health Statistics. *Vital Health Stat 10*. 1993; 1.
10. Hahn B, Lefkowitz D. Annual expenses and sources of payment for health care services. Rockville, MD: Public Health Service, National Expenditure Survey Research Findings 14, Agency for Health Care Policy and Research, Publication No. 93-0007, 1994.
11. Lanza D, Kennedy D. Adult rhinosinusitis defined. *Arch Otolaryngol Head Neck Surg*. 1997; 117(suppl):S1.
12. Chandler JR, Langenbruner DJ, Stevens ER. The pathogenesis of orbital complications in acute sinusitis. *Laryngoscope*. 1970; 80:1414.
13. Gwaltney JM, Sydnor A, Sande MA. Etiology and antimicrobial treatment of acute sinusitis. *Ann Otol Rhinol Laryngol*. 1981; 90:68.
14. Jousimies-Somer HR, Savolainen S, Ylikoski JS. Bacteriological findings of acute maxillary sinusitis in young adults. *J Clin Microbiol*. 1988; 26:1919.
15. Gwaltney JM, Scheld WM, Sande MA, et al. The microbial etiology and antimicrobial therapy of adults with acute community-acquired sinusitis: A fifteen-year experience at the

University of Virginia and review of other selected studies. *J Allergy Clin Immunol.* 1992; 90:457.

16. Peterson KL, Wang M, Canalis RF, Abemayor E. Rhinocerebral mucormycosis: Evolution of the disease and treatment options. *Laryngoscope.* 1997; 107:855.

17. Manning SC, Mabry RL, Shaefer SD, et al. Evidence of IgE-mediated hypersensitivity in allergic fungal sinusitis. *Laryngoscope.* 1992; 103:717.

18. Mabry RL, Manning SC. Radioallergosorbent microscreen and total immunoglobulin E in allergic fungal sinusitis. *Arch Otolaryngol Head Neck Surg.* 1995; 113:721.

19. Bent JP III, Kuhn FA. Diagnosis of allergic fungal sinusitis. *Arch Otolaryngol Head Neck Surg.* 1994; 111:580.

20. Morpeth JF, Rupp NT, Dolen WK, et al. Fungal sinusitis: An update. *Ann Allergy Asthma Immunol.* 1996; 76:128.

21. Benninger MS, Anon J, Mabry RL. The medical management of rhinosinusitis. *Arch Otolaryngol Head Neck Surg.* 1997; 117 (suppl):S41.

22. Cleary KR, Batsakis JG. Sinonasal lymphomas. *Ann Otol Rhinol Laryngol.* 1994; 103:911.

23. Wegener F. Uber eine eigenartige rhinogene Granulomatose mit besonderer Beteiligung des Arteriensystems und der Nieren. *Beitr Pathol Anat.* 1939; 102:36.

24. Vartiainen E, Nuntinen J. Head and neck manifestations of Wegener's granulomatosis. *ENT J.* 1992; 71:423.

25. Kallenberg CG, Mulder AH, Tervaert JW. Antineutrophil cytoplasmic antibodies: a still-growing class of autoantibodies in inflammatory disorders. *Am J Med.* 1992; 93:678.

26. Hoffman GS, Kerr GS, Leavitt RY, et al. Wegener's granulomatosis: an analysis of 158 patients. *Ann Intern Med.* 1992; 116:488.

27. Hyams VJ. Papillomas of the nasal cavity and paranasal sinuses. A clinicopathologic study of 315 cases. *Ann Otol Rhinol Laryngol.* 1971; 80:192.

28. Barnes L, Verbin RS, Gnepp DR. Diseases of the nose, paranasal sinuses, and nasopharynx. In: Barnes L, ed. *Surgical Pathology of the Head and Neck.* Vol 1. New York: Marcel Dekker; 1985:403.

29. Calcaterra TC, Thompson JW, Pagilia DE. Inverting papillomas of the nose and paranasal sinuses. *Laryngoscope.* 1980; 90:53.

30. Myers EN, Fernau JL, Johnson JT, et al. Management of inverted papilloma. *Laryngoscope.* 1990; 100:481.

31. Stankiewicz JA, Girgis SJ. Endoscopic surgical treatment of nasal and paranasal sinus inverted papilloma. *Arch Otolaryngol Head Neck Surg.* 1993; 109:988.

32. McCary WS, Gross CW, Reibel JF, Cantrell RW. Preliminary report: endoscopic vs. external surgery in the management of inverted papilloma. *Laryngoscope.* 1994; 104:415.

33. Schiff M. Juvenile nasopharyngeal angiofibroma: a theory of pathogenesis. *Laryngoscope.* 1959; 9:981.

34. Hamilton W, Mossman H. *Human Embryology: Prenatal Development of Form and Function.* 4th ed. Baltimore: Williams & Wilkins; 1972.

35. Grybauskas V, Parker J, Friedman M. Juvenile nasopharyngeal angiofibroma. *Otolaryngol Clin N Am.* 1986; 19:647.

36. Taxy J. Juvenile nasopharyngeal angiofibroma: an ultrastructural study. *Cancer.* 1977; 39:1044.

37. Economou T, Abemayor E, Ward P. Juvenile nasopharyngeal angiofibroma: an update of the UCLA experience, 1960–1985. *Laryngoscope.* 1988; 98:170.

38. Jacobson M, Petruson B, Svendsen P, et al. Juvenile nasopharyngeal angiofibroma. *Acta Otolaryngol* (Stockh). 1988; 105:132.

39. Fu YS, Perzin KH. Non-epithelial tumors of the nasal cavity, paranasal sinuses and nasopharynx: a clinicopathologic study. I. General features and vascular tumors. *Cancer.* 1974; 33:1275.

40. Zukerberg LR, Rosenberg AE, Randolph G, Pilch BZ, Goodman ML. Solitary fibrous tumor of the nasal cavity and paranasal sinuses. *Am J Surg Pathol.* 1991; 15:126.

41. Witkin GB, Rosai J. Solitary fibrous tumor of the upper respiratory tract: a report of six cases. *Am J Surg Pathol.* 1991; 15:842.

42. Fu YS, Perzin KH. Non-epithelial tumors of the nasal cavity, paranasal sinuses and nasopharynx: a clinicopathologic study. VI. Fibrous tissue tumors. *Cancer.* 1976; 37:2912.

43. Sisson GA, Toriumi DM, Atiyah RA. Paranasal sinus malignancy: a comprehensive update. *Laryngoscope.* 1989; 99:143.

44. Batsakis JG. Cancer of the nasal cavity and paranasal sinuses. In: *Tumors of the Head and Neck: Clinical and Pathological Considerations.* 2nd ed. Baltimore: Williams & Wilkins; 1979:177.

45. Bridger GP, Baldwin M. Anterior craniofacial resection for ethmoid and nasal cancer with free flap reconstruction. *Arch Otolaryngol Head Neck Surg.* 1989; 115:308.

46. Holt GR. Sinonasal neoplasms and inhaled air toxins. *Arch Otolaryngol Head Neck Surg.* 1994; 111:12.

47. Zheng W, McLaughlin JK, Chow WH, Chien HT, Blot WJ. Risk factors for cancers on the nasal cavity and paranasal sinuses among white men in the United States. *Am J Epidemiology.* 1993; 138:965.

48. Kashima HK, Kessis K, Hurban RH, et al. Human papilloma virus in sinonasal papillomas and squamous cell carcinomas. *Laryngoscope.* 1992; 102:973.

49. McGuirt WF. Maxillectomy. *Otolaryngol Clin N Am.* 1995; 28: 1175.

50. American Joint Committee on Cancer. *Manual for Staging of Cancer.* Philadelphia: J.B. Lippincott; 1992.

51. Mosesson RE, Som P. The radiographic evaluation of sinonasal tumors. *Otolaryngol Clin N Am.* 1995; 28:1097.

52. Lund VJ, Lloyd GA, Howard DJ, Chessman AD, Phelps PD. Enhanced magnetic resonance imaging and subtraction techniques in the postoperative evaluation of craniofacial resection for sinonasal malignancy. *Laryngoscope.* 1996; 106:553.

53. Weisman RA, Osguthorpe JD. Pseudotumor of the head and neck masquerading as neoplasia. *Laryngoscope.* 1988; 98:610.

54. Knegt P. Surgery for paranasal sinus cancer. In: Johnson JT, Didolkar MS, eds. *Head and Neck Cancer.* Vol 3. New York: Elsevier Science Publishers; 1993:953.

55. Lawton MT, Spetzler RF. Internal carotid artery sacrifice for radical resection of skull base tumors. *Skull Base Surg.* 1996; 6:119.

56. Lyons BM, Donald PJ. Radical surgery for nasal cavity and paranasal sinus tumors. *Otolaryngol Clin N Am.* 1991; 24: 1499.

57. Richtsmeier WJ, Briggs RJS, Koch WM, et al. Complications and early outcome of anterior craniofacial resection. *Arch Otolaryngol Head Neck Surg.* 1992; 118:913.

58. Osguthorpe JD, Patel S. Craniofacial approaches to sinus malignancy. *Otolaryngol Clin N Am.* 1995; 28:1239.

59. Clayman GL, DeMonte F, Jaffe DM, et al. Outcome and complications of extended cranial base resection requiring microvascular free tissue transfer. *Arch Otolaryngol Head Neck Surg.* 1995; 121:1253.

60. Kraus DH, Shah JP, Arbit E, et al. Complications of craniofacial resection for tumors involving the anterior skull base. *Head Neck.* 1994; 16:307.

61. Bridger GP, Mendelsohn MS, Baldwin M, et al: Paranasal sinus cancer. *Aust NZ J Surg.* 1991; 61:290.

62. Olsen KD, Meland B, Ebersold MJ, et al. Extensive defects of the sino-orbital region. *Arch Otolaryngol Head Neck Surg.* 1992; 118:828.

63. Hochman M. Reconstruction of midfacial and anterior skull base defects. *Otolaryngol Clin N Am.* 1995; 28:1269.

64. McCary WS, Levine PA. Management of the eye in the treatment of sinonasal cancers. *Otolaryngol Clin N Am.* 1995; 28: 1231.

65. Lydiatt DD, Hollins RR. Vascular considerations in approaches to the deep midface. *Head Neck.* 1993; 15:164.

66. Nuss DW, Janecka IP, Sekhar LN, et al. Craniofacial disassembly in the management of skull-base tumors. *Otalaryngol Clin N Am.* 1991; 24:1465.

67. Rice DH. Endonasal surgery for nasal wall tumors. *Otalaryngol Clin N Am.* 1995; 28:1117.

68. Biller HF, Lawson W, Sachdev VP, et al. Esthesioneuroblastoma: surgical treatment without radiation. *Laryngoscope.* 1990; 100:1199.

69. Osguthorpe JD, Weisman RA. Medial maxillectomy for lateral sinus wall neoplasms. *Arch Otalaryngol Head Neck Surg.* 1991; 117:751.

70. Levine PA, Debo RF, Meredith SD, et al. Craniofacial resection at the University of Virginia (1976–1992). *Head Neck.* 1994; 16:574.

71. Catalano PJ, Hecht CS, Biller HF, et al. Craniofacial resection. *Arch Otolaryngol Head Neck Surg.* 1994; 120:1203.

72. Close LG, Mickey B. Transcranial resection of ethmoid sinus cancer involving the anterior skull base. *Skull Base Surg.* 1992; 2:213.

73. Janecka IP, Sen C, Sekhar L, et al. Treatment of paranasal sinus cancer with cranial base surgery. *Laryngoscope.* 1994; 104:553.

74. Catalano P, Sen C. Management of anterior ethmoid and frontal sinus tumors. *Otolaryngol Clin N Am.* 1995; 28:1157.

75. Spiro JD, Soo KC, Spiro RH. Nonsquamous cell malignant neoplasms of the nasal cavities and paranasal sinuses. *Head Neck.* 1995; 17:114.

76. Tran L, Sidrys J, Horton D, Sadeghi A, Parker RG. Malignant salivary gland tumors of the paranasal sinuses. *Am J Clin Oncol.* 1989; 12:387.

77. Maniglia AJ, Phillips DA. Midfacial degloving for the management of nasal, sinus and skull-base neoplasms. *Otolaryngol Clin N Am.* 1995; 28:1127.

78. Har-El G, Lucente FE. Midfacial degloving approach to the nose, sinuses, and skull base. *Am J Rhinol.* 1996; 10:17.

79. Bumpous JM, Maves MD, Gomez SM, et al. Cavernous sinus involvement in head and neck cancer. *Head Neck.* 1993; 15:62.

80. Lawson W, Naidu RK, Le Benger J, et al: Combined median mandibulotomy and Weber-Fergusson maxillectomy. *Arch Otolaryngol Head Neck Surg.* 1990; 116:596.

81. McCaffrey TV, Olsen KD, Yohanan JM, et al. Factors affecting survival of patients with tumors of the anterior skull base. *Laryngoscope.* 1994; 104:940.

82. Raveh J, Laedrach K, Speiser M, et al. The subcranial approach for fronto-orbital and anterioposterior skull base tumors. *Arch Otolaryngol Head Neck Surg.* 1993; 119:385.

83. Pulino AC, Marks JE, Leonetti JP. Postoperative irradiation of patients with malignant tumors of the skull base. *Laryngoscope.* 1996; 106:880.

84. Lund VJ. Malignant melanoma of the nasal cavity and paranasal sinuses. *ENT J.* 1993; 72:285.

85. Nunez F, Suarez C, Alvarez I, et al. Sinonasal adenocarcinoma: epidemiological and clinicopathological study of 34 cases. *J Otolaryngol.* 1993; 22:2.

86. Alvarez J, Suarez C, Rodrigo JP, Nunez F, Caminero MJ. Prognostic factors in paranasal sinus cancer. *Am J Otolaryngol.* 1995; 16:109.

87. Kingdom TT, Kaplan MJ. Mucosal melanoma of the nasal cavity and paranasal sinuses. *Head Neck Surg.* 1995; 17:184.

88. Parsons JT, Kimsey FC, Mendenhall WM, et al. Radiation therapy for sinus malignancies. *Otolaryngol Clin N Am.* 1995; 28:1259.

89. Zappia JJ, Carroll WR, Wolf GT, et al. Olfactory neuroblastoma: the results of modern treatment approaches at the University of Michigan. *Head Neck.* 1993; 15:190.

90. Harrison D. 1990 Ogura Memorial Lecture: Moral dilemmas in head and neck cancer. *Laryngoscope.* 1990; 100:1191.

91. Kraus DH, Sterman BM, Levine HL, et al. Factors influencing survival in ethmoid sinus cancer. *Arch Otolaryngol Head Neck Surg.* 1992; 118:367.

92. Freeman SB, Hamaker RC, Singer MI, et al. Intraoperative radiotherapy of skull base cancer. *Laryngoscope.* 1991; 101: 507.

93. Batsakis JG. The pathology of head and neck tumors: nasal cavity and paranasal sinuses. *Head Neck Surg.* 1980; 2:410.

94. Rafla S. Mucous gland tumors of the paranasal sinuses. *Cancer.* 1970; 24:683.

95. Conley J, Dingman DL. Adenoid cystic carcinoma in the head and neck (cylindroma). *Arch Otolaryngol.* 1974; 100:81.

96. Leafstedt SW, Gaeta JF, Sako K, et al. Adenoid cystic carcinoma of major and minor salivary glands. *Am J Surg.* 1971; 122:756.

97. Spiro H, Huvos AG, Strong EW. Adenoid cystic carcinoma of salivary origin: a clinicopathologic study of 242 cases. *Am J Surg.* 1974; 128:512.

98. Chilla R, Schroth R, Eysholdt U, et al. Adenoid cystic carcinoma of the head and neck. *ORL J Otorhinolaryngol Relat Spec.* 1980; 42:346.

99. Conley J, Pack GT. Melanoma of the mucous membranes of the head and neck. *Arch Otolaryngol.* 1974; 99:315.

100. Batsakis JG, Regezi JA, Solomon AR, et al: The pathology of head and neck tumors: mucosal melanomas. *Head Neck Surg.* 1982; 4:404.

101. Billings KB, Wang MB, Sercarz JA, Fu YS. Clinical and pathologic distinction between primary and metastatic mucosal melanoma of the head and neck. *Otolaryngol Head Neck Surg.* 1995; 112:700.

102. Hyams VJ. Pathology of the nose and paranasal sinuses. In: English GE, ed. *Otolaryngology.* Vol 2. New York: Harper and Row; 1984.

103. Trapp TK, Fu YS, Calcaterra TC. Melanoma of the nasal and paranasal sinus mucosa. *Arch Otolaryngol.* 1987; 113:1086.

104. Mills SE, Frierson HF Jr. Olfactory neuroblastoma: a clinicopathologic study of 21 cases. *Am J Surg Pathol.* 1985; 9:317.

105. Barnes L, Kapdia SB. The biology and pathology of selected skull base tumors. *J Neuro-Oncol.* 1994; 20:213.

106. Ordonez NG, Mackay B. Neuroendocrine tumors of the nasal cavity. *Pathol Ann.* 1993; 23:77.

107. Kadish S, Goodman M, Wang CC. Olfactory neuroblastoma, a clinical analysis of 17 cases. *Cancer.* 1976; 37:1571.

108. Dulguerov P, Calcaterra T. Esthesioneuroblastoma: The UCLA experience 1970–1990. *Laryngoscope.* 1992; 102:843.

109. Tefft M, Fernandez C, Donaldson M, et al. Incidence of meningeal involvement by rhabdomyosarcoma of the head and neck in children: a report of the Intergroup Rhabdomyosarcoma Study. *Cancer.* 1978; 42:253.

110. Raney RB, Tefft M, Newton WA, et al. Improved prognosis with intensive treatment of children with cranial soft tissue sarcomas arising in nonorbital parameningeal sites: a report from the Intergroup Rhabdomyosarcoma Study. *Cancer.* 1987; 59:147.

111. Mark R, Sercarz JA, Tran L, et al. Osteogenic sarcoma of the head and neck: the UCLA experience. *Arch Otolaryngol Head Neck Surg.* 1991; 117:761.

112. Laramore GE, Griffith JT, Boespflug M, et al. Fast neutron radiation therapy for sarcomas—soft tissue, bone and cartilage. *Am J Clin Oncol.* 1989; 12:320.

113. Strickler JG, Meneses MF, Habermann TM, et al. Polymorphic reticulosis: a reappraisal. *Hum Pathol.* 1994; 25:659.

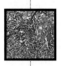

II. MANAGEMENT OF RECURRENT NASOPHARYNGEAL CANCER

■ PAUL DAGUM

■ WILLARD E. FEE, Jr.

Malignant tumors of the nasopharynx can be quite challenging to treat. Although a variety of unusual and metastatic neoplasms have been observed in this region, by far the most common tumors of the nasopharynx are carcinomas. The World Health Organization (WHO) has classified nasopharyngeal carcinomas into three major categories: WHO-I, keratinizing squamous cell carcinoma; WHO-IIA, differentiated nonkeratinizing carcinoma; and WHO-IIB, undifferentiated carcinoma. The last category also covers lymphoepitheliomas. About one third of nasopharyngeal cancers (NPC) in non-Chinese are of the WHO-I type (see reference 23). Herein we emphasize the treatment of NPC with a focus on recurrent disease. Omitted from this discussion is analysis of other tumor types (e.g., chordoma, salivary gland neoplasms).

Nasopharyngeal cancer is the only head and neck nonhematologic cancer that is treated exclusively with radiation therapy. Although all three histologic types of NPC are radiosensitive, the 5-year survival rates are low compared to tumors in other primary sites. It appears that history has played a greater role in dictating the treatment of NPC than the biologic behavior of this disease would dictate.

Nasopharyngeal cancer was recognized as a distinct disease entity in Western society at the end of the 19th century. In 1901, Chevalier Jackson[1] noted that "a careful search of the medical journals in French, German, English, and Italian failed to unearth more than 14 cases," the earliest of those cases reported by Duran Fardel in 1837. One of the earliest accounts of nasopharyngeal cancers treated surgically was in 1911 by Trotter.[2] He reported on 12 patients with tumors of the nasopharynx and advocated "osteoplastic resection of the upper jaw" to expose the nasopharynx for tumor extirpation, claiming that it was "easy to carry out, not dangerous in itself, and leaves no deformity."

In 1916, Norcross[3] reviewed the medical literature and documented 55 reports of nasopharyngeal tumors. The majority of cases were recent, leading Norcross[3] to conclude that tumors of the nasopharynx either had increased in frequency or were being more accurately observed. In 1922, New[4] at the Mayo Clinic in Rochester reported on 79 patients with epitheliomas and lymphosarcomas of the nasopharynx. He observed that early diagnosis of NPC required careful examination of the nasopharynx and recognized that the fossa of Rosenmüller was a common site of primary disease. As late as 1933, there were no reports of keratinizing squamous cell carcinoma arising primarily in the nasopharynx (WHO-I).[5] In contrast, by the 1920s, several researchers had established the exquisite radiosensitivity of differentiated nonkeratinizing and undifferentiated NPC (WHO-IIA and -IIB).[6,7] Primary therapy for small, accessible tumors remained surgical, and radiation therapy was reserved for more extensive disease. Surgical approaches to the nasopharynx varied. These included direct access through the nasal cavity, transmaxillary approaches, and transpalatal approaches. All had been developed in the 1800s by surgeons such as Langenbeck, Dupuytren, Weber, Cheever, and Loeb, to treat choanal atresia or to remove sinonasal polyps.[8] However, due to limited exposure, none of these surgical approaches could be sufficient for true oncologic resection of large tumors.

The first thorough study of the epidemiology and clinical behavior of NPC came from China. In 1930, Kenelm Digby,[9] a British surgeon working at University Surgical Unit of Hong Kong, published his findings of 103 cases of NPC. He reported a male-to-female ratio of 3.1 to 1; the most common age of onset was 41 to 45 years in males and 31 to 35 years in females. These findings have remained stable over generations with similar ratios today. The known association between NPC and certain human leukocyte antigen (HLA) alleles among Chinese (specifically A2, Bw46, and B17) may partially explain these constant ratios.

In his notes, Digby[9] systematically described the clinical presentation of NPC among the Chinese. He recognized the diagnostic inadequacy of nasopharyngoscopy and the difficulty of establishing the diagnosis even after splitting the soft palate. During those years, he treated NPC with "extensive block dissections of both sides of the neck including both anterior and posterior triangles splitting the soft palate in the midline and then diathermising the growth." Ten years later, however, he lamented that "the patients stood the extensive operations fairly well, but recurrence was almost immediate. Deep x-rays hold better prospects of successful treatment, for by using several portals of entry a sufficient dose can be delivered to the lateral relations of the nasopharynx."[10] Delays in diagnosis, early lateral spread of disease that involved the major neurovascular structures, and limited surgical access thus gave way to more frequent radiotherapy treatment of NPC.

RADIATION THERAPY

Several large series of treatment of NPC with radiation therapy have shown 5-year survival rates of approximately 35% to 50% (summarized in Table 6–2). In an analysis of 170 patients, Wang and Meyer[11] showed an overall 5-year survival of 39% and 31% disease-free survival. Hsu et al[12] irradiated 1555 patients and reported a 5-year survival of 47.8%. Similarly, Zhang et al[13] radiated 1302 patients and reported a 5-year survival rate of 47%. In a series of 1882 patients treated at the Hunan Tumor Hospital in China, 1424 treated with a continuous radiation regimen and 458 treated with an 11 to 45 day split course regimen, the overall 5-year survival rate was 34.6%.[14] However, long-term follow-up of NPC has revealed that nonkeratinizing and undifferentiated NPC is best considered a chronic disease, as the risk of death does not plateau beyond 5 years as

it does with squamous cell NPC. Recurrences occurring as late as 10 and 15 years post-treatment are not uncommon. Ten-year survival rates range from 28% to 40%.[12,13,15]

The time to local recurrence of NPC appears to have a bimodal distribution. Several authors have noted that most recurrences occur early with approximately 70% recurring within 2 years and 90% within 3 years.[16–19] Approximately 10% of tumors recur after 5 years.[19,20] Whether early recurrences result from suboptimal radiation doses, insufficient tumor coverage, de novo primaries, or more aggressive biologic behavior is unclear. Late recurrences, however, most certainly arise from de novo primaries. Some authors have observed that the time to recurrence is predictive of the response to reirradiation. Patients who recurred early did not respond as well to reirradiation.[12,17,19] Other studies, however, have failed to verify this relationship.[21]

Several studies have documented a decreased survival rate in patients with squamous cell NPC, as compared to differentiated nonkeratinizing or undifferentiated NPC.[22–24] In contrast, a large series from the National Taiwan University Hospital in Taiwan has not confirmed these observations. There was no statistical difference in 5- and 10-year survival rates between 1501 patients with differentiated nonkeratinizing or undifferentiated NPC and 54 patients with keratinizing squamous cell NPC, all treated with primary radiotherapy.[12] Similarly, in patients treated with radiation therapy at three major U.S. cancer centers no significant difference in recurrence rates among the various histologic types was observed.[18,25,26]

Although histology and recurrence appear unrelated, there is a strong relationship between histology and Epstein-Barr (EB) virus. Neel et al[27] observed that titers of IgG to the diffuse component of early antigen (EA) and IgA antibodies to viral capsid antigen (VCA) were elevated in approximately 85% of patients with nonkeratinizing or undifferentiated NPC. Only 35% of patients with keratinizing squamous cell NPC were positive for anti-EA antibodies and 16% for anti-VCA (IgA). This strong as-

TABLE 6–2	FIVE- AND 10-YEAR SURVIVAL RATES OF PATIENTS WITH NASOPHARYNGEAL CANCER TREATED WITH RADIATION THERAPY				
AUTHOR	YEAR	n	5-YEAR SURVIVAL (%)	10-YEAR SURVIVAL (%)
Wang CC[11]	1971	170	39	NR
Hsu MM[12]	1982	1555	47.8	39.8
Zhang EP[13]	1989	1302	47	33
Chen WZ[15]	1989	1127	NR	28.7
Luo RX[14]	1989	1882	34.6	NR

n, number of patients; NR, not reported

sociation of EB viral titers with disease has led to the suggestion that the virus itself may be a causative agent and lead to tumor chronicity.

Radiotherapy of NPC requires fractionated external beam radiation at doses 66 to 74 Gy, typically delivered through a single nasoanterior portal and opposed lateral portals, designed to limit spinal cord doses to 45 Gy. Treatment doses less than 50 Gy are associated with a high number of early recurrences.[16–19,25,27] Reirradiation for recurrent NPC requires subjecting the nasopharynx and surrounding neurologic structures to doses similar to primary treatment, yielding cumulative radiation doses as high as 120 Gy. These high doses can result in irreversible damage to the optic nerves, brain stem, and temporal lobes. In most series of reirradiated patients, approximately one half of patients are suboptimally treated with doses under 50 Gy.

REIRRADIATION

At the Chinese Academy of Medical Sciences in Beijing, Yan et al[17] described the reirradiation of 219 patients with recurrent NPC. They compared the complication rate at 5 years of reirradiation to the rate after radiation in patients who did not recur. Radiation myelitis, the most serious complication, increased from 9% to 12%. Soft tissue injury—including subcutaneous fibrosis, trismus, and necrosis—increased from 9% to 16%, 11% to 29%, and 2% to 5%, respectively. In their series, complications such as brain injury, cranial nerve paralysis, and osteoradionecrosis were comparable among the two groups. Forty-four percent of patients were treated with less than 50 Gy of radiation, suggesting that awareness of potential complications limited treatment. McNeese and Fletcher[21] reirradiated 30 patients at M.D. Anderson Hospital and noted hearing loss in eight, severe trismus in four, necrosis of the nasopharynx in two, and mandibular necrosis in one patient. One patient died of skull base necrosis, and one patient developed hypopituitarism.

Reirradiation for the treatment of recurrent NPC has a 10% to 25% 5-year survival rate, substantially lower than the survival rate for treatment of a primary occurrence.[16,28,29] Although suboptimal management of recurrences with radiation doses under 50 Gy could explain low retreatment survival rates, more data confirm a low retreatment survival rate regardless of techniques used. Of the 219 recurrences treated by Yan et al,[17] 94 recurrences were localized to the nasopharynx adnexa. Of these, 14/94 (15%) survived 5 years. Zhang et al[13] reirradiated 133 patients with a dosage of 50 to 60 Gy. Five-year survival for reirradiated recurrences was 16.6%.

A few studies report slightly higher survival rates. Fu et al[20] reported on 33 patients reirradiated for recurrent NPC at the University of California in San Francisco over a period of 34 years. Sixteen of those patients (48%) survived 3 years after retreatment, but only five patients (15%) were free of disease at the end of 3 years. Wang and Schultz[19] reported on 35 patients reirradiated for recurrent NPC at the Massachusetts General Hospital over 20 years. Thirty-three of those patients were followed for 5 years, and of these, 12 (36%) were alive and nine (27%) free of disease. In a follow-up series of 38 patients receiving high-dose reirradiation exceeding 60 Gy, Wang[30] reported a 5-year survival of 38% for 32 patients with T1 and T2 recurrent tumors, and 15% for six patients with T3 and T4 recurrences.

CHEMOTHERAPY

Large trials have explored the value of chemotherapy combined with radiotherapy as initial treatment. These trials were motivated by nonrandomized reports that suggested a survival benefit with neoadjuvant chemotherapy in the belief that NPC is chemoresponsive.[31–34] A large international Phase III trial at the Institute Gustave Roussy in France randomized 339 patients with stage IV undifferentiated NPC into two treatment arms.[35] The first group received three cycles of cisplatin, epirubicin, and bleomycin prior to radiation therapy, and the second group received definitive radiotherapy alone. After a median follow-up time of 49 months, a significant difference in disease-free survival was observed in the chemotherapy arm. The rate of tumor progression or recurrence was 32.7% in the chemotherapy arm compared to 54.7% in the radiotherapy arm. However, there was no significant difference in overall survival. In contrast, Chan et al[34] randomized 77 patients with metastatic NPC having a largest nodal diameter greater than 4 cm into treatment with either cisplatin plus 1,5-fluorouracil plus radiotherapy, or radiotherapy alone. After a median follow-up of 28.5 months, they did not find a significant difference in overall survival or disease-free survival between the two groups.

These trials suggest, but do not prove, that chemotherapy may play an important role in treating primary or residual NPC. Larger trials with longer follow-ups will be needed prior to the routine addition of chemotherapy as standard therapy.

SURGERY

Despite the sensitivity of NPC to radiotherapy, management of residual (or recurrent) disease at the primary site continues to challenge clinicians. Residual cervical disease is less problematic and can often be handled with standard lymphadenectomies.

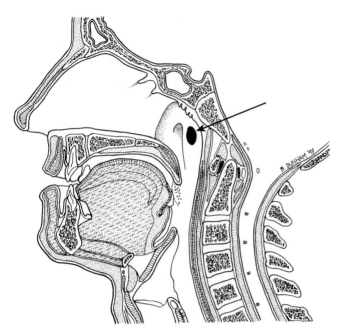

FIGURE 6-7 Sagittal section showing nasopharyngeal cancer originating in the fossa of Rosenmüller (*arrow*).

In 1956, Sooy[36] reported on surgical treatment of recurrent NPC using a combination of electrodesiccation and ^{60}Co irradiation via an intranasal septectomy. Of the 16 patients who were treated, eight died within 2 years. The remaining eight were free of disease, but only three patients were followed for more than 5 years. Whether reirradiation with cobalt, or its combination with electrodessication, was responsible for controlling recurrences is unclear. Nonetheless, Sooy's work was a notable initial effort in surgically treating recurrences in the nasopharynx.

With the refinement of surgical technique, instruments, and radiographic imaging, several successful reports on the surgical management of recurrent NPC were published in the 1980s. These surgical approaches are classified into lateral or anterior approaches. The lateral approach evolved from refinements in temporal bone neurotologic surgery, making possible extensive resections with facial nerve and intratemporal carotid artery preservation. The anterior approach relied on exposure of the nasopharynx via systematic facial skeleton disassembly followed by reassembly using rigid fixation. Whereas a lateral approach provides improved exposure of the pterygomaxillary space and infratemporal fossa, access to the nasopharynx as a whole is limited. Furthermore, the morbidity of a lateral approach is typically greater than that of an anterior approach. When recurrent NPC shows extensive temporal bone involvement, however, only a lateral approach with a total temporal bone resection will offer a chance of cure.

Panje and Gross[37] described their results with eight patients who underwent lateral resection for recurrent T3 or T4 disease. One patient was alive 38 months following resection of the mandibular ramus, posterior maxilla, and temporal bone. Five patients died of primary disease, two with distant metastases and three with local recurrence. Follow-up intervals and the details of the remaining two patients were not reported. It should be noted that surgical morbidity was substantial. All patients required facial nerve rehabilitation and had sensorineural deafness. Five patients had unilateral laryngeal paralysis, six required oral prosthetic restitution, three developed CSF leaks, and three required a gastrostomy for nutrition.

In 1988, Fee et al[38] reported on the treatment of nine patients with recurrent NPC using an anterior approach. This approach combined a transpalatal, transmaxillary, and transcervical exposure of the nasopharynx. Preoperative imaging, using a computed tomography (CT) scan to define bone destruction and a magnetic resonance imaging (MRI) scan to define soft tissue disease extent, allowed careful preoperative planning. Tumors confined to the nasopharyngeal mucosal space, with extension into the pterygomaxillary space, the paranasopharyngeal space, or the sphenoid, clivus, or vertebral bodies, were resected transpalatally (Figs. 6–7, 6–8, and 6–9). The soft palate was resected with the specimen only if it was adjacent to, or invaded by, tumor. In those cases, the posterior half of the palatal bone was submitted as the anterior–inferior margin. After visually confirming the superior, anterior, posterior, lateral, and inferior extent of the tumor, resec-

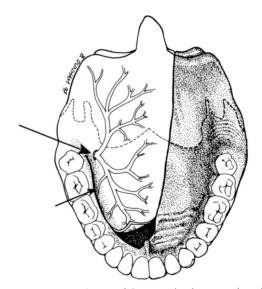

FIGURE 6-8 Surgical view of the transpalatal approach to the nasopharynx. Mucosal incisions (*small arrow*) and mucoperiostal elevation of hard palate mucosa insure preservation of the axial blood supply from the greater palatine artery (*large arrow*).

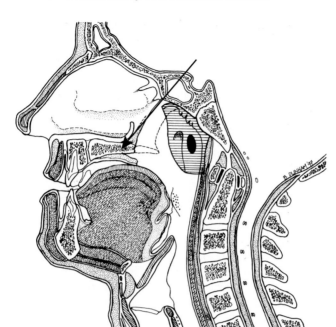

FIGURE 6–9 Transpalatal tumor resection. Adequate exposure of the nasopharynx requires osteotomies of the posterior hard palate, vomer, medial pterygoid plates, and resection of the posterior inferior turbinates (*arrow*). Mucoperiostal flaps are elevated off the posterior nasal septum and the nasal side of the hard palate. Those flaps are coapted together after the resection to separate the oral cavity from the nasal cavity. Resection begins cephalad, with elevation of the mucosa and cancer, and progresses caudally to the first or second vertebral body.

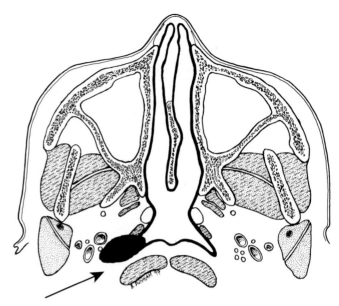

FIGURE 6–10 Nasopharyngeal cancer extending deep into the paranasopharyngeal space and abutting the carotid sheath (*arrow*).

tion proceeded from an inferior to superior direction through the transoral–transpalatal exposure. The posterior margin of the en bloc soft tissue resection included the longus coli muscle and prevertebral fascia extending from the clivus to the first or second cervical vertebral body.

Whereas the transoral–transpalatal approach proves adequate for early recurrences confined to the nasopharyngeal mucosal space, tumor extension into the pterygomaxillary space, sphenoid sinus, clivus, cervical vertebral bodies, or deep paranasopharyngeal space requires greater surgical exposure for complete extirpation. When tumor invades the pterygomaxillary space, these patients undergo transantral maxillary artery ligation followed by a posterior–medial maxillectomy that includes the medial and lateral pterygoid plate to the base of the skull. The soft tissue specimen and attached bony parts of the maxilla are removed en bloc, exposing the clivus and the first and second cervical vertebral bodies. If tumor invades those structures, a large cutting burr is used to resect the involved bone. If tumor invades the sphenoid sinus, that sinus is completely resected anteriorly.

Tumor extension into the paranasopharyngeal space (Fig. 6–10) requires isolation and vascular control of the internal carotid artery and adjacent

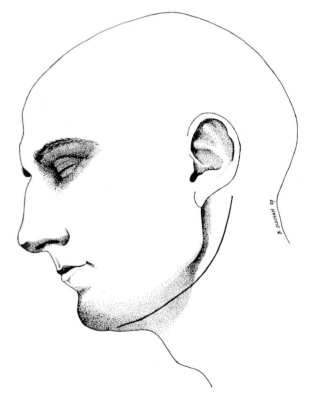

FIGURE 6–11 Transcervical incision. An incision is made 3 cm below the margin of the mandible extending from the mastoid to the submentum.

marks the lateral-most extent of the resection (Fig. 6–13). Lateralizing the internal carotid artery and cranial nerve IX also insures that cranial nerves X, XI, and XII remain lateral to the cotton pledget and allows safe resection of the tumor. Recurrent NPC presenting with new cranial nerve involvement suggests disease extension lateral to the internal carotid artery and is a relative contraindication to surgery.

As noted previously, cervical node recurrence of NPC is treated with a comprehensive cervical lymphadenectomy. Cranial nerve XI is spared only if dictated by the patient's occupation and if safe tumor removal can be accomplished while preserving this nerve.

A review of 41 patients with locally, or locally and regionally, recurrent NPC treated at Stanford University Hospital using an anterior approach nasopharyngectomy reveals 3-year and 5-year survival rates of 55% and 35%, respectively. Disease-free survival rates are 41% and 29% at 3 and 5 years.[39]

Other approaches exist in addition to the anterior nasopharyngectomy developed at Stanford. Tu et al[40] reported on nine patients with recurrences confined to the central paranasopharyngeal mucosal space. Resection proceeded through either a palate fenestration approach or a lateral rhinotomy when tumor intruded into the nasal cavity. Eight patients had pathologically confirmed cancer following resection. Of those eight patients, three survived 5 years, two of them receiving postoperative reirradiation. Wei et al[41] introduced the maxillary swing approach that pedicles the hemimaxilla on a Weber-Ferguson flap. This approach gives excellent exposure of the pterygomaxillary space but inevitably sacrifices the infraorbital nerve and exposes the internal carotid artery to possible damage during the osteotomies.

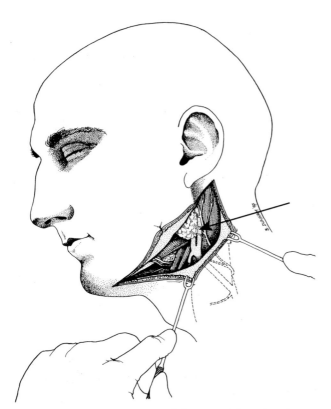

FIGURE 6–12 Deep transcervical dissection. Hypoglossal nerve is identified coursing over the external carotid artery. The internal carotid artery is identified at the carotid bifurcation and dissected superiorly to the skull base (*arrow*).

cranial nerves. A transcervical dissection identifies the internal carotid artery at the skull base (Figs. 6–11 and 6–12). A cotton pledget, placed medially to the internal carotid artery and cranial nerve IX,

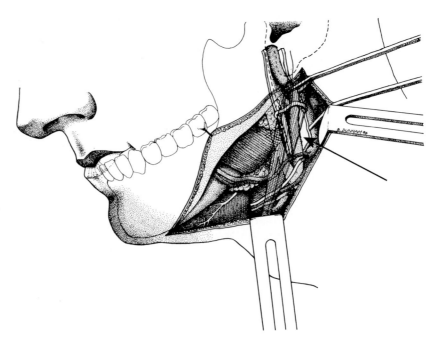

FIGURE 6–13 Internal carotid isolation. The stylopharyngeus and styloglossus muscles have been detached from the styloid process exposing the glossopharyngeal nerve coursing between the internal and external carotid arteries. The internal carotid artery has been circumferentially dissected up to the skull base. A cotton pledget, placed medially and slightly anteriorly to the internal carotid artery, marks the lateralmost extent of safe tumor resection (*arrow*).

Cocker et al[42] report on a transfacial extended maxillotomy and a subtotal maxillectomy for both benign and malignant disease of the nasopharynx.

CONCLUSION

For the most part, NPC is treatable with radiotherapy. However, residual or recurrent disease vexes even the most experienced oncologic team. Evolving experience with surgical treatment of these tumors suggests that oncologic resection of this heretofore inaccessible region is feasible with acceptable morbidity and the potential for long-term care. Nonetheless, the large number of patients who ultimately succumb to their disease serves as a reminder that more focused molecular research is needed for improved disease prevention and cure.

REFERENCES

1. Jackson C. Primary carcinoma of the nasopharynx. A table of cases. *JAMA.* 1901; 37:371.
2. Trotter W. Certain clinically obscure malignant tumours of the nasopharyngeal wall. *Brit Med. J* 1911; 11:1057.
3. Norcross EP. Intrafemoral malignant tumor of the lateral wall of the nasopharynx. *Ann Otol Rhinol Laryngol.* 1916; 25:967.
4. New GB. Syndrome of malignant tumors of the nasopharynx. *JAMA.* 1922; 79:10.
5. Christianson O, McArthur SW. Nasopharyngeal carcinoma. *Arch Surg.* 1933; 27:1109.
6. Crowe SJ, Baylor JW. Benign and malignant growths of the nasopharynx and their treatment with radium. *Arch Surg.* 1923; 6:429.
7. Schmincke A. Ueber lymphoepitheliale Geschwulste. *Beitr F Path Anat.* 1921; 68:161.
8. Wilson CP. Observations on the surgery of the nasopharynx. *Ann Otolaryngol Rhinol Laryngol.* 1957; 66:5.
9. Digby, KH, Thomas GH, Tse HS. Notes on carcinoma of the nasopharynx. *Caduceus.* 1930; 9:45.
10. Digby KH, Fook L, Che YT. Nasopharyngeal carcinoma. *Br J Surg.* 1941; 28:517.
11. Wang CC, Meyer JE. Radiotherapeutic management of carcinoma of the nasopharynx. *Cancer.* 1971; 28:566.
12. Hsu MM, Huang SC, Lynn TC, Hsieh T, Tu SM. The survival of patients with nasopharyngeal carcinoma. *Otolaryngol Head Neck Surg.* 1982; 90:289.
13. Zhang EP, Lian PG, Cai KL, et al. Radiation therapy of nasopharyngeal carcinoma: prognostic factors based on a 10-year follow-up of 1302 patients. *Int J Radiation Oncol Biol Phys.* 1989; 16:301.
14. Luo RX, Tang QX, Huang YW, Liao YP, Mou XD, Hu ZX. Comparison of continuous and split-course radiotherapy for nasopharyngeal carcinoma. *Int J Radiation Oncol Biol Phys.* 1989; 16:307.
15. Chen WZ, Zhou DL, Luo KS. Long-term observation after radiotherapy for nasopharyngeal carcinoma (NPC). *Int J Radiation Oncol Biol Phys.* 1989; 16:311.
16. Hoppe RT, Goffinet DR, Bagshaw MA. Carcinoma of the nasopharynx. *Cancer.* 1976; 37:2605.
17. Yan JH, Hu JH, Gu XZ. Radiation therapy of recurrent nasopharyngeal carcinoma. Report on 219 patients. *ACTA Radiologica Oncology.* 1983; 22:23.
18. Vikram B, Mishra UB, Strong EW, Manolatos S. Patterns of failure in carcinoma of the nasopharynx: I. Failure at the primary site. *Int J Radiation Oncol Biol Phys.* 1985; 11:410.
19. Wang CC, Schulz MD. Management of locally recurrent carcinoma of the nasopharynx. *Radiology.* 1966; 86:900.
20. Fu KK, Newman H, Phillips TL. Treatment of locally recurrent carcinoma of the nasopharynx. *Radiology.* 1975; 117:425.
21. McNeese MD, Fletcher GH. Retreatment of recurrent nasopharyngeal carcinoma. *Radiology.* 1981; 138:191.
22. Chen KY, Fletcher GH. Malignant tumors of the nasopharynx. *Radiology.* 1971; 99:165.
23. Shanmugaratnam K, Chan SH, The GD. Histopathology of nasopharyngeal carcinoma: correlations with epidemiology, survival rates, and other biologic characteristics. *Cancer.* 1979; 44:1029.
24. Hoppe RT, Williams J, Warnke R, Goffinet DR, Bagshaw MA. Carcinoma of the nasopharynx: the significance of histology. *Int J Radiation Oncol Biol Phys.* 1978; 4:199.
25. Mesic JB, Fletcher GH, Goepfert H. Megavoltage irradiation of epithelial tumors of the nasopharynx. *Int J Radiation Oncology Biol Phys.* 1981; 7:447.
26. Meyer JE, Wang CC: Carcinoma of the nasopharynx: factors influencing results of therapy. *Radiology.* 1971; 100:385.
27. Neel HB III, Pearson GR, Weiland LH, et al. Application of Epstein-Barr virus serology to the diagnosis and staging of North American patients with nasopharyngeal carcinoma. *Otolaryngol Head Neck Surg.* 1983; 91:255.
28. Bedwinek JM, Perez CA, Keys DJ. Analysis of failures after definitive irradiation for carcinoma of the nasopharynx. *Cancer.* 1980; 45:2725.
29. Vaeth JM. Radiation therapy of locally recurrent nasopharyngeal cancer. *Radiol Clin North Am.* 1964; 33:72.
30. Wang CC. Reirradiation of recurrent nasopharyngeal carcinoma-treatment techniques and results. *Int J Radiation Oncol Biol Phys.* 1987; 13:953.
31. Atichartakarn V, Kraiphibul P, Clongsusuek P, Pochanugool L, Kulapaditharom B, Ratanatharathorn V. Nasopharyngeal carcinoma: result of treatment with cis-diamminedichloroplatinum II, 5-fluorouracil, and radiation therapy. *Int J Radiation Oncol Biol Phys.* 1988; 14:461.
32. Clark JR, Norris CM, Dreyfuss AI, et al. Nasopharyngeal carcinoma: the Dana-Farber Cancer Institute experience with 24 patients treated with induction chemotherapy and radiotherapy. *Ann Otol Rhinol Laryngol.* 1987; 96:608.
33. Qin D, Hu Y, Yan J, et al. Analysis of 1379 patients with nasopharyngeal carcinoma treated by radiation. *Cancer.* 1988; 61:1117.
34. Chan AT, Teo PM, Leung TW, et al. A prospective randomized study of chemotherapy adjunctive to definitive radiotherapy in advanced nasopharyngeal carcinoma. *Int J Radiation Oncol Biol Phys.* 1995; 33:569.
35. VUMCA I Trial. Preliminary results of a randomized trial comparing neoadjuvant chemotherapy (cisplatin, epirubicin, bleomycin) plus radiotherapy vs. radiotherapy alone in stage iv (> N2, M0) undifferentiated nasopharyngeal carcinoma: a positive effect on progression-free survival. *International Nasopharynx Cancer Study Group.* YUMCA I Trial. *Int J Radiation Oncol Biol Phys.* 1996; 35:463.
36. Sooy FA. Experimental treatment of recurrent carcinoma of the nasopharynx with electrodessication, radioactive cobalt and X-ray radiation. *Ann Otolaryngol Rhinol Laryngol.* 1956; 65: 723.
37. Panje WR, Gross CE. Treatment of tumors of the nasopharynx: surgical therapy. In: Thawley SE, Panje WR, eds. *Comprehensive Management of Head and Neck Tumors.* Vol 1. Philadelphia, PA: W.B. Saunders; 1987: 662.
38. Fee WE Jr, Gilmer PA, Goffinet DR. Surgical management of recurrent nasopharyngeal carcinoma after radiation failure at the primary site. *Laryngoscope,* 1988; 98:1220.
39. Fee WE Jr. The nasopharynx (unpublished observations).
40. Tu G, Hu Y, Xu G, Ye M. Salvage surgery for nasopharyngeal carcinoma. *Arch Otolaryngol Head Neck Surg.* 1988; 114: 328.
41. Wei WI, Lam KH, Sham JST. New approach to the nasopharynx: the maxillary swing approach. *Head Neck.* 1991; 13:200.
42. Cocker EE, Robertson JH, Robertson JT, Crook JP. The extended maxillotomy and subtotal maxillectomy for excision of skull base tumors. *Arch Otolaryngol Head Neck Surg.* 1990; 116:92.

III. PATHOLOGY OF THE NASAL CAVITY, PARANASAL SINUSES, AND NASOPHARYNX

- YAO-SHI FU
- KARL H. PERZIN

Diseases of the nasal cavity, paranasal sinuses, and nasopharynx—especially rhinitis and sinusitis—are relatively common. These inflammatory and infectious diseases require separation from the less common benign and malignant neoplasms. Due to the anatomic proximity of these diseases to the central nervous system and other vital organs, accurate assessment of pathologic specimens by the pathologists plays a major role in assisting clinicians to achieve an optimal management of patients with these diseases.

HANDLING OF SPECIMENS

Depending on anatomic location, lesion size, underlying pathology, and accessibility, the lesion may be biopsied, excised locally, or resected. Specimens from the nasal cavity and paranasal sinuses include the following major categories:

1. Punch biopsy
2. Polypectomy and removal of sinus content and curettage of nasal and sinus mucosa and bony wall
3. Excision through intranasal approach and rhinotomy
4. Resection

If the lesion is accessible only by endoscope, usually only a small portion of the lesion is removed by punch biopsy or forceps—for example, biopsies of the nasopharynx. These specimens are usually small, poorly oriented, and sometimes distorted by crush artifacts. Of all the steps in handling the biopsy specimens, none is more important than orientation of the specimen to assure proper embedding of tissue for perpendicular sectioning through the mucosa. Tangential cuts not only preclude definitive diagnosis but are also the source of over- and underdiagnosis (Fig. 6–14 A and B). The pathologist must be familiar with the appearance of tangentially cut sections and order multiple levels of sectioning or re-embedding when appropriate. In many instances, these maneuvers fail to correct the ill effects of poor orientation and require new biopsies. All small biopsies (less than 5 mm) should have at least three levels to ensure diagnostic tissue is sectioned. To prepare deeper cuts requires remounting the paraffin block and trimming tissue, which often consumes critical diagnostic tissue. For this reason, cutting at least three levels should be a standard laboratory practice.

Multiple pieces of polypoid tissue, turbinates, sinus content, and bony wall are commonly received in the laboratory following polypectomy and endoscopic sinus surgery. Most of the tissues should be submitted for histologic examination. In the case of

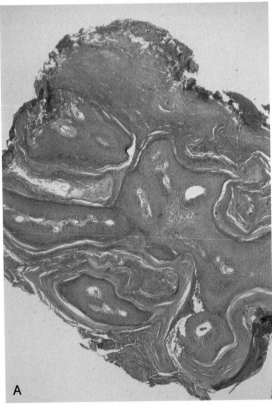
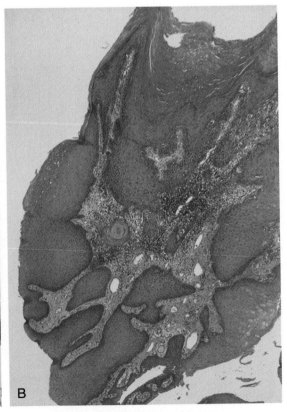

FIGURE 6–14 *A*, Horizontal section through the surface of a hyperkeratotic papilloma. *B*, Reorientation of biopsy cut in a vertical through the lesion demonstrates invasive squamous carcinoma at the base of papilloma characterized by irregular nests of atypical squamous cells.

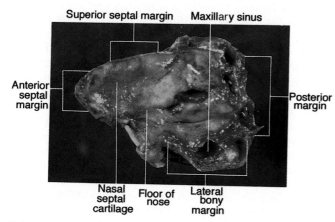

FIGURE 6–15 Partial maxillectomy specimen for chondrosarcoma of nasal septum, anterolateral view.

allergic fungal sinusitis, a correct diagnosis may be missed if the inspissated mucus containing fungal hyphae is not submitted for histologic examination. Another reason for submitting all nasal polyps for histologic examination is that many nasosinus tumors present as polypoid nodules or masses clinically.

Nasosinus tumors are sometimes removed piecemeal by curettage without orientation; such specimens should also be submitted in toto. When the sections are studied, even though the surgical margin cannot be determined, the pathologist should at least examine for the presence of tumor invasion into the bone and other identifiable structures.

In all specimens, the pathologist should examine any pieces of bone that may be included with the curetted tissue. If the inflammatory changes involve bone, this fact should be mentioned in the pathology report. The clinician may wish to correlate the changes seen on radiologic studies with the pathologic findings. If the infection has spread into bone, the possibility exists that it may have extended through the bone into adjacent structures such as the cranial or orbital cavities.

With excision through intranasal approach and rhinotomy, the received tissue is processed in the same manner as outlined in the preceding section. If the excised tumor tissue is oriented, an attempt should be made to determine the status of excision margins.

The pathologist also receives large resection specimens from this area. For example, a radical maxillectomy may have been performed for a biopsy-proven carcinoma. All these specimens should be fixed adequately before sectioning. The gross appearance of the tumor, its dimensions, the patterns of growth, and involvement of adjacent structures should be documented. The slides should show the relationship between tumor and the surgical lines of resection; this relationship can be shown by marking the surgical margins with India ink.

When the pathologist receives a large en bloc resection specimen, the anatomy and orientation of the specimen can be readily determined in many cases because of the presence of structures such as the orbital contents, orbital floor, or lateral wall of the nasal cavity. In other cases, such as a partial maxillectomy, the pathologist may not be able to orient the specimen. In these cases, the clinician and the pathologist should study the specimen together before sections are taken to ensure proper orientation.

Partial maxillectomy is usually performed for tumor located in the inferior portion of the maxilla, such as hard palate or alveolar process. The specimen includes a portion of maxilla that may include part of the alveolar process, palate, and nasal turbinates (Fig. 6–15). Sometimes the incision is extended to include the ethmoid complex and lateral nose for adenocarcinoma of the ethmoid, lateral nasal wall lesion, olfactory neuroblastoma, and chondrosarcoma.

Radical maxillectomy specimen encompasses the entire maxillary wall, usually ethmoid labyrinth, with or without orbital content (Fig. 6–16). The anterior portion includes the entire anterior maxilla, anterolateral portion of the zygomatic process of the frontal bone, the frontal processes of the maxilla, and the medial and inferior walls of the orbit (see Fig. 6–16). Sometimes skin and underlying soft tissue overlying the anterior maxilla are removed. The posterior margin of the specimen includes the pterygoid muscle and, if orbit is removed, optic nerve and orbital content. When viewed from the medial aspect of the specimen, orbital content, turbinates, hard palate, and pterygoid muscle are displayed. The medial margin is composed of the transected hard palate and maxilla (Fig. 6–17). The zygomatic arch is the lateral margin. From the inferior aspect, the alveolar process and hard palate can be visualized. The superior margin includes the exposed orbital soft tissue or, if orbit is not removed, the floor of orbit.

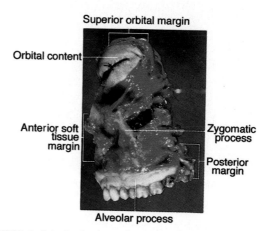

FIGURE 6–16 Radical maxillectomy with orbital exenteration.

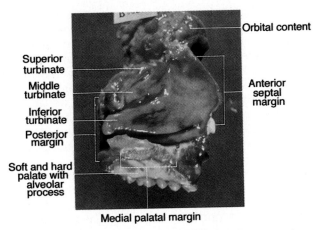

FIGURE 6-17 Medial aspect of a radical maxillectomy with orbital exenteration.

When examining the maxillectomy specimens, inspect any abnormality from outer surface, such as tumor extension into the skin and soft tissues of the anterior maxilla or cheek inferior to the zygoma. The skin may become fixed to the underlying soft tissue or bone to suggest tumor extension. Downward growth of the tumor from the maxillary sinus may result in a mass in the gingivobuccal sulcus or may erode into the oral cavity, creating an oroantral fistula. Tumor mass may be seen on the turbinate or protruding from maxillary antrum. Tumors arising from the maxillary sinus may extend inferiorly into the hard palate, the alveolar process, or the gingivobuccal sulcus. Maxillary sinus tumors may spread upward into the orbital floor (Figs. 6-18 and 6-19). If involved by tumor, the bony wall is soft, fractured, or destroyed. Tumor may extend into the orbital fat and extraocular musculature. Inspect the optic nerve for displacement, thickening, or invasion by the tumor.

Posterolateral extension of the tumor leads to the infratemporal fossa. Posterior extension of the tumor into the pterygoid space has serious clinical implication. Any involvement of the ethmoid sinuses and cribriform plates through the superior and medial extensions should be noted.

After initial inspection and documentation of the specimen dimension, the specimen is fixed in formalin for several hours or overnight. Later, the maxillary antrum is opened to characterize the tumor. Document the tumor size, appearance (color, consistency, hemorrhage, necrosis), local extent, and relationship with adjacent organs, which may be encroached, compressed, or invaded. The involved bone may be thinned like an eggshell, soft, or destroyed altogether. Slowly growing tumors, such as olfactory neuroblastoma, salivary gland tumors, benign tumors, and low-grade sarcomas tend to grow in an expansile fashion.

Because the solutions for decalcification may alter immunoreactivity of the tumor cells, at least some of the tumors should be submitted for histologic examination before decalcification. All surgical margins are marked with ink and dried. Soft tissue at margin that does not require decalcification is submitted first, to be followed by bony sections.

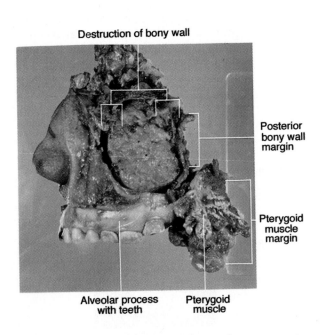

FIGURE 6-18 Radical maxillectomy for maxillary sinus carcinoma, which erodes the upper bony wall of maxillary sinus.

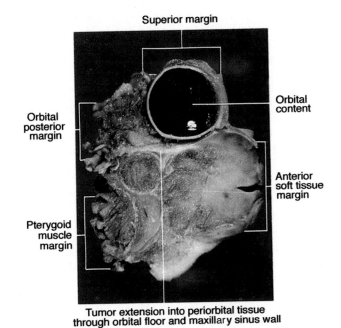

FIGURE 6-19 Cross section of maxillary tumor to demonstrate tumor invasion through the orbital floor. Tumor extends into the pterygoid muscle without involvement of posterior margin.

For routine light microscopy, buffered formalin is the commonest fixative used in the laboratory. Although Bouin's solution provides better preservation of nuclear morphology, it irreversibly damages the nuclear DNA to preclude DNA ploidy analysis and may diminish certain immunohistochemical reactions. In most instances, formalin-fixed tissue is also suitable for most of the immunohistochemical studies; however for B- and T-lymphocyte marker studies of membrane antigens, fresh frozen tissue is needed. Thus, when the differential diagnosis includes lymphoproliferative disorders, it is best to consult the pathologist prior to the biopsy for optimal handling of specimens.

FROZEN SECTIONS

Diagnosis by frozen section is an essential part of clinical management of patients with nasosinus disease. Frozen section diagnosis should be used judiciously to optimize patient management.

The most common indications for the use of frozen section diagnosis in the head and neck region include the following:

To provide immediate treatment under medical emergency. This is exemplified by the confirmation of rhinocerebral form of mucormycosis in a patient with progressive sinusitis. If the diagnosis is confirmed on the frozen section, resection and debridement of necrotic tissue is carried out.

To identify tissue of origin. At the time of resection, surgeons may submit tissue of uncertain origin for frozen section.

To determine the pathology of an excised lesion. During endoscopic surgery for maxillary sinus, a thickened nodular sinus mucosa may be submitted for frozen section to exclude underlying neoplasm. If an inverted papilloma is identified, the surgical approach can be modified.

To ensure adequacy of tissue for diagnosis and ancillary studies. A lesion is biopsied and submitted for frozen section diagnosis to provide adequate amount of tissue for definitive diagnosis. Under these circumstances, the pathologist must determine that the tissue is representative of the lesion, well preserved, and adequate in amount for permanent section. A tissue sample taken from the superficial portion of a deeply seated lesion may include only the capsule and not the lesion itself. The tissue may be necrotic and inadequate for diagnosis. In some instances, the tissue is completely distorted by crush artifacts when obtained by small forceps. Even if the tissue is well-preserved and adequate for diagnosis, be sure to have additional representative nonfrozen tissue available for permanent section. This is because freezing artifacts may interfere with histologic diagnosis. If diagnostic problems are anticipated, tissue is stored in proper preservatives for additional studies. If the frozen section suggests granulomatous

disease or an infectious disease, tissue should be sent for appropriate microbial cultures.

To assess the completeness of surgical resection. From the excised and resected specimens, frozen section diagnosis is often requested to determine the status of surgical margins.

At the time of intraoperative consultation or submitting tissue for permanent section, all excised specimens must be properly oriented anatomically and surgical borders indicated by India ink, sometimes using different colors. Proper embedding and labeling of the tissue are essential. Sometimes a strip of mucosa is submitted separately from a designated margin, in which case the orientation and the side representing the true margin should be identified by the surgeon. In some instances, additional specimens are submitted as extra-margins, and their relationship to the earlier specimens should be clarified.

To avoid an erroneous diagnosis, it is important to have all the pertinent clinical information. This knowledge can minimize overinterpreting the effects of prior diagnostic and therapeutic procedures as neoplasm. Reactive changes and sialometaplasia often follow prior biopsies, and atypical stromal cells are found following radiotherapy. The latter cells have enlarged, hyperchromatic, and irregular nuclei and prominent nucleoli (Fig. 6–20).[1] Within the exuberant granulation, endothelial cells are active and undergo mitosis.

When tissue is taken from soft tissue and bone of the oral cavity, the possibility of embryonic remnants of dental epithelium should be kept in mind. Rests of Malassez are found in the periodontal ligament near the cementum. They are usually seen in the resected specimen as multiple, anastomosing cords, or isolated clusters of round to cuboidal cells with peripheral palisading, commonly about 4 to 20 in number (Fig. 6–21). They are probably the source of periapical cysts, keratocysts, and other odonto-

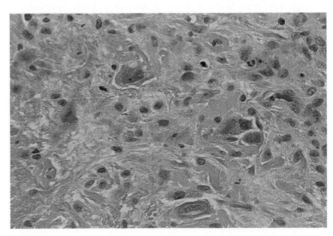

FIGURE 6–20 Frozen section of ulcerated lesion following radiotherapy. Atypical stromal cells with enlarged round-to-oval nuclei and prominent nucleoli are within the ulcer bed covered by fibrinous exudate. History of radiotherapy is helpful to avoid overdiagnosis.

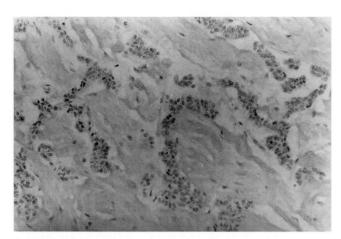

FIGURE 6–21 Rests of Malassez seen adjacent to the resection margin of mandible. Basaloid epithelial cells form connecting cords and nests.

genic tumors.[2] Rests of Serres occur in the region of lamina propria and appear as multiple clusters of polyhedral to squamous epithelial cells, sometimes undergoing cystic degeneration. Peripheral palisading is usually evident. They may simulate recurrent carcinoma or metastatic carcinoma. Rests of Chievits and other unnamed cysts have similar appearance to Rests of Serres.[2]

If dysplastic squamous epithelium is seen, it should be distinguished from invasive carcinoma. In a specimen removed for malignant melanoma, epidermal cells with clear cytoplasm should not be confused with atypical melanocytes. On the other hand, if atypical melanocytes are present on the surgical margins, they should be reported.

In some instances, it is difficult to distinguish reactive cells from neoplastic cells. This problem should be communicated to the surgeons, who may or may not be able to obtain additional margin for frozen section, depending upon the extent of disease and surgical anatomy.

Many factors influence the control of local disease and the recurrence of malignant tumor, especially the tumor size, the tumor differentiation, the local anatomy, and the surgical margin status. Although it has been demonstrated that tumors recur even if the margins are negative, studies have confirmed the status of surgical margins as an independent prognostic factor. Abnormal epithelium detected should be specified as to its histologic type—dysplasia, carcinoma in situ, or invasive carcinoma—and its location—mucosa, stroma, vascular lymphatic channels, perineural space—or both.[3]

Carcinoma of the head and neck recurs locally 70% to 100% when the final surgical margins are positive.[4–6] In the study of Scholl et al,[3] only 15% (32 of 214) of patients whose excision margins were entirely clear of tongue squamous cell carcinoma developed local recurrence. Among those whose surgical margins were positive by intraoperative frozen section but negative at the completion of surgery, the frequency of local recurrence was found to be slightly higher at 17% (7 of 41). But more importantly, 69% (9 of 13) of patients whose margins were positive at the completion of surgery died within 18 months.[3]

Perineural invasion was detected in 5.5% (16 of 268) of patients with tongue carcinoma. Of these, close to 50% had positive surgical margins. It should be noted that perineural invasion by itself did not affect local control (20% of patients with this invasion treated with postoperative radiotherapy recurred and 25% treated by surgery alone recurred, not significant at 5% level).[3]

Zieske et al[7] studied 349 patients, most of whom had tonsillar and hypopharyngeal squamous cell carcinomas. Nine percent of patients had positive margins, of these patients, 94% had Stage III or IV disease. Follow-up data revealed that 26% (84 of 318) with negative margins died of disease, as compared with 77% (24 of 31) with positive margins.[7]

The surgical margins of 70 head and neck cancer specimens were studied by parallel sections or Mohs' chemosurgery. Seventy-five percent of specimens had malignant cells at original margins, which were 1 cm away from the gross tumor. The reasons for local failure include:

1. Specimen not properly oriented and mapped for tumor margins
2. Tumor invaded into bone, which is not suitable for frozen section
3. Failure to see tumor cells on the frozen or permanent section[8]

Other factors include skipped areas of normal tissue with tumor cells spread by vascular lymphatic channels.[8]

In summary, at the time of intraoperative consultation, the pathologists should ask questions for clarification, discuss any diagnostic problems and differential diagnosis, and not hesitate to express uncertainty about the diagnosis. There is ample evidence to support that a positive resection margin with tumor implies lower 5-year survival rates and shorter time for tumor recurrence.[9]

Although formalin-fixed, paraffin-embedded tissue may be used for electron microscopy after deparaffinization, postfixation in gluteraldehyde and osmic acid, and embedding in proper substrate, the preservation of cellular organelles is generally poor due to delay in fixation, protein denaturation, and disruptions of the cell membranes. In the authors' experience, organelles that are likely to be preserved are tonofilaments, neurosecretory granules, and melanosomes. Tissue for electron microscopy is fixed optimally in buffered gluteraldehyde at the time of frozen section consultation in anticipation of diagnostic problems requiring further studies. Sometimes tissue is obtained specifically for electron microscopy after light microscopy and immunohistochemistry have failed to provide definitive diagnosis. Proper fixatives for special studies should be placed in clearly labeled bottles and stored in the refrigerator.

NORMAL HISTOLOGY

The first 2 cm of anterior nares and nasal septum are covered by skin with adnexal tissue in the dermis. Moving further inward, the remaining nasal cavity, paranasal sinuses, nasopharynx, false vocal cord, and subglottic region are lined by ciliated respiratory mucosa with a varying number of goblet cells. The nasosinus mucosa, also referred to as Schneiderian membrane, consists of ciliated cells, columnar cells, goblet cells, and basal cells (Fig. 6–22). The ratio of ciliated cells to goblet cells is about 5:1. The ciliary movement and the secretory product of mucus, lysozyme, immunoglobulin, and interferon help to prevent bacterial and viral invasion.

The specialized olfactory epithelium, extending from the superior turbinate and nasal septum to the roof of the nasal cavity, consists of supporting cells, basal cells, and olfactory cells. Similar to respiratory epithelium, it is pseudostratified and columnar. Embedded among the supporting and basal cells are bipolar olfactory cells or neurons, which send out dendritic processes and olfactory vesicles to the mucosal surface and axon fibers at the base.[10] Because of a mixture of epithelial and neuronal cells in this epithelium, it is not surprising that neoplasms of this site may contain neuronal, epithelial, or both elements.

Although dendritic cells and melanocytes are not readily apparent on hematoxylin and eosin stained sections, their presence in the basal cell layer of squamous mucosa can be demonstrated by immunohistochemistry. This technique also illustrates neuroendocrine cells in the respiratory mucosa and seromucous glands.

Beneath the respiratory and olfactory epithelia are tunica propria with lobules of seromucous glands, blood vessels, lymphatics, nerve fibers, cartilage, and bone. Seromucous glands are minor salivary glands consisting of 90% mucous cells and 10% serous cells (see Fig. 6–22). The secretions drain to the intercalated ducts, striated ducts, excretory ducts, and main duct. Oncocytic and intestinal metaplasia sometimes occur, especially secondary to chronic hypertrophic rhinitis and sinusitis.

In the tunica propria of nasal mucosa are extensive blood vessels in three systems:

1. Subepithelial capillaries located in the submucosal tissue and in the inferior turbinate and anterior nasal septum
2. Periglandular and submucosal capillaries, arterioles, and venules
3. Multiple direct arterial and venous anastomoses, especially around the choanal orifice and posterior nasal septum

These three systems communicate with venous erectile vessels, which are invested with multiple layers of smooth muscle cells and appear irregular in thickness simulating A-V malformation. Some of the vascular spaces are markedly dilated, sometimes simulating cavernous hemangioma. Unlike vascular lesions, the erectile tissue is localized and noninfiltrative. The blood flow is adjusted by throttle vein, periosteal arteries and veins, and sympathetic vasoconstrictor tone to adjust temperature and humidity of the air. The specialized fenestrations between endothelial cells of large subepithelial and periglandular capillaries enhance the transport of fluid and high-molecular-weight substances.

The nasopharynx is bordered by choana and palate anteriorly, sphenoid bone superiorly, the base of occipital bone and the cervical vertebrae posteriorly, and oropharynx inferiorly. The ostium of the eustachian tube opens into the lateral nasopharyngeal wall. A wide, slit-like space around the cranial and dorsal portion of the tubal orifice is referred to as the fossa of Rosenmuller (recessus pharyngeus). Histologically, about 60% of nasopharyngeal mucosa is covered by stratified squamous epithelium, and the remaining mucosa by ciliated columnar epithelium. At the age of adolescence, the latter undergoes squamous metaplasia, which is also called transitional or intermediate epithelium (Fig. 6–23).

In the base of the tongue, nasopharynx, and pharynx, there is abundant lymphoid tissue in the lingual, faucial tonsils, and adenoids—the so-called Waldeyer's ring. Depending upon the location, the epithelium, which lines the mucosa or the clefts, varies from squamous, respiratory, or metaplastic squamous (transitional) in character. The interface with the underlying lymphoid tissue is sometimes

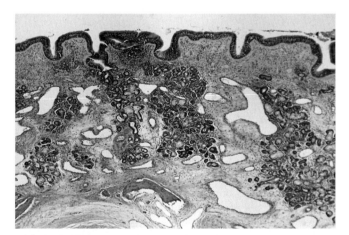

FIGURE 6–22 Normal histology of nasal and paranasal sinus wall consisting of ciliated respiratory mucosa and the underlying laminar propria with seromucous glands, fibrous stroma, and blood vessels of varying sizes. In the turbinate, the bony tissue is immediately beneath the mucosa.

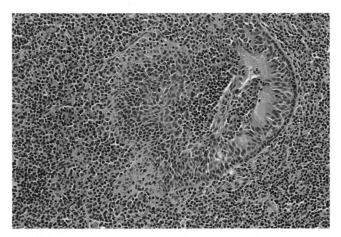

FIGURE 6-23 The respiratory epithelium in nasopharynx undergoes early squamous metaplasia. A well-defined interface between the epithelium and lymphoid stroma helps to avoid overinterpretation as neoplastic cells.

poorly defined and irregular. Loosely cohesive epithelial cells may appear immature, isolated, and intermingled with lymphoid cells. In spite of their immature appearance, the epithelial cells have uniform nuclear morphology, lack mitotic activity, and are not surrounded by desmoplastic stroma. In contrast, nuclear atypia, local infiltration, and stromal reaction are expected in the case of carcinomas.

Throughout the oral cavity and upper respiratory tract, minor salivary glands occur in the submucosal stroma with close to 90% mucinous cells and the remaining 10% serous cells.

INFLAMMATORY, GRANULOMATOUS, AND INFECTIOUS DISEASES

A large proportion of nasal and sinus specimens received in the pathology laboratory are related to the inflammatory and infectious diseases. The clinical presentations are variable. Some have symptoms of allergic reactions, rhinorrhea, nasal obstruction, and epistaxis. Others may present with nasal polyp, tumor masses, or extensive destruction of the midline facial structure with perforation of the nasal septum and palate.

Pathologically, these inflammatory and infectious diseases can be divided into three categories. The first group includes allergic and inflammatory rhinitis and sinusitis. The second category is specific infectious diseases with distinct morphologic changes and causative agents, which can be identified by appropriate stains and cultures. The third group is related to immunologic disorders or unknown etiology, such as sarcoidosis and Wegener's granulomatosis.

In association with these inflammatory and infectious processes, secondary changes occur in the epithelium and stroma. These changes should be distinguished from neoplasms. Mucosal damage often associates with active regeneration, reactive hyperplasia, pseudoepitheliomatous hyperplasia, and squamous metaplasia. The stromal responses with sheets of lymphoid cells or plasma cells may be confused with hematopoietic neoplasms. Fibroblastic and vascular proliferations may similarly present with nuclear atypia and increased mitotic activity to suggest malignancy.

Thus, in dealing with inflammatory and infectious processes of this site, key pathologic decisions involve:

1. Type of inflammatory reaction: allergic, inflammatory, or infectious
2. In the case of suspected infection, performance of appropriate special studies to determine the causative agents
3. Exclusion of additional underlying or coexisting diseases, such as neoplasm
4. Recognition of iatrogenic changes—for example, steroids injected intranasally and myospherulosis following packing of the nasal cavity with petrolatum-based antibiotics.

Acute and Chronic Rhinitis, Sinusitis, and Nasal Polyps

After excluding specific infectious and granulomatous rhinitis, several major types of rhinitis exist: allergic, nonallergic, and atrophic. A correct diagnosis depends on clinical history, physical examination, skin tests, and radioallergosorbent testing (RAST). The diagnosis of allergic rhinitis is made clinically by positive skin and/or RAST tests. The nonallergic inflammatory group includes idiopathic vasomotor rhinitis, hormonal rhinitis, and rhinitis medicamentosa. During pregnancy, elevated estrogen may affect nasal mucosa through increased cholinergic effects. Topical decongestants and various systemic medications are known to cause nasal obstruction and rhinitis medicamentosa. Atrophic rhinitis is a rare, severe, chronic rhinitis caused by *Klebsiella ozaenae* or mixed organisms.

The development of sinusitis is closely related to the local anatomy, respiratory mucosal function and reactivity, and host responses. The anterior ethmoid–middle meatal complex, also referred to as the osteomeatal complex, is believed to be the first location in the development of sinusitis. Local and systemic factors cause mucosal edema, local inflammation, and hypertrophy of this area. These events initiate acute sinusitis secondary to anterior ethmoid cell ostial narrowing, impaired drainage, or stasis of secretions.

Further changes in the local mucociliary transport and ventilation obstruction of the maxillary and frontal sinuses predispose to the further development of chronic sinusitis in more than one site. Sinusitis can be classified as:

1. Acute suppurative sinusitis, 1 day to 4 weeks duration
2. Subacute suppurative sinusitis, 4 weeks to 3 months duration
3. Chronic suppurative sinusitis, more than 3 months
4. Acute and subacute suppurative sinusitis

Gross Pathology

The removed nasal and sinus tissue is usually thickened with varying amount of stromal edema and fibrosis. When the edema is abundant, the tissue appears polypoid and semitransparent. White-grey firm tissue is likely to associate with chronic inflammation and fibrosis.

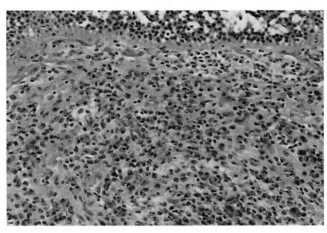

FIGURE 6–25 Nonallergic rhinitis with eosinophilia and abundant inflammatory cells.

Microscopic Pathology

In allergic rhinitis, stromal edema and inflammatory infiltrates, especially eosinophils, are prominent (Fig. 6–24A). In the overlying mucosa and underlying seromucous glands, mucous cells and goblet cells are sometimes hyperplastic (Fig. 6–24B). Similar changes also occur in eosinophilic nonallergic rhinitis, but the patients have negative skin and/or RAST tests (Fig. 6–25). The number of patients affected by allergic and nonallergic rhinitis is almost equal.

Atrophic rhinitis is characterized by atrophy of the surface epithelium and the secretory glands (Fig. 6–26). The chronic inflammatory reaction is usually severe. A variable infiltrate of lymphocytes and plasma cells may be found within the secretory glands, associated with acinar atrophy. Hyperplastic changes may be seen within small ducts, leading to

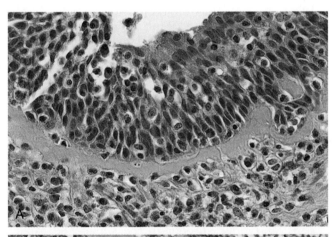

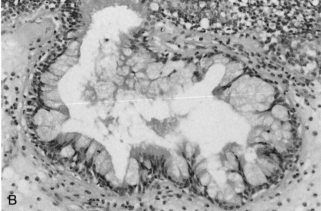

FIGURE 6–24 Allergic rhinitis. A, Respiratory mucosa is hyperplastic with proliferation of basal cells. The basement membrane is thickened. Eosinophils are abundant. B, Hyperplastic mucous cells and goblet cells in the seromucous glands.

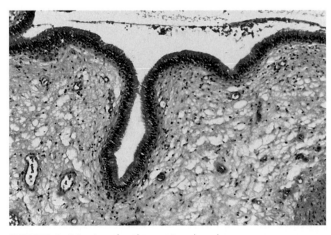

FIGURE 6–26 Atrophic rhinitis. Atrophic, thin respiratory mucosa and underlying dense fibrous tissue devoid of seromucous glands.

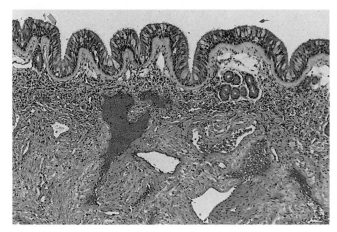

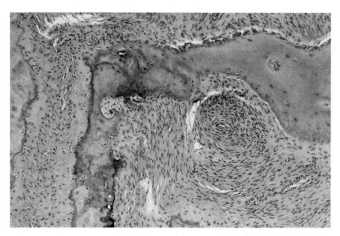

FIGURE 6–27 Vasomotor rhinitis is characterized by marked stromal edema, multiple dilated congested blood vessels, and limited inflammatory cells.

FIGURE 6–28 Marked fibrosis of bony wall with hypercellularity may mimic fibrous neoplasm.

almost solid plugging of these ducts with epithelial and possibly myoepithelial cells. Squamous metaplasia is common. Nasal moisture is reduced, cilia are destroyed, and crusts are formed. The turbinates are atrophic. Possible etiologies include bacterial infections, deficiency in vitamin A and iron, and secondary atrophy following sinus surgery for chronic sinusitis.

Vasomotor rhinitis is related to overreactive parasympathetic stimulation of the nasal mucosa causing vasodilation, edema, and hypersecretion of mucus. Symptoms include nasal obstruction, profuse rhinorrhea, infrequent sneezing, stuffiness, facial pressure and headache. The clinical diagnosis of vasomotor rhinitis is made by excluding other types of rhinitis. Microscopically, stromal edema is a prominent feature. Capillaries and thick-walled blood vessels are often dilated and increased in number, and sometimes come close to the mucosal surface (Fig. 6–27). Eosinophils, lymphocytes, and plasma cells are usually limited in number. Mast cells and basophils may be abundant. Seromucous glands are mildly hyperplastic.

Complications of Rhinitis and Sinusitis

By the time surgery is performed for long-standing rhinitis and sinusitis, the removed tissue may demonstrate additional secondary changes superimposed on the primary disease. For these reasons, precise classification of rhinitis and sinusitis may not be possible. For example, vasomotor rhinitis may be complicated by infectious rhinitis and sinusitis. In most instances, the respiratory mucosa and the underlying seromucous glands are hyperplastic with an increase of goblet cells. The basement membrane beneath the respiratory mucosa is thickened. The number of inflammatory cells varies. In the case of allergic rhinitis, eosinophilic infiltrates and stromal edema are prominent. Lymphocytes and plasma

cells are abundant in the case of nonallergic rhinitis, while limited in the case of vasomotor rhinitis. In severe sinusitis, inflammatory infiltrates are associated with fibrosis and vascular proliferation, sometimes extending into bone (Fig. 6–28).

When the openings of seromucous glands are obstructed, retention cysts result from accumulation of fluid in the submucosal seromucous glands. These cysts are most commonly found in the floor of the maxillary antrum. When the drainage of the sinus content into the nasal cavity is impeded by swollen mucosa at the ostia, mucus and debris fill the sinus in the form of a mucocele (Fig. 6–29). The expanded mucoceles cause thinning, atrophy, and destruction of the bony sinus wall. Ruptured retention cysts can result in a histologic appearance quite similar to the mucocele of the lip. The released mucous material is surrounded by granulation tissue and abundant foamy macrophages with mucin in the cytoplasm. Other causes of mucoceles include osteoma, trauma, polyps, and prior surgery to the sinus. The frontal

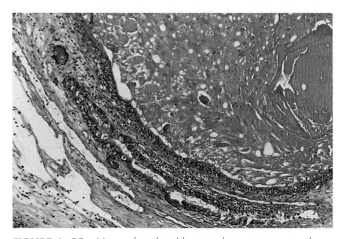

FIGURE 6–29 Mucocele is lined by atrophic respiratory epithelium and filled with mucus and cellular debris.

sinus is most commonly affected, followed by the ethmoid and maxillary sinuses. Sphenoid sinus mucoceles are rare.

Because the ethmoid sinus is separated from the orbit by a thin layer of bone, lamina papyracea, an inflammatory process readily extends into the adjacent organs causing orbital and periorbital cellulitis and abscesses. Osteomyelitis is prone to occur in the frontal bones and maxilla. Intracranial complications, although rare, may include epidural and subdural abscess, meningitis, brain abscess, and cavernous sinus thrombosis. The cranial nerves may also become affected.

Nasal Polyps

Nasal polyps are soft, edematous, semitranslucent polypoid masses of tissue most often affecting both nasal cavities and the ethmoid region, usually associated with rhinitis and sinusitis (Fig. 6–30). Sometimes polyps occur in the posterior nasal cavity, so-called choanal polyps.

Microscopically, the ciliated respiratory epithelium of the nasal polyps, similar to rhinitis and sinusitis, may undergo squamous metaplasia and hyperplasia with proliferation of basal cells and goblet cells. Squamous dysplasia and carcinoma in situ occur in 1.1% of nasal polyps.[11] Thickened basement membrane occurs beneath the respiratory mucosa. Ulcerated and damaged respiratory mucosa is followed by a metaplastic squamous epithelium (Fig. 6–31). The mucosa is occasionally atrophic, especially in the presence of retention cysts and mucoceles. The underlying seromucous glands can be hyperplastic with enlarged lobules, within which mucous cells are increased in number, and the cytoplasm is distended with mucin. In other cases, the seromucous glands are atrophic. The ducts leading to the glands are often cystically dilated, producing retention cysts.

In the nasal polyps, edema is prominent in the

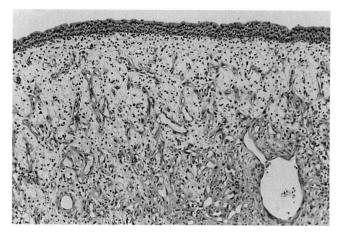

FIGURE 6–31 The stroma of the polyp is marked by edema and vascular proliferation.

lamina propria. Eosinophilic, proteinaceous fluid sometimes accumulates as microcystic spaces. A variable number of neutrophils, eosinophils, lymphocytes, and plasma cells is seen. The presence of numerous eosinophils indicates that the lesion probably has an allergic etiology. The inflammatory infiltrate sometimes extends into the bony wall. The bony trabeculae react and deposit new osteoid material on the outer borders.

The stroma may contain large, bizarre, pleomorphic spindle-shaped cells having hyperchromatic nuclei, and prominent nucleoli may be observed in the stroma.[12] Rare mitotic figures also occur. These atypical stromal cells may lead the pathologist to suspect the presence of a malignant tumor such as an embryonal rhabdomyosarcoma; however, these atypical cells are usually seen in the context of inflamed granulation tissue and are thought to represent bizarre reactive myofibroblasts (Fig. 6–32). The presence of these cells does not indicate that the lesion will recur or behave in a malignant manner.[12]

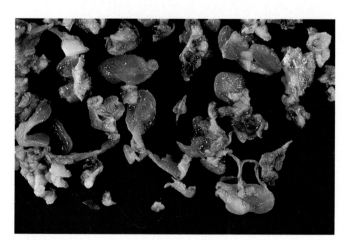

FIGURE 6–30 Multiple nasal polyps with edematous, grey-white, semitransparent appearance. Some polyps have fibrous stalks.

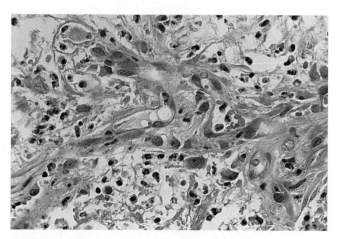

FIGURE 6–32 Atypical stromal cells are characterized by enlarged round to oval nuclei with prominent nucleoli. The nuclei are similar to each other without nuclear irregularity or pleomorphism.

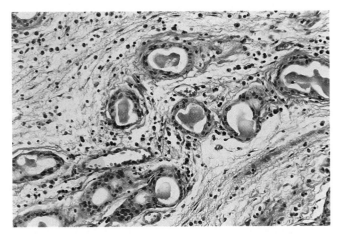

FIGURE 6-33 Nasal polyp in cystic fibrosis is typified by atrophic seromucous glands and dilated ducts containing inspissated mucous material.

About 5% to 10% of the patients with mucoviscidosis (cystic fibrosis) develop polyps in the nasal cavity and paranasal sinuses.[13] The characteristic feature is the accumulation of inspissated, dense mucoid material in the acini and ducts of seromucous glands (Fig. 6–33). This material is primarily acid mucin, which is blue-purple in color by alcian blue/PAS stain. The neutral mucin seen in ordinary inflammatory polyps is red-purple in color.[14]

Differential Diagnosis

Hyperplastic respiratory mucosa with polypoid projections and infoldings may simulate nasosinus papilloma, especially on tangential cuts. A form of hyperplasia is described by Wenig and Heffner[15] under the name of adenomatoid hamartoma in association with nasal polyp, rhinitis, and sinusitis. In their series of 27 men and four women (mean age 58 years), polypoid nodules up to 4.9 cm in size occur in the nasosinus and nasopharynx, most commonly on the posterior nasal septum. Microscopically, multiple dilated, branching and crowded glandular spaces are lined by two to three layers of hyperplastic ciliated epithelium (Figs. 6–34 *A* and *B*). Nuclear atypia is minimal or absent. Some of the submitting pathologists made the diagnosis of papilloma and adenocarcinoma for this newly recognized hamartoma.

Hyperplastic respiratory mucosa and early squamous metaplasia with proliferating basal cells arranged vertically can simulate dysplastic change, especially when the immature cells also present with enlarged nuclei and increased nuclear cytoplasmic ratios (Figs. 6–35 *A–C*). The mitotic activity is rare and limited to the deep layers. Nuclear irregularity and hyperchromasia are absent. Ciliated cells often remain on the surface.

In association with rhinitis, sinusitis, and nasal polyps, squamous metaplasia of the respiratory mu-

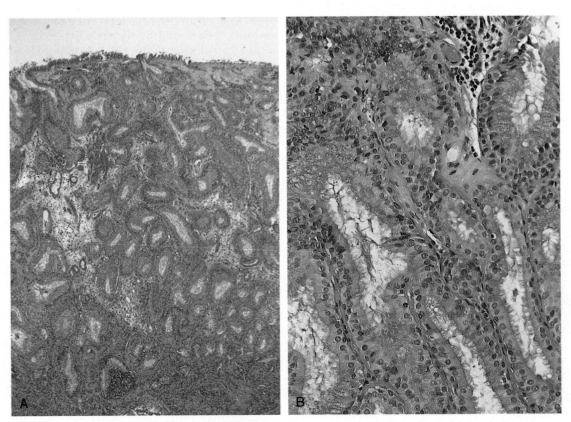

FIGURE 6-34 Adenomatoid hamartoma. *A,* Branching, budding, and overcrowded glands are located beneath the respiratory surface. *B,* These hyperplastic glands are lined by ciliated and nonciliated mucus-secreting cells.

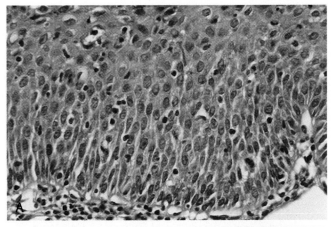

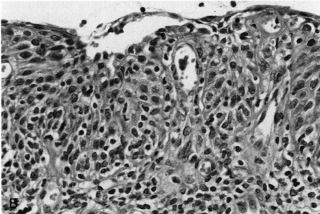

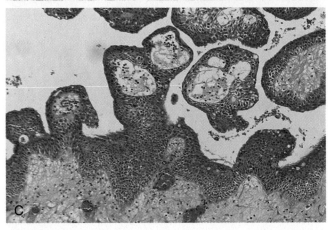

FIGURE 6-35 *A,* Squamous metaplasia with proliferation of basal cells and maturation in the upper layers. Although the cells appear immature, the cellular polarity is maintained. The cells appear monotonous with uniform nuclei. The mitotic activity is low to absent. *B,* Reactive squamous metaplasia with mild nuclear irregularity. *C,* Squamous metaplasia with polypoid hyperplasia simulates nasal papilloma. In papilloma, the fibrovascular stalk is thin and delicate.

cosa is common. Less commonly, squamous metaplasia occurs in the underlying seromucous glands in the form of necrotizing sialometaplasia. This entity was first described in the palate associated with mucosal ulcer and necrosis, secondary to inflamma-

tion, local injury, ischemia, and medical interventions. Maisel et al[16] reported a 68-year-old woman who presented with recurrent epistaxis and required resection of the posterior inferior turbinate. The nasal mucosa was ulcerated and associated with chronic inflammation. Squamous metaplasia involved both the mucosa and the underlying seromucous gland. The latter was interpreted as squamous cell carcinoma, and this diagnosis led to a partial maxillectomy.

It is important to recognize this benign reparative change because of its close resemblance to squamous cell carcinoma and mucoepidermoid carcinoma. The damaged seromucous glands undergo squamous metaplasia, resulting in a mixed population of mucous secreting cells and squamous cells. The latter have immature and reactive appearance with enlarged nuclei, prominent nucleoli, and rare mitotic figures. Similar changes can also extend to the damaged ducts. Tangential cuts through the excretory ducts near the mucosal surface result in irregular tongue-like protrusions to further imitate invasive squamous carcinoma. The preservation of the lobular architecture; the lack of nuclear hyperchromasia, irregularity and pleomorphism; and the surrounding inflammatory response should suggest the possibility of necrotizing sialometaplasia (Fig. 6–36).

Pseudoepitheliomatous hyperplasia in the nasosinus region is most commonly associated with mucosal ulcer with or without prior medical interventions. Less commonly, this change occurs over the underlying disease, such as rhinoscleroma, fungal infection, and neoplastic disease. The latter includes granular cell tumor, malignant lymphoma, and fibrohistiocytic tumors.[17] The elongated and thickened rete pegs extend into the underlying connective tissue and have smooth, sharp, and sometimes pointed borders. The constituent cells resemble each other and have uniform nuclei without nuclear atypia. Rare mitotic figures occur. Invasive squamous cell carcinoma has irregular, confluent rete pegs, in which the component cells disclose varying degrees of nuclear atypia and abnormal differentiation, including dyskeratosis and keratin pearls. The surrounding stroma has the myxoid, desmoplastic appearance with fibroblastic proliferation and chronic inflammation.

In specimens with severe chronic rhinitis and sinusitis, the lymphoid or plasmacytic infiltrates may be heavy and diffuse to raise the question of lymphoma or plasmacytoma. The infiltrates tend to be heterogeneous and lack nuclear atypia. The background capillaries are proliferative and lined by plump endothelial cells. A helpful finding is the presence of Russell bodies, whose presence suggests a benign process. In contrast, plasmacytomas are composed of immature cells that have large, atypical, pleomorphic nuclei and demonstrate numerous mitoses. Russell bodies are rarely seen.

Inflammatory pseudotumor associated with marked fibroblastic proliferations may present with

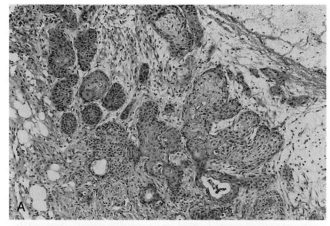

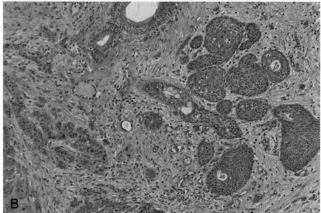

FIGURE 6–36   Sialometaplasia. *A*, The seromucous glands and ducts are replaced by solid nests of immature squamous metaplasia. Notice the preservation of the lobular pattern and smooth borders. The fibrous stroma is infiltrated by chronic inflammatory cells. *B*, This sialometaplasia (*right field*) is coexisting with invasive squamous carcinoma (*left field*). Note the irregular nests of tumor cells with moderate nuclear atypia.

nuclear atypia and increased mitotic activity to suggest malignancy. Severe hemorrhage and necrosis can also lead to inflammatory pseudotumor[18] and cholesterol granuloma. (See later section on cholesterol granuloma.)

In some specimens, aggregates of inspissated mucus are mixed with eosinophils, Charcot-Leyden crystals, acute and chronic inflammatory cells. This is typically found in children or young adults, who present with chronic sinusitis and opacified sinus without bony destruction on radiograph, especially the maxillary antrum. The curetted tissue has a rubbery consistency and translucent appearance. In extreme cases, the texture of mucus is so dense as to simulate chondroid matrix, raising the possibility of mixed tumor (Fig. 6–37), chondroid tumor, and even rhabdomyosarcoma.[19] This inspissated mucus can also be seen in the case of allergic fungal sinusitis with numerous eosinophils and Charcot-Leyden crystals in the background. A correct diagnosis depends on the demonstration of fungal organisms by

special stains or by culture. (See later section on allergic fungal sinusitis.)

Rarely, children or young adults with storage diseases may present with nasal polyps and airway obstruction. In the case of mucopolysaccharidosis, numerous foamy histiocytes accumulate in the stroma. Endothelial cells and the surrounding stromal cells contain vacuolated material, which reacts weakly with periodic acid–Schiff (PAS) and alcian blue stains (Fig. 6–38). Inflammatory infiltrates are minimal in amount. Determination of the specific metabolic disorder requires biochemical assay of the serum or urine.[20]

Infectious diseases of the upper respiratory tract are rare and usually seen in patients with immunologic deficiency and those coming from the endemic areas. However, these diseases are actually more common than expected because of the increase of immigrants and ease of worldwide travel.

Tuberculosis

Tuberculosis may involve the skin of the nose, the mucocutaneous junction, the nasal cavity, and the

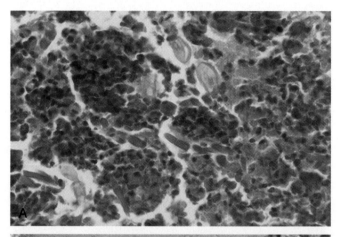

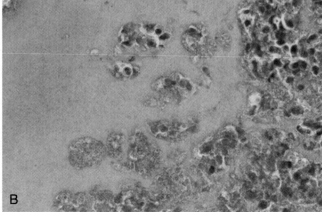

FIGURE 6–37   *A*, Dense secretion with abundant eosinophils and Charcot-Leyden crystals. *B*, Inspissated mucus simulates cartilaginous tissue.

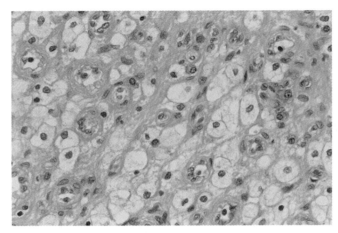

FIGURE 6–38 Nasal polyps in association with fusidosis. The most distinct feature is the collection of abundant foamy histiocytes.

remainder of the upper resiratory tract, especially the larynx. The erythematous, ulcerative, polypoid lesion may destroy the underlying cartilage, resulting in perforation of the nasal septum.[21] Most biopsies yield characteristic caseating granulomas consisting of epithelioid cells, Langhans giant cells, lymphocytes and plasma cells (Fig. 6–39). Special stains are used to identify acid-fast organisms.

Leprosy

Leprosy of the nose, nasal cavity, and nasopharynx most commonly affects the septum and inferior turbinate. Most infections are lepromatous type. The tuberculoid form with well-formed granuloma is rare and limited to the skin. In the early stage, the chronic inflammatory reaction, consisting of lymphocytes, plasma cells and macrophages, appears nonspecific. Later, large foamy histiocytes (lepra cells) predominate to form nodules and become more characteristic for leprosy. With the Wade Fite stain, numerous *Mycobacterium leprae* can usually be found in the cytoplasm of lepra cells and endothelial cells. The disease apparently ends with fibrosis.[21]

In tuberculoid form and borderline cases, nodules of epithelioid cells and giant cells are mixed with lymphocytes and plasma cells; however, no acid-fast bacilli can be identified.[22] The use of polymerase chain reaction has improved the detection of *M. leprae*. A rare complication of leprosy patients is the nasal infection with maggots, so-called myiasis.[22]

Rhinoscleroma

Rhinoscleroma is seen mainly among individuals living and coming from the endemic areas of this disease (parts of Eastern Europe, the Mediterranean area, the Middle East, Central Africa, Pakistan, Indonesia, and Latin America).[21–23]

Gross Pathology

Rhinoscleroma initially affects the mucous membranes of the nasal cavity and later may extend into the nasopharynx and larynx. The polypoid lesions gradually become firm, indurated, and nodular. The mucosa is white, thickened, and covered by exudates, usually not ulcerated. Large masses may eventually cause airway obstruction.

Microscopic Pathology

The overlying epithelium is usually intact, but squamous metaplasia and pseudoepitheliomatous hyperplasia may be seen (Fig. 6–40A). A correct diagnosis can be reached by performing fine needle aspiration or biopsy of the lesion. The first impression on inspecting the biopsy is a diffuse infiltration of plasma cells, with the differential diagnosis of plasma cell granuloma or plasmacytoma (Fig. 6–40B). On further examination, a variable number of foamy histiocytes occurs from area to area. These histiocytes have abundant, somewhat foamy cytoplasm. This should raise the possibility of Mikulicz cells by ordering special stains (Fig. 6–40C). Because of the numerous histiocytes with abundant cytoplasm, leprosy and sinus histiocytosis with massive lymphadenopathy should be considered in the differential diagnosis. The inflammatory process usually does not involve the underlying cartilage and bone.

On PAS, silver, and Gram stains, gram-negative short bacilli (*Klebsiella rhinoscleromatis*) can be demonstrated in the cytoplasm of histiocytes, thus confirming the diagnosis of rhinoscleroma (Fig. 5–40D). A specific identification of the organisms can be achieved by immunoperoxidase technique using rabbit anti-Klebsiella capsular antigen III. It has been found to improve the specificity of histochemical stains and to detect lesions that are otherwise negative by cultures or other special stains.[24]

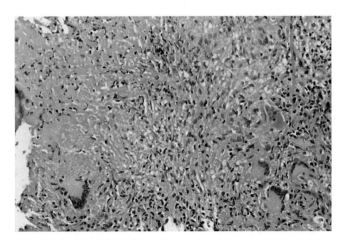

FIGURE 6–39 Tuberculosis. Extensive caseating necrosis surrounded by multinucleated Langhans giant cells and epithelioid cells.

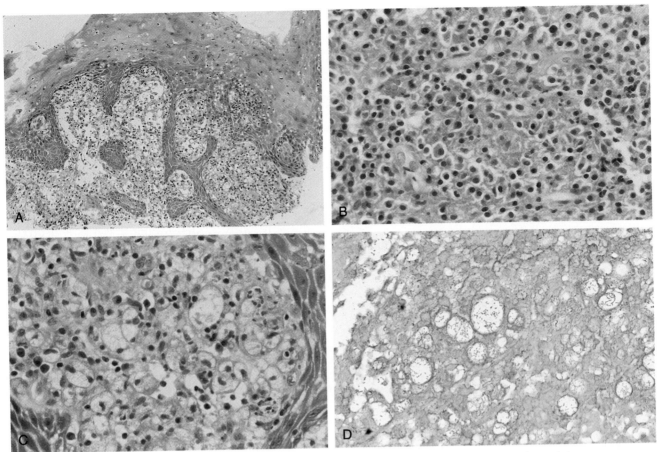

FIGURE 6-40 Rhinoscleroma. *A*, Pseudoepitheliomatous hyperplasia of the overlying squamous mucosa. *B*, The underlying stroma contains numerous plasma cells mixed with foamy histiocytes. *C*, Higher magnification of histiocytes revealing vacuolated or granular cytoplasm. *D*, Gram stain demonstrates numerous coccobacilli within the cytoplasm of foamy histiocytes confirming the diagnosis of rhinoscleroma and Mikulicz cells.

Differential Diagnosis

When faced with chronic inflammatory process with granulomatous reaction or abundant histiocytes, special stains and culture should be performed to exclude Mikulicz cells and lepra cells. If infectious organisms are absent and the histiocytes have dense eosinophilic cytoplasm, the possibility of sinus histiocytosis with massive lymphadenopathy (Rosai-Dorfman disease) should be considered. Although this disease typically involves cervical lymph nodes in young individuals, extranodal manifestations are common. In a series of more than 400 cases, 43% of patients have extranodal involvement, especially in the skin (49 cases), nasosinuses (48 cases), soft tissue (38 cases), eyelid/orbit (36 cases), bone (33 cases), salivary gland (22 cases), central nervous system (21 cases), and oral cavity (12 cases).[25] It should be noted that some patients present primarily with extranodal disease and that lymphadenopathy is minimal or unapparent. Involvement of multiple sites is also common. Thus, in biopsy from the head and neck region, this disease should always be kept in mind.

When sinus histiocytosis with massive lymphadenopathy occurs in the nasal cavity and nasopharynx, clinical findings include a tumor mass of the nasal cavity, maxillary antrum, or cheek; less common symptoms include hearing loss and cranial nerve deficits. The most distinct histologic feature is a sheet-like proliferation of histiocytes intermixed with lymphocytes simulating sinus histiocytosis of the lymph node (Fig. 6–41*A*). Stromal fibrosis and hyalinization can be marked in some cases (Fig. 6–41*B*). Individual histiocytes have large round to oval nuclei, prominent nucleoli, and abundant eosinophilic granular cytoplasm. Vacuolated cytoplasm is also common. Phagocytosis of lymphocytes, nuclear debris, and red blood cells is sometimes evident (Fig. 6–41*C*). Plasma cells and eosinophils are numerous in some cases. This mixed cellular infiltrate combined with large histiocytes having lobated nuclei and prominent nucleoli suggests Hodgkin's disease (Fig. 6–41*D*). Special stains for bacterial, acid-fast, and fungal organisms have been negative. By immunohistochemistry, the histiocytes express S-100 protein and pan-macrophage antigen (such as Leu-M3), which suggest activated macrophages.[26]

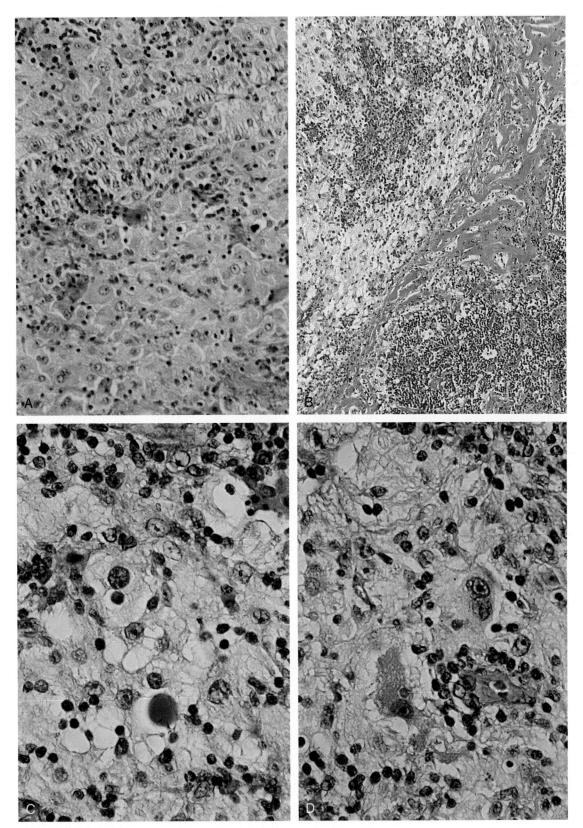

FIGURE 6–41   Rosai-Dorfman disease. *A,* Sheets of histiocytes are mixed with lymphocytes and plasma cells. These histiocytes have abundant eosinophilic cytoplasm. *B,* In this case, hyalinization of the stroma is a prominent feature. *C,* Phagocytosis of lymphocytes by histiocytes. *D,* Some histiocytes have irregular nuclei and prominent nucleoli simulating Reed-Sternberg cells. Erythrophagocytosis is also evident.

Syphilis

Congenital and all stages of syphilis may rarely cause rhinitis, necrosis, deformity, and masses of the nose. The cellular infiltrates of plasma cells, lymphocytes, epithelioid cells, and rare Langhans giant cells are not specific and are difficult to distinguish from other midline destructive disease. Warthin-Starry stain may demonstrate the *Treponema pallidum.*

Leishmaniasis

Nasal leishmaniasis is extremely rare, except in patients coming from the endemic area; the presentation is typically nasal ulceration or fine nodularity, sometimes extending into the nasopharynx. In the biopsy, the key findings include perivascular lymphocytic infiltration and vascular proliferation with plump endothelial cells containing protozoa parasites. These parasites are also found in histiocytes, neutrophils, and fibroblasts with the aid of PAS or Giemsa stain.[22]

Fungal Sinusitis

Four types of fungal sinusitis exist: (1) Noninvasive in the form of fungus ball, (2) invasive and destructive, (3) allergic, and (4) noninvasive but destructive.[27]

NONINVASIVE

Noninvasive fungal sinusitis exists in the form of mycetoma and is most commonly caused by aspergillus, which is normally found in the air and may be inhaled. These organisms normally occur on the mucosal surfaces of the nasal cavity and paranasal sinuses but only rarely produce disease. In patients with chronic sinusitis and poor drainage, aspergilli may proliferate in the sinus lumen and produce a fungus ball, called an aspergilloma, which may be identified in curettings from the involved sinus. The ball is usually composed of hyphae, but conidiospores may also be seen.

Aspergillus (fumigatus and flavus) consists of uniform septate hyphae that branch at 45-degree angles and measure 3 to 6 microns in diameter (Fig. 6–42). Sporulating structures (conidial heads or conidiospores) ranging up to 30 microns in diameter may be seen in nature, on culture media, or within air spaces of the body, such as paranasal sinuses and bronchi.

INVASIVE

Invasive fungal sinusitis occurs in two major forms: acute fulminant (affecting immunosuppressed or immunocompromised patients or those with neoplastic, metabolic, or debilitating disease) and chronic indo-

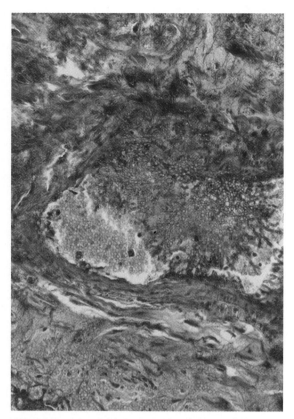

FIGURE 6–42 Aspergillosis. Fungus ball consists of branching and budding hyphae evident even on the H&E slide.

lent form in immunocompetent individuals. The most serious complication of the acute fulminant form is spread to the central nervous system, the so-called rhinocerebral form, which is most commonly associated with phycomycosis (murcormycosis) and followed by aspergillus.[28–30] Phycomycosis refers to an infection caused by the class Phycomycetes, which includes the orders Mucorales (genera Rhizopus, Mucor, and Absidia) and Entomophthorales. Entomophthorales may, rarely, cause indolent chronic granulomatous infection of the sinuses or skin.

Most phycomycotic infections are produced by members of the Mucorales group. They are normally identified as saprophytic organisms on the mucosal surfaces of the nasal cavity and paranasal sinuses. Under certain circumstances, these fungi may invade the underlying tissues, causing a serious and often rapidly fatal rhinocerebral form of mucormycosis. Conditions that predispose to invasive mucormycosis include:

1. Poorly controlled diabetes mellitus (most common)
2. Lymphomas, leukemias, and other malignant neoplasms
3. Immunosuppressed states under immunosuppressive therapy or chemotherapy.

This disease is also expected to increase among recipients of organ and bone marrow transplants.[28,29]

In fulminating invasive mucormycosis, the fungi extend directly into the underlying tissues and have a marked tendency to invade blood vessels, especially arteries, leading to thrombosis of vessels and necrosis of the involved tissue (Fig. 6–43 A and B). As a result, the nasal and/or ethmoid mucosa appears pale or brown-black. From the site of invasion, the organisms may extend into the orbital cavity, producing the clinical picture of a rapidly spreading orbital cellulitis, or into the cranial cavity, causing meningoencephalitis. Progressive tissue necrosis may involve the skin of the eye, the nose, and the maxillary areas.

When fulminating invasive mucormycosis is suspected, the clinician should biopsy the nasal or ethmoid mucosa and alert the pathologist about the suspected diagnosis. Special stains for fungi (PAS, silver-methenamine, or others) should be ordered. These organisms usually can be seen in routine sections but may be identified only with the special stains, especially if only a few fungi are present. Since Mucorales organisms have a special affinity for blood vessels, the pathologist should concentrate on examining blood vessel walls and their lumina, especially in areas where inflammation and necrosis are observed. Mucorales has a typical morphology, consisting of broad, branching, nonseptate hyphae, varying in width from 6 to 50 microns and in length from 100 to 200 microns (see Fig. 6–43 A and B). Curettings from inflamed and necrotic nasal or sinus tissue may be submitted without an adequate history. The pathologist should suspect mucormycosis in any case in which blood vessel thrombosis and extensive tissue necrosis are observed and special stains for fungi should be ordered under these circumstances. Improvement in survival is attributed to early diagnosis followed by aggressive radical resection of affected tissues and systemic amphotericin B therapy.[29] The extent of disease has been shown to be related to the host immune response, especially the serum fungistatic activity.

Invasive fungal sinusitis in the immunocompetent is chronic and indolent. In this case the disease tends to be more localized. The histologic findings vary considerably. In the case of aspergillosis, an acute inflammatory reaction with numerous neutrophils and even abscess formation is produced. In other cases fibrosis and chronic inflammation are seen, sometimes associated with caseating and non-caseating granulomas. Giant cells of various types may be observed. Oxalate crystals may be seen. Special stains for acid-fast bacteria and fungi should

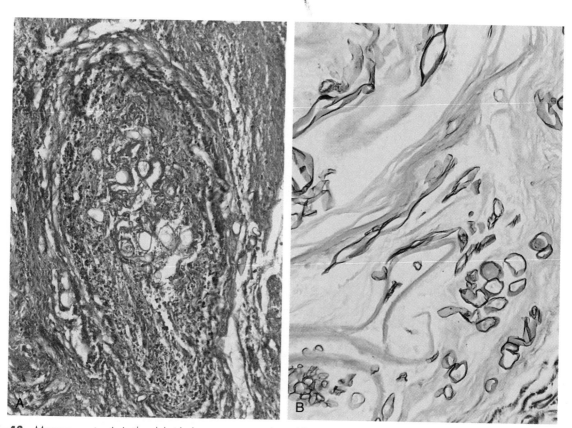

FIGURE 6–43 Mucormycosis. A, In the debrided necrotic tissue, fungal hyphae penetrate through the vessel wall and extend into the vascular lumen. These fungal organisms are characterized by thick pseudohyphae. B, Gomori methenamine silver stain reveals nonseptate hyphae of varying thickness characteristic of mucormycosis.

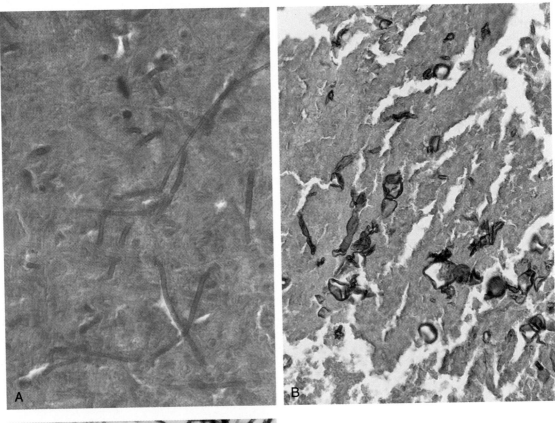

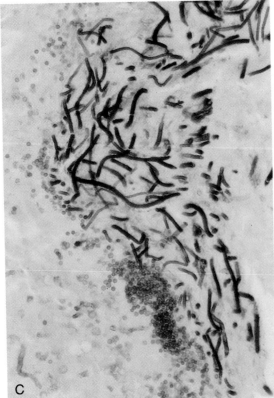

FIGURE 6-44 Allergic sinusitis associated with Demati-aceae organisms (phaeohyphomycosis). *A,* On the H&E slide, the branching hyphae are yellow-brown in color. *B,* Some hyphae are degenerated and appear pleomorphic and variable in thickness. *C,* Fontana stain demonstrates melanin pigment in the hyphae, which are not pigmented on H&E stain.

always be ordered when histologic study of any lesion of the nasal cavity and paranasal sinuses demonstrates granuloma formation.

ALLERGIC

Most patients with allergic fungal sinusitis are young and asthmatic. Nasal polyps are usually present. The sinuses are filled with dense mucoid material described earlier. Facial pain and eye infection may occur. A correct morphologic diagnosis requires histologic examination of the secretion, because the sinus wall merely demonstrates the chronic inflammation and eosinophilia without fungal organisms. Within the secretion, numerous eosinophils are mixed with desquamated respiratory mucosal cells, cell debris, Charcot-Leyden crystals, and fungal hyphae. Under these conditions, special stains for fungal organisms should be requested because the number of fungi may be limited or obscured by thick mucus on routine hematoxylin and eosin-stained section.

The fungal organisms identified include Aspergillus, Dematiaceae family (Bipolaris, Curvularia, Alternaria, and Exserohilum), and Chrysosporium (a Hyphomycetes of which Candida is a member).[31-33] Infections caused by dematiacious molds are also referred to as phaeohyphomycosis. In contrast to the Aspergillus organisms, which have straight thin hyphae branching at right angles, Dematiaceae in phaeohyphomycosis are characterized by septate hyphae, which are yellow-brown in color (Fig. 6–44A). As the hyphae become degenerated, they appear pleomorphic, ribbon-like, and swollen (Fig. 6–44B). Spores may be seen. Not all the hyphae are pigmented by hematoxylin and eosin stain, and the pigment can be demonstrated by Fontana-Masson stain (Fig. 6–44C).

NONINVASIVE, DESTRUCTIVE

Rowe-Jones and Moore-Gillon[34] described a rare form of chronic, destructive sinusitis in the absence of invasive aspergillus.

Rhinosporidiosis

Rhinosporidiosis is a chronic infection caused by the fungus Rhinosporidium seeberi.[23,35,36] Rhinosporidiosis is seen in endemic areas, such as India. Patients present with multiple broad-based or polypoid lesions involving the nasal cavity and, less commonly, the nasopharynx. The endospores are transmitted through contaminated dust and water and infect the nasal mucosa, most commonly on the inferior turbinate. Grossly, the lesion is polypoid, usually small, single or multiple.

Microscopic Pathology

In the biopsy, the organisms are characterized by large spores with a thick, glistening, double-contoured wall (Fig. 6–45 A and B). The spores vary from 100 to 400 microns in diameter. Within the spores are variable numbers of endospores, about the size of red blood cells, (see Fig. 6–45B). The surrounding chronic inflammatory reaction usually consists of lymphocytes and plasma cells. Sometimes histiocytes and foreign-body giant cells may be associated with poorly preserved, distorted sporocysts. Rarely, an acute inflammatory response with neutrophils and microabscesses occurs. These organisms can be demonstrated by special fungal stains.

Differential Diagnosis

The rhinosporidiosis organisms resemble Coccidioides immitis, because both have spores and endospores. Coccidiodomycosis organisms are smaller, however. The endospores are about 2 to 5 microns in diameter, as compared with 6 to 10 microns for rhinosporidiosis. Chrysosporiosis always involves

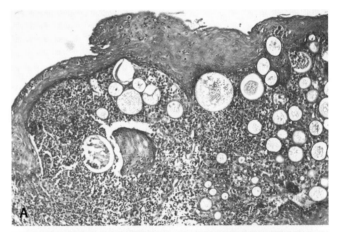

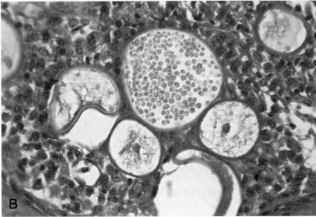

FIGURE 6–45 Rhinosporidosis. A, The large spores have a thick glistening capsule and contain numerous endospores. B, Degeneration and necrosis of the endospores result in the vacuolated and granular appearance in the large spores.

the lung. Within the microcystic spaces of cylindrical cell papilloma, the accumulated mucous material may assume the appearance of spores. At closer examination, no real cell wall or endospores can be seen.

Sarcoidosis

About 5% of patients with generalized sarcoidosis have similar disease in the upper aerodigestive tract.[37] In the study by Neville et al,[38] 38 (4.6%) of 818 patients with sarcoidosis have involvement of the nose and upper respiratory tract, including 32 lupus pernio and 21 mucosal disease.[39] In these patients, nasal mucosa is most commonly involved, especially the nasal septum and inferior turbinates. The next level of involvement is epiglottis, larynx, and pharynx.

Gross Pathology

Sarcoidosis first appears as small granular lesions, becomes coalescent, and forms nodules with mucosal erosion and crusting. Septal perforation may rarely ensue.[22,39]

Microscopic Pathology

The histologic features of sarcoidosis involving the mucous membranes of the nasal cavity and paranasal sinuses are similar to those seen in other organs and tissues. Nodules of epithelioid cells and multinucleated Langhans giant cells are surrounded by lymphocytes and plasma cells (Fig. 6–46A). Laminated calcified bodies, so-called Schaumann bodies, tend to occur in the giant cells of longstanding disease (Fig. 6–46B). Necrosis is usually limited and focal. Sarcoid granulomas are sometimes found in the nasal mucosa without clinical abnormality.[40]

Differential Diagnosis

Other sarcoid-like granulomas include Crohn's disease and orofacial granulomatosis. In the latter, patients with Melkersson-Rosenthal syndrome and cheilitis granulomatosa present with diffuse facial and lip swelling, oral ulcers, gingival overgrowth, mucosal tags, and sometimes facial palsy. The oral biopsy reveals edema, lymphangiectasia, and granuloma.[39]

Wegener's Granulomatosis

The clinical presentation and gross pathology of Wegener's granulomatosis (WG) are characterized by extensive nasosinus mucosal erosion, ulceration, and necrosis. Septal perforation, nasal collapse, and sec-

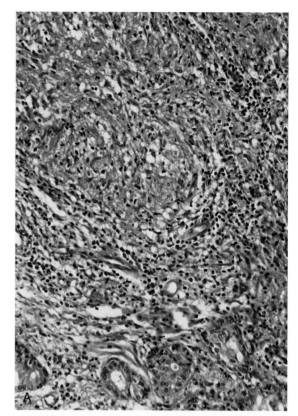

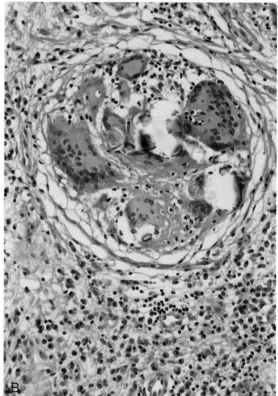

FIGURE 6–46 Sarcoidosis of nasal cavity. *A,* Well-circumscribed granulomatous reaction consists of epithelioid cells, multinucleated giant cells, and peripheral lymphocytes and plasma cells. *B,* Calcifications in multinucleated giant cells (Schaumann bodies).

ondary skin changes with swelling, edema, and erythema are common in severe cases. These clinical features have been referred to as lethal midline granuloma, and the underlying causes include a variety of infectious, neoplastic, and immunologic diseases. Thus, the clinical and pathologic differential diagnosis is broad, including Wegener's granulomatosis, malignant lymphoma, squamous cell carcinoma, tuberculosis, leprosy, syphilis, osteomyelitis, various bacterial and fungal infections, pemphigus, and cocaine use.[21,39,41,42]

Microscopic Pathology

Although the diagnostic criteria of WG are well known and well established, pathologic diagnosis based on small biopsies continues to pose a challenge. First, it is still a disease by exclusion, because infectious diseases can have all the histologic features associated with WG. Second, biopsies may reveal only some, but not all, of the histologic criteria required for the diagnosis of WG. Third, the clinical manifestations are highly variable. The disease may first appear in the head and neck regions and be localized to this area with or without developing disease elsewhere. The disease may involve the lungs, kidneys, skin, eyes, ears, joints, nervous system, or heart.[43] The upper respiratory tract is reported to be involved in 60% to 95% of the cases.[44] At the time of diagnosis, the disease may be localized in only one site. WG involving only trachea and larynx has been reported.[45]

Wegener's granulomatosis of the upper respiratory tract most commonly involves the nasal cavity and paranasal sinuses, and less commonly the larynx. Oral cavity, periorbital tissue, mastoid and middle ear, and salivary gland are occasionally affected. The nasal turbinate and septum are particularly susceptible. It begins with the development of ulcers, followed by granulation tissue, crusts, swelling, and ultimately destruction and further extension into the surrounding tissues, including facial skin and perforation of nasal septum or palate. The involved oral gingiva appears hyperplastic with exuberant, granular, and friable gums. The radiographs of the sinuses reveal mucosal thickening and varying degrees of opacification.

The triads of histologic criteria are necrosis, granulomatous reaction, and vasculitis.[46–48]

Areas of necrosis in the early stage appear in the form of micro-abscesses and later become surrounded by giant cells. Areas of necrosis apparently enlarge, coalesce, and often become quite broad and extensive. This development seems to be a late event and occurs in severe cases. A distinct type of necrosis, often referred to as geographic necrosis, has irregular serpiginous borders and basophilic, liquified appearance in the center (Fig. 6–47A). Less commonly, it has the character of coagulative or fibrinoid necrosis with eosinophilic material and nuclear

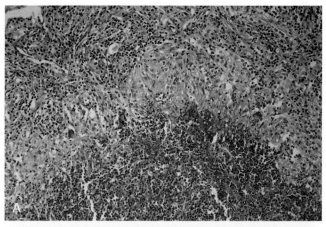

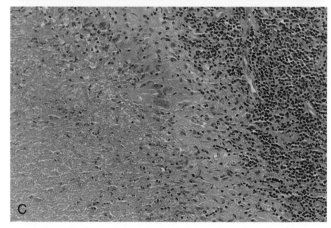

FIGURE 6–47 Wegener's granulomatosis with different types of necrosis. *A,* Liquified necrosis with abundant nuclear debris simulating abscess. *B,* Extensive fibrinoid necrosis with irregular, serpiginous borders. *C,* The necrosis is surrounded by epithelioid cells, multinucleated giant cells, lymphocytes and plasma cells.

debris in the background (Fig. 6–47B). Neutrophils, sometimes degenerated, can be seen. The borders of necrosis are lined by palisaded epithelioid histiocytes and multinucleated giant cells (Fig. 6–47C).

The granulomatous reaction varies from a few giant cells to clusters of histiocytes and giant cells and

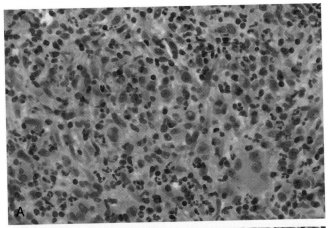

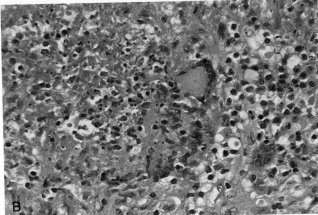

FIGURE 6-48 Wegener's granulomatosis with different granulomatous reactions. *A,* Early granulomatous reaction consisting of epithelioid cells and rare multinucleated giant cells mixed with eosinophils and lymphocytes. *B,* Well-formed granulomatous reaction associated with central necrosis, epithelioid cells, multinucleated giant cells with horseshoe configuration and outer rim of lymphocytes and plasma cells.

to well-formed necrotizing granulomas (Fig. 6–48). These histiocytes are accompanied by lymphocytes, plasma cells, and eosinophils. Eosinophils are invariably present, but quite prominent in 5% of cases.[46,47] Some lymphoid cells have enlarged lobulated nuclei and small nucleoli, but they do not appear atypical or neoplastic. Nodules of sarcoid type noncaseating granuloma are rarely found in WG.

One should recognize that foreign-body granulomatous reaction unrelated to WG can be seen, secondary to necrosis, or previous diagnostic and therapeutic procedures. These foreign-body giant cells may contain birefringent material or brownish structures resembling myospherules.[47]

All stages of vasculitis can be present ranging from acute to chronic. Small to medium-sized arteries and veins are most likely to be affected. The involved blood vessels may be entirely necrotic (Fig. 6–49A), and the endothelial cells are damaged and sometimes associated with thrombus. The vascular lumens are obliterated by necrotic debris and acute

inflammatory cells, making it difficult to recognize vasculitis (Fig. 6–49B). Granulomatous reaction occurs in some of the vessel walls (Fig. 6–49C). Scar formation and onion-skinning pattern of perivascular fibrosis characterize the chronic vasculitis (Fig. 6–49D). An elastic stain is helpful to confirm destroyed elastic interna, which may remain locally in the vessel wall.

According to Devaney et al,[47] infiltration of vessel wall by chronic inflammatory cells is most common. This is followed by acute inflammatory infiltrates. Fibrinoid necrosis, granulomatous reaction, and cicatrical change are less common.

Biopsies from the head and neck areas most commonly reveal nonspecific, mixed acute and chronic inflammation, and mucosal ulcerations without granuloma, necrosis, or vasculitis.[47] Only 16% of head and neck biopsies demonstrated necrosis, granuloma, and vasculitis. Vasculitis and granuloma were found in 21%, and vasculitis and necrosis in 23% of biopsies. Among the individual histologic features, granulomas with scattered giant cells were most commonly identified (42%), followed by necrosis (33%) and vascular changes (26%). At least one of the histologic triads was found in 55% of sinus biopsies, in 20% of nasal biopsies, and in 18% of laryngeal biopsies.[47] Thus, if radiographic abnormalities of sinus exist, biopsies of paranasal sinus are preferred.

Differential Diagnosis

The differential diagnosis of WG includes a wide range of infectious, inflammatory, and lymphoproliferative diseases. Special stains and culture for infectious organisms are essential diagnostic steps. What constitutes sufficient evidence for WG? In the opinion of Fienberg,[46] the presence of distinct necrosis and its association with vasculitis is sufficient for the diagnosis of WG, even though granuloma is absent.

Devaney et al[47] proposed a set of criteria for WG based on clinical evidence and head and neck biopsies with the prerequisite that infectious agents be excluded by culture and special stains.

Diagnostic: If (1) the histologic triad of necrosis, granuloma, and vasculitis are accompanied by clinical disease in the lung, kidney, or head and neck region; or (2) two of three histologic triad plus typical clinical disease in three sites (lung, kidney, and head and neck)

Probable: Two of three histologic triads and clinical involvement of kidney or lung

Suggestive: One of three histologic triads and clinical disease in three sites (lung, kidney, and head and neck)

Suspicious: One of three histologic triads and clinical lung or kidney disease

Nonspecific: None of histologic triads, even in the presence of clinical disease in three sites

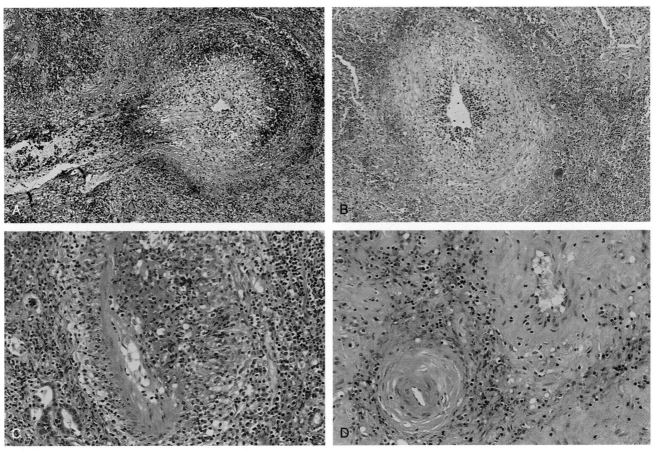

FIGURE 6–49 Wegener's granulomatosis with different types of vasculitis. *A,* Extensive necrosis and destruction of vessel walls. *B,* Fibrotic thickened blood vessel with inflammatory cells in the subintimal layer. *C,* Characteristic granulomatous reaction involves the medial and advantial layers. *D,* Blood vessels with features of chronic vasculitis. The medial and advantial layers are fibrotic and laminated in appearance.

In recent years, a positive test for antineutrophil cytoplasmic antibodies (ANCA) has been found to have a specificity for WG in 85% to 98% of cases.[49,50] These antibodies are detected in patients with active WG. Patients with limited form of WG are negative for this antibody, however.[49] In patients with less than diagnostic biopsies, a positive ANCA test provides strong support for the possibility of WG.

Lymphoid granulomatosis and polymorphic reticulosis/nasal angiocentric lymphoma can simulate WG clinically, because these diseases may spread to lung, kidney, skin, or other organs and frequently involve blood vessels. They differ from WG by the presence of atypical lymphoid cells and mitotic figures. Other evidence of malignancy includes infiltration of the nerve, skeletal muscle, and bone. Lymphocyte marker studies by immunohistochemistry are reported to be useful in separating WG from lymphomas.[51] A more detailed discussion on polymorphic reticulosis/nasal angiocentric lymphoma will appear in a later section (see pages 219–223).

In the case of allergic angiitis and granulomatosis (Churg-Strauss syndrome), most patients have asthma, pulmonary infiltrates, peripheral eosino-philia, and systemic vasculitis.[52] The latter two are uncommon in WG. Patients with Churg-Strauss syndrome often present with nasal polyps, which are rare in WG. Biopsies reveal necrotizing granuloma and prominent eosinophilia. Although esosinophils are seen in two thirds of biopsies with WG, only 5% of specimens have prominent eosinophilia.[52] The necrotizing, granulomatous angiitis typically affects medium-sized arteries in many organs.[53]

The entity of eosinophilic angiocentric fibrosis, described by Roberts et al,[54] is histologically similar to Kimura's disease. The involved nasal septum and larynx reveal perivascular infiltration of eosinophils associated with lymphoid hyperplasia. This is followed by fibrosis in the perivascular space and stroma. There is no granuloma, vasculitis, or necrosis.

Idiopathic midline destructive disease (IMDD) can be difficult or impossible to separate from WG. The predominant features are acute and chronic inflammation (Fig. 6–50 *A* and *B*). Rare giant cells or granulomas are found in about 10% of cases.[55] Foci of necrosis and perivascular inflammation are seen in occasional specimens without vasculitis. Clinically,

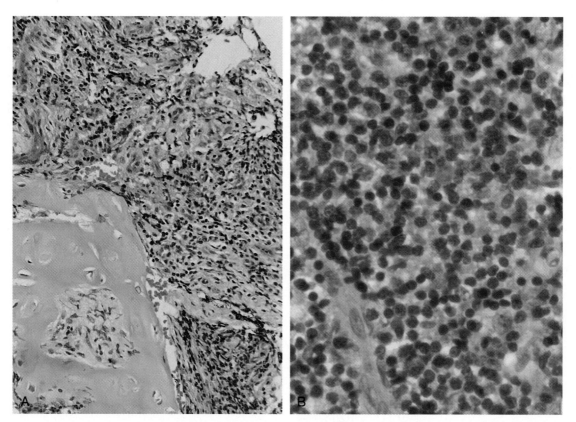

FIGURE 6–50   Idiopathic midline destructive disease. *A*, Extension of chronic inflammatory tissue into the bone associated with midline facial destructive process. *B*, The predominant lymphocytes are mixed with a small number of eosinophils and plasma cells.

IMDD is confined to the upper respiratory tract and presents with obvious destructive process or sinusitis. Wegener's granulomatosis does not erode through facial skin, but this is common in IMDD.

Changes related to cocaine use are similar to IMDD. Nasal septal perforation may be related to vasoconstriction, leading to ischemic necrosis.[41,42]

Prognosis

With cyclophosphamide (usually combined with steroid), long-term remissions are reported in more than 80% of patients.[43,44] The most common causes of death are uremia and respiratory failure.[39]

Granulomas Secondary to Steroid Injection

A distinctive type of granulomatous lesion involving the nasal mucous membranes may be found after injection of prednisolone acetate (Hydeltra TBA), which is sometimes used to relieve nasal obstruction due to vasomotor rhinitis, nasal edema, or nasal polyps. This steroid preparation is only slightly soluble and is long-acting. The granulomas are found when the patients are subsequently treated by polypec-

tomy or curettage. These granulomas may be solitary or confluent, have a central zone of amorphous, basophilic, and/or birefringent crystalline material and are surrounded by a layer of palisading histiocytes with foreign-body-type giant cells (Fig. 6–51*A* and *B*). Wolff[56] first described this entity and postulated that the granulomas were of the foreign-body type, induced by the injected material that is not absorbed. The pathologist should be familiar with this type of granuloma, which should be differentiated from other granulomatous lesions.

Myospherulosis

This change was first described as myospherulosis-like organisms involving the nasal cavity, paranasal sinuses, and middle ear.[57] These structures were characterized by "parent bodies" ranging in size from 20 to 120 microns. Spherules measuring 5 to 7 microns were found within the parent bodies and also scattered within the tissues (Fig. 6–52).[57] Myospherulosis is now widely accepted as the result of altered red blood cells following hemostatic packing with gauze containing petrolatum-based ointments and antibiotics.[58] This iatrogenically induced change has also been described outside the nasal cavity and

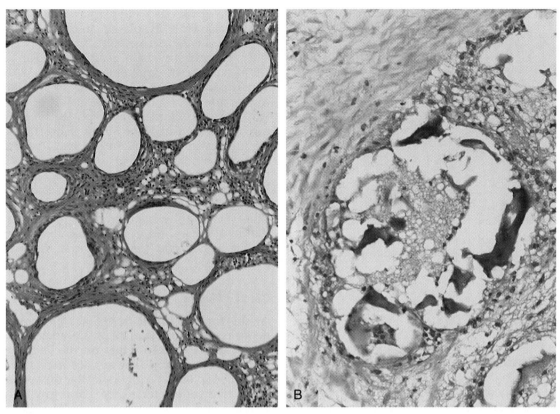

FIGURE 6–51 Granuloma following injection of long-acting steroid. *A,* Multiple oval empty spaces are surrounded by multinucleated giant cells and foamy histiocytes. *B,* Residual injected material has a basophilic, homogeneous appearance.

paranasal sinuses, including breast and soft tissues, where similar packing was used.

Necrobiotic Granuloma Following Surgical Procedure

Tissue reactions following biopsy or resection include a granulomatous change that simulates rheumatoid nodule with central fibrinoid necrosis and palisaded histiocytes, lymphocytes, and plasma cells in the periphery. Such reactions also occur after surgery in the uterine cervix, urinary bladder, and prostate.

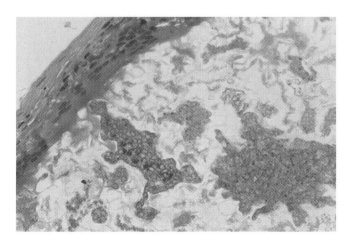

FIGURE 6–52 Myospherulosis aggregates of circular endospore-like structures surrounded by lipid material. The outer rim has collections of multinucleated giant cells. These endospore-like particles represent altered red blood cells.

Cholesterol Granuloma

Cholesterol granuloma results from hemorrhage. Cholerosterol needle-like crystals are surrounded by hemosiderin-laden macrophages and foreign-body multinucleated giant cells. When associated with chronic sinusitis, the adjacent fibrous tissue is infiltrated by varying numbers of lymphocytes, plasma cells, and foamy histiocytes (Fig. 6–53). In the series of Friedman and Osborn,[22] the change is limited to the maxillary sinus, especially in individuals during the first two decades of life, presenting with nasal discharge, obstruction, or pain. Rarely, the sinus epithelium undergoes keratinization with accumulation of abundant keratin debris simulating middle-ear cholesteatoma.[59] Cholesterol granulomas also occur in the middle ear and upper jaw following dental extraction.

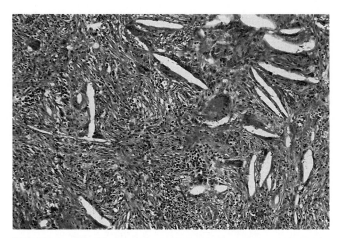

FIGURE 6–53 Cholesterol granuloma. In the stroma, cholesterol clefts are surrounded by multinucleated giant cells, lymphocytes, and fibroblasts.

BENIGN PAPILLOMAS

Hyperkeratotic Squamous Papilloma

Hyperkeratotic squamous papilloma occurs in the anterior nares, nasal vestibule, or nasal septum as a small papillary lesion, usually less than 1 cm. It is hyperkeratotic with prominent granular cell layers. The papillary fronds are supported by delicate fibrovascular cores. The rete pegs reveal varying degrees of enlargement and elongation. The maturation process is maintained. Nuclear atypia is absent. These papillomas are microscopically similar to verruca vulgaris that also occurs in the larynx.[60] These papillomas may rarely progress to invasive squamous cell carcinoma.

Nasosinus Papilloma

Nasosinus papilloma is a benign neoplasm arising from either the squamous epithelium of the anterior nasal cavity or the respiratory mucosa of the remaining nasosinus. Many terms have been used for this lesion, including inverted papilloma, Schneiderian papilloma, and transitional cell papilloma. Other authors favor the term papillomatosis, because of the multifocal nature and combined inverted and exophytic growth patterns.[61] Although the etiology of nasosinus papilloma is controversial, recent studies using molecular techniques have found human papillomavirus DNA in the majority of nasosinus papillomas to support a close relationship between papillomavirus infection and papilloma. With in situ hybridization technique, HPV type 6/11 was found in eight of nine (89%) fungiform papillomas.[62] Using a similar method, a rare HPV type 57B was detected in six of seven (86%) fungiform papillomas, six of

eight (75%) inverted papillomas, one of three (33%) papillomas with dysplasia, and two of four (50%) papillomas with carcinoma.[63]

By polymerase chain reaction (PCR), four of 26 (15%) squamous papillomas, seven of 29 (24%) inverted papillomas, and one of 24 (4%) squamous cell carcinomas were positive for HPV, including type 6 and 11 in papillomas and type 18 in squamous cell carcinoma.[64] In another study using PCR, 13 of 20 (65%) inverted papillomas had sequences for Epstein-Barr virus (EBV) genomes and nine (45%) had HPV type 6/11/16/18.[65] Five (25%) had both EBV and HPV sequences. The detected HPV types occur primarily in the genital areas to raise the possibility of autoinoculation from the genital tract to the nasal cavity. Fu et al[62] presented seven patients having concurrent genital warts and nasal septal papillomas.

Clinical Findings and Gross Pathology

At the time of initial detection, the majority of patients present with unilateral polypoid nasal masses or thickened mucosa either on the lateral nasal wall or the nasal septum. The surface may appear granular and papillary. With time, the disease spreads to more than one site in the nasal cavity, paranasal sinuses, and nasopharynx, including the eustachian tube. Thus, symptoms resulting from papillomas include not only those related to the nasosinuses, but also the middle ear problems.

About one third to one half arise in the lateral nasal wall and the remainder between nasal septum or sinuses. In the latter, maxillary antrum is most common, followed by ethmoid. The nasal septal papillomas are asymptomatic, flat and wartlike, with finely lobulated grey-white surfaces. Papillomas of other locations are polypoid, bulky, elastic firm, opaque, white, and sometimes papillary on the surface (Fig. 6–54). About 15% of patients with papillo-

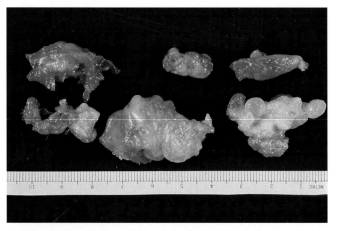

FIGURE 6–54 Gross appearance of inverted papilloma. Some of the nodules have the appearance of nasal polyps. Others appear thickened and indurated with a few papillary projections.

mas have allergic symptoms, and their lesions may simulate nasal polyps with marked stromal edema and translucent appearance. If the bony wall is removed, it is important to study histologic evidence of bony erosion, new bone formation, and destruction.

Microscopic Pathology

Hyams[66] classified the nasosinus papillomas into three major types: fungiform, inverted, and cylindrical. Age of patients varied from 11 to 85 years, predominantly 30 to 50 years (median 35 years). Fungiform papilloma tends to involve more younger patients than inverted papilloma. Papillomas are rare in individuals under 21 years, and male-to-female ratio is five to one.[66]

The fungiform or exophytic type in Hyams' series comprising 50% of papillomas arises almost exclusively in the nasal septum and a few from the lateral nasal wall.[66] The proliferating cells form papillary fronds supported by delicate fibrovascular cores. The component cells in fungiform papillomas

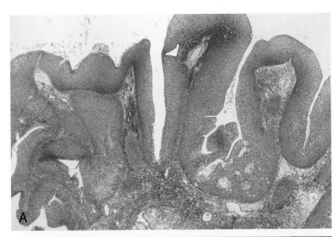

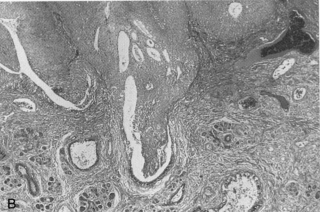

FIGURE 6–55 Fungiform papilloma. A, Papillary fronds supported by delicate fibrovascular cores. The lining epithelium is thickened. B, Papilloma extend directly into the underlying ducts of the seromucous glands.

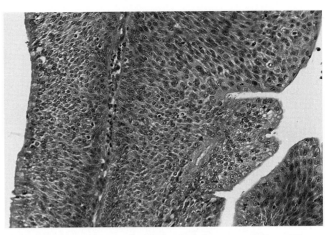

FIGURE 6–56 The papillomatous epithelium is more than 10 layers thick. Beneath the ciliated columnar cells are basal cells and intermediate cells.

are similar to those of inverted papilloma, including mature squamous cells, basal cells, and cells intermediate between columnar and squamous cells (also referred to as transitional cells) (Fig. 6–55A). When mature squamous cells predominate, hyperkeratosis and koilocytosis are evident. These areas closely resemble genital and skin warts. If there are seromucous glands underneath, fungiform papillomas often extend directly into the ducts of these glands (Fig. 6–55B).[67,68]

The majority of inverted papillomas have exophytic and inverted growth patterns (Fig. 6–56).[61] They constitute 47% of nasosinus papillomas and most commonly originate from the respiratory mucosa of lateral nasal wall and paranasal sinuses.[66] From the mucosal surface, the proliferating cells grow into the stroma by invagination or direct extension into the underlying seromucous glands as bulky solid sheets. Depending on the degree of maturation, the component cells may resemble basal cells (see Fig. 6–56), transitional cells, or mature squamous cells (Fig. 6–57). The overlying ciliated and nonciliated columnar cells often persist. Mature squamous cells sometimes have clear cytoplasm filled with glycogen or resemble koilocytes with perinuclear halos, nuclear hyperchromasia, and bi- or multinucleation (Fig. 6–58). With increasing thickness of papillomatous epithelium, the overlying ciliated cells eventually become desquamated. In the deep layers, occasional mitotic figures occur (Fig. 6–59).

The least common type, cylindrical cell papilloma, comprising 3% of papillomas, occurs mostly on the lateral nasal wall, maxillary sinus, and ethmoid sinus in a way similar to the inverted type.[66] The proliferating cells form microcysts and complex cribriform glands and papillary projections on the mucosal surface and the underlying stroma (Fig. 6–60 A and B). The principal cells are ciliated and

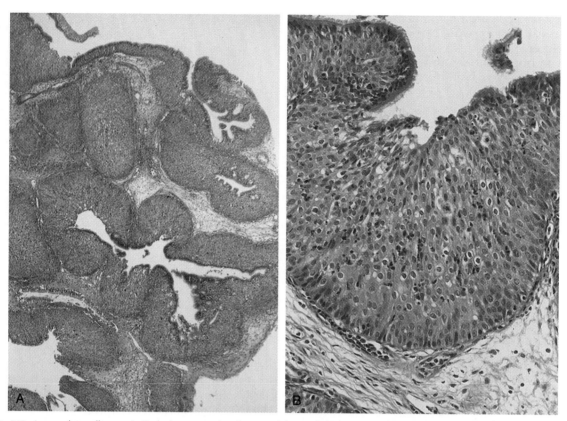

FIGURE 6–57   Inverted papilloma. *A,* Both the mucosal surface and the underlying inverted spaces are occupied by thickened hyperplastic epithelium. *B,* The proliferating mature squamous cells have relatively uniform nuclei. Ciliated cells are preserved on the surface.

nonciliated tall columnar cells and goblet cells normally found in the upper layers of respiratory epithelium. Sometimes oncocytic cells predominate; such lesions are designated as oncocytoid papillomas (Fig. 6–61).[69] Within the microcystic spaces, condensed mucinous secretions, granular material, and nuclear debris sometimes resemble endospores of rhinosporidiosis. A closer examination fails to demonstrate thick capsule or spores as expected in the case of rhinosporidiosis. The closely apposed back-to-back glands with nuclear stratification can become quite confluent and broad to suggest an adenocarcinoma. Rarely, goblet cells, mucinous cells, and epidermoid cells proliferate in solid sheets (Fig. 6–62 *A* and *B*).

In the majority of nasosinus papillomas, both exophytic and inverted patterns occur.[67] Papillomas arising from the skin of nasal vestibule are similar

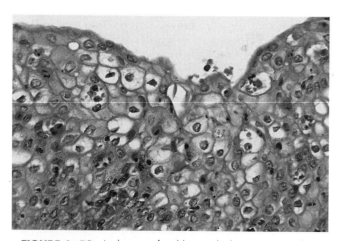

FIGURE 6–58   In the superficial layers, koilocytes are evident.

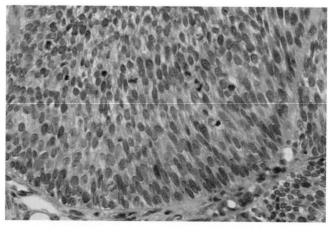

FIGURE 6–59   Immature basal cells reveal occasional mitotic figures.

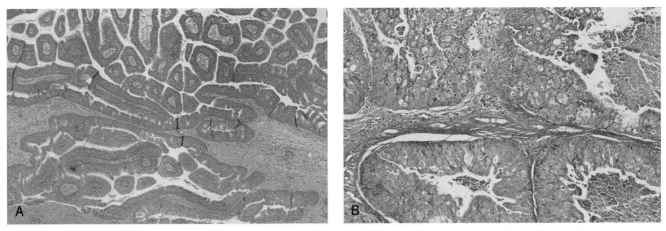

FIGURE 6–60   Cylindrical cell papilloma. *A,* Low-power view showing multiple papillary projections on the surface. *B,* This oncocytoid variant has both exophytic and inverted growth patterns.

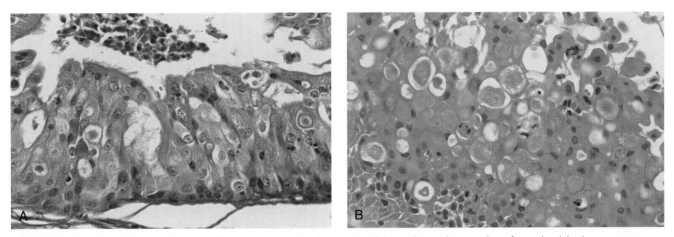

FIGURE 6–61   Oncocytic papilloma. *A,* Oncocytes with abundant eosinophilic and granular cytoplasm form glandular lumens containing eosinophilic secretions. *B,* Microcystic spaces contain dense eosinophilic material and basophilic mucus that may suggest rhinosporidiosis.

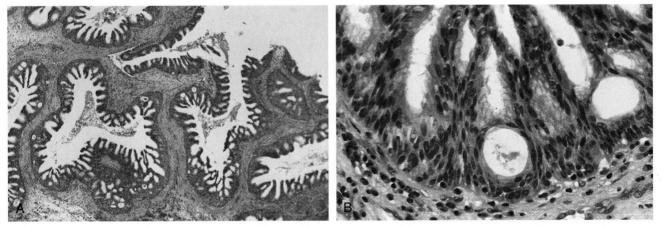

FIGURE 6–62   Variant of cylindrical cell papilloma. *A,* Complex papillary projections occur within the inverted, dilated glandular spaces. *B,* The proliferating cells include tall columnar ciliated cells and non-ciliated mucus-secreting cells.

to skin warts and verruca vulgaris. Papillomas arising from the mature squamous mucosa of the nasal septum and anterior nasal cavity have predominantly exophytic growth in a manner similar to genital warts and laryngeal squamous papilloma. An inverted growth results from downward extension of papilloma into the underlying seromucous glands or invagination into the stroma. In the sinus wall, inverted papilloma may extend into the periosteum and bony wall to cause reactive new bone formation. This expansile papillomatous growth can be distinguished from invasive carcinoma by well-defined borders and lack of nuclear atypia. The background stroma may be edematous, vascular, and infiltrated by varying numbers of inflammatory cells.

The mitotic activity in the majority of nasosinus papillomas is less than two mitoses per ten high-power fields. Only 15% have greater than 10 mitotic figures per 10 high-power fields.[70] The level of mitotic activity has no impact on tumor recurrence.[69] Nuclear atypia is usually minimal in the absence of dysplastic and malignant changes.

Differential Diagnosis

Reactive hyperplasia of squamous and respiratory epithelia can be difficult to distinguish from papilloma. Papilloma should have excessive cellular proliferation, usually more than eight to 10 cell layers and an exophytic or inverted growth, or both.

The reported frequency of squamous dysplasia and carcinoma in situ in a series of 61 inverted papillomas is 6% and 3%, respectively.[69] The dysplastic epithelium covers pre-existing papilloma, thus the configuration may be papillary or inverted, or both. The hallmarks of squamous dysplasia/carcinoma in situ include

1. Cellular disorganization with predominant vertical nuclear arrangement and loss of horizontal arrangement in the superficial layers
2. Cellular immaturity with increased nuclear cytoplasmic ratio as compared to the cells in the comparable level
3. Increased cellular proliferation with mitotic activity and sometimes abnormal mitotic figures
4. Nuclear irregularity, hyperchromasia, and altered chromatin patterns (Fig. 6–63 A and B).

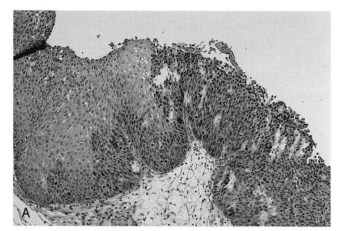

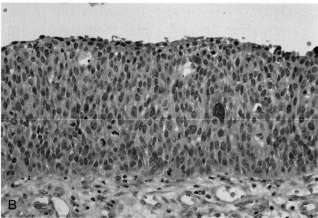

FIGURE 6–63 *A,* Inverted papilloma (*left*) associated with squamous cell carcinoma in situ (*right*). The latter has a higher cellularity and nuclear hyperchromasia, and undermines the base of papilloma. *B,* This squamous cell carcinoma in situ is characterized by cellular disorganization, nuclear pleomorphism, and numerous mitotic figures.

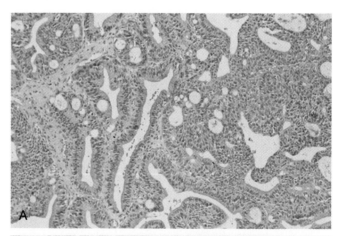

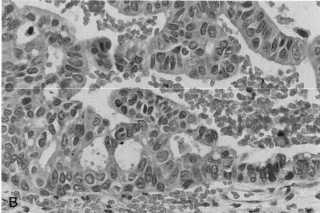

FIGURE 6–64 Cylindrical cell papilloma with dysplastic change. *A,* The glandular spaces become complex and closely apposed to each other. There are also solid areas. *B,* Glandular cells demonstrate nuclear irregularity, hyperchromasia, and mitotic figures.

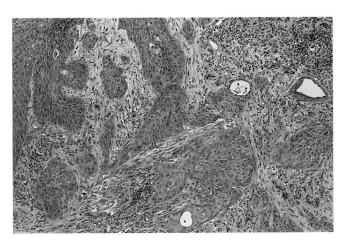

FIGURE 6-65 Invasive squamous cell carcinoma occurs at the base of inverted papilloma. Irregular configuration of the tumor cell nests associated with desmoplastic stroma differs from the smooth borders expected for papilloma or squamous cell carcinoma in situ.

Based on the severity of these changes, the lesion is graded as mild, moderate, or severe dysplasia or carcinoma in situ.

Glandular dysplasia within the cylindrical cell papilloma is characterized by complex papillary architecture, back-to-back overcrowded glandular arrangement, nuclear atypia, and increased mitotic activity (Fig. 6-64 A and B).

The majority of invasive carcinoma associated

with inverted papilloma are squamous type, usually poorly differentiated. In early squamous cell carcinoma, tongue-like processes break through the base of dysplastic papilloma (Fig. 6-65). Osborn[71] reported "transitional" cell variant of squamous cell carcinoma, characterized by broad sheets of high-grade dysplastic cells surrounded by hyaline membranes and fibrous stroma. Conventional stromal invasion in the form of small epithelial nests is difficult to discern even in the resected specimen (Fig. 6-66 A and B). Osborn[71] stated that "if sheets of atypical cells demonstrate nuclear anaplasia, the lesion should be considered as invasive." A more detailed discussion on this group of neoplasm is presented in the later section (see page 173).

Immunohistochemical stain for cell adehsion molecule, CD44, may help to distinguish between inverted papilloma, papilloma with squamous cell carcinoma in situ, and invasive squamous cell carcinoma. In the study by Ingle et al,[72] all 76 nasosinus inverted papillomas expressed CD44 with strong membranous staining in 83% and moderate or weakening staining in the remaining 17%. Two specimens with squamous cell carcinoma in situ in papilloma were strongly positive for CD44. In contrast, CD44 expression was entirely absent in six of 10 invasive squamous cell carcinomas. In the remaining four tumors, two each were focally and diffusely stained.[72]

In the excised papillomas, coexisting invasive car-

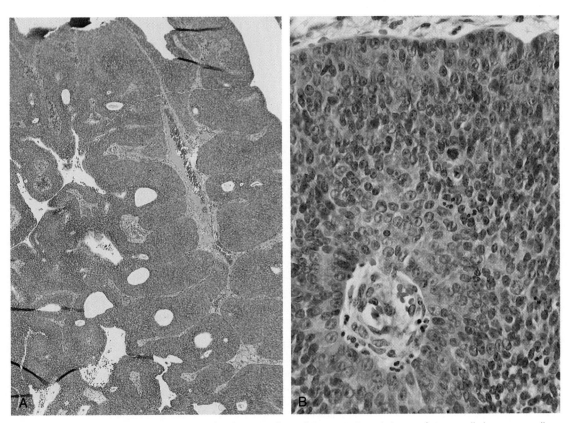

FIGURE 6-66 Transitional cell carcinoma associated with inverted papillomas. A, Broad sheets of tumor cells have a papillary growth pattern on the surface. The interface with the stroma is smooth, simulating squamous cell carcinoma in situ. B, The tumor cells have anaplastic appearance and increased mitotic activity.

cinoma is found in 7% to 8%.[73,74] An additional 3% to 6% of patients developed invasive carcinoma subsequent to papilloma excision.[68,70,75]

Of the nine oncocytic papillomas with concurrent carcinoma, six are squamous cell type, two poorly differentiated mucoepidermoid carcinoma, and one undifferentiated carcinoma.[76] Most invasive carcinomas coexisting with papilloma are unilateral, but bilateral and multifocal involvement has been reported in immunocomprised hosts.

Prognosis

All three types of papillomas have comparable rates for local recurrence—about 50%.[68-70] Most recurrences are detected within the first 5 years after surgery. However, recurrences may occur 5 or more years later.[61] The frequency of recurrence is closely related to the extent of surgery performed. In a review of literature, 64% of patients experienced recurrence following limited local excisions, as compared to 11% after more complete resection.[75] In one study, the presence of dysplasia increases the local recurrence.[61] The prognosis of patients with concurrent invasive carcinoma depends on the histologic grade and the extent of the tumor.

SQUAMOUS CELL CARCINOMA AND UNDIFFERENTIATED CARCINOMA

Squamous Dysplasia and Carcinoma In Situ

In specimens removed for rhinitis, sinusitis, or nasal polyp, dysplasia may be found incidentally. In nickel workers, the nasal respiratory mucosa undergoes squamous metaplasia with loss of ciliated cells.

Cells in the deep layers proliferate with budding rete pegs. In mild and moderate dysplasia, increased mitotic activity and nuclear abnormalities (enlargement, hyperchromasia, and irregularity) occur in the deep layers (Fig. 6–67A).[77] In severe dysplasia and carcinoma in situ, abnormal cells occupy most of the epithelium (Fig. 6–67B). The degree of severity correlates with the amount and the duration of nickel exposure.[77]

Squamous Cell Carcinoma of Nasal Vestibule

Carcinomas of the nasal vestibule are rare; most are squamous type and rarely basal cell carcinoma. Taxy[78] reported five cases of squamous cell carcinoma involving four men and one woman, age 52 to 82 years at diagnosis. The tumors were located within the nasal vestibule or mucocutaneous junction of the nasal septum and were 1–3 cm in size. Ulceration and keratinization were common and tumor cells sometimes invaded into the perichondrium or bone of the nasal septum (Fig. 6–68 A and B). The clinical course was indolent, and most patients were treated by local excision or radiotherapy, or both. Nodal metastasis occurred in less than 10% of patients. The 5-year survival rates in the literature were close to 70% to 80%.[78]

Overview of Carcinoma of Nasal Cavity and Paranasal Sinuses

About 3% of head and neck malignancies occur in the nasal cavity and paranasal sinuses. Of these, 58% to 67% affect the maxillary sinus, 16% to 31% originate in the nasal cavity, 10% to 19% involve the ethmoid sinus, and less than 1% to 3% arise in

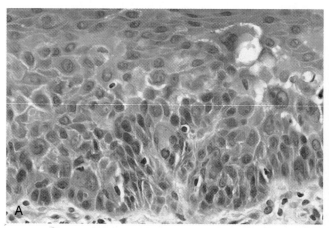 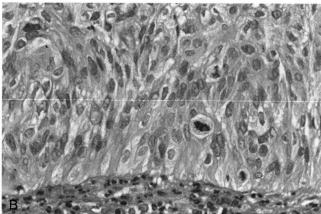

FIGURE 6–67 *A,* Moderate squamous dysplasia with proliferation of atypical cells in the parabasal and intermediate layers. *B,* Severe squamous dysplasia/carcinoma in situ with cellular disorganization and immature cells occupying the entire thickness of the epithelium. The mitotic figures occur throughout the epithelium.

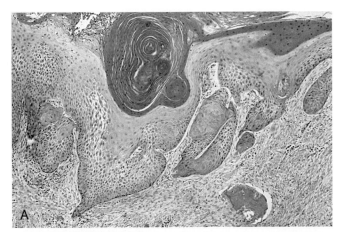

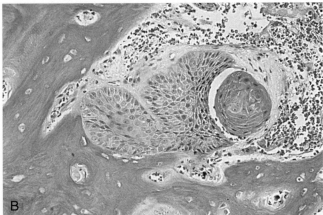

FIGURE 6-68 *A, Squamous cell carcinoma, keratinizing type and well-differentiated, of nasal vestibule. B, Tumor extension into bone.*

the sphenoid and frontal sinuses (Table 6–3).[79–82] The types of tumors encountered are diverse, with the majority being squamous cell carcinoma and its variants (57%), followed by nonepithelial neoplasms (17%), glandular tumors (15%), undifferentiated carcinoma (7%), and unclassified and miscellaneous tumors (4%) (Table 6–4).

The majority of nasosinus carcinomas occur during the sixth to seventh decades of life. Male-to-female ratio is two to one. Patients with nasal cavity carcinoma are at increased risk for developing a second primary tumor, especially in the other head and neck regions, lung, breast, and gastrointestinal tract.[83]

Over 90% of invasive carcinomas arising from mucosa of the upper aerodigestive tract fall into the spectrum of squamous cell carcinoma and its variants.[84] Those having recognizable squamous differentiation by light microscopy are classified as keratinizing and nonkeratinizing types. Special variants of squamous cell carcinoma include verrucous, papillary, and basaloid types. Undifferentiated carcinomas are divided into small cell and large cell types. Glandular neoplasms of the nasosinus and nasopharynx are discussed together in the later section.

Squamous Cell Carcinoma and Variants

The clinical appearance of nasosinus squamous cell carcinoma is characterized by exophytic, friable, necrotic, and ulcerated mass obstructing the nasal cavity. In the resected specimen, some of the tumors grow as well-circumscribed masses filling the sinus cavity in an expansile fashion with erosion of the bony wall and limited local infiltration. Others are friable, necrotic, hemorrhagic, and destructive. The latter are likely to be poorly differentiated, rapid in growth, and aggressive.

The original Broders' histologic grade for squamous cell carcinoma used skin cancer as a model, grouped into four grades. Most authors use a three-grade system based on (1) extent of keratinization, (2) mitotic acitivity, and (3) nuclear features. This grading method correlates to some extent with the tumor behavior. Squamous cell carcinoma is also subclassified by cell type.

KERATINIZING TYPE

In invasive keratinizing squamous cell carcinomas, the tumor cells exhibit keratinization, intercellular

TABLE 6 – 3	SITES INVOLVED BY MALIGNANT TUMORS OF THE NASAL CAVITY AND PARANASAL SINUSES		
	JACKSON ET AL[80]	LEWIS AND CASTRO[79]	HOPKIN ET AL[81]
Maxillary sinus	77 (67%)	451 (58%)	295 (53%)[b]
Nasal cavity	19 (16%)	237 (31%)	147 (26%)
Ethmoid sinus	15 (13%)	75 (10%)	107 (19%)
Frontal sinus	3 (3%)	6 (0.6%)	7 (1.2%)
Sphenoid sinus	1 (1%)	3 (0.4%)	5 (0.9%)
Total	115	772[a]	561

[a] Includes 538 primary tumors (69%) and 234 secondary neoplasms (31%)
[b] Includes 77 patients (14%) who also had involvement of ethmoid sinus

TABLE 6–4	TYPES OF MALIGNANT TUMORS REPORTED IN THE NASAL CAVITY AND PARANASAL SINUSES			
	JACKSON ET AL[80]	LEWIS AND CASTRO[79]	HOPKIN ET AL[81]	TOTAL
Squamous cell carcinoma and variants	63 (55%)	496 (64%)	261 (47%)	820 (57%)
Undifferentiated carcinoma	11 (10%)		92 (17%)	103 (7%)
Glandular Neoplasms	17 (15%)	129 (17%)	70 (12%)	216 (15%)
Adenoid cystic carcinoma	8 (7%)		30 (5%)	
Adenocarcinoma	7 (6%)	129 (17%)	40 (7%)	
Papillary adenocarcinoma	2 (2%)			
Nonepithelial Neoplasms	24 (21%)	110 (14%)	112 (20%)	246 (17%)
Malignant melanoma	7 (6%)	34 (4%)	39 (7%)	
Malignant lymphoma	3 (3%)	40 (5%)	35 (6%)	
Plasmacytoma	2 (2%)	13 (2%)	8 (1%)	
Olfactory neuroblastoma	5 (4%)		3 (1%)	
Neuroblastoma	1 (1%)			
Fibrosarcoma	3 (3%)		11 (2%)	
Angiosarcoma	1 (1%)			
Chondrosarcoma	1 (1%)			
Carcinosarcoma	1 (1%)			
Other sarcomas		23 (3%)	16 (3%)	
Unclassified and other tumors		37 (5%)	25 (5%)	62 (4%)
Total	115	772	561	1148 (100%)

bridges, and "pearls." Tumor cells usually have enlarged, hyperchromatic nuclei, but the degree of nuclear anaplasia and mitotic activity is variable. Stromal invasion is indicated by the presence of irregular nests and cords of cells in a desmoplastic stroma, which is often associated with chronic inflammatory response (Fig. 6–69A). In superficial biopsies, the only sign of stromal invasion may be in

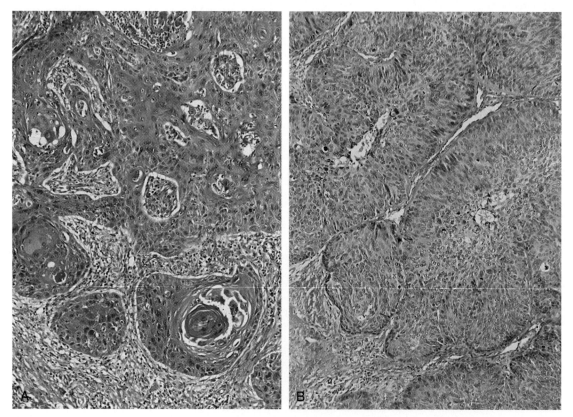

FIGURE 6–69   Squamous cell carcinoma. *A*, Keratinizing type. Tumor cells form keratin pearls. *B*, Transitional cell variant of nonkeratinizing carcinoma. Tumor cells form broad sheets, which have smooth borders and are surrounded by basement membrane–like material. Conventional stromal invasion is not evident.

the form of single cells becoming isolated from the base of rete pegs or the tip of tongue-like protrusions. The configuration of the nests and the character of the cells should be carefully assessed to determine the invasive nature.

NONKERATINIZING TYPE

A nonkeratinizing type of squamous cell carcinoma tends to form solid nests of variable sizes. These masses may have relatively smooth borders. Individual tumor cells reveal uniform large, round, or oval nuclei with prominent nucleoli. The cytoplasm varies from pale acidophilic to amphophilic to vacuolated. The cells may have distinct borders. Occasionally, individual cell keratinization may be identified consistent with squamous cell carcinoma. Some nonkeratinizing poorly differentiated tumors may contain focal spindle cells or resemble lymphoepithelioma of the nasopharynx. When the spindle cells predominate, this group of tumor is referred to as spindle cell carcinoma, which will be discussed in the later section.

Some of the nonkeratinizing squamous cell carcinomas may have a papillary or endophytic growth pattern. The papillary type will be discussed in the section on papillary squamous carcinoma. When inverted, these poorly differentiated squamous cell carcinomas have been designated as "transitional cell" carcinoma, or "Schneiderian" carcinoma.[71] The tumor cells are arranged in broad sheets, which have smooth borders and are surrounded by basement membrane–like material (Fig. 6–69B). Irregular nests of conventional stromal invasion are usually absent, especially in small biopsies. Because of this, the lesion is likely to be underdiagnosed as squamous carcinoma in situ. A combination of peripheral palisading in the tumor nests and surrounding basement membrane may suggest ameloblastoma.

VERRUCOUS TYPE

About 5% of head and neck squamous cell carcinomas are extremely well-differentiated verrucous carcinoma, which is recognized as a separate entity because of its distinct clinical and pathologic features. Of the 105 cases reported by Kraus and Perez-Mesa,[85] the anatomic locations include 73% in oral cavity, 11% larynx, 4% nasal cavity, and the remaining 12% in the genital tract. Rarely, the tumor involves nasal septum.[86] It affects males in their sixth to eighth decades, especially in the buccal mucosa and the glottis of larynx. It is rare before the age of 35 years.[87]

Grossly, it is warty, papillary, and ranging in size from 1 cm to bulky—exceeding 5 cm. The adjacent mucosa may be hyperplastic or leukoplakic. Microscopically, the surface is thickened with marked hyperkeratosis. In deep biopsy with full thickness, pushing, sharply defined borders are evident. The bulky rete pegs are often confluent. Keratin pearls and cysts may be seen. In tangential cuts, they appear as solid nests with smooth borders. In addition, the tumor cells maintain normal maturation having only mild nuclear atypia. The mitotic activity is low. A heavy lympho-plasmacytic infiltration is typical, and granulomatous reaction to keratin debris is sometimes seen in the stroma. In about 10% of verrucous carcinomas, there are areas of conventional invasive squamous carcinoma. Such tumors may have a more aggressive behavior.

PAPILLARY TYPE

The entity of papillary squamous neoplasms was described by Crissman et al[88] and Ishiyama et al.[89] In their series, these tumors were found predominantly in the oral cavity, tonsillar fossa, oropharynx, and larynx and rarely in the nasosinus. The clinical appearance simulates squamous papilloma and verrucous carcinoma.

In biopsies, the severely dysplastic epithelium appears in broad papillary fronds, which are supported by delicate fibrovascular cores. The usual diagnosis rendered is a papillary squamous carcinoma in situ. In contrast to verrucous carcinoma, the tumor cells demonstrate cytologically malignant immature cells occupying most of the epithelium. The nuclei are enlarged, hyperchromatic, variable in size and shape, and mitotically active with abnormal forms. In biopsy specimen, stromal invasion may be absent. Thus, a correct diagnosis requires excision of the tumor base to determine stromal invasion.

SPINDLE CELL TYPE

This tumor most commonly occurs in the oral cavity, upper respiratory tract, and occasionally in the esophagus and skin of the head and neck region. Almost all present with a polypoid or exophytic mass, varying in size from a few cm to more than 5 cm in size. In the two series combined,[90,91] 43% of cases occurred in the larynx, 40% oral cavity, 20% hypopharynx and pyriform sinus, 14% sinonasal tract, and 11% oropharynx. In one series, 95% of patients used tobacco, 32% had prior radiotherapy, and 24% consumed excess alcohol.[91] When occurring in the nasosinus and nasopharynx, the common presentation is a fungating, ulcerative, and infiltrative mass.[92]

The histologic features are highly variable and polymorphic. The predominant features are spindle cells forming interlacing bundles simulating fibrosarcoma or leiomyosarcoma. Storiform, microcystic, and pericytomatous patterns may be focal or prominent. Some areas may resemble angiosarcoma with slit-like spaces. The stroma may be myxoid or highly collagenized with broad areas of hyalinization simulating osteoid tissue. Tumor giant cells and osteoclast-type giant cells may also present, resembling osteosarcoma.

Individual cells are elongated, or round to oval in shape. The cytoplasm is usually abundant, eosinophilic, fibrillar, or vacuolated. The nuclei have the hallmarks of malignancy with hyperchromasia, coarsely granular chromatin, pleomorphism, high mitotic activity, and prominent nucleoli (Fig. 6–70A). Some may mimic rhabdomyoblasts. It should be noted that in a minority of cases, the spindle cells lack nuclear atypia similar to those seen in a benign reactive fibroblastic proliferation or aggressive fibromatosis. Thus, many spindle cell lesions have to be considered in the differential diagnosis.

Some tumors contain readily recognizible areas of conventional squamous cell carcinoma with nests of keratinized cells. Such foci may be limited in amount and require a diligent search or may be entirely absent, especially in small biopsies. The polypoid tumor may be largely ulcerated with a limited amount of intact mucosa usually at the base tumor, where a dysplastic squamous epithelium is evident.[19] The carcinomatous components usually have the appearance of poorly differentiated squamous carcinoma, but adenosquamous carcinoma and verrucous squamous carcinoma have also been reported.[93]

In biopsies from the head and neck region containing spindle cell tumor, squamous cell carcinoma should be considered and appropriate immunohisto-chemical stains should be performed. If cytokeratin is detected, the diagnosis of carcinoma is confirmed (Fig. 6–70B). However, not all spindle cell carcinomas express cytokeratin.[90,94,95] Thus, additional immunohistochemical stains are necessary to exclude spindle cell sarcoma and melanoma.[96,97]

Spindle cell squamous carcinoma generally behaves more aggressively than the conventional squamous cell carcinoma of comparable clinical stage. In addition to its local extent of disease, the anatomic location also affects the prognosis. Of the 13 patients with nasosinus spindle cell squamous carcinoma, 77% died of disease, as compared to 60% with oral tumor and 33% with laryngeal tumor.[98] In addition to local recurrence, metastasis to the cervical lymph node and lung is common.

BASALOID TYPE

Basaloid squamous cell carcinoma has distinct histologic features to be recognized as a separate entity. The tumor affects more males than females, especially in their sixth to seventh decades of life. The most common tumor sites are base of tongue, hypopharynx, and supraglottic larynx. Rare tumors also involve palate, tonsil, buccal mucosa, floor of mouth, and nasal cavity.[99]

Histologically, it contains conventional squamous

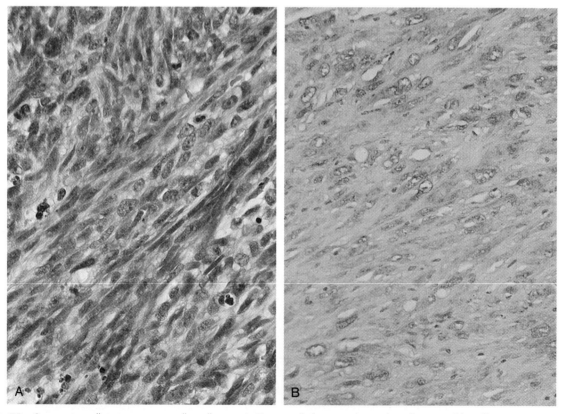

FIGURE 6–70 Squamous cell carcinoma, spindle cell type. *A,* Tumor cells form interlacing bundles resembling fibrosarcoma. Nuclear hyperchromasia, irregularity, and mitotic figures are apparent. *B,* Immunohistochemical stain for cytokeratin is positive.

cell carcinoma and basaloid components that resemble basal cell carcinoma of the skin. The latter consists of solid nests of basaloid cells with scant cytoplasm, hyperchromatic nuclei, inconspicuous nucleoli, and high mitotic activity. Peripheral palisading is a distinct feature. A microcystic pattern resulting from cellular degeneraton and necrosis may suggest a glandular neoplasm. Deposits of hyalinized material are sometimes abundant enough to consider salivary gland tumors, such as high-grade adenoid cystic carcinoma. Indeed some authors consider basaloid squamous cell carcinoma to have originated from the minor salivary glands. But the occurrence of squamous cell carcinoma in situ in 50% of basaloid squamous cell carcinomas favors a mucosal origin.[100]

Basaloid squamous cell carcinoma is more difficult to separate from squamous cell carcinoma containing cells with neuroendocrine differentiation. This distinction is best based on the immunoreactivity with antibodies of neuron-specific enolase, chromogranin, synaptophysin, and neuroendocrine markers.

Basaloid squamous cell carcinoma is an aggressive tumor. It is usually locally advanced and bulky. At presentation cervical lymph node metastasis is present in 60% to 80% of cases.[99,100] Distant metastases occurred in 40 to 60% of cases, mostly to the lung, skin, bone, and brain.[100,101] Surgical resection is often combined with radiotherapy and chemotherapy to achieve maximal effects.

SMALL CELL ANAPLASTIC CARCINOMA

Small cell anaplastic carcinoma, histologically similar to pulmonary counterpart, rarely involves the nasosinus. The small tumor cells have round to oval to elongated nuclei, punctate chromatin, indistinct nucleoli, and scant cytoplasm (Fig. 6–71A). Mitotic figures and cell necrosis are easily seen. Neuroendocrine markers may be positive by immunohistochemistry (Fig. 6–71B).

A separate small cell undifferentiated neoplasm was reported following radiotherapy for retinoblastoma.[102] By immunohistochemistry, the tumor cells express not only neuroendocrine markers but also keratin, S-100 protein, epithelial membrane antigen, and muscle markers. Based on a small number of reported cases, both of these small cell tumors have strong propensity for local and distant spread.[102] The key differential diagnosis is the less aggressive olfactory neuroblastoma, which have more abundant cytoplasm and lower mitotic activity. The distinction

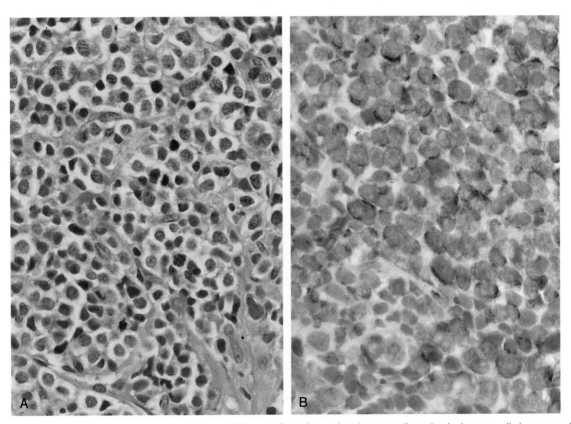

FIGURE 6–71 Small cell anaplastic carcinoma. A, Broad sheets of small round malignant cells. Individual tumor cells have round to oval, hyperchromatic nuclei and scant cytoplasm. An epithelial nesting pattern is suggested. B, Immunohistochemical stain for synaptophysin is positive.

between small cell anaplastic carcinoma and poorly differentiated neuroendocrine carcinoma is more difficult, and these two tumors are probably related.

Large Cell Undifferentiated Carcinoma

Large cell undifferentiated carcinoma of the nasosinus has been recognized as a distinct entity.[103,104] The majority of patients have bony, cranial, or orbital involvement at diagnosis. The tumor cells vary from medium to large in size, have polygonal configuration, and form irregular nests and sheets without luminal formation. The nucleoli are large (Fig. 6–72 A and B). The mitotic activity is high, exceeding 10 mitotic figures per 10 high-power fields. The amphophilic cytoplasm does not disclose keratinization. Scattered isolated cell necrosis is a prominent feature. Immunohistochemical stains for cytokeratin and epithelial membrane antigen are positive in the majority of cases; some additionally express neuron-specific enolase.[104] Other immunohistochemical stains and electron microscopy are helpful to differentiate these tumors from malignant lymphoma, melanoma, and rhabdomyosarcoma. One third of

patients developed metastasis in the cervical lymph nodes. The survival rate at 3 years is about 30%. Rarely, poorly differentiated carcinomas may contain spindle cell sarcoma[105] or endodermal sinus tumor.[106]

Prognosis

Most carcinomas arising in the nasal cavity and paranasal sinus grow readily into adjacent structures. At the time of diagnosis, most of these tumors have extensive local infiltration. Patients with locally advanced T3 and T4 tumors, positive surgical margin on resected specimen, and extension into the skull base, dura, and brain have poor outcome.[107,108] Less than 15% to 20% of nasal cavity and sinus carcinomas metastasize to the cervical lymph nodes.[80] Lymphatics draining the anterior nasal cavity lead to submandibular nodes. From the entire nasal cavity, lymphatics drain to retropharyngeal and anterior jugular nodes. Metastases from the maxillary antrum may be seen in submandibular and other anterior cervical nodes. After surgery, radiotherapy, or both, the 5-year survival rate for nasal carcinoma ranges from 38% to 63% and for max-

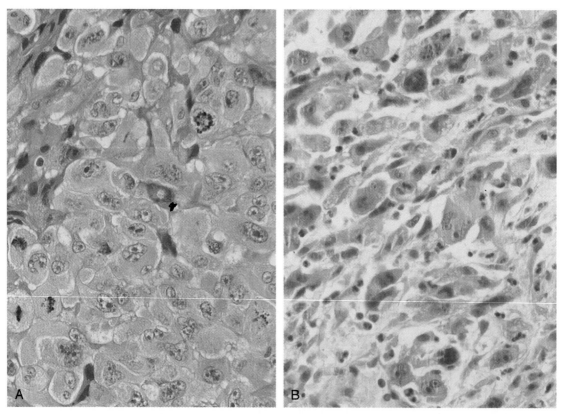

FIGURE 6–72 Large cell undifferentiated carcinoma. A, Tumor cells have round to oval to irregular nuclei containing prominent nucleoli. The cytoplasm is eosinophilic and abundant. Immunohistochemical stains confirm the presence of cytokeratin and the absence of S-100 protein and melanoma specific antigen by antibodies, HMB-45 and KBA-62. B, Large sarcomatoid cells vary from round to oval to elongated in shape. The nuclear pleomorphism and prominent nucleoli are also apparent.

illary carcinoma from 13% to 35%.[82] Patients with localized nasal carcinoma have more favorable outcome, with 10-year survival rates close to 80%.[108] Most nasal vestibular carcinomas are well-differentiated squamous carcinoma and have excellent prognosis.

NASOPHARYNGEAL TUMORS

Benign and malignant tumors of the nasopharynx fall into three majority categories: (1) nasopharyngeal carcinomas, (2) salivary gland tumors, and (3) nonepithelial neoplasms. In Hong Kong, where nasopharyngeal carcinoma is prevalent, 93% of nasopharyngeal malignancies are carcinoma, followed by malignant lymphoma (5%) and miscellaneous tumors (2%), such as adenocarcinoma and rhabdomyosarcoma.[109]

Nasopharyngeal Carcinoma

Nasopharyngeal carcinoma (NPC) differs from carcinomas arising in the nasal cavity and paranasal sinuses in several important respects: clinical, etiologic, and histologic. Males outnumber females by a ratio of 2.5 to 3.0.[110] Due to the anatomic location, carcinoma may remain silent for some time. Thirty-two percent to 44% of patients present initially with metastasis in the cervical lymph node.[111]

Gross Pathology

Nasopharyngeal carcinoma arises most frequently in the superior wall or vault, followed by the pharyngeal recess in the lateral wall. By nasopharyngoscope, tumors have the following appearance: (1) bulging (elevated, full), (2) infiltrative, (3) exophytic and lobulated, and (4) ulcerative.[112] In some cases, no lesion is seen with certainty, and the carcinoma is identified by random blind biopsies of the nasopharynx.

From the primary site, the tumor spreads directly to the base of skull, the pterygoid fossa, the paranasal sinuses, or oropharynx. Metastatic disease may be found in cervical lymph nodes, lungs, skeleton, and viscera.

Microscopic Pathology

According to the World Health Organization (WHO) histologic typing system, NPCs are classified into: type I, keratinizing, and type II, nonkeratinizing. Type II tumors are further subclassified into A, differentiated, and B, undifferentiated.[113] The latter includes the lymphoepithelioma, anaplastic, clear cell, and spindle cell variants.[113] Acantholysis may occur rarely in squamous carcinomas producing a pseu-

doglandular pattern.[114] In terms of the distribution of histologic types, there is a remarkable variation from different geographic areas. In Singapore, the frequency of keratinizing, differentiated nonkeratinizing, and undifferentiated carcinomas is 20%, 33%, and 47%, respectively.[109] In Hong Kong, the ratio of keratinizing, differentiated nonkeratinizing, and undifferentiated tumors is 3%, 9%, and 88%, respectively.[109] At the Armed Forces Institute of Pathology, 14% of NPCs are keratinizing type, 4% differentiated nonkeratinizing type, and 82% undifferentiated type.[19]

This WHO classification of NPC offers that a correlation exists between the histologic type and the presence of antibodies against Epstein-Barr viral capsid antigens and early antigens. These antibodies are detected in 85% of North American patients with differentiated nonkeratinizing or undifferentiated carcinoma. In contrast, antiviral capsid antigen is found in 16% and anti-early antigen in 35% of those having keratinizing tumors.[111] In patients whose metastatic carcinoma in a cervical lymph node suggests NPC, but in whom triple biopsy fails to detect the primary tumor, elevated serum titers for anti-EBV capsid antigen and anti-early antigen provide strong support for the diagnosis of primary NPC.

Keratinizing and differentiated nonkeratinizing squamous carcinomas rarely occur in children, who develop mainly undifferentiated carcinoma. Patients with undifferentiated carcinoma have shown a bimodal age distribution peaked at second and sixth decades of life.[115,116]

In the keratinizing type, the tumor cells have demonstrable intercellular bridges and keratin formation (Fig. 6–73A), while the tumor cells of differentiated nonkeratinizing type present with eosinophilic cytoplasm and well-defined cell borders suggestive of squamous differentiation (Fig. 6–73B). They grow in the compact nests rather than syncytial loose cohesive aggregates. The predominant tumor cells in the undifferentiated type have oval or round vesicular nuclei, prominent nucleoli, and indistinct cell borders arranged in a syncytial pattern (Fig. 6–74A). Spindle cells may be present focally or predominantly (Fig. 6–74B).

In the Regaud type of undifferentiated carcinoma, the tumor cells appear in irregular and well-defined nests mixed with abundant lymphoid cells and plasma cells (see Fig. 74 A and B). This is in contrast to the Schmincke type, in which the neoplastic cells are arranged in loosely cohesive aggregates, strands, or single cells homogeneously intermingled with lymphoid cells, simulating large cell lymphoma and Hodgkin's disease (Fig. 6–75 A and B). By immunohistochemical stains, carcinoma cells are positive for cytokeratin and negative for common leucocyte antigen (Fig. 6–75C).

The WHO classification provides prognostic information. Among patients with keratinizing carcinomas, the survival rates are 30% at 3 years and less

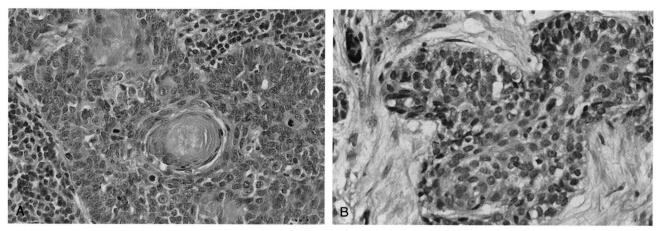

FIGURE 6–73   Squamous cell carcinoma of nasopharynx. *A,* Keratinizing type. Keratin pearl formation in the midst of poorly differentiated squamous cells. *B,* Differentiated nonkeratinizing type. Tumor cells are arranged in broad sheets and contain eosinophilic cytoplasm suggestive of individual cell keratinization.

than 20% at 5 years. Of those having differentiated nonkeratinizing or undifferentiated carcinomas, 70% survived 3 years and 59% 5 years.[111] These differences in survival rates are believed to reflect radiosensitivity of the tumors, with the keratinizing carcinomas being less responsive than others.

Hsu et al[117] have found the degree of nuclear atypia to influence prognosis. Their designated type A tumors included those nonkeratinizing and undifferentiated carcinomas having marked nuclear anaplasia/pleomorphism (Fig. 6–76 *A* and *B*). These type A neoplasms are more aggressive than type B

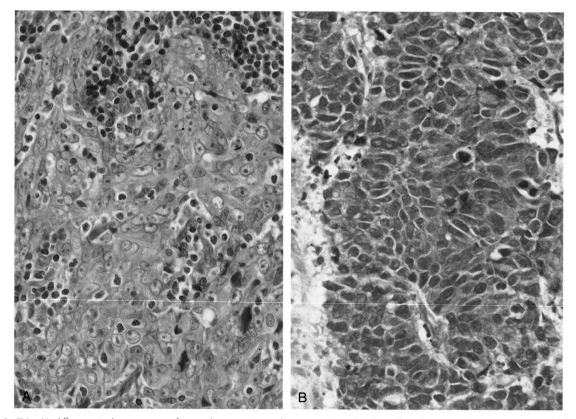

FIGURE 6–74   Undifferentiated carcinoma of nasopharynx, Regaud type. *A,* Broad sheets of malignant cells are characterized by round to oval nuclei containing a single, prominent nucleolus. *B,* Tumor cells are arranged in a trabecular pattern and have oval to elongated, hyperchromatic nuclei.

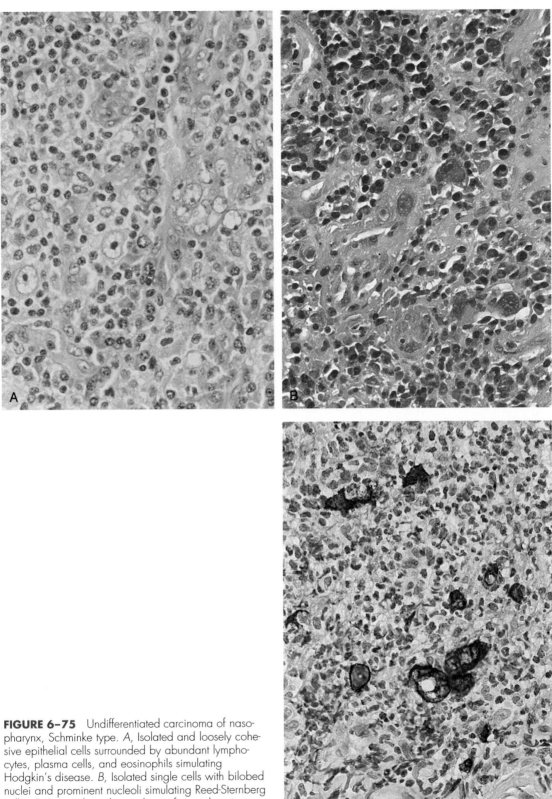

FIGURE 6-75 Undifferentiated carcinoma of nasopharynx, Schminke type. *A,* Isolated and loosely cohesive epithelial cells surrounded by abundant lymphocytes, plasma cells, and eosinophils simulating Hodgkin's disease. *B,* Isolated single cells with bilobed nuclei and prominent nucleoli simulating Reed-Sternberg cells. *C,* Immunohistochemical stain for cytokeratin is positive in the tumor cells.

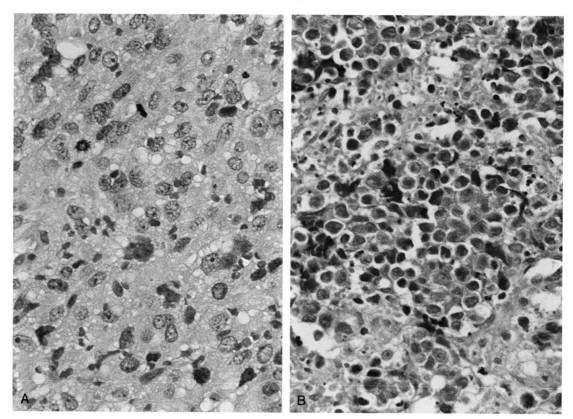

FIGURE 6–76　Undifferentiated carcinoma of nasopharynx. *A,* Round cells with high-grade nuclear anaplasia. *B,* Tumor cells have scant cytoplasm resembling small cell carcinoma. Extensive tumor necrosis is evident. Compared to the small cell anaplastic carcinoma the nucleoli are more prominent in this undifferentiated carcinoma.

neoplasms, which have only moderate or little anaplasia. NPC with predominantly spindle cells also have a worse prognosis (Fig. 6–77). Based on these findings NPC can be grouped into (1) high-grade malignancy: keratinizing carcinoma with a 5-year survival rate of 21%, (2) intermediate malignancy:

type A carcinomas, 5-year survival 30% to 40%, and (3) low-grade malignancy: type B carcinomas, 5-year survival 60% to 72%.[117] Finally, the precursor lesions of NPC were described as resembling severe dysplasia/carcinoma in situ of the uterine cervix (Fig. 6–78).

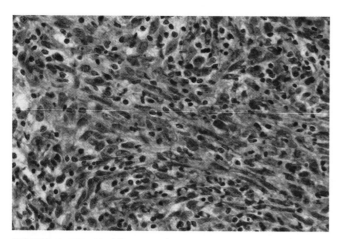

FIGURE 6–77　Undifferentiated carcinoma consisting predominantly of spindle cells simulating sarcoma, such as synovial sarcoma.

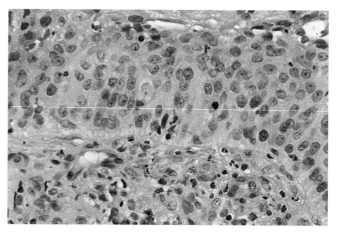

FIGURE 6–78　Squamous cell carcinoma in situ of nasopharynx made up of round to oval malignant cells occupying the entire thickness of the mucosa.

Differential Diagnosis

Nasopharyngeal biopsies can be quite difficult to interpret, because of the crush artifact or only a small number of tumor cells available for study. Immunohistochemical stains should be applied when faced with a possible malignant neoplasm.

Immunohistochemistry and Electron Microscopy

Electron microscopic studies of NPC have shown a varying number of tonofibrils, keratin-like structures, and desmosomal junctions, suggestive of squamous differentiation.[118] In a study of 10 undifferentiated carcinomas, tonofilaments could not be identified in two neoplasms; the only evidence of epithelial differentiation was the presence of cell junctions.[118]

Using commercially available antibody against a broad spectrum of keratin, positive staining was found in all carcinomas of the keratinizing type, 88% of the nonkeratinizing type, 90% of the undifferentiated type and 50% of adenocarcinomas.[119] Common leucocyte antigen was absent in the malignant cells. In another study of 69 nonkeratinizing and undifferentiated carcinomas stained for cytokeratin and common leucocyte antigen, all but three were positive for cytokeratin to confirm the diagnosis of carcinoma. Two of the three cytokeratin-negative tumors were common leucocyte antigen positive, supporting the diagnosis of lymphoma. There was only one neoplasm where diagnosis could not be determined.[120] Thus, most nasopharyngeal neoplasms can be diagnosed by the use of multiple immunohistochemical stains.

Prognosis

Most reports have shown the clinical stage of tumor to be the most important prognostic factor.[121,122] Survival figures vary considerably, depending on the method of staging used in the study. When the carcinoma is confined to the nasopharynx, the prognosis is relatively good. When the tumor has metastasized to cervical lymph nodes, the chance of cure is diminished. Involvement of bone and/or cranial nerves is associated with a poor prognosis.

BENIGN AND MALIGNANT GLANDULAR TUMORS

Malignant glandular neoplasms of this region can originate from the respiratory epithelium or the underlying seromucous glands. The former group of tumors tends to occur high in the nasal cavity and ethmoid sinus, while the salivary gland neoplasms, exemplified by adenoid cystic carcinoma, develop more commonly from the lower nasal cavity and maxillary sinus.

In a series of 37 mucous gland neoplasms arising in the upper respiratory passages, Rafla[123] found the following distribution: adenoid cystic carcinoma, 16; adenocarcinoma, 14; mucoepidermoid carcinoma, two; malignant mixed tumor, two; anaplastic adenocarcinoma, two; and pleomorphic adenoma, one. Thus, about 40% of glandular neoplasms arise from the respiratory epithelium and the remaining 60% from seromucous glands.

In the nasopharynx, glandular neoplasms are uncommon. The majority originate from the seromucous glands, such as oncocytic cystadenoma, acinic cell carcinoma, and mucoepidermoid carcinoma.

Salivary Gland Tumors

Benign salivary gland tumors are rarely seen in the nasal cavity and the paranasal sinuses. Benign mixed tumors (pleomorphic adenomas), myoepithelioma, oncocytic metaplasia, papillary cystadenoma, and oncocytomas have been reported.

Benign mixed tumors of the nasal cavity most commonly originate from the bony or cartilaginous nasal septum, and rarely the turbinate.[124] These neoplasms grow by expansion, vary from less than 1 cm to 7 cm in size, and may extend into an adjacent paranasal sinus. They appear as a polypoid, exophytic, dome-shaped mass, usually covered by an intact mucosa.

The microscopic features are similar to mixed tumors of the major salivary glands. The cellularity, however, is high with closely packed oval epithelial cells arranged in nests and sheets. Ducts, tubules, and stromal components are less common (Fig. 6–79 A and B). In a study of 40 cases of intranasal mixed tumors, local recurrence was found in three patients (7.5%) following surgical excision.[124]

Myoepithelioma, a rare variant of monomorphic adenoma, consists of uniform, spindle-shaped cells arranged in bundles or in sheets. The cells lack pleomorphism and mitotic activity. Less commonly, the tumor cells have a plasmacytoid appearance. One of the distinct helpful features is the presence of hyaline membranes in the stroma. The differential diagnosis includes schwannoma, leiomyoma, fibroma, and myxoma. Myoepithelial differentiation can be demonstrated by immunohistochemical expression of S-100 protein and smooth muscle actin.[125,126]

Adenoid cystic carcinoma (ACC) is the most common malignant tumor to arise from the minor salivary glands; it is particularly prone to occur in the oral cavity and nasal and paranasal sinus areas. The clinical presentation is a submucosal, infiltrative firm mass, usually greater than 2 cm.

Histologically, these tumors are similar to ACC of the major salivary glands. Small basaloid cells with hyperchromatic nuclei and scant cytoplasm are arranged in tubules, cribriform glands, and solid sheets. The latter two patterns predominate in ACC arising in the upper respiratory tract.[127] The cribri-

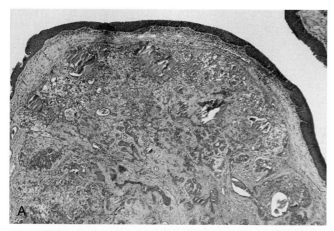

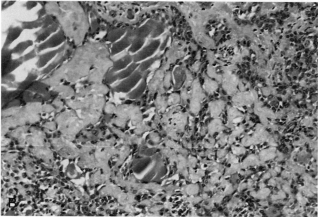

FIGURE 6–79 Benign mixed tumor of nasal cavity. *A,* Beneath the squamous epithelium is a well-circumscribed tumor consisting of irregular epithelial cords and nests. *B,* Areas of hyalinized and chondroid stroma.

form spaces contain mucinous or hyaline material. Local infiltration and perineural invasion are usually evident to exclude a benign mixed tumor (Fig. 6–80). Predominantly solid ACC can be distinguished from undifferentiated small cell carcinomas and basaloid squamous cell carcinoma by its low mitotic activity. The demonstration of myoepithelial cell differentiation by immunohistochemistry also supports the diagnosis of ACC.

ACC widely infiltrates bone, involves nerves, and has usually spread beyond the resection margins. The latter should be carefully documented for therapeutic and prognostic considerations.

Mucoepidermoid carcinoma involved the upper respiratory passages in eight (13%) of 60 mucoepidermoid carcinomas from all sites.[128] Of these, seven occurred in the maxillary sinus and one in the nasal cavity. Such tumors can also arise in the nasopharynx. Histologically, these neoplasms have a distinct pattern and heterogeneous cell population. In well- and moderately differentiated tumors, mucous cells, epidermoid cells, and intermediate cells form cystic and glandular structures (Fig. 6–81A). In addition, clear cells, oxyphilic cells, and spindle cells occur in varying numbers (Fig. 6–81B). Poorly differentiated

lesions grow in solid nests with a predominance of epidermoid cells. Rare glandular cells have a signet-ring appearance and require mucicarmine and PAS stains for positive identification.

Tumors designated as "adenosquamous" carcinoma involving the nasal, oral, and laryngeal cavities most likely represent variants of mucoepidermoid carcinoma and behave like a poorly differentiated mucoepidermoid carcinoma.[129]

Malignant mixed tumor (MMT) is rarely found in the upper respiratory passages. In a series of 47 MMTs, one involved this area. These lesions have been extensively discussed by LiVolsi and Perzin.[130]

Acinic cell carcinomas have been reported in the nasosinus and nasopharynx.[131,132] Tumor cell cytoplasm may appear eosinophilic, basophilic, granular, or clear (Fig. 6–82 *A* and *B*). The nuclei are uniform, and nucleoli may be conspicuous. The differential diagnosis includes rhabdomyoma, chordoma, paraganglioma, melanoma with balloon cells, alveolar soft part sarcoma, and ganglioneuroma.[132] The diagnosis of acinic cell carcinoma can be confirmed by immunoperoxidase stain (positive for amylase) and electron microscopy (presence of zymogen granules).[132]

Low-grade polymorphic papillary adenocarcinoma may rarely occur in the nasosinus and nasopharynx. Wenig et al[133] reported nine cases of primary nasopharyngeal low-grade papillary adenocarcinoma in five males and four females, who were 11 to 64 years old (mean 37 years). The tumor size varied from 0.5 cm to 3.5 cm. Histologically, the tumor cells form complex papillae and cribriform glands, which are lined by a few pseudostratified layers of columnar to cuboidal cells (Fig. 6–83A). They have optically clear nuclei and reveal moderate nuclear atypia, small nucleoli, and rare to absent mitotic activity (Fig. 6–83B). Psammoma bodies occur in 20% of cases. All tumors involve the mucosal surface. By special stains, mucinous material and PAS diastase–resistant granules accumulate in the cytoplasm. By

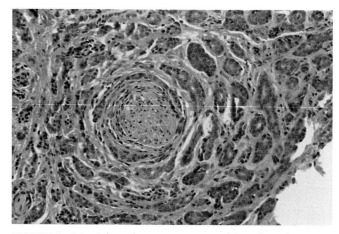

FIGURE 6–80 Adenoid cystic carcinoma of the ethmoid sinus with perineural invasion. Tumor cells form predominantly tubules with basaloid appearance. Some of the cells have small pyknotic nuclei suggestive of myoepithelial cell differentiation.

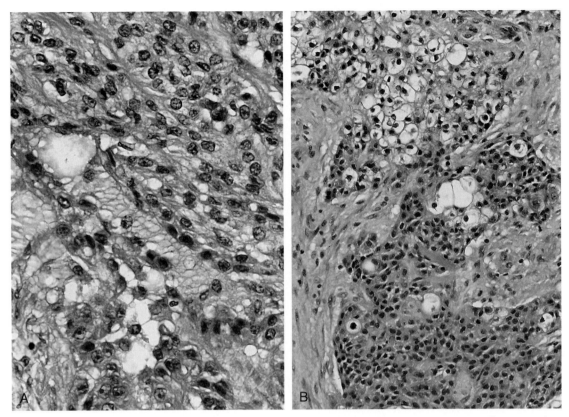

FIGURE 6-81 Mucoepidermoid carcinoma of nasopharynx. *A*, Glandular spaces lined by mucous-secreting cells. *B*, Irregular nests and sheets of heterogeneous cells. Some cells have clear cytoplasm and distinct cell borders, others have the appearance of intermediate cells.

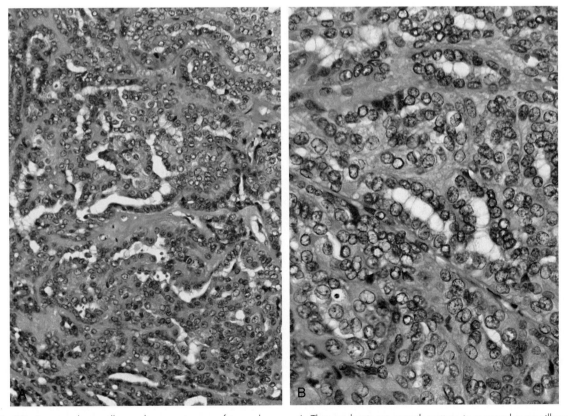

FIGURE 6-82 Low-grade papillary adenocarcinoma of nasopharynx. *A*, The predominant growth pattern is a complex papillary architecture. Less commonly, the tumor cells form closely apposed glands. *B*, The uniform nuclei have optically clear appearance resembling those seen in papillary carcinoma of the thyroid gland.

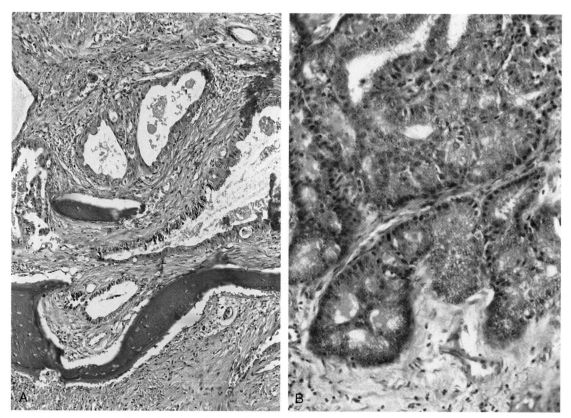

FIGURE 6–83   Adenocarcinoma of maxillary sinus, low grade. *A,* Irregular cystic spaces are lined by well-differentiated glandular cells that invade into bony wall. *B,* Tumor cells form cribriform glands and have low-grade nuclear atypia.

immunohistochemistry, the tumor cells express diffuse epithelial membrane antigen and focal carcinoembryonic antigen on the luminal borders. S-100 protein and glial filament acidic protein are entirely negative.

Because of the predominant papillary arrangement, optically clear nuclei, and formation of psammoma bodies, the possibility of metastatic papillary thyroid carcinoma to the nasopharynx was raised in some cases, but thyroglobulin was negative in all cases.

Wenig et al[133] believe that these nasopharyngeal papillary tumors originate from the respiratory mucosa and can be distinguished from polymorphic low-grade adenocarcinoma of the minor salivary gland. The latter are submucosal in location, rarely reaching to the mucosa surface. The growth patterns are variable, and the cytoplasm lacks mucinous and PAS diastase–resistant material. About 90% of tumors demonstrate myoepithelial differentiation by showing S-100 protein and glial filament acidic protein by immunohistochemistry.[134]

In the series of Wenig et al,[133] none of their nine cases of nasopharyngeal papillary adenocarcinoma recurred following complete local excision. Mills et al[134] reported a papillary variant of polymorphic low-grade adenocarcinoma arising from the palatal minor salivary glands. The tumor cells also exhibit

optically clear nuclei. Six of 14 (43%) patients developed cervical lymph node metastasis. These tumors appear more aggressive than the low-grade papillary of the nasopharynx described by Wenig et al.[133] Distinction of these two papillary adenocarcinomas can be difficult and requires immunohistochemical stains.

Nonsalivary Gland Tumors

Gross Pathology

Clinical examination reveals papillary, sessile, or smooth ill-defined masses. Cut surfaces have grey, translucent, mucoid appearance.

Microscopic Pathology

The predominant growth patterns vary from small acini, tubular glands, cribriform glands, and papillary structures to solid nests and sheets. Very often several different patterns coexist. The types of cells also differ from tumor to tumor and within the same tumor. To simplify the classification, Heffner et al[135] divided the adenocarcinomas into low grade and high grade, based on growth patterns, nuclear features, and mitotic activity. Low-grade tumors consist of uniform cells arranged in acini, glands, cystic spaces, and papillae (see Fig. 6–70 A and B).

The high-grade neoplasms include about an equal number of intestinal type carcinomas and poorly differentiated solid tumors. The intestinal or colonic

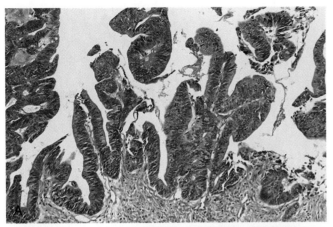

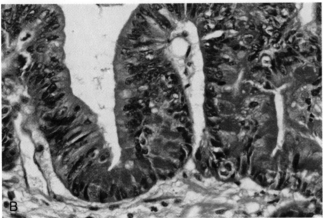

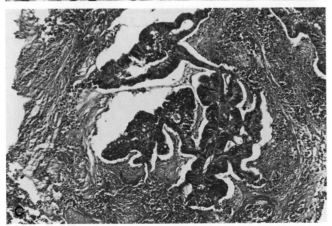

FIGURE 6–84 Adenocarcinoma of ethmoid sinus, colonic type. A, The papillary pattern and tall columnar lining cells resemble villous adenoma of the colon. Even on this low power, some cells have densely eosinophilic cytoplasm to suggest paneth cells. B, Higher magnification to illustrate picket fence arrangement of the nuclei, occasional mitosis, and paneth cells with abundant granular, eosinophilic cytoplasm. C, Areas of abundant mucinous material and inflammatory cells.

variant of adenocarcinomas are made up of absorptive cells and goblet cells forming glands, nests, and abundant mucin. The degree of differentiation varies. Some are extremely well-differentiated, having the appearance of a colonic adenoma with villous pattern and minimal nuclear atypia (Figure 6–84A). Paneth cells and enterochromaffin cells occur at the base of glands, which are sometimes surrounded by a few layers of smooth muscle cells simulating muscularis mucosae (Fig. 6–84B).

In small biopsies evidence of stromal invasion may be absent. The presence of mucous pools and necrotic debris in the stroma should lead to a careful survey of the entire specimen to exclude the possibility of malignancy (Fig. 6–84C). In all cases, the patient should be examined for evidence of intestinal tumor before the neoplasm is accepted as a primary lesion of the upper respiratory passages.

Heffner's classification offers useful prognostic information. Among the patients with low-grade tumors, 78% had no evidence of disease, 13% were alive with disease, and 9% died of disease. In contrast, only 7% in the high-grade group had no evidence of disease, 15% were alive with disease, and 78% had died of disease, including 29% with distant metastases.[135] Other authors also found the degree of differentiation to correlate with prognosis.[136]

The intestinal variant in the Heffner's series[135] was classified as high grade, because most patients with this type died of disease within 3 years of diagnosis. In more recent studies the behavior of intestinal type of tumors was found to be most closely related to the extent of disease and growth patterns.[137–140] Well-differentiated tumors with predominantly papillary and tubular structures have better prognosis than those poorly differentiated counterparts.[139,140]

Based on a review of 213 cases of intestinal type carcinoma reported in the literature, 60% of patients died of disease (80% of these died in 3 years), 53% had local recurrences, 8% had cervical lymph node metastases, and 13% had distant metastases.[138] When this tumor is associated with wood dust exposure, it affects males and ethmoid sinus and has a better prognosis than sporadic cases, which tend to affect women and maxillary sinus.[138]

BENIGN AND MALIGNANT NONEPITHELIAL TUMORS

In a series of 264 benign and malignant nonepithelial tumors and tumor-like conditions, 156 (60%) benign lesions were predominantly vascular tumors and osseous and fibro-osseous lesions. The 108 malignant nonepithelial neoplasms in the order of frequency are malignant lymphoma, fibromatosis/fibrosarcoma, rhabdomyosarcoma, bone sarcomas, and plasmacytoma.[141] Neurogenic tumors, including schwannoma, neurofibroma, and olfactory neuroblastoma, are encountered occasionally.

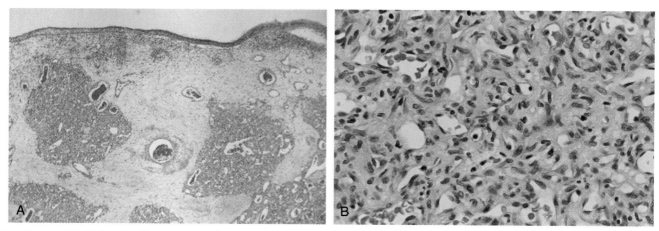

FIGURE 6–85 *A,* Capillary hemangioma of nasal cavity consisting of well-circumscribed lobules of capillaries and large feeding vessels. *B,* Solid area with small vascular spaces.

The clinical presentations of these nonepithelial tumors are similar to those caused by epithelial neoplasms. Except in a few instances, no specific findings are identified on physical or radiologic examination. In most cases the correct diagnosis is made by histologic examination of the excised tissue. These nonepithelial tumors are seen much less frequently than epithelial neoplasms and constitute only about 10% to 20% of all tumors found in the nasal cavity, paranasal sinuses, and nasopharynx.

Vascular Tumors

HEMANGIOMA

Hemangiomas are found most often in the anterior nasal septum, followed by the turbinates and the vestibule. Grossly, they are polypoid, grey to purple, lobulated, and less than 2 cm in size. Microscopically, capillary hemangiomas are seen most frequently and have a distinct lobular pattern (Fig. 6–85). When the vascular spaces remain unopen and solid, they are also referred to as benign hemangioendotheliomas. Cavernous hemangiomas, venous hemangiomas, and angiomatoses are less common. Their histologic appearance is similar to those occurring elsewhere.[141] Vascular malformations may easily be overlooked in multiple pieces of curetted tissue. In contrast to normal vascular channels and to the vessels in hemangiomas, vascular malformations contain numerous closely packed tortuous blood vessels of variable sizes and configurations.

These vascular tumors and malformations are prone to develop organizing thrombi in the form of Masson's intravascular vegetating hemangioendothelioma (intravenous granuloma pyogenicum). Ingrowth of active endothelial cells into the fibrin clot produces irregular villous projections sometimes simulating angiosarcoma (Fig. 6–86A). Further organization results in hyaline and fibrous cores (Fig. 6–86B). A similar process of organization also occurs in the hematoma and infarcted tissues.

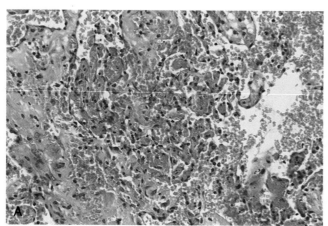
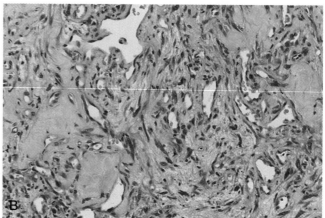

FIGURE 6–86 Thrombus formation is common in all types of hemangiomas. *A,* Early organizing thrombus. Ingrowth of endothelial cells into the fibrinous material. Some endothelial cells are hyperplastic with plump nuclei. *B,* Hyalinized thrombus with irregular recanalized capillaries.

Pyogenic granuloma is generally considered to be pseudotumor with mucosal ulceration and lobulated vascular proliferation. When the following features are encountered, a neoplastic process should be suspected: lobular pattern replaced by solid growth, presence of high mitotic activity, proliferation of spindle cells between blood vessels, intervascular stromal fibrosis, and epithelioid appearance of endothelial cells.[142]

ANGIOFIBROMA

Angiofibroma develops in the nasopharynx of teenaged boys; young children and adults may be affected. Although rare cases of angiofibroma were reported in females, the accuracy of diagnosis is questioned. Clinically, angiofibromas produce nasal obstruction, epistaxis, and sometimes massive hemorrhage. It presents as a bulging nasopharyngeal mass, which may extend into the posterior nasal cavity. These tumors may infiltrate locally to involve adjacent structures, including the pterygoid region, sphenoid sinus, base of skull, orbital cavity, hard and soft palate, cheek, and temple.[143]

Angiofibromas have a sessile or polypoid appearance, grey-white to purple-red color, and firm rubbery consistency (Fig. 6–87). The mucosa may be focally hemorrhagic or eroded. Microscopically, these tumors are composed of a characteristic fibrous stroma in which are found numerous blood vessels of varying sizes and shapes. Smaller vascular channels are surrounded only by the fibrous stroma. Larger vessels may have an irregular or incomplete smooth muscle coat. Elastic fibers usually cannot be found in the vessel walls, either with elastic tissue stains or with the electron microscope. Stromal cells vary from mature fibrocytes with small, dense nuclei to fibroblasts, which have larger, round to oval nuclei with a fine chromatin pattern (Fig. 6–88A). Mast cells, multinucleated giant cells, and plump cells with abundant eosinophilic cytoplasm also occur

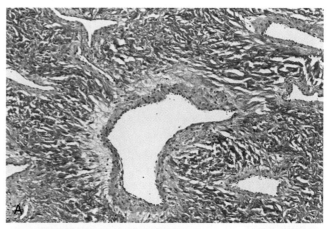
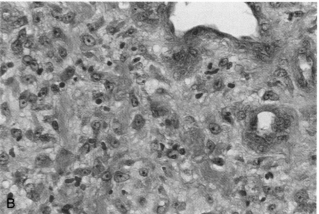

FIGURE 6–88 *A,* Irregular vascular spaces are lined by smooth muscle cells of varying thickness. In the collagenous stroma are mature fibroblasts. *B,* Some stromal cells have plump round to oval nuclei and small nucleoli.

(Fig. 6–88*B*). The collagenous stroma may be myxomatous.

By ultrastructural study and immunohistochemistry, most of the stromal cells appear to be fibrocytes or fibroblasts, but smooth muscle cells and myofibroblasts have been identified.[141]

In most cases, angiofibromas can be easily diagnosed histologically. Occasionally, the stroma may show focal areas of moderate to marked hypercellularity, suggestive of fibromatosis or fibrosarcoma. The stromal cells in angiofibromas, however, usually still have regular nuclei without pleomorphism or hyperchromatism. Only a few mitoses may be identified. A tumor that demonstrates marked stromal cellularity with numerous mitoses is more likely a sarcoma. Malignant soft tissue tumors arising in the nasal cavity tend to have a more vascular stroma than similar neoplasms growing elsewhere. However, the blood vessels found in these sarcomas are relatively small compared with the larger vessels seen in angiofibromas. The smaller vascular channels of angiofibromas may become compressed by the stroma, producing a picture reminiscent of hemangiopericytoma, but the vessels rarely exhibit the slit-like pattern that is found in pericytic tumors.

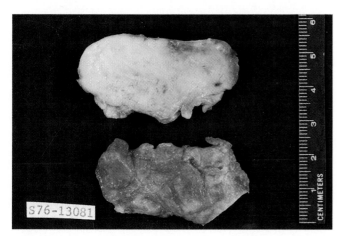

FIGURE 6–87 Angiofibroma of nasopharynx. Grossly, it has a multinodular appearance without a capsule. The cut surface reveals punctate vascular spaces in a homogenous fibrous stroma.

Recurrence after surgical resection varies from 7% to 14%.[143,144] In some cases, the lesion regresses after puberty. Rare example of sarcomatous transformation of angiofibroma typically follows radiotherapy to the area.[145,146]

GLOMUS TUMOR AND HEMANGIOPERICYTOMA

These tumors occur in the nasal cavity and paranasal sinuses as a polypoid mass, which bleeds easily on contact. Histologically, glomus tumor consists of round to oval cells with round to oval nuclei and eosinophilic cytoplasm. The tumor cells proliferate in bundles or in clusters around the capillaries (Fig. 6–89) and sometimes merge with the smooth muscle cells of the vessel walls. Areas of hyalinization and myxoid change may be extensive to suggest a benign mixed tumor.

Most of the nasosinus hemangiopericytomas are composed of uniform, round to spindle-shaped cells proliferating around the capillaries in a whorl-like or compartmentalized fashion (Fig. 6–90 A and B). Perivascular fibrosis and cuffing occur between the endothelial cells and pericytes.[147] Nuclear atypia is usually mild and the mitotic activity is low. Rarely hemangiopericytoma may contain mature lipocytes in single form, clusters, or lobules, the so-called lipomatous hemangiopericytoma.[148] Malignant hemangiopericytoma is usually large, mitotically active, necrotic, and widely infiltrative.

HEMANGIOPERICYTOMA-LIKE INTRANASAL TUMORS

These neoplasms have vascular channels that are not dispersed uniformly throughout. These blood vessels resemble the normal capillaries seen in the nasosinus and do not have the typical compressed

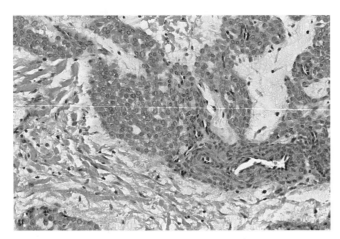

FIGURE 6–89 Glomus tumor of nasal cavity. The epithelioid tumor cells wrap around the blood vessels. The stroma is sometimes quite myxoid to simulate a benign mixed tumor.

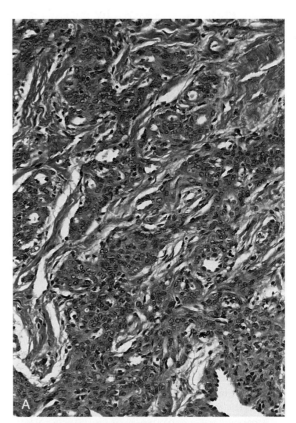

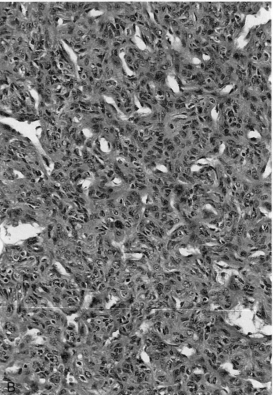

FIGURE 6–90 Hemangiopericytoma of nasal cavity. A, Whorl-like proliferation of uniform tumor cells around the capillaries. B, Irregular capillaries are surrounded by tufts of elongated tumor cells.

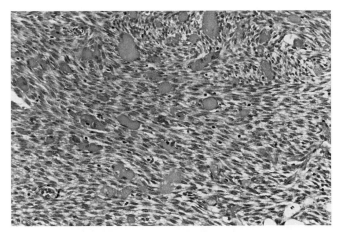

FIGURE 6–91   Hemangiopericytoma-like tumor of nasal cavity. Monotonous population of spindle cells and scattered dilated capillaries. The spindle cells have uniform nuclei without atypia or increased mitotic activity. The cytoplasm is scant. Note the lack of whorl-like pattern seen in typical hemangiopericytomas.

irregular and slit-like vessels found in typical hemangiopericytomas (Fig. 6–91).[149] In addition, the spindle-shaped cells are arranged in uniform interlacing bundles. None of the 23 patients with nasal hemangiopericytoma-like neoplasm recurred.[149] This is in contrast to four of 11 (36%) hemangiopericytomas of the nasosinus recurred after excision.[147] Whether hemangiopericytoma-like tumors are true hemangiopericytomas, fibrous tumors, or some other type of neoplasm remains to be determined.

MALIGNANT HEMANGIOENDOTHELIOMA AND ANGIOSARCOMA

This author encountered a patient who developed a nasal low-grade malignant hemangioendothelioma 15 years after radiotherapy for nasopharyngeal carcinoma. The proliferating cells have histiocytoid and signet-ring appearance. These vacuolated cells form small aggregates simulating embryonic angioblasts (Fig. 6–92 A–C).

Both well-differentiated and poorly differentiated angiosarcomas were reported in the nasosinus.[141,150,151] The prognosis is poor.[151] Immunohistochemical stains for factor VIII are valuable in the confirmation of endothelial origin, especially in epithelioid angiosarcoma, in which anaplastic tumor cells are difficult to separate from carcinoma.

Fibrous Tumors

SOLITARY FIBROUS TUMORS

These neoplasms, similar to that found in the pleura, were reported in the nasosinus as a rubbery, firm, grey-white mass up to 7 cm in size.[152,153] Most are found in the turbinate, nasal septum, maxillary antrum, and nasopharynx.

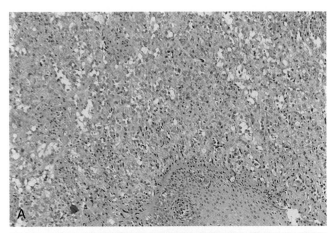

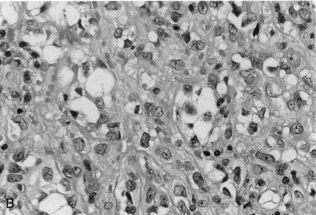

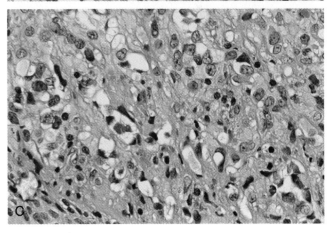

FIGURE 6–92   Low-grade hemangioendothelioma of posterior nasal cavity following radiotherapy for nasopharyngeal carcinoma. *A*, Sheets of tumor cells forming irregular spaces. *B*, Some spaces are lined by atypical cells with vacuolated cytoplasm and signet-ring appearance. *C*, Signet-ring tumor cells attempt to form small vascular spaces simulating angioblasts. Factor VIII is demonstrated by immunohistochemical stain.

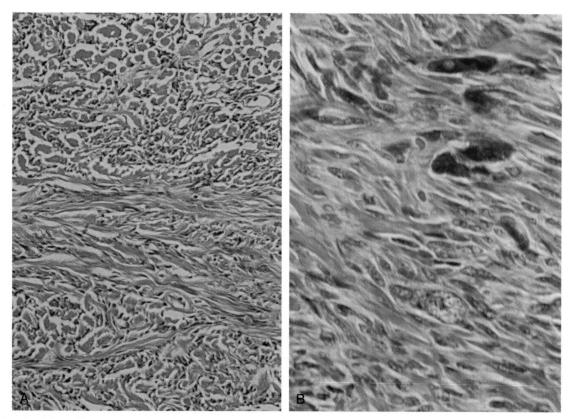

FIGURE 6-93 Solitary fibrous tumor of nasal turbinate. *A,* Mature fibrocytes are arranged in a nondescript pattern. The background stroma is heavily collagenized. *B,* Some of the tumor cells have large, hyperchromatic, and irregular nuclei. Mitotic activity in this tumor is low to absent.

Microscopically, plump fibroblasts infiltrate the adjacent seromucous glands without encapsulation. They are typically arranged in bundles and whorls (Fig 6-93*A*). Most tumor cells have uniformly oval to elongated nuclei and scant cytoplasm, but nuclear hyperchromasia and irregularity may be seen (Fig. 6-93*B*). Mitotic activity is low to absent. In one case, the mitotic activity was found focally up to 1 to 2 mitotic figures per 10 high-power fields. The stroma is rich in scattered, branching capillaries simulating hemangiopericytoma. Hyalinized fibrous stroma is a prominent feature. Immunohistochemical expression of CD34 is helpful to confirm the diagnosis. Local resection resulted in cure in all but one case.[152,153] This patient had a persistent nasopharyngeal fibrous tumor 4 years following local resection and tumor embolization.[153]

FIBROMATOSIS

Fibromatosis of the nasosinus affects young children, as well as adults in their seventh decade. Maxillary sinus and turbinates are most commonly involved by a white, firm, polypoid mass, ranging from 1 to 5 cm in size. The cut surface has a whorl-like appearance. Mature fibroblasts form interlacing bundles and have uniform nuclei and indistinct nucleoli. Local infiltration into the adjacent soft and bony tissue helps to separate fibromatosis from a benign process (Fig. 6-94). Their mild to moderate cellularity, minimal nuclear atypia, rich collagenous matrix, and low to absent mitotic activity differ from fibrosarcoma.[154] Fibromatosis of the head and neck region may be multicentric and undergoing spontaneous regression.[154]

FIBROSARCOMA

Fibrosarcoma of the nasosinus occurs most frequently in the maxillary sinus, nasal cavity, and ethmoid region during the fifth and sixth decades of life. In the resection specimen, the tumor varies from 3 to 6 cm in size and has a polypoid, fleshy, white, homogeneous appearance. It grows by expansion or by infiltration (Fig. 6-95).

The cellularity in fibrosarcoma is high, and the tumor cells are arranged in a distinct herringbone pattern (Fig. 6-96*A*). Although the elongated nuclei are relatively uniform in size and shape, there is evidence of nuclear atypia, altered chromatin patterns, small nucleoli, and increased mitotic activity in some part of the tumor (Fig. 6-96*B*). In one study, the number of mitotic figures per 50 high-power fields is reported as less than five mitoses in 66%, five to eight mitoses in 19%, and more than 10 mitoses in 15% of cases.[155] A low mitotic activity

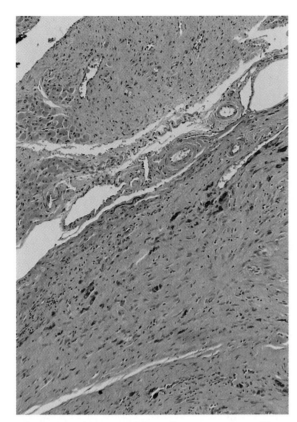

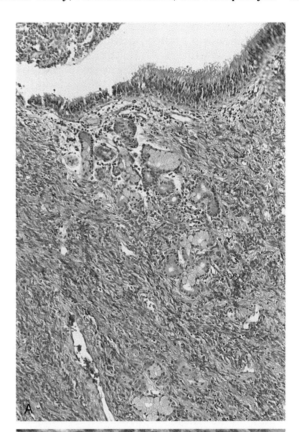

FIGURE 6-94   Fibromatosis of maxillary sinus. Mature fibrous tissue consists of interlacing bundles of mature fibroblasts with minimal nuclear atypia and low mitotic activity. Infiltration into skeletal muscle is evident.

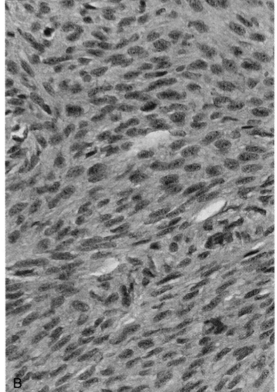

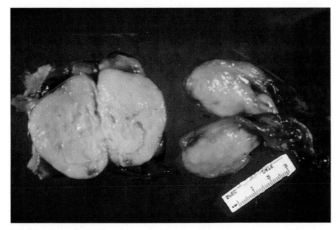

FIGURE 6-95   Fibrosarcoma of maxillary sinus. This polypoid mass, although well-circumscribed, extends into the surrounding soft tissue and bone.

FIGURE 6-96   Well-differentiated fibrosarcoma. *A*, Beneath the respiratory mucosa, tumor cells infiltrate the seromucous glands. *B*, Higher magnification to reveal nuclear hyperchromasia, mild irregularity, and rare mitotic figures.

combined with minor nuclear atypia contributes to the underdiagnosis of fibrosarcoma as fibroma and schwannian cell tumors.[155] Poorly differentiated fibrosarcoma is more readily diagnosed with apparent nuclear anaplasia, high mitotic activity, and scant collagenous stroma. The majority of nasosinus fibrosarcomas, however, are well-differentiated.[154,155]

An unusual finding associated with nasosinus fibrosarcoma is the proliferation and entrapment of surface respiratory mucosa simulating inverted papilloma in 31% of fibrosarcomas.[155] The stroma may be vascular with scattered capillaries mimicking hemangiopericytoma.

Differential Diagnosis

Fibrous tumors should be distinguished from inflammatory pseudotumors that may infiltrate the surrounding tissues. The latter lesions consist of hyalinized fibrous tissue mixed with varying numbers of lymphocytes and neutrophils resembling Riedel's thyroiditis, sclerosing mediastinitis, and retroperitoneal fibrosis. In the head and neck region this lesion has been reported to occur in the parotid gland, maxillary sinus, nasal cavity, orbit, and parapharyngeal space and is usually controlled by surgical excision.[156]

Because of its mature appearance, fibromatosis is sometimes classified as scar tissue, especially in biopsies. The stroma may be myxoid, leading to the consideration of myxoma or embryonal rhabdomyosarcoma. In fibromatosis, the component cells are bipolar in shape, as compared to the stellate cells in myxomas. In embryonal rhabdomyosarcoma, the cellularity and the nuclear atypia are more apparent than fibromatosis.

Fibrosarcoma may be underdiagnosed as benign fibroma, atypical polyp, or neurogenic tumor, because of low mitotic activity and limited nuclear atypia. But the high cellularity and local infiltration should suggest a malignant process.

Fibrosarcoma should be distinguished from other spindle cell sarcomas, most effectively with the use of immunohistochemical stains. Synovial sarcoma rarely occurs in the nasopharynx.[157,158] The monophasic variant can be difficult to separate from fibrosarcoma and other spindle cell sarcomas. The nondescript, diffuse or whorl-like architecture, pericytomatous pattern, and calcification are characteristic of synovial sarcoma. The biphasic variant contains additional epithelial elements in the form of glands, clefts, papillae, and solid sheets (Fig. 6–97A). Squamous cells and osteoid metaplasias may be extensive (Fig. 6–97B).[158] In small biopsies, these epithelial components may dominate to simulate carcinoma (Fig. 6–97C). Immunohistochemical stain for cytokeratin is useful to visualize epithelial differentiation in monophasic and biphasic synovial sarcomas.

Various osseous and fibro-osseous lesions, especially fibrous dysplasia, ossifying fibroma, and oste-

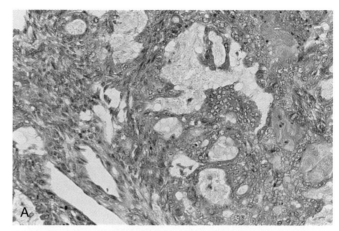

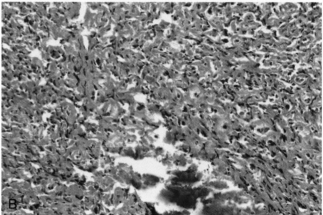

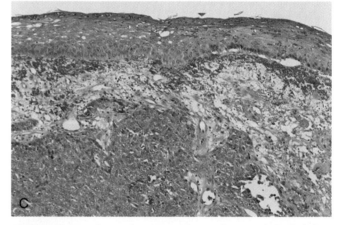

FIGURE 6–97 Synovial sarcoma of nasopharynx. *A,* Epithelial cells forming cribriform spaces with proteinaceous material in the lumen, simulating glandular neoplasm. The background spindle cells, although small in number, should raise the suspicion of synovial sarcoma. *B,* Fibrous stroma with calcification may simulate osteosarcoma. *C,* Beneath the squamous mucosa are sheets of epithelioid tumor cells, simulating nasopharyngeal carcinoma.

osarcoma, have areas of bony and fibroblastic proliferations. Although reactive new bone formation can occur in the periphery of fibromatosis and fibrosarcoma, osteoid or bone formation should not be seen in the substance of these lesions. Fibrosarcomatous areas may be recognized in many soft tissue tumors, including osteosarcoma, chondrosarcoma, leiomyosarcoma, synovial sarcoma, malignant schwannoma, and fibrous histiocytoma. In general, differentiation toward another type of tissue should lead to a diagnosis other than fibrous tissue neoplasm. Fibromatosis and fibrosarcomas should contain only rare multinucleate giant cells or cells with large, bizarre, or highly pleomorphic nuclei. If such cells are found, the tumor can usually be identified as some other type of neoplasm.

The use of immunohistochemical stains is recommended to distinguish spindle cell neoplasms. In a series of 42 nasosinus "fibrosarcomas", 10 (24%) neoplasms were positive for S-100 protein to support the diagnosis of malignant schwannoma. Five of these additionally expressed rhabdomyoblastic markers for the diagnosis of Triton tumor.[155] Without immunohistochemical stains, a correct diagnosis may not be made.

Prognosis

Fibromatosis has potential for recurrence if incompletely excised. En bloc resection with clear surgical margins minimizes tumor recurrence. A careful examination of the surgical margin is important for management and prognosis of patients.

The majority of nasosinus fibrosarcomas are well-differentiated and associated with favorable outcome.[154,155] In the study of Fu and Perzin,[154] all patients treated initially by local excision had local recurrence. Most patients treated with radical maxillectomy and en bloc resection with clear surgical margins have done well. Only one (9%) of 11 patients developed distant metastasis. In the series of Heffner and Gnepp,[155] 15 of 67 (22%) patients died of tumor who had large tumor, more extensive local disease, and increased mitotic activity, greater than four mitoses per 50 high-power fields. Tumor metastasized most commonly to the lung, bone, and liver. The remaining 52 cases (78%) have had no evidence of tumor at the last follow-up, although 20 (38%) of these 52 patients had one or more tumor recurrence.[155] Tumor recurrence was closely related to the type of surgical treatment. Complete local resection had the lowest recurrence, as compared to limited excision. Thus, treatment should be aimed to achieve complete excision. Tumors localized to the nasal cavity also have better prognosis than those extending into the paranasal sinuses.

Fibrous Histiocytoma

Both benign and malignant fibrous histiocytomas occur in the upper respiratory passages, producing the same clinical features that are associated with fibrous tumors. These neoplasms are histologically similar to fibrous histiocytomas found elsewhere, with the majority being storiform-pleomorphic type and rarely inflammatory type.[159,160] Local recurrence (42%) and distant metastasis (25%) are common, but cervical lymph node metastasis is rare.[160]

Myxoma

Myxoma growing in this area appears to arise in bone. On gross examination these tumors usually consist of a grey to white multinodular tissue with a soft, gelatinous to firm consistency. The tumor borders are smooth without capsule. Microscopically, myxomas are composed of avascular myxoid matrix in which lie scattered spindle-shaped and stellate cells.[161] The cells contain small, dark, elongated or ovoid nuclei and usually demonstrate elongated cytoplasmic tails. In focal areas, a more fibrous stroma may be seen in which the cells exhibit the appearance of fibrocytes. Following curettage and incomplete local excision of the lesion, the tumor is likely to recur. En bloc resection offers the best chance of cure.

Skeletal Muscle Tumors

Adult type of *rhabdomyoma* may rarely be found in this area.[162,163] The fetal variant of rhabdomyoma typically occurs in the pre- and post-auricular region and, less commonly, in the pharynx, larynx, and oral cavity. Immature spindle mesenchymal cells and elongated, fetal rhabdomyoblasts are found in a myxoid stroma. The latter have eosinophilic fibrillar cytoplasm, but cross striations are rarely seen. Rare rhabdomyoblasts have a round, strap-like, or spindle shape.[164] The well circumscription of the mass and the lack of nuclear atypia and mitotic activity allow separation from rhabdomyosarcoma.

Rhabdomyosarcoma arising in the upper respiratory tract usually occurs in the first and second decades, and rarely in young adults.[162] The frequency in decreasing order in the head and neck region is orbit, nasopharynx, middle ear, and nasosinus.[165]

Rhabdomyosarcoma, when small, has the appearance of a solid nodule with a vascular pink-red smooth surface. With increasing size, especially in the nasal cavity, paranasal sinuses, and/or nasopharynx, these tumors produce bulky polypoid masses simulating multiple nasal polyps (Fig. 6–98).[162]

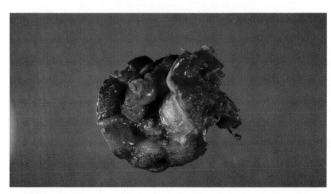

FIGURE 6-98 Sarcoma botryoides of nasopharynx and palate. Polypoid exophytic nodules involving the mucosal surface.

Rhabdomyosarcomas of the nasosinus are predominantly of the embryonal type (80%), and the remaining 20% alveolar or spindle cell variants.[166] Sarcoma botryoides, a variant of embryonal rhabdomyosarcoma, presents with multiple polypoid nodules projecting into the lumen. Microscopically, three distinct zones are apparent: the submucosal hypercellular cambium layer, the middle myxoid hypocellular tissue, and the deeper immature, primitive hypercellular sarcomatous tissue, which is often myxomatous and similar to embryonal rhabdomyosarcoma (Fig. 6–99).

Embryonal rhabdomyosarcomas are composed of round to spindle-shaped mesenchymal cells that contain hyperchromatic nuclei and variable number of mitoses. Elongated strap-shaped cells and/or small round "tadpole" cells, both having acidophilic (eosinophilic) cytoplasm, are usually recognized. Cross striations may be identified. A myxoid stroma may be seen in focal areas (Fig. 6–100).

The tumor cells in alveolar rhabdomyosarcomas appear as loosely cohesive cells in spaces formed by fibrous septa, simulating a glandular neoplasm or lymphoma (Fig. 6–101A). The possibility of rhabdomyoblasts is suggested by a rim of eosinophilic,

sometimes striated, cytoplasm around the nucleus (Fig. 6–101B). This alveolar architecture may be seen focally in embryonal rhabdomyosarcomas. In the pleomorphic variant, tumor cells exhibit large, bizarre, single or multiple nuclei and abundant eosinophilic cytoplasm (Figs. 6–102 A and B).

A spindle cell variant of rhabdomyosarcoma was reported in the nasosinus.[167,168] The tumor cells are arranged in interlacing bundles simulating leiomyosarcoma (Fig. 6–103 A and B). In other areas, tumor cells form storiform patterns and are separated by abundant collagenous stroma resulting in hypocellularity. Because areas of typical embryonal rhabdomyosarcoma tend to occur in the periphery of the tumor, some authors consider this to be a variant of embryonal rhabdomyosarcoma (Fig. 6–103C).[168] Rhabdomyoblastic differentiation is suggested by a densely eosinophilic, sometimes refractile, cytoplasm and cross striations (Fig. 6–103D).

The pathologist may encounter difficulty in establishing the diagnosis of rhabdomyosarcoma, especially in small specimens in which characteristic rhabdomyoblasts cannot be identified. By multiple immunohistochemical stains, 90% of rhabdomyosarcomas express one or more muscle cell markers, such as myoglobin, desmin, and muscle-specific actin.[166]

With current combined treatment modalities the 5-year survival rates have improved to 44% for nasosinus rhabdomyosarcomas.[168] For rhabdomyosarcoma of the orbit and other head and neck regions, the survival rates are even higher—in the range of 90% and 75%, respectively.[165]

Smooth Muscle Tumors

Smooth muscle tumors of the nasosinus are rare. In a review of literature up to 1990, 30 cases of leiomyosarcoma were reported, whereas only a few examples of leiomyoma were recorded.[169,170] In the nasosinus, about one third of leiomyosarcomas were confined to the nasal cavity, and the remaining two thirds involved either the paranasal sinus or both the nasal cavity and paranasal sinuses, usually maxillary sinus.[170] The patients presented with small, 2 cm pedunculated, polypoid nodules or bulky masses, which had grey-red whorled cut surfaces.

The tumor cells are arranged in 90-degree interlacing bundles with nuclear palisading and blunt-ended nuclei in longitudinal cuts. On cross section, clear halos surround the nuclei. Fibrillar eosinophilic cytoplasm is evident by hematoxylin and eosion and trichrome stains (Fig. 6–104 A and B on page 198). Mitotic figures are numerous.[169] In one study, one to 13 mitotic figures were found per 10 high-power fields.[170] By immunohistochemistry, muscle specific actin, and desmin were positive in 86%

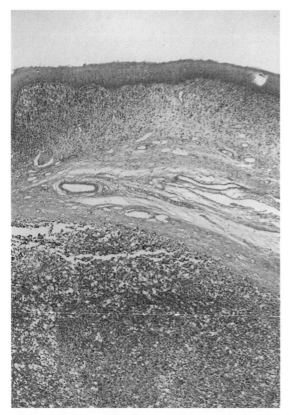

FIGURE 6–99 Sarcoma botryoides of nasopharynx. Beneath the squamous epithelium are three distinct zones: the hypercellular cambium zone immediately beneath the squamous epithelium, myxoid hypocellular tissue, and deeper pleomorphic sarcoma.

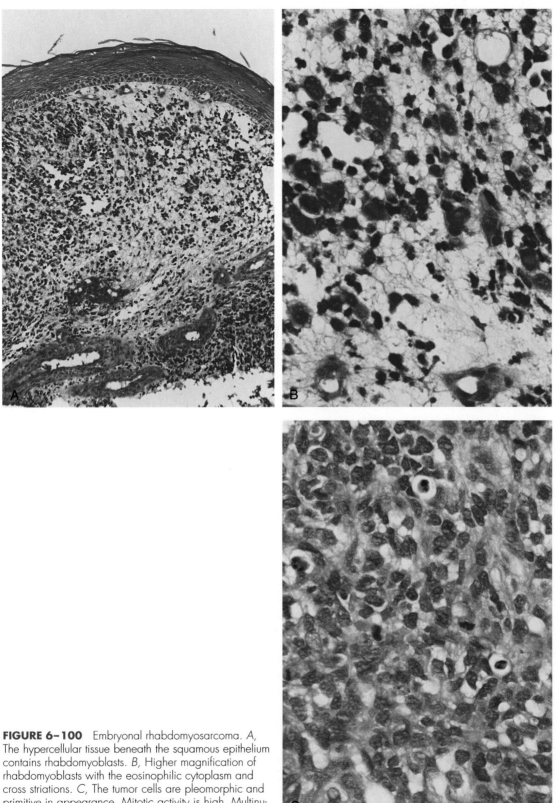

FIGURE 6-100   Embryonal rhabdomyosarcoma. *A,* The hypercellular tissue beneath the squamous epithelium contains rhabdomyoblasts. *B,* Higher magnification of rhabdomyoblasts with the eosinophilic cytoplasm and cross striations. *C,* The tumor cells are pleomorphic and primitive in appearance. Mitotic activity is high. Multinucleated giant cells and rhabdomyoblasts may be seen.

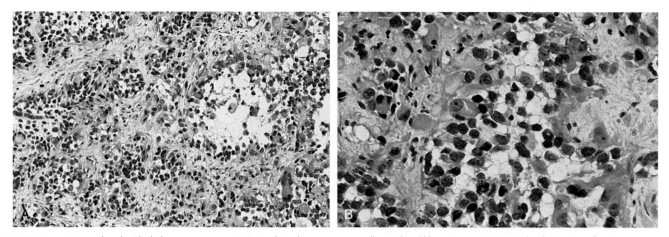

FIGURE 6–101   Alveolar rhabdomyosarcoma. *A,* Loosely cohesive tumor cells in gland-like spaces. Even on this low magnification, some of the cells have identifiable eosinophilic cytoplasm. *B,* Higher magnification to demonstrate rhabdomyoblasts with eosinophilic cytoplasm.

(six of seven) and 14% (one of seven) of cases, respectively.[170]

In most cases, surgical resection is followed by radiotherapy and/or chemotherapy for locally advanced tumor. The prognosis is excellent if the tumor is localized to the nasal cavity, with all cases reported to be free of tumor recurrence.[170] In contrast, in the presence of sinus involvement, 70% of patients had tumor recurrence, 10% died of tumor, and only 15% were disease free.[170]

Fatty Tumors

These tumors are rarely seen in the nasosinus.[171,172] In the head and neck region, well-differentiated and

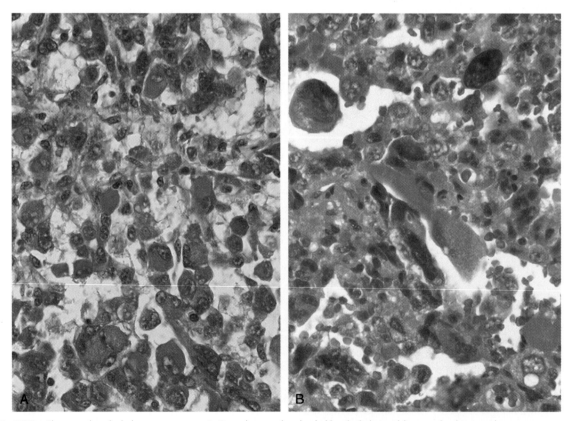

FIGURE 6–102   Pleomorphic rhabdomyosarcoma. *A,* Round to oval tadpole-like rhabdomyoblasts with pleomorphic eccentric nuclei, prominent nucleoli, and abundant eosinophilic cytoplasm. *B,* Pleomorphic cells with gigantic nuclei and cross striations. Some are multinucleated.

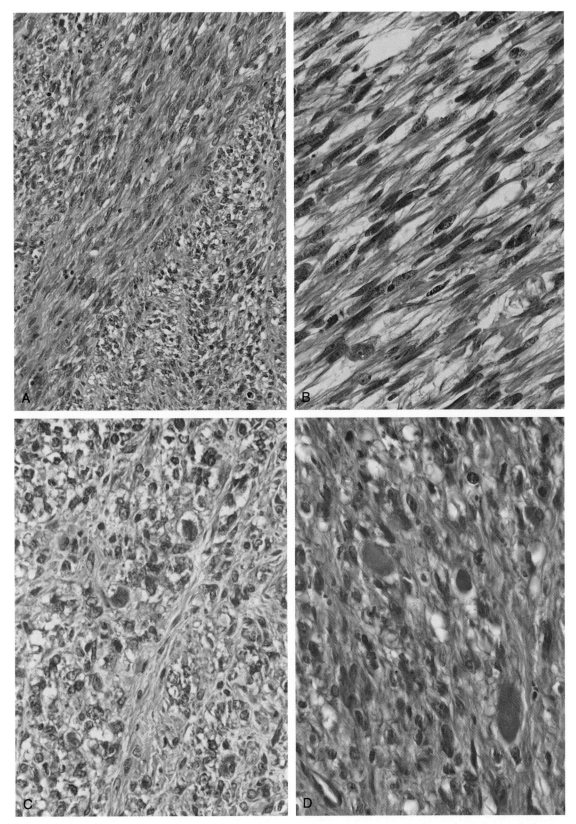

FIGURE 6–103 Spindle cell variant of rhabdomyosarcoma. *A,* Tumor cells form interlacing bundles with 90-degree angles resembling smooth muscle tumors. *B,* Tumor cells have longitudinal fibrillar cytoplasm and blunted nuclei. *C,* Rhabdomyoblastic differentiation. *D,* Rhabdomyoblasts with cross striations.

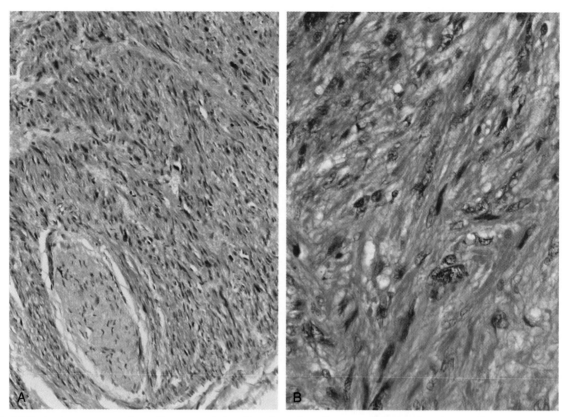

FIGURE 6-104 Leiomyosarcoma of maxillary sinus. *A,* Bundles of spindle cells surround the peripheral nerve fibers. *B,* Individual cells have irregular, hyperchromatic nuclei and fibrillar eosinophilic cytoplasm that is positive for desmin by immunohistochemistry supporting smooth muscle origin.

myxoid liposarcomas have lower risk for local recurrence and distant metastasis than round cell and pleomorphic liposarcomas.

Neural and Neuroectodermal Tumors

NASAL GLIOMA

Nasal glioma is a congenital malformation, in which displaced glial tissue occurs without intracranial connection, and the meningeal continuity to the brain has closed during embryonic development. In contrast, encephalocele results from herniation of brain tissue and leptomeninges through a bony defect of the skull. The excised tissue has the appearance of normal brain with connection to ventricle or subarachnoid space. Degeneration may result in loss of neurons. In such cases distinction from nasal glioma will require other clinical findings.[173]

Nasal gliomas usually are found in infants but occasionally may be identified in older children and adults. The majority of these lesions (approximately 60%) present as small, firm subcutaneous nodules at or near the bridge of the nose. About 30% produce intranasal masses that are usually attached to the

upper part of the nasal cavity and often have a polypoid appearance. A few have been described in the paranasal sinuses (frontal, maxillary), tongue, palate, tonsillar region, and nasopharynx.[174] Approximately 10% are found within both the nasal cavity and the subcutaneous tissue. The intranasal masses may produce symptoms of nasal obstruction. Lesions thought to be nasal gliomas may be resected by local surgical excision. This should be avoided if an encephalocele is connected to the cranial cavity as seen by imaging techniques.

Nasal gliomas grow slowly, apparently at the same rate as normal brain tissue. Histologically, nests and masses of fibrillary neuroglial tissue form a prominent network of glial fibers. Astrocytic cells may show gemistocytic changes (Fig. 6-105). Neuronal cells are rarely identified. Large astrocytic cells may be misinterpreted as histiocytes. Choroid plexus, ependymal cells, and pigmented cells with retinal differentiation have also been reported.[166,173] Recurrence after excision is found in 4% to 10% of cases.[162,172] Rare cases of heterotopic brain tissue have been reported to occur in the nasopharynx, including one giving rise to oligodendroglioma.[174,175]

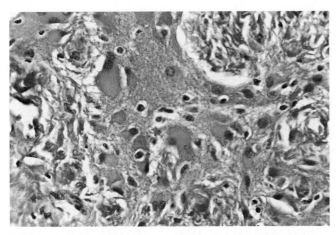

FIGURE 6–105 Nasal glioma with gliosis and gemistocytic astrocytes.

MENINGIOMA

Meningiomas are derived from meningeal arachnoid cells, which are generally considered to be neuroectodermal in origin. Rarely, meningiomas may arise outside the cranial cavity in such sites as the nasal cavity, paranasal sinuses, middle ear, temporal bone, parotid gland, and orbital cavity.[176] These ectopic tumors are thought to originate in arachnoid cells that are trapped within or outside bone when the various cranial bones develop and fuse.

In a series of 12 nasal and sinus meningiomas, about half had evidence of cranial involvement.[176] In these patients the meningiomas probably originated intracranially, infiltrated locally, and first manifested clinically outside the cranial cavity. Other patients have no demonstrable intracranial lesion, and the tumor can be accepted as an ectopic meningioma. Within the nasal cavity and paranasal sinuses, meningiomas may grow as polyps or space-occupying masses. In these cases the pathologist usually receives curetted pieces of firm, grey tissue. Histologically these lesions have the appearance of intracranial meningiomas. Meningotheliomatous form is most commonly found in the nasosinus meningiomas. Psammoma bodies may or may not be present. Unless the pathologist remembers that meningiomas may be seen in this area, these lesions may be misdiagnosed as some type of epithelial or soft tissue neoplasm. They may be confused particularly with the psammomatous type of ossifying fibroma, especially in frozen sections. Immunohistochemical characters include frequent positivity for vimentin and epithelial membrane antigen and coexpression of cytokeratin and S-100 protein in some meningiomas.[177]

PITUITARY TUMOR

Pituitary tumors may occasionally infiltrate locally through the sellar bone and extend into the sphe-noid sinus, posterior nasal cavity, and/or superior nasopharynx, there producing polypoid lesions or space-occupying masses leading to nasal obstruction. Some of these tumors may arise in ectopic pituitary tissue, misplaced during the migration of anterior pituitary cells from Rathke's pouch, an evagination from the nasopharyngeal roof. Both invasive and ectopic adenomas may be locally destructive and aggressive.[178]

Histologically, these neoplasms are composed of nests and cords of cells, producing an epithelial pattern and sometimes extending into the bone (Fig. 6–106 A–C). Most of the tumor cells are chromophobic type with abundant amphophilic or vacuolated cytoplasm (see Fig. 6–106A). Occasional cells have acidophilic cytoplasm with fine or coarse granules (see Fig. 6–106B). Tumor cells may show a moderate degree of nuclear pleomorphism and mitotic activity, leading to the diagnosis of carcinoma or plasmacytoma (Fig. 6–106D). Immunohistochemical stains are helpful to identify pituitary hormones. A few tumors have produced prolactin, TSH, or ACTH with Cushing's syndrome.[179]

PARAGANGLIOMA

Paragangliomas rarely occur in the nasal cavity and paranasal sinuses. In a series of 73 paragangliomas of the head and neck region, three were reported in the nasal cavity.[180] Symptoms include epistaxis and/or nasal obstruction. These lesions may produce polypoid or space-occupying masses and may locally infiltrate into adjacent bone. Histologically, these neoplasms have the typical appearance of paragangliomas: small nests of uniform chief cells and occasional sustentacular cells lying in a richly vascular stroma. Irregular, large, hyperchromatic nuclei may be seen. Paragangliomas are usually benign and not functional; rare examples of ACTH production with Cushing's syndrome and malignant behavior have been reported.[180,181] The differential diagnosis includes olfactory neuroblastoma. Paraganglioma cells have more abundant cytoplasm, form compact cell balls throughout the tumor, and reveal rare, if any, mitotic activity.

SCHWANN CELL TUMOR

Schwann cell tumors may arise from branches of the trigeminal nerve and autonomic nervous system to involve the nasal cavity and paranasal sinuses.[182] The Schwann cell tumors arising in this area exhibit the same histologic features as those seen elsewhere. Neurilemomas (schwannomas) are more common than neurofibromas and present as encapsulated nodules. Compact bundles of Schwann cells with nuclear palisading are intermingled with hypocellular myxoid stroma (Fig. 6–107A). In neurofibromas, bundles of schwannian cells have comma-shaped nuclei in a myxoid stroma. Large, hyperchromatic,

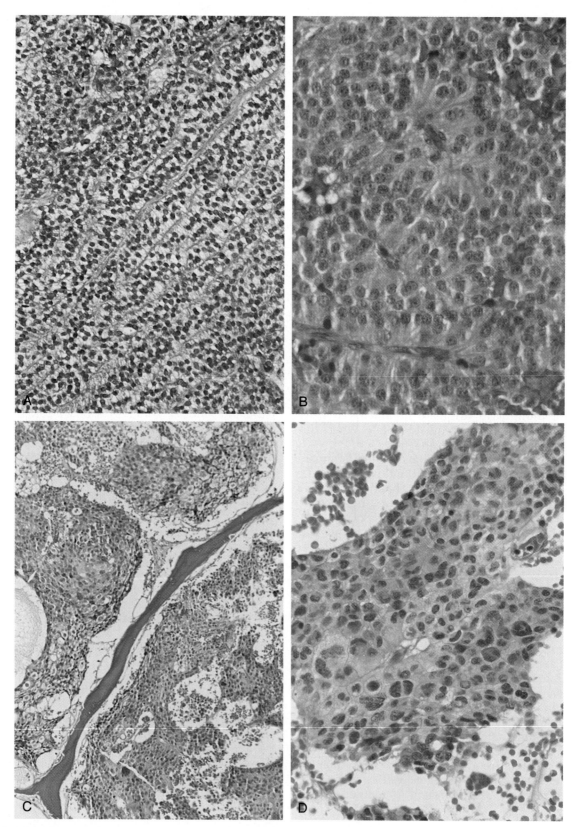

FIGURE 6–106 Pituitary adenoma presenting as nasopharyngeal mass. *A,* Sheet of monotonous epithelial cells having uniform nuclei and vacuolated cytoplasm. *B,* A close association with capillaries suggests an organoid, pseudorosette pattern seen in neuroendocrine neoplasms. *C,* Infiltration of bone by sheets of tumor cells resembling a metastatic carcinoma. *D,* Nuclear atypia may occur in pituitary adenoma.

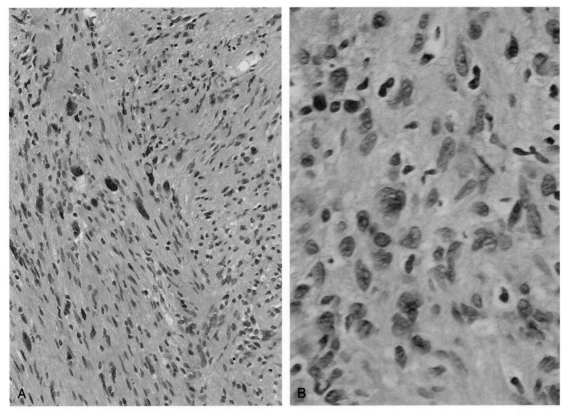

FIGURE 6-107 Schwannoma of nasal cavity. *A*, Schwannian cells form interlacing bundles with nuclear palisading. *B*, Nuclear hyperchromasia and irregularity are common in schwannomas and neurofibromas.

irregular nuclei are commonly found in schwannomas and neurofibromas (Fig. 6–107B). This feature alone is not indicative of malignancy.

MALIGNANT SCHWANNOMA

Malignant schwannomas have high cellularity, increased mitotic activity, and nuclear atypia (Fig. 6–108 A and B).[183] These tumors are highly aggressive with an overall survival of 15% following surgery and radiotherapy.[184,185] However, Heffner and Gnepp[155] reported a group of malignant schwannoma having uniform cells resembling well-differentiated fibrosarcoma, low mitotic activity, and low-grade malignant behavior. Five of 10 malignant schwannoma contained rhabdomyoblastic elements, the so-called Triton tumors (Fig. 6–108 C and D). Because in the nasosinus skeletal muscle cells normally occur only in the posterior nasal choanae (palatal muscle), orbit, and facial muscle in the subcutaneous tissue of nose, these skeletal muscle cells in the malignant schwannoma are considered part of the tumor.

OLFACTORY NEUROBLASTOMA

Olfactory neuroblastomas are thought to arise from the specialized sensory neuroepithelial (neuroecto-dermal) cells that are normally found in the upper part of the nasal cavity, including the superior nasal concha, the upper part of septum, the roof of nose, and the cribriform plate of ethmoid.[186,187] These specialized cells, in addition to giving rise to neuroblastomas, are the likely progenitor of "neuroendocrine" carcinomas and mixed neuroblastoma and carcinoma.[188–190]

Olfactory neuroblastomas may occur in any age group but most often after the age of 40 years.[186] These tumors most commonly cause nasal obstruction, epistaxis, and a mass high in the nasal cavity and ethmoid region. Rare examples of functional olfactory neuroblastomas with secretion of vasopressin causing hypertension and severe hyponatremia have been reported.[191,192]

The excised tumors vary from a small polypoid nodule less than 1 cm in size to a large mass involving ethmoids and nasal cavity bilaterally with extension into the adjacent paranasal sinuses. The smooth surface appears grey-tan to pink-red and hypervascular (Fig. 6–109).

The histologic appearance of olfactory neuroblastomas varies by differentiation. The well-differentiated tumors are usually composed of cellular nests surrounded by fine fibrovascular septa in an organoid fashion. These relatively uniform cells, which are slightly larger than lymphocytes, lie in a finely

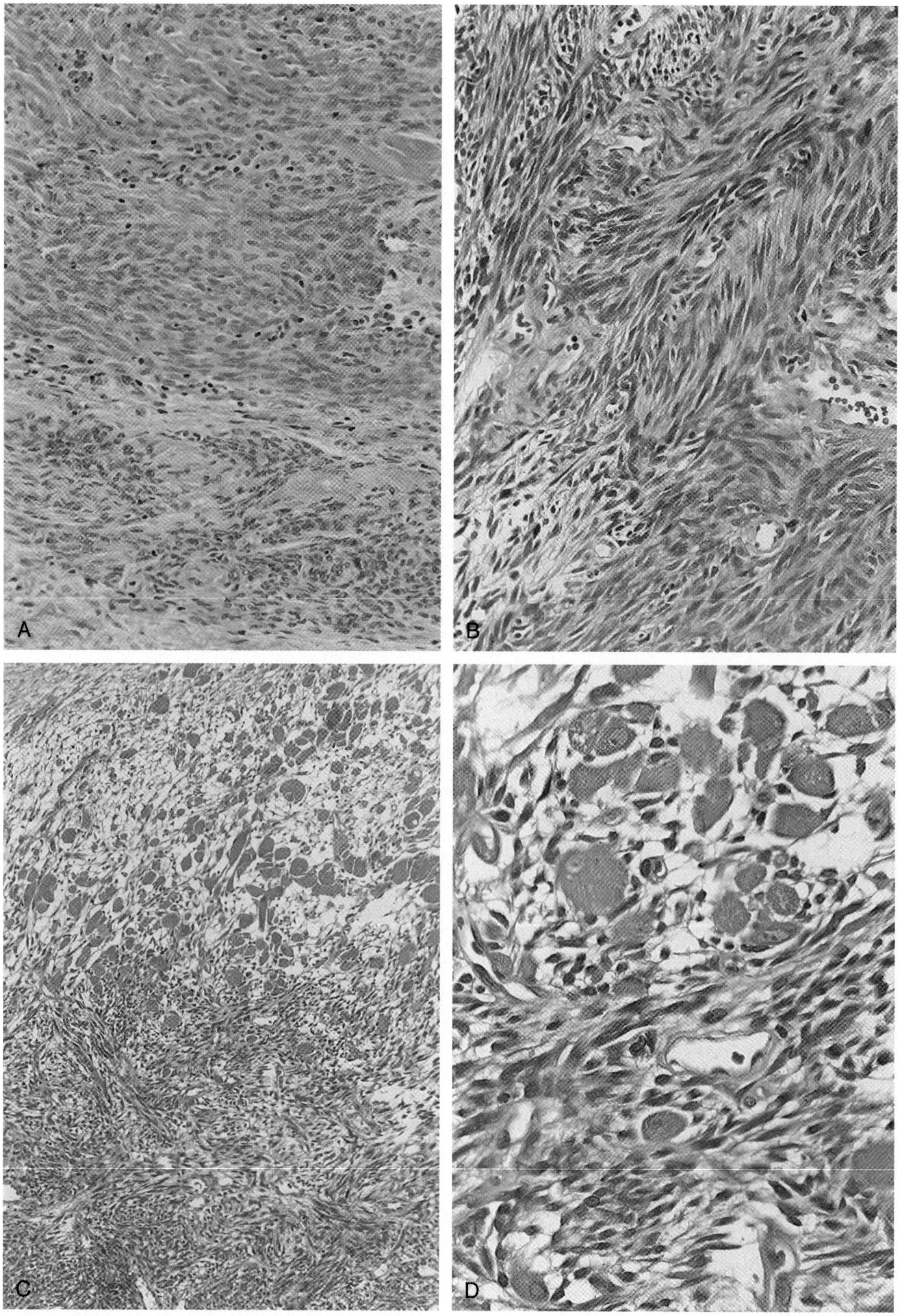

FIGURE 6–108   Malignant schwannoma. *A*, Tumor cells form a whorl-like pattern. *B*, Tumor cells form interlacing bundles with nuclear palisading and a herringbone pattern. *C*, Triton tumor. Spindle cells form storiform pattern and interlacing bundles. Mature rhabdomyoblasts can be identified even on this low power. *D*, Higher magnification to show mature rhabdomyoblasts with cross striations.

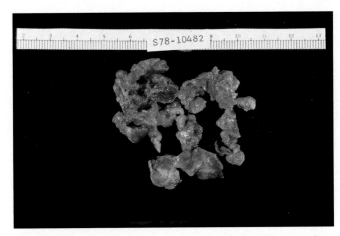

FIGURE 6–109 Olfactory neuroblastoma of ethmoid sinus. It has a multinodular, vascular appearance.

By immunohistochemistry, neuron-specific enolase and synaptophysin are positive in more than 80% of olfactory neuroblastomas[193] and expressed in a diffuse pattern.[189] A small number of cells in the periphery of tumor nests react with the antibodies against S-100 protein and glial filament acidic protein (GFAP) to indicate Schwann cell differentiation.[193,194] This focal and peripheral distribution helps to distinguish olfactory neuroblastoma from malignant melanoma, which contain more diffuse S-100 protein positive cells and also cells containing melanoma antigen demonstrable by antibody HMB-45. It is interesting that olfactory neuroblastoma cells are negative for Ewing's sarcoma associated MIC2 antigen.[189] Thus, this antigen can be used to separate olfactory neuroblastoma from Ewing's sarcoma and primitive neuroectodermal tumors.

Differential Diagnosis

In a small biopsy specimen of an olfactory neuroblastoma in which considerable crush artifact has occurred, the pathologist may see nests of somewhat dark-staining cells. The neurofibrillar stroma may not be easily recognized. As a result the olfactory neuroblastoma may be misinterpreted as some type of poorly differentiated or undifferentiated carcinoma. Immunohistochemical stains may not be conclusive, because low-molecular-weight cytokeratin can be positive in one third of olfactory neuroblastomas,[193] and neuroendocrine markers are positive in some of the undifferentiated carcinomas.[188,193] In general, poorly differentiated and undifferentiated carcinomas have higher mitotic activity, more distinct nucleoli, and obvious necrosis.

Conversely, other types of nasal tumors may be misinterpreted as olfactory neuroblastoma, including undifferentiated carcinomas, various poorly differentiated adenocarcinomas, malignant lymphomas, and even embryonal rhabdomyosarcomas. Multiple immunohistochemical stains are needed to come to a correct diagnosis. Finally, the discussion of neuroendocrine carcinoma is covered in a later section.

Prognosis

Olfactory neuroblastomas grow slowly into the adjacent structures and recur in 30% of cases after surgical excision. Localized nasal tumors have a better prognosis than those involving the adjacent sinuses and structures. Cervical lymph node metastases are seen in about 20% of cases.[186] If distant metastases are included, the overall rates of metastasis in different series increase to 38%[186] to 62%.[191] The 5-year survival rates are in the range of 58%, but the actual cure rate is lower, because these tumors may recur many years after initial treatment.[186] Most reports recommend that these neoplasms be treated with a combination of surgical resection and radiotherapy.[186,191]

fibrillar stroma (Fig. 6–110A). Homer Wright pseudorosettes are characterized by rings of neoplastic cells with finely fibrillar or granular material in the center (Fig. 6–110B). True rosettes of Flexner variant, defined as duct-like spaces lined by nonciliated columnar cells with basally placed nuclei, are only rarely identified (Fig. 6–110C). The cells have round to oval nuclei with a uniformly distributed fine or coarse chromatin pattern (Fig. 6–110D). Only occasional prominent nucleoli may be seen. Nuclear pleomorphism is minimal. Mitotic activity is variable, but generally low. In a small number of cases, rare mature and immature ganglion cells may be seen. Occasionally, the adjacent seromucous glands undergo hyperplasia or oncocytic metaplasia. When neuroblastoma cells infiltrate into the oncocytes, an oncocytic carcinoid tumor or neuroendocrine carcinoma is suggested (Fig. 6–110E). By immunohistochemical stains, neuroendocrine differentiation is evident in the tumor cells, but negative in the glandular cells (Fig. 6–110F).

As the olfactory neuroblastomas become less mature and poorly differentiated, pseudorosettes and fibrillar stroma occur rarely. The tumor cells form large, solid sheets and reveal anaplastic, round to oval nuclei with high mitotic activity, small nucleoli, and coarse chromatin (Fig. 6–111 A and B). Tumor cells undergo necrosis. Their neural differentiation requires immunohistochemistry or electron microscopy to confirm (Fig. 6–111C).

By ultrastructural study, membrane-bound dense core neurosecretory granules are present in the cytoplasm and in nerve processes, which additionally contain neurotubules and neurofilaments. The diameter of the granules is 90 to 240 μm. The fibrillary stroma corresponds to immature nerve processes.[188] Cells lining the true rosettes provide evidence of olfactory differentiation with olfactory vesicles and microvilli on apical borders.[188]

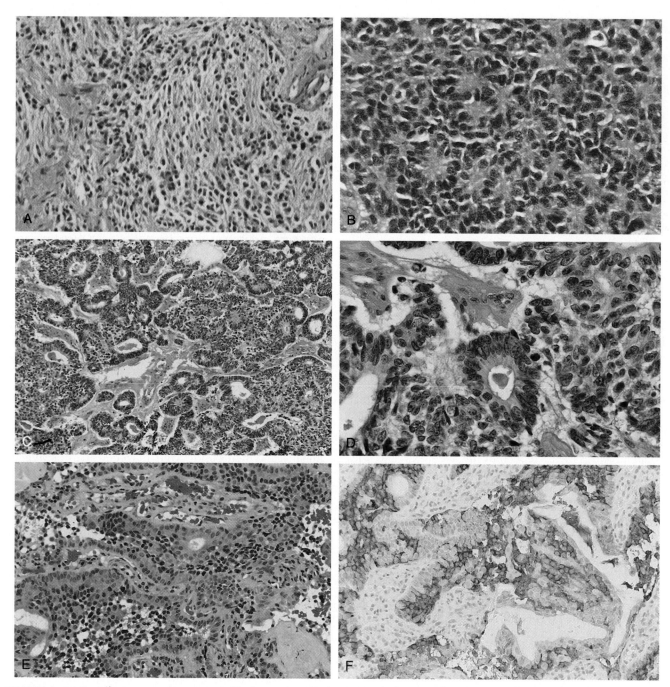

FIGURE 6–110 Olfactory neuroblastoma. *A,* Fibrillar matrix in the background of tumor cells. *B,* Tumor cells are arranged in a pseudorosette pattern. *C,* Flexner type of rosettes and glandular spaces. Notice the background vascular stroma. *D,* Higher magnification of a Flexner rosette merging with the background neuroepithelial cells, a useful feature to distinguish from glandular tumors. In addition the nucleoli are indistinct. Cells of nasosinus adenocarcinoma usually have more prominent nucleoli. *E,* Tumor cells infiltrate the adjacent hyperplastic seromucous glands with lumens, which may simulate tumor rosettes. *F,* Immunohistochemical stain for synaptophysin is positive in the tumor cells and negative in the glandular cells.

NEUROENDOCRINE CARCINOMA

Neuroendocrine carcinomas are nasal tumors that on light microscopic examination have a histologic spectrum from carcinoid tumors to small cell neuroendocrine carcinomas.[188] Some tumor cells may have an oncocytic appearance with abundant eosinophilic granular cytoplasm.[195] In spite of variation in the degree of nuclear atypia and mitotic activity, these tumors share the following features: a distinct organoid arrangement, punctate chromatin pattern, and inconspicuous nucleoli. Nuclei are oval or elongated (Fig. 6–112 *A* and *B*). Some authors reported functional neuroendocrine carcinomas with secretion of

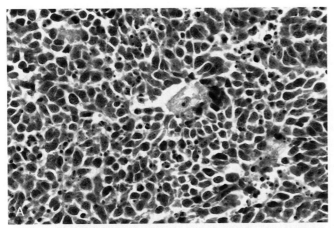

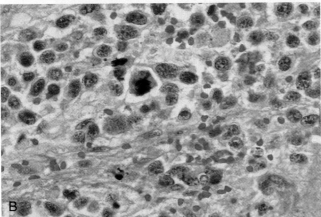

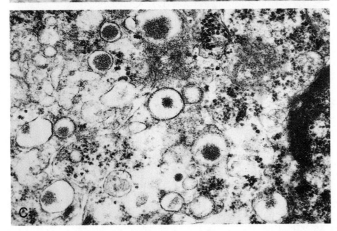

FIGURE 6-111 Poorly differentiated olfactory neuroblastoma. *A,* Diffuse small cells undergoing individual cell necrosis. *B,* Tumor cells have coarsely granular chromatin, indistinct nucleoli, bizarre mitosis, and fibrillar matrix. *C,* Membrane-bound neuroendocrine granules with dense cores and outer clear halos.

corticotropin, calcitonin, or beta-melanocyte–stimulating hormone.[196]

By immunohistochemical stains most neuroendocrine carcinomas express cytokeratin.[189] Neuroendocrine markers, such as neuron specific enolase, synaptophysin, and chromogranin, are focal (Fig. 6–112 *C* and *D*).[188] This is in contrast to a more diffuse and intense immunoreactivity seen in olfactory neuro-

blastomas.[189] Additionally, cytokeratin is more diffuse and prominent in neuroendocrine carcinomas than olfactory neuroblastomas.[189]

Ultrastructurally, cells of neuroendocrine carcinomas contain neurosecretory granules, but they differ from olfactory neuroblastoma by having desmosomal junctions and tonofilaments, and lacking neurofilaments and neuritic processes.[188,196] However, because of the morphologic continuum between olfactory neuroblastoma and neuroendocrine carcinoma, the distinction cannot be made in all cases. Prognosis has not been clearly defined because of the small number of cases reported. The prognosis is reported to correlate with the degree of differentiation, nuclear anaplasia, and mitotic activity.[188]

MIXED NEUROBLASTOMA AND CARCINOMA

Olfactory neuroblastoma may rarely coexist with adenocarcinomas, squamous carcinomas, or undifferentiated carcinomas (Fig. 6–113 *A* and *B*).[190] It has been suggested that these mixed neoplasms arise from the basal cells of the olfactory epithelium.[190]

PRIMITIVE NEUROECTODERMAL TUMORS

Primitive neuroectodermal tumors (PNET) may rarely involve the head and neck region as primary or secondary tumor.[197,198] Similar to other round cell tumors, the neoplastic cells have predominantly round to oval nuclei and scant cytoplasm. Occasional nuclei are elongated. They grow in a diffuse infiltrative pattern and undergo active mitosis. The histologic distinction from malignant schwannoma, olfactory neuroblastoma, and Ewing's sarcoma can be difficult and requires immunohistochemical stains. In the majority of PNETs, the tumor cells express vimentin and mic2 glycoproteins. S-100 protein and neuroendocrine markers may be positive in some cells. Olfactory neuroblastoma cells are generally negative for vimentin and mic2 glycoproteins.[189] Malignant schwannoma and Ewing's sarcoma do not express neuroendocrine differentiation.

Melanocytic Lesions and Tumors

MELANOSIS AND NEVI

These are rarely found in this area. When present, the nasal vestibule is most commonly affected, followed by the nasal mucosa. In association with nasosinus malignant melanomas, melanocytic hyperplasia and melanin pigment may be seen in the respiratory mucosa and underlying seromucous glands (Fig. 6–114).[199]

MALIGNANT MELANOMAS

A group of 52 malignant melanomas arising in the mucous membranes of the head and neck had the

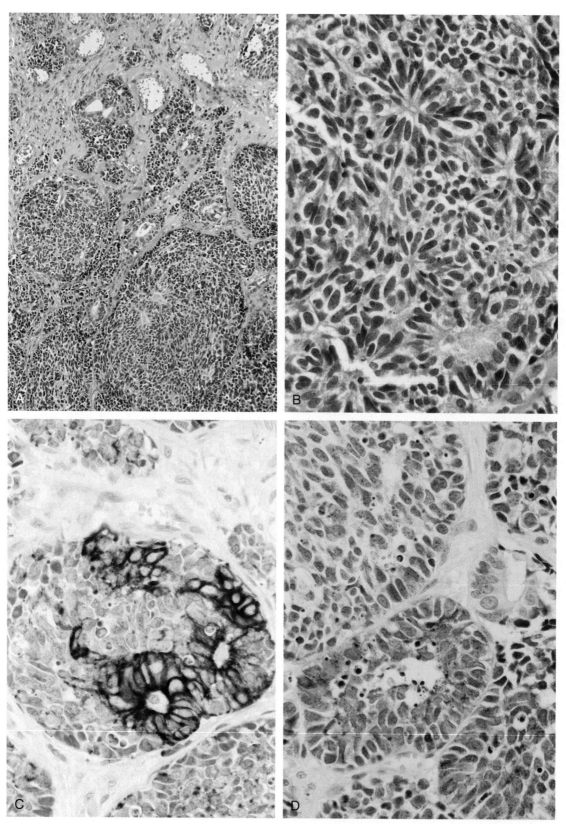

FIGURE 6–112 Neuroendocrine carcinoma. *A,* Broad sheets of tumor cells form occasional glandular spaces. *B,* The predominant cells have elongated nuclei with rosette-like arrangement. Tumor cells have finely granular chromatin and indistinct nucleoli. *C,* Immunohistochemical stain for cytokeratin is positive in tumor cells forming the glandular lumens, whereas the surrounding neuroepithelial-like cells are negative. *D,* Immunohistochemical stain for chromagranin is positive in some of the neuroepithelial cells.

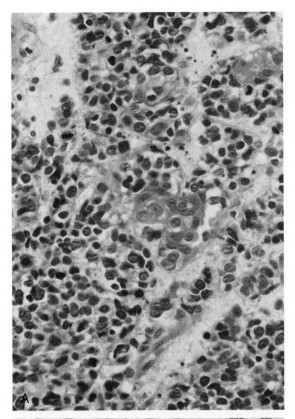

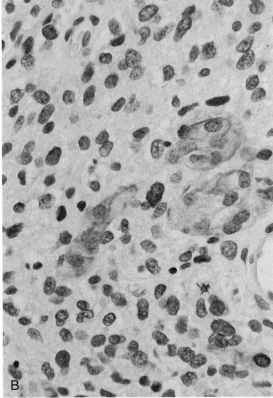

FIGURE 6–113 Mixed olfactory neuroblastoma and squamous cell carcinoma. *A,* Clusters of malignant squamous cells with eosinophilic cytoplasm. *B,* Immunohistochemical stain for cytokeratin is positive in the squamous cells, but negative in the neuroblastic cells.

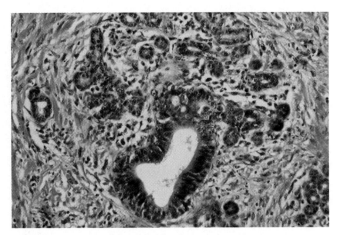

FIGURE 6–114 Melanosis of seromucous glands adjacent to a malignant melanoma.

following distribution: oral cavity, 26 (50%); nasal cavity and sinuses, 18 (35%) (including nasal cavity eight, maxillary antrum four, floor of nose two, ethmoid sinus two, vestibule one, and turbinate one); and pharyngolarynx, eight (15%).[200] Within the nasal cavity, malignant melanomas most commonly involve the nasal septum, followed by the inferior and middle turbinates.[200] Clinically, the majority of patients have symptoms of nasal obstruction and/or epistaxis.

Gross Pathology

Nasal melanomas at the time of diagnosis have usually reached a few centimeters in size, have a polypoid appearance, and vary in color from white to grey, brown, or black. The consistency has been described as firm, friable, or gelatinous.

Microscopic Pathology

Nasosinus malignant melanomas have a wide spectrum of changes seen in other melanomas. A helpful diagnostic feature is the presence of junctional activity and epidermal migration (Fig. 6–115*A*). Most nasosinus melanomas grow in sheets or nests of variable sizes. Polygonal cells of variable sizes may have vesicular nuclei and prominent nucleoli (Fig. 6–115*B*). In a small number of cases, spindle cells predominate (Fig. 6–115*C*). The amount of melanin pigment varies considerably. In a series of 14 nasosinus melanomas, the predominant features are small blue cells in eight cases (Fig. 6–115*D*), spindle cells in three neoplasms, epithelioid cells in two tumors, and pleomorphic cells in one case.[201] Thus, the differential diagnosis includes a wide range of tumors, including olfactory neuroblastoma, neuroendocrine carcinoma, undifferentiated carcinoma, lymphoma, and sarcoma.

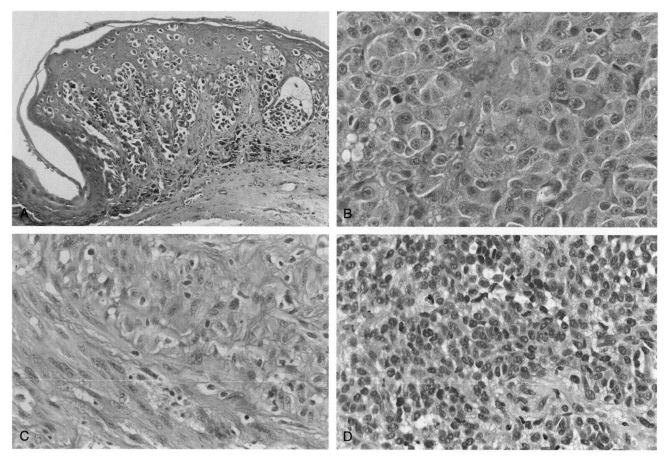

FIGURE 6–115 Malignant melanoma. *A,* Superficial spreading type of anterior nasal septum showing junctional activity and pagetoid migration of the epidermis by atypical melanocytes. *B,* Epithelioid melanoma cells with abundant eosinophilic cytoplasm, prominent nucleoli, and mitotic figures. *C,* Spindle cell variant. *D,* Small cell variant. Diffuse, loosely cohesive small round cells simulate malignant lymphoma.

Useful immunohistochemical stains include vimentin in 14 (100%) cases, melanoma antigen by HMB-45 in 13 (93%) neoplasms, and S-100 protein in 12 (86%) tumors.[201] Rare tumor cells may express epithelial membrane antigen and cytokeratin. Melanomas presenting as myxoid, botryoid mass[202] and metastatic melanoma to the nasosinus have been described.[203]

The prognosis of malignant melanomas arising in the nasosinus is generally poor because of advanced local disease. In one study only those patients whose melanomas measured less than 8 mm in thickness survived.[204] The reported 5-year survival rates are in the range of 25% to 30%.[204]

Dermoid Cyst, Teratoma, and Teratoid Carcinosarcoma

DERMOID CYST

Dermoid cysts have also been referred to as teratoid cysts, dermoid tumors, hamartoma, choristoma, and hairy polyps. They occur in the nasopharynx and are developmental anomalies of the first branchial arch in which ectodermal and mesodermal tissues are malformed rather than true neoplasms.[166] These lesions are usually recognized at birth but may be found somewhat later. Clinical problems include difficulty in breathing, sucking, or swallowing. These lesions may produce pedunculated masses attached to the lateral nasopharyngeal wall or to the nasopharyngeal portion of the soft palate. Sessile masses or those with short stalks may lead to complete obstruction of the nasopharynx.

Histologically, various tissues have been described, including skin, accessory skin structures, fibrous and adipose tissue, smooth muscle, skeletal muscle, cartilage, and bone. Minor salivary glands may be seen, but they may merely be entrapped glands. Treatment consists of surgical excision.

TERATOMA

True teratomas contain trigerminal elements and are found mainly in the nasopharynx of newborns and young infants (Fig. 6–116 *A* and *B*). The majority are mature teratomas. Even in the presence of im-

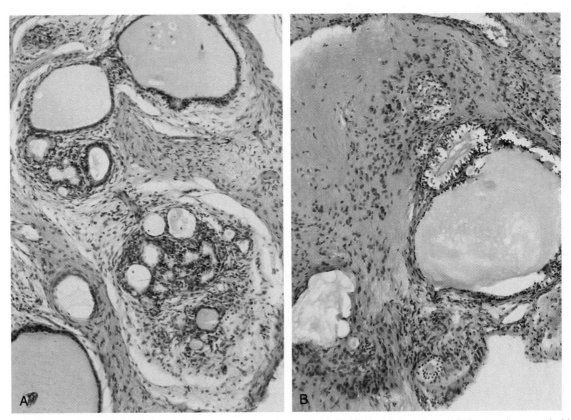

FIGURE 6–116 Immature teratoma of nasopharynx. *A,* Multiple cystic spaces lined by immature gut epithelium and surrounded by smooth muscle cells. *B,* Immature gut-like epithelium surrounded by central nervous tissue.

mature elements, tumor recurrence rarely occurs after surgical excision. In contrast, teratomas with carcinomatous elements or endodermal sinus tumor behave in a malignant fashion. Epignathi are teratomas that have differentiated into a parasitic fetus and are usually attached to the sphenoid bone.[166,205]

TERATOID CARCINOSARCOMA

Teratoid carcinosarcoma contains both carcinomatous and sarcomatous tissues.[206,207] The epithelial elements usually consist of mature glycogenated squamous cells and immature intestinal or respiratory epithelium (Fig. 6–117 *A–D*). Primitive neuroepithelial elements with rosettes, pseudorosettes, or neurofibrillary matrix often predominates in these tumors (Fig. 6–118 *A–C*). The stromal elements include hypercellular embryonal tissue with spindle cells embedded in a myxoid matrix, islands of cartilage and bone, smooth muscle, and skeletal muscle in varying degrees of maturation (Fig. 6–118*D;* see also Fig. 6–117 *A–D*). Although these carcinosarcomas histologically resemble immature teratomas, none contain seminoma, embryonal carcinoma, or choriocarcinoma. Their occurrence in adults with a median age of 60 years also differs from conventional germ cell tumor. An aggressive behavior is evident by the development of cervical lymph node metastases in 35% of patients and death in 60% of patients in 3 years.[206]

Osseous and Fibro-osseous Lesions and Tumors

Craniofacial bones develop directly from mesodermal cells through intramembranous ossification. Osteoid is first deposited in the stroma and developed into a woven fibrous bone. Later, osteoblasts line the borders of woven bone to form lamellar bone with regular cement lines. Craniofacial bones continue to grow into adult life and are in direct contact with dental structures and involved with adjacent inflammatory and infectious diseases. These special environments explain the development of unique lesions rarely seen in the long bones.

OSTEOMA

Osteomas of nasosinus involve predominantly the frontal sinus, especially the ostium at the junction of the frontal sinus and the anterior ethmoid air cells. Ethmoid and maxillary sinuses are less commonly

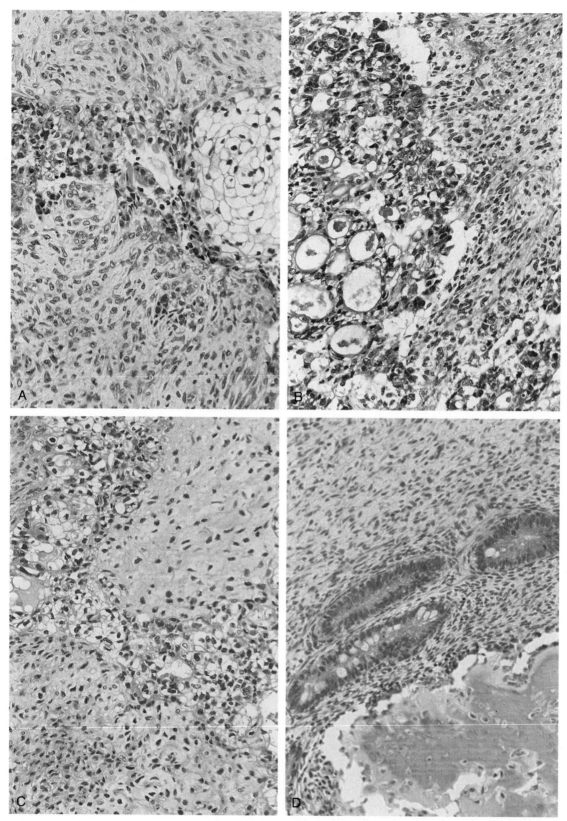

FIGURE 6–117   Teratoid carcinosarcoma. *A,* A nest of teratoid glycogenated squamous cells and myxoid hypercellular sarcomatous tissue. *B,* Glandular tissue surrounded by immature mesenchymal tissue. *C,* Chondroid differentiation. *D,* Immature gut-like epithelium surrounded by hypercellular mesenchymal and osteoid tissues.

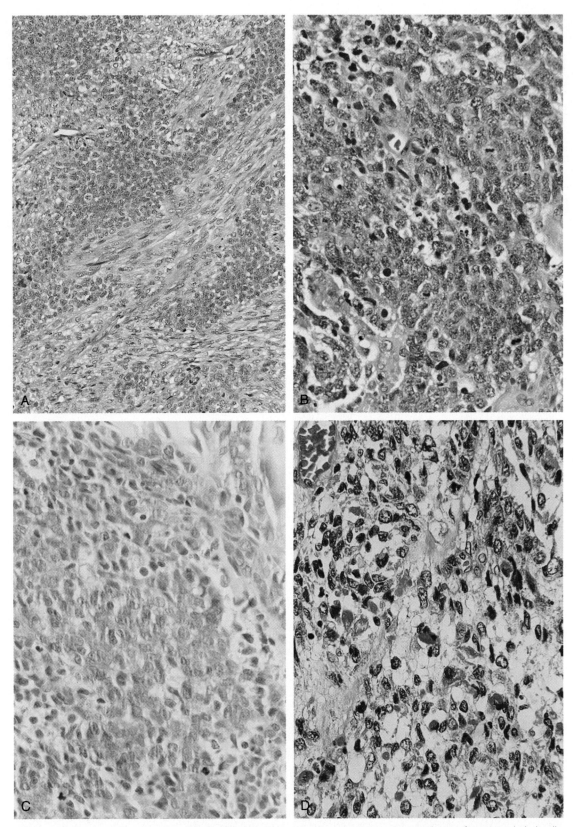

FIGURE 6-118   Teratoid carcinosarcoma. *A,* Neuroepithelial and mesenchymal components. *B,* Sheets of neuroepithelial cells consisting of small round cells with scant cytoplasm and active mitosis. *C,* Immunohistochemical stain for synaptophysin is diffusely positive to confirm neuroepithelial cells. *D,* Rhabdomyoblastic elements.

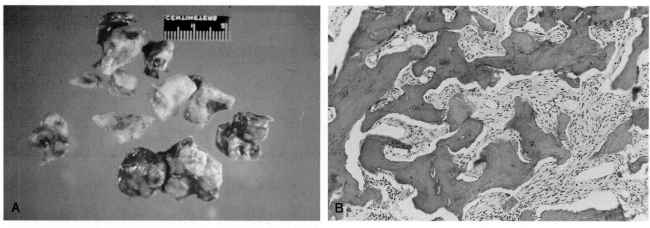

FIGURE 6–119 Mature osteoma of frontal sinus. *A,* Multiple nodules of sclerotic bone. *B,* Mature, thick lamellar bone and fibrous stroma.

affected.[208,209] Most patients are asymptomatic and the lesions are detected by radiographic studies. These osteomas vary in size from 1.5 mm to 30 mm (Fig. 6–119*A*) and consist of sclerotic bone with absence of Haversian canals (ivory type), mature lamellar bone (compact type), and bone and fibrous tissue (mixed type) (Fig. 6–119*B*).[208,209]

FIBROUS DYSPLASIA

Fibrous dysplasia represents a benign neoplasm or a hamartoma, in which osseous maturation is arrested at the woven bone stage, thus the lamellar bone is usually not seen.[208] Histologically, these lesions are composed of fibrous and osseous tissue in varying proportions (Fig. 6–120*A*). The moderately to highly

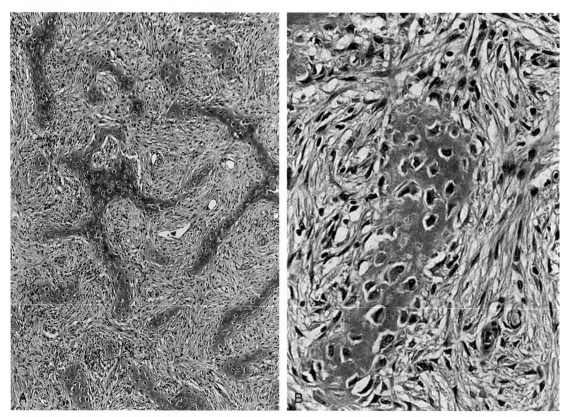

FIGURE 6–120 Fibrous dysplasia of maxillary sinus. *A,* Irregular woven bone surrounded by cellular fibrous stroma. *B,* Deposit of osteoid material by specialized mesenchymal cells results in the woven bone. However, there is no further maturation to the formation of lamellar bone and osteoblastic rimming. The background fibroblasts have uniform nuclei.

cellular fibrous stroma consists of relatively mature spindle-shaped fibroblasts, which usually do not show nuclear hyperchromasia, pleomorphism, or mitotic activity.

The osseous component contains irregular trabeculae of woven bone without osteoblasts or regular cement lines (Fig. 6–120B). With polarized light, woven bone with irregular birefringent fibers may be identified. In most cases the diagnosis poses no difficulty. However, foci of reactive new bone formation with trabeculae of lamellar bone lined by osteoblasts may be seen on the edges of the lesion, where it merges with the pre-existing bone. Similar reactive change may be found within recurrent lesions of fibrous dysplasia, sometimes obscuring the diagnostic foci of woven bone.

Rare cases of fibrous dysplasia may present with rapid growth simulating sarcoma or be complicated by mucocele and aneurysmal bone cyst.[210] Areas of giant cell reparative granuloma sometimes predominate the lesion, making a correct diagnosis difficult.

Fibrous dysplasia grows slowly and is usually treated with conservative local curettage or excision. Several surgical excisions may be required for cosmetic reasons. Radiotherapy is contraindicated because of the possibility of inducing sarcoma in the irradiated bone.

OSSIFYING FIBROMA

Ossifying fibroma behaves clinically as a locally aggressive neoplasm, invading locally and destroying adjacent bone. After local excision, recurrences are frequently seen, and more extensive resection may be required.[208] Histologically, ossifying fibromas are composed of fibrous tissue and lamellar bone with osteoblastic rimming, the former usually predominating (Fig. 6–121). The fibrous stroma varies from moderately to highly cellular. The spindle-shaped fi-

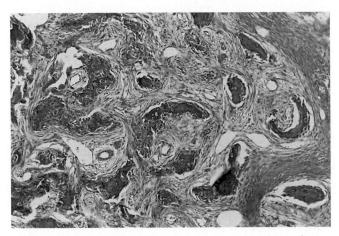

FIGURE 6–121 Ossifying fibroma, usual type, consisting of irregular, lamellar bone rimmed by osteoblasts. The fibrous stroma is mildly to moderately cellular.

broblastic cells usually show only minimal pleomorphism and mitotic activity.

In the juvenile variant of ossifying fibroma (JOF), the osseous components consist of cellular osteoid strands, "psammoma-like" islands, or cementum-like material. In the latter case, some authors apply the term cemento-ossifying fibroma. Other authors consider JOF a variant of fibrous dysplasia. In spite of different terms given to JOF, the clinical and pathologic features are distinct enough to be recognized as a separate entity.

The psammoma-like ossicles are laminated and rimmed by pink osteoid material and osteoblasts. Transitional stages between osteoid, psammoma-like bone, and more fully developed lamellar bone may be found.[208,211,212] The fibrous stroma is usually cellular with oval to elongated fibroblasts forming compact, whorl-like syncytium (Fig. 6–122 A–C). The mitotic activity and nuclear atypia are minimal. In the stroma, collections of osteoclasts, hemorrhage, and myxoid change indistinguishable from myxoma are sometimes prominent. Cystic spaces and aneurysmal bone cyst have also been reported.

Over 90% of facial juvenile ossifying fibromas occur in the paranasal sinuses, especially ethmoid sinus and nasal turbinates (one third), supra-orbital frontal region (one third), maxillary sinus (20%), mandible (10%), and sphenoid sinus (rare).[211] The reported mean age of the patients varies from 11.8 years[210] to 21 years.[212] At the time of surgery 60% of cases are under 19 years.[212] Male and females are equally affected. The frequency of polyostotic involvement varies from 5% to 46%.[211,212] Most patients present with a slowly growing facial mass, but depending on the locations, ocular symptoms with impaired vision, blindness, proptosis, and displacement of eyeball may occur. Following currettage, about 30% of cases recur and require resection of the lesion.[211,212]

Based on the anatomic location and morphologic spectrum, it is suggested that juvenile ossifying fibroma results from overgrowth of mucoperiosteum of sinus walls, especially those septa that lengthen during facial deveopment.[212] Familiarity with the distinct bone formation and cellular stroma helps to avoid overinterpretation of juvenile ossifying fibroma as fibromatosis, well-differentiated fibrosarcoma, or osteosarcoma.

GIANT CELL TUMORS

Both benign and malignant giant cell tumors have been reported in the nasosinus and base of skull.[208] Numerous osteoclast-type giant cells are evenly distributed throughout the lesion. The number of nuclei per giant cell is high and constant (Fig. 6–123A). The nuclei maintain round to oval configuration, which is also shared by the stromal cells (Fig. 6–123B). Secondary to hemorrhage, necrosis, and reactive new bone formation, fibroblasts proliferate. In

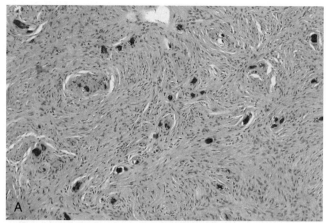

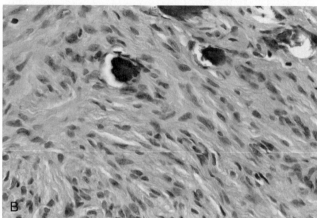

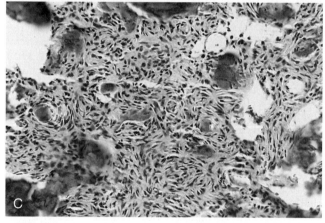

FIGURE 6–122   Ossifying fibroma, juvenile type. *A,* Scattered calcified psammoma-like bodies in a cellular fibrous tissue. *B,* Higher magnification of psammoma-like bodies. *C,* Psammoma-like structures are surrounded by hypercellular fibrous stroma, in which spindle cells are arranged in a storiform pattern. Nuclear atypia and mitotic activity are not evident.

the well-preserved areas, giant cells and stromal cells share the same nuclear features—a helpful point to separate giant cell tumor from other giant cell–rich lesions, including giant cell "reparative" granulomas, aneurysmal bone cyst, "brown tumors" of hyperparathyroidism, and fibrous histiocytomas.

GIANT CELL GRANULOMA AND ANEURYSMAL BONE CYST

Giant cell granuloma (Fig. 6–124) and aneurysmal bone cyst (Fig. 6–125) are considered to be morphologically identical.[213] Both affect teenagers and young adults, and the recurrent rates for both are similar in the range of 10% to 20%.[213] Giant cell tumor is rare before the age of 25. The predominant features are fibrous stroma, scattered giant cells, dilated vascular spaces, and reactive new bone. Within the fibrous stroma, fibroblasts are reactive in appearance with elongated nuclei, rather than the round to oval stromal cells seen in giant cell tumor (see Fig. 6–124).

In summary, although some authors consider all giant cell–rich craniofacial lesions to be the same disease,[214] others have observed aggressive giant cell tumors in these bones.[208,214] Whether or not giant cell lesions occurring in craniofacial Paget's disease represent true neoplasms is controversial.

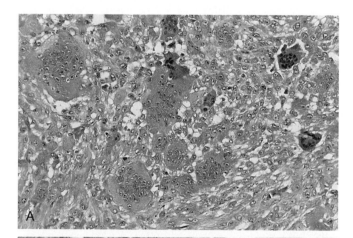

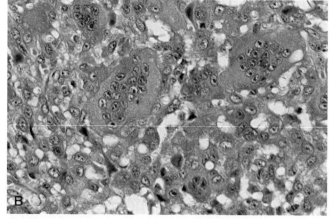

FIGURE 6–123   Giant cell tumor of maxilla. *A,* Osteoclastic giant cells contain many round to oval nuclei and medium-sized nucleoli. *B,* The background stromal cells share the same nuclear features as osteoclastic giant cells.

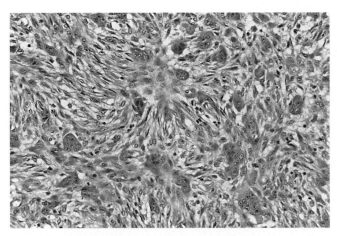

FIGURE 6-124 Giant cell reparative granuloma consisting of multinucleated osteoclasts and cellular fibrous stroma with a storiform pattern. The number of nuclei per osteoclast is variable and generally small.

OSTEOSARCOMA (OSTEOGENIC SARCOMA)

Osteosarcomas are composed histologically of overtly malignant spindle-shaped mesenchymal cells associated with immature osteoid and bone (Figs. 6-126 A–D).[208] Some patients developed osteosarcoma many years following radiotherapy for retinoblastoma. The age of patients is about 2 decades older than that of long bones cases. Overall, 33% of patients with osteosarcoma of the head and neck region were disease-free for more than 5 years, and those who received combined treatment modality had the lowest recurrent rates.[215]

Cartilaginous Tumors

CHONDROMA

Kilby and Ambegaokar[216] reported 128 nasal chondromas with the following distribution: ethmoids and nasal cavity, 50%; nasal septum, 17%; maxilla and maxillary antrum, 18%; hard palate, 6%; nasopharynx, sphenoid sinus, and eustachian tube, 6%; and alar cartilage, 3%. Most of these chondromas are small, less than 2 cm in size and likely to be hamartomas.[216,217] They have the appearance of well-circumscribed, mature, lobulated hyaline cartilage with mild increase of cellularity (Fig. 6-127). Nuclear atypia is absent. Focal calcification, ossification, and mucinous degeneration occur rarely.

Enzinger et al[218] described a group of subcutaneous and soft tissue tumors under the name of "ossifying fibromyxoid tumor of soft part." Most of these tumors occurred in the upper and lower extremities and trunk. About 14% involved the head and neck region. This author encountered one such tumor in the nasal vestibule. This well-circumscribed 1.5 cm nodule consisted of lobulated fibromyxoid stroma

with focal osteoid deposits (Fig. 6-128A). Oval to elongated fibroblasts were arranged in bundles and cords. The nuclei were uniform or slightly irregular in shape (Fig. 6-128B). The cytoplasm was scant without demonstrable glycogen by PAS stains. Mitotic activity was low, averaging one to two mitotic figures per 10 high-power fields. The osteoid material appeared as lace-like eosinophilic material or large trabeculae. The cellularity was focally high enough to raise the suspicion of sarcoma. One of the most distinctive features is a shell-like mature bone beneath the capsule. By immunohistochemistry, 74% of tumors express S-100 protein to suggest cartilaginous or neural origin.[218] After local excision, 27% of patients developed one or more recurrences, but none died of tumor.[218]

McDermott et al[219] reported seven examples of nasal chondromesenchymal hamartoma, which is similar to the chest wall mesenchymal hamartoma. Except for one patient, who was 7 years old at diagnosis, all others were 3 months old or younger. These nasal tumors may extend into the ethmoid region and cranial fossa. The most distinct feature is the well-circumscribed islands of mature cartilage surrounded by spindle cell stroma. The latter can be highly cellular and myxoid. Blood-filled spaces are lined by osteoclasts to simulate aneurysmal bone cyst. The spindle cells have uniform nuclei and low mitotic activity. In the periphery of the tumor, reactive new bone formation occurs. Five of seven patients have done well following excision without recurrence for 2 to 50 months. Two patients have persistent disease, including one with continued growth in the superior nasal cavity.[219]

CHONDROSARCOMA

Chondrosarcoma occurs in the nasal septum, ethmoid sinus, and nasopharynx as a raised, thickened,

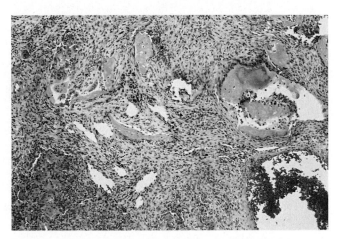

FIGURE 6-125 Aneurysmal bone cyst, solid type. Vascular spaces, osteoid trabeculae with osteoblasts, cellular fibrous stroma, and osteoclasts characterize this lesion.

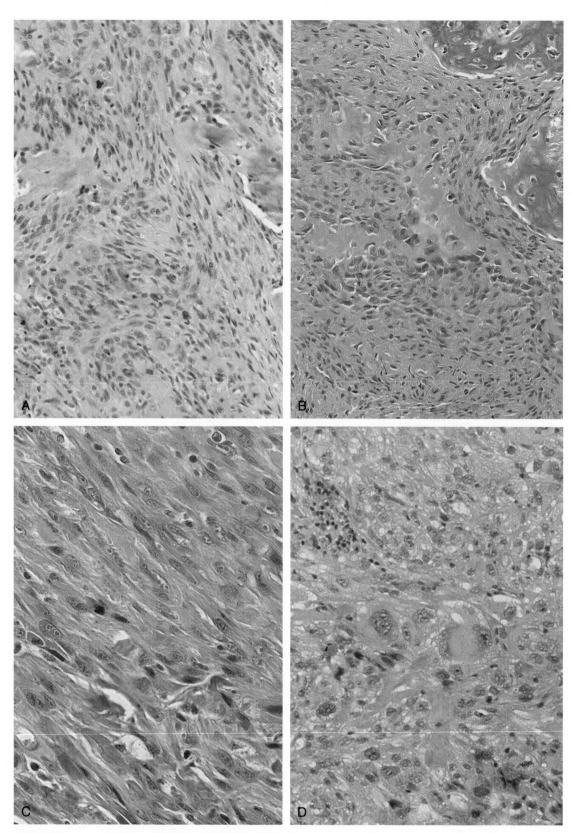

FIGURE 6-126 Osteosarcoma of maxillary sinus. *A*, Highly cellular fibrous stroma with deposit of osteoid material. *B*, Formation of irregular woven bone. *C*, Spindle cells with nuclear atypia and mitotic activity. *D*, Pleomorphic and bizarre stromal cells with osteoid stroma.

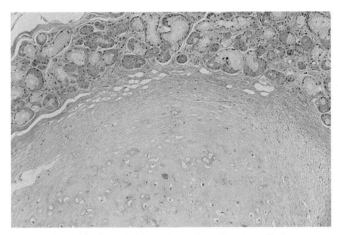

FIGURE 6-127 Chondroma of nasal septum. A well-circumscribed hyaline cartilaginous nodule compressing seromucous glands. The cellularity is mild.

the periphery of hyaline cartilage, spindle cells proliferate. In poorly differentiated chondrosarcomas, spindle cell sarcoma predominates. Mesenchymal chondrosarcoma rarely occurs in this region.[217]

In biopsy specimens, a correct diagnosis is often difficult, because the stroma may be extensively myxoid, simulating myxoma, chondromyxoid fibroma, and benign mixed tumor. In the hyaline cartilage, cellularity and nuclear atypia are minimally abnormal. The best evidence of malignancy depends on the permeation of bony trabeculae (Fig. 6–129C) and radiographic evidence of bony destruction. The possibility of chordoma should be excluded by immunohistochemical stains. In the presence of osteoid matrix, the likelihood of osteogenic sarcoma should be considered.

The prognosis of chondrosarcoma in this region is closely related to the degree of differentiation, tumor size, anatomic location, and surgical resectability.[220,221]

firm, and sometimes ulcerated mass with grey, translucent cut surfaces (Fig. 6–129A). Histologically, the majority are well-differentiated, lobulated hyaline cartilage with increased cellularity, nuclear hyperchromasia, atypia, bi- or multinucleation, mucinous degeneration, and necrosis (Fig. 6–129B). Areas of calcification occur with some frequency. In

DIFFERENTIAL DIAGNOSIS

Without knowing the clinical and radiographic findings, benign fibro-osseous lesions may be classified as fibromatosis or sarcoma. Fibrosarcomas growing in the upper respiratory tract may invade pre-existing bone and, in these foci, malignant spindle cells

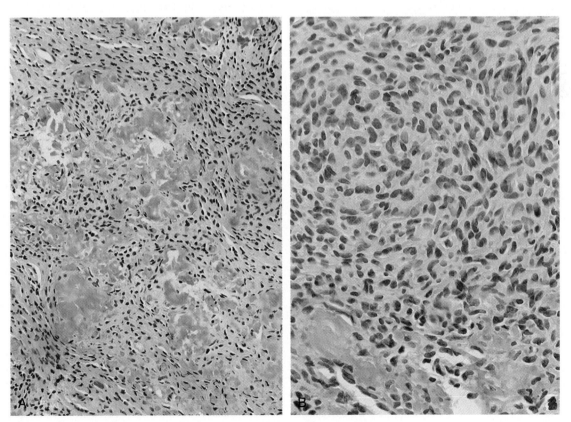

FIGURE 6-128 Ossifying fibromyxoid tumor of nasal septum. A, Lobules of eosinophilic, chondroid material are surrounded by fibrous stroma. B, In the cellular fibrous stroma, the stromal cells reveal mild nuclear irregularity.

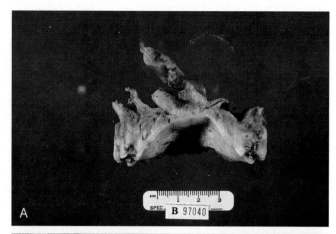

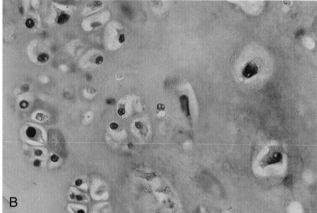

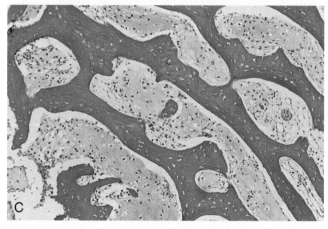

FIGURE 6–129 Chondrosarcoma of nasal septum. A, The nasal septum and the floor of maxilla are replaced by lobulated myxoid cartilaginous tissue. B, Atypical chondrocytes reveal nuclear enlargement, irregularity, hyperchromasia, and binucleation. C, Even though this cartilaginous lesion is well-differentiated, mildly atypical, and slightly hypercellular, permeation of the adjacent bone is diagnostic for chondrosarcoma.

may be surrounded by irregular and disrupted bone to simulate osteosarcoma.[208] Conversely, a small specimen may show only fibrosarcoma, but the resection specimen may demonstrate unquestionable areas of malignant osteoid or bone. Most reports indicate that osteosarcomas with predominantly chondrosarcomatous elements have a slightly better prognosis than ordinary osteosarcomas.[208]

Chordoma and Other Bone Tumors

CHORDOMA

Chordoma occurs mainly in the sacrococcygeal and spheno-occipital regions. In the latter site these tumors involve the posterior nasal cavity, sphenoid sinus, sphenoid bone, nasopharynx, and base of skull. Histologically, tumor cells grow in sheets, nests, and cords, often with a lobulated pattern. The characteristic cell, the physaliferous cell, contains a vacuolated cytoplasm, producing a bubble-like appearance. Some of these cells have multiple fine vacuoles in their cytoplasm, others exhibit a signet-ring appearance, and some have a clear cytoplasm (Fig. 6–130A). With PAS and mucicarmine stains these spaces usually are empty, but a rim of mucin-positive material may be found at the borders of vacuoles. Additional cells have a more dense eosinophilic cytoplasm. Many tumor cells also contain glycogen.[222]

In most chordomas the cells show little pleomorphism, hyperchromatism, or mitotic activity. However, in a few cases tumor cells become less differentiated and assume a sarcomatous appearance. These lesions can only be classified as chordoma when more typical areas are recognized. Some chordomas growing in this area contain cartilaginous tissue having the features of chondroma or well-differentiated chondrosarcoma (Fig. 6–130B). These tumors have been diagnosed as "chondroid chordoma." If physaliferous cells are found in a lesion, a diagnosis of chordoma should be made even though cartilaginous or sarcomatous features are identified.

By immunohistochemical stains, tumor cells in the chondroid components of chordoma express cytokeratin (83%), epithelial membrane antigen (77%), and S-100 protein (58%). In contrast, low-grade chondrosarcomas are negative for cytokeratin and epithelial membrane antigen and positive for S-100 protein.[223] These immunostains appear useful for diagnosis.

Chordomas of this region grow slowly, infiltrate locally, and rarely metastasize. Following surgery and radiotherapy, long-term survival is possible in spite of multiple recurrences.[222]

EWING'S SARCOMA

Rare examples of Ewing's sarcoma have been reported to occur in the mandible and the maxilla as aggressive, destructive tumors.[224] Diffuse sheets and nests of small round cells contain scant vacuolated cytoplasm and round to oval, small to medium-sized nuclei, and fine chromatin. Nucleoli are usually small. The presence of glycogen and mic2 glycoprotein support the diagnosis.

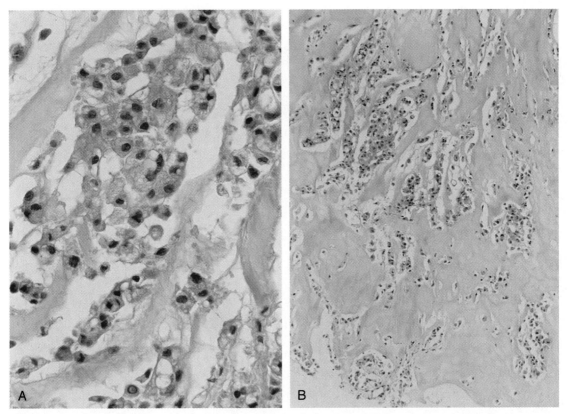

FIGURE 6-130 *Chordoma of skull base. A, Tumor cells have abundant vacuolated cytoplasm. Nuclear atypia is mild. The background matrix has a mucinous appearance. B, Clusters and cords of epithelioid tumor cells are surrounded by abundant hyaline cartilaginous stroma.*

Malignant Lymphoma

Malignant lymphoma is the most common malignant nonepithelial neoplasm found in the upper respiratory tract and most commonly involves the nasal cavity, the maxillary sinus, and the nasopharynx.[141] Nasosinus lymphomas are divided into conventional non-Hodgkin's lymphoma and nasal T- or natural killer cell lymphoma (NT/NKCL).[225-227]

Most malignant lymphomas of the nasosinus and nasopharynx are non-Hodgkin's lymphomas. In the western countries, such as the United States, nasosinus lymphomas comprise about 1.5% of all lymphomas and are equally divided between B-cell and T-cell types.[228] In Asia and South America (Peru), nasosinus lymphomas are much more common (6.8% to 8% of all lymphomas), predominantly T-cell type, and associated with Epstein-Barr virus (EBV).[228,229]

Gross Pathology

A raised polypoid unilateral lesion in the early stage develops progressively into an ulcerated and necrotic mass, which may become bilateral. Some patients develop clinical features of lethal midline granuloma. Cut surface reveals grey-white, friable, homogeneous tissue.

Microscopic Pathology

In a series of 120 conventional non-Hodgkin's lymphomas reported from Armed Forces Institute of Pathology, more males than females were affected with a ratio of 1.35 to 1. About 60% of patients were in their sixth to eighth decades of life.[228] Those with low-grade lymphomas presented with obstruction symptoms, while high-grade lymphomas tended to associate with nonhealing ulcer, cranial nerve involvement, facial swelling, epistaxis, or pain. High-grade B-cell lymphomas typically caused soft tissue or bony destruction.[228]

Nasosinus non-Hodgkin's lymphomas have a broad spectrum of morphology and cellular differentiation. Most are diffuse; nodular lymphomas are only rarely seen.[228] The predominant histologic types include: 44 cases of diffuse mixed small and large cell type, with 41 T-cell and three B-cell; 39 cases of diffuse sheets of large B cells, with 29 follicular center and 10 immunoblastic cells; nine cases of diffuse small, noncleaved cell lymphoma; and four of Burkitt's lymphoma (Fig. 6-131 *A-C*). In terms of the phenotype, nasal lymphomas are equally divided between B-cell (39 cases) and T-cell (34 tumors) types. Of the 39 sinus lymphomas, B-cell type predominate (77%) (Fig. 6-132 *A-D*). With lymphomas

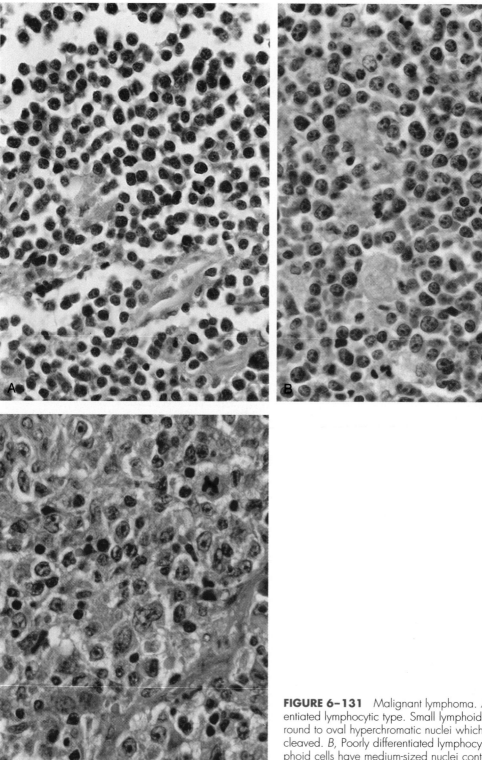

FIGURE 6–131 Malignant lymphoma. *A,* Well-differentiated lymphocytic type. Small lymphoid cells with round to oval hyperchromatic nuclei which are noncleaved. *B,* Poorly differentiated lymphocytic type. Lymphoid cells have medium-sized nuclei containing multiple nucleoli and coarse chromatin. *C,* Large cell lymphoma characterized by large lymphoid cells with irregular cleaved nuclei, prominent nucleoli, and a moderate amount of cytoplasm.

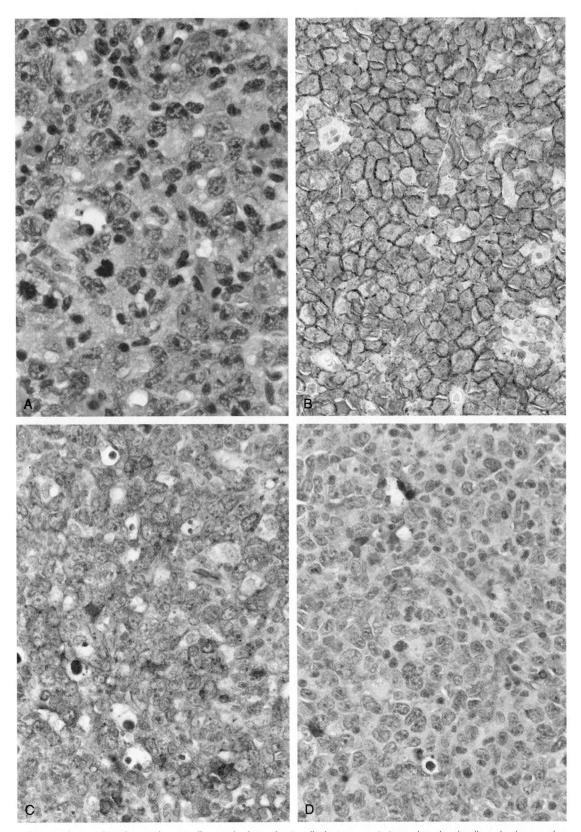

FIGURE 6–132   Malignant lymphoma, large cell type, high-grade, B-cell phenotype. *A,* Large lymphoid cells with pleomorphic nuclei, coarse chromatin, and prominent nucleoli. *B,* Immunohistochemical stain for B-cell marker, L-26, is diffusely positive. *C,* Diffusely positive for lambda light chain. *D,* Entirely negative for kappa light chain.

involving both nasal cavity and paranasal sinus, the majority are T-cell type (10/12, 83%).[228]

NT/NKCL differs clinically and histologically from ordinary lymphomas. Patients are prone to develop extensive swelling of nasal, facial, and periorbital tissues; mucosal ulceration; tissue necrosis; bone destruction; and fistula formation, producing the clinical picture of "lethal midline granuloma."[225] Nasal septal perforation and collapse of the nasal bridge may be seen.

Histologically, the most common features of NT/NKCL are angiocentricity and necrosis (Fig. 6–133 A and B). Tumor cells surround the blood vessels and infiltrate into blood vessel walls, which are sometimes destroyed and thrombosed with fibrin clots. These infiltrative features are required for angiocentricity, which is detected in only about 60% of specimens. For this reason, angiocentricity is not required for the diagnosis of NT/NKCL. Blood vessels surrounded by neoplastic cells alone does not meet the criterion for angiocentricity.[225,227]

Necrosis is present in almost all the biopsies and has the appearance of coagulative type. Apoptotic cells are common. The presence of nuclear debris and neutrophils sometimes simulates abscesses. As to the cause of necrosis, in addition to ischemia secondary to vascular damage, other possibilities include the effects of tumor necrosis factor and cytokines secreted by the tumor cells.[225]

NT/NKCL has a wide morphologic spectrum. The predominant lymphoid cells may be small, medium, or large (Fig. 6–133C). A mixture of the preceding cell types also occurs. In such cases, an inflammatory or infectious disease is suggested, especially when other inflammatory cells are present. Features indicative of lymphoid neoplasm include nuclear atypia and mitotic activity.

By working formulation NT/NKCL falls in the category of diffuse large cell lymphoma or diffuse mixed small and large cell lymphoma with intermediate grade of malignancy.[229] By in situ hybridization over 80% of NT/NKCL lesions have detectable EBV associated nuclear RNA 1/2 (EBER 1/2). Other frequently detected markers are T-cell receptor associated complex (CD3) and natural killer cell–related marker (CD56) (neural cell adhesion molecular) (Fig.

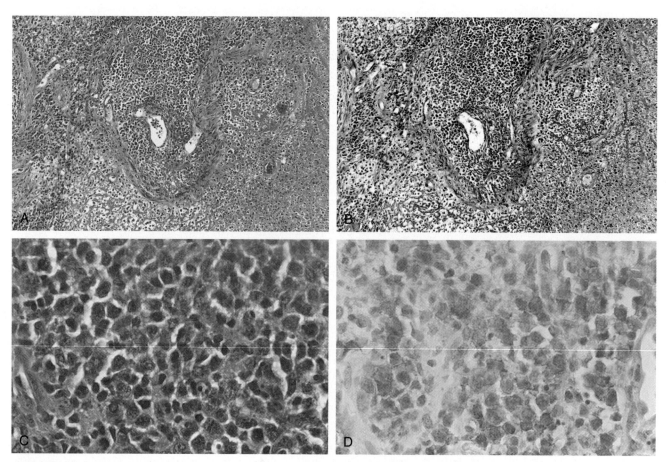

FIGURE 6–133 Nasal T/natural killer cell lymphoma. *A,* Angiocentric and angioinvasive patterns with lymphoid cells concentrate around the blood vessel and infiltrate the vessel wall. A rim of residual media layer is suggested. *B,* Elastic stain confirms the elastic interna in the media layer. *C,* A homogeneous population of lymphoid cells with medium-sized irregular nuclei with finely granular chromatin and small nucleoli. *D,* Tumor cells are diffusely positive for CD56. Courtesy of Dr. Bruce Wenig.

6–133D). However, CD16, CD57, and T-cell receptor beta-chain gene rearrangement are negative.[225,229,230]

Differential Diagnosis

Inflammatory and infectious lesions and Wegener's granulomatosis are key considerations when faced with lymphoid process. In benign conditions, nuclear atypia and mitotic activity are absent or minimal. Immunohistochemical stains and in situ hybridization for EBV-related nuclear RNA are helpful to confirm NT/NKCL.

Lymphomatoid granulomatosis (LYG) and NT/NKCL share several clinical and morphologic similarities. Upper respiratory tract, skin, and gastrointestinal tract are favored sites of both diseases. NT/NKCL is more likely to spread to testis, while kidney and brain are favored by LYG. Morphologically, LYG also demonstrates angiocentricity, necrosis, cellular atypia, and increased mitotic activity (Fig. 6–134 A and B). The cellular infiltrates in LYG are mixed, including mature and immature lymphocytes, immunoblasts, plasma cells, eosinophils, epithelioid histiocytes, and large atypical cells. In the latter, the nuclei appear irregular, bilobed and contain prominent nucleoli, resembling Reed-Sternberg cells (Fig. 6–134 C and D).

Jaffe et al[227] proposed the term angiocentric immunoproliferative lesion to include both NT/NKCL and LYG, and developed a grading system based on cellular elements, cytologic atypia, and necrosis. Using this system, the majority of lymphomatoid granulomatosis lesions have grade 1 or 2 atypia, whereas NT/NKCL is more likely to have grade 3 atypia and more aggressive behavior.

In a study of four cases of lymphomatoid granulomatosis of the lung, atypical medium to large B cells were found in a background of T cells and the EBV sequences were localized to B cells. Ig heavy chain gene rearrangement may be monoclonal, polyclonal, or oligoclonal. These findings suggest lymphomatoid granulomatosis is a T-cell rich EBV related B-cell lymphoproliferative disease, in which T cells are abundant and reactive in nature.[231] In contrast, NT/NKCL is a T-cell lymphoproliferative disorder, in which EBV occurs in T and NK cells.[229,230]

Prognosis

Prognosis of nasosinus lymphoma is closely related to the extent of local disease. Following radiotherapy and chemotherapy, 11 (17%) of 66 patients developed nodal and extranodal spread. With a median follow-up of 3 years, 24 (36%) died of disease, 17 (26%) alive without disease, 13 (20%) alive with disease, and 12 (18%) died of other causes.[228] In other series, the overall 5-year survival rates range from 45% to 56%.[232,233] The majority of patients who died developed systemic lymphoma.[234]

It appears that cases of NT/NKCL have better outcome than those of conventional lymphomas. Following radiotherapy, the 5- and 15-year survival rates are reported to be 63% and 50%, respectively.[230] Patients with LYG have variable outcome and in general are more indolent than NT/NKCL. One of the serious complications for patients with NT/NKCL and LYG is the development of hemophagocytic syndrome leading to a rapid fatality. This syndrome is probably related to EBV.

Plasmacytoma

Plasmacytomas most often occur within bone. Occasionally these tumors may arise in extraosseous sites, most commonly in the upper respiratory tract.[235] In this area plasmacytomas usually produce raised, smooth-surfaced lesions. Histologically these neoplasms are composed of a pure population of plasma cells, usually growing in solid sheets, cords, and single files (Fig. 6–135 A–D). Most of the cells show atypical features including large pleomorphic nuclei, high nuclear/cytoplasmic ratios, large coarse chromatin clumps, and mitotic activity.[235]

In the upper respiratory tract, some inflammatory lesions may contain sheets of numerous plasma cells ("plasma cell granulomas"). The presence of the following features favors a reactive lesion: (1) numerous small blood vessels lined by large but uniform endothelial cells, (2) mature plasma cells, (3) other types of inflammatory cells, (4) Russell bodies, and (5) polyclonality by immunohistochemistry. Occasionally, a plasmacytoma, in which the cells contain relatively little cytoplasm, may be misinterpreted as a malignant lymphoma. Some plasmacytomas grow in clusters of cells and may be misdiagnosed as a pituitary tumor or some other epithelial neoplasm.

When a diagnosis of extramedullary plasmacytoma is made, the patient should be examined for evidence of plasma cell disease elsewhere. If none is found, the tumor should be treated as a primary extraosseous lesion. Some patients are free of disease following surgery or radiotherapy, while others develop local recurrence or multiple myeloma. Rarely, plasmacytomas may metastasize to cervical lymph nodes.[235]

METASTATIC TUMORS

The majority of metastatic tumors seen in the nasosinus have known primary tumor elsewhere. Less commonly, a metastasis to the nasosinus is the first manifestation of the disease. Overall, renal cell carcinoma is the most common primary site, followed by lung, breast, and colon.[236] Malignant lymphomas and leukemias may also involve this area as part of generalized disease. Many metastatic tumors are poorly differentiated and require clinical information and immunohistochemistry to reach a correct diagnosis.

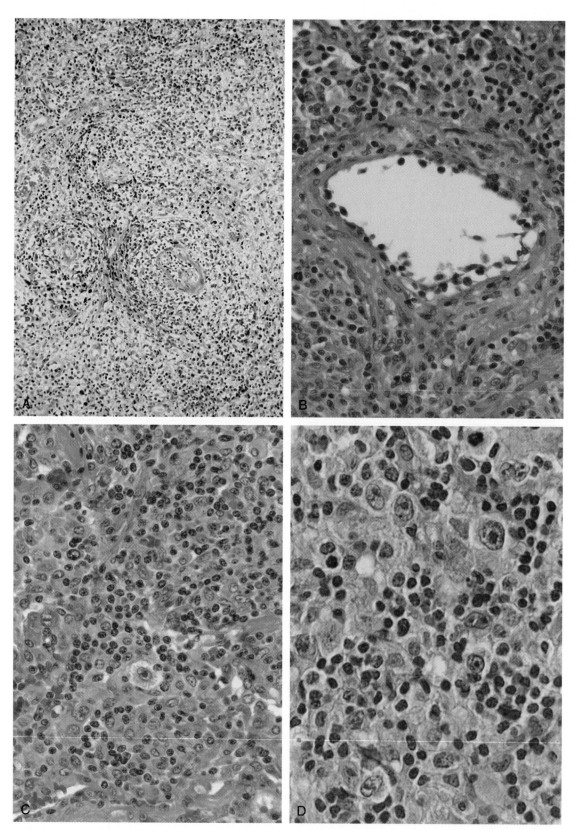

FIGURE 6–134 Lymphomatoid granulomatosis. *A,* Angiocentric pattern. Several vessel walls are destroyed and infiltrated by lymphoid cells. Only the endothelial cells and subintimal layer remain recognizible. *B,* The entire thickness of vessel wall is invaded by atypical lymphoid cells. *C,* A heterogeneous population of small lymphocytes, plasma cells, and atypical mononuclear cells and background lymphocytes and plasma cells. *D,* Large atypical mononuclear cells with lobulated nuclei and prominent nucleoli simulate Reed-Sternberg cells.

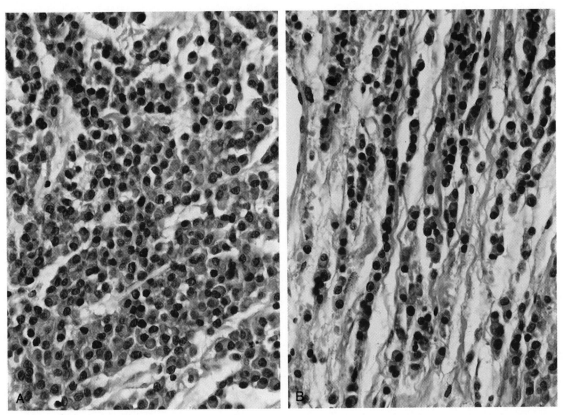

FIGURE 6-135 Plasmacytoma. *A,* Sheets of plasmacytoid cells have eccentric nuclei and basophilic cytoplasm. *B,* Plasmacytoid cells arranged in single files simulating metastatic carcinoma.

REFERENCES

1. Weidner N, Askin FB, Berthrong M, Hopkins MB, Kute TE, McGuirt FW. Bizarre (pseudomalignant) granulation-tissue reactions following ionizing-radiation exposure. A microscopic, immunohistochemical, and flow-cytometric study. *Cancer.* 1987; 59:1509–1514.
2. Dunlap CL, Barker BF. Diagnostic problems in oral pathology. *Semin Diag Pathol.* 1985; 2:16–30.
3. Scholl P, Byers RM, Batsakis JG, Wolf P, Santini H. Microscopic cut-through of cancer in the surgical treatment of squamous carcinoma of the tongue. Prognostic and therapeutic implications. *Am J Surg.* 1986; 152:354–360.
4. Shah JP, Cendon RA, Farr HW, Strong EW. Carcinoma of the oral cavity. *Am J Surg.* 1976; 132:504–507.
5. Looser KG, Shah JP, Strong EW. The significance of "positive" margins in surgically resected epidermoid carcinomas. *Head Neck Surg.* 1978; 1:107–111.
6. Pittam MR, Thornton H, Palmer BV, Chapman P, Shaw HJ. Results and prognostic factors in salvage surgery for squamous carcinoma of the tongue. *Br J Surg.* 1982; 69:188–190.
7. Zieske LA, Johnson JT, Myers EN, Thearle PB. Squamous cell carcinoma with positive margins. Surgery and postoperative irradiation. *Arch Otolaryngol Head Neck Surg.* 1986; 112: 863–866.
8. Davidson TM, Nahum AM, Haghighi P, Astarita RW, Saltzstein SL, Seagren S. The biology of head and neck cancer. *Arch Otolaryngol.* 1984; 110:193–196.
9. Cook JA, Jones AS, Phillips DE, Soler-Lluch E. Implications of tumour in resection margins following surgical treatment of squamous cell carcinoma of the head and neck. *Clinical Otolaryngol.* 1993; 18:37–41.
10. Jafek BW. Ultrastructure of human nasal mucosa. *Laryngoscope.* 1983; 93:1576–1599.

11. de la Cruz MA, Sanchez Lopez MJ, Merino Royo E, Requena L. Premalignant changes in nasal and sinus polyps: A retrospective 10 year study (1979–1988). *J Laryngol Otol.* 1990; 104:210–212.
12. Compagno J, Hyams VJ, Lepore ML. Nasal polyposis with stromal atypia. Review of follow-up study of 14 cases. *Arch Pathol Lab Med.* 1976; 100:224–226.
13. Brihaye P, Clement PA, Dab I, Desprechin B. Pathological changes of the lateral nasal wall in patients with cystic fibrosis (mucoviscidosis). *Int J Ped Otorhinolaryngol.* 1994; 28:141–147.
14. Oppenheimer EH, Rosenstein BJ. Differential diagnosis of nasal polyps in cystic fibrosis and atopy. *Lab Invest.* 1979; 40: 445–449.
15. Wenig BM, Heffner DK. Respiratory epithelial adenomatoid hamartomas of the sinonasal tract and nasopharynx: A clinicopathologic study of 31 cases. *Ann Otol Rhinol Laryngol.* 1995; 104:639–645.
16. Maisel RH, Johnston WH, Anderson HA, Cantrell RW. Necrotizing sialometaplasia involving the nasal cavity. *Laryngoscope.* 1977; 87:429–434.
17. Krasne DL, Warnke RA, Weiss LM. Malignant lymphoma presenting as pseudoepitheliomatous hyperplasia. A report of two cases. *Am J Surg Pathol.* 1988; 12:835–842.
18. Takimoto T, Kathoh T, Ohmura T, Kamide M, Nishimura T, Umeda R. Inflammatory pseudotumour of the maxillary sinus mimicking malignancy. *Rhinology.* 1990; 28:123–127.
19. Hyams VJ: Unusual Tumors and Lesions. In: Gnepp DR, ed. *Pathology of the Head and Neck.* New York: Churchill Livingstone; 1988:459–495.
20. Bredenkamp JK, Smith ME, Dudley JP, Williams JC, Crumley RL, Crockett DM. Otolaryngologic manifestations of the mucopolysaccharidoses. *Ann Otol Rhinol Laryngol.* 1992; 101: 472–478.

21. Friedmann I. Ulcerative/necrotizing diseases of the nose and paranasal sinuses. *Curr Diag Pathol.* 1995; 2:236–255.
22. Friedmann I, Osborn DA. *Pathology of Granulomas and Neoplasms of the Nose and Paranasal Sinuses.* Edinburgh: Churchill Livingstone; 1982.
23. Batsakis JG, El-Naggar AK. Rhinoscleroma and rhinosporidiosis. *Ann Otol Rhinol Laryngol.* 1992; 101:879–882.
24. Meyer PR, Shum TK, Becker TS, Taylor CR. Scleroma (rhinoscleroma). *Arch Pathol Lab Med.* 1983; 107:377–383.
25. Foucar E, Rosai J, Dorfman R. Sinus histiocytosis with massive lymphadenopathy (Rosai-Dorfman disease): Review of the entity. *Sem Diag Pathol.* 1990; 7:19–73.
26. Eisen RN, Buckley PJ, Rosai J. Immunophenotypic characterization of sinus histiocytosis with massive lymphadenopathy (Rosai-Dorfman disease). *Sem Diag Pathol.* 1990; 7:74–82.
27. Saeed SR, Brookes GB. Aspergillosis of the paranasal sinuses. *Rhinology.* 1995; 33:46–51.
28. Nussbaum ES, Hall WA. Rhinocerebral mucormycosis: changing patterns of disease. *Surg Neurol.* 1994; 41:152–156.
29. Parfrey NA. Improved diagnosis and prognosis of mucormycosis. Clinicopathologic study of 33 cases. *Medicine.* 1986; 65:113–123.
30. McGill TJ, Simpson G, Healy GB. Fulminant aspergillosis of the nose and paranasal sinuses: A new clinical entity. *Laryngoscope.* 1980; 90:748–754.
31. Sobol SM, Love RG, Stutman HR, Pysher TJ. Phaeohyphomycosis of the maxilloethmoid sinus caused by Drechslera spicifera: a new fungal pathogen. *Laryngoscope.* 1984; 94:620–627.
32. Padhye AA, Ajello L, Wieden MA, Steinbronn KK. Phaeohyphomycosis of the nasal sinuses caused by a new species of Exserohilum. *J Clin Microbiol.* 1986; 24:245–249.
33. Zieske LA, Kopke RD, Hamill R. Dematiaceous fungal sinusitis. *Otolaryngol Head Neck Surg.* 1991; 105:567–577.
34. Rowe-Jones JM, Moore-Gillon V. Destructive noninvasive paranasal sinus aspergillosis: component of a spectrum of disease. *J Otolaryngol.* 1994; 23:92–96.
35. Gori S, Scasso A. Cytologic and differential diagnosis of rhinosporidiosis. *Acta Cytol.* 1994; 38:361–366.
36. Thianprasit M, Thagerngpol K. Rhinosporidiosis. *Curr Top Med Mycol.* 1989; 3:64–85.
37. Gordon WW, Cohn AM, Greenberg SD, Komorn RM. Nasal sarcoidosis. *Arch Otolaryngol.* 1976; 102:11–14.
38. Neville E, Mills RGS, James DG. Prognostic factors predicting the outcome of sarcoidosis. An analysis of 818 patients. *Quart J Med.* 1983; 52:525–533.
39. Batsakis JG, Luna MA. Midfacial necrotizing lesions. *Semin Diag Pathol.* 1987; 4:90–116.
40. Miglets AW, Viall JH, Kataria YP. Sarcoidosis of the head and neck. *Laryngoscope.* 1977; 87:2038–2048.
41. Deutsch HL, Millard DR Jr. A new cocaine abuse complex. Involvement of nose, septum, palate, and pharynx. *Arch Otolaryngol Head Neck Surg.* 1989; 115:235–237.
42. Sercarz JA, Strasnick B, Newman A, Dodd LG. Midline nasal destruction in cocaine abusers. *Otolaryngol Head Neck Surg.* 1991; 105:694–701.
43. Hoffman GS, Kerr GS, Leavitt RY, et al. Wegener's granulomatosis: an analysis of 158 patients. *Ann Intern Med.* 1992; 116:488–498.
44. Kornblut AD, Wolff SM, DeFries HO, Fauci AS. Wegener's granulomatosis. *Laryngoscope.* 1980; 90:1453–1465.
45. Hellman D, Laing T, Petri M, et al. Wegener's granulomatosis: isolated involvement of the trachea and larynx. *Ann Rheum Dis.* 1987; 46:628–632.
46. Fienberg R. The protracted superficial phenomenon in pathergic (Wegener's) granulomatosis. *Hum Pathol.* 1981; 12:458–467.
47. Devaney KO, Travis WD, Hoffman G, Leavitt R, Lebovics R, Faucci AS. Interpretation of head and neck biopsies in Wegener's granulomatosis. *Am J Surg Pathol.* 1990; 14:555–564.
48. Mark EJ, Matsubara O, Tan-Liu NS, Fienberg R. The pulmonary biopsy in the early diagnosis of Wegener's (pathergic) granulomatosis: A study based on 35 open lung biopsies. *Hum Pathol.* 1988; 19:1065–1071.
49. Gross WL, Ludemann G, Kiefer G, et al. Anticytoplasmic antibodies in Wegener's granulomatosis. *Lancet.* 1986; 1:806.
50. Fienberg R, Mark EJ, Goodman M, et al. Correlation of antineutrophil cytoplasmic antibodies with extrarenal histopathology of Wegener's (pathergic) granulomatosis and related forms of vasculitis. *Hum Pathol.* 1993; 24:160–168.
51. Noorduyn LA, Torenbeek R, van der Valk P, et al. Sinonasal non-Hodgkin's lymphomas and Wegener's granulomatosis: a clinicopathological study. *Virchows Archiv. a, Pathological Anatomy and Histopathol.* 1991; 418:235–240.
52. Olsen KD, Neel HB III, Deremee RA, Weiland LH. Nasal manifestations of allergic granulomatosis and angiitis (Churg-Strauss syndrome). *Arch Otolaryngol Head Neck Surg.* 1980; 88:85–89.
53. Sasaki A, Hasegawa M, Nakazato Y, Ishida Y, Saitoh S. Allergic granulomatosis and angiitis (Churg-Strauss syndrome). Report of an autopsy case in a nonasthmatic patient. *Acta Pathol (Jpn).* 1988; 38:781–788.
54. Roberts PF, McCann BG. Eosinophilic angiocentric fibrosis of the upper respiratory tract: a mucosal variant of granuloma faciale? A report of three cases. *Histopathology.* 1985; 9:1217–1225.
55. Tsokos M, Fauci AS, Costa J. Idiopathic midline destructive disease (IMDD): A subgroup of patients with the "midline granuloma" syndrome. *Am J Clin Pathol.* 1982; 77:162–168.
56. Wolff M. Granulomas in nasal mucous membrane following local steroid injections. *Am J Clin Pathol.* 1974; 62:775–782.
57. Kyriakos M. Myospherulosis of the paranasal sinuses, nose and middle ear. *Am J Clin Pathol.* 1977; 67:118–130.
58. Rosai J. The nature of myospherulosis of the upper respiratory tract. *Am J Clin Pathol.* 1978; 69:475–481.
59. Storper IS, Newman AN. Cholesteatoma of the maxillary sinus. *Arch Otolaryngol Head Neck Surg.* 1992; 11B:975–977.
60. Barnes L, Yunis EJ, Krebs F III, Sonmez-Alpan E. Verruca vulgaris of the larynx. Demonstration of human papillomavirus types 6/11 by in situ hybridization. *Arch Pathol Lab Med.* 1991; 115:895–899.
61. Synder RN, Perzin KH. Papillomatosis of nasal cavity and paranasal sinuses (inverted papilloma, squamous papilloma). *Cancer.* 1972; 30:668–690.
62. Fu YS, Hoover L, Franklin M, Cheng L, Stoler M. Human papillomavirus identified by nucleic acid hybridization in concomitant nasal and genital papillomas. *Laryngoscope.* 1992; 102:1014–1019.
63. Wu TC, Trujillo JM, Kashima HK, Mounts P. Association of human papillomavirus with nasal neoplasia. *Lancet.* 1993; 341:522–524.
64. Kashima HK, Kessis T, Hruban RH, Wu TC, Zinreich SJ, Shah KV. Human papillomavirus in sinonasal papillomas and squamous cell carcinoma. *Laryngoscope.* 1992; 102:973–976.
65. Macdonald MR, Le KT, Freeman J, Hui MF, Cheung RK, Dosch HM: A majority of inverted sinonasal papillomas carries Epstein-Barr virus genomes. *Cancer.* 1995; 75:2307–2312.
66. Hyams VJ. Papillomas of the nasal cavity and paranasal sinuses. A clinicopathologic study of 315 cases. *Ann Otol Rhinol Laryngol.* 1971; 80:192–207.
67. Fu YS. Histopathology of inverted papillomas and surgical implications. *Am J Rhinol.* 1995; 2:75–76.
68. Kelly JH, Joseph M, Carroll E, et al. Inverted papilloma of the nasal septum. *Arch Otolaryngol.* 1980; 106:767–771.
69. Barnes L, Bedetti C. Oncocytic Schneiderian papilloma: a reappraisal of cylindrical cell papilloma of the sinonasal tract. *Hum Pathol.* 1984; 15:344–351.
70. Christensen WN, Smith RR. Schneiderian papillomas: A clinicopathologic study of 67 cases. *Hum Pathol.* 1986; 17:393–400.
71. Osborn DA. Nature and behavior of transitional tumors in the upper respiratory tract. *Cancer.* 1970; 25:50–60.
72. Ingle R, Jennings TA, Goodman ML, Pilch BZ, Bergman S, Ross JS. CD 44 expression in sinonasal inverted papillomas and associated squamous cell carcinoma. *Am J Clin Pathol.* 1998; 109:309–314.

73. Phillips PP, Gustafson RO, Farcer GW. The clinical behavior of inverting papilloma of the nose and paranasal sinuses: Report of 112 cases and review of literature. *Laryngoscope.* 1990; 100:463–469.

74. Kristensen S, Vorre P, Elbrond O, et al. Nasal Schneiderian papillomas: A study of 83 cases. *Clin Otolaryngol.* 1985; 10: 125–134.

75. Calcaterra TC, Thompson JW, Paglia DE. Inverting papillomas of the nose and paranasal sinuses. *Laryngoscope.* 1980; 90:53–60.

76. Kapadia SB, Barnes L, Pelzman K, Mirani N, Heffner DK, Bedetti C. Carcinoma ex oncocytic schneiderian (cylindrical cell) papilloma. *Am J Otolaryngol.* 1993; 14:332–338.

77. Trojussen W, Solberg LA, Hogetveit AC. Histopathologic changes of nasal mucosa in nickel workers. A pilot study. *Cancer.* 1979; 44:963–974.

78. Taxy JB. Squamous carcinoma of the nasal vestibule. An analysis of five cases and literature review. *Am J Clin Pathol.* 1997; 107:698–703.

79. Lewis JS, Castro EB. Cancer of the nasal cavity and paranasal sinuses. *J Laryngol Otol.* 1972; 86:255–262.

80. Jackson RT, Fitz-Hugh GS, Constable WC. Malignant neoplasms of the nasal cavities and paranasal sinuses. *Laryngoscope.* 1977; 87:726–736.

81. Hopkin N, McNicoll W, Dalley VM, Shaw HJ. Cancer of the paranasal sinuses and nasal cavities. Part I. Clinical features. *J Laryngol Otol.* 1984; 98:585–595.

82. Bosch A, Vallecillo L, Frias Z. Cancer of the nasal cavity. *Cancer.* 1976; 37:1458–1463.

83. Barnes L, Verbin RS, Gnepp DR. Diseases of the nose, paranasal sinuses, and nasopharynx. In: Barnes L, ed. *Surgical Pathology of the Head and Neck.* New York: Marcel Dekker; 1985: 403–451.

84. Kraus DH, Roberts JK, Medendorp SV, et al. Nonsquamous cell malignancies of the paranasal sinuses. *Ann Otol Rhinol Laryngol.* 1990; 99:5–11.

85. Kraus FT, Perez-Mesa C. Verrucous carcinoma: clinical and pathologic study of 105 cases involving oral cavity, larynx and genitalia. *Cancer.* 1966; 19:26.

86. Hanna GS, Ali MH. Verrucous carcinoma of the nasal septum. *J Laryngol Otol.* 1987; 101:184–187.

87. Luna MA, Tortoledo ME. Verrucous carcinoma. In: Gnepp DR, ed. *Pathology of the Head and Neck.* New York: Churchill Livingstone; 1988: 459–495.

88. Crissman JD, Kessis T, Shah KV, et al. Squamous papillary neoplasia of the adult aerodigestive tract. *Hum Pathol.* 1988; 19:1387–1396.

89. Ishiyama A, Eversole LR, Ross DA, et al. Papillary squamous neoplasms of the head and neck. *Laryngoscope.* 1994; 104: 1446–1452.

90. Zarbo RJ, Crissman JD, Venkat H, Weiss, MA. Spindle-cell carcinoma of the upper aerodigestive tract mucosa. An immunohistologic and ultrastructural study of 18 biphasic tumors and comparison with seven monophasic spindle-cell tumors. *Am J Surg Pathol.* 1986; 10:741–753.

91. Leventon GS, Evans HL. Sarcomatoid squamous cell carcinoma of the mucous membranes of the head and neck: A clinicopathologic study of 20 cases. *Cancer.* 1981; 48:994–1003.

92. Hyams VJ, Batsakis JG, Michaels L. *Tumors of the Upper Respiratory Tract and Ear.* Washington, DC: Armed Forces Institute of Pathology; 1986.

93. Boulay CES, Isaacson P. Carcinoma of the esophagus with spindle cell features. *Histopathology.* 1981; 5:403–414.

94. Ellis GL, Langloss JM, Heffner DK, Hyams VJ. Spindle-cell carcinoma of the aerodigestive tract. An immunohistochemical analysis of 21 cases. *Am J Surg Pathol.* 1987; 11:335–342.

95. Weidner N. Sarcomatoid carcinoma of the upper aerodigestive tract. *Semin Diag Pathol.* 1987; 4:157–168.

96. Nakhleh RE, Zarbo RJ, Ewing S, et al. Myogenic differentiation in spindle cell (sarcomatoid) carcinomas of the upper aerodigestive tract. *Appl Immunihistochem.* 1993; 1:58–68.

97. Nappi O, Wick MR. Sarcomatoid neoplasms of the respiratory tract. *Semin Diag Pathol.* 1993; 10:137–147.

98. Batsakis JG, Rich DH, Howard DR. The pathology of head and neck tumors: spindle-cell lesions (sarcomatoid carcinomas, nodular fasciitis, and fibrosarcoma) of the aerodigestive tracts, part 14. *Head Neck Surg.* 1982; 4:499–513.

99. Banks ER, Frierson HF Jr, Mills SE, et al. Basaloid squamous cell carcinoma of the head and neck. A clinicopathologic and immunohistochemical study of 40 cases. *Am J Surg Pathol.* 1992; 16:939–946.

100. Wain SL, Kier R, Vollmer RT, Bossen EH. Basaloid-squamous carcinoma of the tongue, hypopharynx, and larynx: report of 10 cases. *Hum Pathol.* 1986; 17:1158–1166.

101. Raslan WF, Barnes L, Krause JR, Contis L, Killeen R, Kapadia SB. Basaloid squamous cell carcinoma of the head and neck: a review of the English literature. *Am J Otolaryngol.* 1994; 15:204–211.

102. Frierson HF Jr, Ross GW, Stewart FM, Newman SA, Kelly MD. Unusual sinonasal small-cell neoplasms following radiotherapy for bilateral retinoblastomas. *Am J Surg Pathol.* 1989; 13:947–954.

103. Helliwell TR, Yeoch LH, Stell PM. Anaplastic carcinoma of the nose and paranasal sinuses. Light microscopy, immunohistochemistry and clinical correlation. *Cancer.* 1986; 58:2038–2045.

104. Frierson HF Jr, Mills SE, Fechner RE, Taxy JB, Levine PA. Sinonasal undifferentiated carcinoma. An aggressive neoplasm derived from schneiderian epithelium and distinct from olfactory neuroblastoma. *Am J Surg Pathol.* 1986; 10: 771–779.

105. Piscioli F, Aldovini D, Bondi A, Eusebi V. Squamous cell carcinoma with sarcoma-like stroma of the nose and paranasal sinuses: report of two cases. *Histopathology.* 1984; 8:633–639.

106. Manivel C, Wick MR, Dehner LP. Transitional (cylindric) cell carcinoma with endodermal sinus tumor-like features of the nasopharynx and paranasal sinuses. Clinicopathologic and immunohistochemical study of two cases. *Arch Pathol Lab Med.* 1986; 110:198–202.

107. Alvarez I, Suarez C, Rodrigo JP, Nunez F, Caminero MJ. Prognostic factors in paranasal sinus cancer. *Am J Otolaryngol.* 1995; 16:109–114.

108. Ang KK, Jiang GL, Frankenthaler RA, et al. Carcinomas of the nasal cavity. *Radiotherapy and Oncology.* 1992; 24:163–168.

109. McGuire LJ, Lee JC. The histopathologic diagnosis of nasopharyngeal carcinoma. *Ear Nose Throat J.* 1990; 69:229–236.

110. Shanmugaratuam K, Chan SH, de-The G, et al. Histopathology of nasopharyngeal carcinoma. *Cancer.* 1979; 44:1029–1044.

111. Neel HB III. Nasopharyngeal carcinoma. Clinical presentation, diagnosis, treatment, and prognosis. *Otolaryngol Clin North Am.* 1985; 18:479–490.

112. Woo JKS, Sham CL. Diagnosis of nasopharyngeal carcinoma. *Ear Nose Throat J.* 1990; 69:241–251.

113. Shamugaratnam K, Sobin LH. Histological Typing of Upper Respiratory Tract Tumor. *International Histological Classification of Tumors,* 2nd ed. Geneva, Switzerland: World Health Organization; 1991.

114. Zaatari GS, Santoianni RA. Adenoid squamous cell carcinoma of nasopharynx and neck region. *Arch Pathol Lab Med.* 1986; 110:542.

115. Hawkins EP, Krischer JP, Smith BE, Hawkins HK, Finegold MJ. Nasopharyngeal carcinoma in children—a retrospective review and demonstration of Epstein-Barr viral genomes in tumor cell cytoplasm: a report of the pediatric oncology group. *Hum Pathol.* 1990; 21:805–810.

116. Sham JST, Poon YF, Wei WI, Choi D. Nasopharyngeal carcinoma in young patients. *Cancer.* 1990; 65:2606–2610.

117. Hsu HC, Chen CL, Hsu MM, Lynn TC, Tu SM, Huang SC. Pathology of nasopharyngeal carcinoma. Proposal of a new histologic classification correlated with prognosis. *Cancer.* 1987; 59:945–951.

118. Taxy JB, Hidvegi EF, Battifora H. Nasopharyngeal carcinoma: antikeratin immunohistochemistry and electron microscopy. *Am J Clin Pathol.* 1985; 83:320–325.

119. Kamino H, Huang SJ, Fu YS. Keratin and involucrin immu-

nohistochemistry of nasopharyngeal carcinoma. *Cancer.* 1988; 61:1142–1148.

120. Oppedal BR, Bohler PJ, Marton PF, Brandtzaeg P. Carcinoma of the nasopharynx with supplementary immunohistochemistry. *Histopathology.* 1987; 11:1161–1169.

121. Fedder M, Gonzalez MF. Nasopharyngeal carcinoma. A brief review. *Am J Med.* 1985; 79:365.

122. Baker SR, Wolfe RA. Prognostic factors in nasopharyngeal malignancy. *Cancer.* 1982; 49:163–169.

123. Rafla S: Mucous gland tumors of paranasal sinuses. *Cancer.* 1970; 24:683–691.

124. Compagno J, Wong RT. Intranasal mixed tumors (pleomorphic adenomas): a clinicopathologic study of 40 cases. *Am J Clin Pathol.* 1977; 68:213–218.

125. Begin LR, Rochon L, Frenkiel S. Spindle cell myoepithelioma of the nasal cavity. *Am J Surg Pathol.* 1991; 15:184–190.

126. Dardick I. Malignant myoepithelioma of parotid salivary gland. *Ultrastruct Pathol.* 1985; 9:163–168.

127. Perzin KH, Gullane P, Clairmont AC. Adenoid cystic carcinomas arising in salivary glands: a correlation of histologic features and clinical course. *Cancer.* 1978; 42:265–282.

128. Healey WV, Perzin KH, Smith L. Mucoepidermoid carcinoma of salivary gland origin: classification, clinical-pathologic correlation, and results of treatment. *Cancer.* 1970; 26: 368–388.

129. Gerughty RM, Hennigar GR, Brown FM. Adenosquamous carcinoma of the nasal, oral and laryngeal cavities. *Cancer.* 1968; 22:1140–1155.

130. LiVolsi VA, Perzin KH. Malignant mixed tumors arising in salivary glands. *Cancer.* 1977; 39:2209–2230.

131. Perzin KH, Cantor JO, Johannessen JV. Acinic cell carcinoma arising in nasal cavity: report of a case with ultrastructural observations. *Cancer.* 1981; 47:1818–1822.

132. Ordonez NG, Batsakis JG. Acinic cell carcinoma of the nasal cavity: electron-optic and immunohistochemical observations. *J Laryngol Otol.* 1986; 100:345–349.

133. Wenig BM, Hyams VJ, Heffner DK. Nasopharyngeal papillary adenocarcinoma. A clinicopathologic study of a low-grade carcinoma. *Am J Surg Pathol.* 1988; 12:946–953.

134. Mills SE, Garland TA, Allen MS. Low grade papillary adenocarcinoma of palatal salivary gland origin. *Am J Surg Pathol.* 1984; 8:367–374.

135. Heffner DK, Hyams VJ, Hauck KW, Lingeman C. Low-grade adenocarcinoma of the nasal cavity and paranasal sinuses. *Cancer.* 1982; 50:312–322.

136. Alessi DM, Trapp TK, Fu YS, Calcaterra TC. Nonsalivary sinonasal adenocarcinoma. *Arch Otolaryngol Head Neck Surg.* 1988; 114:996–999.

137. Klintenberg C, Ologsson J, Hellquist H, Sokjer H. Adenocarcinoma of the ethmoid sinuses. A review of 28 cases with special reference to wood dust exposure. *Cancer.* 1984; 54: 482–488.

138. Barnes L. Intestinal-type adenocarcinoma of the nasal cavity and paranasal sinuses. *Am J Surg Pathol.* 1986; 10:192–202.

139. Kleinsasser O, Schroeder HG. Adenocarcinoma of the inner nose after exposure to wood dust. Morphological findings and relationship between histopathology and clinical behavior in 79 cases. *Arch Otorhinolaryngol.* 1988; 245:1–15.

140. Franquemont DW, Fechner RE, Mills SE. Histologic classification of sinonasal intestinal-type adenocarcinoma. *Am J Surg Pathol.* 1991; 15:368–375.

141. Fu YS, Perzin KH. Non-epithelial tumors of the nasal cavity, paranasal sinuses and nasopharynx: A clinicopathologic study. I. General features and vascular tumors. *Cancer.* 1974; 33:1275–1288.

142. Kapadia SB, Heffner DK. Pitfalls in the histopathologic diagnosis of pyogenic granuloma. *Eur Arch Otorhinolaryngol.* 1992; 249:195–200.

143. Wit TR, Shah JP, Sternberg SS. Juvenile nasopharyngeal angiofibroma. A 30 year clinical review. *Am J Surg.* 1983; 146: 521–525.

144. Bremer JW, Neel HB, DeSanto LW, Jones GC. Angiofibroma: treatment trends in 150 patients during 40 years. *Laryngoscope.* 1986; 96:1321–1329.

145. Makek MS, Andrews JC, Fisch U. Malignant transformation of a nasopharyngeal angiofibroma. *Laryngoscope.* 1989; 99: 1088–1092.

146. Spagnolo DV, Papadimitriou JM, Archer M. Postirradiation malignant fibrous histiocytoma arising in juvenile nasopharyngeal angiofibroma and producing alpha-1-antitrypsin. *Histopathology.* 1984; 8:339–352.

147. Eichhorn JH, Dickersin GR, Bhan AK, Goodman ML. Sinonasal hemangiopericytoma. A reassessment with electron microscopy, immunohistochemistry, and long-term follow-up. *Am J Surg Pathol.* 1990; 14:856–866.

148. Nielsen GP, Dickersin GR, Provenzal JM, Rosenberg AE. Lipomatous hemangiopericytoma. A histologic, ultrastructural and immunohistochemical study of a unique variant of hemangiopericytoma. *Am J Surg Pathol.* 1995; 19:748–756.

149. Compagno J, Hyams VJ. Hemangiopericytoma-like intranasal tumors. A clinicopathologic study of 23 cases. *Am J Clin Pathol.* 1976; 66:672–683.

150. Yasuoka T, Okumura Y, Okuda T, Oka N. Hemangioma and malignant hemangioendothelioma of the maxillary sinus: Case reports and clinical consideration. *J Oral Maxillofac Surg.* 1990; 48:877–881.

151. Mark RJ, Tran LM, Sercarz J, Fu YS, Calcaterra TC, Juillard GF. Angiosarcoma of the head and neck. The UCLA experience 1955 through 1990. *Arch Otolaryngol Head Neck Surg.* 1993; 119:973–978.

152. Zukerberg LR, Rosenberg AE, Randolph G, Pilch BZ, Goodman ML. Solitary fibrous tumor of the nasal cavity and paranasal sinuses. *Am J Surg Pathol.* 1991; 15:126–130.

153. Witkin GB, Rosai J. Solitary fibrous tumor of the upper respiratory tract. A report of six cases. *Am J Surg Pathol.* 1991; 15:842–848.

154. Fu YS, Perzin KH. Non-epithelial tumors of the nasal cavity, paranasal sinuses and nasopharynx: A clinicopathologic study. VI. Fibrous tissue tumors. *Cancer.* 1976; 37:2912–2928.

155. Heffner DK, Gnepp DR. Sinonasal fibrosarcomas, malignant schwannomas, and "Triton" tumors. A clinicopathologic study of 67 cases. *Cancer.* 1992; 70:1089–1101.

156. Wold LE, Weiland LH. Tumefactive fibro-inflammatory lesions of the head and neck. *Am J Surg Pathol.* 1983; 7:477–482.

157. Numez-Alonso C, Gashti EN, Christ ML. Maxillofacial synovial sarcoma. *Am J Surg Pathol.* 1979; 3:23–30.

158. Milchgrub S, Ghandur-Mnaymneh L, Dorfman HD, Albores-Saavedra J. Synovial sarcoma with extensive osteoid and bone formation. *Am J Surg Pathol.* 1994; 17:357–363.

159. Perzin KH, Fu YS. Non-epithelial tumors of the nasal cavity, paranasal sinuses and nasopharynx: A clinicopathologic study. XI. Fibrous histiocytoma. *Cancer.* 1980; 45:2616–2626.

160. Barnes L, Kanbour A. Malignant fibrous histiocytoma of the head and neck. A report of 12 cases. *Arch Otolaryngol Head Neck Surg.* 1988; 114:1149–1156.

161. Fu YS, Perzin KH. Non-epithelial tumors of the nasal cavity, paranasal sinuses and nasopharynx: A clinicopathologic study. VII. Myxomas. *Cancer.* 1977; 39:195–203.

162. Fu YS, Perzin KH. Non-epithelial tumors of the nasal cavity, paranasal sinuses and nasopharynx: A clinicopathologic study. V. Skeletal muscle tumors (rhabdomyoma and rhabdomyosarcoma). *Cancer.* 1976; 37:364–376.

163. Gale N, Rott T, Kambic V. Nasopharyngeal rhabdomyoma. Report of case (light and electron microscopic studies) and review of the literature. *Pathol Res Pract.* 1984; 178:454–460.

164. Kapadia SB, Meis JM, Frisman DM, Ellis GL, Heffner DK, Hyams VJ. Adult rhabdomyoma of the head and neck: A clinicopathologic and immunophenotypic study. *Hum Pathol.* 1993; 24:608–617.

165. Sutow WW, Lindberg RD, Gehan EA, et al. Three-year relapse-free survival rates in childhood rhabdomyosarcoma of the head and neck. Report from the intergroup rhabdomyosarcoma study. *Cancer.* 1982; 49:2217–2221.

166. Kapadia SB, Popek EJ, Barnes L. Pediatric otorhinolaryngic pathology: diagnosis of selected lesions. *Pathology Annual.* 1994; 29(Pt 1): 159–209.

167. Cavazzana AO, Schmidt D, Ninfo V, et al. Spindle cell rhabdomyosarcoma. A prognostically favorable variant of rhabdomyosarcoma. *Am J Surg Pathol.* 1992; 16:229–235.

168. Callender TA, Weber RS, Janjan N, et al. Rhabdomyosarcoma of the nose and paranasal sinuses in adults and children. *Arch. Otolaryngol Head Neck Surg.* 1995; 112:252–257.

169. Fu YS, Perzin KH. Non-epithelial tumors of the nasal cavity, paranasal sinuses and nasopharynx: A clinicopathologic study. IV. Smooth muscle tumors (leiomyoma and leiomyosarcoma). *Cancer.* 1975; 35:1300–1308.

170. Kuruvilla A, Wenig BM, Humphrey DM, Heffner DK. Leiomyosarcoma of the sinonasal tract. A clinicopathologic study of nine cases. *Arch Otolaryngol Head Neck Surg.* 1990; 116:1278–1286.

171. Fu YS, Perzin KH. Non-epithelial tumors of the nasal cavity, paranasal sinuses and nasopharynx. A clinicopathologic study. VIII. Lipoma and liposarcoma. *Cancer.* 1977; 40:1314–1317.

172. McCulloch TM, Makielski KH, McNutt MA. Head and neck liposarcoma. A histopathologic reevaluation of reported cases. *Arch Otolaryngol Head Neck Surg.* 1992; 118:1045–1049.

173. Patterson K, Kapur S, Chandra RS. "Nasal gliomas" and related brain heterotopias: a pathologist's perspective. *Pediatr Pathol.* 1986; 5:353–362.

174. Seibert RW, Seibert JJ, Jimenez JF, Angtuaco EJ. Nasopharyngeal brain heterotopia—a cause of upper airway obstruction in infancy. *Laryngoscope.* 1984; 94:818–819.

175. Bossen EH. Oligodendroglioma arising in heterotopic brain tissue of the soft palate and nasopharynx. *Am J Surg Pathol.* 1987; 11:571–574.

176. Perzin KH, Pushparaj N. Nonepithelial tumors of the nasal cavity, paranasal sinuses, and nasopharynx: A clinicopathologic study. XIII. Meningiomas. *Cancer.* 1984; 54:1860–1869.

177. Winek RR, Scheithauer BW, Wick MR. Meningioma, meningeal hemangiopericytoma (angioblastic meningioma), peripheral hemangiopericytoma, and acoustic schwannoma. *Am J Surg Pathol.* 1989; 13:251–261.

178. Iwai Y, Hakuba A, Khosla VK, et al. Giant basal prolactinoma extending into the nasal cavity. *Surg Neurol.* 1992; 37:280–283.

179. Lloyd RV, Chandler WF, Kovacs K, Ryan N. Ectopic pituitary adenomas with normal anterior pituitary glands. *Am J Surg Pathol.* 1986; 10:546–552.

180. Lack EL, Cubilla AL, Woodruff JM, Farr HW. Paragangliomas of the head and neck region. *Cancer.* 1977; 39:397–409.

181. Apple D, Kreines K. Cushing's syndrome due to ectopic ACTH production by a nasal paraganglioma. *Am J Med Sci.* 1982; 283:32–35.

182. Nguyen QA, Gibbs PM, Rice DH. Malignant nasal paraganglioma: A case report and review of the literature. *Arch Otolaryngol Head Neck Surg.* 1995; 113:157–161.

183. Perzin KH, Panyu H, Wechter S. Nonepithelial tumors of the nasal cavity, paranasal sinuses and nasopharynx: A clinicopathologic study. XII. Schwann cell tumors (neurilemoma, neurofibroma, malignant schwannoma). *Cancer.* 1982; 50:2193–2202.

184. Fernandez PL, Cardesa A, Bombi JA, Palacin A, Traserra J. Malignant sinonasal epithelioid schwannoma. *Virchows Archiv. a, Pathol Anat Histopath.* 1993; 423:401–405.

185. Bailet JW, Abemayor E, Andrews JC, Rowland JP, Fu YS, Dawson DE. Malignant nerve sheath tumors of the head and neck: A combined experience from two university hospitals. *Laryngoscope.* 1991; 101:1044–1049.

186. Mills SE, Frierson HF Jr. Olfactory neuroblastoma. A clinicopathologic study of 21 cases. *Am J Surg Pathol.* 1985; 9:317–327.

187. Barnes L, Kapadia SB. The biology and pathology of selected skull base tumors. *J Neuro-Oncol.* 1994; 20:213–240.

188. Ordonez NG, Mackay B. Neuroendocrine tumors of the nasal cavity. *Pathol Ann.* 1993; 28(2):77–111.

189. Argani P, Perez-Ordonez B, Xiao H, Caruana SM, Huvos AG, Ladanyi M. Olfactory neuroblastoma is not related to the Ewing family of tumors. Absence of EWS/FLI1 gene fusion and MIC2 expression. *Am J Surg Pathol.* 1998; 22:391–398.

190. Miller DC, Goodman ML, Pilch BZ, et al. Mixed olfactory neuroblastoma and carcinoma. A report of two cases. *Cancer.* 1984; 54:2019–2028.

191. Olsen KD, DeSanto LW. Olfactory neuroblastoma. Biologic and clinical behavior. *Arch Otolaryngol.* 1983; 109:797–802.

192. Singh W, Ranage C, Best P, Angus B. Nasal neuroblastoma secreting vasopressin. A case report. *Cancer.* 1980; 45:961–966.

193. Frierson HF Jr, Ross GW, Mills SE, Frankfurter A. Olfactory neuroblastoma. Additional immunohistochemical characterization. *Am J Clin Pathol.* 1990; 94:547–553.

194. Choi HS, Anderson PJ. Immunohistochemical diagnosis of olfactory neuroblastoma. *J Neuropathol Exp Neurol.* 1985; 44:18–31.

195. Siwersson U, Kindblom LG. Oncocytic carcinoid of the nasal cavity and carcinoid of the lung in a child. *Pathol Res Pract.* 1984; 178:562–569.

196. Kameya T, Shimosato Y, Adachi I, Abe K, Ebihara S, Ono I. Neuroendocrine carcinoma of the paranasal sinus. *Cancer.* 1980; 45:330–339.

197. Kushner BH, Hajdu SI, Gulati SC, Erlandson RA, Exelby PR, Liberman PH. Extracranial primitive neuroectodermal tumors. *Cancer.* 1991; 67:1825–1829.

198. Dehner LP. Primitive neuroectodermal tumor and Ewing's sarcoma. *Am J Surg Pathol.* 1993; 17:1–13.

199. Cove H. Melanosis, melanocytic hyperplasia and primary malignant melanoma of the nasal cavity. *Cancer.* 1979; 44:1424–1433.

200. Conley J, Pack GT. Melanoma of the mucous membrane of the head and neck. *Arch Otolaryngol.* 1974; 99:315–319.

201. Franquemont DW, Mills SE. Sinonasal malignant melanoma. A clinicopathologic and immunohistochemical study of 14 cases. *Am J Clin Pathol.* 1991; 96:689–697.

202. Chetty R, Slavin JL, Pitson GA, Dowling JP. Melanoma botryoides: a distinctive myxoid pattern of sino-nasal malignant melanoma. *Histopathol.* 1994; 24:377–379.

203. Billings KR, Wang MB, Sercarz JA, Fu YS. Clinical and pathologic distinction between primary and metastatic mucosal melanoma of the head and neck. *Arch Otolaryngol Head Neck Surg.* 1995; 112:700–706.

204. Trapp TK, Fu YS, Calcaterra TC. Melanoma of the nasal and paranasal sinus mucosa. *Arch Otolaryngol.* 1987; 113:1086–1089.

205. Lack EE. Extragonadal germ cell tumors of the head and neck region: Review of 16 cases. *Hum Pathol.* 1985; 16:56–64.

206. Heffner DK, Hyams VJ. Teratocarcinosarcoma (malignant teratoma?) of the nasal cavity and paranasal sinuses. A clinicopathologic study of 20 cases. *Cancer.* 1984; 53:2140–2154.

207. Shindo ML, Stanley RB Jr, Kiyabu MT. Carcinosarcoma of the nasal cavity and paranasal sinuses. *Head and Neck.* 1990; 12:516–519.

208. Fu YS, Perzin KH. Non-epithelial tumors of the nasal cavity, paranasal sinuses and nasopharynx: A clinicopathologic study. II. Osseous and fibro-osseous lesions, including osteoma, fibrous dysplasia, ossifying fibroma, osteoblastoma, giant cell tumor and osteosarcoma. *Cancer.* 1974; 33:1289–1305.

209. Earwaker J. Paranasal sinus osteomas: A review of 46 cases. *Skeletal Radiol.* 1993; 22:417–423.

210. Shapeero LG, Vanel D, Ackerman LV, et al. Aggressive fibrous dysplasia of the maxillary sinus. *Skeletal Radiol.* 1993; 22:563–568.

211. Slootweg PJ, Panders AK, Koopmans R, Nikkels PG. Juvenile ossifying fibroma. An analysis of 33 cases with emphasis on histopathological aspects. *J Oral Pathol Med.* 1994; 23:385–388.

212. Johnson LC, Yousefi M, Vinh TN, Heffner DK, Hyams VJ, Hartman KS: Juvenile active ossifying fibroma. Its nature, dynamics and origin. *Acta Otolaryngol.* 1991; 488(suppl):1–40.

213. Stolovitzky JP, Waldron CA, McConnel FMS. Giant cell lesions of the maxilla and paranasal sinuses. *Head Neck.* 1994; 16:143–148.

214. Fechner RE. Problematic lesions of the craniofacial bones. *Am J Surg Pathol.* 1989; 13(suppl):17–30.

215. Mark RJ, Sercarz JA, Tran L, Dodd LG, Selch M, Calcaterra TC. Osteogenic sarcoma of the head and neck. The UCLA experience. *Arch Otolaryngol Head Neck Surg.* 1991; 117:761–766.

216. Kilby D, Ambegaokar AG. The nasal chondroma. *J Laryngol Otol.* 1977; 91:415–426.

217. Fu YS, Perzin KH. Non-epithelial tumors of the nasal cavity, paranasal sinuses and nasopharynx: A clinicopathologic study. III. Cartilaginous tumors (chondroma and chondrosarcoma). *Cancer.* 1974; 34:453–463.

218. Enzinger FM, Weiss SW, Liang CY. Ossifying fibromyxoid tumor of soft parts. *Am J Surg Pathol.* 1989; 13:817–827.

219. McDermott MB, Ponder TB, Dehner LP. Nasal chondromesenchymal hamartoma. An upper respiratory tract analogue of the chest wall mesenchymal hamartoma. *Am J Surg Pathol.* 1998; 22:425–433.

220. Mark RJ, Tran LM, Sercarz J, Fu YS, Calcaterra TC, Parker RG. Chondrosarcoma of the head and neck. The UCLA experience, 1955–1988. *Am J Clin Oncol.* 1993; 16:232–237.

221. Koka V, Vericel R, Lartigau E, Lusinchi A, Schwaab G. Sarcomas of nasal cavity and paranasal sinuses: chondrosarcoma, osteosarcoma and fibrosarcoma. *J Laryngol Otol.* 1994; 108:947–953.

222. Perzin KH, Pushparaj N. Nonepithelial tumors of the nasal cavity, paranasal sinuses, and nasopharynx: A clinicopathologic study. XIV. Chordomas. *Cancer.* 1986; 57:784–796.

223. Wojno KJ, Hruban RH, Garin-Chesa P, Huvos AG. Chondroid chordomas and low-grade chondrosarcomas of the craniospinal axis. An immunohistochemical analysis of 17 cases. *Am J Surg Pathol.* 1992; 16:1144–1152.

224. Lane S, Ironside JW. Extra-skeletal Ewing's sarcoma of the nasal fossa. *J Laryngol Otol.* 1990; 104:570–573.

225. Fu YS, Perzin KH. Non-epithelial tumors of the nasal cavity, paranasal sinuses and nasopharynx: A clinicopathologic study. X. Malignant lymphomas and midline malignant reticulosis. *Cancer.* 1979; 43:611–621.

226. Jaffe ES. Pathologic and clinical spectrum of post-thymic T-cell malignancies. *Cancer Invest.* 1984; 2:415–426.

227. Jaffe ES, Chan JKC, Su IJ, et al. Report of the workshop on nasal and related extranodal angiocentric T/NK-cell lymphomas: definition, differential diagnosis and epidemiology. *Am J Surg Pathol.* 1996; 20:103–111.

228. Abbondanzo SL, Wenig BM. Non-Hodgkin's lymphoma of the sinonasal tract. A clinicopathologic and immunophenotypic study of 120 cases. *Cancer.* 1995; 75:1281–1291.

229. van Gorp J, Weiping L, Jacobse K, et al. Epstein-Barr virus in nasal T-cell lymphomas (polymorphic reticulosis/midline malignant reticulosis) in western China. *J Pathol.* 1994; 173: 81–87.

230. Strickler JG, Meneses MF, Habermann TM, et al. Polymorphic reticulosis: a reappraisal. *Hum Pathol.* 1994; 25:659–665.

231. Wilson WH, Kingma DW, Raffeld M, Wittes RE, Jaffe ES. Association of lymphomatoid granulomatosis with Epstein-Barr viral infection of B lymphocytes and response to interferon-alpha2b. *Blood.* 1996; 87:4531–4537.

232. Frierson HF Jr, Mills SE, Innes DJ Jr. Non-Hodgkin's lymphomas of the sinonasal region: histologic subtypes and their clinicopathologic features. *Am J Clin Pathol.* 1984; 81:721–727.

233. Robbins KT, Fuller LM, Vlasak M, et al. Primary lymphomas of the nasal cavity and paranasal sinuses. *Cancer.* 1985; 56: 814–819.

234. Kapadia SB, Barnes L, Deutsch M. Non-Hodgkin's lymphoma of the nose and paranasal sinuses: A study of 17 cases. *Head Neck Surg.* 1981; 3:490–499.

235. Fu YS, Perzin KH. Non-epithelial tumors of the nasal cavity, paranasal sinuses and nasopharynx: A clinicopathologic study. IX. Plasmacytoma. *Cancer.* 1978; 42:2399–2406.

236. Bernstein JM, Montgomery WW, Balogh K. Metastatic tumors to the maxilla, nose and paranasal sinuses. *Laryngoscope.* 1966; 76:621–650.

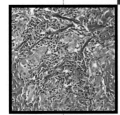

CHAPTER 7

Major Salivary Glands

I. CLINICAL CONSIDERATIONS FOR THE DISEASES OF THE SALIVARY GLANDS

■ MICHAEL KAPLAN

■ ELLIOT ABEMAYOR

The presence of a mass in the vicinity of the parotid or submandibular gland is not an unusual clinical finding; however, it can be a highly challenging problem given the spectrum of disease processes as well as the variety of benign and malignant tumors such a mass may represent: Is this a cyst, tumor or a lymph node? Is it part of a systemic inflammatory or autoimmune problem? If a tumor, is it benign or malignant? What is the role of fine needle aspiration (FNA), magnetic resonance imaging (MRI), and computed tomography (CT)? Are other evaluation tools useful, such as radionuclide scanning or ultrasound? For lesions of the parotid, in whom should a parotidectomy be done? In whom may it be avoided? These are just some of the questions confronting the clinician in this setting. This chapter reviews the surgical anatomy of the major salivary glands and the clinical presentation of various lesions; it also examines various treatment options. More comprehensive discussions of the relevant anatomy are given elsewhere.[1,2]

SURGICAL ANATOMY

The major salivary glands consist of the parotid, submandibular, and sublingual glands. Since 85% of salivary gland diseases appear in the parotid, discussion concentrates on this major gland. Where differences with other salivary glands arise, these are discussed as well.

The parotid gland is easily palpable overlying the ramus of the mandible anterior to the tragus of the ear. The inferior-most part of the gland (the "tail") is palpable between the mastoid process of the temporal bone posterosuperiorly and the angle of the mandible anteroinferiorly. The masseter muscle overlying the ramus of the mandible and the internal pterygoid muscle deep to the mandible form the anterior border of the parotid compartment. Posteriorly, the bony and cartilaginous external auditory canal, the mastoid process, and the base of the styloid process form the upper posterior border of the compartment. The sternocleidomastoid and posterior belly of the digastric muscle form the lower posterior border of the compartment, and the zygomatic arch forms the superior border. The deep portion of the parotid ("deep lobe") extends between the stylomandibular ligament and the mandible to lie on the styloid muscles and carotid sheath. A tumor involving the isthmus of the parotid extending through this constricture is sometimes referred to as a "dumbbell" tumor; tumors may also arise solely in the deep lobe and are occasionally referred to as "round" tumors. As this space is just lateral to the lateral pharyngeal space, deep lobe parotid tumors may be palpable intraorally, displacing the soft palate and tonsillar fossa anteromedially.

The parotid gland is unilobular with numerous processes and lacks true superficial and deep lobes; however, the presence of the facial nerve makes it clinically useful to subdivide this gland's anatomy. Near the isthmus, the facial nerve enters the gland and subsequently divides at the so-called pes anserinus ("goose foot") into its major branches. It is in this way that the gland may be thought of as that portion lateral to the plane of the facial nerve branches (the superficial lobe) and a deep portion medial to the facial nerve. These are the product of surgical dissection and not true separate anatomic units.

Three to five processes of the parotid gland often exist, making it extremely difficult to perform a true total parotidectomy. The three superficial processes are the condylar process (near the temporomandibular joint), the meatal process (in the medial area of the incisura of the external auditory canal), and the posterior process (projecting between the mastoid and the sternocleidomastoid muscle). Two deep processes are the glenoid process, which rests on the vaginal process of the tympanic portion of the temporal bone, and the stylomandibular process, which projects anteromedially above the stylomandibular ligament.

The parotid is drained by Stensen's duct, which is 4 to 7 cm long and found along the anterior border of the parotid inferior to the zygoma, crossing the masseter and buccal fat pad, and then penetrating the buccinator muscle before opening intraorally opposite the second maxillary molar.

The blood supply of the parotid gland is from branches of the external carotid artery. The retromandibular vein drains the gland. Lymphatic drainage is via intraglandular and extraglandular lymph nodes, of which there may be as many as 20 such periparotid nodes. These are all located in the superficial lobe and drain into the deep jugular chain.

Facial Nerve

The facial nerve exits the temporal bone through the stylomastoid foramen, which is immediately posterior to the base of the styloid process and immediately anterior to the attachment of the posterior belly of the digastric muscle at the digastric ridge of the mastoid tip. If not identifiable from a more distal location, the facial nerve may be identified at the stylomastoid foramen after removing the mastoid tip. If tumor precludes this approach as well, then the descending portion of the facial nerve may be found by drilling into the mastoid itself.

From the stylomastoid foramen, the facial nerve travels anterolaterally toward the parotid gland, sending off branches to the posterior auricular muscle, the posterior belly of the digastric muscle, and the stylohyoid muscle. The facial nerve then enters the parotid gland posterior to the facial vein and soon branches at the pes anserinus into an upper temporal facial division and a lower cervical facial division. It subsequently branches in variable fashion to innervate facial muscles of expression. The plane of these branches is superficial to the external carotid artery and facial vein. The particular course of the major branches of the facial nerve is variable; the surgeon must locate and dissect those branches in the area of the tumor in order to safely extirpate tumor.

Submandibular Gland

In contrast to the parotid, which contains only serous glands, the submandibular gland contains both serous and mucous glands. This difference in histology is important in considering the types of benign and neoplastic disorders to which the latter gland is subject.

The submandibular or submaxillary gland lies inferomedial to the body of the mandible. Most of the gland is superficial to the mylohyoid muscle, but a deep extension lies between the mylohyoid and the hyoglossus muscle. The stylomandibular ligament separates the submandibular gland from the parotid gland. The 5 cm submandibular duct (Wharton's duct) courses between the mylohyoid and hyoglossus muscles along the genioglossus muscle to enter the floor of the mouth near the midline lingual frenulum. The hypoglossal nerve lies below the duct, and the lingual nerve lies above it. The lingual nerve is best seen by medially retracting the mylohyoid muscle. The marginal mandibular and cervical branches of the facial nerve run in the fascia superficial to the submandibular gland in a course superficial to the anterior facial vein. The lingual and facial arteries supply the gland with the facial artery, creating a groove in the gland's deep portion; the anterior facial vein drains it, and lymphatic drainage is into the submandibular nodes to the deep jugular nodes.

Sublingual Gland

The smallest of the major salivary glands, the sublingual gland, weighing only 2 gm, lies in the sublingual depression on the inner surface of the mandible near the symphysis. Eight to 20 ducts exit its superior surface in the sublingual fold of the floor of the mouth. The sublingual branch of the lingual artery and submental branch of the facial artery supply the gland. Lymphatic drainage goes to the submental and submandibular nodes. Primary tumors of the sublingual gland are rare. Along with minor salivary gland tumors, this area is covered clinically in the chapter on oral cavity tumors.

CLINICAL PRESENTATION

A thorough history and physical examination are fundamental in order to be able to formulate an initial differential diagnosis and management plan. Certain clinical parameters are unique to the salivary glands and need to be evaluated in turn (Table 7–1).

A complete history usually allows a clinician to distinguish between infection or tumor. For example, a short history (days) of pain and swelling in an otherwise healthy adult, associated with physical signs of inflammation such as tenderness, suggest an infectious or obstructive etiology. In the submandibular gland, stones with subsequent ductal obstruction are the likeliest cause for this scenario, since 80% of salivary stones occur in this gland. In an older patient, similar signs and symptoms in the parotid gland suggest acute suppurative sialadenitis as the etiology. If pus can be expressed from the duct, initial empiric antibiotics are prescribed, making sure to cover the usual upper airway pathogens as well as staphylococcal organisms. Needle aspiration may also be appropriate in order to obtain material for culture; an abscess should generally be incised and drained. Although rare today, mumps usually presents in children as painful bilateral parotid enlargement.

A history of recurrent episodes of inflammation in an adult suggests chronic sialadenitis, often secondary to sialolithiasis, duct dilatation, or prior sialadenitis with fibrosis. A first branchial cleft may also present as a localized area of infection or generalized parotitis. This is because the cyst tract courses through the parotid. In some children, recurrent juvenile parotitis can similarly present in this fashion. However, in this latter group, there is no known etiologic agent and surgery is contraindicated.

Unlike infection, most tumors have had a longer history, usually measured in weeks or months, with a discrete palpable mass prompting the initial consultation. Pain is an ominous clinical accompaniment to a tumor and is usually present in the group with adenoid cystic carcinoma; however, its absence does not preclude the presence of a malignancy. Growth is usually slow and steady, without intervening fluctuations in size. A rapid increase in size of a previously small, painless mass may occur secondary to cystic degeneration, infection, or hemorrhage. Another form of clinical presentation is one of diffuse glandular enlargement, without a discrete mass or associated signs of inflammation. This suggests an infiltrative, noninflammatory etiology such as sialadenosis. Alcohol and a number of medications are associated with such a process. Lymphoepithelial lesions may present with diffuse enlargement or as a distinct mass simulating a tumor. If there is a history of autoimmune diseases, Sjögren's is a leading candidate in the differential diagnosis. A patient who is HIV-positive is prone to developing parotid cysts as well as generalized lymphadenopathy.[3,4]

In organizing one's thoughts and choosing among management options, it is helpful to distinguish three general types of lesions presenting in the major salivary glands: (1) non-neoplastic lesions, (2) lymphoepithelial lesions, and (3) tumors. These may be further classified as shown in Tables 7–2 and 7–3.

PREOPERATIVE EVALUATION OF A MASS LESION

A mass in or near the parotid gland unaccompanied by an inflammatory history may be a congenital, benign, or malignant tumor. Our discussion focuses on the parotid area, as lesions there are most common. However, similar principles apply to other salivary glands with appropriate adaptations for the relevant anatomy. Diffuse, bilateral lesions of short duration or in the context of systemic disease are more likely related to the primary disease process

T A B L E 7 – 1	**CLINICAL PARAMETERS**
CATEGORY	**EXAMPLE**
Age	Neonate
	Child
	Adult
	Geriatric
Ethnicity	Southern Chinese
	African-American
Past medical history/ associated illnesses	Autoimmune or infiltrative diseases
	HIV status/AIDS/immunocompromised
	Prior malignancy
	Medications/drugs/alcohol
Duration of symptoms	Days
	Weeks
	Months
Systemic signs/ symptoms	Fever
	Weight loss
	Anemia
Local signs/symptoms	Size and changes in size
	Evidence of ductal obstruction (pain, tenderness)
	Local inflammation (fever, erythema, palpable nodes)
	Evidence of disease extension
	Facial nerve paresis or paralysis
	Skin involvement
	Palpable lymphadenopathy
	Trismus

TABLE 7 – 2	CLASSIFICATION OF MAJOR SALIVARY GLAND MASSES

NON-NEOPLASTIC

Congenital

First branchial cleft cyst
Lymphatic malformation/(lymphangioma)
Hemangioma/vascular malformation

Granulomatous Diseases

Sarcoidosis
Tuberculosis
Other (Actinomycosis, cat-scratch disease, etc.)

Infections

Viral infections
    Mumps
    Hepatitis C
    Other (CMV, adenovirus, etc.)
Bacterial sialadenitis

Noninflammatory or Unknown Etiology

Sialadenosis
Sialolithiasis (see also bacterial sialadenitis)
Recurrent parotitis of children
    (Juvenile recurrent parotitis)

LYMPHOEPITHELIAL LESIONS

Benign Lymphoid Proliferation

Autoimmune: Sjögren's
Benign lymphoepithelial lesion (BLEL), myoepithelial sialadenitis (MESA)
HIV(+)/AIDS-related cysts

Lymphomas[15]

Mucosa-associated lymphoid tumors (MALToma):low-grade B-cell lymphomas
Intraparotid nodal lymphomas

TUMORS

Benign

Pleomorphic adenoma (including myoepithelioma)
    Recurrent pleomorphic adenoma
    Metastasizing pleomorphic adenoma (very rare)
Basal cell adenoma
Oncocytoma (and clear cell adenoma)
Cystadenoma
    Warthin's tumor (papillary cystadenoma lymphomatosum, adenolymphoma)
    Other: sebaceous lymphadenoma, papillary cystadenoma

Malignant (see Table 7–3)

itself rather than intrinsic salivary gland dysfunction. Therefore, further discussion of nonmass lesions is omitted.

The management of a small nontender mass in the parotid that has been present for more than 6 weeks is straightforward: lack of inflammatory signs and the longer history make a tumor etiology most likely. In adult nonimmunocompromised patients without prior malignancy, 80% of such masses are benign. Most clinicians would agree that, in an otherwise medically healthy patient, a superficial parotidectomy with dissection and preservation of the facial nerve by an experienced surgeon is the appropriate next step in management. Many would do no further evaluation of the mass (other than chest x-ray and perioperative laboratory tests), reasoning that the surgical procedure would not be changed. Even if the mass proves malignant on permanent histology, the lesion with a cuff of normal tissue will have been removed, and the only consideration is whether postoperative irradiation should be added. In the unlikely event that enlarged nodes are noted in the immediate area, they would have been biopsied intraoperatively and, if found to be malignant, a neck dissection would be considered either at that time (if discussed preoperatively with the patient) or as a secondary procedure. The same reasoning applies in the submandibular area, except that a smaller percentage (50% to 60%) are benign and a suprahyoid or supraomohyoid neck dissection are considerations.

When should additional preoperative evaluation be indicated? Several factors, such as an unusual location of the lesion, difficulty in clinically assessing deep extension, multiplicity, or a history of prior malignancy may be indications for further evaluation. If the clinician feels that more than a straightforward parotidectomy may be needed, he or she may want more preoperative cytologic or radiologic information. Such information may also be helpful to a patient in understanding the possible need for a more extensive procedure.

A diagnostic fine needle aspiration (FNA) helps the clinician and patient decide when—or even if—surgery is indicated. For example, in a patient with a known history of a prior malignancy, the FNA would be helpful in excluding metastatic tumor. In an HIV-positive individual, the FNA could differentiate between a parotid cyst or a lymphoma. If the latter is suspected, safer biopsy of a cervical lymph

TABLE 7 – 3	MALIGNANT MAJOR SALIVARY GLAND TUMORS BY BEHAVIOR

Low Grade

Mucoepidermoid carcinoma, low and intermediate grade
Acinic cell carcinoma
Adenocarcinoma, not otherwise specified, low grade
Epithelial myoepithelial carcinoma
Basal cell adenocarcinoma

High Grade

Mucoepidermoid carcinoma, high grade
Adenoid cystic carcinoma
Adenocarcinoma, not otherwise specified, high grade
Salivary duct carcinoma
Carcinoma ex pleomorphic adenoma
Squamous cell carcinoma
Undifferentiated and neuroendocrine carcinoma

node would be warranted for diagnostic purposes rather than subjecting the patient to a facial nerve dissection with its attendant possible morbidity. Similarly, FNA diagnosis of a benign tumor in an elderly, medically frail patient could safely preclude surgical exploration—as would the diagnosis of a reactive intraparotid lymph node in a young, robust individual.

The predictive accuracy of FNA is contingent on user expertise and experience. When properly practiced by an experienced cytopathologist, the procedure is well-tolerated and safe. Results correlate with the final histology at least as well as intraoperative frozen section analysis.[5,6] Fine needle aspiration of salivary lesions, as elsewhere in the head and neck, requires close communication between clinician and pathologist. An accurate diagnosis may not always be possible, as, for example, in the face of a difficult or rare underlying histology. In such instances, a descriptive report is given. This description may or may not be helpful to the clinician, but it is rarely misleading. For instance, suggesting a benign lesion is malignant, or vice-versa, is unusual. Cystic or lymphoid lesions, mucoepidermoid carcinoma, and cellular mixed tumors without stroma or with nuclear atypia are the more common situations posing difficulties for the cytopathologist attempting to make a complete and accurate diagnosis. Numer-

ous reviews over the past 15 years suggest that, in satisfactory specimens reviewed by experienced cytopathologists, the false-negative rate in benign lesions is less than 2% to 5%, and the false-positive rate in malignant ones is similarly low.[7-10] Predictive values are generally greater than 90%. If the cytological diagnosis seems inconsistent with clinical judgment, this dichotomy should lead to further thought and investigation before deciding on appropriate treatment.

Radiologic evaluation is helpful in larger tumors (greater than 3 to 4 cm) where the possibility of malignancy or deep lobe involvement is higher. Magnetic resonance imaging (MRI) with contrast is the radiologic examination of choice, as this provides multiplanar imaging and better tissue contrast as compared to computed tomography (CT). Other imaging techniques play little role in the evaluation of salivary tumors and are of only historical interest. Although Warthin's tumors and oncocytomas can be detected with technetium-99 radionuclide imaging, FNA is more specific.

Benign tumors usually demonstrate low signal intensity on T1-weighted MRI images and high signal intensity on T2-weighted images (reflecting their higher seromucinous secretions); such masses are usually well-circumscribed with smooth margins (Fig. 7–1). Low-grade malignancies may be indistinguishable

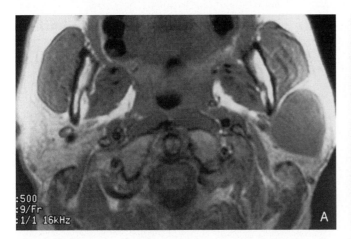

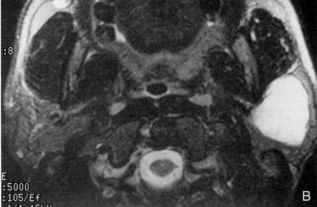

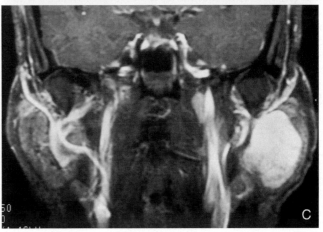

FIGURE 7–1   A 28-year-old male presents with a slowly enlarging mass in the left parotid region. *A*, An axial T1-weighted image shows a rounded, well-circumscribed, smoothly marginated mass in the left parotid gland. Overlying subcutaneous fat and skin are normal. *B*, An axial fast spin-echo T2-weighted image with fat suppression shows that the mass is homogeneously hyperintense compared with normal gland and with muscle. *C*, A coronal postgadolinium T1-weighted image with fat suppression shows intense, homogeneous enhancement of the smoothly marginated mass. A pleomorphic adenoma was confirmed surgically.

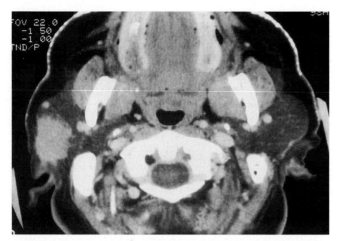

FIGURE 7–2 A 68-year-old female presents with a slowly enlarging mass in the right parotid region. An axial image from a contrast-enhanced CT scan demonstrates a homogeneously enhancing soft-tissue mass in the right parotid gland. The margins are spiculated, and irregular soft tissue extends into the subcutaneous fat overlying the right parotid gland. An acinic cell carcinoma was identified at surgery.

from benign tumors, though the margins are often more spiculated.

Malignant tumors often have more poorly defined or spiculated margins and are often low in signal intensity on both T1 and T2 images. The CT appearance also likely shows more spiculated margins (Fig. 7–2). The value of MRI lies not so much in discerning whether a tumor is malignant, but rather in anatomically delineating the extent of disease (Fig. 7–3) and the presence of abnormal cervical nodes. MRI may also demonstrate central nonenhancement consistent with necrosis within the mass (Fig. 7–4).

When there are overt signs of malignancy (e.g., skin involvement, facial nerve paralysis, or enlarged firm nodes), MRI, in addition to helping plan surgical approaches, may assist the radiation oncologist in delineating the areas to be included in postoperative irradiation. Defining the histology via an FNA may also provide information as to whether further evaluation is needed (such as chest CT in a patient with adenoid cystic carcinoma to exclude the high probability of pulmonary metastases).

TREATMENT

Table 7–4 delineates the current American Joint Commission on Cancer staging system for salivary gland malignancies. Table 7–5 summarizes the treatment approach for malignant tumors of the major salivary glands that present without distant metastases. Benign tumors are treated similarly to stage I malignancies (complete resection of the tumor with preservation of motor nerves), except that radiation

is one option for recurrent pleomorphic adenomas where reoperation would significantly jeopardize facial nerve function (to be discussed later). The surgical techniques of facial nerve dissection, as well as selective or comprehensive neck dissections, are reviewed elsewhere. Here we discuss certain controversial issues and the management of difficult problems.

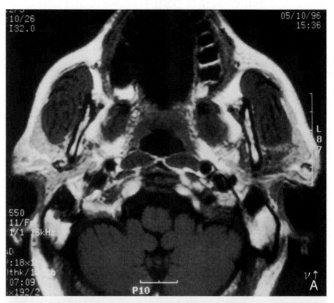

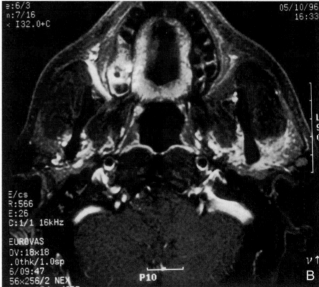

FIGURE 7–3 A 69-year-old male has noted a history of left periparotid pain and weakness of his face lasting several months. *A,* An axial T1-weighted image demonstrates an irregularly marginated, infiltrative soft-tissue mass in the left parotid gland. Though this process closely abuts the mandible, the cortex appears intact, and the marrow space has normal fatty signal intensity. *B,* Following gadolinium administrations, an axial T1-weighted image with fat saturation demonstrates enhancement of this process, which appears to involve the posterior aspect of the left masseter muscle. A fine-needle aspirate showed a poorly differentiated malignancy, and squamous cell carcinoma was diagnosed at surgery.

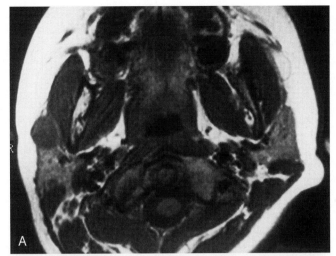

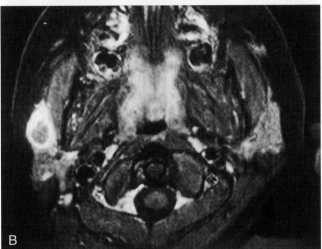

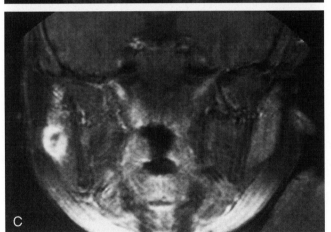

FIGURE 7–4 A 10-year-old male recently noted the development of a small lump in the right parotid region. *A*, An axial T1-weighted image shows a small, round mass in the right parotid gland with apparently well-defined margins. The overlying subcutaneous fat and skin are unremarkable. *B*, Post-gadolinium, an axial T1-weighted image with fat saturation demonstrates central nonenhancement of the mass consistent with necrosis. In addition, the margins of the mass now appear slightly irregular. *C*, A post-gadolinium T1-weighted image with fat saturation in the coronal plane is motion degraded, but better demonstrates the irregular, spiculated margins of the lesion. At surgery, an acinic cell carcinoma, microcystic type, was identified.

T A B L E 7 – 4	STAGING OF MAJOR SALIVARY GLAND MALIGNANCIES

Tx	Primary tumor cannot be assessed
T0	No evidence of primary tumor
T1	Tumor ≤2 cm in greatest dimension
T2	Tumor 2–4 cm in greatest dimension
T3	Tumor 4–6 cm in greatest dimension
T4	Tumor >6 cm in greatest dimension
	All categories are subdivided: (a) no local extension, (b) local extension. (Local extension is clinical/macroscopic invasion of skin, soft tissue, bone, or nerve. Microscopic evidence alone is not local extension for classification purposes.)
Nx	Regional nodes cannot be assessed
N0	No regional lymph mode metastases
N1	Single ipsilateral node <3 cm in diameter
N2a	Single ipsilateral node 3–6 cm in diameter
N2b	Multiple ipsilateral nodes, none >6 cm
N2c	Bilateral or contralateral nodes, none >6 cm
N3	Metastasis in a lymph node >6 cm
Mx	Presence of distant metastases cannot be assessed
M0	No distant metastases
M1	Distant metastases

Stage	T	N	M
Stage I	T1a	N0	M0
	T2a	N0	M0
Stage II	T1b	N0	M0
	T2b	N0	M0
	T3a	N0	M0
Stage III	T3b	N0	M0
	T4a	N0	M0
	Any T (except T4b)	**N1**	**M0**
Stage IV	T4b	Any N	Any M
	Any T	**N2, N3**	Any M
	Any T	Any N	**M1**

American Joint Commission on Cancer, 1988

ISSUES IN OPERATIVE MANAGEMENT

Adequate Operation for Parotid Tumor

Proper exposure, identification of relevant anatomic landmarks, and meticulous hemostasis are key to the successful execution of any variety of parotidectomy. The facial nerve may be found in several ways, including following distal branches retrograde or finding the nerve descending within the mastoid or at the stylomastoid foramen. By far, the most common method used is to locate the nerve in the small triangle bounded by the tympanomastoid suture superiorly, digastric muscle posteriorly, and the styloid process anteriorly. The nerve usually lies 4 to 8 mm inferior to the bony suture, running an anterior-inferior course. Adjacent tissue is serially dissected, tested with a VII stimulator if there is any question, and bleeding controlled with fine bipolar cautery. The nerve is located and dissected distally by lifting tissue lateral to it, with bipolar electrocau-

TABLE 7 – 5	MANAGEMENT PRINCIPLES FOR TREATMENT OF SALIVARY GLAND MALIGNANCIES			

	STAGE HISTOLOGY			
MANAGEMENT ISSUES	I, Low grade (0–4 cm, no local extension)	I, High grade	II–IV w/ N0M0 (Local extension and/ or >4 cm)	Any T, N1–3 (Positive nodes)
Surgical procedure (extent of parotidectomy)	Superficial (partial) or total as needed	Superficial (partial) or total as needed	To fit disease: may require mastoid tip, mandible, muscles	To fit disease
(If submandibular tumor)	Submandibular triangle resection	Wide excision submandibular triangle	Supraomohyoid neck dissection is likely; skin, muscles to fit disease	Radical or modified radical neck dissection; skin, muscles to fit disease
Management of VII nerve (For submandibular tumors management of V, XII nerves)	Preserve	Preserve	Preserve functioning branches if possible[a]	Preserve functioning branches if possible[a]
Neck dissection?	No	No[b]	No[b]	Yes
Postoperative RT?	No, unless positive margins	Yes	Yes[c]	Yes[c]

[a] Resected VII branches requiring reconstruction should be reconstructed immediately, usually with a cable graft.

[b] If positive nodes are found at surgery, neck dissection is indicated. In SCC, some would include a neck dissection; others would not as postoperative RT is to be included.

[c] High-LET radiation, such as fast neutron irradiation, should be considered when there are macroscopic positive margins, in unresectable tumors, and for previously irradiated tumors.

tery used for hemostasis and division. Interfering as little as possible with the blood supply to the nerve branches minimizes the risk of postoperative facial weakness.

Most surgeons agree that it is sufficient to remove a parotid tumor by leaving a cuff of normal tissue around and attached to it during the dissection rather than simply enucleating the tumor from the glandular bed. This en bloc excision may, at times, require dissection between two or more branches of the facial nerve in order to remove tumor extending medially toward the masseter muscle. Whether a tumor is located in the superficial lobe of the parotid or extends medially, its dissection from the underlying facial nerve implies that the tumor mass lies immediately adjacent to a branch of the nerve. Thus, the closest margin of resection is in reality the nerve itself. When reviewing the fixed tissue, an unsuspecting pathologist may conclude that a close or "positive margin" exists since tumor on the microscope slide will approach the inked resection margin. However, this positive or close margin does not require further therapy since sacrifice of a normally functioning branch of the facial nerve is contraindicated. As in many areas of the head and neck, close communication is mandatory between pathologist and clinician in order to determine if further therapy is warranted.

Frozen Section Diagnosis

Frozen sections share the same difficulty as FNA in the evaluation of parotid lesions with problematic histology. As discussed earlier, an FNA is likely the best choice for preoperative evaluation. Cohen et al[11] in 1990 compared FNA with frozen section diagnoses. Difficulties for one technique were also noted for the other technique. An overall accuracy rate of 71% for frozen section was observed when compared to 88% for FNA. Layfield et al[5] similarly reported FNA as being somewhat superior: an 11% false-negative rate for frozen section diagnosis compared to a 4.7% for FNA, particularly for malignancies. A surgeon may encounter a situation where histologic confirmation of malignancy would be helpful but not available preoperatively. Noting the possibility of a misleading result, a frozen section may be helpful in confirming a clinical suspicion. For example, frozen section confirmation of perineural invasion could assist in the decision to sacrifice a particular facial nerve branch. If a nearby lymph node appears to be involved with disease, an excisional biopsy can confirm nodal spread. A conservative alternative is to limit the procedure solely to a parotidectomy and await permanent section diagnosis. Even the most experienced pathologist may find it difficult to interpret salivary gland frozen section material—a process that must be accomplished quickly.

Facial Nerve Monitoring

Facial nerve monitoring using a two-channel device may assist a surgeon in avoiding injury to the facial nerve but is no substitute for meticulous dissection and experience. It is usually sufficient to have a disposable facial nerve monitor at hand. Experienced surgeons often find even a disposable monitor unnecessary in patients without prior surgery who have small tumors. In recurrent cases, where finding the nerve may be challenging, external facial nerve monitoring is often extremely helpful; electrical stimulation may be the only indication of where a branch lies.

Indications for Neck Dissection

It is prudent to palpate adjacent nodes in the parotid field and to biopsy any that are hard or enlarged (greater than 10 mm). Larger tumors or those associated with facial nerve paralysis are more likely to have positive regional lymphadenopathy, as are certain histologies such as squamous cell carcinoma (SCC) or high-grade mucoepidermoid carcinoma. A modified radical neck dissection is indicated if nodes are involved in SCC, high-grade mucoepidermoid carcinoma, adenocarcinoma, melanoma, or undifferentiated carcinoma. In general, many feel that elective neck dissection can be omitted in necks showing clinically negative results if postoperative irradiation is likely to be used.

POSTOPERATIVE TREATMENT

Other than for surgical complications and recurrence, there are no additional treatment issues for benign tumors. For treatment of malignant tumors, the major issue is the need for postoperative adjuvant therapy—radiation plus or minus chemotherapy.

To address the indications for irradiation, it is helpful to first review the factors that affect prognosis in salivary gland malignancies. These include: (1) histopathology (high grade vs. low grade); (2) tumor size; (3) extraparotid extension (clinical/macroscopic invasion of skin, soft tissue, bone, or nerve); and (4) lymph node involvement. These parameters are incorporated into the staging system and treatment plan (see Tables 7–4 and 7–5).

Histopathology

The next part of this chapter reviews the pathology of the major salivary gland tumors. Table 7–9 of that part and Table 7–3 in this part list the more common malignancies encountered, as well as some of the rarer ones. It is helpful to discuss as a group the few low-grade carcinomas from the more numerous high-grade ones. Low- and intermediate-grade tumors include acinic cell carcinoma and low-grade mucoepidermoid carcinoma. Most other malignant tumors commonly encountered in the major salivary glands are high-grade. The 10-year survival rate for low-grade mucoepidermoid carcinoma is over 90%, and for acinic cell carcinoma over 80%.[1] In contrast, for the high-grade tumors (high-grade mucoepidermoid carcinoma, adenoid cystic carcinoma, high-grade adenocarcinoma, carcinoma ex-pleomorphic adenoma, and squamous cell carcinoma), the 5-year survivals are generally reported to be 50% to 75% (occasionally lower in some series), and the 10-year survival rates 25% to 60%. Undifferentiated carcinomas have an even lower survival rate. The low-grade tumors have less than 15% incidence of lymph node metastases, the high-grade ones 20% to 45%, with high-grade mucoepidermoid carcinoma and squamous cell carcinoma being the highest.

Numerous studies have shown that the larger a malignant parotid tumor, the worse the prognosis. This, in turn, is reflected in the staging system and treatment paradigms. Stage I tumors have less than a 2% incidence of distant metastases, whereas a 39% rate is seen among Stage III tumors.[12] Larger tumors have a higher recurrence rate as well.

Irradiation

Retrospective evidence strongly suggests that irradiation reduces the incidence of recurrence and improves locoregional control rates. Conventional fractionation using photons or 4meV electrons to a dose of 60 to 65 Gy is commonly employed. For patients with grossly positive margins—or in whom the tumor is unresectable or who are poor surgical risks—at least one study supports the superiority of neutrons over photons, with 2-year locoregional control of 67% versus 17%.[13]

The indications for regional postoperative irradiation can be simply summed up: all major salivary gland malignancies should receive postoperative irradiation except low-grade Stage I tumors that are resected with clear margins. Thus, only low-grade malignancies less than 4 cm resected with a cuff of normal tissue should be clinically observed without postoperative irradiation. A histologically low-grade tumor that is large or that infiltrates extraparotid tissue is included in the group for which irradiation is recommended. The treatment of draining lymph nodes is similarly recommended if the tumor is high grade, large, or has a greater than 30% chance of exhibiting nodal metastases. As discussed previously, whether the neck is treated with postoperative radiation therapy or a prophylactic neck dissection is controversial.

Chemotherapy

There is little experience in multi-institution trials for the efficacy of chemotherapy in treating salivary gland tumors. For adenoid cystic carcinoma there are isolated cases of the use of certain drugs such as cisplatin, adriamycin, ifosfamide, and vincristine showing complete response rates of less than 10%. Most agree that the role of chemotherapy is limited to palliation for metastatic or recurrent cases. Resection of minimal pulmonary metastases of adenoid cystic carcinoma should be strongly considered.

RECURRENT DISEASES

Recurrent malignant tumors present a problem for which there are only inadequate solutions. Usually, the area has already been irradiated. If an MRI suggests the tumor is resectable, this should be strongly considered. This may require sacrifice of the facial nerve with proximal margins obtainable only via a temporal bone resection. If the carotid artery is encased in tumor, cure or local control with carotid resection and bypass are quite unlikely. The possible role of intraoperative irradiation for recurrent cases is not yet known. The use of neutrons as reirradiation has been reported, with about a 20% incidence of severe late complications.

The presence of a mass in the parotid in a patient who has previously undergone a parotidectomy for pleomorphic adenoma is not unusual. The incidence of recurrent pleomorphic adenoma is estimated to be 2% to 30%, with most recurrences occurring years following initial surgery. Of tumors that recur once, over 25% reoccur, often with increasingly shorter intervals between recurrences. This is challenging since the risk of facial nerve paresis is notably greater in subsequent operations. The possibility of carcinoma ex pleomorphic adenoma should be evaluated by FNA, especially if nonsurgical treatment is being considered. For recurrent pleomorphic adenoma there are three management options: (1) re-resection with facial nerve monitoring, (2) irradiation with or without repeat surgery, and (3) careful clinical follow-up without intervention. An MRI is extremely helpful in delineating the extent of disease. The MRI is helpful in planning surgery, especially as multicentric recurrence is not rare—particularly in reoccuring cases. If irradiation is planned, the MRI is helpful in planning fields. If no intervention is planned immediately, then the MRI serves as an objective baseline for comparison of future growth. If surgery is performed, either the tumor alone is resected, or a total parotidectomy is per-

formed. As would be expected, the incidence of postoperative paresis is high. Hence, irradiation as a nonoperative approach should be discussed. It appears effective in retarding subsequent growth, but adverse effects—including a low rate of radiation-induced malignancy—must be considered. The third option is "watchful waiting," an especially attractive option when tumor appears adherent to a functioning facial nerve. Periodic clinical and radiological follow-up examinations are done, with intervention postponed until the rate of tumor growth indicates intervention or VII involvement becomes evident. The choice selected for a particular patient depends upon overall health, occupation, desires, and tolerance for the different risks. Considerable work is currently being done on the genetics of pleomorphic adenoma. It is possible that in the future the correlation between cytogenetic subgroups of pleomorphic adenoma and their respective clinical courses may suggest that patients with selected pleomorphic adenomas might benefit from postoperative irradiation initially or that they might receive a disproportional benefit from radiation therapy for recurrences.

COMPLICATIONS OF TREATMENT

Prevention of complications from salivary gland surgery begins with understanding the pathophysiology of inflammatory and infectious processes and the management principles for treating the tumors that arise. Familiarity with the roles and limitations of FNA and MRI is necessary when the diagnosis is uncertain, for large tumors, or when a tumor is likely malignant. Parotid and submandibular gland surgery can be done with low morbidity by an experienced surgeon. Wound infections are unusual. Most perioperative complications are managed conservatively.

Following removal of the drains within a few days of surgery, subsequent swelling may be noted, with or without pain. This may be due to a sialocele or seroma. Aspiration of the fluid may need to be done more than once. Occasionally, it may be necessary to open the inferior part of the incision minimally and to place a pressure dressing for a few days, and occasionally longer.

Postoperative infection is not common. Cellulitis is treated empirically: numerous antibiotic choices such as second-generation cephalosporins, first-generation cephalosporins plus metronidazole, or clindamycin are all satisfactory. If there is pus, antibiotics that cover staphylococcus species are usually best.

Some patients may note the symptoms of gustatory sweating months after surgery (Frey's syndrome). With starch-iodine testing, this can be demonstrated in essentially all patients. Antiperspirant applied to the area before meals should be tried as an initial intervention in those few patients whose symptoms are severe enough to warrant intervention. This postoperative result should be anticipated, as well as other phenomena such as earlobe numbness. Many surgical interventions have been proposed over the years to manage Frey's syndrome, suggesting that none have proven consistently helpful.

The most critical postoperative complication is facial paralysis. The key to the prevention of facial paralysis is identification and preservation of the branches of the facial nerve. This is easiest when the tumor is small and there is no prior inflammation, surgery, or irradiation. Techniques of finding and dissecting the nerve without injuring it are reviewed extensively elsewhere.

When a major branch of the facial nerve or the nerve itself proximal to the pes is transected intraoperatively (e.g., to resect a malignant tumor), consideration should be given to repair at the end of the procedure. Paralysis of the marginal mandibular branch and the branches to the orbicularis oculi are most likely to be symptomatic. Paralytic ectropion, conjunctivitis, exposure keratitis, and epiphora result from paralysis of the obicularis oculi muscle. Incomplete lower lip depression, leading to possible lip-biting and oral incompetence with drooling result from marginal mandibular nerve weakness. If the two ends can be approximated without tension, a neurorrhaphy should be done. More likely, a cable graft will be needed, using, for example, the greater auricular nerve, if available. If the facial nerve was involved by tumor, it is wise to check by frozen section the proximal and distal ends before proceeding with the neurorrhaphy. Supplementary rehabilitative procedures including fascial slings, muscle transfers, and hypoglossal-facial nerve anastamoses are discussed in numerous surgical texts.

Transient facial nerve paralysis is the most common postoperative complication that requires treatment. Maintaining ocular lubrication is key in preventing corneal complications. Artificial tears or a transparent plastic bubble are commonly used. If recovery is expected to be delayed (such as after a cable graft), an upper-lid gold weight may be placed during, or soon after, surgery. Ophthalmologic consultation is sought if the patient notes a scratchy foreign-body sensation or blurred vision, or if neovascularization of the cornea, conjunctivitis, or keratitis are noted.

REFERENCES

1. Kaplan MJ, Johns ME. Salivary glands: Malignant neoplasms. In: Cummings CW, et al., eds. *Otolaryngology—Head and Neck Surgery*. St. Louis: Mosby; 1993:1043.
2. Graney DE, Jacobs JR, Kern R. Salivary glands: Anatomy. In: Cummings CW, et al., eds. *Otolaryngology—Head and Neck Surgery*. St. Louis: Mosby; 1993:977.
3. Holliday RA, Cohen WA, Schinella RA, et al. Benign lymphoepithelial parotid cysts and hyperplastic cervical adenopathy in AIDS-risk patients: A new CT appearance. *Radiology*. 1988; 168:439.
4. Shugar JM, Som PM, Jacobson AL, Ryan JR, Bernard PJ, Dickman SH. Multicentric parotid cysts and cervical adenopathy in AIDS patients. A newly recognized entity: CT and MR manifestations. *Laryngoscope*. 1988; 98:772.
5. Layfield LJ, Tan P, Glasgow BJ. Fine needle aspiration salivary glands: Comparison with frozen sections and histologic findings. *Arch Pathol Lab Med*. 1987; 111:346.
6. Wheelis RF, Yarington CT Jr. Tumors of the salivary glands: Comparison of frozen section diagnosis with final pathologic diagnosis. *Arch Otolaryngol*. 1984; 110:76.
7. Abele JS, Miller TR, Knoll R. Fine needle aspiration diagnosis of salivary glands. In: Abele JS, Miller TR, eds. *Seventh Annual Symposium on Fine Needle Aspiration*. San Francisco: University of California; 1987:283.
8. Quzilbash AH, Siamos J, Young JEM, Archibald SD. Fine needle aspiration biopsy cytology of major salivery glands. *Acta Cytol*. 1985; 29:503.
9. Nettle WJ, Orrell SR. Fine needle aspiration in the diagnosis of salivary gland lesions. *Aust NZ J Surg*. 1989; 59:47.
10. Jayaram N, Ashin D, Raajwanshi A, Radhika S, Banerjee CK. The value of fine-needle aspiration biopsy in the cytodiagnosis of salivary gland lesions. *Diag Cytopathol*. 1989; 5:345.
11. Cohen MB, Fisher PE, Holly EA, Ljung B-M, Lowhagen T, Bottles K. Fine needle aspiration biopsy diagnosis of mucoepidermoid carcinoma. Statistical analysis. *Acta Cytol*. 1990; 34:43.
12. Spiro RH, Huvos AG, Strong EW. Cancer of the parotid gland. *Am J Surg*. 1975; 13:452.
13. Griffin TW, Pajak TF, Laramore GE, et al. Neutron vs photon irradiation of inoperable salivary gland tumors: results of an RTOG-MRC cooperative randomized study. *Int J Radiat Oncol Biol Phys*. 1988; 15:1085.

BIBLIOGRAPHY

Kaplan MJ, Johns ME. Malignant neoplasms (of the major salivary glands). In: Cummings CW, et al., eds. *Otolaryngology–Head and Neck Surgery*. 2nd ed. St. Louis: Mosby; 1992:1043.
Eisele DW, Johns ME. Complications of surgery of the salivary glands. In: Eisele DW, ed. *Complications in Head and Neck Surgery*. St. Louis: Mosby; 1993:183.
Kaplan MJ. Complications of salivary gland surgery. In: Weissler MC, Pillsbury HC III, eds. *Complications of Head and Neck Surgery*. St. Louis: Mosby; 1995:172.

II. SALIVARY GLAND PATHOLOGY

■ L E W I S   E V E R S O L E

The salivary tree is composed of many differentiated cell types (Fig. 7–5). The secretory bulb or acinus is represented by an outer basket of myoepithelial cells that encase the mucous, serous, or seromucous secretory cells (Fig. 7–6 A–C). The acinar secretions drain into the terminal or intercalated ducts composed of low cuboidal cells that are also enveloped by myoepithelia (see Fig. 7–7A). The intercalated ducts then progress proximally into the striated ducts, which are characterized by columnar eosinophilic cells that are rich in mitochondria (see Fig. 7–7B). Neither intercalated nor striated ducts are simple conduits; both serve secretory and ion-exchange functions. These intralobular ducts leave the lobule and progress to the major ductal drainage system as extralobular ducts composed of basal reserve cells and pseudostratified columnar cells. Near the oral epithelial orifices, these ducts are composed of a basal cell layer, stratified squamous keratinocytes and luminally oriented cuboidal or columnar cells that give way to squames at the ductal exit into the surface oral epithelium. Specific tumors, both benign and malignant, are made up of epithelial cells that simulate these normal differentiated cell types, either singularly or in various combinations.

The major salivary glands share common histologic features in their ductal conduits yet vary in their acinar cell populations. The parotid acini are exclusively serous, with prominent amylase positive zymogen granules; the submandibular gland consists of both serous and mucous acini, the latter

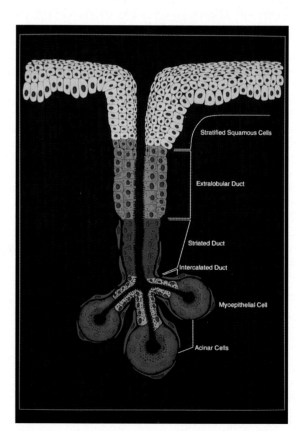

FIGURE 7–5 Diagrammatic representation of the salivary tree showing acini, myoepithelial cells, and ductal system.

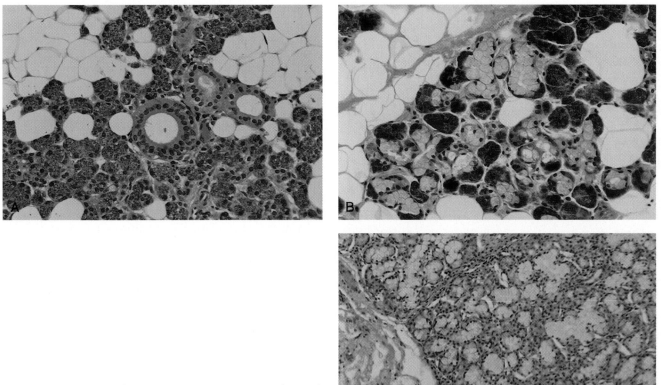

FIGURE 7–6 A, Parotid acini, prominent zymogen granules, and adipose infiltration (H&E, × 150). B, Submandibular gland showing mucous acini capped by serous demilunes (H&E, × 150). C, Sublingual gland is predominantly mucous with seromucous demilunes (H&E, × 100).

frequently capped by serous demilunes (see Fig. 7–6 A and B). The sublingual gland, like many minor salivary glands of the oral and sinonasal-tracheal mucosa, is composed of seromucous and mucous acinar cells; zymogen granule serous acinar cells are rare.

In the aging patient, adipose deposition is a common finding and does not compromise secretory function (see Fig. 7–6A). Both acinar and ductal cells may become engorged with mitochondria, producing strikingly eosinophilic acini and ductal cells (termed oncocytes, similar to Hürthle cells of the thyroid epithelium) (Fig. 7–8). Glycogen accumulation in salivary epithelium may evolve, and such cells exhibit copious clear cytoplasm (clear cell oncocytes).

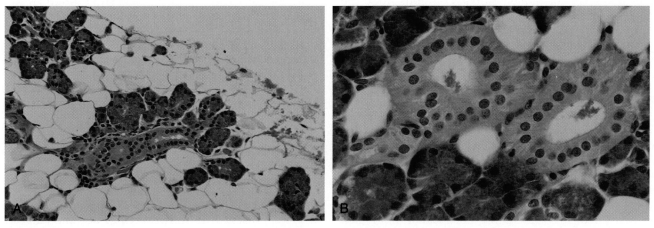

FIGURE 7–7 A, Intercalated duct with a cluster of serous acini and surrounding adipocytes (H&E, × 150). B, Striated ducts are prominently eosinophilic (H&E, × 350).

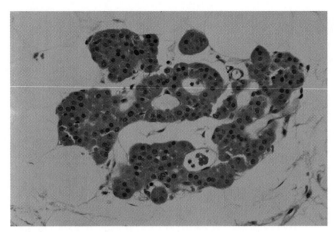

FIGURE 7–8   Ductal and acinar oncocytes in parotid gland (H&E, × 150).

Histochemical stains are not usually required for the diagnosis of most salivary diseases, yet such stains often may help confirm an interpretation based on H&E stains alone. Ductal cells, being simple epithelia, stain for low-molecular-weight cytokeratins (CK 8, 14, 18, 19). Myoepithelial cells are characterized by the immunohistochemical (IHC) markers vimentin and smooth muscle actin (in neoplasms, they may also stain for S-100 protein). Mucous cells stain with alcian blue or mucicarmine, while serous cells are PAS-positive, failing to digest with diastase yet losing positivity after neuraminidase digestion. IHC staining of acinar cells in formalin-fixed tissue is usually negative for cytokeratins yet positive for lysozyme or amylase.

BIOPSY, TISSUE HANDLING, AND FROZEN SECTIONS

The diagnosis of major salivary lesions may be made clinically for suspected inflammatory or immunopathologic diseases. Histopathologic diagnosis is usually, although not exclusively, reserved for salivary masses suspected to represent neoplasms. Lower lip minor salivary gland biopsy for the diagnosis of Sjögren's syndrome is preferred to parotid biopsy. Open biopsies are rarely undertaken for major gland tumefactions, because seeding of tumor cells is a risk. Less invasive diagnostic methods, including needle core biopsy and FNA, are available and reliable.

Core biopsies should be embedded longitudinally in order to sample the largest populations of cells. Keep in mind that histopathologic diagnosis is based on many features—including encapsulation, or lack thereof, and cell growth patterns. Cytologic features of pleomorphism, atypical mitoses, and hyperchro-

matism are not commonly encountered in many of the salivary gland malignancies. Therefore, when specimens are received in the laboratory they must be examined carefully to assess tumor margins for encapsulation or invasion of parenchyma. Most salivary gland tumors are treated by surgical excision in continuity with normal gland. These resections may include total or partial sialectomy; for parotid tumors the resection may be restricted to the superficial lobe alone. The pathologist should discuss the orientation of the specimen with the surgeon, and any resected nerve segments should be labeled. If cervical lymph nodes are taken in continuity or separately, they should be oriented from uppermost to lowermost nodes.

In rare instances of lumpectomy, it is advisable to ink the outer margin of the tumor prior to sectioning. For large masses, sections for pathology should be taken from both central and peripheral (marginal) regions, sampling as many areas as possible in order to obtain representative areas. Recall that mixed tumors may contain a regional focus of carcinomatous transformation, and acinic cell carcinomas may harbor foci of dedifferentiation. The remaining tissue can be stored in fixative should additional sampling be deemed appropriate.

When FNA suggests lymphoma, touch preps should be obtained from the cut surface of the mass, securing enough slides for immunophenotyping.

For instances that include lymph node dissection, the nodes should be grouped according to anatomic location and each group of nodes placed in a separate cassette for embedding. Findings should be reported for which node groups contain tumor.

Frozen sections should be obtained at the time of surgery, especially if FNA findings are equivocal. For subtotal sialectomy, it is also advisable to obtain frozen sections on the margins at the time of excision. For neurotropic lesions such as adenoid cystic carcinoma, facial nerve segments should be examined by cross section to assess for perineural space extension. Multiple sequential samples may be requested, and the surgeon may continue to procure samples up to the skull base. Positive findings may result in the decision to undertake a partial temporal bone resection.

Massive invasive salivary gland malignancies may invade contiguous osseous tissues. These osseous tissues should be labeled according to bone and site, and samples should be placed into decalcification solution. Osseous extension has a significant negative impact on prognosis.

DEVELOPMENTAL DISEASES

Salivary gland developmental disorders (Table 7–6) may be present from birth, yet not become clinically evident until late childhood or early adulthood. Adenomatous hyperplasia is of unknown cause and is

TABLE 7-6	DEVELOPMENTAL DISEASES OF THE SALIVARY GLANDS

Adenomatous hyperplasia
Dysgenic cysts
Sialocysts
Sebaceous rests, choristomas, and hamartomas

most often encountered in the palatal minor glands.[1-5] Dysgenic cysts are familial lesions of the major glands, whereas single sialocysts are more often encountered in the minor glands. The single or multilocular sialocysts may be true developmental cysts; however, duct blockage by a coagulated mucinous plug is the probable causative factor. This condition would not engender true cysts, but rather, aneurysmal-like cystic sialectasis.[6-21] The histopathologic features of sialocysts are therefore detailed under the obstructive diseases.

Adenomatous Hyperplasia[1-5]

Gross Pathology

The gland is grossly enlarged but otherwise of normal color and consistency.

Microscopic Pathology

The entire mass or nodule is composed of normal acini and ducts, identical to those of the parent gland. Occasionally there will be foci of lymphocytic or plasma cell infiltration within the intralobular stroma.[1,3] Most instances have been described in the palate where the acini are pure mucous (Fig. 7–9).

Differential Diagnosis

Acinic cell carcinoma may be an initial consideration; however, on closer examination, the presence of intercalated, striated, and intralobular excretory ducts allows for identification of normal glandular features.

Dysgenic Cysts of Major Glands[6-21]

Gross Pathology

The parotid gland is compressed by the presence of large cystic spaces filled with serous fluid. The cysts are variable in size and multifocal. Some are only a few millimeters in diameter, others may be 3 to 4 cm. They may distend the capsule, but are more often randomly scattered within the substance of the gland.

Microscopic Pathology

Salivary parenchyma is normal in most areas. Glandular tissue adjacent to the cystic areas may exhibit acinar degeneration with periductal fibrosis. Inflammatory cell infiltration is minimal or absent. The cysts are lined by ductal columnar, cuboidal, stratified squamous cells, or combinations of these cell types.[13-15] They may be small or quite large and contain a pale secretion product.

Differential Diagnosis

The differential diagnosis includes ductal ectasia secondary to chronic inflammatory obstructive disease, papillary cytadenoma lymphomatosum, intraparotid branchial cleft cyst, and HIV-associated cystic disease of major salivary glands. In obstructive sialadenitis, the ectatic ducts may appear identical to dysgenic cysts; yet there will be a large number of smaller ducts involved by ectasia, and the adjacent parenchyma will exhibit diffuse inflammation or acinar degeneration and periductal fibrosis. Warthin's tumor is distinctive, with the cystic spaces showing papillary projections into the lumens and lined by tall columnar oncocytes. The papillary projections overlie sheets of lymphocytes with germinal centers.

Benign lymphoepithelial or branchial cleft cysts are usually located in the lateral neck, but sometimes are localized within the substance of the parotid gland. The histologic features are the same as in the neck, being lined by stratified squamous epithelium with a surrounding wall of lymphoid tissue containing germinal centers.[16-18] HIV-associated cysts are large and lined by stratified squamous epithelium. The entire parenchyma is effaced by infiltrating intermediate and large-sized lymphocytes. Lastly, dysgenic cysts should be suspected when there are no symptoms of obstruction and bilateral parotid enlargements are cystic and present since childhood or early adulthood.

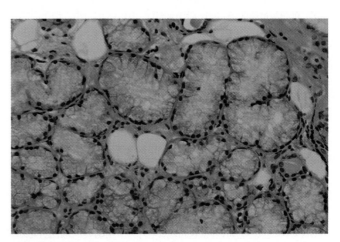

FIGURE 7–9 Mucous acini appear normal in adenomatous hyperplasia of the palate (H&E, × 300).

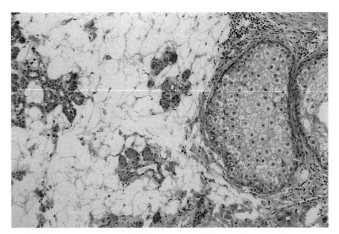

FIGURE 7-10 Sebaceous rest within the parotid gland (H&E, × 33).

Sebaceous Rests, Choristomas, and Hamartomas

Embryologically, the parotid salivary primordium arises from stomadial ectoderm. In the same region of the primitive buccal mucosa, sebaceous glands arise that are known, in adult oral mucosa, as Fordyce's granules. The cognate nature of these two structures in the same embryologic site probably accounts for the frequency of sebaceous lesions that may be encountered in the parotid glands to the exclusion of the other major glands (see Neoplasms). Sebaceous acinar rests or multilobular foci of sebaceous differentiation can be encountered in normal glands.[6,7,19] Another benign change in parotid parenchyma is oncocytosis. Oncocytes, also known as oxyphilic cells, begin to accumulate with advancing age.

Gross Pathology

Rests, sebaceous choristomas, and oncocyotsis are not associated with clinically identifiable swelling and are therefore encountered in normal tissue coincidentally adjacent to other lesions that may have been surgically removed.

Microscopic Pathology

Focal sebaceous rests are characterized by formation of acinar lobules identical to those found in normal skin adnexa (Fig. 7-10). When these acini are multiple, they may connect to stratified squamous ducts, which in turn are contiguous with salivary excretory ducts. Such lesions are considered to be choristomas. Oncocytosis may occur alone or lie adjacent to a tumorous nodule of oncocytic cells (oncocytoma). Oncocytes are characterized by small, round, often pyknotic, centrally placed nuclei with voluminous pale homogeneous eosinophilic cytoplasm, which on

electron microscopy are found to be mitochondria-rich (see Fig. 7-8). These cells may transform from either acinar or ductal cells and may be isolated or occur as multifocal clones.

Differential Diagnosis

Sebaceous neoplasms should be considered in the differential diagnosis of choristoma. The former show distinctive histopathologic features and include sebaceous lymphadenoma and sebaceous carcinoma. Oncocytosis is differentiated from oncocytoma by an absence of a well-defined tumor mass.

INFLAMMATORY AND IDIOPATHIC DISEASES

Inflammatory lesions of the major salivary glands include post-obstructive sialadenitis, infectious sialadenitis, and noninfectious sialadenitis, which includes the benign lymphoepithelial lesion of Sjögren's syndrome. The characteristic features common to all of the sialadenitides, with only a few exceptions, are acinar degeneration and replacement by infiltrating inflammatory cells. Sialadenosis is a nonspecific hypertrophy of acini that may accompany a variety of systemic illnesses. Table 7-7 lists the classification of salivary inflammatory disorders.

TABLE 7 - 7	CLASSIFICATION OF SALIVARY INFLAMMATORY DISORDERS

Obstructive Sialadenitis
Sialolithiasis
Retention cysts
Mucus extravasation (mucocele, ranula)
Sclerosing polycystic adenosis

Necrotizing Sialometaplasia

Infectious Sialadenitis
Cytomegalovirus (inclusion disease)
Mumps
Bacterial sialadenitis
Tuberculosis

HIV-Associated Cystic Sialadenitis

Sarcoidosis

Cystic Fibrosis

Autoimmune Sialadenitis (Benign lymphoepithelial lesion)

Amyloidosis

Sialadenosis

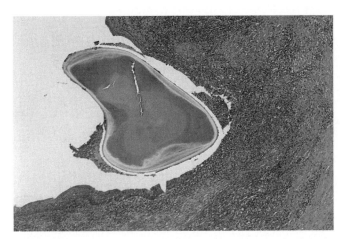

FIGURE 7-11 Sialolith within a dilated duct showing periductal inflammation (H&E, × 33).

Obstructive Sialadenitis[22-37]

The most common cause of salivary obstruction is the formation of intraductal sialoliths, a phenomenon usually encountered in the submandibular gland that may also affect other glands. Formation of viscous mucous plugs can occur in the extralobular ducts of both major and minor glands and result in obstructive changes.[22-26] Obstructive salivary inflammatory disease may also be seen when neoplasms compress and shut off salivary flow to large ducts. Focal obstructions due to trauma or inflammation that cause ductal stricture may result in the formation of aneurysmal dilatation of ducts, referred to as retention cysts or sialocysts. Some of these lesions may be developmental; others may be caused by formation of mucous plugs in the ducts. Ductal severage results in extravasation of mucin with pooling in the connective tissues.[34,36] A localized nodular form of parenchymal sclerosis, which clinically presents as a tumor, has been recently described and is termed *sclerosing polycystic adenosis*.[37]

Gross Pathology

Sialolithiasis is characterized by formation of salivary calculi from a nidus of pooled mucinous proteins. They are usually white or grey and may vary considerably in size from a few millimeters to 3 cm. The obstructed gland maintains its lobular architecture with a yellow-white appearance and is firm on cut section if considerable fibrosis is extant. Glands obstructed secondary to mucous plugs or strictures may show cystic sacculations, or a single cystic duct may be evident. Mucoceles are identified as submucosal cystic nodules with gelatinous contents. In sclerosing polycystic adenosis, a localized nodule with a spongy appearance is evident.

Microscopic Pathology

Decalcification and processing of sialoliths discloses a laminated onionskin pattern of basophilic calcified amorphous material (Fig. 7–11). The gland will show acinar degeneration with lymphocyte and plasma cell infiltration. The ducts are dilated, sialodochitis is a feature, and the ductal epithelium surrounding the stone often shows squamous and mucous metaplasia.[31] Respiratory ciliated epithelium is also commonly seen in duct cells adjacent to, or in the vacinity of, a sialolith. More established obstructive disease is characterized by fibrosis; indeed, lobules may be composed of hyalinized stromal scarification with multiple dilated ducts lined by compressed cuboidal cells and containing eosinophilic inspissated proteinaceous secretion product. This appearance connotes an end-stage gland and is termed *chronic sclerosing sialadenitis* (Fig. 7–12). Glands obstructed for many years may also contain extensive foci of dystrophic calcifications. In chronic polycystic adenosis, the process appears as an encapsulated nodule with multifocal ectasias.

Retention cysts, or *sialocysts*, are found in both major and minor glands and may be unilocular or multilocular.[8-12] The cells lining the dilated cystic structures are cuboidal, flattened squamous, or columnar oncocytes (Fig. 7–13 A–C). There may be papillary projections into the lumens (Fig. 7–13D). The obstructed gland is chronically inflamed or shows sclerosing sialadenitis. In *mucus extravasation phenomena* (mucocele, ranula), pooled mucin is seen in the connective tissue; this zone of mucus extravasation is walled off by granulation tissue infiltrated by histiocytes.[34,35] Trapped within the pooled mucin are foam cells and neutrophils (Fig. 7–14). The gland underlying the severed duct shows obstructive sialadenitis with fibrosis.

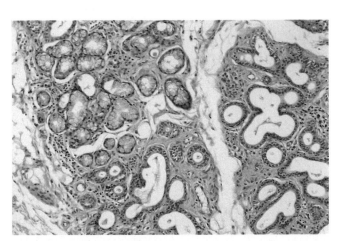

FIGURE 7-12 Chronic sclerosing sialadenitis showing acinar degeneration, ductal ectasia, fibrosis, and mononuclear inflammatory cell infiltration. These changes are encountered in obstructive disease (H&E, × 33).

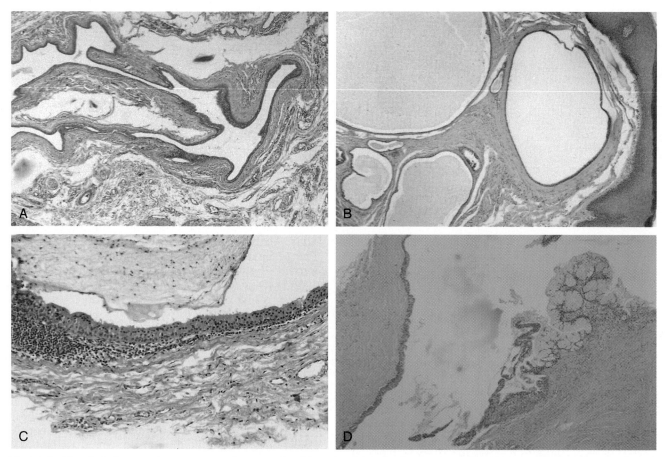

FIGURE 7–13 *A,* Sialocyst with a tortuous configuration, lined by cuboidal and columnar duct cells (H&E, × 13). *B,* Sialocyst, multiocular cysts are lined by cuboidal duct cells (H&E, × 13). *C,* Duct blockage cystic structure with oncocytic metaplasia (H&E, × 33). *D,* Sialocyst, mucopapillary variant may be mistaken for low-grade mucoepidermoid carcinoma (H&E, × 13).

Differential Diagnosis

Obstructive sialadenitis is usually associated with a clinically or historically evident etiology, and the inflammatory changes are chronic and nonspecific. The other forms of chronic sialadenitis are histo-

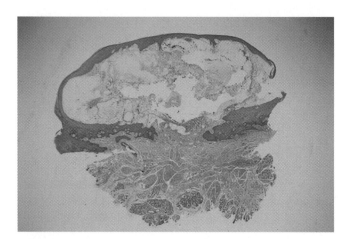

FIGURE 7–14 Mucus extravasation phenomenon (mucocele). Pooled mucin distends the epithelium of the lower lip (H&E, × 10).

pathologically unique and should not be confused with typical obstructive sialadenitis. The sialocysts and mucous-plug-associated sialodochitis/cystic dilatations may be confused with dysgenic cysts or cystadenomas, particularly when mucous metaplasia and papillary projections are encountered. Minor gland obstructive sialocysts of the lip and buccal mucosa often show oncocytic metaplasia, and when sialodochitis is present as well, they have been erroneously classified as Warthin's tumors. Kimura's disease may involve salivary parenchyma as well as parotid lymph nodes and may be confused with obstructive sialadenitis. The distinction may be made by the distinct vascular proliferation with plump endothelial cells and lymphoid aggregates with germinal center formation and tissue eosinophilia.

Necrotizing Sialometaplasia[38–42]

Thought to be a lesion secondary to arterial occlusion, necrotizing sialometaplasia (NSM) is most commonly encountered as a chronic ulcer of the palate.[38,39] Other glands can be affected, but the lesion is rarely seen in the major salivary glands.

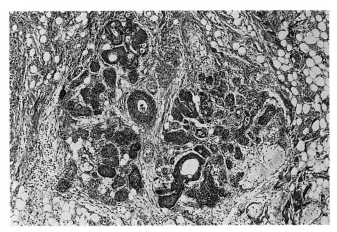

FIGURE 7–15 Necrotizing sialometaplasia. Coagulation necrosis of acini is seen inferiorly; acinar and ductal elements show squamous metaplasia (H&E, × 33).

Gross Pathology

Most instances of necrotizing sialometaplasia occur in minor salivary glands, particularly the palate. On gross examination of a mucosal biopsy, a deep-seated ulcer is seen with a grey ulcer bed. On cut section, the deeper tissues are also grey and soft or friable.

Microscopic Pathology

Since most cases arise from oral or sinonasal submucosal glands, a mucosal biopsy is observed. A deep-seated ulcer is encountered with underlying necrotic salivary tissue. At the inferior margin, lobular architecture is preserved, as are the remnants of acinar structures, a feature of ischemic or coagulative necrosis. Interposed between the foci of salivary gland necrosis and the ulcer bed are salivary ducts in which the lumens exhibit varying degrees of obliteration (Fig. 7–15). The process of ductal squamous metaplasia has replaced the luminal cuboidal or columnar cells with spinous layer cells. These metaplastic ducts are always oval or round.[38,40,42] Some ducts remain intact, and a few mucous or seromucous acini are intact or show signs of degeneration in which the acini are ductualizing.

Differential Diagnosis

Necrotizing sialometaplasia has been mistaken for squamous cell carcinoma and mucoepidermoid carcinoma, both clinically and histopathologically.[38] The lesion is easily differentiated from these carcinomas. There is no keratin pearl formation, and the metaplastic ducts are always round or oval without finger-like invasive extensions or linear cords. The metaplastic squamous cells do not form keratin pearls or squamous eddies, and cytologic atypia is absent. Finally, the foci of coagulative necrosis can usually be identified in the acinar lobules underlying the metaplastic ducts.

Infectious Sialadenitis[43–48]

Gross Pathology

The usual lobular structure of normal glands is often maintained, but the normal grey color is replaced in a chronically inflamed gland by red, pink, or yellow friable material on cut section.[38] Cystic liquefactive foci are seen when abscess formation occurs. Similar findings are seen in endemic parotitis (mumps). In CMV salivary disease, the glands appear grossly normal. In acute parotitis with abscess formation, cystic foci with yellow exudate may occur in focal areas of the parenchyma. Tuberculous sialadenitis is characterized by multiple granulomas within the parenchyma appearing as miliary fibrotic foci or white nodules with internal foci of necrotic caseous material.

Microscopic Pathology

Acute streptococcal or staphylococcal sialadenitis may evolve by retrograde infection in an obstructed gland. Acinar degeneration is seen along with interstitial mixed neutrophilic and round cell inflammatory cell infiltrates. Multiple or single abscess are often seen in acute glands with cystic foci filled with necrotic amorphous debris and sheets of neutrophils. Endemic parotitis is rarely examined microscopically since it is diagnosed clinically. The lobular architecture is maintained with an interstitial subacute infiltrate, and the acini are vacuolated or manifest cloudy swelling. Salivary inclusion disease rarely shows inflammatory changes. The glands are normal, and evidence of CMV infection may be found in either acinar or ductal nuclei (Fig. 7–16). The classic large, smudged amphophilic intranuclear inclusion bodies are rimmed by a pale halo.

Tuberculous sialadenitis, akin to tuberculous lymphadenitis (scrofula), evinces the usual caseating granulomas with peripheral epithelioid cells and

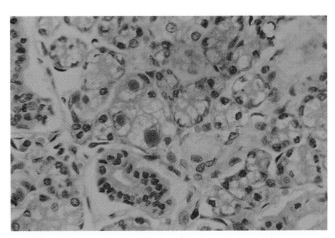

FIGURE 7–16 Salivary inclusion disease. Cytomegalovirus inclusions can be found in both acinar and ductal cells in an otherwise normal appearing gland (H&E, × 130).

Langerhans giant cells. The granulomas may be localized to intraglandular lymph nodes or may replace salivary parenchyma. Acid-fast staining will confirm the presence of tubercle bacilli.[43]

Differential Diagnosis

Differentiating mumps from bacterial sialadenitis is not always possible on histopathologic assessment alone. Culture for bacterial organisms may be required to confirm a bacterial etiology. Salivary inclusion disease shows pathognomonic inclusions and can also be confirmed by IHC or DNA in situ hybridization for identification of CMA DNA sequences.

When tuberculosis is suspected, other granulomatous inflammatory lesions to be considered include sarcoidosis and cat scratch fever, both of which may affect the parotid or other major and minor salivary glands. Caseation is not a feature of sarcoidosis, and the lesions will be negative for acid-fast bacilli. In cat scratch fever, the epithelioid histiocytes form stellate palisading borders that encircle caseous necrosis; on Warthin-Starry staining, the characteristic pleomorphic bacilli will be identified.[45,46]

HIV-Associated Cystic Sialadenitis[49–62]

Gross Pathology

The parotid glands are affected bilaterally and are grossly enlarged. On cut section, lobular architecture is preserved, and the gland has a yellow lymphoid appearance with large and small cystic foci.

Microscopic Pathology

The normal parenchyma is effaced with diffuse infiltration by a mixed population of large and medium-sized lymphocytes.[55,56] Residual salivary ducts may be seen with few, if any, remnants of acini. Interposed cysts are numerous, lined by stratified squamous epithelium or a hybrid ductal columnar/squamous type lining. Epimyoepithelial islands are seen, yet are dominated by the well-defined cysts. In many instances, germinal centers are present and show enlargement with the presence of intrafollicular macrophages, many of which have phagocytized tingible bodies, and by large clear follicular center cells with reniform nuclei.

Histochemical Findings

The lymphocyte population in HIV sialadenitis is unique and can be distinguished from that of the benign lymphoepithelial lesion (BLEL). Immunomarkers disclose that the lymphoid cells are predominantly T cells as opposed to the B-cell predominance of BLEL.[58] When germinal centers are present, T cells may accompany the normal resident B cells. Thus, mantle zone cells and the primary population stain for UCHL1 whereas follicles contain both UCHL1 and L26 positive lymphocytes.

Differential Diagnosis

Benign lymphoepithelial lesion and mucosa-associated lymphoid tissue lymphoma (MALToma) are the chief entities to be considered in the differential diagnosis. In BLEL there are no cysts; rather, the typical epimyoepithelial islands are seen within a sea of mature lymphocytes. In MALToma, the lymphoid element is diffusely populated with small follicular center cells exhibiting monocytoid or plasmacytoid cytologic characteristics. These cells stain positively for the L26 B-cell marker. Benign lymphoepithelial cyst, or branchial cleft cyst, may appear similar, but it is not multifocal and is typically found in the lateral neck rather than in the substance of the parotid gland.

Sarcoidosis

Sarcoidosis is a systemic noncaseating granulomatous disease that tends to affect many organs with a predilection for lymphoid tissue, particularly the hilar lymph nodes.[63–75] Nonlymphoid tissue may also be affected. Bilateral involvement of the parotid gland has been referred to as the Heerfordt syndrome—a disease that may clinically resemble Mikulicz's or Sjögren's syndrome. *Orofacial granulomatosis* includes the Melkerson-Rosenthal syndrome and cheilitis granulomatosa, in which sarcoid-like granulomas occur within the lobules of minor salivary glands of the lips.[66–70]

Gross Pathology

The salivary gland remains encapsulated and is stippled with multiple round or oval, individual or confluent white nodules that on cross section give the gland a steppingstone appearance. The entire parenchyma may be involved, and in the parotids the glands are enlarged.

Microscopic Pathology

The salivary parenchyma is replaced by clearly defined round or oval granulomas that look as if they had been molded by a cookie cutter. There may be only remnants of normal parenchyma evident, and this glandular tissue usually exhibits evidence of acinar degeneration and ectasia of remaining ducts. The granulomas are composed of epithelioid histiocytes that are both spindled and ovoid with large pale reniform or prolate nuclei. Multinucleated giant cells are randomly dispersed throughout, and some may contain intracytoplasmic asteroid bodies (Fig. 7–17). In the minor glands of the lip, in instances of

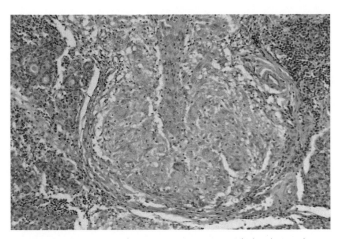

FIGURE 7-17 Sarcoidosis. Noncaseating epithelioid granulomas replace normal glandular parenchyma (H&E, × 33).

cheilitis granulomatosa, the granulomas replace salivary lobules and are multifocal and widespread throughout the submucosa of the lip.[68,69]

Differential Diagnosis

Usually the cookie-cutter granulomas with a multinodular pattern are unique to sarcoid or other forms of noninfectious orofacial granulomatosis. Included in the differential diagnosis is tuberculosis, particularly the noncaseating atypical forms such as *Mycobacterium avium intracellulare* as seen in HIV-seropositive subjects. Cat scratch disease may arise in a parotid lymph node, but the granulomas are typically necrotizing. In sarcoid or sarcoid-like lesions of salivary parenchyma, special stains for micro-organisms are negative.

Cystic Fibrosis

Inherited as an autosomal recessive disease in children, cystic fibrosis is a disorder of glandular fluid electrolyte transport, with the most severe complications occurring in the lungs and gastrointestinal tract where secretions are thick and viscous, culminating in malabsorption and chronic obstructive pulmonary disease.[76-78] The palmar sweat test reveals sodium and chloride elevations.

Gross Pathology

Salivary glands in mucoviscidosis appear similar to those in chronic obstructive sialadenitis, with the submandibular and sublingual glands being the more severely involved owing to the presence of mucous secreting cells. These glands are small, fibrotic, and white to yellow on cut section with microcystic foci.[77] The cysts contain thick homogeneous proteinaceous material.

Microscopic Pathology

Acini, especially mucous acini, are replaced by fibrous tissue, and the remaining ducts are ectatic. Mononuclear inflammatory cell infiltration is usually encountered. The ectatic ducts may form microcysts that contain a hyalinized eosinophilic secretion product, and some of the intraductal protein plugs may become calcified.

Differential Diagnosis

The histopathologic features of cystic fibrosis are those of a sclerosing sialadenitis. The bilateral involvement, predilection for mucous secreting glands in the clinical setting of malnutrition, intestinal disease, and pulmonary obstructive disease are important features in the diagnosis since sialolithiasis may cause similar, if not identical, changes.

Autoimmune Sialadenitis/Benign Lymphoepithelial Lesion[79-99]

Gross Pathology

In the early stages of Sjögren's syndrome, lobular architecture is preserved; the gland may appear normal or yellow. In latter stages, lobules are effaced, and the entire gland may appear yellow with a cut surface resembling lymph node tissue.

Microscopic Pathology

Lobular architecture may be maintained in benign lymphoepithelial lesion (BLEL) in early stages, whereas in older lesions inflammation may obliterate or efface the lobular fibrous septa.[79,82] In the evolving lesion, intact acini are evident at one end of the lobule, while at the opposite pole a virtual sea of lymphocytes encroaches upon the parenchyma, causing acinar obliteration with preservation of ductal structures. As the lesion becomes established, all acini are destroyed and replaced by mature small lymphocytes. The ducts enlarge as both ductal and myoepithelial hyperplasia occurs, obscuring any remnants of a lumen. Lymphocytes transmigrate into these large and irregular "epimyoepithelial islands" (Fig. 7-18 *A* and *B*). In late stage Sjögren's syndrome, the classic BLEL can undergo progressive fibrosis and hyalinization.

Minor salivary glands, particularly those of the lower lip, are often biopsied to obtain a lymphocyte focus score.[92-94] Five to eight lobules should be procured and examined for focal lymphocytic sialadenitis. The lymphoid infiltrates occur in aggregates of 50 or more lymphocytes, and while they may be periductal, epimyoepithelial islands are not generally encountered. If there is one lymphoid aggregate in each lobule, Sjögren's syndrome should be suspected. When there are two or more aggregates, the score is subjectively uprated, depending on the ex-

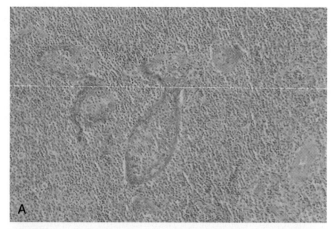

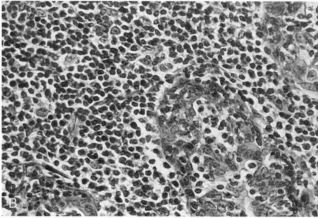

FIGURE 7-18 *A,* Benign lymphoepithelial lesion. Epimyoepithelial islands arise from residual ducts and associated myoepithelia, while the acini are totally replaced by infiltrating lymphocytes, most of which are T cells. (H&E, × 33). *B,* Benign lymphoepithelial lesion. Small lymphocytes infiltrate the epithelial islands (H&E, × 150).

tent of the lymphocyte infiltration. Such findings are highly correlated with BLEL in the parotid gland.

Differential Diagnosis

The benign lymphoepithelial lesion may be confused with chronic nonspecific sialadenitis. In BLEL, unlike chronic nonspecific sialadenitis or post-obstructive sialadenitis, the infiltrate is purely lymphocytic. In the other conditions, there is usually a mixture of mononuclear cell types, including plasma cells, lymphocytes, and macrophages with occasional scattered neutrophils. Also, in nonspecific sialadenitis, total replacement of all acini is not usually encountered. Sebaceous lymphadenoma has a pattern similar to BLEL, being a lymphoid lesion with epithelial islands showing sebaceous differentiation. Malignant lymphoma is also a major entity to consider in the differential diagnosis. Non-Hodgkin's lymphomas arise from intraparotid lymph nodes, and there are rare to no glandular structures or epimyoepithelial

islands to be seen. MALTomas, however, show the classic morphologic features of BLEL, with sheets of infiltrating lymphocytes replacing acini accompanied by the formation of epimyoepithelial islands. The distinguishing feature lies with the lymphocyte cell population. The lymphocytes of MALTtoma are small- to medium-sized marginal zone cells; some have a monocytoid or plasmacytoid appearance, owing to their significant amount of eosinophilic cytoplasm. Epimyoepithelial islands may also be encountered in HIV sialadenitis, yet large cysts are present as well.

Amyloidosis[100-105]

The pathologic starch-like protein, amyloid, is deposited in many tissues and tumors, and these deposits may interfere with function by replacing normal cells. The amyloid proteins are varied but share a β-pleated chain. Amyloid deposition may be unifocal, yet in the salivary glands it is usually a manifestation of systemic multifocal amyloidosis. The chief disease associations are myeloma, chronic infectious diseases, and hereditary forms.

Gross Pathology

The parotid glands are grossly enlarged. On sectioning, they show white-tan diffuse fibrosis with loss of lobular architecture.

Microscopic Pathology

Acini and ducts are replaced by globular and diffuse sheets of acellular eosinophilic hyaline material (Fig. 7–19A). Remaining ducts are compressed, and adjacent parenchyma shows signs of chronic obstructive disease with mononuclear inflammatory cell infiltration, fibrosis, and ductal ectasia.[100,103] Congo red staining and examination by polarized light will disclose green birefringence in the hyalizied foci (Fig. 7–19B). Amyloid is also strongly positive for the thioflavin T fluorochrome.

Differential Diagnosis

The microscopic features are distinctive and should not be confused with other entities. Although obstructive sialadenitis may be associated with fibrosis, diffuse or globular deposits of hyaline material, replacing large regions of parenchyma, are not seen in nonspecific obstructive disease. Congo red staining will confirm the diagnosis, after which the underlying disease associations must be pursued.

Sialadenosis[106-109]

Salivary enlargement, particularly of the parotid glands, may be seen in a variety of systemic condi-

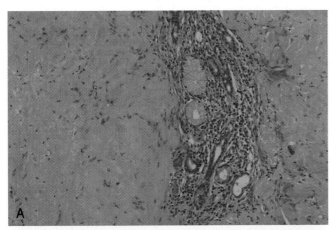

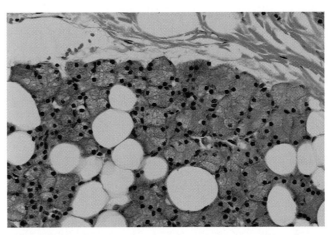

FIGURE 7–20 Sialadenosis in diabetes. Cloudy swelling of parotid acini with loss of granular definition (H&E, × 33).

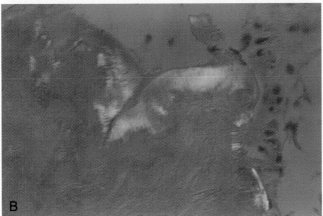

FIGURE 7–19 A, Amyloidosis of parotid gland replacing acini (H&E, × 33). B, Benign lymphoepithelial lesion. Small lymphocytes infiltrate the epithelial island (H&E, × 150).

tions including endocrinopathies, diabetes mellitus, neuropathies, malnutrition, liver disease, and alcoholism.[106,107] This ill-defined entity is usually not accompanied by any significant symptoms other than the physical finding of diffuse, soft bilateral enlargement.

Gross Pathology

The parotid glands are grossly enlarged and are otherwise unremarkable on sectioning. Those with fatty infiltration will appear yellow and lose the usual glandular lobularity.

Microscopic Pathology

There are no specific histopathologic changes in sialadenosis other than cytoplasmic swelling and a cloudy appearance of the parotid secretory granules (Fig. 7–20). In alcoholism and diabetes mellitus acinar degeneration may be evident, characterized by fatty infiltration, loss of acini, and retention of ducts.[108,109]

Differential Diagnosis

Regardless of the underlying systemic cause, all forms of sialadenosis show common histopathologic features. The differential diagnosis is then based on identification of the characteristic clinical and laboratory findings that typify each of the associated systemic illnesses.

NEOPLASTIC DISEASES

General Considerations[110–163]

Neoplasms arising from salivary gland parenchyma assume myriad patterns of growth and differentiation. Although there has been considerable speculative discussion on specific cells of origin for each tumor entity, research employing both animal models and human tissue has disclosed that virtually all cell types of the normal salivary gland secretory tree are capable of entering the cell cycle.[110–112] For the surgical pathologist, it is perhaps more important to recognize what normal salivary tissues are being emulated by the tumor rather than attempting to muse over which specific cell type gave rise to the tumor.[114–116]

Tumor stromal changes are, like the epithelial tumor component, often variable. Both benign and malignant lesions often manifest stromal inductive effects. Myxoid stroma is populated by myoepithelial cells; alternatively, many salivary gland tumors demonstrate foci of marked hyalinization representing zones of basal lamina duplication.

It is noteworthy that the tumor cells of the more common salivary gland malignancies do not exhibit significant cytologic atypia in the form of nuclear pleomorphism and high mitotic activity. Differentiating one tumor from another requires directing attention to two major histopathologic parameters: (1) cellular differentiation patterns and (2) growth patterns in relation to the surrounding normal tissues. Cytodifferentiation features are detailed for each specific entity. In the context of the growth pattern, perhaps the single most important feature that distinguishes benign from malignant neoplasia is encapsulation, or clearly defined demarcation from the neighboring tissues. Malignant salivary gland tumors lack encapsulation; the tumor cells and cell nests invade contiguous glandular and connective tissues.

The histomorphologic patterns observed by the surgical pathologist emulate cellular arrangements encountered in normal glands, yet the pathologic cellular architecture is predictably aberrant.[139,141,142,147] Tumors harbor cuboidal, columnar, acinar, myoepithelial, squamous, and undifferentiated polygonal cells; some contain distinctly clear cytoplasm.[110,111] There are some basic patterns of growth that occur in each individual tumor that provide the salient features allowing for a specific diagnosis. These cellular mosaics are illustrated in Figure 7–21. Polygonal tumor cells may form solid islands; microcystic spaces without luminal type cu-

boidal or columnar cells; macrocystic structures that are lined by cuboidal, columnar, or mucous goblet cells; or elongated tubular or trabecular arrangements. Other patterns show small ductal structures, many of which may be surrounded by spindled, stellate, or hyalinized myoepithelial cells. These may cluster or extend diffusely into a myxoid stroma; yet others exhibit papillary projections into luminal cell–lined cystic spaces, form clusters with aggregates of microcystic structures termed a cribriform pattern, orient themselves in single cell linear arrays (so-called Indian-file), or form anastomosing cords in a retiform arrangement. Some tumors are monotonous, others are polymorphic, exhibiting combinations of these patterns.

Benign Neoplasms

The benign tumors of salivary gland origin are typically encapsulated, or at least well-demarcated grossly. Most are uninodular, although some may be multinodular, indicative of multiple growth centers. Such tumors may show small pseudopod-like exten-

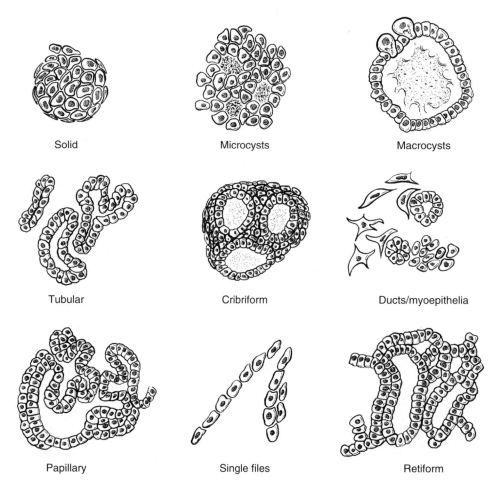

Solid   Microcysts   Macrocysts

Tubular   Cribriform   Ducts/myoepithelia

Papillary   Single files   Retiform

FIGURE 7–21 Histopathologic cell group organization in salivary gland tumors.

TABLE 7–8	CLASSIFICATION OF MAJOR SALIVARY GLAND ADENOMAS

Pleomorphic Adenoma (Mixed tumor)

Myoepithelioma
  Plasmacytoid (hyaline) cell type
  Spindle cell type

Basal Cell Adenoma and Canalicular Adenoma

Membranous variant

Oncocytoma

Clear cell variant

Cystadenomas

Papillary cystadenoma lymphomatosum (Warthin's tumor)
Sebaceous lymphadenoma
Papillary cystadenoma

Papillomas

Sialadenoma papilliferum
Intraductal papilloma
Inverted ductal papilloma

terns observed in both the epithelial and the stromal components of pleomorphic adenoma. The term "mixed tumor" comes from the early impression that these tumors were proliferations of both epithelial and mesenchymal germ layers. Now, however, it seems that the mesenchymal components of pleomorphic adenomas are primarily derived from myoepithelia; however, adipose, chondroid, and osseous elements are sometimes evident in these tumors.[175,177]

Pleomorphic adenoma is, by far, the most common neoplasm of the parotid and minor salivary glands, being quite rare in the submandibular and sublingual glands. Most cases arise in the third and fourth decades with a female predilection.

Gross Pathology

The mixed tumor may be uninodular or multinodular; the latter is more common in recurrent tumors that have been previously operated. The tumors are well-demarcated, usually encapsulated, and solid white or grey on cut section (Fig. 7–22 *A*

sions that invade the capsule of the main tumor cell population, which then form a new tumor cell nidus histologically identical to the parent tumor. This feature is more often encountered in tumors that recur after incomplete excision.

The cellular components of the benign tumors are quite varied, yet they are usually well-differentiated without any atypia.[111,112] As stated previously, these tumors tend to occur in adults, and there is a slight female predilection for most of them. Many of the benign lesions that arise in the major glands are rarely, if ever, found to arise from the minor salivary glands of the oral cavity or from mucous glands of the sinonasal and tracheal aerodigestive tract. The benign tumors fall into one of two broad categories: (1) pleomorphic adenomas characterized by a plethora of cell types and (2) monomorphic adenomas in which the cell population is relatively homogeneous. The classification of benign salivary gland tumors is found in Table 7–8.

PLEOMORPHIC ADENOMA[164–199]

The so-called mixed tumor or pleomorphic adenoma manifests the largest array of histopatholgic patterns of any salivary tumor; indeed, it may be the most diverse tumor in the entire human body.[163–199] The marked variability in microscopic appearance is attributed to the diverse cell types that participate in the neoplastic process, as well as the multivariant potential of these cells. Thus, the term "pleomorphic" does not refer to cytologic features of atypia characteristic of malignancy; rather, pleomorphic refers to the diversity of benign histopathologic pat-

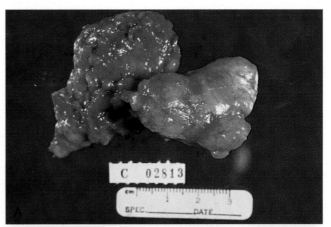

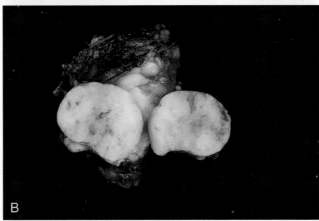

FIGURE 7–22 *A*, Gross appearance of encapsulated pleomorphic adenoma in the parotid gland. *B*, Gross appearance of hemisected, encapsulated pleomorphic adenoma of the parotid glands.

FIGURE 7-23 Encapsulation is evident in this pleomorphic adenoma of the palate (H&E, × 10).

and *B*). Foci of bluish mucin may be seen. Hemorrhage and necrosis are rarely seen except in cases that have been subjected to fine needle aspiration cytology.

Microscopic Pathology

No other salivary gland tumor shows as many patterns and cell types as the pleomorphic adenoma. The classic appearance is that of a neoplasm with a fibrous capsule, although tumor islands are commonly found within the substance of the capsule (Fig. 7–23). At low magnification, the tumor shows admixed foci of loose myxoid stroma traversed by small caliber vascular channels and sheets of polygonal cells with microcytic foci and clearly defined ductal structures (Fig. 7–24 *A–D*). Isolated ductal islands are scattered within the myxoid regions and show inner cuboid or columnar luminal cells with an outer mantle of myoepithelial cells that are polygonal, clear, or spindle in appearance. The spindle cells give the impression that they are spinning off from the ducts into the stroma. In fact, the spindle cells of the myxoid matrix are myoepithelial cells. The more solid sheets are made up of undifferentiated epithelial cells that lack cohesiveness, although many are probably myoepithelial; scattered about are ductal structures composed of cuboidal cells arranged around a glycocalyx and a central pool of acellular eosinophilic secretion product.

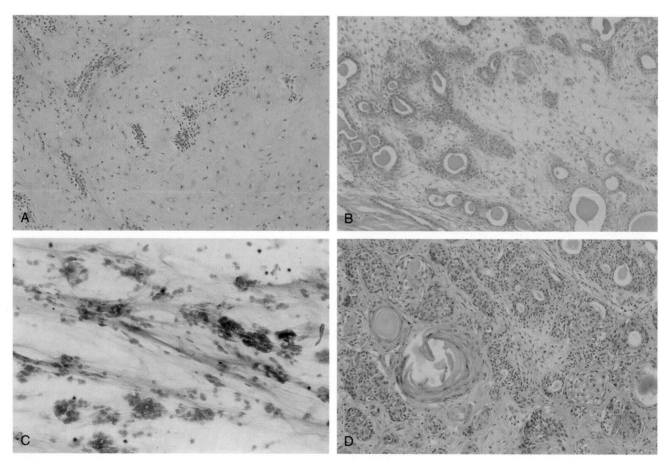

FIGURE 7-24 *A,* Pleomorphic adenoma. Ductal structures within a chondroid stroma (H&E, × 33). *B,* Pleomorphic adenoma. Ductal structures lined by cuboidal cells with outer layer of spindling myoepithelial cells that extend into the myxoid stroma (H&E, × 33). *C,* Pleomorphic adenoma. FNA showing mucoid background with spindle myoepithelial cells and small epithelial clusters (× 100). *D,* Pleomorphic adenoma. Cuboidal cell-lined ducts and islands with keratin pearls (H&E, × 33).

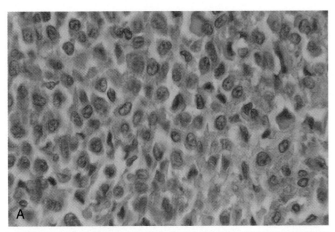

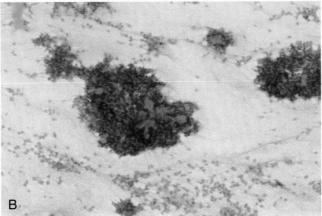

FIGURE 7-25 A, Pleomorphic adenoma. Plasmacytoid or hyaline myoepithelial cells (H&E, × 66). B, Pleomorphic adenoma. FNA of hyaline myoepithelial cells (H&E, × 100).

Many variations accompany or replace this basic configuration of ductal, polygonal, and myoepithelial cells, and a variety of connective tissue elements may be encountered in the stroma. Included as stromal variations are extensive hyalinization surrounding the epithelial component and synthesis of adipose, chondroid, and osseous tissues.

The epithelial cells of pleomorphic adenoma can assume a variety of appearances as well. The polygonal and spindle cell myoepithelial cells can be replaced by a unique plasmacytoid or hyaline cell. These myoepithelial cells are oval or round with a small eccentric nucleus displaced by homogeneous, hyalinized, prominently eosinophilic cytoplasm.[177,178] When these cells dominate the tumor, it may be referred to as *hyaline cell* or *plasmacytoid myoepithelioma* (Fig. 7–25 A and B). If the entire tumor is composed of monomorphic spindle cells (often arranged in a multinodular pattern) and if the appropriate IHC markers are demonstrable, *spindle cell myoepithelioma* is the diagnosis.[195] Many pathologists consider these myoepithelial tumors to be variants of mixed tumor or monomorphic adenoma and not entities unto themselves.

Oncocytic changes, foci of squamous and mucous cell metaplasia, can also be seen in pleomorphic adenomas, yet they do not obscure the ductal and myoepithelial elements. Occasionally, a benign pleomorphic adenoma contains cytologically disturbing epithelial cells. Such cells are usually dispersed throughout the tumor. While they have pleomorphic nuclei, mitotic figures are absent, and there is no evidence of invasion into adjacent parenchyma or contiguous connective tissues. Such tumor is likely to behave like a pleomorphic adenoma rather than a malignant mixed tumor.

Various types of crystals may be deposited in these tumors. It is of interest that tyrosine crystals, characterized by eosinophilic refractive florets, are more common in mixed tumors removed from black patients. Collagen crystalloids, typified by needle-shaped, radially arranged, nonrefractile structures and oxalate crystals may also be seen (Fig. 7–26).

Histochemical Findings

The tumor cells are negative for mucin and PAS stains unless foci of true mucous cells are evident. The glycocalyx and secretion products found within ductal lumina are usually PAS positive. The epithelial ductal structures stain positively with low-molecular-weight cytokeratins, particularly CK 14, 8, 18, and 19. Spindle, polygonal, and plasmacytoid myoepithelial cells stain with vimentin and smooth muscle actin and will sometimes show positivity for S-100 protein.[184,194] Although IHC markers are rarely needed for diagnosis, they are important in the spindle cell lesions thought to be myoepithelioma, smooth muscle actin being a significant finding in such tumors located within a salivary gland.

Differential Diagnosis

The differential diagnosis of mixed tumor may occasionally include chordoma when the tumor is pre-

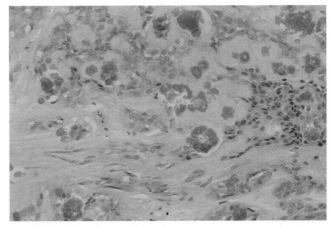

FIGURE 7-26 Pleomorphic adenoma. Numerous crystal rosettes are evident (H&E, × 66).

dominantly myxoid. The classic physaliferous cell is absent in mixed tumors. The spindle cell myoepithelial variant may be confused with meningioma, nerve sheath tumor, and myofibroblastic spindle cell tumors. The latter may react with anti–smooth muscle actin antisera. The presence of cytologic atypia may suggest carcinoma ex mixed tumor. If pleomorphism is present in only a few cells located throughout the tumor, is not marked, and there are no foci of invasion, then the tumor should still be classified as benign pleomorphic adenoma.

BASAL CELL ADENOMA AND CANALICULAR ADENOMA[200–220]

A monomorphic adenoma, the basal cell adenoma is most often encountered in the parotid gland and is relatively uncommon in other major and minor glands.[202,211] Conversely, canalicular adenoma, another monomorphic adenoma, is found predominantly in the minor glands of the upper lip and buccal mucosa. It is very rare in the major glands.[200,210] A clinicopathologic variant of major gland basal cell adenoma is the membranous type that may be associated with familial cutaneous cylindromas (turban tumors).[215,216]

Gross Pathology

The basal cell adenoma is well-circumscribed or encapsulated, round to oval, and on cut section is solid tan or pink. These tumors have the consistency of a lymph node. The membranous variant may be multinodular or even multifocal within the parotid parenchyma. Similarly, canalicular adenomas of the lip minor glands may be multiple.

Microscopic Pathology

Histologically, basal cell adenomas show a striking similarity to cutaneous basal cell carcinomas as well as to solid variants of ameloblastoma.[206,209] Oval and linear islands are enveloped by an outer stratum of polarized basal cells; cells making up the center population are monotonous with round nuclei, scant cytoplasm, and indistinct cell borders (Fig. 7–27). The nuclei contain evenly dispersed chromatin in most tumors, yet sometimes they are speckled with a vesicular and granular appearance. As a rule, squamous differentiation is lacking, although occasionally keratin pearls are noted in the center of the islands. The stroma is fibrous and clearly separates the tumor cell nests from one another. The *membranous variant* or *dermal analog tumor* occurring in conjunction with cutaneous turban tumors shows similar histology to basal cell adenoma with the additional appearance of peripheral basal lamina duplication in the form of hyalin rims.[207]

Variations occur; not all tumors are purely solid

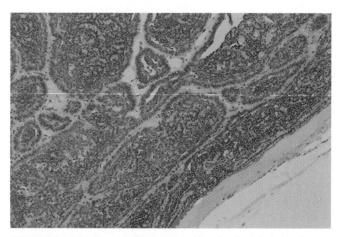

FIGURE 7–27 Basal cell adenoma. Islands of epithelial cells show a prominent outer basal cell stratum with inner basaloid cells and foci of ductal structures (H&E, × 33).

and basaloid. The *tubular pattern* is composed of basilar cell islands that show extensive ductal differentiation with lumina containing eosinophilic secretion products. In the *trabecular pattern*, the basilar cells are arranged in linear cords of monomorphic cells, some of which arborize to create a retiform pattern.[203,213] In yet other tumors both tubular and trabecular patterns can coexist, and in some basal cell adenomas, solid areas are interspersed with these variant patterns as well.

Canalicular adenoma is a discrete form of monomorphic adenoma rarely found in major glands; most instances are located in the minor glands of the upper lip where they can be single or multiple.[210,212] Indeed, in situ foci of canalicular adenoma can often be detected in otherwise normal salivary gland tissue lying adjacent to the tumor mass. Canalicular adenoma exhibits a unique histologic appearance of double-row columnar cells arranged in arborizing ribbons (Fig. 7–28). The unique stroma is hypocellular and mucinous without collagen fibers. Within the mucinous stroma is an extensive capillary network. The epithelial cell ribbons anastomose and form dilated ductal structures simulating canals through which one might envision the passage of a Venetian gondolier—hence the term "canalicular." There are often large cystic spaces in these tumors, and solid basaloid islands may be interposed between the canalicular element. Cribriform patterns may also be encountered yet are rarely dominant.

Histochemical Findings

Basal cell adenomas are cytokeratin positive and most of the epithelial cells are S-100 negative, unlike canalicular adenomas that are also positive for low-molecular-weight cytokeratin as well as S-100 protein positive. The tubulotrabecular basal cell lesions also stain with S-100 protein.[218]

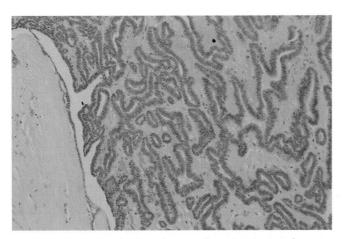

FIGURE 7-28 Canalicular adenoma. Interconnecting retiform arrays of ductal canals prevail (H&E, × 33).

Differential Diagnosis

Basal cell adenomas are unique. Although the histopathologic features are shared with cutaneous basal cell carcinoma and certain ameloblastomas, localization to the parotid gland is sufficient to exclude these impostors. In the palate, ameloblastoma should be excluded by imaging studies to rule out evidence of intraosseous disease. Basal cell adenocarcinoma must be considered in the differential diagnosis and can be excluded when there is no evidence of parenchymal invasion; otherwise, cytologic features of malignancy are not helpful since basal cell adenocarcinomas can appear identical cytologically to basal cell adenoma. Thus encapsulation versus invasion is the chief distinguishing feature.

Canalicular adenoma will often show cribriform patterns causing confusion with adenoid cystic carcinoma and polymorphous low-grade adenocarcinoma. Again, circumscription and encapsulation are important features of this benign tumor. Furthermore, localization to the upper lip and the typical canalicular reteform pattern will be evident in other regions of the tumor.

ONCOCYTOMA[221-237]

Of all the salivary adenomas, this monomorphic tumor is the only one with a marked predilection for the elderly, is more common in females, and is essentially a major gland neoplasm with only a sporadic case located in minor glands.[226] Oncocytosis is a common event in the aged parotid gland, and oncocytes may be found in normal glands adjacent to oncocytoma. These tumors are mitochondria-rich and are slow growing with limited potential for progressive proliferation. It is assumed that most oncocytomas reach a given size and then lose their potential for further growth, thereby relegating them

to the status of hamartoma. It must be realized, however, that a malignant counterpart exists, although malignant transformation from a pre-existing benign oncocytoma probably does not occur.

Gross Pathology

Oncocytomas are encapsulated smooth nodules and can be multifocal or multinodular. On sectioning, they are white or grey and homogeneous.

Microscopic Pathology

The classic cell is the oxyphil cell or oncocyte. These cells are cuboidal with finely stippled, strikingly eosinophilic cytoplasm with round nuclei exhibiting homogeneous cytoplasm (Fig. 7-29A). These cells may be arranged in diffuse sheets, trabeculae, doughnut-shaped duct-like structures; they may assume organoid patterns.[233] Common to all oncocytomas is the lack of a collagenous stroma. Rather, the oncocytic clusters regardless of their pattern are sep-

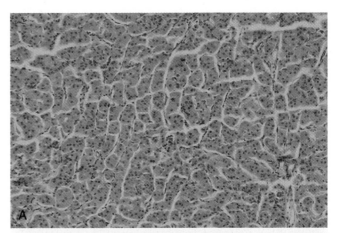

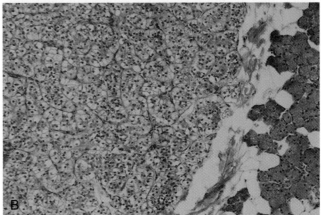

FIGURE 7-29 A, Oncocytoma. Sheets of oncocytic ductal appearing cells lie wtihin a stroma-less capillary background (H&E, × 33). B, Clear cell oncocytoma. Clear cells form organoid or acinar clusters with a sparse stroma (H&E, × 33).

arated by fine fibrovascular septae. *Clear cell oncocytoma* is a variant and may be accompanied by diffuse clear cell oncocytosis in the neighboring gland.[237] Clear oncocytes are monomorphic and show completely clear vacuolated cytoplasm with centrally placed, small, monomorphic, homogeneously stained nuclei (Fig. 7–29B). As with oxyphilic oncocytomas, they are well encapsulated; however, adjacent foci of clear cell oncocytic change in normal glandular parenchyma may yield a false impression of invasion.

Histochemical Findings

By enzyme histochemistry on fresh frozen sections, these tumors will be markedly positive for such mitochondrial-associated oxidative enzymes as cytochrome oxidase, succinic dehydrogenase, and diaphorases. Oncocytes are also cytoplasmically positive for phosphotungstic acid hematoxylin (PTAH). IHC markers are not necessary for diagnosis. The oncocytes are cytokeratin positive and negative for myoepithelial markers such as smooth muscle actin and S-100 protein.

Differential Diagnosis

The differential diagnosis for oxyphilic oncocytomas is quite limited since their histopathologic features are readily identifiable. Acinic cell carcinoma, metastatic oncocytic tumors, and pleomorphic adenomas with oxyphilic elements must be included in the differential diagnosis. Acinic cell adenocarcinoma can usually be excluded handily since these tumors tend to be heterogeneous and to harbor cells with cytoplasmic granularity or mucinous material. Furthermore, they usually show microcystic or papillary patterns, features foreign to oncocytoma. The clear cell variant offers a greater challenge since many organs may manifest clear cell variants of carcinoma and must be differentiated from clear cell oncocytes. Finally, mucoepidermoid carcinoma and clear cell carcinoma of the salivary gland must be excluded. These latter two salivary primary tumors are sufficiently unique to allow differentiation (see the following sections).

CYSTADENOMAS[238–277]

Papillary cystadenoma lymphomatosum, or Warthin's tumor, is by far the most common of the cystadenomas and almost exclusively a parotid gland tumor. Although it has been reported to arise in minor glands, most of these cases are probably reactive oncocytic metaplasia of ducts with a secondary lymphocytic infiltrative response. Other rare benign adenomas are cystic in appearance and are distinct from Warthin's tumor.

Gross Pathology

Papillary cystadenoma lymphomatosum shows a classic gross anatomical appearance. The tumor mass is round with a thin tenacious capsule (Fig. 7–30). On hemisection, the tumor is reddish-grey with a spongy microcystic consistency.[239,240] The cystic spaces are occasionally large; sometimes only a single cystic cavity is seen. These cysts contain a serous or viscous mucinous secretion product, yet sometimes the secretions are thick or caseous. Other cystadenomas are also encapsulated tumors with a spongy character containing serous secretions in the microcystic spaces.

Microscopic Pathology

The *papillary cystadenoma lymphomatosum* is a monomorphic tumor with a single epithelial cell type. The tumor is encapsulated and exhibits a classic, easily recognized pattern.[240,243] Multiple cystic spaces are penetrated by papillary projections that are lined by columnar oncocytes with a basilar nuclear stratum and a luminal staggered nuclear layer (Fig. 7–31 A and B). Within the cystic spaces is an eosinophilic coagulum. The second characteristic finding lies in the stroma. Supporting the epithelial fronds is a lymphocytic stroma that includes germinal centers. *Sebaceous lymphadenoma* bears a resemblance to Warthin's tumor; diffuse lymphocytic infiltration is evident and although not cystic, epithelial islands are present throughout and show sebaceous acini (Fig. 7–32).[264,267]

The other papillary cystic adenomas do not show a lymphoid stroma. Benign cystadenomas are composed of both macro- and micro-cystic spaces, many of which may show papillary projections (Fig. 7–33 A–C). The lining cells are columnar ductal type cells that may be oncocytic with eosinophilic cytoplasm,

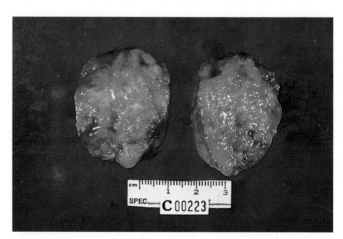

FIGURE 7–30 Papillary cystadenoma lymphomatosum. Gross appearance on hemisection.

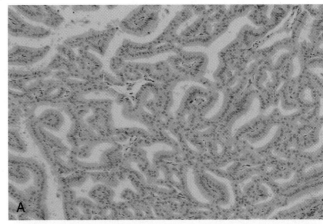

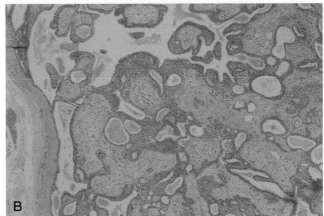

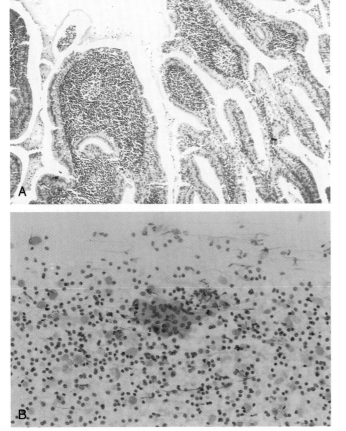

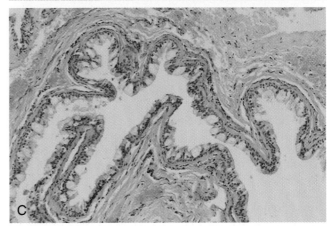

FIGURE 7-31 *A,* Papillary cystadenoma lymphomatosum. Cystic spaces are lined by papillary projections of columnar oncocytes possessing a double row of nuclei. The supportive fronds are made up of lymphocytes with foci or germinal center formation. (H&E, × 33). *B,* Papillary cystadenoma lymphomatosum. FNA showing lymphocytes and "glassy" epithelial cells (PAP, × 100).

FIGURE 7-33 *A,* Papillary cystadenoma. Papillary configurations of columnar cells overlying thin fibrovascular fronds (H&E, × 33). *B,* Papillary cystadenoma with abundant stroma (H&E, × 33). *C,* Papillary mucous cystadenoma. Cystic spaces are lined by tall mucus-secreting columnar cells with intracystic papillary projections (H&E, × 66).

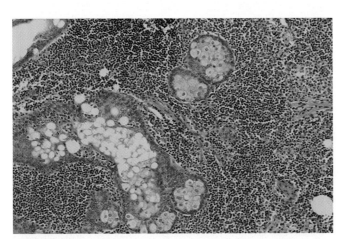

FIGURE 7-32 Sebaceous lymphadenoma. The architecture resembles that of benign lymphoepithelial lesion. Squamous, ductal, and sebaceous epithelial cells are identifiable within a stromal background of lymphocytes (H&E, × 33).

or they may be more basophilic, resembling pseudostratified columnar epithelium of the sinonasal tract, yet lacking cilia.[169,170] The nuclei are oval and vesicular without molding or crowding and there is no evidence of cytologic atypia. *Cystadenomas* and *papillary cystadenomas* both show mature fibrous stromal elements between cystic cavities.

Histochemical Findings

IHC markers are not required for diagnosis. The epithelial cells stain with low-molecular-weight cytokeratins in both papillary cystadenoma lymphomatosum and other cystadenomas. There are no myoepithelial cell markers in the epithelial cells. Lymphoid cells label for T cells and B-cell markers are positive in germinal centers.

Differential Diagnosis

Papillary cystadenoma lymphomatosum is unique and easily recognizable. In minor glands, most masses—particularly those in the buccal mucosa—are reactive foci of duct obstruction with oncocytic metaplasia, and some may show foci of lymphoid infiltration. These lymphoid infiltrates do not form the classic supportive fronds of the epithelial projections of Warthin's tumor. Papillary cystadenoma must be differentiated from its malignant counterpart, papillary cystadenocarcinoma. The latter shows similar papillary cystic configuration; however, the lining cells show nuclear crowding, molding, and pleomorphism with increased mitotic activity. Lack of invasive foci is also a differentiating feature of the benign cystadenomas.

PAPILLOMAS[278-296]

Papillomas of salivary origin arise from the excretory ducts at the ductal orifice with oral mucosa, while a few cases have been observed in sinonasal glands. These benign papillary proliferations can be exophytic or endophytic within the major duct (i.e., inverted).

Gross Pathology

Exophytic lesions show clear gross evidence of papillary projections. The intraductal and inverting ductal papillomas are usually encountered in intraoral minor glands, which on cut section are cystic or solid white or grey in appearance and are clearly demarcated or even cup-shaped on cut section.

Microscopic Pathology

There are three variant forms of salivary ductal papilloma. *Sialadenoma papilliferum* is a rare tumor that involves the parotid or oral cavity minor glands.[278,280] The surface papillary projections are lined by stratified squamous epithelium that merges inferiorly with typical ductal cells; these ductal elements are confluent with normal underlying large excretory ducts (Fig. 7–34A). The ductal cells lining

the papillary stalks are pseudostratified columnar cells.

Another type of papilloma is the *intraductal papilloma*. Most cases are seen in minor glands, also at the excretory orifice.[286,288] A dilated cystic space is evident and projecting into this space are papillary projections lined by monomorphic psuedostratified columnar cells (Fig. 7–34B). The third type of papilloma is the *inverted ductal papilloma*. These rare

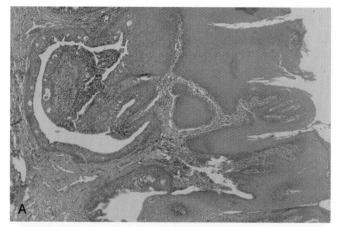

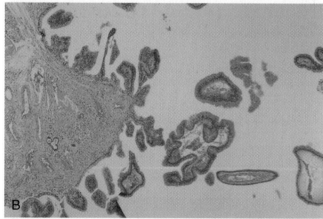

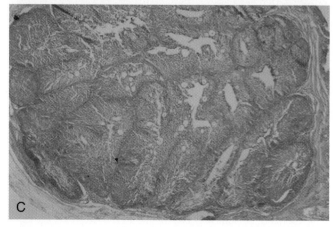

FIGURE 7–34 *A,* Sialadenoma papilliferum. Papillary projections are seen along the surface as well as within dilated ducts (H&E, × 13). *B,* Intraductal papilloma (H&E, × 33). *C,* Inverted ductal papilloma (H&E, × 33).

lesions bear a resemblance to sinonasal inverted papillomas (Fig. 7–34C). There is a layer of surface stratified squamous epithelium with a dilated ductal invagination.[291,294] This duct is cup-shaped and lined by acanthomatous stratified squamous epithelium arranged in lobular inverted rete ridge-like projections that push their way (as opposed to invasion) into the underlying connective tissue. The luminal surface of these inverting squamous projections is often represented by columnar and mucous cells.

Histochemical Findings

There are no unique IHC features for these lesions. The squamous elements are positive for both low- and high-molecular-weight cytokeratins.[294] Mucous cells located at the luminal aspect of inverted papillomas are alcian blue and mucicarmine positive.

Differential Diagnosis

These papillary lesions are sufficiently distinct histopathologically to distinguish them from other papillary lesions such as squamous papilloma, laryngeal papillomatosis, and condyloma. None of these lesions harbor ductal or salivary type cells. Papillary cystadenomas can be excluded on the basis of size and their diffuse proliferative nature.

Malignant Neoplasms

The most common site for major gland epithelial malignancies is the parotid, followed by the submandibular gland. Rarely, tumors are located in the sublingual gland. The more common malignancies include mucoepidermoid carcinoma (28%), acinic cell carcinoma (23%), adenocarcinoma not otherwise specified (16%), adenoid cystic carcinoma (9%), malignant mixed tumor (8%), and squamous cell carcinoma (6%), with many rare forms of adenocarcinoma collectively making up the remainder (10%) of the tumors arising in major glands. Thirty percent of tumors in the parotid gland, 40% in the submandibular gland, and 70% in the sublingual gland are malignant.[111,112] Table 7–9 lists the malignant epithelial tumors of major salivary glands.

Malignant epithelial tumors of the major glands are typically invasive, although some low-grade malignancies may be partially delineated from surrounding tissues. Most arise de novo; yet, occasionally, carcinomas arise from pre-existing benign neoplasms, usually from pleomorphic adenomas. In early stages these tumors may be encapsulated; yet, with time, foci of capsular invasion can be demonstrated both grossly and microscopically.

Cytologic atypia with pleomorphism, increased and abnormal mitotic figures, and nuclear enlargement are frequently lacking in low- or intermediate-grade salivary carcinomas. Therefore, the diagnosis rests with recognizing characteristic histomorphologic patterns and observing marginal invasion of the

TABLE 7–9	CLASSIFICATION OF MAJOR SALIVARY GLAND ADENOCARCINOMAS

Mucoepidermoid Carcinoma
Low, intermediate, high grade
Clear cell variant

Adenoid Cystic Carcinoma
Tubular, cribriform, solid

Acinic Cell Carcinoma
Solid, microcystic, papillary cystic, follicular

Adenocarcinoma, not otherwise specified (NOS)

Polymorphous Low-grade Adenocarcinoma

Carcinoma ex Mixed Tumor

Rare Carcinomas
Squamous cell carcinoma
Clear cell carcinoma
Epithelial-myoepithelial carcinoma
Basal cell adenocarcinoma
Undifferentiated and neuroendocrine carcinomas
Sialoblastoma of infancy
Malignant pleomorphic adenoma
Carcinosarcoma
Cystadenocarcinoma
Salivary duct carcinoma
Sebaceous carcinoma and lymphadenocarcinoma
Oncocytic adenocarcinoma
Mucinous adenocarcinoma
Adenosquamous carcinoma

contiguous normal salivary tissue or connective tissue stroma.[134,139,141]

Most of the malignant tumors that arise in the major glands are encountered in minor salivary and mucous glands as well; however, acinic cell carcinoma, epithelial-myoepithelial carcinoma of intercalated ducts, and carcinoma ex mixed tumor are rarely reported to occur in minor glands. Polymorphous low-grade adenocarcinoma, on the other hand, is a minor gland malignancy that tends not to occur in the major glands.[111,112]

MUCOEPIDERMOID CARCINOMA[296–326]

Mucoepidermoid carcinomas (MECA), first described by Stewart, Foote, and Becker, are found in both major and minor glands; as the term implies, the tumor is characterized by cells that emulate the proximal (ductal orifice) excretory ducts, being stratified squamous accompanied by mucous secreting cells.[301] These neoplasms occur at any age, with an approximate 15% prevalence per decade, spanning the third to the seventh decades. There is a slight predilection for females. About 50% of all MECA arise in the parotid; among the three major glands, almost 88% are parotid, 10% submandibular, and only 2% arise from the sublingual glands. Less than 0.5% arise from ectopic parotid epithelium enclaved within a cervical lymph node. Importantly, such a lesion could represent a metastatic focus, necessitating re-evaluation of the ipsilateral major gland, both clinically and by imaging techniques.[312]

Gross Pathology

There are varying degrees of cellularity in MECA, some being ostensibly solid, others being cystic. Most appear relatively well-circumscribed or partially encapsulated; however, the opposite pole of the mass may blend imperceptibly into the contiguous glandular tissue. On sectioning, solid areas appear firm yellow or tan. Cystic areas contain mucinous, viscous, or myxomatous secretion products that are translucent and grey or bluish. The cystic foci may be diffuse and small or large and focal. Recurrent neoplasms may be multifocal or nodular, indurated, and infiltrative. Brown hemorrhagic foci are commonly noted as well. Smaller tumors are usually enveloped within either the superficial or deep lobe, while larger neoplasms may invade the capsule and may be bound to adjacent connective tissues. When accompanied by lymph node dissec-

tion, all nodes should be sampled for micrometastases. Grossly involved nodes are solid or multicystic and are usually larger than 1 cm.

Microscopic Pathology

There are many variations in cell types and growth patterns of MECA. These patterns are of prognostic significance, being subdivided into low, intermediate, and high grades.[298,300,311] The former rarely metastasize locally, but the high-grade tumors behave more similarly to head and neck squamous cell carcinomas, often eventuating in nodal or hematogenous metastases. Importantly, in the major glands, all these tumors are capable of metastasis. Common to all types of MECA is the presence of the squamous or "epidermoid" cells, mucous secreting cells, and intermediate cells.

Low-grade tumors are composed of macrocystic tumor foci with intraluminal papillary projections (Fig. 7–35A). The cystic spaces are lined by stratified squamous, cuboidal, columnar, and mucous secreting cells. In these low-grade neoplasms, the mucous cells may be single goblet cells or may form acinar-

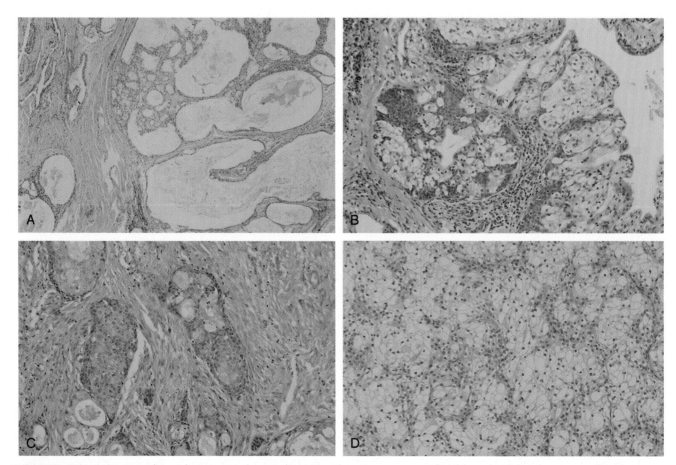

FIGURE 7–35 *A,* Mucoepidermoid carcinoma, low-grade variety. There are macrocysts lined by cuboidal and mucous cells with a paucity of squamous (epidermoid) cells (H&E, × 13). *B,* Mucoepidermoid carcinoma, low-grade variety. Mucous and clear and small foci of epidermoid cells are present (H&E, × 33). *C,* Mucoepidermoid carcinoma, intermediate-grade variety. Both mucous and squamous cells are present in solid islands with macrocystic foci (H&E, × 33). *D,* Mucoepidermoid carcinoma, clear cell variant. Sheets of clear cells are divided by capillary septa surrounded by condensations of squamoid cells (H&E, × 33).

like aggregates that line the papillary projections (Fig. 7–35B). These macrocysts are enveloped by mature collagenous stroma that is rarely inflamed although lymphoid aggregates, often with germinal center formation, are located around the periphery. The peripheral zone is well-demarcated; it may even have a pseudocapsule along a portion of the tumor margins, while the opposite pole is infiltrative. Cytologically, the nuclei are bland and monomorphic. Mitotic figures are not evident.[313]

High-grade MECA, in contrast to the low-grade variety, is solid with very few cystic loci.[326] Solid nests of squamous keratinocytes are seen, as are isolated foci of mucous secreting cells. Polygonal basaloid cells, termed intermediate cells, are interposed between the other cell types. A prominent clear cell component may also be evident. There is usually some degree of cytologic atypia; indeed, it may be marked with pleomorphism, hyperchromatism, and many mitotic figures—but not always. The preponderance of solid sheets of epidermoid cells and the lack of a macrocystic element are the key features of the high-grade lesion. Along the tumor margins are histologically identifiable foci of invasion into normal glandular parenchyma.

The intermediate-grade variant of MECA logically falls midway between the low- and high-grade forms in reference to histopathologic features. Thus, both solid nests of epidermoid and intermediate cells with only occasional mucous cells are evident and are intermixed with islands exhibiting microcyst formation, lined by stratified squamous, ductal, and mucous cells (Fig. 7–35C). Some margins are demarcated, others are invasive, and perilesional lymphoid aggregates are sometimes seen. Most intermediate-grade tumors have a relatively equal distribution of solid and cystic foci, and cytologic atypia is not usually observed.

Some MECAs are made up almost entirely of clear cells and have been referred to as the clear cell variant (Fig. 7–35D). The clear cells form diffuse sheets that may resemble clear cell or glycogen-rich adenocarcinomas.[305,311] A unique histomorphologic feature is the clustering of compressed squamous foci interposed among the clear cells, particularly along the margin of the tumor cell nests. Pure clear cell variants should probably be classified as intermediate-grade tumors with a moderate propensity for nodal metastasis. In total, the majority of MECAs are of the low and intermediate grades, with only 20% to 25% being high-grade.

For grading MECAs, Auclair et al[326] have developed a scoring system based on the following parameters: less than 20% of intracystic component (2 points), presence of neural invasion (2 points), presence of necrosis (3 points), four or more mitoses per 10 high-power fields (3 points), and having cellular anaplasia (4 points). Those tumors having a total score of 0–4 points are classifed as low grade, 5–6 points as intermediate grade, and 7 or more points as high grade. This grading system correlates well with the prognosis of most MECAs, with a possible exception of those involving the submandibular gland. The mortality rates for low-grade, intermediate-grade, and high-grade MECAs of all major and minor salivary glands combined are 3%, 10%, and 46% respectively.[112] However, 13% of patients with low-grade MECA of the submandibular gland have died of disease.[112]

Histochemical Findings

Mucicarmine and alcian blue-PAS stains may be employed to demonstrate the presence of mucous cells, although in low- and intermediate-grade tumors, such cells are readily identifiable on routine H&E stains. Therefore, if there is a question as to whether a lesion is squamous cell carcinoma of salivary gland origin versus high-grade MECA, such stains may be diagnostically helpful. There are no immunomarker studies that are of diagnostic importance. Luminal cells stain with cytokeratin 14, 18, and/or 19, while squamous cells stain with high molecular weight cytokeratins.

Differential Diagnosis

Low-grade tumors may be confused with cystadenoma, papillary cystadenoma, and cystadenocarcinomas, whereas high-grade lesions may show features of squamous cell carcinoma. In all MECAs, some foci or squamous differentiation should be encountered, whereas cystadenomas are composed exclusively of cuboidal, columnar, and mucous cells. High-grade tumors can be differentiated from squamous cell carcinomas by finding mucous secreting cells. This may be facilitated by application of mucicarmine or alcian blue pH2.5/PAS staining when mucous cells are few and far between.[311,326] The clear cell variant of MECA must be differentiated from clear cell carcinoma and metastatic renal cell carcinoma (hypernephroma). In the former, condensed fusiform groups of squamous cells are interposed between the clear cell nests, but prominent vascularity as seen in the clear cell type of renal cell carcinoma is not seen in MECA. Furthermore, most MECA clear cell tumors contain foci or more classic regions with both squamous and mucous cells. Other salivary gland tumors that may contain abundant clear cells are listed in Table 7–10.

TABLE 7–10	SALIVARY TUMORS WITH PROMINENT CLEAR CELL COMPONENT

Oncocytoma
Clear cell carcinoma
Mucoepidermoid carcinoma
Epithelial-myoepithelial carcinoma
Acinic cell carcinoma

Perhaps the most significant entity in the differential diagnosis of MECA is the benign condition, necrotizing sialometaplasia (NSM). NSM is more commonly encountered in the oral cavity, particularly in the soft and hard palate minor salivary glands than in major glands. NSM is characterized by diffuse foci of acinar coagulative necrosis with the acinar outlines ghosted, yet identifiable without stainable nuclei. Adjacent to the necrotic foci are oval zellballen of squamous cells that represent squamous metaplasia of ducts. Importantly, these cellular nodules fail to show anaplastic or atypical features, and mucous goblet cells are not often seen.

ADENOID CYSTIC CARCINOMA[327-351]

The so-called cylindroma was first described by Billroth,[333] its name derived from its multiple cylindric appearance on gross sectioning of the tumor. The currently accepted terminology, adenoid cystic carcinoma, comes from its histopathologic appearance for the classic cribriform pattern. In reality, three distinct cellular arrangements—cribriform, tubular, and solid—are encountered in these tumors. The preponderance of one particular pattern over the others has been shown in some (but not all) investigations to have prognostic implications. These tumors arise in both major and minor glands of the aerodigestive tract. They are notorious for local recurrence and persistence, with favorable short-term—but very poor long-term—survivals.[350]

The majority arise in the fifth through seventh decades, and there is a slight female predilection. Adenoid cystic carcinoma is the fourth common malignancy of the major glands and may arise in minor glands, the palate being the favored site.

Gross Pathology

The tumor is usually relatively well circumscribed, yet on sectioning no capsule can be identified, and the tumor margins are infiltrative. The tumor is pink or tan and often exhibits a mottled surface with minute cylindric foci. Cystic foci are not encountered unless necrosis has occurred, an uncommon event in adenoid cystic carcinoma.

Surgeons often sacrifice the facial nerve and label it in relation to tumor. Because of the marked neurotropism for this salivary malignancy, sections should be taken along the course of the nerve to the proximal cranial base segment to examine for microscopic evidence of perineural space spread.

Microscopic Pathology

There are three distinct morphologic patterns in adenoid cystic carcinoma, all of which share similar cytologic features.[343,348,349] The cribriform pattern is a hallmark of this tumor yet may be found in other salivary tumors as well. In cribriform tumor islands, cells with round hyperchromatic, round, oval, or angulated nuclei, and scant cytoplasm with indistinct cell borders assume a Swiss-cheese pattern of microcysts, usually filled with eosinophilic hyalinized secretion product (Fig. 7–36A). Larger cystic structures may contain basophilic mucin. Duplicated basal lamina also forms hyalinized stroma around the cribriform islands, and this hyalinized matrix may merge and be confluent with that found within the microcysts. The luminal cells do not form well-defined cuboidal or columnar ductal structures. FNA shows solid clusters of small, dark, round nucleated cells with sparse cytoplasm. When a cribriform nest is aspirated, characteristic oval hyaline structures are surrounded by these hyperchromatic round cells.

The second pattern is tubular (Fig. 7–36B). The tumor cells are basaloid or cuboid and are arranged in linear arrays with back-to-back cells. These tubules may be solid, without lumina, or they may exhibit dilatations with duct-like formations. The surrounding stroma is loose, often myxoid; it can also be hyalinized.

The third pattern is solid (Fig. 7–36C). Basaloid monomorphic sheets and islands are rimmed by either polygonal or basal cells that show no ductal or squamous differentiation, although infrequently, some squamous eddies may be seen. The basaloid cells are either small and hyperchromatic or larger and oval with stippled chromatin. Often, both cell types occur in the same solid nests. Mitotic activity is low in the cells of tubular and cribriform glands but it is increased in solid areas, sometimes by more than five mitoses per 10 high-power fields.[112]

Many pathologists grade adenoid cystic carcinoma on the basis of pattern predominance.[350] It should be noted that any one tumor may harbor one, two, or all three patterns. Clinicopathologic studies have disclosed that recurrence, metastatic rate, and survival can be related to grade of malignancy; a preponderant tubular pattern carries a better prognosis than a cribriform variant, which in turn fares more favorably than those with a solid pattern. There are, however, conflicting opinions on the issue of grading. In general, tubular predominance is grade I, cribriform is grade II, and solid is grade III.

Wherever nerves pass through the areas of tumor invasion, perineural invasion can be seen (Fig. 7–36D). Laminated concentric tumor strands or even large sheets are seen to wrap around nerve fibers, and in some cases tumor cells are encased within the nerve proper.

Histochemical Findings

Both ductal and myoepithelial cells are identified with IHC markers. Epithelial membrane antigen (EMA) and low-molecular-weight cytokeratins 14, 18, and 19 are positive in the luminally oriented cells. Vimentin, cytokeratin, and muscle-specific actin myoepithelial cells are found in the outer strata of tumor islands in all three morphologic patterns of

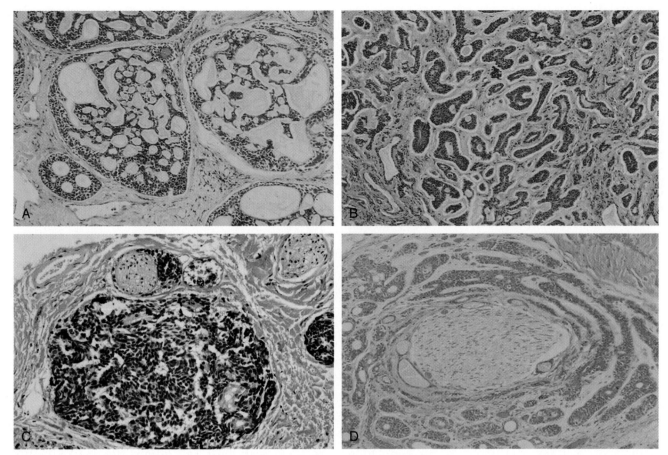

FIGURE 7–36 *A,* Adenoid cystic carcinoma. Cribriform pattern (H&E, × 33). *B,* Adenoid cystic carcinoma. Tubular pattern (H&E, × 33). *C,* Adenoid cystic carcinoma. Solid pattern with perineural invasion (H&E, × 33). *D,* Adenoid cystic carcinoma. Perineural invasion (H&E, × 33).

adenoid cystic carcinoma. Many cells are also CEA positive.

Differential Diagnosis

The solid pattern of adenoid cystic carcinoma, if it is the sole pattern, must be differentiated from neuroendocrine carcinoma and basal cell adenocarcinoma.[328–330] The former may show rosette structures and will usually stain with such neuroendocrine markers as NSE, synaptophysin, and chromogranin. Basal cell adenocarcinomas usually are distinctive with highly polarized basilar cells, squamous eddies, and minimal stroma hyalinization.

The cribriform pattern so typical of adenoid cystic carcinoma and the tubular pattern are also encountered in canalicular adenoma and polymorphous low-grade adenocarcinoma, both of which occur in minor glands and are almost never seen in the major salivary glands. These tumors have other features that allow for their separation from adenoid cystic carcinoma. Perineural invasion is commonly encountered in polymorphic low-grade adenocarcinoma and epimyoepithelial carcinoma of intercalated ducts.

ACINIC CELL ADENOCARCINOMA[352–384]

Of all salivary malignancies, acinic cell carcinomas show the most favorable prognosis and survival.[353–355] The tumor does, however, sometimes exhibit aggressive tendencies with late recurrence and metastasis. In the major glands, 90% occur in the parotid; this tumor arises uncommonly in minor glands. About 60% of acinic cell carcinomas occur in females, arising with almost equal distribution from the second to the seventh decades. These neoplasms are so named because the cell populations resemble serous, mucous, or seromucous acinar cells, and ductal structures are not a prominent component.

Gross Pathology

Acinic cell tumors that have not been surgically treated previously are usually less than 5 cm and are uninodular with well-defined or partially encapsulated borders (Fig. 7–37). Multinodularity is more often encountered in recurrent tumors. The cut surface is grey to pink to white and may be friable with small cystic spaces containing mucinous material. Large cystic spaces are sometimes encountered.

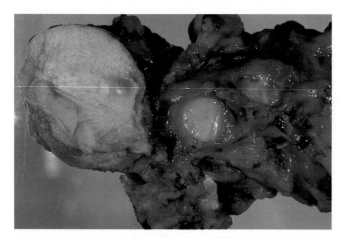

FIGURE 7–37 Gross appearance of recurrent acinic cell carcinoma shows multiple yellow-tan nodules.

Microscopic Pathology

As with other salivary gland tumors, acinic cell adenocarcinomas show many cellular patterns, both between tumors and within tumors. The predominant patterns as detailed by Abrams and Melrose[362] are the solid, microcystic, papillary microcystic, and follicular types. Any given tumor may be of one histomorphologic type exclusively or may exhibit a combination of patterns, yet there is no correlation between pattern and prognosis. As mentioned previously, the tumor derives its name from its cytologic features in which individual cells emulate acinar secretory cells. These cells may resemble mature adult serous, mucous, or seromucous acinar cells, or they may be hybrid cells with clear or vacuolated cytoplasms and a lack of acinar cluster or bulb morphology.[364,365]

The solid type is made up of acinar cell sheets (Fig. 7–38A). The least common acinar type is the serous cell with clearly defined zymogen granules; more often the cells are a hybrid mucinous or clear cell type. All have distinct plasma membranes and occur in broad sheets with fine small caliber vascular stromal septa. Mature collagenous stroma is seen only around the peripheral aspects of the tumor mass.

The microcystic variant also lacks collagenous stroma, and the clear or mucinous cells are arranged around small lumina (Fig. 7–38B). These luminal cells assume a cobblestone or hobnail appearance with a more apocine appearance, rather than being ductal, cuboidal, or columnar cell types. Only in the follicular variant are true ductal structures seen.

The papillary cystic form of acinic cell adenocarcinoma, as is seen in Warthin's tumor, shows multiple large cystic spaces into which extend papillary projections of acinar type cells that also harbor microcystic spaces lined by hobnail luminal cells (Fig. 7–38C). The stroma is delicate. The cystic spaces may be large or small.

The follicular variant, so named because of its resemblance to follicular carcinoma of the thyroid, is uncommon. Acinar sheets comprised of hybrid clear or mucinous cells are infused with multiple ducts lined by prominent cuboidal cells.

Although well-demarcated, acinic cell adenocarcinomas have only pseudocapsules, and microscopic evidence of invasion into the parotid parenchyma can usually be noted. Rarely, foci of anaplastic carcinoma can be found in otherwise ordinary acinic cell neoplasms. Another common feature is the presence of perilesional lymphoid aggregates, many of which contain germinal centers. This common stromal reaction has been erroneously interpreted as lymph node metastasis.

Rarely, a less differentiated clone of cells will evolve in an otherwise bland acinic cell carcinoma. This *dedifferentiated variant* of acinic cell tumor carries a much worse prognosis.[381] The tumor cells are arranged in cords, trabeculae, and ducts with pleomorphic or large vesicular nuclei (Fig. 7–38D).

Histochemical Findings

Mucosubstance staining is positive in acinic cell lesions, particularly with PAS, although predominantly clear cell populations may stain negatively since their glycogen was washed away during processing. Such clear cell lesions are markedly PAS-positive on frozen sections. Alcian blue and mucicarmine stains are also usually positive in the microcytic spaces, yet tumor cells are only occasionally stained with these acidic mucin stains. With IHC, some of the acinic cell neoplasms will stain positively for lactoferrin, amylase, and lysozyme. Cytokeratin and vimentin may also be localized to some of the cells in these tumors. In general, IHC offers little or no benefit in the diagnosis of acinic cell adenocarcinoma variants.

Differential Diagnosis

Acinic cell adenocarcinoma may resemble mucoepidermoid carcinoma, particularly intermediate-grade MECA with microcystic foci. Usually MECA has foci of squamous and intermediate cells, a feature not encountered in acinic cell lesions. Clear cell carcinoma is also in the differential diagnosis. Although acinic cell neoplasms may harbor clear cell nests, they are not exclusively made up of such cells as is clear cell adenocarcinoma of salivary origin.[384] It is unlikely for follicular thyroid carcinoma to metastasize to the lower pole of the thyroid, yet in the lateral neck node, metastatic thyroid versus follicular variant of acinic cell carcinoma may become an issue. Thyroidglobulin IHC may be helpful in such instances, and of course a history of primary thyroid or parotid tumor should be explored before making a final diagnosis.

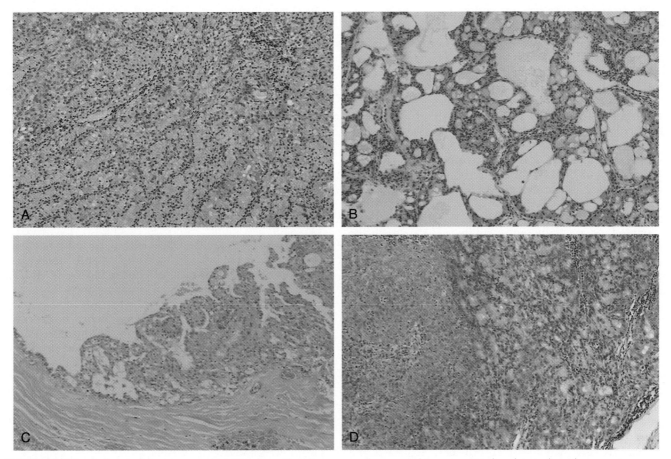

FIGURE 7–38 *A,* Acinic cell carcinoma. Solid pattern with acinar type cells arranged in compact trabecular cords and sparse stroma (H&E, × 33). *B,* Acinic cell carcinoma. Microcystic pattern is seen with cells showing eosinophilic and mucinous cytoplasm (H&E, × 33). *C,* Acinic cell carcinoma. In the papillary cystic pattern lining cells assume a hobnail appearance (H&E, × 33). *D,* Dedifferentiated acinic cell carcinoma. Typical well-differentiated acinic cell carcinoma on the right and anaplastic carcinomatous cell population on the left (H&E, × 33).

ADENOCARCINOMA NOT OTHERWISE SPECIFIED[385–398]

When a tumor is encountered that does not possess histomorphologic features of the herein-described salivary tumor variants, yet shows adenoid differentiation with invasive or cytologically atypical features, the neoplasm is referred to as adenocarcinoma, not otherwise specified (NOS).[391] As a group of unclassifiable salivary adenocarcinomas, the majority arise in the fifth to eighth decades with a peak in the seventh decade. Eighty percent involve the parotid, 20% the submandibular gland, and less than 1% arise in the sublingual gland. In regard to all sites, minor glands are the site for adenocarcinoma NOS in 40% of cases, the major glands in 60%. There is no significant sexual predilection for these carcinomas.

Gross Pathology

The tumor is often clearly demarcated in some, clearly infiltrative in others, and a combination of encapsulation with foci of extension into contiguous parenchyma or capsule may be observed. On cut section, these tumors are quite variable, but are usually greyish-white or pink with or without foci of hemorrhage. Large and small cystic spaces are uncommon, yet are seen in some tumors.

Microscopic Pathology

The characteristic feature of this group of tumors is ductal differentiation without histopathologic characteristics that would allow for a specific diagnosis for the other specified malignant tumors of salivary epithelia. It is, therefore, a diagnosis by exclusion.[385,387,388] The patterns of growth are highly variable both between and within tumors. Solid sheets, trabecular cords, ductal structures, Indian-file arrangements, and microcystic spaces may be seen. The cytologic features are also varied and include polygonal, cuboidal, mucinous, clear, and basaloid cells. Cytologic atypia is more commonly seen in this group of tumors than the other salivary carcinomas and includes hyperchromatism, pleomorphism, and mitotic figures (Fig. 7–39). Indeed, based upon degree of atypia, the tumors may be graded with low-grade types being the least common. High-grade (grade III) adenocarcinoma NOS harbors pleomorphic or large anaplastic nuclei, tumor giant cells, and a high mitotic index. The tumors are predominantly solid and one must sometimes search many fields to find ductal structures—although microcysts, often mucicarmine or alcian blue positive, are usually identifiable. Intermediate-grade (grade II) adenocarcinoma NOS is more easily recognized for its glandular/ductal differentiation, and cytologic atypia is not as pronounced. Low-grade (grade I) tumors are well-circumscribed, have recognizable cuboidal luminal cells, and are generally well-demarcated or partially encapsulated. Because of the extreme variation in this group of tumors, grading is quite subjective; however, distinction between low- and high-grade tumors is usually not problematic.[391–394] It should also be noted that adenocarcinoma NOS may contain fields that simulate other well-recognized salivary tumors; yet, these isolated foci are not pervasive.

Histochemical Findings

As stated previously, alcian blue/PAS and mucicarmine stains may be helpful, particularly for high-grade, poorly differentiated adenocarcinomas. Cytoplastic and microcystic mucin positivity may be seen in only a few isolated foci but will establish the diagnosis. IHC staining offers no diagnostic advantage.

Differential Diagnosis

There may be foci that resemble adenoid cystic, acinic cell, or epithelial-myoepithelial carcinoma; however, the vast majority of tumor cells do not

share features in common with other salivary tumor types. In this context, the possibility of metastatic adenocarcinoma from a distant site must be considered in the differential diagnosis.

Also to be considered in the differential diagnosis is carcinoma ex mixed tumor. The entire tumor must be perused to determine whether or not a focus of typical pleomorphic adenoma is present, since the malignant component of carcinoma ex mixed tumor is typically an adenocarcinoma NOS.

POLYMORPHOUS LOW-GRADE ADENOCARCINOMA[399–418]

This salivary gland tumor is essentially localized to minor glands.[411] Only a few instances have been reported to occur in the parotid gland, relegating polymorphous low-grade adenocarcinoma (PMLGA) to the list of rare tumors of major glands. In minor glands, PMLGA is second only to mucoepidermoid carcinoma in terms of prevalence, being more common than adenoid cystic carcinoma, a tumor that is microscopically similar. PMLGA consisting predominantly or exclusively of papillary elements is best classified as papillary cystadenocarcinoma because this papillary variant is more aggressive than the typical PMLGA.[411]

Gross Pathology

In minor glands, the tumor is surfaced by mucous membrane; it is rarely ulcerated. The tumor is solid, grey to white, and well-circumscribed without a demonstrable capsule.

Microscopic Pathology

The tumor is relatively well-demarcated yet not encapsulated. It invades the adjacent salivary gland or soft tissue. The cells are arranged in solid lobular islands, diffuse sheets, islands with internal ductules, and cribriform and papillary arrangements (Fig. 7–40 A–C). This polymorphous architecture is intermixed, and around the periphery are slender Indian-file strands of hyperchromatic cells.[401,403,405] The nuclei are typically large and show peppered chromatin. Nucleoli and mitotic activity are rare or absent. When nerves are in the vicinity of the tumor, perineural invasion may be seen (Fig. 7–40D). The stroma is mature, without significant hyalinization or duplicated basal lamina.

Histochemical Findings

Cytokeratin cocktails label the epithelial cells. S-100 protein and EMA are also positive. Smooth muscle actin and CEA are expressed in some cells and negative in others.[407] Thus, there is no clearly evident

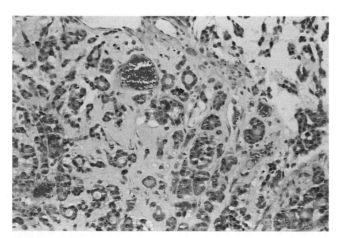

FIGURE 7–39 Adenocarcinoma NOS. Ductal patterns are evident, yet the pattern does not conform to other recognized salivary carcinomas (H&E, × 33).

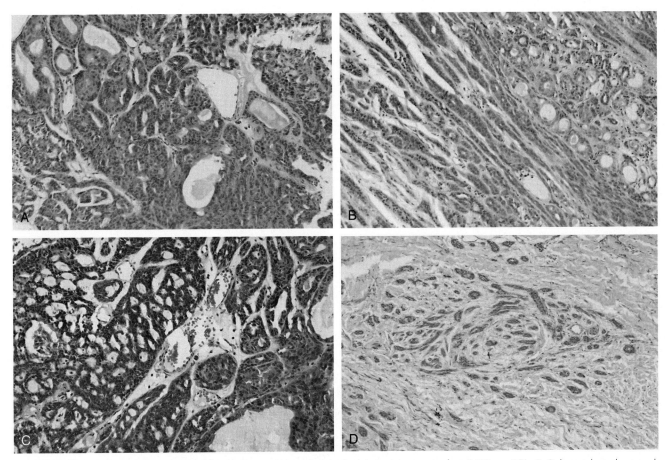

FIGURE 7-40 *A,* Polymorphous low-grade adenocarcinoma. Solid, ductal, and microcytic foci (H&E, × 33). *B,* Polymorphous low-grade adenocarcinoma. Indian-file and tubular patterns (H&E, × 33). *C,* Polymorphous low-grade adenocarcinoma. Solid lobules and cribriform patterns with dense fibrous stroma (H&E, × 33). *D,* Polymorphous low-grade adenocarcinoma. Perineural and intraneural invasion (H&E, × 33).

myoepithelial element; most cells react similarly to the terminal or intercalated ducts.

Differential Diagnosis

The three lesions to be considered in the differential diagnosis are basal cell form of monomorphic adenoma, basal cell adenocarcinoma, and adenoid cystic carcinoma, all of which show cellular patterns that overlap with those of PMLGA. Basal cell adenomas are well-circumscribed and usually encapsulated with smooth borders, while PMLGA shows invasion around the periphery. The basal cell adenoma is also more monotonous and the nuclei are small. Basal cell adenocarcinoma is a major salivary gland lesion, whereas PMLGA is a minor salivary gland tumor. Microscopically, the solid lobules of PMLGA may resemble those of basal cell adenocarcinoma; yet the latter is more monotonous, shows prominent basal cell polarization, and may exhibit basal lamina duplication. The major dilemma for the surgical pathologist is differentiation from adenoid cystic carcinoma (ACCA). Both tumors show solid, tubular, and cribriform patterns, and perineural invasion is encountered in both lesions as well. The main distinguishing features for PMLGA include:

1. Nuclei are large and pale staining, while in ACCA they are hyperchromatic and angulated.
2. While cribriform patterns are encountered in both, PMLGA does not tend to show significant hyalinization typically associated with cribriform patterns in ACCA.
3. The peripheral Indian-file strands are typical for PMLGA.

Although enigmatic, it is interesting to note that the propensity for perineural invasion in PMLGA does not predispose to local recurrence, particularly at skull base as seen with ACCA.

CARCINOMA EX MIXED TUMOR[419-429]

Pleomorphic adenomas may occasionally undergo adenocarcinomatous transformation.[420] This transformation event occurs in fewer than 3% of all mixed tumors, and the chance for adenocarcinomatous change increases with the number of recurrences of the original benign pleomorphic adenoma. Some are encountered after four or five recurrences. Importantly, one must realize that the typical features of benign mixed tumor often prevail; the adenocarcinomatous component is focal and may not be the predominant finding. Therefore, it is incumbent upon the surgical pathologist to examine all the sections carefully, particularly in recurrent lesions, to search out a focus of malignant transformation. This same caveat holds true when fine aspiration cytology is performed on recurrent mixed tumor. Sampling error would be expected to yield false-negative findings for malignancy given that the needle sample may not access the focus of adenocarcinomatous transformation.

The parotid is the site for 80% of major gland carcinoma ex mixed tumor, the remainder occurring in the submandibular and minor glands. Most cases arise during the sixth to eighth decades. Females are slightly more likely than males to develop this form of cancer. Carcinomatous transformation has also been reported in other benign salivary tumors (e.g., Warthin's tumor), but such an event is extremely rare.

Gross Pathology

The tumors are usually twice as large as benign mixed tumors. They are grey to white and may have myxoid or mucinous foci. The margins are often partially encapsulated, with foci of invasive cords that extend into the parenchyma or glandular capsule. Some will be fixed to and invade contiguous connective tissues in the neck.

Microscopic Pathology

The ratio of benign mixed tumor loci to adenocarcinomatous foci is quite variable from one tumor to another. Conceptually, only a single focus or clone of cells undergoes adenocarcinomatous transformation in an otherwise benign pleomophic adenoma. In many instances the bulk of the tumor mass is represented by classic mixed tumor patterns (see previous discussion, pleomorphic adenoma), with only a small area of adenocarcinoma.[423,428,429] In other cases, the adenocarcinomatous element is dominant and pervasive. It is truly uncommon to encounter typical salivary adenocarcinoma variants in carcinoma ex mixed tumor; rather, the malignant element is epithelial and more typical of adenocarcinoma, NOS. The malignant cell patterns are decidedly glandular, with most tumors exhibiting tubular, trabecular, and ductal patterns (Fig. 7–41). Some may have solid loci with or without microcystic/ductal elements or even sheets of mucinous or clear cells. Common to all of these patterns are local infiltration and cytopathologic evidence of malignancy to include nuclear anaplasia (i.e., large nuclei with nucleoli), pleomorphism, hyperchromasia, and in-

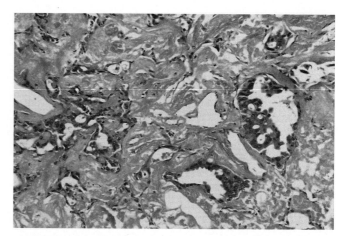

FIGURE 7–41 Carcinoma arising from pleomorphic adenoma. Typical mixed tumor morphology with a focus of glandular islands exhibiting cytologic atypia (H&E, × 33).

creased and bizarre mitotic figures. Loss of cohesiveness with Indian-filing and individual cells in the stroma may also be featured. On fine needle aspiration, fortuitous samples may show features of both benign mixed tumor and clusters of cells with cytologic atypia (e.g., mucinous background, cell clusters with feathered myoepithelial satellites accompanied by clustered groups that may show ductal groups with hyperchromatic, large nuclei). In tumors with only a small focus of malignant transformation, only the typical pleomorphic adenoma pattern will prevail, and the diagnosis of carcinoma ex mixed tumor will not be attainable until surgical specimens are processed.

Histochemical Findings

There are no characteristic histochemical or IHC markers for carcinoma ex mixed tumor. The myxoid stroma is alcianophilic and intraductal mucins are stainable. The luminal cells stain for cytokeratins and the myoepithelial element is usually both vimentin and smooth muscle actin positive.

Differential Diagnosis

Benign mixed tumor is the most significant entity in the differential histopathologic diagnosis. As stated previously, sections must be carefully examined for a focus of malignancy. Alternatively, when encountering a clear case of malignancy in a case with a history of pre-existent mixed tumor, one should search for evidence of pleomorphic adenoma. Recurrent benign mixed tumor presents with multiple well-circumscribed nodules. Cells reveal minimal cytologic atypia and rare mitotic activity. Carcinosarcoma is easily differentiated from carcinoma ex mixed tumor in that both the epithelial and mesenchymal components show unequivocal cytologic evidence of malignant neoplasia. Metastasizing mixed tumor is an otherwise benign mixed tumor that metastasizes yet continues to manifest histopathologic features of benignity. Such lesions are comparable to the rare basal cell carcinoma that metastasizes to regional nodes or the otherwise benign ameloblastoma that, on rare occasions, undergoes regional or hematogenous spread.

RARE SALIVARY GLAND TUMORS

There are many rare variations of salivary malignancies, each tumor type representing less than 1% to 2% of all salivary malignancies. Most arise in the parotid gland, with the minority being evenly distributed between the submandibular and minor glands. There are, however, some rare major gland variants that are not so rare in the minor glands, particularly those of the oral cavity. Polymorphous low-grade adenocarcinoma almost never occurs in major glands, yet is the second most prevalent malignant salivary tumor of oral minor glands. Adenosquamous carcinoma is also generally limited to minor salivary glands where it occurs in the vicinity of the excretory ductal orifice. Conversely, there are major gland adenocarcinomas that are rarely found in minor glands. Basal cell adenocarcinoma and epithelial-myoepithelial carcinoma are examples. Each of these rare variants will be described in brief here. The reader is referred to the text by Ellis, Auclair, and Gnepp or the AFIP fascicle on Salivary Gland Tumors for more detailed explication on these entities.

Gross Pathology

These rare adenocarcinoma variants are all potentially invasive and infiltrative yet may show partial encapsulation. Depending upon the tumor they are grey, pink, or white solid masses with indistinct margins. Rarely, some will show necrotic foci or hemorrhage; others may have a bluish mucinous appearance.

Microscopic Pathology

The histopathologic features of each of these rare variants will be described preceded by a brief clinicopathologic overview. This is a group of tumors with diverse behavioral patterns, some being low-grade tumors, others being extremely aggressive with high metastatic rates and poor prognosis.
Squamous Cell Carcinoma.[430–434] Malignant tumors characterized by classic squamous differentiation without any glandular or ductal differentiation are encountered in the parotid and other salivary glands. Since excretory ducts at the ductal orifice of the oral mucosa are essentially lined by typical nonkeratinized stratified squamous epithelium, it is understandable that squamous cancer can arise in both major and minor glands. Histopathologically, squamous cell carcinoma of salivary tissues is identical to that of surface epithelium (Fig. 7–42 *A* and *B*). The tumor cells are arranged in islands and cords

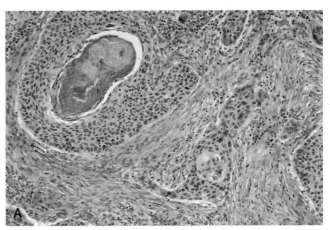
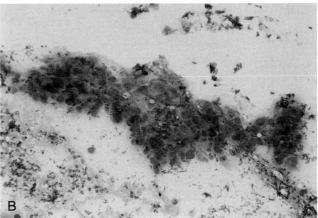

FIGURE 7–42 *A,* Squamous cell carcinoma of salivary origin. Keratin pearl formation is evident (H&E, × 33). *B,* FNA of salivary gland squamous cell carcinoma (H&E, × 100).

with an outer basal cell layer and an inner spinous layer.[429–431] The cells show classic cytologic features of malignancy, including pleomorphism, hyperchromatism, increased nuclear size, and variable degrees of keratin differentiation. Unlike mucoepidermoid carcinoma, there are no glandular formations and no mucous cells. Squamous cell carcinoma invades adjacent salivary parenchyma and tends to metastasize to regional nodes. In the differential diagnosis, one must consider metastatic spread to an intraparotid lymph node from an upper aerodigestive tract mucosal primary tumor.
Clear Cell Carcinoma.[435–446] Salivary gland tumors composed of a monotonous population of clear cells have been classified as glycogen-rich adenocarcinomas or, more appropriately, simply clear cell carcinoma of salivary gland origin.[439] The tumor cells are arranged in large lobular sheets without intervening fibrous stroma. Rather, the oval islands are separated by fine vascular septa (Fig. 7–43). These tumors show a lack of encapsulation with invasion of adjacent salivary parenchyma. The individual cells are bland without significant cytologic atypia, although some instances may harbor pleomorphic nu-

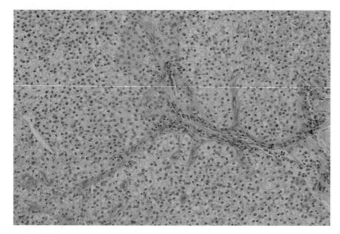

FIGURE 7–43 Clear cell carcinoma. The clear cells are arranged in large lobular sheets with fine capillary septa (× 33).

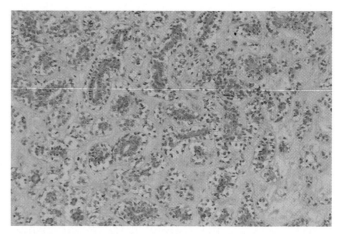

FIGURE 7–44 Epithelial-myoepithelial carcinoma of intercalated ducts. Cuboidal cells line ducts and are enveloped by an outer stratum of clear myoepithelial cells (H&E, × 33).

clei with increased mitotic activity. Therefore, despite a bland cytologic appearance, the tumors may be aggressive and metastasize regionally. Invasion and lack of encapsulation are the hallmarks of malignancy.[435–438] The differential diagnosis includes metastatic renal cell carcinoma, the clear cell variant of which shows small organoid clusters of cells with copious vascularization.[439–441] Clear cell variant of mucoepidermoid carcinoma exhibits squamoid condensations and foci of mucicarminophilic cells, while the clear cells of epithelial-myoepithelial carcinoma surround ductal luminal cells, features not seen in the pure clear cell adenocarcinoma of salivary gland origin.

Epithelial-Myoepithelial Carcinoma.[447–455] The histologic and cytologic features of this variant are sufficiently unique to allow a straightforward diagnosis in most instances. The tumor is often well-demarcated with foci of parenchymal invasion. Tumor cells are arranged in diffuse sheets with a unique internal architecture. Many small ducts, resembling the intercalated ducts, are evident and are surrounded by a ring of clear cells that, on electron microscopy, show features of glycogen-rich myoepithelial cells (Fig. 7–44).[452] The combination of luminal ductal cuboidal epithelial cells and surrounding clear myoepithelia account for the term given to this rare tumor. Most arise in the parotid gland yet a few cases have been described in other major glands as well as minor glands.[450–452] Occasionally, cribriform patterns are encountered in epithelial-myoepithelial carcinoma, a feature that has caused some pathologists to consider adenoid cystic carcinoma.

Basal Cell Adenocarcinoma.[456–464] Like its benign counterpart the basal cell adenoma, basal cell adenocarcinoma is made up of sheets and islands of basaloid cells.[459] Certainly the outer strata of cells are cuboidal basal cells, with the inner group also showing a polygonal basaloid appearance (Fig. 7–45). In various regions, there is usually some attempt, in the

sea of monotony, for ductal differentiation. The main feature connoting potential for metastasis, thereby warranting a diagnosis of adenocarcinoma, is the lack of encapsulation seen in basal cell adenoma. The adenocarcinoma variant shows clear evidence of invasion into adjacent parenchymal and connective tissues. Mitotic figures are seen, yet are not frequent, and the cells are monomorphic, without any significant cytologic atypia. The chief entities in the differential diagnosis are basal cell and membranous adenoma and solid variant of adenoid cystic carcinoma.[463,464] In the former, the tumor is encapsulated; in the latter, the cells are anaplastic and hyperchromatic, and a search of all sections will usually disclose some cribriform or tubular architecture.

Undifferentiated and Neuroendocrine Carcinomas.[465–477] Undifferentiated tumors arise in many sites of the body. Occasionally tumors with the features of neuroendocrine carcinoma, primitive neuroectodermal

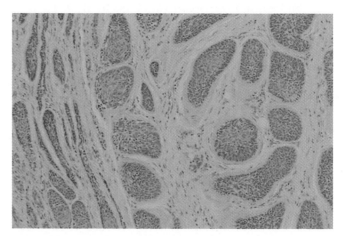

FIGURE 7–45 Basaloid cell adenocarcinoma. Basaloid nests infiltrating a mature and often hyalinized stroma (H&E, × 33).

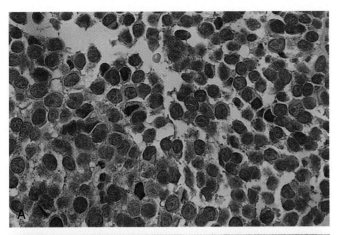

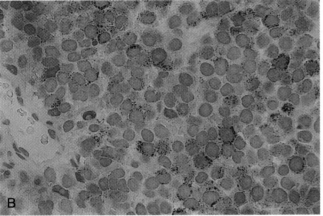

FIGURE 7-46 *A,* Small cell undifferentiated carcinoma of salivary origin (H&E, × 200). *B,* Small cell undifferentiated carcinoma of salivary origin. Positive immunostain for cytokeratin 20 (IHC, DAB, × 200).

tumor (PNET), extraskeletal Ewing's sarcoma, and large cell undifferentiated carcinoma arise in the salivary glands, usually the parotid.[473] Such tumors are characterized by islands of round cells lacking distinct cytoplasmic borders (Fig. 7-46 *A* and *B*). Like other neuroendocrine tumors, the nuclei are often represented by speckled chromatin with nuclear molding and grooving.[470,474] The large cell undifferentiated carcinomas are indistinguishable from the undifferentiated variety of nasopharyngeal carcinoma, except the cells tend to be arranged in islands separated by fibrous stroma rather than showing the diffuse sheeting with lymphocyte infiltration so typical of nasopharyngeal carcinomas. Interestingly, many of these undifferentiated tumors of salivary origin are populated by both large anaplastic and small hyperchromatic cells.

A unique form of undifferentiated carcinoma, the so-called malignant lymphoepithelial lesion, is encountered primarily among American, Canadian, and Greenland Eskimos. It arises in the parotid gland and shares features with the benign lymphoepithelial lesion of Sjögren's syndrome.[473] Importantly, the epimyoepithelial island component, al-

though surrounded by mature lymphocytes, is cytologically atypical with anaplastic large nuclei and nuclear pleomorphism. This latter tumor is found almost exclusively among Eskimos. In non-Eskimos, both small and large cell undifferentiated carcinomas may arise in the major salivary glands and must be considered after a search has ruled out small cell carcinoma derived from another site (i.e., nasopharyngeal carcinoma, oat cell carcinoma of the lung, or other sites metastatic to the salivary glands). In addition, the differential diagnosis must take into consideration lymphoma, neuroblastoma, esthesioneuroblastoma, sinonasal undifferentiated carcinoma, and melanoma. Immunostains, particularly common leukocyte antigen, rule out intraparotid lymphoma (see following). Many of these primary undifferentiated salivary tumors are positive for neuroepithelial markers including neuron specific enolase, synaptophysin, and chromogranin and cytokeratin 20. Electron microscopic studies have revealed the presence of neurosecretory granules. Ultimately the diagnosis is made by exclusion, subsequent to a negative metastatic work-up.

Sialoblastoma of Infancy.[478-485] The only malignant tumor typically found in newborns and infants is sialoblastoma.[479] Only a handful of these cases have been reported. They typically arise shortly after birth as a lobulated parotid enlargement. The tumor is characterized by oval islands of undifferentiated round cells (Fig. 7-47). The cells are large with speckled chromatin and prominent nucleoli, and the cytoplasm is sparse without plasma membranes. There is no evidence of glandular differentiation.[483,485] The differential diagnosis should include embryonal rhabdomyosarcoma and neuroblastoma/ PNET, both of which can be eliminated with immunomarker studies (e.g., desmin for rhabdomyosarcoma; NSE, synaptophysin, or chromogranin for neuroendocrine tumors).

Malignant Pleomorphic Adenoma and Carcinosarcoma.[486-504] The most common form of malignant

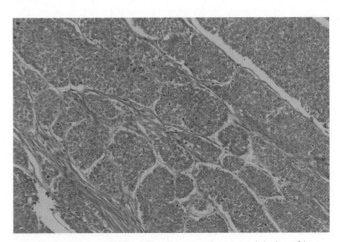

FIGURE 7-47 Sialoblastoma. Organoid nests or lobules of basaloid cells reside within a sparse stroma (H&E, × 33).

mixed tumor, as detailed earlier, is carcinoma ex mixed tumor, an adenocarcinoma that arises in a pre-existing benign pleomorphic adenoma. The rarest of these lesions is the metastasizing mixed tumor that coincidentally metastasizes. This type of mixed tumor fails to show any histopathologic evidence of malignancy; rather, it is a classic pleomorphic adenoma in every sense, clinically and histopathologically.[486–489] By some fluke, they manage to place themselves in the realm of carcinomas by entering vessels and seeding into a cervical node, the lung, or even distant osseous sites, an event likened to that of the rare metastasizing basal cell carcinoma of skin. Surgical manipulation is likely a predisposing factor since nearly all reported instances of metastasizing mixed tumor occurred subsequent to surgical excision of the primary lesion. The metastases usually harbor both epithelial and stromal components. Even though these lesions appear benign, histologically, 40% of patients die from disease.

Another form of malignant mixed tumor is the lesion that exhibits both epithelial and mesenchymal malignant neoplasia. These extremely rare tumors are referred to as *carcinosarcomas*. The epithelial islands, trabeculae, or cords may show ductal formations with unequivocal atypical cytologic features including hyperchromasia, pleomorphism, nuclear enlargement, and mitotic figures; yet simultaneously, the stroma is clearly sarcomatous (Fig. 7–48A). The spindle cells of the stroma, which can be mesenchymal or myoepithelial, are also pleomorphic and show mitotic activity. The sarcomatous component is usually represented by spindle cells yet may exhibit features of malignant fibrous histiocytoma with pleomorphic giant cells. It may show other aspects of differentiation including malignant osteoblasts and atypical bone formation (i.e., osteosarcoma).[499,503] The epithelial element is cytokeratin positive whereas the sarcoma component is positive for vimentin (Fig. 7–48B).

The third form of malignant mixed tumor is a lesion that shows all the myxoid or chondroid stromal variations associated with typical myoepithelial proliferation in mixed tumors. However, the epithelial and ductal elements exhibit focal cytologically malignant cells. The carcinomatous cells are confined within the capsule. This variant has been referred to as noninvasive carcinoma ex mixed tumor[491] or carcinoma in situ ex mixed tumor.[424] The prognosis is excellent and similar to that for benign mixed tumor.[424]

Cystadenocarcinoma.[505–515] The benign cystadenoma or papillary cystadenoma has cystadenocarcinoma as its malignant counterpart. The benign form does not progress into a malignant variant; rather, the cystadenocarcinoma merely shows an architectural pattern in common with its benign counterpart, yet is malignant from its inception. Large cystic spaces are evident and many of these tumors have intracystic papillary projections.[507,509,512] The lining cells are cuboidal, columnar, or mucinous and show clear evi-

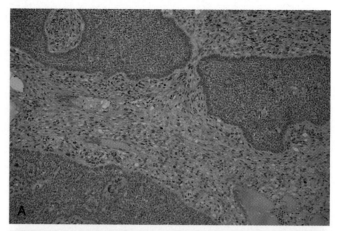

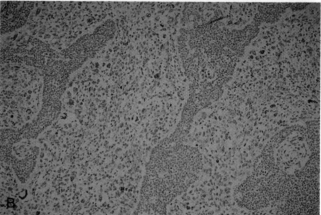

FIGURE 7–48 *A,* Carcinosarcoma. Basaloid carcinoma element with a pleomorphic spindle cell element (H&E, × 33). *B,* Carcinosarcoma. Vimentin positivity in spindle cell element (IHC, DAB, × 33).

dence of nuclear atypia (hyperchromatism, pleomorphism). Mitotic figures are variable in these tumors. They fail to show encapsulation, and while they may be well-demarcated, foci of invasion are readily demonstrable. Low-grade mucoepidermoid carcinomas are to be considered in the differential diagnosis; however, they fail to show cytologic atypia and MECA will have loci of epidermoid or squamous cells. As a group, cystadenocarcinomas and their papillary subvariants have a relatively good prognosis after parotidectomy.[514]

Salivary Duct Carcinoma.[516–530] Of all salivary adenocarcinoma variants, salivary duct carcinoma is perhaps the most cytologically malignant (Fig. 7–49). The tumor is characterized by large oval islands composed of hyperchromatic and pleomorphic nuclei. Mitotic activity can be brisk.[516,520,522] These islands typically show comedonecrosis and the surrounding cells are arranged in ducts. The stroma is typically mature collagen. These tumors demonstrate a very poor prognosis and metastasize both nodally and distantly. The microscopic features are distinct, and only adenocarcinoma NOS would be considered in the differential diagnosis.

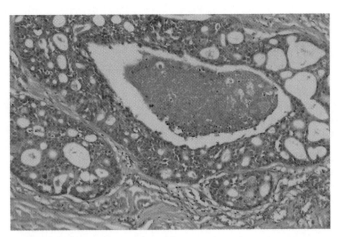

FIGURE 7–49 Salivary duct carcinoma. Ductal structures surrounded by pleomorphic epithelial cells arranged in microcystic pattern and comedonecrosis (H&E, × 33).

Sebaceous Carcinoma and Lymphadenocarcinoma.[523–530] Sebaceous differentiation is occasionally seen in the normal parotid and is a feature of certain benign lymphoepithelial lesions. Sebaceous carcinoma is identical histopathologically to those tumors located in the skin or on the eyelids. Solid sheets and islands forming sebaceous acinar clusters are seen to blend with foci of squamous differentiation emulating sebaceous gland ducts (Fig. 7–50). Typically the sebocytes have an eccentric nucleus with microlobulated, bubbly cytoplasm. The tumor islands are invasive, and the nuclei show clear evidence of malignancy—including increased size, pleomorphism, hyperchromatism, and mitotic figures.[522,528] When sebaceous adenocarcinomatous elements are enmeshed in a lymphoid stroma giving a low-power impression of benign lymphoepithelial lesion, the term sebaceous lymphadenocarcinoma is applied.

Oncocytic Adenocarcinoma.[531–537] The rare malignant counterpart of oncocytoma is oncocytic or oxyphilic adenocarcinoma of salivary glands. Malignant oncocytomas are also known to arise in other glands including the thyroid. In salivary glands, the parotid is the favored site, although the tumor is occasionally found in the oral or sinonasal glands.[532,536] The tumor cells are invasive and arranged in confluent zellballen yielding an organoid pattern. The nuclei are large, vesicular, and pleomorphic. The characteristic oxyphilic, mitochondria-rich cytoplasm is copious. Mitotic figures are often encountered. The stroma, as in benign oncocytoma, is sparse with only small vascular septa between the tumor cells. The differential diagnosis includes acinic cell adenocarcinoma, carcinoid, and paraganglioma; the latter two can be ruled out on the basis of IHC demonstration of neuroendocrine markers.

Mucinous Adenocarcinoma.[538–539] Adenocarcinomas of other sites are sometimes literally swimming in a sea of mucin; they are therefore regarded as mucinous adenocarcinomas (Fig. 7–51). This pattern is also encountered in the major salivary glands.[538] The tumor cells are arranged in cords or trabeculae; the nuclei are large and vesicular or pleomorphic and hyperchromatic. These cords are swirled yet do not exhibit any significant arborization or retiform arrangement. They appear as small worms in a basophilic mucinous sea divided into lobules by thin fibrous septa.

Adenosquamous Carcinoma.[541–544] A minor salivary gland tumor, adenosquamous carcinoma is localized to the mucosal exit of an extralobular duct. Remnants of normal duct may be encountered and are surrounded by invasive islands and cords of tumor cells showing a combination of squamous and ductal differentiation patterns (Fig. 7–52). There is usually a significant degree of pleomorphism and hyperchromatism. On lower magnification, the appearance is that of a squamous cell carcinoma that

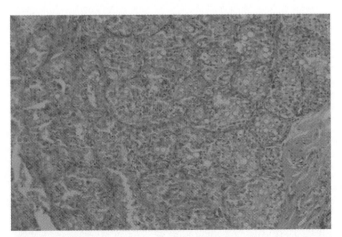

FIGURE 7–50 Sebaceous carcinoma of salivary origin. Organoid islands with typical bubbly sebaceous cytoplasm (H&E, × 33).

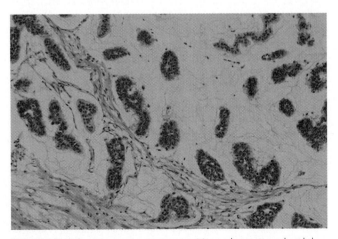

FIGURE 7–51 Mucinous carcinoma. Hyperchromatic cuboidal and columnar cell clusters are surrounded by large lobules of mucoid stroma with fibrous septa (H&E, × 33).

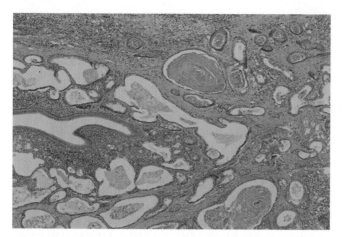

FIGURE 7-52 Adenosquamous carcinoma. Squamous islands are located near the epithelial surface mucosa with deeper islands showing glandular differentiation (H&E, × 33).

T A B L E 7 – 1 1	CLASSIFICATION OF SALIVARY STROMAL NEOPLASMS

Angiomas

Cellular and capillary hemangiomas
Lymphangioma

Other Benign and Malignant Stromal Tumors

Adult stromal tumors (nerve sheath, adipose, fibroblastic, myofibroblastic tumors, etc.)

Malignant Lymphoma and MALToma

appears to be arising from both the surface and the proximal region of the excretory duct. On further examination, foci of ductal differentiation in the neoplastic islands can be seen.[542,543] Mucoepidermoid carcinoma and necrotizing sialometaplasia exhibit similar patterns of growth, yet do not show significant cytologic atypia as seen in adenosquamous carcinoma. Pseudoglandular squamous cell carcinoma or adenoacanthoma must be included in the differential diagnosis. This tumor does not arise from salivary ducts.

STROMAL TUMORS

Most stromal tumors arise during infancy or early childhood, with the exception of intrasalivary malignant lymphoma.[545,546] They clinically simulate glandular tumors, owing to their diffuse enlargements that are typically located in the parotid gland. Rarely, the submandibular gland is the site for stromal neoplasms. In adults, nerve sheath and myofibroblastic tumors are the most common benign neoplasms, while vasoformative sarcomas are the most commonly encountered malignant stromal tumors.[546–548] The histopathologic features of these soft-part neoplasms that may arise within the major salivary glands do not differ from those arising in other locations. It is important to realize that soft-part benign and malignant tumors do, albeit rarely, arise in the salivary gland proper. The classification for the rare stromal neoplasms of salivary glands is given in Table 7–11.

ANGIOMAS[545,547,549–552]

Gross Pathology

The gross findings vary depending on the type of angioma. Cellular and capillary hemangiomas are red or pink and relatively solid, while cavernous hemangiomas are spongy and hemorrhagic. A lobular pattern is usually evident in both.

Microscopic Pathology

Infantile lesions are usually cellular without clearly defined vascular channels.[545] The acini are replaced by oval and elongated nuclei without any collagen fibers in the background. These mesenchymal cells are evenly scattered with a lobular configuration, and residual ductal structures are sparsely distributed throughout the lesion. One can usually spot a few lumina surrounding a few erythrocytes (Fig. 7–53). Capillary hemangiomas probably evolve from these more cellular precursor lesions. They also replace acini, spare many of the normal ducts, and show clear evidence of lumina. These lumina are surrounded by endothelial cells and pericytic cells. Cavernous hemangiomas, as seen in other sites, are made up of dilated vascular channels containing aggregates of erythrocytes; some of the vessels may show thrombosis and even phlebolithiasis. These cavernous lesions tend to occur in an older age group on into adult life.

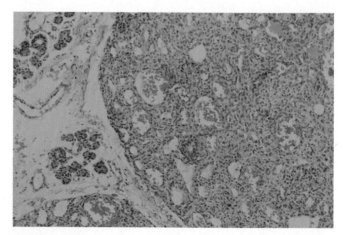

FIGURE 7-53 Capillary hemangioma of the parotid parenchyma in a child (H&E, × 33).

Lymphangioma also tends to occur in infants and children and is less commonly seen than hemangioma.[552] These intraglandular lymphatic vessel hamartomas may be of small caliber or may be composed of dilated cystic cavernous channels (cystic hygroma). Typically, the lumens contain an eosinophilic lymphatic proteinaceous coagulum and only rarely contain a few scattered red blood cells.

Histochemical Findings

Special stains are not required when vascular channels are easily identifiable. The cellular hemangiomas with minimal lumina formation can be identified by vimentin and markers for endothelial cell differentiation (factor VIII, CD31, CD34).

Differential Diagnosis

These lesions are readily recognizable on routine histologic examination. The only lesion that may be confused with other tumors is the cellular variant, which may resemble other connective tissue tumors yet can be segregated out on the basis of endothelial cell marker positivity.

OTHER BENIGN AND MALIGNANT STROMAL TUMORS[546,548,553-576]

Gross Pathology

The benign nerve sheath and connective tissue tumors are well-demarcated or encapsulated. Most are white or grey and solid, while myxomatous and adipose tumors are soft and mucoid or yellow. Sarcomas are infiltrative and invasive.

Microscopic Pathology

As mentioned previously, the tumors of salivary gland stroma are not histopathologically unique; they are identical to those arising in other sites. For this reason, detailed explication will not be given here. It is sufficient to mention that the most common benign tumors are, in decreasing order of frequency, vasoformative hamartomas, neurilemmoma, nodular fasciitis, and neurofibroma.[554-556] Lipoma, extracranial meningioma, fibrous histiocytoma, fibromatosis, angioleiomyoma, granular cell tumor, and soft tissue giant cell tumor have all been reported to arise in the substance of the parotid gland. Intraglandular sarcomas include hemangiopericytoma, neurogenic sarcoma, fibrosarcoma, malignant fibrous histiocytoma, and rhabdomyosarcoma. Other sarcomas are extremely rare.

Histochemical Findings

The plethora of connective tissue tumor markers is too voluminous to detail here. The reader is referred to textbooks of head and neck soft tissue tumors.

Differential Diagnosis

With few exceptions, the stromal tumors are spindle cell lesions. Therefore, they must be distinguished from benign and malignant spindle cell variant of myoepithelioma. IHC positivity for vimentin and smooth muscle actin is often helpful in this regard, although nodular fasciitis and myofibromatosis will react similarly. Some myoepithelial tumors show foci of glandular (ductal) differentiation whereas others are pure spindle cell tumors.

MALIGNANT LYMPHOMA AND MALTOMA[577-592]

The parotid as well as other major and minor salivary glands harbor many foci of lymphocytes. The parotid gland, within its parenchyma, has as many as 20 lymph nodes. In addition, periductal lymphoid aggregates, representing components of the mucosa associated lymphoid tissue (MALT), are seen throughout all major and minor glands. B-cell lymphomas are most common and some arise from intraparotid node. Other unique and well-differentiated lymphomas with plasmacytoid or monocytoid features arise from MALT cells and are classified as intrasalivary MALTomas. A unique form of MALToma is encountered in the minor glands of the palate. It was known in the past as atypical lymphoproliferative disease of the palate. Lastly, it must be emphasized that patients with Sjögren's syndrome with benign lymphoepithelial lesion of the parotid are 40 times more likely than the general population to develop lymphoma, though it may not arise from BLEL (i.e., extrasalivary nodal sites).

Gross Pathology

The tumor arising de novo in the gland is round or oval, uni- or multinodular, and firm tan or white on cut section. Lymphomas arising in glands with pre-existing benign lymphoepithelial lesion are not as clearly defined since the entire gland is firm and pale.

Microscopic Pathology

Since lymphomas can arise from parotid lymph nodes, they show conventional features identical to the variants of Hodgkin's and non-Hodgkin's type lesions encountered in other lymph nodes throughout the body.[577] Extranodal mucosa-associated lymphoid tissue in the parotid gland, akin to gut-associated lymphoid tissue, may give rise to marginal zone low-grade B-cell lymphomas.[585,592] The parenchyma is replaced by sheets of lymphocytes, all with a monomorphic character (Fig. 7–54). These lymphoid cells resemble small lymphocytes and centrocyte-like cells with cleaved nuclei. Some MALTomas may contain monocytoid B cells, which have a significant amount of eosinophilic cytoplasm with a round to oval, small or intermediate-sized

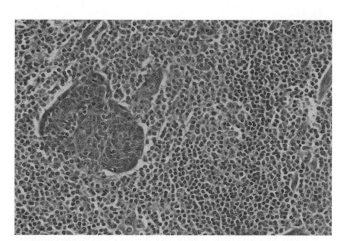

FIGURE 7-54 MALT lymphoma with epimyoepithelial island closely resembles benign lymphoepithelial lesion. The lymphocytes in MALToma are monocytoid and labeled with B lymphocyte markers (H&E, × 66).

nucleus that may be centrally or eccentrically placed (monocytoid, plasmacytoid). Dispersed throughout are epimyoepithelial islands which appear as solid nests of vacuolated epithelial cells infiltrated by lymphocytes. There are often some ductal elements as well. Progression from low-grade MALToma to a higher grade lymphoma may occur.

Histochemical Findings

The histochemical findings are helpful in that the lymphoid element is monoclonal and stains with L26, a B-cell marker. On frozen sections, Ig monoclonality may be demonstrable for light or heavy chain restriction.

Differential Diagnosis

The differential diagnosis for MALToma includes benign lymphoepithelial lesion, sebaceous lymphadenoma, and HIV polycystic lymphocytic infiltration. There is a lack of sebaceous differentiation and cyst formation in MALToma. The monotony of the infiltrate, with monocytoid cytologic features, disfavors benign lymphoepithelial lesion, which is polyclonal and predominantly consists of T lymphocytes.

REFERENCES

1. Giansanti JS, Baker GO, Waldron CA. Intraoral mucinous, minor salivary gland lesions presenting clinically as tumors. *Oral Surg Oral Med Oral Pathol.* 1971; 32:918–922.
2. Devildos LR, Langlois CC. Minor salivary gland lesion presenting clinically as tumor. *Oral Surg Oral Med Oral Pathol.* 1976; 41:657–659.
3. Arafat A, Brannon RB, Ellis GL. Adenomatoid hyperplasia of mucous salivary glands. *Oral Surg Oral Med Oral Pathol.* 1981; 52:51–55.
4. Aufdemorte TB, Ramzy I, Holt GR, Thomas JR, Duncan DL. Focal adenomatoid hyperplasia of salivary glands: A differential diagnostic problem in fine needle aspiration biospy. *Acta Cytol.* 1985; 29:23–28.
5. Brannon RB, Houston GD, Meader CL. Adenomatoid hyperplasia of mucous salivary glands: A case involving the retromolar area. *Oral Surg Oral Med Oral Pathol.* 1985; 60:188–190.
6. Micheau C. Les glandes dites sebecees de la parotide et de la sousmaxillaire. *Ann Pathol.* 1969; 14:119–126.
7. Lee CM Jr. Intraparotid sebaceous glands. *Ann Surg.* 1949; 129:152–156.
8. Richardson GS, Clairmont AA, Erickson ER. Cystic lesions of the parotid gland. *Plast Reconstr Surg.* 1978; 61:364–369.
9. Work WP. Cysts and congenital lesions of the parotid gland. *Otolaryngol Clin North Am.* 1977; 10:339–343.
10. Pieterse AS, Seymour AE. Parotid cysts: An analysis of 16 cases and suggested classification. *Pathology.* 1981; 13:225–234.
11. Cohen MN, Rao U, Shedd DP. Benign cysts of the parotid gland. *J Surg Oncol.* 1984; 27:85–88.
12. Batsakis JG, Raymond AK. Sialocysts of the parotid glands. *Ann Otol Rhinol Laryngol.* 1989; 98:487–489.
13. Seifert G, Thomsen ST, Donath K. Bilateral dysgenetic polycystic parotid glands. Morphological analysis and differential diagnosis of a rare disease of the salivary glands. *Virchows Arch [A].* 1981; 390:273–288.
14. Dobson CM, Ellis HA. Polycystic disease of the parotid glands: Case report of a rare entity and review of the literature. *Histopathology.* 1987; 11:953–961.
15. Batsakis JG, Bruner IM, Luna MA. Polycystic (dysgenetic) disease of the parotid glands. *Arch Otolaryngol Head Neck Surg.* 1988; 114:1146–1148.
16. Cunningham WE. Branchial cysts of the parotid gland. *Ann Surg.* 1929; 90:114–119.
17. Leonard JR, Maran AG, Huffman WC. Branchial cleft cysts in the parotid gland: Facial nerve anomaly. *Plast Reconstr Surg.* 1968; 41:493–496.
18. Sisson GA, Summers GW. Branchiogenic cysts within the parotid gland: Report of a case. *Arch Otolaryngol.* 1972; 96:165–167.
19. Gnepp DR, Sporck TF. Benign lymphoepithelial parotid cyst with sebaceous differentiation—cystic sebaceous lymphadenoma. *Am J Clin Path.* 1980; 74:683–687.
20. Scott R. Branchial cysts in the parotid gland. *J R Coll Surg Edinb.* 1987; 32:336–338.
21. Wong PNC, Djamshidi M. Gigantic parotid retention cyst. *J Oral Maxillofac Surg.* 1984; 42:618–620.
22. Fein S, Mohnac AM. Submandibular gland extravasation cyst: Report of an unusual case. *J Oral Surg.* 1973; 31:551–552.
23. Anneroth G, Eneroth CM, Isacsson G. Morphology of salivary calculi: The distribution of the inorganic component. *J Oral Pathol Med.* 1975; 4:257–265.
24. Levy DM, ReMine WH, Devine KD. Salivary gland calculi: Pain, swelling associated with eating. *JAMA.* 1962; 181:1115–1119.
25. Jensen JL, Howell FV, Rick GM, Correll RW. Minor salivary gland calculi: A clinicopathologic study of forty-seven new cases. *Oral Surg Oral Med Oral Pathol.* 1979; 47:44–50.
26. Langlais RP, Kasle MJ. Sialolithiasis: The radiolucent ones. *Oral Surg Oral Med Oral Pathol.* 1975; 40:686–690.
27. Murphy JB. Dystrophic calcification of the submandibular gland. *Oral Surg Oral Med Oral Pathol.* 1989; 67:362.
28. Narang R, Dixon RA. Surgical management of submandibular sialadenitis and sialolithiasis. *Oral Surg Oral Med Oral Pathol.* 1977; 43:201–210.
29. Galili D, Marmary Y. Juvenile recurrent parotitis: Clinicoradiologic follow-up study and the beneficial effect of sialography. *Oral Surg Oral Med Oral Pathol.* 1986; 61:550–556.
30. Schnitt SJ, Antonioli DA, Jaffe B, Peppercorn MA. Granulomatous inflammation of minor salivary gland ducts: A new oral manifestation of Crohn's disease. *Hum Pathol.* 1987; 18:405–407.
31. Blitzer A. Inflammatory and obstructive disorders of salivary glands. *J Dent Res.* 1987; 66:675–679.
32. Rubin MM, Cozzi G. Acute transient sialadenopathy associ-

ated with anesthesia. *Oral Surg Oral Med Oral Pathol.* 1986; 61:227–229.

33. Busuttil A. Irradiation-induced changes in human salivary glands. *Clin Otolaryngol.* 1977; 2:199–206.

34. Standish SM, Shafer WG. The mucus retention phenomenon. *J Oral Surg.* 1959; 17:15–22.

35. Bhaskar SN, Bolden TE, Weinmann JP. Pathogenesis of mucoceles. *J Dent Res.* 1956; 35:863–874.

36. Zafarulla MYM. Cervical mucocele (plunging ranula): An unusual case of mucous extravasation cyst. *Oral Surg Oral Med Oral Pathol.* 1986; 62:63–66.

37. Smith BC, Ellis GL, Slater LJ, Foss RD. Sclerosing polycystic adenosis of major salivary glands. A clinicopathologic analysis of nine cases. *Am J Surg Pathol.* 1996; 20:161–170.

38. Abrams AM, Melrose RJ, Howell FV. Necrotizing sialometaplasia: A disease simulating malignancy. *Cancer.* 1973; 32: 130–135.

39. Dunlap CL, Barker BE. Necrotizing sialometaplasia: Report of five additional cases. *Oral Surg Oral Med Oral Pathol.* 1974; 37:722–727.

40. Mesa ML, Gertler RS, Schneider LC. Necrotizing sialometaplasia: Frequency of histologic misdiagnosis. *Oral Surg Oral Med Oral Pathol.* 1984; 57:71–73.

41. Johnston WH. Necrotizing sialometaplasia involving the mucous glands of the nasal cavity. *Hum Pathol.* 1977; 8:589–592.

42. Grillion GL, Lallv ET. Necrotizing sialometaplasia: literature review and presentation of five cases. *J Oral Surg.* 1981; 39: 747–753.

43. Stanley RB, Fernandez JA, Peppard SB. Cervicofacial mycobacterial infections presenting as major salivary gland disease. *Laryngoscope.* 1983; 93:1271–1275.

44. Van der Wall JD, Leake J. Granulomatous sialadenitis of the major salivary glands: A clinicopathological study of 57 cases. *Histopathology.* 1987; 11:131–144.

45. Wear DJ, Margileth AM, Hadfield TL, Fischer GW, Schlagel CJ, King FM. Cat scratch disease: A bacterial infection. *Science.* 1983; 221:1403–1405.

46. Watkinson JC, Hornung EA, Fagg NLK. Cat-scratch disease: An unusual cause of parotid pain (a case report with a literature review). *J Laryngol Otol.* 1988; 102:562–564.

47. Myer C, Cotton RF. Salivary gland disease in children: A review. *Clin Pediatr.* 1986; 25:314–322.

48. Seifert G, Miehlke A, Haubrich J, Chilla R. *Diseases of the Salivary Glands: Pathology–Diagnosis–Treatment–Facial Nerve Surgery.* Stuttgart, Germany: Georg Thieme Verlag; 1986: 110–163.

49. Gordon JI, Golbus J, Kurtides ES. Chronic lymphadenopathy and Sjögren's syndrome in a homosexual man. *N Engl J Med.* 1984; 311:1441–1442.

50. Couderc L-J, D'Agay M-F, Danon F, Harzic M, Brocheriou C, Clauvel J-P. Sicca complex and infection with human immunodeficiency virus. *Arch Intern Med.* 1987; 147:898–901.

51. Ioachim HL, Lerner CW, Tapper ML. The lymphoid lesions associated with the acquired immunodeficiency syndrome. *Am J Surg Pathol.* 1983; 7:543–553.

52. Ewing EP Jr, Chandler FW, Spira TJ, Brynes RK, Chan WC. Primary lymph node pathology in AIDS and AIDS-related lymphadenopathy. *Arch Pathol Lab Med.* 1985; 109:977–981.

53. Smith FB, Rajdeo H, Panesar N, Bhuta K, Stahl R. Benign lymphoepithelial lesion of the parotid gland in intravenous drug users. *Arch Pathol Lab Med.* 1988; 112:742–745.

54. Ryan JR, Loachim HL, Marmer J, Loubeau M. Acquired immune deficiency syndrome-related lymphadenopathies presenting in salivary gland lymph nodes. *Arch Otolaryngol.* 1985;111: 554–556.

55. Holliday RA, Cohen WA, Schinelia RA, et al. Benign lymphoepithelial parotid cysts and hyperplastic cervical adenopathy in AIDS risk patients: A new CT appearance. *Radiology.* 1988; 168:439–441.

56. Finer MD, Schinella RA, Rothstein SG, Persky MS. Cystic parotid lesions in patients at risk for the acquired immunodeficiency syndrome. *Arch Otolaryngol Head Neck Surg.* 1988; 114:1290–1294.

57. Ulirsch RC, Jaffe ES. Sjögren's syndrome-like illness associated with the acquired immuno-deficiency syndrome-related complex. *Hum Pathol.* 1987; 18:1063–1068.

58. Kornstein MJ, Parker GA, Mills AS. Immunohistology of the benign lymphoepithelial lesion in AIDS-related lymphadenopathy: A case report. *Hum Pathol.* 1988; 19:1359–1361.

59. DiGiuseppe JA; Wu TC; Corio RL. Analysis of Epstein-Barr virus-encoded small RNA 1 expression in benign lymphoepithelial salivary gland lesions. *Mod Pathol.* 1994; 7:555–559.

60. Labouyrie E, Merlio JP, Beylot-Barry M, et al. Human immunodeficiency virus type 1 replication within cystic lymphoepithelial lesion of the salivary gland. *Am J Clin Path.* 1993; 100:41–46.

61. Schiodt M, Dodd CL, Greenspan D, et al. Natural history of HIV-associated salivary gland disease. *Oral Surg Oral Med Oral Pathol.* 1992; 74:326–331.

62. Schiodt M. HIV-associated salivary gland disease: A review. *Oral Surg Oral Med Oral Pathol.* 1992; 73:164–167.

63. James DG, Williams WJ. *Sarcoidosis and Other Granulomatous Disorders.* Philadelphia: WB Saunders; 1985:21–246.

64. Nessan VJ, Jacoway JR. Biopsy of minor salivary glands in the diagnosis of sarcoidosis. *N Engl J Med.* 1979; 301:922–924.

65. Eveson JW. Granulomatous disorders of the oral mucosa. *Sem Diag Pathol.* 1996; 13:118–127.

66. Rogers RS III. Melkersson-Rosenthal syndrome and orofacial granulomatosis. *Dermatol Clin.* 1996; 14:371–379.

67. MacFadyen EE, Ferguson MM. Pitcairne's disease: an historical presentation of orofacial granulomatosis. *J Royal Soc Med.* 1996; 89:77–78.

68. Armstrong DK, Burrows D. Orofacial granulomatosis. *Int J Dermatol.* 1995; 34:830–833.

69. Takeshita T, Koga T, Yashima Y. Case report: Cheilitis granulomatosa with periodontitis. *J Dermatol.* 1995; 22:804–806.

70. Miralles J, Barnadas MA, de Moragas JM. Cheilitis granulomatosa treated with metronidazole. *Dermatology.* 1995; 191: 252–253.

71. Kung ITM, Gibson IB, Bannatyne PM. Kimura's disease: A clinicopathological study of 21 cases and its distinction from angiolymphoid hyperplasia with eosinophilia. *Pathology.* 1984; 16:39–44.

72. Rosai J, Gold J, Landy R. The histiocytoid hemangiomas: A unifying concept embracing several previously described entities of skin, soft tissue, large vessels, bone and heart. *Hum Pathol.* 1979; 10:707–730.

73. Googe PB, Harris PB, Mihm MC Jr. Kimura's disease and angiolymphoid hyperplasia with eosinophilia: Two distinct histopathological entities. *J Cutan Pathol.* 1987; 14:263–271.

74. Goldman RL, Klein HZ. Subcutaneous angiolymphoid hyperplasia with eosinophilia: Report of a case masquerading as a salivary gland tumor. *Arch Otolaryngol.* 1976; 102:440–441.

75. Tham K-T, Leung P-C, Saw D, Gwi E. Kimura's disease with salivary gland involvement. *Br J Surg.* 1981; 68:495–497.

76. Quinton PM. Defective epithelial ion transport in cystic fibrosis. *Clin Chem.* 1989; 35:726–730.

77. Buchwald M, Tsui L-C, Riordan JR. The search for the cystic fibrosis gene. *Am J Physiol.* 1989; 257:147–152.

78. Shwachman H. Cystic fibrosis. In: Petersdorf RG, Adams RD, Braunwald E, Isselbacher KJ, Martin JB, Wilson JD, eds. *Harrison's Principles of Internal Medicine.* 10th ed. New York: McGraw Hill; 1983:1542–1544.

79. Mikulicz J. *Uber eine eigenartige symmetrische Erkrankung der Tränen- und Mundspeicheldrüsen.* Stuttgart, Germany: Beitr z Chir Fetscr f Theodor Billroth; 1892:610–630.

80. Mikulicz, J. Concerning a peculiar symmetrical disease of the lacrimal and salivary glands. *Medical Classics.* 1937; 2:165–186.

81. Ferlito A, Cattai N. The so-called "benign lymphoepithelial lesion." *J Laryngol Otol.* 1980; 94:1189–1197.

82. Godwin IT. Benign lymphoepithelial lesion of the parotid gland (adenolymphoma, chronic inflammation, lymphoepithelioma, lymphocytic tumor, Mikulicz disease): Report of eleven cases. *Cancer.* 1952; 5:1089–1103.

83. Morgan WS. The probable systemic nature of Mikulicz's disease and its relation to Sjögren's syndrome. *N Engl J Med*. 1954; 251:5–10.

84. Batsakis, JG. Lymphoepithelial lesion and Sjögren's syndrome. *Ann Otol Rhinol Laryngol*. 1987; 96:354–355.

85. Saku T, Okabe IT. Immunohistochemical and ultrastructural demonstration of keratin in epimyoepithelial islands of autoimmune sialadenitis in man. *Arch Oral Biol*. 1984; 29: 687–689.

86. Kjörell U, Ostberg Y, Virtanen I, Thornell L-E. Immunohistochemical analyses of autoimmune sialadenitis in man. *J Oral Pathol Med*. 1988; 17:374–380.

87. Bernier JL, Bhaskar SN. Lymphoepithelial lesions of salivary glands. *Cancer*. 1958; 11:1156–1179.

88. Nelson WR, Kay S, Sally JJ. Mikulicz's disease of the palate. *Ann Surg*. 1963; 157:152–156.

89. Clark PM, Gamble JW. Mikulicz disease of a minor salivary gland. *J Oral Surg*. 1978; 36:895–897.

90. Bhaskar SN, Bernier JL. Mikulicz's disease; clinical features, histology, and histogenesis; report of seventy-three cases. *Oral Surg Oral Med Oral Pathol*. 1960; 13:1387–1399.

91. Bloch KJ, Buchanan WW, Wohl MJ, Bunim JJ. Sjögren's syndrome: A clinical, pathological and serological study of sixty-two cases. *Medicine*. 1965; 44:187–231.

92. Chisholm DM, Lyell A, Haroon TS, Mason DK, Beeley JA. Salivary gland function in sarcoidosis. *Oral Surg Oral Med Oral Pathol*. 1971; 31:766–771.

93. Tarpley TM, Anderson L, Lightbody P, Sheagren JN. Minor salivary gland involvement in sarcoidosis. *Oral Surg Oral Med Oral Pathol*. 1972; 33:755–762.

94. Daniels TE. Labial salivary gland biopsy in Sjögren's syndrome: Assessment as a diagnostic criterion in 362 suspected cases. *Arthritis Rheum*. 1984; 27:147–156.

95. Zulman J, Jaffe R, Talal N. Evidence that the malignant lymphoma of Sjögren's syndrome is a monoclonal B-cell neoplasm. *N Engl J Med*. 1975; 299:1215–1220.

96. Daniels TE. Salivary histopathology in diagnosis of Sjögren's syndrome. *Scand J Rheumatol*. 1986; 61(suppl):36–43.

97. Chisholm DM, Mason DK. Labial salivary gland biopsy in Sjögren's syndrome. *J Clin Pathol*. 1968; 21:656–660.

98. Andrade RE, Hagen KA, Manivel JC. Distribution and immunophenotype of the inflammatory cell population in the benign lymphoepithelial lesion (Mikulicz disease). *Hum Pathol*. 1988; 19:932–941.

99. Speight PM, Cruchley A, Williams DM. Epithelial HLA-DR expression in labial salivary glands in Sjögren's syndrome and non-specific sialadenitis. *J Oral Pathol Med*. 1989; 18:178–183.

100. Schima W, Amann G, Steiner E, Steurer M, Vormittag W, Steurer L. Case report: Sicca syndrome due to primary amyloidosis. *Brit J Radiol*. 1994; 67:1023–1025.

101. Hachulla E, Janin A, Flipo RM, et al. Labial salivary gland biopsy is a reliable test for the diagnosis of primary and secondary amyloidosis. A prospective clinical and immunohistologic study in 59 patients: *Arthritis Rheum*. 1993; 36:691–697.

102. Schlesinger I. Multiple myeloma and AL amyloidosis mimicking Sjögren's syndrome. *South Med J*. 1993; 86:568–569.

103. Myssiorek D, Alvi A, Bhuiya T. Primary salivary gland amyloidosis causing sicca syndrome. *Ann Otol Rhinol Laryngol*. 1992; 101:487–490.

104. Franklin, E. Immunopathology of amyloid disease. *Hosp Pract*. 1980; 14:70–75.

105. Glenner, G. Amyloid deposits and amyloidosis: The beta-fibrilloses. *N Engl J Med*. 1980; 302:1283–1333.

106. Tandler B. Salivary gland changes in disease. *J Dent Res*. 1987; 66:398–406.

107. Hasler JF. Parotid enlargement: A presenting sign in anorexia nervosa. *Oral Surg Oral Med Oral Pathol*. 1982; 53:567–573.

108. Donath K, Seifert G. Ultrastructural studies of the parotid glands in sialadenosis. *Virchows Arch [A]*. 1975; 365:119–135.

109. Batsakis JG. Pathology consultation: sialadenosis. *Ann Otol Rhinol Laryngol*. 1988; 97:94–95.

110. Dardick I. *Color Atlas/Text of Salivary Gland Tumor Pathology*. New York: Igakyu-Shoin Med Pub; 1996.

111. Ellis GL, Auclair PL, Gnepp DR. *Surgical Pathology of the Salivary Glands*. Philadelphia: WB Saunders; 1992.

112. Ellis GL, Auclair PL. *Atlas of Tumor Pathology: Tumors of the Salivary Glands*. Washington, DC: Armed Forces Institute of Pathology; 1995.

113. Batsakis JG, Regezi JA. The pathology of head and neck tumors: Salivary glands. Part 1. *Head Neck Surg*. 1978; 1:59–68.

114. Eversole LR. Histogenic classification of salivary gland tumors. *Arch Pathol Lab Med*. 1971; 92:433–443.

115. Regezi JA, Batsakis JG. Histogenesis of salivary gland neoplasms. *Otolaryngol Clin North Am*. 1977; 10:297–307.

116. Batsakis JG. Salivary gland neoplasia: An outcome of modified morphogenesis and cyto-differentiation. *Oral Surg Oral Med Oral Pathol*. 1980; 49:229–232.

117. Dardick I, Byard RW, Carnegie JA. A review of proliferative capacity of major salivary glands and the relationship to current concepts of neoplasia in salivary gland. *Oral Surg Oral Med Oral Pathol*. 1990; 69:53–67.

118. Walker NI, Gobe GC. Cell death and cell proliferation during atrophy of the rat parotid gland induced by duct obstruction. *J Pathol*. 1987; 153:333–344.

119. Geiger S, Geiger B, Leitner O, Marshak G. Cytokeratin polypeptide expression in different epithelial elements in human salivary glands. *Virchows Arch [A]*. 1987; 410:403–414.

120. Leoncini P, Cintorino M, Vindigni C, et al. Distribution of cytoskeletal and contractile proteins in normal and tumour-bearing salivary and lacrimal glands. *Virchows Arch [A]*. 1988; 412:329–337.

121. Born LA, Schwechheimer K, Maier H, Otto HE. Cytokeratin expression in normal salivary glands and in cystadenolymphomas demonstrated by monoclonal antibodies against selective cytokeratin polypeptides. *Virchows Arch [A]*. 1987; 411:588–589.

122. Dardick I, Rippstein P, Skimming L, Boivin M, Dairkee SH. Immunohistochemistry and ultra-structure of myoepithelium and modified myoepithelium of the ducts of human major salivary glands: Histogenetic implications for salivary gland tumors. *Oral Surg Oral Med Oral Pathol*. 1987; 64:703–715.

123. Dardick I, Parks WR, Little J, Brown DL. Characterization of cytoskeletal proteins in basal cells of human parotid salivary gland ducts. *Virchows Arch [A]*. 1988; 412:525–532.

124. Batsakis JG, Kraemer B, Sciubba, JJ. The pathology of head and neck tumors: The myoepithelial cell and its participation in salivary gland neoplasia, part 17. *Head Neck Surg*. 1983; 5: 222–233.

125. Dardick I, van Nostrand AWP. Myoepithelial cells in salivary gland tumors—revisited. *Head Neck Surg*. 1985; 7:395–408.

126. Dardick I, van Nostrand AWP. Morphogenesis of salivary gland tumors: A prerequisite to improving classification. *Pathol Annu*. 1987; 22(pt 1):I53.

127. Dardick I, Jeans MTD, Sinnott NM, Wittkuhn JF, Kahn HJ, Baumal R. Salivary gland components involved in the formation of squamous metaplasia. *Am J Pathol*. 1985; 119:33–43.

128. Chang WWL. Cell population changes during acinus formation in the postnatal rat submandibular gland. *Anat Rec*. 1974; 178:187–202.

129. Klein RM. Acinar cell proliferation in the parotid and submandibular salivary glands of the neonatal rat. *Cell Tissue Kinet*. 1982; 15:187–195.

130. Sharawy M, O'Dell NL. Regeneration of submandibular salivary gland autografted in the rat tongue. *Anat Rec*. 1981; 201: 499–511.

131. Dardick I, van Nostrand AWP, Phillips MJ. Histogenesis of salivary gland pleomorphic adenoma (mixed tumor) with an evaluation of the role of the myoepithelial cell. *Hum Pathol*. 1982; 13:62–75.

132. Alos L, Cardesa A, Bombi JA, Mallofre C, Cuchi A, Traserra J. Myoepithelial tumors of salivary glands: A clinicopathologic, immunohistochemical, ultrastructural and flow cytometric study. *Sem Diag Pathol*. 1996; 13:138–147.

133. Seifert, G. Classification and differential diagnosis of clear and basal cell tumors of the salivary glands. *Sem Diag Pathol.* 1996; 13:95–103.

134. Foote FW Jr, Frazell EL. Tumors of the major salivary glands. *Cancer.* 1953; 6:1065–1133.

135. Rawson AJ, Howard JM, Royster HP, Horn RC Jr. Tumors of the salivary glands: A clinicopathologic study of 160 cases. *Cancer.* 1950; 3:445–458.

136. Thackray AC, Sobin LH. *Histological Typing of Salivary Gland Tumors.* Geneva, Switzerland: World Health Organization; 1972.

137. Sharkey FE. Systematic evaluation of the World Health Organization classification of salivary gland tumors. *Am J Clin Pathol.* 1977; 67:272–278.

138. Spitz MR, Batsakis, JG. Major salivary gland carcinoma. Descriptive epidemiology and survival of 498 patients. *Arch Otolaryngol.* 1984; 110:45–48.

139. Eveson JW, Cawson RA. Salivary gland tumours. A review of 2410 cases with particular reference to histological types, site, age and sex distribution. *J Pathol.* 1985; 146:51–58.

140. Eveson JW, Cawson RA. Tumors of the minor (oropharyngeal) salivary glands: A demographic study of 136 cases. *J Oral Pathol Med.* 1985; 14:500–509.

141. Thackray T, Lucas RB. Tumors of the major salivary glands, fascicle 10. *Atlas of Tumor Pathology,* 2nd series. Washington DC: Armed Forces Institute of Pathology; 1974.

142. Morgan MN, Mackenzie DH. Tumors of salivary glands. A review of 204 cases with 5-year followup. *Br J Surg.* 1968; 55:284–288.

143. Yu GY, Ma DQ. Carcinoma of the salivary gland: A clinicopathologic study of 405 cases. *Semin Surg Oncol.* 1987; 3:240–244.

144. Bhargava S, Sant MS, Arora MM. Histomorphologic spectrum of tumours of minor salivary glands. *Indian J Cancer.* 1982; 19:134–140.

145. Isacsson G, Shear M. Intraoral salivary gland tumors: A retrospective study of 201 cases. *J Oral Pathol.* 1983; 12:57–62.

146. Fitzpatrick PJ, Theriault C. Malignant salivary gland tumors. *Int J Radiat Oncol Biol Phys.* 1986; 12:1743–1747.

147. Seifert G, Rieb H, Donath K. Classification of the tumours of the minor salivary glands. Pathohistologic analysis of 160 cases. *Laryngol Rhinol Otol.* 1980; 59:379–400.

148. Friedman M, Levin B, Grybauskas V, et al. Malignant tumors of the major salivary glands. *Otolaryngol Clin North Am.* 1986; 19:625–636.

149. Fu KK, Leibel SA, Levine ML, Friedlander LM, Boles R, Phillips TL. Carcinoma of the major and minor salivary glands. Analysis of treatment results and sites and causes of failure. *Cancer.* 1977; 40:2882–2890.

150. Spiro RH. Salivary neoplasms: Overview of a 35-year experience with 2807 patients. *Head Neck Surg.* 1986; 8:177–184.

151. Castro EB, Huvos AG, Strong EW, Foote FW Jr. Tumors of the major salivary glands in children. *Cancer.* 1972; 29:312–317.

152. Krolls SO, Trodahl JN, Boyers RC. Salivary gland lesions in children. A survey of 430 cases. *Cancer.* 1972; 30:459–469.

153. Myer C, Cotton RT. Salivary gland disease in children: A review. Part 1: Acquired non-neoplastic disease. *Clin Pediatr.* 1986; 25:314–322.

154. Seifert G, Okabe H, Caselitz J. Epithelial salivary gland tumors in children and adolescents. Analysis of 80 cases (Salivary Gland Registry 1965–1984). *ORLJ.* 1986; 48:137–149.

155. Gnepp DR, Heffner DK. Mucosal origin of sinonasal tract adenomatous neoplasms. *Mod Pathol.* 1989; 2:365–371.

156. Neville BW, Damm DD, Weir JC, Fantasia JE. Labial salivary gland tumors. *Cancer.* 1988; 61:2113–2116.

157. Owens OT, Calcaterra TC. Salivary gland tumors of the lip. *Arch Otolaryngol.* 1982; 108:45–47.

158. Goldblatt LI, Ellis GL. Salivary gland tumors of the tongue. Analysis of 55 new cases and review of the literature. *Cancer.* 1987; 60:74–81.

159. Kessler DJ, Mickel RA, Calcaterra TC. Malignant salivary gland tumors of the base of the tongue. *Arch Otolaryngol.* 1985; 111:664–666.

160. Devries EJ, Johnson JT, Myers EN, Barnes EL, Mandell-Brown M. Base of tongue salivary gland tumors. *Head Neck Surg.* 1987; 9:329–331.

161. Roper PR, Wolf PF, Luna MA, Goepfert H. Malignant salivary gland tumors of the base of the tongue. *South Med J.* 1987; 80:605–608.

162. Goepfert H, Giraldo AA, Byers RM, Luna MA. Salivary gland tumors of the base of tongue. *Arch Otolaryngol.* 1976; 102:391–395.

163. Spiro RH, Huvos AG, Strong EW. Cancer of the parotid gland. A clinicopathologic study of 288 primary cases. *Am J Surg.* 1975; 130:452–459.

164. Sweeney EC, McDermott M. Pleomorphic adenoma of the bronchus. *J Clin Pathol.* 1996; 49:87–89.

165. Olsha O, Gottschalk-Sabag S. Metastatic pleomorphic adenoma. *Inv Met.* 1995; 15:163–166.

166. Dardick I. Myoepithelioma: Definitions and diagnostic criteria. *Ultrastruct Pathol.* 1995; 19:335–345.

167. Chidzonga MM, Lopez Perez VM, Portilla-Alvarez AL. Salivary gland tumours in Zimbabwe: Report of 282 cases. *Int J Oral Maxillofac Surg.* 1995; 24:293–297.

168. Klijanienko J, Vielh P. Fine-needle sampling of salivary gland lesions. I. Cytology and histology correlation of 412 cases of pleomorphic adenoma. *Diag Cytopathol.* 1996; 14:195–200.

169. Seifert G, Donath K. Multiple tumours of the salivary glands—terminology and nomenclature. Oral Oncology. *Eur J Cancer.* 1996; 32B:3–7.

170. Malone B, Barker SR. Benign pleomorphic adenomas in children. *Ann Otol Rhinol Laryngol.* 1984; 93:210–214.

171. Nigro MF, Spiro RH. Deep lobe parotid tumors. *Am J Surg.* 1977; 134:523–527.

172. Som PM, Shugar JMA, Sacher M, Stollman AL, Biller HF. Benign and malignant pleomorphic adenomas: CT and MR studies. *J Comp Asst Tomog.* 1988; 12:65–69.

173. Miricti DR, McArdle CB, Kulkarni MV. Benign pleomorphic adenomas of the salivary glands: Surface coil MR imaging versus CT. *J Comp Asst Tomog.* 1987; 11:620–623.

174. Batsakis JG. Recurrent mixed tumors: *Ann Otol Rhinol Laryngol.* 1986; 95:543–544.

175. Lee PS, Sabbath-Solitare M, Redondo TC, Ongcapin EH: Molecular evidence that the stromal and epithelial cells in pleomorphic adenomas of salivary gland arise from the same origin: Clonal analysis using human androgen receptor (HUMARA) assay. *Hum Pathol.* 2000; 31:498–503.

176. Batsakis JG, Kraemer B, Sciubba J. The pathology of head and neck tumors: The myoepithelial cell and its participation in salivary gland neoplasia. *Head Neck Surg.* 1983; 5:222–233.

177. Guerra MF, Gonzalez FJ, Campo FR, deLlano MA: Giant pleomorphic adenoma of the lacrimal gland. *J Oral Maxillofac Surg.* 2000; 58:569–572.

178. Lomax-Smith JD, Azzopardi JG. The hyaline cell: A distinctive feature of "mixed" salivary tumors. *Histopathology.* 1978; 2:77–92.

179. Buchner A, David R, Hansen LS. "Hyaline" cells in pleomorphic adenomas of salivary gland origin. *Oral Surg Oral Med Oral Pathol.* 1981; 52:506–512.

180. Thomas K, Hutt MS. Tyrosine crystals in salivary gland tumors. *J Clin Pathol.* 1981; 34:1003–1005.

181. Campbell WG Jr, Priest RE, Weathers DR. Characterization of two types of crystalloids in pleomorphic adenomas of minor salivary glands: A light microscopic, electron microscopic and histochemical study. *Am J Pathol.* 1985; 118:194–202.

182. Dyke PL, Haidu SI, Strong EW, Erlandson RA, Fleisher M. Mixed tumor of parotid containing oxylate crystals. *Arch Pathol Lab Med.* 1971; 91:89–92.

183. Erlandson RA, Cardon-Cardo C, Higgins PJ. Histogenesis of benign pleomorphic adenoma (mixed tumor) of the major salivary glands: An ultrastructural and immunohistochemical study. *Am J Surg Pathol.* 1984; 8:803–820.

184. Mori M, Tsukitani K, Minomiya T, Okada Y. Various expressions of modified myoepithelial cells in pleomorphic ade-

noma: Immunohistochemical studies. *Pathol Res Pract.* 1987; 182:632–646.

185. Sato M, Hayashi Y, Yoshida H, Yanagawa T, Yura Y, Nitta T. Search for specific markers of neoplastic epithelial duct and myoepithelial cell lines established from human salivary gland and characterization of their growth in vitro. *Cancer.* 1984; 54:2959–2967.

186. Krolls SO, Boyers RC. Mixed tumors of salivary glands. Long term follow-up. *Cancer.* 1972; 30:276–281.

187. Maran AG, Machenzie IJ, Stanley RE. Recurrent pleomorphic adenomas of the parotid gland. *Arch Otolaryngol Head Neck Surg.* 1984; 110:167–171.

188. Eneroth C-M, Franzen S, Zajicek J. Cytologic aspirates from 1000 salivary gland tumors. *Acta Otolaryngol.* 1967; 224:168–172.

189. O'Dwyer P, Farrar WB, James AG, Finkelmeir W, McCabe DP. Needle aspiration biopsy of major salivary gland tumors: Its value. *Cancer.* 1986; 57:554–557.

190. LiVolsi VA, Perzin KH. Malignant mixed tumors arising in salivary gland. I. Carcinomas arising in mixed tumors: A clinicopathologic study. *Cancer.* 1977; 39:2209–2230.

191. Ryan RE Jr, Desanto LW, Weiland LH, DeVine KD, Beahrs OH. Cellular mixed tumors of the salivary glands. *Arch Otolaryngol.* 1978; 104:451–453.

192. Sheldon WH: So-called mixed tumors of salivary glands. *Arch Pathol.* 1943; 35:1–20.

193. Simpson RH, Jones H, Beasley P. Benign myoepithelioma of the salivary glands: A true entity? *Histopathology.* 1995; 27:1–9.

194. Alos L, Carrillo R, Ramos J, et al. High-grade carcinoma component in epithelial-myoepithelial carcinoma of salivary glands: Clinicopathological, immunohistochemical and flow-cytometric study of three cases. *Virchows Arch [A].* 1999; 434: 291–299.

195. Sciubba JJ, Brannon RB. Myoepithelioma of salivary glands: Report of 23 cases. *Cancer.* 1982; 49:562–572.

196. Chaudhry AP, Satchidanad S, Peer R, Cutler LS. Myoepithelial adenoma of the parotid gland: A light and ultrastructural study. *Cancer.* 1982; 49:288–293.

197. Batsakis JG. Myoepithelioma. *Ann Otol Rhinol Laryngol.* 1985; 94:523–524.

198. Dardick I, Thomas MJ, van Nostrand AWP. Myoepithelioma—new concepts of histology and classification: A light and electron microscopic study. *Ultrastruct Pathol.* 1989; 13: 187–224.

199. Barnes L, Appel BN, Perez H, El-Attar AM. Myoepitheliomas of the head and neck: Case report and review. *J Surg Oncol.* 1985; 28:21–28.

200. Davis WM, Davis WM Jr. Canalicular adenoma: Report of case. *J Oral Surg.* 1971; 29:500–502.

201. Christ TF, Crocker D. Basal cell adenoma of minor salivary gland origin. *Cancer.* 1972; 30:214–219.

202. Bernacki EG, Batsakis JG, Johns ME. Basal cell adenoma: Distinctive tumor of salivary glands. *Arch Otolaryngol.* 1974; 99:84–87.

203. Crumpler C, Scharfenberg JC, Reed RI. Monomorphic adenomas of salivary glands: Trabecular, tubular, canalicular, and basaloid variants. *Cancer.* 1976; 38:193–200.

204. Fantasia JE, Neville BW. Basal cell adenomas of the minor salivary glands. *Oral Surg Oral Med Oral Pathol.* 1980; 50:433–440.

205. Batsakis JG, Brannon RB, Sciubba JJ. Monomorphic adenomas of major salivary glands: A histologic study of 96 tumors. *Clin Otolaryngol.* 1981; 6:129–143.

206. Mintz GA, Abrams AM, Melrose RJ. Monomorphic adenomas of the major and minor salivary glands: Report of twenty-one cases and review of the literature. *Oral Surg Oral Med Oral Pathol.* 1982; 53:375–380.

207. Batsakis JG, Brannon RB. Dermal analogue tumors of major salivary glands. *J Laryngol Otol.* 1981; 95:155–164.

208. Nagao K, Matsuzaki O, Saiga H, et al. Histopathologic studies of basal cell adenoma of the parotid gland. *Cancer.* 1982; 50:736–745.

209. Gardner DG, Daley TD. The use of the terms monomorphic adenoma, basal cell adenoma, and canalicular adenoma as applied to salivary gland tumors. *Oral Surg Oral Med Oral Pathol.* 1983; 56:608–615.

210. Daley TD, Gardner DG, Smout MS. Canalicular adenoma: Not a basal cell adenoma. *Oral Surg Oral Med Oral Pathol.* 1984; 57:181–188.

211. Batsakis JG. Basal cell adenoma of the parotid gland. *Cancer.* 1972; 29:226–230.

212. Nelson JF, Jacoway JR. Monomorphic adenoma (canilicular type): Report of 29 cases. *Cancer.* 1973; 31:1511–1513.

213. Kratochvil FJ, Auclair PL, Ellis GE. Clinical features of 160 cases of basal cell adenoma and 121 cases of canalicular adenoma. *Oral Surg Oral Med Oral Pathol.* 1990; 70:605.

214. Strychalski I. Basal cell adenoma of intraoral minor salivary gland origin. *J Oral Surg.* 1974; 32:595–600.

215. Headington JT, Bataskis JG, Beals TF, Campbell TE, Simmons JL, Stone WD. Membranous basal cell adenoma of parotid gland, dermal cylindromas, and trichoepitheliomas: Comparative histochemistry and ultrastructure. *Cancer.* 1977; 39:2460–2469.

216. Reingold IM, Keasbey LE, Graham JH. Multicentric dermal type cylindromas of the parotid glands in a patient with florid turban tumor. *Cancer* 1977; 40:1702–1710.

217. Herbst EV, Utz W. Multifocal dermal type basal cell adenomas of parotid glands with coexisting dermal cylindromas. *Virchows Arch [A].* 1984; 95–102.

218. Dardick I, Kahn HJ, van Nostrand AWP, Baumal R. Salivary gland monomorphic adenoma: Ultrastructural, immunoperoxidase, and histogenetic aspects. *Am J Pathol.* 1984; 115:334–348.

219. Chen KT. Carcinoma arising in monomorphic adenoma of the salivary gland. *Am J Otolaryngol.* 1985; 6:39–41.

220. Luna MA, Batsakis JG, Tortoledo ME, Deljunco GW. Carcinomas ex monomorphic adenoma of salivary glands. *J Laryngol Otol.* 1989; 103:756–759.

221. Schaffer J. Beitrage zur Histologie Menischlicher Organe. IV. Zunge. V. Mundhohle-Schlundkopf. VI. Oesophagus VII. Cardia. Sitzungsber. d. Kais. Akad. d. Wissensch., Math. naturwiss. Classe, Abth. III 1897; 106:353–357.

222. Zimmermann KW. Die Speicheldrusen der Mundhohle und die Bauchspeicheldruse. In: Von Motlendorff W. *Handbuch der Mikroskopischen Anatomie der Menschen.* Berlin, Germany: Julius Springer; 1927:5–128.

223. Hamperl IT. Onkocyten und Geschwulste der Spei cheldrusen. *Virchows Arch [A].* 1931; 282:724–736.

224. Hamperl H. Ober das Vorkomnien von Onkocyten in verschiedenen Organen und ihren Geschwulsten. *Virchows Arch [A].* 1936; 298:327–375.

225. Meza-Cliavez L. Oxyphilic granular cell adenoma of the parotid gland (oncocytoma): Report of five cases and study of the oxyphilic granular cells (oncocytes) in normal parotid glands. *Am J Pathol.* 1949; 25:523–537.

226. Eneroth CW. Oncocytoma of major salivary gland. *J Laryngol Otol.* 1965; 79:1064–1072.

227. Boley JO, Robinson DW. Bilateral oxyphilic granular cell adenoma of the parotid. *Arch Pathol Lab Med.* 1954; 58:564–567.

228. Codington JB. Oxyphilic granular cell adenoma of the parotid gland. *Am J Surg.* 1959; 97:333–338.

229. Hamperl H. Benign and malignant oncocytoma. *Cancer.* 1962; 15:1019–1027.

230. Tandler B, Hutter R, Erlandson R. Ultrastructure of oncocytoma of the parotid gland. *Lab Inv.* 1970; 23:567–580.

231. Das S, Sengupta P, Chatterjee SK, Sarkar SK. Oncocytoma of tongue in a child. *J Pediatr Surg.* 1976; 11:113–114.

232. Zipermam HH, Capers TH. Oxyphilic cell adenoma of the tongue. *US Armed Forces Med J.* 1955; 6:1039–1042.

233. Hastrup N, Bretlau P, Kroudahl A, Metchiors H. Oncocytomas of the salivary glands. *J Laryngol Otol.* 1982; 96:1027–1032.

234. Batsakis JG, Martz DG. Oxyphilic cell tumor of the submaxillary gland. *US Armed Forces Med J.* 1960; 11:1383–1386.

235. Chan MNY, Radden BG. Intraoral benign solid oncocytoma. *Int J Oral Maxillofac Surg.* 1986; 15:503–506.

236. Damm DD, White DK, Geissler RH, Drummond JF, Henry BB. Benign solid oncocytoma of intraoral minor salivary glands. *Oral Surg Oral Med Oral Pathol.* 1989; 67:84–86.

237. Ellis GL. "Clear cell" oncocytoma of salivary gland. *Hum Pathol.* 1988; 19:862–867.

238. Hildebrad O. Veber angeborne epitheliale Cysten und Fisteln des Halse. *Arch F Kim Chir.* 1895; 49:167–192.

239. Albrecht H, Arzt L. Beitrage zur frage der gewebsrerirrung gapillare cystadenome lymphdrusen. *Frankfurt Ztsch F Path.* 1910; 4:47–69.

240. Warthin AS. Papillary cystadenoma lymphomatosum: A rare teratoid of the parotid region. *J Cancer Res Clin Oncol.* 1929; 14:116–125.

241. Chaudhry AD, Gorlin RI. Papillary cystadenoma lymphomatosum. *Am J Surg.* 1958; 95:923–931.

242. Jaffe RH. Adenolymphoma (onkocytoma) of parotid gland. *Am J Cancer* 1932; 16:1415–1423.

243. Martin H, Ehrlich HE. Papillary cystadenoma lymphomatosum (Warthin's tumor) of the parotid gland. *Surg Gynecol Obstet.* 1944; 79:611–623.

244. Kurreja HK, Jain HK. Adenolymphoma of submandibular salivary gland. *J Laryngol Otol.* 1972; 85:1201–1203.

245. Fantasia JE, Miller AS. Papillary cystadenoma lymphomatosum arising in minor salivary gland. *Oral Surg Oral Med Oral Pathol.* 1981; 52:411–416.

246. Baden E, Pierce M, Selmon AJ, Roberts TW, Doyle. Intra-oral papillary cystadenoma lymphomatosum. *J Oral Surg.* 1976; 34:533–541.

247. Singh RS. Adenolymphoma presenting as pharyngeal tumour. *J Laryngol Otol.* 1966; 80:199–203.

248. Foulsham CK, Snyder GG, Carpenter RJ. Papillary cystadenoma lymphomatosum of the larynx. *Otolaryngol Head Neck Surg.* 1981; 89:960–964.

249. Kennedy TL. Warthin's tumor: A review indicating no male predominance. *Laryngoscope.* 1983; 93:889–891.

250. Lamelas J, Terry IH, Alfonso AE. Warthin's tumor: Multicentricity and increasing incidence in women. *Am J Surg.* 1987; 154:347–351.

251. Eveson IW, Cawson RA. Warthin's tumor (cystadenolymphoma) of salivary glands: A clinicopathologic investigation of 278 cases. *Oral Surg Oral Med Oral Pathol.* 1986; 61:256–262.

252. Kavka SJ. Bilateral simultaneous Warthin's tumors. *Arch Otolaryngol.* 1970; 91:302–303.

253. Beck LD, Maguda TA. Papillary cystadenoma lymphomatosum (Warthin's tumor): A multicentric benign tumor. *Laryngoscope.* 1967; 77:1840–1847.

254. Lumeran H, Freedman P, Caracciolo P, Remigio PS. Synchronous malignant mucoepidermoid tumor of the parotid gland and Warthin's tumor in adjacent lymph node. *Oral Surg Oral Med Oral Pathol.* 1975; 39:954–958.

255. Astacio JN. Papillary cystadenoma lymphomatosum associated with pleomorphic adenoma of the parotid gland. *Oral Surg Oral Med Oral Pathol.* 1974; 38:91–95.

256. Tanaka N, Chen WC. A case of bilateral papillary cystadenoma lymphomatosum. (Warthin's tumor) of the parotid complicated with mucoepidermoid tumor. *Gann.* 1953; 44:229–231.

257. McClatchy KD, Appelblat NH, Langin JL. Carcinoma in papillary cystadenoma lymphomatosum (Warthin's tumor). *Laryngoscope.* 1982; 92:98–99.

258. Baker M, Yuzon D, Baker BH. Squamous cell carcinoma arising in benign adenolymphoma (Warthin's tumor) of the parotid gland. *J Surg Oncol* 1980; 15:7–10.

259. Nakashima N, Goto K, Takeuchi, J. Malignant papillary cystadenoma lymphomatosum. *Virchows Arch [A].* 1983; 399:207–219.

260. Miller R, Yanagihara ET, Aaron AD, Lukes RI. Malignant lymphoma in a Warthin's tumor. *Cancer.* 1982; 50:2948–2950.

261. Howard DR, Bagley C, Batsakis JG. Warthin's tumor: A functional immunologic study of the lymphoid cell component. *Am J Otolaryngol.* 1982; 3:15–19.

262. Tandler B, Shipkey FH. Ultrastructure of Warthin's tumor. *J Ultrastruc Mol Struct Res.* 1964; 11:292–305.

263. Korsrud FR, Brandtzaeg P. Immunohistochemical studies on epithelium and lymphoid components of Warthin's tumor. *Acta Otolaryngol* 1979; 360(suppl):221–224.

264. Rawson AI, Horn RC. Sebaceous glands and sebaceous gland containing tumors of the parotid salivary gland. *Surgery.* 1950; 27:93–101.

265. Gnepp DR, Sporck FT. Lymphoepithelial cyst with sebaceous differentiation (cystic sebaceous lymphadenoma). *Am J Clin Pathol.* 1980; 74:683–687.

266. Gnepp DR, Brannon R. Sebaceous neoplasms of salivary gland origin, report of 21 cases. *Cancer.* 1984; 53:2155–2170.

267. Wasan SM. Sebaceous lymphadenoma of the parotid gland. *Cancer.* 1971; 28:1019–1022.

268. Baratz M, Loewenthal M, Rozin M. Sebaceous lymphadenoma of the parotid gland. *Arch Pathol Lab Med.* 1976; 100:269–270.

269. Whittaker JS, Turner EP. Papillary tumors of the minor salivary glands. *J Clin Pathol.* 1976; 29:795–805.

270. Skorpil F. Iber das Cystadenoma papillare der grosen und kleinen Speicheldrusen. *Frankfurt Z Path.* 1941; 5:39–59.

271. Akin RK, Kreller AI, Walters PI: Papillary cystadenoma of the lower lip: Report of a case. *J Oral Maxillofac Surg.* 1973; 31:808–860.

272. Brooks HW, Hiebert AE, Pullman NK, Stofer BE. Papillary cystadenoma of the palate: Review of the literature and report of two new cases. *Oral Surg.* 1956; 9:1047–1050.

273. Goldman RR. Melanogenic papillary cystadenoma of the soft palate. *Am J Clin Pathol.* 1967; 48:49–52.

274. Kerpel WM, Freedman PD, Lumerman H. The papillary cystadenoma of minor salivary gland origin. *Oral Surg Oral Med Oral Pathol.* 1978; 46:820–826.

275. Kroe DJ, Pitcock JA, Cocke EW. Oncocytic papillary cystadenoma of the larynx. *Arch Pathol.* 1967; 84:429–432.

276. Donald PJ, Krause CJ. Papillary cystadenoma of the larynx. *Laryngoscope.* 1973; 83:2024–2028.

277. Eversole LR, Sabes WR. Minor salivary gland duct changes due to obstruction. *Arch Otolaryngol.* 1971; 94:19–24.

278. Abrams AM, Finck FM. Sialadenoma papilliferum: A previously unreported salivary gland tumor. *Cancer.* 1969; 24:1057–1063.

279. Castigliano SG, Gold L. Intraductal papilloma of the hard palate. *Oral Surg Oral Med Oral Pathol.* 1954; 7:232–238.

280. Crocker DJ, Christ TF, Cavalaris CJ. Sialadenoma papilliferum: Report of case. *J Oral Surg.* 1972; 30:520–521.

281. Maiorano E, Favia G, Ricco R. Sialadenoma papilliferum: An immunohistochemical study of five cases. *J Oral Pathol Med.* 1996; 25:336–342.

282. van der Wal JE; van der Waal I. The rare sialadenoma papilliferum. Report of a case and review of the literature. *Int J Oral Maxillofac Surg.* 1992; 21:104–106.

283. Jensen JL, Reingold IM. Sialadenoma papilliferum of the oral cavity. *Oral Surg Oral Med Oral Pathol.* 1973; 35:521–525.

284. Soofer SB, Tabbara S: Intraductal papilloma of salivary gland. A report of two cases with diagnosis by fine needle aspiration biopsy. *Acta Cytol.* 1999; 43:1142–1146.

285. Shirastina K, Watatani K, Miyazaki T. Ultrastructure of a sialadenoma papilliferum. *Cancer.* 1984; 53:468–474.

286. Abbey LM. Solitary intraductal papilloma of the minor salivary glands. *Oral Surg Oral Med Oral Pathol.* 1975; 40:135–140.

287. Shiotani A, Kawaura M, Tanaka Y, Fukuda H, Kanzaki J. Papillary adenocarcinoma possibly arising from an intraductal papilloma of the parotid gland. *ORLJ.* 1994; 56:112–115.

288. Ishikawa T, Imada S, Ijuhin N. Intraductal papilloma of the anterior lingual salivary gland. Case report and immunohistochemical study. *Int J Oral Maxillofac Surg.* 1993; 22:116–117.

289. Rouse RV, Soetikno RM, Baker RJ, Barnard IC, Triadafilopoulos G, Longacre TA. Esophageal submucosal gland duct adenoma. *Am J Surg Pathol.* 1995; 19:1191–1196.

290. Alho OP, Kristo A, Luotonen J, Autio-Harmainen H. Intra-

ductal papilloma as a cause of a parotid duct cyst. A case report. *J Laryngol Otol.* 1996; 110:277–278.

291. White DK, Miller AS, McDaniel RK, Rothman BN. Inverted ductal papilloma: A distinctive lesion of minor salivary gland. *Cancer.* 1982; 49:519–524.

292. Wilson DF, Robinson BW. Oral inverted ductal papilloma. *Oral Surg Oral Med Oral Pathol.* 1984; 57:520–523.

293. Greer RO. Inverted oral papilloma. *Oral Surg Oral Med Oral Pathol.* 1973; 36:400–403.

294. de Sousa SO, Sesso A, de Araujo NS, de Araujo VC. Inverted ductal papilloma of minor salivary gland origin: Morphological aspects and cytokeratin expression. *Eur Arch Otorhinolaryngol.* 1995; 252:370–373.

295. Hegarty DJ, Hopper C, Speight PM. Inverted ductal papilloma of minor salivary glands. *J Oral Pathol Med.* 1994; 23: 334–336.

296. Eversole LR, Sabes WR. Minor salivary gland duct changes due to obstruction. *Arch Otolaryngol Head Neck Surg.* 1971; 94:19–24.

297. el-Naggar AK, Lovell M, Killary AM, Batsakis JG. Genotypic characterization of a primary mucoepidermoid carcinoma of the parotid gland by cytogenetic, fluorescence in situ hybridization, and DNA ploidy analysis. *Cancer Gen Cytogen.* 1996; 89:38–43.

298. Plambeck K, Friedrich RE, Hellner D, Donath K, Schmelzle R. Mucoepidermoid carcinoma of the salivary glands: Clinical data and follow-up of 52 cases. *J Cancer Res Clin Oncol.* 1996; 122:177–180.

299. Wenig BM, Adair CF, Heffess CS. Primary mucoepidermoid carcinoma of the thyroid gland: A report of six cases and a review of the literature of a follicular epithelial–derived tumor. *Hum Pathol.* 1995; 26:1099–1108.

300. Hicks MJ, el-Naggar AK, Flaitz CM, Luna MA, Batsakis JG. Histocytologic grading of mucoepidermoid carcinoma of major salivary glands in prognosis and survival: A clinicopathologic and flow cytometric investigation. *Head Neck.* 1995; 17: 89–95.

301. Stewart FW, Foote FW, Becker WE. Mucoepidermoid tumors of salivary glands. *Ann Surg.* 1945; 122:820–844.

302. Masson P, Berger L. Epitheliomas a double metaplasie, del la partoide. *Bull Assoc Franc L'etude du Cancer.* 1924; 13:366–373.

303. Volkmann R. Ceber endotheliale Geschwülste zugleich ein Beitrag zu den Speicheldrilsen-und Gaumentumoren. *Deutsche Zeitschrift fur Chirurqie.* 1895; 41:1–180.

304. Krompecher E. Ideber den Ausgang und Einteilung der Epitheliome der Speichel-und Schleimdriisen. *Beitrage zur pathologischen Anatomie und zur Allgemeinen Pathologie.* 1922; 70: 489–509.

305. Spiro RH, Huvos AG, Berk R, Strong EW. Mucoepidermoid carcinoma of salivary gland origin: A clinicopathologic study of 367 cases. *Am Surg.* 1978; 136:461–468.

306. Evans HL. Mucoepidermoid carcinoma of salivary glands: A study of 69 cases with special attention to histologic grading. *Am J Clin Pathol.* 1984; 81:696–701.

307. Healey WV, Perzin KH, Smith L. Mucoepidermoid carcinoma of salivary gland origin: Classification, clinical-pathologic correlation, and results of treatment. *Cancer.* 1970; 26: 368–388.

308. Woolner LB, Petter JR, Kirklin JW. Mucoepidermioid tumors of major salivary glands. *Am J Clin Pathol.* 1954; 24:1350–1362.

309. Nascimento AG, Amaral AL, Prado LA, Kligerman J, Silveira RP. Mucoepidermoid carcinoma of salivary glands: A clinicopathologic study of 46 cases. *Head Neck Surg.* 1986; 8:409–417.

310. Melrose RJ, Abrams AM, Howell FV. Mucoepidermoid tumors of the intraoral minor salivary glands: A clinicopathologic study of 54 cases. *J Oral Pathol.* 1973; 2:314–325.

311. Bhaskar SN, Bernier JL. Mucoepidermoid tumors of major and minor salivary glands; clinical features, histology, variations, natural history and results of treatment for 144 cases. *Cancer.* 1962; 15:801–817.

312. Eversole LR. Mucoepidermoid carcinoma: A review of 815 cases. *J Oral Maxillofac Surg.* 1970; 28:490–494.

313. Eneroth CM, Hjertman L, Moberger G, Soderberg G. Mucoepidermoid carcinomas of the salivary glands, with special reference to the possible existence of a benign variety. *Acta Otolaryngol.* 1972; 73:68–74.

314. Chomette G, Auriol M, Tereau Y, Vaillant IM. Mucoepidermoid tumors of minor salivary glands. Clinical and pathologic correlations. Histoenzymologic and ultrastructural studies. *Ann Pathol.* 1982; 2:29–40.

315. Jakobsson PA, Blanck C, Eneroth CM. Mucoepidermoid carcinoma of the parotid gland. *Cancer.* 1968; 22:111–124.

316. Eversole LR, Rovin S, Sabes WR. Mucoepidermoid carcinoma of minor salivary glands: Report of 17 cases with follow-up. *J Oral Surg.* 1972; 30:107–112.

317. Eversole LR. Glycoprotein heterogeneity in mucoepidermoid carcinoma. A histochemical evaluation. *Arch Otolaryngol.* 1972; 96:426–432.

318. Kumasa S, Yuba R, Sagara I, Okutomi I, Okada Y, Mori M. Mucoepidermoid carcinomas: Immunohistochemical studies on keratin, S-100 protein, lactoferrin, lysozyme and amylase. *Bas Appl Histochem.* 1988; 32:429–441.

319. Hamper K, Schimmelpenning H, Caselitz J, et al. Mucoepidermoid tumors of the salivary glands. Correlation of cytophotometrical data and prognosis. *Cancer.* 1989; 63:708–717.

320. Jensen OJ, Poulsen T, Schiodt T. Mucoepidermoid tumors of salivary glands: A long term followup study. *APMIS.* 1988; 96:421–427.

321. Dardick I, Dava D, Hardie I, van Nostrand AWP. Mucoepidermoid carcinoma: Ultrastructural and histogenetic aspects. *J Oral Pathol.* 1984; 13:342–358.

322. Spiro RH, Koss LG, Hajdu SI, Strong EW. Tumors of minor salivary origin. A clinicopathologic study of 492 cases. *Cancer.* 1973; 31:117–129.

323. Thorvaldsson SE, Beahrs OH, Woolner LB, Simons JH. Mucoepidermoid tumors of the major salivary glands. *Am J Surg.* 1970; 120:432–438.

324. Conley J, Tinsley PP. Treatment and prognosis of mucoepidermoid carcinoma in the pediatric age group. *Arch Otolaryngol.* 1985; 111:322–324.

325. Connell HC, Evans JC. Mucoepidermoid carcinoma of the salivary glands. *Am J Surg.* 1972; 124:519–521.

326. Auclair PL, Goode RK, Ellis GL. Mucoepidermoid carcinoma of intraoral salivary glands. Evaluation and application of grading criteria in 143 cases. *Cancer.* 1992; 69:2021–2030.

327. Haddad A, Enepekides DJ, Manolidis S, Black M. Adenoid cystic carcinoma of the head and neck: A clinicopathologic study of 37 cases. *J Otolaryngol.* 1995; 24:201–205.

328. Seifert G. Classification and differential diagnosis of clear and basal cell tumors of the salivary glands. *Sem Diag Pathol.* 1996; 13:95–103.

329. Fonseca I, Soares J. Basal cell adenocarcinoma of minor salivary and seromucous glands of the head and neck region. *Sem Diag Pathol.* 1996; 13:128–137.

330. Stanley MW, Horwitz CA, Rollins SD, et al. Basal cell (monomorphic) and minimally pleomorphic adenomas of the salivary glands. Distinction from the solid (anaplastic) type of adenoid cystic carcinoma in fine-needle aspiration. *Amer J Clin Pathol.* 1996; 106:35–41.

331. Papadaki H, Finkelstein SD, Kounelis S, Bakker A, Swalsky PA, Kapadia SB. The role of p53 mutation and protein expression in primary and recurrent adenoid cystic carcinoma. *Hum Pathol.* 1996; 27:567–572.

332. Vuhahula EA, Nikai H, Ogawa I, et al. Correlation between argyrophilic nucleolar organizer region (AGNOR) counts and histologic grades with respect to biologic behavior of salivary adenoid cystic carcinoma. *J Oral Pathol Med.* 1995; 24:437–442.

333. Billroth T. Beobachtungen uber Geschwulste der Speicheldrusen. *Virchows Arch [A].* 1859; 17:357–375.

334. Foote FW Jr, Frazell EL. Tumors of the major salivary glands. *Cancer.* 1953; 6:1065–1133.

335. Foote FW Jr, Frazell EL, eds. Tumors of the major salivary glands, section IV, fascicle 11. In: *Atlas of Tumor Pathology.* Washington, DC: Armed Forces Institute of Pathology, 1954.

336. Waldron CA, El-Mofty SK, Gnepp DR. Tumors of the intraoral minor salivary glands: A demographic and histologic study of 426 cases. *Oral Surg Oral Med Oral Pathol.* 1988; 66: 323–333.

337. Perzin KH, Gullane P, Clairmont AC. Adenoid cystic carcinoma arising in salivary glands: A correlation of histologic features and clinical course. *Cancer.* 1978; 42:265–282.

338. Tarpley TM, Giansanti JS. Adenoid cystic carcinoma. *Oral Surg Oral Med Oral Pathol.* 1976; 41:484–497.

339. Krolls SO, Trodahl JN, Boyers RC. Salivary gland lesions in children: A survey of 430 cases. *Cancer.* 1972; 30:459–469.

340. Castro EB, Huvos AG, Strong EW, Foote FW Jr. Tumors of the major salivary glands in children. *Cancer.* 1972; 29:312–317.

341. Eneroth C-M, Hjertman L. Adenoid cystic carcinoma of the submandibular gland. *Laryngoscope.* 1966; 76:1639–1661.

342. Goldblatt LI, Ellis GL. Salivary gland tumors of the tongue. Analysis of 55 new cases and review of the literature. *Cancer.* 1987; 60:74–81.

343. Nascimento AG, Amaral ALP, Prado LAF, Kligerman J, Silveira TRP. Adenoid cystic carcinoma of salivary glands: A study of 61 cases with clinicopathologic correlation. *Cancer.* 1986; 57:312–319.

344. Eneroth C-M, Zajicek J. Aspiration biopsy of salivary gland tumors. IV. Morphologic studies on smears and histologic sections from 45 cases of adenoid cystic carcinoma. *Acta. Cytol* 1969; 13:59–63.

345. Chen JC, Gnepp DR, Bedrossian, WM. Adenoid cystic carcinoma of the salivary glands: An immunohistochemical study. *Oral Surg Oral Med Oral Pathol.* 1988; 65:316–326.

346. Hoshino M, Yamamoto I. Ultrastructure of adenoid cystic carcinoma. *Cancer.* 1970; 25:186–198.

347. Chaudhry AP, Leifer C, Cutler LS, Satchidanand S, Laday GR, Yamane GM. Histogenesis of adenoid cystic carcinoma of the salivary glands: Light and electron-microscopic study. *Cancer.* 1986; 58:72–82.

348. Eby LS, Johnson DS, Baker HW. Adenoid cystic carcinoma of the head and neck. *Cancer.* 1972; 29:1160–1168.

349. Conley J, Dingman DL. Adenoid cystic carcinoma in the head and neck (cylindroma). *Arch Otolaryngol.* 1974; 100:81–90.

350. Matsuba HM, Spector CJ, Thawley SE, Simpson R, Mauney M, Pikul FJ. Adenoid cystic salivary gland carcinoma: A histopathologic review of treatment failure patterns. *Cancer.* 1986; 57:519–524.

351. Blanck C, Eneroth C-M, Jacobsson F, Jakobsson PA. Adenoid cystic carcinoma of the parotid gland. *Acta Radiol.* 1967; 177–196.

352. Nasse D. Die Geschwulste der Speicheldrusen und verwandte Tumoren des Kopfes. *Arch Klin Chir.* 1892; 44:233–302.

353. Godwin IT, Foote FW Jr, Frazell EL. Acinic cell adenocarcinoma of the parotid gland: Report of twenty-seven cases. *Am J Pathol.* 1954; 30:465–477.

354. Skalova A, Leivo I, Von Boguslawsky K, Saksela E. Cell proliferation correlates with prognosis in acinic cell carcinomas of salivary gland origin. Immunohistochemical study of 30 cases using the MIB 1 antibody in formalin-fixed paraffin sections. *J Pathol.* 1994; 173:13–21.

355. Timon CI, Dardick I, Panzarella T, Thomas J, Ellis G, Cullane P. Clinicopathological predictors of recurrence for acinic cell carcinoma. *Clin Otolaryngol.* 1995; 20:396–401.

356. Yoshihara T, Shino A, Shino M, Ishii T. Acinic cell tumour of the maxillary sinus: An unusual case initially diagnosed as parotid cancer. *Rhinol.* 1995; 33:177–179.

357. Rosenbaum PS, Mahadevia PS, Goodman LA, Kress Y. Acinic cell carcinoma of the lacrimal gland. *Arch Ophthalmol.* 1995; 113:781–785.

358. Napier SS, Herron BT, Herron BM. Acinic cell carcinoma in Northern Ireland: A 10–year review. *Br J Oral Maxillofac Surg.* 1995; 33:145–148.

359. Ferreiro JA, Kochar AS. Parotid acinic cell carcinoma with undifferentiated spindle cell transformation. *J Laryngol Otol.* 1994; 108:902–904.

360. Timon CI, Dardick I, Panzarella T, et al. Acinic cell carcinoma of salivary glands. Prognostic relevance of DNA flow cytometry and nucleolar organizer regions. *Arch Otolaryngol Head Neck Surg.* 1994; 120:727–733.

361. Fox NM Jr, ReMine WH, Woolner LB. Acinic cell carcinoma of the major salivary glands. *Am J Surg.* 1963; 106:860–867.

362. Abrams AM, Melrose RI. Acinic cell tumors of minor salivary gland origin. *Oral Surg Oral Med Oral Pathol.* 1978; 46:220–233.

363. Eveson JW, Cawson RA. Salivary gland tumors: A review of 2410 cases with particular reference to histological types, site, age and sex distribution. *J Pathol.* 1985; 146:51–58.

364. Batsakis JG, Chinn EK, Weimert TA, Work WP, Krause CI. Acinic cell carcinoma:. A clinicopathologic study of thirty-five cases. *J Laryngol Otol.* 1979; 93:325–340.

365. Abrams AM, Scofield HH, Hansen LS. Acinic cell adenocarcinoma of the minor salivary glands: A clinicopathologic study of 77 cases. *Cancer.* 1965; 18:1145–1162.

366. Bhaskar SN. Acinic cell carcinoma of salivary glands: Report of twenty-one cases. *Oral Surg Oral Med Oral Pathol.* 1964; 17:62–74.

367. Erlandson RA, Tandler B. Ultrastructure of acinic cell carcinoma of the parotid gland. *Arch Pathol Lab Med.* 1972; 93:130–140.

368. Chomette G, Auriol M, Vaillant JM. Acinic cell tumors of salivary glands. Frequency and morphological study. *J Biol Buccale.* 1984; 12:157–169.

369. Chaudhry AP, Cutler LS, Leifer C, Satchidanand S, Labay G, Yamane G. Histogenesis of acinic cell carcinoma of the major and minor salivary glands: An ultrastructural study. *J Pathol.* 1986; 148:307–320.

370. Warner TF, Seo IS, Azen EA, Hafez GR. Zarling Immunocytochemistry of acinic cell carcinomas and mixed tumors of salivary glands. *Cancer.* 1985; 56:2221–2227.

371. Gorlin RJ, Chaudhry A. Acinic cell tumor of the major and minor salivary glands. *J Oral Surg.* 1957; 15:304–306.

372. Spiro RH, Huvos AG, Strong EW. Acinic cell carcinoma of salivary origin: A clinicopathologic study of 67 cases. *Cancer.* 1978; 41:924–935.

373. Peiziti KH, LiVolsi VA. Acinic cell carcinomas arising in salivary glands: A clinicopathologic study. *Cancer.* 1979; 44:1434–1457.

374. Ellis GL, Corio RL. Acinic cell adenocarcinoma: A clinicopathologic analysis of 294 cases. *Cancer.* 1983; 52:542–549.

375. Chen S-Y, Brannon RB, Miller AS, White DK, Hooker SP. Acinic cell adenocarcinoma of minor salivary glands. *Cancer.* 1978; 42:678–685.

376. Ferlito A. Acinic cell carcinoma of minor salivary glands. *Histopathology.* 1980; 4:331–343.

377. Castellanos JL, Lally ET. Acinic cell tumor of the minor salivary glands. *J Oral Maxillofac Surg.* 1982; 40:428–431.

378. Gustafsson H, Carlsoo B. Multiple acinic cell carcinoma: Some histological and ultrastructural features of a case. *J Laryngol Otol.* 1985; 99:1183–1193.

379. Nelson DW, Nichols RD, Fine G. Bilateral acinous cell tumors of the parotid gland. *Laryngoscope.* 1978; 88:1935–1941.

380. Eneroth C-M, Jakobsson PA, Blanck C. Acinic cell carcinoma of the parotid gland. *Cancer.* 1966; 19:1761–1772.

381. Stanley RJ, Weiland LH, Olsen KD, Pearson BW. Dedifferentiated acinic cell (acinous) carcinoma of the parotid gland. *Otolaryngol Head Neck Surg.* 1988; 98:155–161.

382. Caselitz J, Seifert G, Grenner G, Schmidtberger R. Amylase as an additional marker of salivary gland neoplasms: An immunoperoxidase study. *Pathol Res Pract.* 1983; 176:276–283.

383. Dardick I, George D, Jeans D, et al. Ultra-structural morphology and cellular differentiation in acinic cell carcinoma. *Oral Surg Oral Med Oral Pathol.* 1987; 63:325–334.

384. Echevarria RA. Ultrastructure of the acinic cell carcinoma and clear cell carcinoma of the parotid gland. *Cancer.* 1967; 20:563–571.

385. Fonesca I, Felix A, Soares J. Dedifferentiation in salivary carcinomas. *Am J Surg Pathol.* 2000:469–471.

386. Thackray AC, Lucas RB. Tumors of the major salivary

glands. Fascicle 10. In: *Atlas of Tumor Pathology*, 2nd series. Washington, DC: Armed Forces Institute of Pathology; 1974.

387. Spiro RH. Salivary neoplasms: Overview of a 35-year experience with 2807 patients. *Head Neck Surg.* 1986; 8:177–184.

388. Rosenfeld L, Sessions DG, McSwain B, Graves H Jr. Malignant tumors of salivary gland origin: 37 year review of 184 cases. *Ann Surg.* 1966; 163:726–735.

389. Sharkey FE. Systematic evaluation of the World Health Organization classification of salivary gland tumors. *Am J Clin Pathol.* 1977; 67:272–278.

390. Chaudhry AP, Vickers RA, Godin RJ. Intraoral minor salivary gland tumors: Analysis of 1414 cases. *Oral Surg Oral Med Oral Pathol.* 1961; 14:1194–1226.

391. Auclair PL, Ellis GL. Adenocarcinoma, not otherwise specified. In: Ellis GL, Auclair PL, Gnepp DR, eds. *Surgical Pathology of the Salivary Glands.* Philadelphia: WB Saunders; 1991: 318–332.

392. Bauer WH, Bauer JD. Classification of glandular tumors of salivary glands. Study of one hundred forty-three cases. *Arch Pathol.* 1953; 55:328–346.

393. Eveson JW, Cawson RA. Salivary gland tumours: A review of 2410 cases with particular reference to histological types, site, age and sex distribution. *Pathol.* 1985; 146:51–58.

394. Bissett RI, Fitzpatrick PJ. Malignant submandibular gland tumors: A review of 91 patients. *Am J Clin Oncol.* 1988; 11: 46–51.

395. Spiro RH, Huvos AG, Strong EW. Adenocarcinoma of salivary origin: Clinicopathologic study of 204 patients. *Am J Surg.* 1982; 144:423–431.

396. Seifert G, Okabe H, Caselitz J. Epithelial salivary gland tumors in children and adolescents: Analysis of 80 cases (Salivary Gland Registry 19651984). *ORLJ.* 1986; 48:137–149.

397. Burbank PM, Dockerty MB, Devine KD. Clinico-pathologic study of 43 cases of glandular tumor of the tongue. *Surg Gynecol Obstet.* 1959; 109:573–582.

398. Reddy SP, Marks JE. Treatment of locally advanced high-grade, malignant tumors of major salivary glands. *Laryngoscope.* 1988; 98:450–454.

399. Aberle AM, Abrams AM, Bowe R, Melrose RJ, Handlers JR. Lobular (polymorphous low-grade) carcinoma of minor salivary glands. A clinicopathologic study of twenty cases. *Oral Surg Oral Med Oral Pathol.* 1985; 60:387–395.

400. Anderson C, Krutchkoff D, Pedersen C, Cartun R, Berman M. Polymorphous low grade adenocarcinoma of minor salivary gland: A clinicopathologic and comparative immunohistochemical study. *Mod Pathol.* 1990; 3:76–82.

401. Batsakis JG, Pinkston GR, Luna M, Byers RM, Sciubba JJ, Tillery GW. Adenocarcinomas of the oral cavity: A clinicopathologic study of terminal duct carcinomas. *J Laryngol Otol.* 1983; 97:825–835.

402. Evans HL, Batsakis JG. Polymorphous low-grade adenocarcinoma of minor salivary glands. A study of 14 cases of a distinctive neoplasm. *Cancer.* 1984; 53:935–942.

403. Freedman PD, Lumerman H. Lobular carcinoma of intraoral minor salivary gland origin. Report of twelve cases. *Oral Surg Oral Med Oral Pathol.* 1983; 56:157–165.

404. Frierson HF Jr, Mills SE, Garland TA. Terminal duct carcinoma of minor salivary glands. A nonpapillary subtype of polymorphous low-grade adenocarcinoma. *Am J Clin Pathol.* 1985; 84:8–14.

405. Gnepp DR, Chen JC, Warren C. Polymorphous lowgrade adenocarcinoma of minor salivary gland. An immunohistochemical and clinicopathologic study. *Am J Surg Pathol.* 1988; 12:461–468.

406. Miliauskas JR. Polymorphous low-grade (terminal duct) adenocarcinoma of the parotid gland. *Histopathology.* 1991; 19: 555–557.

407. Regezi JA, Zarbo PJ, Stewart JC, Courtney RM. Polymorphous low-grade adenocarcinoma of minor salivary gland. A comparative histologic and immunohistochemical study. *Oral Surg Oral Med Oral Pathol.* 1991; 71:469–475.

408. Ritland F, Lubensky I, LiVolsi VA. Polymorphous lowgrade adenocarcinoma of the parotid salivary gland. *Arch Pathol Lab Med.* 1993; 117:1261–1263.

409. Simpson RH, Clarke TJ, Sarsfield PT, Gluckman PG, Baba-

jews AV. Polymorphous low-grade adenocarcinoma of the salivary glands: A clinicopathological comparison with adenoid cystic carcinoma. *Histopathology.* 1991; 19:121–129.

410. Slootweg PJ. Low-grade adenocarcinoma of the oral cavity: Polymorphous or papillary? *J Oral Pathol Med.* 1993; 22:327–330.

411. Wenig BM, Gnepp DR. Polymorphous low-grade adenocarcinoma of minor salivary glands. In: Ellis GL, Auclair PL, Gnepp DR, eds. *Surgical Pathology of the Salivary Glands.* Philadelphia: WB Saunders; 1991:390–411.

412. Thomas KM, Cumberworth VL, McEwan J. Orbital and skin metastases in a polymorphous low grade adenocarcinoma of the salivary gland. *J Laryngol Otol.* 1995; 109:1222–1225.

413. Clayton JR, Pogrel MA, Regezi JA. Simultaneous multifocal polymorphous low-grade adenocarcinoma. Report of two cases. *Oral Surg Oral Med Oral Pathol.* 1995; 80:71–77.

414. Tanaka F, Wada H, Inui K, et al. Pulmonary metastasis of polymorphous low-grade adenocarcinoma of the minor salivary gland. *Thorac Cardiovasc Surg.* 1995; 43:178–180.

415. Miller AS, Hartman GG, Chen SY, Edmonds PR, Brightman SA, Harwick RD. Estrogen receptor assay in polymorphous low-grade adenocarcinoma and adenoid cystic carcinoma of salivary gland. *Oral Surg Oral Med Oral Pathol.* 1994; 77:36–40.

416. Ritland F, Lubensky I, LiVolsi VA. Polymorphous low-grade adenocarcinoma of the parotid salivary gland. *Arch Pathol Lab Med.* 1993; 117:1261–1263.

417. de Araujo VC, de Sousa SO. Expression of different keratins in salivary gland tumours. Oral Oncology. *Eur J Cancer.* 1996; 32B:14–18.

418. Toth AA, Daley TD, Lampe HB, Stitt L, Veinot L. Schwann cell differentiation of modified myoepithelial cells within adenoid cystic carcinomas and polymorphous low-grade adenocarcinomas: Clinicopathologic assessment of immunohistochemical staining. *J Otolaryngol.* 1996; 25:94–102.

419. Duck SW, McConnel FM. Malignant degeneration of pleomorphic adenoma-clinical implications. *Am J Otolaryngol.* 1993; 14:175–178.

420. Eneroth CM, Blanck C, Jakobsson PA. Carcinoma in pleomorphic adenoma of the parotid. *Acta Otolaryngol (Stockh).* 1968; 66:477–492.

421. Eneroth CM, Zetterberg A. Malignancy in pleomorphic adenoma. A clinical and microspectrophotometric study. *Acta Otolaryngol (Stockh).* 1974; 77:426–432.

422. Gerughty RM, Scofield HH, Brown FM, Hennigar GR. Malignant mixed tumors of salivary gland origin. *Cancer.* 1969; 24:471–486.

423. Gnepp DR. Malignant mixed tumors of the salivary glands: A review. *Pathol Annu.* 1993; 28(Pt 1):279–328.

424. LiVolsi VA, Perzin KH. Malignant mixed tumors arising in salivary glands. 1. Carcinomas arising in benign mixed tumors: A clinicopathologic study. *Cancer.* 1977; 39:2209–2230.

425. Moberger JG, Eneroth CM. Malignant mixed tumors of the major salivary glands. Special reference to the histologic structure in metastases. *Cancer.* 1968; 21:1198–1211.

426. Nagao K, Matsuzaki O, Saiga H, et al. Histopathologic studies on carcinoma in pleomorphic adenoma of the parotid gland. *Cancer.* 1981; 48:113–121.

427. Shrikhande SS, Talvalkar GV. Malignant mixed salivary gland tumors—a clinicopathological study of 48 cases. *Indian J Cancer.* 1979; 16:9–12.

428. Spiro RH, Huvos AG, Strong EW. Malignant mixed tumor of salivary origin: A clinicopathologic study of 146 cases. *Cancer.* 1977; 39:388–396.

429. Tortoledo ME, Luna M, Batsakis JG. Carcinomas ex pleomorphic adenoma and malignant mixed tumors. Histomorphologic indexes. *Arch Otolaryngol Head Neck Surg.* 1984; 110:172–176.

430. Batsakis JG. Primary squamous cell carcinomas of major salivary glands. *Ann Otol Rhinol Laryngol.* 1983; 92:97–98.

431. Batsakis JG, McClatchey KD, Johns M, Regezi J. Primary squamous cell carcinoma of the parotid gland. *Arch Otolaryngol.* 1976; 102:355–357.

432. Shemen LJ, Huvos AG, Spiro RH. Squamous cell carcinoma of salivary gland origin. *Head Neck Surg.* 1987; 9:235–240.

433. Marks MW, Ryan RF, Litwin MS, Sonntag BV. Squamous cell carcinoma of the parotid gland. *Plast Reconst Surg.* 1987; 79:550–554.

434. Gaughan RK, Olsen KD, Lewis JE. Primary squamous cell carcinoma of the parotid gland. *Arch Otolaryngol Head Neck Surg.* 1992; 118:798–801.

435. Batsakis JG, el-Naggar AK, Luna MA. Hyalinizing clear cell carcinoma of salivary origin. *Ann Otol Rhinol Laryngol.* 1994; 103:746–748.

436. Rajab E, Akmal SN, Nasir AM. Glycogen-rich clear cell carcinoma in the tongue. *J Laryngol Otol.* 1994; 108:716–718.

437. Cassidy M, Connolly CE. Clear cell carcinoma arising in a pleomorphic adenoma of the submandibular gland. *J Laryngol Otol.* 1994; 108:529–532.

438. Shrestha P, Yang LT, Liu BL, et al. Clear cell carcinoma of salivary glands: Immunohistochemical evaluation of clear tumor cells. *Anticancer Res.* 1994; 14:825–836.

439. Eversole LR. On the differential diagnosis of clear cell tumours of the head and neck. Oral Oncology. *Eur J Cancer.* 1993; 29B:173–179.

440. Hayashi A, Ohtsuki Y, Sonobe H, et al. Glycogen-rich clear cell carcinoma arising from minor salivary glands of the uvula. A case report. *Acta Pathol Jpn.* 1988; 38:1227–1234.

441. Melnick SJ, Amazon K, Dembrow V. Metastatic renal cell carcinoma presenting as a parotid tumor: A case report with immunohistochemical findings and a review of the literature. *Hum Pathol.* 1989; 20:195–197.

442. Milchgrub S, Gnepp DR, Vuitch F, Delgado R, Albores Saavedra J. Hyalinizing clear cell carcinoma of salivary gland. *Am J Surg Pathol.* 1994; 18:74–82.

443. Mohamed AH, Cherrick HM. Glycogen-rich adenocarcinoma of minor salivary glands. A light and electron microscopic study. *Cancer.* 1975; 36:1057–1066.

444. Ogawa I, Nikai H, Takata T, et al. Clear cell tumors of minor salivary gland origin. An immunohistochemical and ultrastructural analysis. *Oral Surg Oral Med Oral Pathol.* 1991; 72:200–207.

445. Simpson RH, Sarsfield PT, Clarke T, Babajews AV. Clear Cell carcinoma of minor salivary glands. *Histopathology.* 1990; 17:433–438.

446. Uri AK, Wetmore RF, Iozzo RV. Glycogen-rich clear cell carcinoma in the tongue. A cytochemical and ultrastructural study. *Cancer.* 1986; 57:1803–1809.

447. Batsakis JG, el-Naggar AK, Luna A. Epithelialmyoepithelial carcinoma of salivary glands. *Ann Otol Rhinol Laryngol.* 1992; 101:540–542.

448. Chen KT. Clear cell carcinoma of the salivary gland. *Hum Pathol.* 1983; 14:91–93.

449. Collina G, Gale N, Visona A, Betts CM, Cenacchi V, Eusebi V. Epithelial-myoepithelial carcinoma of the parotid gland: A clinico-pathologic and immunohistochemical study of seven cases. *Tumori.* 1991; 77:257–263.

450. Corio RL, Sciubba JJ, Brannon RB, Batsakis JG. Epithelialmyoepithelial carcinoma of intercalated duct origin. A clinicopathologic and ultrastructural assessment of sixteen cases. *Oral Surg Oral Med Oral Pathol.* 1982; 53:280–287.

451. Daley TD, Wysocki GP, Smout MS, Slinger RR. Epithelialmyoepithelial carcinoma of salivary glands. *Oral Surg Oral Med Oral Pathol.* 1984; 57:512–519.

452. Donath K, Seifert G, Schmitz R. Diagnose und ultrastruktur des tubultiren speichelgangcareinoms. Epithelial-myoepitheliales schaltstijstuckcarcinom. *Virchows Arch [A].* 1972; 356:16–31.

453. Fonseca I, Soares J. Epithelial-myoepithelial carcinoma of the salivary glands. A study of 22 cases. *Virchows Arch [A].* 1993; 422:389–396.

454. Hamper K, Briigmann M, Koppermann R, et al. Epithelialmyoepithelial duct carcinoma of salivary glands: A follow-up and cytophotometric study of 21 cases. *J Oral Pathol Med.* 1989; 18:299–304.

455. Palmer RM. Epithelial-myoepithelial carcinoma: An immunocytochemical study. *Oral Surg Oral Med Oral Pathol.* 1985; 59:511–515.

456. Adkins GF. Low grade basaloid adenocarcinoma of salivary gland in childhood—the so-called hybrid basal cell adenoma-adenoid cystic carcinoma. *Pathology.* 1990; 22:187–190.

457. Atula T, Luemi PJ, Donath K, Happonen RP, Joensuu H, Grenman R. Basal cell adenocarcinoma of the parotid gland: A case report and review of the literature. *J Laryngol Otol.* 1993; 107:862–864.

458. Batsakis JG, Luna NM. Basaloid salivary carcinoma. *Ann Otol Rhinol Laryngol.* 1991; 100:785–787.

459. Ellis GL, Wiscovitch JG. Basal cell adenocarcinomas of the major salivary glands. *Oral Surg Oral Med Oral Pathol.* 1990; 69:461–469.

460. Hyma BA, Scheithauer BW, Weiland LH, Irons GB. Membranous basal cell adenoma of the parotid gland. Malignant transformation in a patient with multiple dermal cylindromas. *Arch Pathol Lab Med.* 1988; 112:209–211.

461. Klima M, Wolfe K, Johnson PE. Basal cell tumors of the parotid gland. *Arch Otolaryngol.* 1978; 104:111–116.

462. Lo AK, Topf JS, Jackson IT, Silberberg B. Minor salivary gland basal cell adenocarcinoma of the palate. *J Oral Maxillofac Surg.* 1992; 50:531–534.

463. Murty GE, Welch AR, Soames JV. Basal cell adenocarcinoma of the parotid gland. *J Laryngol Otol.* 1990; 104:150–151.

464. Williams SB, Ellis GL, Auclair PL. Immunohistochemical analysis of basal cell adenocarcinoma. *Oral Surg Oral Med Oral Pathol.* 1993; 75:64–69.

465. Hui KK, Luna MA, Batsakis JG, Ordonez NG, Weber R. Undifferentiated carcinomas of the major salivary glands. *Oral Surg Oral Med Oral Pathol.* 1990; 69:76–83.

466. Kraemer BB, Mackay B, Batsakis JG. Small cell carcinomas of the parotid gland. A clinicopathologic study of three cases. *Cancer.* 1983; 52:2115–2121.

467. Nagao K, Matsuzaki O, Saiga H, et al. Histopathologic studies of undifferentiated carcinoma of the parotid gland. *Cancer.* 1982; 50:1572–1579.

468. Batsakis JG, Luna MA. Undifferentiated carcinomas of salivary glands. *Ann Otol Rhinol Laryngol.* 1991; 100:82–84.

469. Cleary KR, Batsakis JG. Undifferentiated carcinoma with lymphoid stroma of the major salivary glands. *Ann Otol Rhinol Laryngol.* 1990; 99:236–238.

470. Gnepp DR, Corio RL, Brannon RB. Small cell carcinoma of the major salivary glands. *Cancer.* 1986; 58:705–714.

471. Gnepp DR, Wick MR. Small cell carcinoma of the major salivary glands. An immunohistochemical study. *Cancer.* 1990; 66:185–192.

472. Hamilton-Dutoit SJ, Therkildsen MH, Neilsen NH, Jensen H, Hansen JP, Pallesen G. Undifferentiated carcinoma of the salivary gland in Greenlandic Eskimos: Demonstration of Epstein-Barr virus DNA by in situ nucleic acid hybridization. *Hum Pathol.* 1991; 22:811–815.

473. Eversole LR, Gnepp DR, Eversole GM. Undifferentiated carcinoma. In: Ellis GL, Auclair PL, Gnepp DR, eds. *Surgical Pathology of the Salivary Glands.* Philadelphia: WB Saunders; 1991:422–440.

474. Brown DH, Illman J, MacMillan C. Small cell anaplastic carcinoma of the parotid gland. *J Otolaryngol.* 1997; 26:332–334.

475. Gnepp DR, Ferlito A, Hyams VJ. Primary anaplastic small cell (oat cell) carcinoma of the larynx: Review of the literature and report of 18 cases. *Cancer.* 1983; 51:1731–1745.

476. Chan JK, Suster S, Wenig BM, Tsang WY, Chan JB, Lau AL. Cytokeratin 20 immunoreactivity distinguishes Merkel cell (primary cutaneous neuroendocrine) carcinomas and salivary gland small carcinomas from small cell carcinomas of various cites. *Am J Surg Pathol.* 1997; 21:226–234.

477. Takata T, Caselitz J, Seifert G. Undifferentiated tumours of salivary glands: Immunocytochemical investigations and differential diagnosis of 22 cases. *Pathol Res Pract.* 1987; 182:161–168.

478. Adkins GF. Low grade basaloid adenocarcinoma of salivary gland in childhood—the so-called hybrid basal cell adenoma-adenoid cystic carcinoma. *Pathology.* 1990; 22:187–190.

479. Batsakis JG, Brannon RB, Sciubba JJ. Monomorphic adenomas of major salivary glands: A histologic study of 96 tumours. *Clin Otolaryngol.* 1981; 6:129–143.

480. Batsakis JG, Mackay B, Ryka AF, Seifert RW. Perinatal sali-

vary gland tumours (embryomas). *J Laryngol Otol.* 1988; 102: 1007–1011.

481. Canalis RF, Mok MW, Fishman SM, Hemenway WG. Congenital basal cell adenoma of the submandibular gland. *Arch Otolaryngol Head Neck Surg.* 1980; 106:284–286.

482. Danzinger H. Adenoid cystic carcinoma of the submaxillary gland in an 8-month-old infant. *Can Med Assoc J.* 1964; 91: 759–761.

483. Harris MD, McKeever P, Robertson JM. Congenital tumours of the salivary gland: A case report and review. *Histopathology.* 1990; 17:155–157.

484. Hsueh C, Gonzalez-Crussi F. Sialoblastoma: A case report and review of the literature on congenital epithelial tumors of salivary gland origin. *Pediatr Pathol.* 1992; 12:205–214, 6311.

485. Taylor GP. Congenital epithelial tumor of the parotid: Sialoblastoma. *Pediatr Pathol.* 1988; 8:447–452.

486. Chen KT. Metastasizing pleomorphic adenoma of the salivary gland. *Cancer.* 1978; 42:2407–2411.

487. Collina G, Eusebi V, Carasoli PT. Pleomorphic adenoma with lymph-node metastases report of two cases. *Pathol Res Pract.* 1989; 184:188–193.

488. Cresson DH, Goldsmith M, Askin FB, Reddick RL, Postma DS, Siegal GP. Metastasizing pleomorphic adenoma with myoepithelial cell predominance. *Pathol Res Pract.* 1990; 186: 795–800.

489. el-Naggar A, Batsakis JG, Kessler S. Benign metastatic mixed tumours or unrecognized salivary carcinomas? *J Laryngol Otol.* 1988; 102:810–812.

490. Freeman SB, Kennedy KS, Parker GS, Tatum SA. Metastasizing pleomorphic adenoma of the nasal septum. *Arch Otolaryngol Head Neck Surg.* 1990; 116: 1331–1333.

491. Gnepp DR, Wenig BM. Malignant mixed tumors. In: Ellis GL, Auclair PL, Gnepp DR, eds. *Surgical Pathology of the Salivary Glands.* Philadelphia: WB Saunders; 1991:350–368.

492. Moberger JG, Eneroth CM. Malignant mixed tumors of the major salivary glands. Special reference to the histologic structure in metastases. *Cancer.* 1968; 21:1198–1211.

493. Youngs GR, Scheuer PJ. Histologically benign mixed parotid tumour with hepatic metastasis. *J Pathol.* 1973; 109:171–172.

494. Crissman JD, Wirman JA, Harris A. Malignant myoepithelioma of the parotid gland. *Cancer.* 1977; 40:3042–3049.

495. Dardick I. Malignant myoepithelioma of parotid salivary gland. *Ultrastruct Pathol.* 1985; 9:163–168.

496. Singh R, Cawson RA. Malignant myoepithelial carcinoma (myoepithelioma) arising in a pleomorphic adenoma of the parotid gland: An immunohistochemical study and review of the literature. *Oral Surg Oral Med Oral Pathol.* 1988; 66:65–70.

497. Alvarez-Canas C, Rodilla IG. True malignant mixed tumor (carcinosarcoma) of the parotid gland. Report of a case with immunohistochemical study. *Oral Surg Oral Med Oral Pathol.* 1996; 81:454–458.

498. Carson HJ, Tojo DP, Chow JM, Hammadeh R, Raslan WF. Carcinosarcoma of salivary glands with unusual stromal components. Report of two cases and review of the literature. *Oral Surg Oral Med Oral Pathol.* 1995; 79:738–746.

499. Gandour-Edwards RF, Donald PJ, Vogt PJ, Munn R, Min KW. Carcinosarcoma (malignant mixed tumor) of the parotid: Report of a case with a pure rhabdomyosarcoma component. *Head Neck.* 1994; 16:379–382.

500. Spraggs PD, Rose DS, Grant HR, Gallimore AP. Post-irradiation carcinosarcoma of the parotid gland. *J Laryngol Otol.* 1994; 108:443–445.

501. Bleiweiss IJ, Huvos AG, Lara J, Strong EW. Carcinosarcoma of the submandibular salivary gland. Immunohistochemical findings. *Cancer.* 1992; 69:2031–2035.

502. Garner SL, Robinson RA, Maves MD, Barnes CH. Salivary gland carcinosarcoma: True malignant mixed tumor. *Ann Otol Rhinol Laryngol.* 1989; 98:611–614.

503. Rumnong V, Banerjee AK, Joshi K, Kataria RN. Carcinosarcoma of parotid gland having osteosarcoma as sarcomatous component: A case report. *Indian J Pathol Microbiol.* 1993; 36: 492–494.

504. Toynton SC, Wilkins MJ, Cook HT, Stafford ND. True malignant mixed tumor of a minor salivary gland. *J Laryngol Otol.* 1994; 108:76–79.

505. Spiro RH, Huvos AG, Strong EW. Adenocarcinoma of salivary origin: Clinicopathologic study of 204 patients. *Am J Surg.* 1982; 144:423–430

506. Pisharodi LR. Low grade papillary adenocarcinoma of minor salivary gland origin. Diagnosis by fine needle aspiration cytology. *Acta Cytol.* 1997; 41:1407–1411.

507. Allen MS Jr, Fitz-Hugh GS, March WL Jr. Low-grade papillary adenocarcinoma of the palate. *Cancer.* 1974; 33:153–158.

508. Fliss DM, Zirkin H, Puterman M, Tovi F. Low-grade papillary adenocarcinoma of buccal mucosa salivary gland origin. *Head Neck Surg.* 1989; 11:237–241.

509. Mills SE, Garland TA, Allen MS Jr. Low-grade papillary adenocarcinoma of palatal salivary gland origin. *Am J Surg Pathol.* 1984; 8:367–374.

510. Slootweg PJ, Muller H. Low-grade adenocarcinoma of the oral cavity: A comparison between the terminal duct and the papillary type. *J Craniomaxillofac Surg.* 1987; 15:359–364.

511. Seifert G, Miehlke A, Haubrich J, Chilla R. *Diseases of the Salivary Glands: Pathology-Diagnosis-Treatment-Facial Nerve Surgery.* Suttgart, Germany: Georg Thieme Verlag; 1986: 248–252

512. Attar A, Scheffer P, Roucayrol AM, Blanchard P. Papillary cystadenocarcinoma of the submaxillary gland. A rare diagnosis. *Rev Stomatol Chir Maxillofac.* 1989; 90:330–333.

513. Blanck C, Eneroth CM, Jakobsson PA. Mucus-producing adenopapillary (non-epidermoid) carcinoma of the parotid gland. *Cancer.* 1971; 28:676–685.

514. Chen NM. Papillary cystadenocarcinoma of the salivary glands: Clinicopathologic analysis of 22 cases. *Chung Hua Kou Chiang Hsueh Tsa Chih.* 1990; 25:102–104, 126.

515. Danford M, Eveson JW, Flood TR. Papillary cystadenocarcinoma of the sublingual gland presenting as a ranula. *Br J Oral Maxillofac Surg.* 1992; 30:270–272.

516. Chen KTK, Hafez GR. Infiltrating salivary duct carcinoma: A clinicopathologic study of five cases. *Arch Otolaryngol.* 1981; 107:37–39.

517. Garland TA, Innes DI, Fechner RE. Salivary duct carcinoma: An analysis of four cases with review of literature. *Am J Clin Pathol.* 1984; 81:436–441.

518. Hui KK, Batsakis JG, Luna MA, Mackay B, Byers RM. Salivary duct adenocarcinoina: A high grade malignancy. *J Laryngol Otol.* 1986; 100:105–114.

519. de Araujo VC, de Souza SOM, Sesso A, Sotto MN, de Araujo NS. Salivary duct carcinoma: Ultrastructural and histogenetic considerations. *Oral Surg Oral Med Oral Pathol.* 1987; 63:592–596.

520. Afzelius LE, Cameron WR, Svensson C. Salivary duct carcinomas: Clinicopathologic study of 12 cases. *Head Neck Surg.* 1987; 9:151–156.

521. Simpson RH, Clarke TJ, Sparsfield PT, Babajews AV. Salivary duct adenocarcinoma. *Histopathology.* 1991; 18:229–235.

522. Barnes L, Rao U, Krause J, Contis L, Schwartz A, Scalamogna P. Salivary duct carcinoma. Part I. A clinicopathologic evaluation and DNA image analysis of 13 cases with review of the literature. *Oral Surg Oral Med Oral Pathol.* 1994; 78:64–73.

523. Gnepp DR, Brannon R. Sebaceous neoplasms of salivary gland origin: Report of 21 cases. *Cancer.* 1984; 53:2155–2170.

524. Gnepp DR. Sebaceous neoplasms of salivary gland origin: A review. In: Sommers S, Rosen PP, eds. *Pathol Annu,* Part 1. 1983; 18:71–102.

525. Batsakis JG, Littler ER, Leahy MS. Sebaceous cell lesions of the head and neck. *Arch Otolaryngol.* 1972; 95:151–157.

526. Silver H, Goldstein MA. Sebaceous cell carcinoma of the parotid region: A review of the literature and a case report. *Cancer.* 1966; 19:1773–1779.

527. Mathis VH. Beitrag zur kenntnis der sialome. *Dtsch Zahn-Mund Kiefer.* 1968; 50:205–208.

528. MacFarland JK, Vilori JB, Palmer JD. Sebaceous cell carcinoma of the parotid gland. *Am J Surg.* 1975; 130:499–501.

529. Shulman J, Waisman J, Morledge D. Sebaceous carcinoma of the parotid gland. *Arch Otolaryngol.* 1973; 98:417–421.

530. Housholder MS, Zeligman I. Sebaceous neoplasms with visceral carcinomas. *Arch Derm.* 1980; 116:61–64.

531. Sikorowa L. Oncocytoma malignum. *Nowotworg.* 1957; 7:125–131.

532. Hamperl IT. Benign and malignant oncocytoma. *Cancer.* 1962; 15:1019–1027.

533. Baziz-Malik G, Gupta DN. Metastasizing (malignant) oncocytoma of the parotid gland. *Z Krebsforch.* 1968; 70:193–197.

534. Fayemi AO, Toker C. Malignant oncocytoma of the parotid gland. *Arch Otolaryngol.* 1974; 99:375–376.

535. Gray SR, Cornog JL, Seo IS. Oncocytic neoplasms of salivary glands: A report of 15 cases including 2 malignant oncocytomas. *Cancer.* 1976; 38:1306–1317.

536. Goode RK, Corio RL. Oncocytic adenocarcinoma of salivary glands. *Oral Surg Oral Med Oral Pathol.* 1988; 65:61–66.

537. DiMaio SI, DiMaio VJM, DiMaio TM, Nicastri AD, Chen CK. Oncocytic carcinoma of the nasal cavity. *South Med J.* 1980; 73:803–806.

538. Luna MA, Batsakis JG, Ordonez NG, Mackay B, Tortoledo ME. Salivary gland adenocarcinomas: A clinicopathologic analysis of three distinctive types. *Semin Diagn Pathol.* 1987; 4:117–135.

539. Balin AK, Fine RM, Golitz LE. Mucinous carcinoma. *J Dermatol Surg Oncol.* 1988; 14:521–524.

540. Reed DN Jr, Hassan AA, Wilson RF. Primary mucinous adenocarcinoma of the trachea: The case for complete surgical resection. *J Surg Oncol.* 1985; 28:29–31.

541. Damiani IM, Damiani KK, Hauck K, Hyams VJ. Mucoepidermoid-adenosquamous carcinoma of the larynx and hypopharynx: A report of 21 cases and a review of the literature. *Otolaryngol Head Neck Surg.* 1981; 89:235–243.

542. Gerughty RM, Hennigar GR, Brown RM. Adeno-squamous carcinoma of the nasal, oral and laryngeal cavities: A clinicopathologic survey of ten cases. *Cancer.* 1968; 22:1140–1155.

543. Siar CH, Ng KIT. Adenosquamous carcinoma of the floor of the mouth and lower alveolus: A radiation-induced lesion? *Oral Surg Oral Med Oral Pathol.* 1987; 63:216–220.

544. Sanner JR. Combined adenosquamous carcinoma and ductal adenoma of the hard and soft palate: Report of case. *J Oral Surg.* 1979; 37:331–334.

545. Batsakis J. Vascular tumors of the salivary glands. *Ann Otol Rhinol Laryngol.* 1986; 95:649–650.

546. Krolls SO, Trodahl JN, Borgers RC. Salivary gland lesions in children: A survey of 430 cases. *Cancer.* 1972; 30:459–469.

547. Tresserra L, Martinez-Mora J, Boix-Ochoa J. Hemangiomas of the parotid gland in children. *J Maxillofac Surg.* 1977; 5:238–241.

548. Baum RK, Perzik SL. Tumors of the parotid gland in children: Review of 40 cases. *Am Surg.* 1965; 31:719–723.

549. Stevenson EW. Hemangioma of the salivary gland: Review of the literature and report of a rare lesion in the submaxillary area. *South Med J.* 1966; 59:1187–1190.

550. Totsuka Y, Fukuda H, Toniita K. Compression therapy for parotid hemangioma in infants: A report of three cases. *J Craniomaxillofac Surg.* 1988; 16:366–370.

551. Noone RB, Brown HJ. Cystic hygroma of the parotid gland. *Am J Surg.* 1970; 120:404–407.

552. Crawford AP. Lymphangioma of the parotid gland. *Med J Aust.* 1981; 2:141–142.

553. Kavanaugh KT, Panje WR. Neurogenic neoplasms of the seventh cranial nerve presenting as a parotid mass. *Am J Otolaryngol.* 1982; 3:53–56.

554. Roos DB, Byars LT, Ackerman LV. Neurilemmomas of the facial nerve presenting as parotid gland tumors. *Ann Surg.* 1956; 144:258–262.

555. Weitzner S. Plexiform neurofibroma of major salivary glands in children. *Oral Surg Oral Med Oral Pathol.* 1980; 50:53–57.

556. Wolff M, Rankow RM. Meningioma of the parotid gland: An insight into the pathogenesis of extracranial meningiomas. *Hum Pathol.* 1971; 2:453–459.

557. Nilsen R, Lind O. Benign fibrous xanthoma of the parotid gland: A case report. *Br J Oral Surg.* 1978–1979; 16:111–114.

558. Ferrari PG, Viva E, Derada TG, Girardi E. Rare case of a fibrous histiocytoma located in the parotid. *Minerva Stomatol.* 1982; 31:693–696.

559. Fata JJ, Rabuzzi DD. Aggressive juvenile fibromatosis presenting as a parotid mass. *Ear Nose Throat J.* 1988; 67:678–684.

560. Majmudar S, Winiarski N. Desmoid tumor presenting as a parotid mass. *JAMA.* 1978; 239:337–339.

561. Baker SE, Jensen JL, Correll RW. Lipomas of the parotid gland. *Oral Surg Oral Med Oral Pathol.* 1981; 52:167–171.

562. Janecka IP, Conley J, Perzin KH, Pitman G. Lipomas presenting as parotid tumors. *Laryngoscope.* 1977; 87:1007–1010.

563. Joner JK, Kuo TT, Griffiths CM, Itharat S. Multiple granular cell tumors. *Laryngoscope.* 1980; 90:1646–1651.

564. Duhig JT, Ayer JP. Vascular leiomyoma: A study of sixty-one cases. *Arch Pathol.* 1959; 68:424–430.

565. Auclair PL, Limgloss IM, Weiss SW, Corio RL. Sarcomas and sarcomatoid neoplasms of the major salivary gland regions: A clinicopathologic and immunohistochemical study of 67 cases and review of the literature. *Cancer.* 1986; 58:1305–1315.

566. Volpe R. Primary sarcomas of the parotid gland: A clinicopathologic report of two cases. *Pathologica.* 1981; 73:541–546.

567. Sandhyamani S, Mahapatra AK, Kapur BM. Leiomyosarcoma of the parotid gland. *Aust NZ J Surg.* 1983; 53:179–181.

568. Benjamin E, Wells S, Fox H, Reeve NL, Knox F. Malignant fibrous histiocytoma of salivary glands. *J Clin Pathol.* 1982; 35:946–953.

569. Seifert G, Oehne H. Mesenchymal (nonepithelial) salivary gland tumors: Analysis of 167 cases of the salivary gland register. *Laryngol Rhinol Otol* (Stuttg). 1986; 65:485–491.

570. Piscioli F, Antolini M, Pusiol T, Dalri P, Lo-Bello MD, Mair K. Malignant schwannoma of the submandibular gland: A case report. *ORLJ.* 1986; 48:156–161.

571. Cernea P, Debry D, Laudenbacli P, et al. Hemangiopercytome de la parotide. *Rev Stomatol Chir Maxillofac.* 1969; 70: 132–135.

572. Neal TF, Starke WR. Hemangiopericytoma of the parotid gland: A case report with autopsy. *Laryngoscope.* 1973; 83: 1953–1958.

573. Yeh C-K, Fox PC, Fox CH, Travis WD, Lane HC, Baum BJ. Kaposi's sarcoma of the parotid gland in acquired immunodeficiency syndrome. *Oral Surg Oral Med Oral Pathol.* 1989; 67:308–312.

574. Manning JT, Raymon AK, Batsakis JG. Extraosseous osteogenic sarcoma of the parotid gland. *J Laryngol Otol.* 1986; 100:239–242.

575. Jones JK, Baker HW. Liposarcoma of the parotid gland: Report of a case. *Arch Otolaryngol.* 1980; 106:497–499.

576. Takata T, Caselitz J, Seifert G. Undifferentiated tumours of salivary glands. *Pathol Res Pract.* 1987; 182:161–168.

577. Gleeson MJ, Bennett MH, Cawson RA. Lymphomas of salivary glands. *Cancer.* 1986; 58:699–704.

578. Hyman GA, Wolff M. Malignant lymphomas of the salivary glands: Review of the literature and report of 33 new cases, including four cases associated with the lymphoepithelial lesion. *Am J Clin Pathol.* 1976; 65:421–438.

579. Schmid U, Helbron D, Lennert K. Primary malignant lymphomas localized in salivary glands. *Histopathology.* 1982; 6: 673–687.

580. Schmid U, Helbron D, Lennert K. Development of malignant lymphoma in myoepithelial sialadenitis (Sjögren's syndrome). *Virchows Arch [A].* 1982; 395:11–43.

581. Bienenstock J. Gut and bronchus associated lymphoid tissue: An overview. *Adv Exp Med Biol.* 1982; 149:471–477.

582. Isaacson P, Wright DH. Malignant lymphoma of mucosa-associated lymphoid tissue: A distinctive type of B-cell lymphoma. *Cancer.* 1983; 52:1410–1416.

583. Isaacson P, Wright DH. Extranodal malignant lymphoma arising from mucosa-associated lymphoid tissue. *Cancer.* 1984; 53:2515–2524.

584. Isaacson PG, Spencer J. Malignant lymphoma of mucosa-associated lymphoid tissue. *Histopathology.* 1987; 11:445–462.

585. Hyjek E, Smith WJ, Isaacson PG. Primary B-cell lymphoma

of salivary glands and its relationship to myoepithelial sialadenitis. *Hum Pathol.* 1988; 19:766–776.

586. Sheibani K, Burke JS, Swartz WG, Nademanee A, Winberg CD. Monocytoid B-cell lymphoma: Clinicopathologic study of 21 cases of a unique type of low-grade lymphoma. *Cancer.* 1988; 62:1531–1538.

587. Schmid U, Lennert K, Gloor F. Immunosialadenitis (Sjögren's syndrome) and lymphoproliferation. *Clin Exp Rheumatol.* 1989; 7:175–180.

588. Watkin CT, MacLennan KA, Hobsley M. Lymphomas presenting as lumps in the parotid region. *Br J Surg.* 1984; 71: 701–702.

589. Kassan S, Thomas T, Moutsopoulos HM, et al. Increased risk of lymphoma in sicca syndrome. *Ann Intern Med.* 1978; 89: 888–892.

590. Colby TV, Dorfman RF. Malignant lymphomas involving the salivary glands. *Pathol Ann.* 1979; 14:307–324.

591. Kerrigan DP, Irons J, Chen I-M. bcl-2 gene rearrangement in salivary gland lymphoma. *Am J Surg Pathol.* 1990; 14:1133–1138.

592. Takahashi H, Cheng J, Fujita S, et al. Primary malignant lymphoma of the salivary gland: A tumor of mucosa associated lymphoid tissue. *J Oral Pathol Med.* 1992; 21:318–325.

CHAPTER 8

Larynx, Hypopharynx, and Trachea

I. CLINICAL CONSIDERATIONS FOR NON-NEOPLASTIC LESIONS OF THE LARYNX

■ PEAK WOO

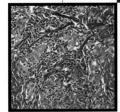

REACTIVE EPITHELIAL CHANGES

Several clinical forms of benign reactive epithelial changes can involve the vocal fold, including cysts, sulcus vocalis, mucosal bridge, benign keratosis, and vascular ectasia. Although cysts and sulcus vocalis are considered by Bouchayer et al[1] to be congenital in origin, it is likely that epithelial reaction to voice abuse and environmental exposure contribute to their development in adults. They are seen more frequently in voice professionals and those with chronic laryngitis than in the general population.[2]

The squamous epithelium of the vocal cord is capable of a variety of morphologic reactions in response to inflammation, irritation, and usage. The epithelial changes in patients with sulcus vocalis and mucosal bridge cannot be differentiated from those of chronic hyperplastic laryngitis. These changes include hyperplasia of the prickle layer, parakeratosis, and hyperkeratosis. Deep to the epithelium there is fibrosis of the superficial lamina propria with inflammatory cellular infiltrate. The lack of pathologic differentiation between hyperplasia and hyperkeratosis and the clinical entities of sulcus vocalis and hyperplastic laryngitis has contributed to some confusion in the diagnosis of sulcus vocalis and its incidence. In Europe and Japan, sulcus vocalis appears to be a far more common diagnosis than in the United States. However, this trend may be reversing with improved recognition that glottal furrow is a common finding seen during videoendoscopy and microlaryngoscopy.[3–5]

Vocal cord cysts affect adults primarily and children occasionally. These cysts may be congenital or acquired. The cyst wall may be lined by squamous epithelium or by respiratory or glandular epithelium. The cyst's contents are determined by the cyst lining and may range from cheesy keratin to watery saliva. The lined cysts have variable degrees of cyst wall reaction and fibrosis, which contribute to the ease with which they can be managed surgically. Cysts may develop as a result of microtrauma and displacement of the squamous epithelium into Reinke's space. Alternatively, mucous cysts may develop in Reinke's space secondary to microtrauma with obstruction of the ductal elements of minor salivary glands.

It is generally agreed that chronic inflammation and irritation represent important factors in the etiology of chronic hyperplastic laryngitis. Epithelial hyperplasia represents one form of tissue reaction to chronic irritation and inflammation. Clinical terms that have been used to describe this condition in the larynx include laryngitis sicca, chronic hyperplastic laryngitis, pachydermia of the larynx, leukoplakia, benign keratosis, and others. Histologic examination of tissue often fails to differentiate between these clinical forms. Chronic hyperplastic laryngitis may be thought of as a variant of a chronic inflammatory disorder that has progressed to vocal fold epithelial changes.

Clinical Presentation

Sulcus Vocalis

Patients with sulcus vocalis present with voice fatigue and chronic, unremitting hoarseness of prolonged duration. Left untreated, the voice quality may deteriorate slowly over a period of months to years until voice complaints prompt a referral. Affected patients may have been evaluated by multiple physicians and have been diagnosed as having chronic laryngitis, muscular tension dysphonia, or laryngeal edema. The lack of visible lesions on the vocal folds is associated with pressure and strain on phonation with a rough, coarse voice quality. Breathiness may be mixed with the rough voice quality if there is glottal incompetence. Dysphonia resulting from increased muscular tension in the larynx and neck is associated with (1) palpably increased phonatory muscle tension in the extralaryngeal and suprahyoid muscles; (2) elevation of the larynx in the neck on increasing vocal pitch; (3) an open posterior glottic chink between the arytenoid cartilages on phonation, and (4) variable degrees of mucosal changes.[6]

Cysts

Patients with vocal cord cysts have a husky, veiled voice that is difficult to differentiate from the voice changes caused by nodules and polyps. Cysts are often confused with vocal nodules because they may be difficult to differentiate when small. Unlike nodules, cysts do not respond to behavioral voice therapy to reduce contact stress. Videostroboscopic examination of vocal fold vibration is highly diagnostic in those patients with a differential diagnosis of vocal nodules who have not shown improvement with behavioral therapy.

Vascular Ectasia and Varicose Veins of the Vocal Cord

Vascular ectasia and varicose veins of the vocal cord are unusual lesions that involve the vocal fold edge and are most commonly found in women. Occasionally, dilated vessels appear on the vocal folds following trauma, such as that induced by radiation therapy or surgical stripping. The patients at risk for varices are female performers and voice professionals who are subject to considerable vocal strain. The dilated vessels may increase the risk of vocal fold hemorrhage by varix rupture. More commonly, the varix becomes problematic as a result of its dilation during voice warm-up exercises, interfering with performance by its effect on vocal fold vibration.[7]

Hyperplastic Laryngitis

Hyperplastic laryngitis is a condition characterized by chronic inflammation, squamous cell metaplasia, and epithelial keratinization. The cause of this condition is chronic inflammation. Thus, it is seen largely in male patients, in smokers, and in those exposed to industrial pollutants. Gastroesophageal reflux disease (GERD) has been implicated as contributing to chronic hyperplastic laryngitis. Other terms used to describe this entity include pachydermia laryngica, laryngitis sicca, and leukoplakia. The combination of heavy smoking, exposure to chronic laryngeal irritants, and vocal abuse contributes to the development of this entity, although its exact pathogenesis is not known.

The malignant potential of chronic hyperplastic laryngitis cannot be determined by cytologic study or physical examination alone. The presence of hyperplastic laryngitis must be considered to be a possible cofactor for cancerous degeneration despite the low incidence of this degeneration.[8] Affected patients may present with hoarse voice; chronic dry cough; and dry, crusted, or rarely, blood-tinged sputum.

Symptoms and Signs

Sulcus Vocalis

The vocal function of 126 patients with sulcus vocalis was evaluated by Hirano et al[5] using a test battery of multidimensional evaluation items. Of the 126 patients, 31 had a unilateral sulcus and 95 had bilateral lesions. The voice of most patients had a mild degree of hoarseness with a breathy quality. An incomplete glottic closure, a small vibratory amplitude, and a small mucosal wave were frequently observed during the stroboscopic examination. The maximal phonation time, fundamental frequency range, and sound pressure-level range of phonation were decreased, whereas the airflow during phonation was increased.[5] If the sulcus vocalis has a distinct groove, it may be seen on deep inspiration as a vocal cord duplication or a glottal furrow. Smaller sulci may be hidden on the undersurface of the vibrating edge and may not be discovered until microlaryngoscopy is performed. The stroboscopic features of spindle-shaped vocal cord closure with bowing of the affected vocal cord and reduced vibratory amplitude are characteristic of sulcus vocalis. In cases in which a sulcus vocalis is suspected, diagnostic microlaryngoscopy is useful in establishing a definitive diagnosis.

During microlaryngoscopy, it is very important to use a blunt probe to palpate the vocal fold edge. A linear sulcus may thus be identified during palpation as an epithelium-lined groove or a slit that attaches deeply to the vocal ligament. The base of the sulcus may be thickened by keratin or may be white and fibrous, and devoid of the usual Reinke's space (Fig. 8–1).

Cysts

Cysts of the vocal fold are usually solitary, although multiple cysts (Fig. 8–2) and complex cysts (Fig. 8–3) may be seen. The diagnosis is easily established during microlaryngoscopy using magnification and palpation. There may be a small depression on the contralateral vocal fold, or there may be epithelial thickening over the cyst. However, small cysts cause a characteristic bump on the edge of the vocal fold

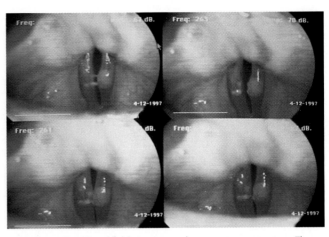

FIGURE 8–2 Vocal fold cyst on stroboscopic examination. The cyst causes a bulge of the affected vocal fold and, consequently, poor closure. There is reduced vocal fold vibratory amplitude and loss of the mucosal wave.

and can be confirmed easily by cordotomy and direct inspection.

Vascular Ectasia and Varix

Vascular ectasia may be easily identified if it is on the superior surface of the vocal fold (Fig. 8–4), especially if the vessels are dilated and cause a nodular irregularity. However, the ectasia may involve the undersurface of the vocal fold, in which case it may be exceedingly difficult to diagnoses. Because the fluctuating size of the varix depends on voice use, it may be necessary to stress the varix by asking the speaker or singer to perform at maximal performance levels prior to examination with videostroboscopy. Examination of the undersurface of the vocal folds may be facilitated by asking the patient to sing or speak in a loud, low voice. This will enhance the phase difference between the upper and the lower

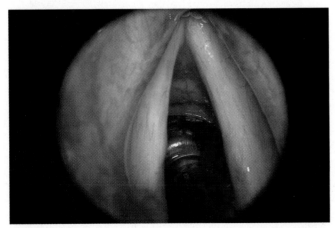

FIGURE 8–1 Sulcus vocalis. The mid-cord glottal furrow is white, and adehsion to the vocal ligament is obvious on palpation. During microlaryngoscopy, the examiner should carefully palpate and probe the vocal folds, as these may be on the undersurface of the vocal fold.

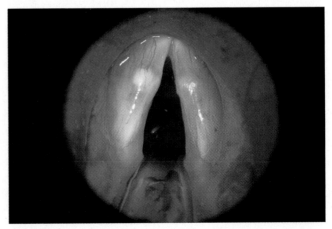

FIGURE 8–3 Bilateral vocal fold cysts. These lesions were misdiagnosed as vocal cord nodules for many months owing to the patient's clinical appearance.

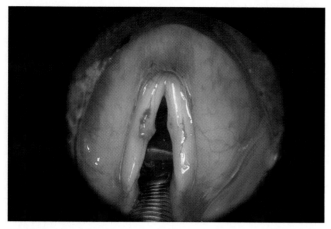

FIGURE 8-4 Vascular ectasia of the vocal folds. There are multiple, dilated, ectatic vessels on the superior surface of the vocal folds. The vocal folds show reactive nodular changes at the membranous contact point.

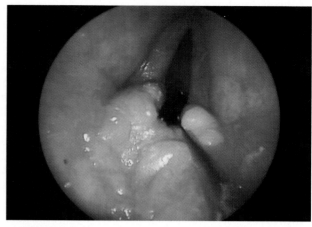

FIGURE 8-5 Pachydermia laryngica. The patient had chronic laryngitis and a posterior glottis that was obliterated by thick, keratotic tissue. The vocal folds are hyperemic, dry, and have a frosted glass appearance.

edge of the vocal folds and permit the examination of the lower lip of the vocal fold during closure, while the upper lip is still in the abducted phase.

Hyperplastic Laryngitis

The most common symptom of hyperplastic laryngitis is chronic hoarseness, which may show some fluctuation. The patient may complain of chronic sore throat, chronic throat clearing, throat irritation, and chronic cough. The degree of involvement of the larynx may be variable but is usually diffuse. Early in the disease process, the larynx looks dry and the vocal fold mucous cover and light reflecting off the mucosa is broken, giving the appearance of a "salt and pepper" larynx. Involvement of the larynx and vocal fold may be characterized by a "frosted glass" appearance as the submucosa becomes increasingly swollen and red. Early epithelial changes may be subtle. Examination of the larynx by a magnified telescope offers the best view. The vocal fold epithelium has a frosted glass appearance, along with edema and surface stippling (Fig. 8–5). These changes may be patchy or localized and may occur over several sites within the larynx. When viewed by mirror examination, early vocal fold thickening may be difficult to distinguish from retained, thick mucus. Conversely, thickened mucus that is retained on one side of the vocal folds may be easily misinterpreted as a white lesion. In these patients, stroboscopic examination is most useful.

Early in the disease process, the vocal fold cover continues to vibrate and show vibratory amplitude. Later, with increased inflammation and keratinization, the vibratory amplitude is lost (Fig. 8–6). The patient must strain to produce simple tones. There is progressive loss of dynamic range in both amplitude and frequency. The hypertrophic changes over the true cords are usually associated with increased,

thick, inspissated mucus over the larynx and trachea. The false vocal fold usually hypertrophies as the patient strains to use false vocal fold vibration as the new vocal sound source, producing voice by ventricular phonation. The differential diagnosis of chronic hyperplastic laryngitis should include carcinoma, granulomatous laryngitis, systemic infiltration of the larynx by amyloidosis, and chronic staphylo-

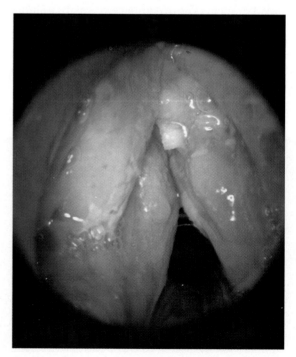

FIGURE 8-6 Severe chronic hyperplastic laryngitis. The sites of involvement include the true and false vocal folds. This iron worker is a heavy smoker and worked within a blasting foundry. The biopsy showed mild dysplasia with acute and chronic inflammation.

coccal or tuberculous laryngitis. In some patients, a definitive diagnosis can be established only by microlaryngoscopy, culture, and biopsy studies.

Treatment

Speech therapy and surgery are two modalities that have been used to treat sulcus vocalis. Primary speech therapy alone is usually unsuccessful owing to the firm tethering of epithelia to vocal ligament. Surgical management has included microlaryngoscopy, microlaryngoscopy with steroid injection, microlaryngoscopy with fat injection, and laryngeal framework surgery. The practice of treating sulcus vocalis by vocal fold stripping is neither necessary nor recommended. Bouchayer's method[1] of microdissection and excision of a small sulcus vocalis has been used with success by this author, although the extent of vibratory restoration has been variable. The technique utilizes microsurgical instruments with magnification. It involves (1) meticulous dissection of the epithelium from the dense attachment to the vocal ligament; (2) excision of the sulcus vocalis; (3) redraping of the mucosa over the vocal fold edge; and (4) injection of steroids to reduce fibrosis. As with a scar excision of the vocal fold, this technique works well with small defects and a small sulcus. Ford et al[2] have analyzed the various problems associated with sulcus vocalis repair and have correctly concluded that there is no one best treatment technique. Other techniques have been proposed, including slicing mucosa, followed by intensive vocal rehabilitation. The aim of the surgery is to detach the mucosa of the sulcus and to interrupt the longitudinal fibrotic tension lines.[9] To facilitate the dissection of the epithelium from the vocal ligament, the submucosal infusion technique described by Kass et al[10] may be used. Although the submucosal infusion technique is most helpful when the vocal fold epithelium requires resection and/or when extensive dissection in the superficial lamina propria is necessary, the infusion technique can help to identify the site of the tethering better than blunt dissection alone.[10] Endoscopic microsuture repair of vocal fold defects can also be used to rotate the sulcus edge after resection to a noncritical vibratory segment.[11] If the defect in the vocal fold remains after endoscopic repair, alternative methods of surgical rehabilitation include phonosurgery by laryngoplasty and fat augmentation. The author has treated a large sulcus vocalis by a combination of endoscopic microflap elevation, excision of the sulcus vocalis, and lipoinjection. Voice improvement was documented by improved voice and vocal fold vibration. After surgery, aggressive postoperative rehabilitation by a voice therapist knowledgeable in scarred vocal fold rehabilitation is necessary to restore vibration to the stiffened vocal folds.

Vocal fold cysts (see Fig. 8–3) are best treated without the laser, using fine microlaryngeal instruments. Because these pathologic lesions lie in the subepithelial layer, a microflap technique or cordotomy that allows the removal of the lesion while sparing the overlying mucosa results in a superior functional outcome. The technique of cordotomy has been described by Bouchayer and others.[1,12,13] Care must be taken to remove the epithelial lining and sac in order to prevent recurrence. The small mucosal incision on the superior surface of the vocal fold should be made over the offending lesion; identification of the lesion as a cyst or polyp may be accomplished by careful dissection of the overlying epithelium. Cysts are dissected from the vocal ligament attachments and the superficial layer of the lamina propria by blunt and sharp dissection under microscopic control (Fig. 8–7). After a cyst is evacuated, the mucosal flap is replaced. The minimal mucosal incision should heal without severe disturbance. Occasionally, fibrin glue is used to weld the tissue flaps together, although this has not been necessary in the author's experience.

Vocal fold varix and vascular ectasia may require surgical treatment if there is an impairment of performance that cannot be compensated for by singing or rehabilitation methods. Surgery should also be

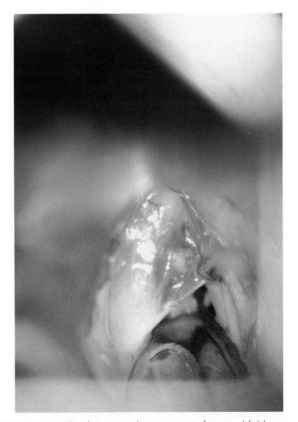

FIGURE 8–7 Cordotomy and evacuation of a vocal fold cyst. The incision is made on the superior surface of the vocal fold. Dissection to delineate the cyst wall is done with fine picks and elevators and the cyst is removed.

considered in patients with recurrent vocal fold hemorrhages secondary to the offending varix. The use of a microspot CO_2 laser and microcautery are two techniques that have been described for the coagulation of small vessels. If the vascular ectasia is large, it is best treated by excision using microscissors (Fig. 8–8). Care should be taken to excise a small length of the offending feeding vessel so as to prevent vascular leakage and reformation of the varix.

Chronic hyperplastic laryngitis is difficult to treat because: (1) it is difficult to achieve an excellent functional voice result owing to the involvement of Reinke's space by chronic inflammation; and (2) the process is often diffuse and the epithelium that remains for resurfacing the excised mucosa is poor in quality. Treatment of chronic hyperplastic laryngitis begins by removal of the identifiable mucosal irritants and reversal of chronic inflammation. Strategies include smoking cessation, reduction of industrial irritants, control of GERD by empirical treatment with proton pump inhibitors, and voice therapy to reduce abuse. Inhalation of steam and use of systemic and inhaled mucokinetic drugs can do much to reduce the symptoms of chronic hoarseness. By optimizing local mucosal hygiene, the effects of surgical scarring may be minimized.

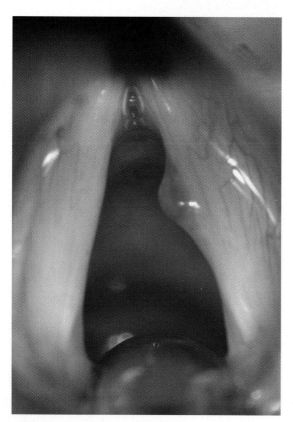

FIGURE 8–8   Large, ectatic vessel causing polyp formation in a young female patient.

After surgery, voice rest, aggressive hydration, mucolytic drugs, antibiotics, and antacids are prescribed. The patient should be monitored closely and should not return to work in a dusty, loud environment before the proper healing has been completed.

Operative removal of chronic hyperplastic laryngitis has several goals:

1. Operative biopsy of the abnormal mucosa to establish a histologic diagnosis
2. Operative removal of the offending mass to restore normal voice patterns, provided adequate healing can occur by ingrowth of more normal epithelium
3. Prevention of neoplastic degeneration in cases of hyperplasia with dysplasia

The microlaryngeal techniques for lesion removal may be facilitated by laser technology. Vasoconstrictors may be infused into the subepithelial layer before surgery, and may be applied during the surgery, to improve hemostasis and margin control.[10]

The treatment of hyperplastic laryngitis incorporates surgical and medical modalities. Biopsy-proven benign keratosis is best treated by microlaryngoscopy and careful removal of the affected epithelium. Using modern microlaryngeal surgical techniques, it is often possible to find a plane between the abnormal epithelium and the normal subepithelial layer. The importance of selected epithelial removal while leaving intact the jelly-like Reinke's layer should be emphasized. Vocal fold stripping should no longer be used in the treatment of hyperplastic laryngitis. Unlike vocal stripping, careful epithelial removal using modern microsurgical instruments and techniques leaves intact the vocal ligament and the superficial layer of the lamina propria.

The surgical technique for resection of epithelial lesions has been well described by Kleinsasser[13] and others. The author's preferred technique is to make an incision, grasp the lesion with microforceps, and gently tease the epithelial layer away with a sharp pick. When the abnormal epithelium has been dissected free, microscissors are used to remove the epithelium for histologic examination. The residual epithelial mucosal tags are then trimmed with microscissors or a CO_2 laser in microspot mode. This creates a linear vocal fold edge and allows smooth epithelial resurfacing.

In the postoperative period, careful avoidance of trauma, irritants, and edema is necessary to decrease scarring and fibrosis. Steroids and antibiotics are given in the postoperative period to reduce vocal fold inflammation and edema. Voice rest for a period of 1 week is advisable. Antireflux and antitussive agents to reduce cough and throat clearing are routinely prescribed to reduce the risk of further laryngeal trauma.[14]

Careful removal of epithelial lesions offers the best chance for functional voice return. Despite such careful surgical approaches, some residual vocal disabilities can be anticipated after epithelial cover resection. Some decrement in vibratory amplitude can occur despite excellent healing and a normal epithelium. The voice quality usually improves, but it may remain decreased in loudness and dynamic range. Such results should be anticipated and discussed with the patient prior to surgical treatment. The presence of mucosal vibratory changes in these patients should not be construed as a poor surgical result.

The patient with recurrent benign mucosal lesions after previous surgical removal represents an especially challenging problem. These patients may have already undergone multiple microlaryngeal excisions for benign vocal fold lesions. Despite this, epithelial lesions may continue to develop. If laryngeal irritants have been adequately removed and the mucosal hygiene has been maximized, the decision as to whether to perform repeat laryngeal excision must be individualized. Although complete removal of the offending lesion offers the best chance for cure, involvement of the anterior commissure and subglottic areas may make complete resection difficult without risk of web and scar formation. In some patients with benign keratosis, it is reasonable to monitor the lesion by selected biopsy studies rather than to repeat vocal fold cover resection. Such an approach demands careful follow-up examinations and frequent visits by a compliant patient.

Radiologic and other diagnostic tests are usually not indicated in the work-up. Endolaryngeal cytologic study has been advocated but does not replace histologic diagnosis based on biopsy studies. In the patient with chronic hyperplastic laryngitis, the suspicion of granulomatous laryngitis and other systemic illness with laryngeal findings will dictate the extent of radiographic work-up.

Prognosis

The prognosis for voice restoration and subsequent voice improvement in patients with sulcus vocalis, vascular ectasia, or vocal cord cyst is excellent. The prognosis for restoration of normal voice in patients with chronic hyperplastic laryngitis is guarded.

Controversies

Controversy exists as to the malignant potential of hyperplastic lesions of the vocal folds. In patients with chronic hyperplastic laryngitis, repeated vocal cord stripping is not indicated unless dysplasia or carcinoma in situ has been identified. Careful endoscopic surveillance, conservative biopsy studies, removal of gross lesions, and, in some patients, enrollment in a chemoprevention protocol using retinoic acid therapy have been used by the author for selected patients.

VOCAL CORD POLYPS, NODULES, AND REINKE'S EDEMA

Clinical Presentation

Vocal cord polyps are common benign vocal cord lesions that come to attention because of chronic hoarseness. The duration of hoarseness may be variable depending on the awareness of the patient and the tolerance of the individual to voice disturbance. Occasionally, large vocal cord polyps present with obstruction and stridor. Sudden airway obstruction due to pedunculated laryngeal polyps has been reported.[15] Vocal cord polyps tend to occur more frequently in male adults and tend to be unilateral, but may occasionally be bilateral. Development of isolated polyps is associated with vocal fold trauma, such as that caused by voice abuse or violent coughing. A variety of polyps has been described based on clinical description, including hemorrhagic polyps, sessile or pedunculated polyps, fibromatous polyps, edematous polyps, myxomatous polyps, and hemangiomatous polyps. All are related to the pathophysiology of microtrauma to the subepithelial layer, vascular disruption, hemorrhage, and vascular leakage followed by inflammation and repair. These lesions are, therefore, never true tumors, although occasionally, the pathologic results may suggest a hemangioma rather than a vocal cord polyp. The polyps develop from submucosal vessel hemorrhage, inflammatory response, and repair and, thus, are often associated with a large feeding vessel or groups of vessels (Fig. 8–9).

True vocal cord nodules are almost exclusively a disorder affecting females (Fig. 8–10). The nodules

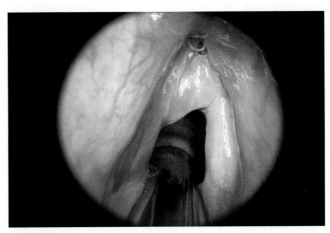

FIGURE 8–9 Vocal cord polyp. This large, unilateral, vocal cord polyp is associated with vocal fold hemorrhage.

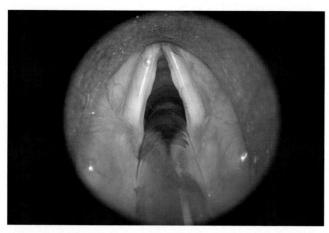

FIGURE 8-10 Bilateral vocal fold nodules. This pubescent female cheerleader had a history of chronic hoarseness. Note the symmetry of the lesion, with thickening at the midmembranous fold. Although most vocal fold nodules respond to speech therapy, larger fibrotic nodules can be treated efficiently with surgery followed by behavioral therapy.

are always bilateral and occur at the contact point of the vocal folds during phonation. The mid-membranous vocal fold is the most common site of vocal nodules. Rarely, multiple bilateral nodules can be seen on the vocal fold edge. Many patients without true nodules, but with polyps or cysts, are diagnosed as having vocal nodules. Thus, true vocal nodules are defined as bilateral, epithelial, and subepithelial injury secondary to microtrauma from voice abuse. The true vocal nodule, then, is a phonologic disorder that secondarily causes organic changes in the vocal fold.

Patients at risk for vocal nodules are those with voice professions that demand overuse or abuse of voice. Teachers, singing students, receptionists, and others with vocally challenging professions requiring them to perform vocal tasks in loud environments are especially at risk. The clinical presentation is similar to that of vocal cord polyps. Chronic hoarseness and early vocal fatigue are typical. The patient may complain of a voice that improves after vocal rest but is unable to be sustained through the day. If the patient is a singer, the voice may be normal in the speaking range but deficient in soft, gentle phonation.

Reinke's edema is a clinical entity that is distinct from vocal cord polyps and vocal nodules (Fig. 8-11). Polypoid corditis and polypoid degeneration are other terms used for this lesion. Most patients with Reinke's edema are smokers. Females present with a pitch disturbance that often causes them to be mistaken for males when talking on the phone. Chronic hoarseness and voice loss may prompt an otolaryngologic consultation. The boundaries of Reinke's space are limited to the condensation of the conus elasticus fibers onto the vocal fold edge. The squamous epithelium of the vocal cord (and its transition to the respiratory epithelium above and below) is loosely draped over the vocal fold ligament, and there is a potential space between the fibrous vocal ligament and the epithelial cover. This potential space is restricted to the triangular subepithelial space, and is limited by the superior and inferior arcuate lines. Excessive accumulation of fluid and protein in this space results in laryngeal edema and polypoid tissue formation.

The different pathophysiologic characteristics of these entities have recently been investigated by new histologic methods. Gray et al[16] have examined benign laryngeal lesions for patterns of injury indicated by deposition of fibronectin and collagen type IV. An immunoperoxidase technique has been used to compare 33 fresh or paraffin-embedded tissues with regard to their staining of monoclonal antibodies directed against fibronectin and collagen type IV. Two types of patterns have been recognized. One pattern shows intense fibronectin deposition in the superficial layer of the lamina propria, often coupled with basement membrane zone injury, as indicated by thick, collagen type IV bands. The other pattern shows rare basement membrane zone injury and very little fibronectin deposition. The first pattern correlates most closely with nodules, whereas the second pattern is more closely linked with Reinke's edema. The practical implications of differentiating between these clinical entities is that vocal fold nodules are attributable to microtrauma, which may be reversible, whereas vocal polyps and Reinke's edema are caused by submucosal stromal hemorrhage and deposition, which may require surgical correction.

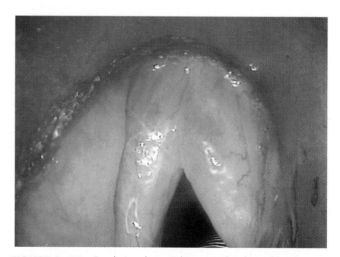

FIGURE 8-11 Reinke's edema (also termed polypoid corditis and polypoid degeneration). This 63-year-old female smoker wanted to undergo surgery to correct her voice because it was frequently mistaken for a man's voice. The massive vocal folds caused a lowered pitch and a husky voice characterized by vocal fry.

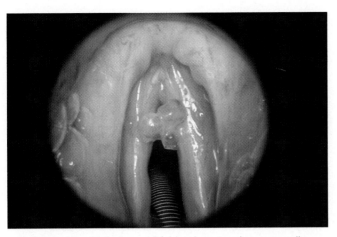

FIGURE 8-12 Multiple vocal fold polyps mistaken as papillomas of the larynx in a voice abuser and teacher.

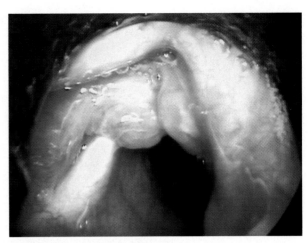

Figure 8-13 Supraglottic polyps. Bilateral herniation of the false vocal folds into the glottic aperture produced dysphonia despite normal vocal folds. CO_2 laser excision was successful.

Diagnosis

The diagnosis of vocal cord polyps may be easily established by office endoscopy and videostroboscopy. Large, pedunculated lesions can be appreciated with a mirror. The location of vocal cord polyps may be variable, but is generally limited to the membranous portion of the vocal fold (Fig. 8-12). Occasionally, a pedunculated polyp may be seen to arise from the subglottic or the supraglottic surface of the vocal fold (Fig. 8-13). Most commonly, however, the vocal fold polyp is seen at or close to the vibratory margin of the vocal fold edge. Smaller lesions and those that are difficult to differentiate from vocal fold cysts or nodules are most easily diagnosed by videostroboscopy. One of the most useful indications for stroboscopic examination is in the differential diagnosis of benign mucosal lesions and the early detection of small lesions of the vocal fold cover that cannot easily be visualized (Fig. 8-14). The clinical implication of accurate differentiation between cysts, nodules, and polyps lies in their management and the choice of surgical treatment. Vocal cord nodules are treated very effectively by speech therapy alone. By contrast, vocal fold cysts should be removed by microlaryngoscopy using a cordotomy and microflap approach. Vocal cord polyps are treated efficiently by microsurgery and voice therapy, and occasionally by voice therapy alone. The isolated polyp has an asymmetric appearance, causing reduced vibratory amplitude of the vocal fold with reduction in mucosal wave. The amount of disturbance is often limited to the vocal fold edge. Because of the exophytic or pedunculated appearance, the disturbance of the mucosal vibratory margin of the affected vocal fold may be minimal (Fig. 8-15).

Vocal fold nodules have a symmetric appearance. They are variable in size and stiffness and may have superficial keratin deposits on the surface. Small vocal nodules are easily missed by mirror examination

if the larynx is viewed in abduction. On phonation, the preferential contact of the nodal point is easily detected if the larynx is viewed with stroboscopic light. When the vocal fold nodules are small and soft, the vocal fold edge is pale and translucent. The vocal folds oscillate with good vibratory amplitude and the mucosal wave propagates across the nodule. Excessive air leakage through the glottis is heard as husky voice quality. The vocal cords adduct, assuming an hourglass appearance. More organized vocal cord nodules of longer duration are associated with a worse voice and have poorer rehabilitation potential with voice therapy alone. Videostroboscopy shows the nodules to be independent masses that may not vibrate on phonation. The mature nodes

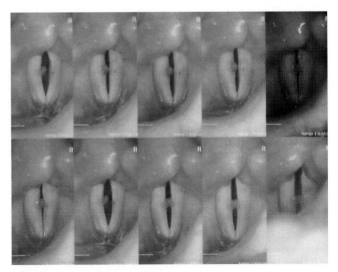

FIGURE 8-14 Hemorrhagic polyp in a folk singer. Stroboscopic examination of the glottal cycle shows irregular, incomplete closure. There is reduced amplitude of vibration and mucosal wave on the vocal fold on the side of the polyp.

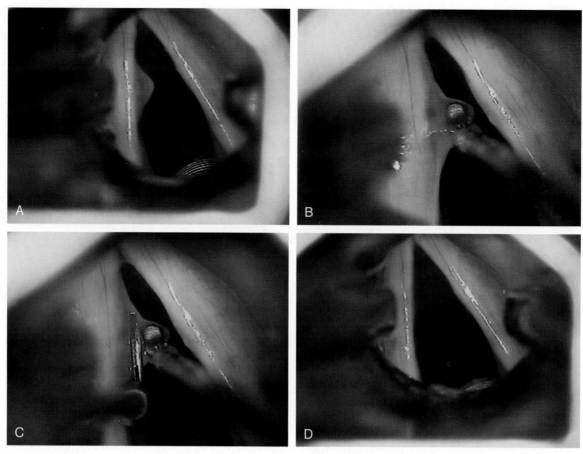

FIGURE 8–15 Surgical excision of a simple polyp by microlaryngoscopy without CO_2 laser. *A,* The polyp is identified. *B,* Gentle retraction medially with small cup forceps shows the cleavage plane and the attachment site of the polyp. *C,* Forward-angled scissors are used to define the angle of excision and the amount of resection. Note that care is taken to "leave a little extra" on the vocal fold to avoid overexcision of the vocal fold cover. *D,* At completion, the surgery should result in a straight vocal fold.

have increased stiffness and cause a greater reduction of vibratory amplitude and mucosal wave. This is associated with increased fibrosis under the basement membrane and increased keratin on the surface. Rarely is surgical treatment necessary for nodules. Recent reports have suggested a correlation between vocal nodules and failed voice training with anterior commissure microwebs.[17,18]

Reinke's edema, once it has progressed to polypoid change, can easily be appreciated with mirror laryngoscopy and/or fiberoptic laryngoscopy. This lesion is characterized by a pale, bluish appearance due to the degree of excessive superficial lamina propria. The vocal folds have increased mass and vibrate at a lowered fundamental frequency. Because of the symmetric involvement, the vocal folds vibrate symmetrically.

Muscle tension dysphonia, associated with polyps, vocal nodules, chronic laryngitis, or polypoid degeneration, is often present.[19] Because of the association of smoking and voice abuse in patients with laryngeal polyps, there is often evidence of poor mucosal hygiene of the vocal fold cover. Dehydration, mild chronic laryngitis, and thick, inspissated mucus are often noted on endoscopic examination of patients with vocal cord polyps. When there is evidence of chronic laryngeal inflammation, reflux laryngitis and nonspecific laryngitis should be evaluated in conjunction with the more obvious diagnosis of laryngeal polyps.

Radiologic Evaluation

Because of the ease with which lesions of the vocal folds can be appreciated using modern office and operative laryngoscopic instrumentation, radiographic examination is not indicated in most patients with vocal nodes, polyps, or cysts. Large polyps arising from the false vocal cords and subglottic masses should be included in the differential diagnosis. Diagnostic studies for these entities should include appropriate soft-tissue films of the neck and computed tomography (CT) scanning of the larynx. Among the major technologic improvements in diagnostic laryngoscopic equipment for the office and endoscopy suite are quartz and xenon light sources, flexible laryngoscopes, fiberoptic rod lighting, special-purpose laryngoscopes, and rigid telescopes.[20]

These, combined with videoendoscopy and stroboscopy, should allow the clinician to differentiate between most benign vocal cord lesions prior to definitive surgery or treatment.

Treatment

Because the lesions just discussed are benign, aggressive surgical excision of every vocal fold lesion may be avoided. The rationale for a conservative yet safe approach takes into account the likelihood of neoplasm and the likelihood that the lesion will resolve without surgery. This approach is used because: (1) the cause of the underlying tissue disturbance may be behavioral; thus, surgery may have a short effect in alleviating dysphonia; (2) the results of surgery may be unpredictable, and scarring may result in a voice quality that is less than desirable; and (3) the voice quality of the patient with a benign vocal lesion may impart a distinctive character to the patient's voice. This is especially true in voice professionals. The office-based examination should never be used to make a histologic diagnosis. In patients with a lesion that is atypical and that fails to improve with a brief course of conservative treatment, histologic examination is mandatory. In patients with more typical benign lesions, the goals of treatment must be tailored to the individual patient's needs. To this end, a more efficient approach may be to conduct a multidisciplinary evaluation and to decide on a course of management for voice disorders in conjunction with otolaryngology and speech pathology professionals and, if indicated, singing teachers. The goal of management of benign vocal fold lesions is to use the most conservative yet efficient methods of treatment to return the patient to full function.[21] Treatment options comprise medical, behavioral, rehabilitative, and surgical methods, or a combination of methods.

It is important for patients to understand fully the cause of the disorder and the characteristics of the behavioral and environmental abuses that contribute to the lesion. Speech therapy evaluation, even when surgery is indicated, is important for: (1) reducing the contact stress of the vocal lesions during the perioperative period; (2) instituting voicing behaviors and strategies that will carry over to the postoperative period; (3) reviewing good mucosal hygiene care of the vocal tract; and (4) monitoring and guiding voice recovery during the rehabilitation period.

Surgery for benign vocal fold lesions should involve the use of the most precise instrumentation with the least disruption of normal vocal fold structure. Besides the choice of instrumentation, clinical experience with regard to the surgical technique and the extent of surgery can be guided by careful evaluation of postsurgical results. In most patients, the surgical goals for phonomicrosurgery are not simply anatomic restoration of grossly normal-appearing vocal folds, but the restoration of normal vocal fold vibration and function.[22]

Vocal Cord Polyps

The vocal cord polyps that are unlikely to respond to conservative therapy are pedunculated or hemorrhagic. Large, unilateral, fusiform polyps are also unlikely to respond to conservative measures alone. These lesions may be treated efficiently by microlaryngoscopy followed by a brief period of voice therapy. The precision of suspension microlaryngoscopy and bimanual instrumentation performed under general anesthesia cannot be equaled by office-based techniques,[13] although some authors have advocated indirect techniques that can be done under local anesthesia.[23] Pedunculated polyps are grasped by the edge of the lesion using small microinstruments and are excised along a plane parallel to the vocal fold edge. The small defect that remains generally closes rapidly. If there is a large feeding vessel to the polyp, short, pulsed, CO_2 laser energy may be used to coagulate the vessel.

Postsurgical voice rest of 1 week's duration is advisable. This is followed by reintroduction of voice use depending on vocal function needs. Consultation with a speech pathologist may be helpful in preventing muscular tension dysphonia in the postoperative period.

Reinke's Edema

The preferred treatment for polypoid corditis is the submucosal evacuation of Reinke's edema via a cordotomy approach. This approach places the incision on the superolateral surface of the vocal fold. The cordotomy is carried into the superficial layer of the lamina propria. The excess gelatinous material is evacuated by suction and carefully removed with cup forceps. The mucosa is then draped over the vocal fold ligament and the excessive mucosa is trimmed back to permit edge-to-edge approximation. If necessary, a microsuture of 6-0 chromic gut or fibrin glue is used to improve mucosal edge approximation. Courey et al[12] have described both medial and lateral microflap approaches for the treatment of subcordal lesions, such as cysts, nodules, and polyps. However, the advantages of sparing mucosa and limiting surgical trauma must be balanced by surgical experience in the application of these techniques. Postoperative monitoring of smoking habits, reflux, and mucosal hygiene is important in preventing a recurrence.

Vocal Cord Nodules

Surgical treatment of vocal cord nodules is usually not necessary. If surgery is necessary, it should be incorporated into the total rehabilitation program, which includes a period of preoperative voice therapy followed by surgery, followed by postoperative voice therapy. The surgery for bilateral vocal cord nodules should be conservative and should remove only the fibrous, exophytic portion of the lesion. No attempt should be made to excise all abnormal tissue if the tissue removal will result in incompetence of the vocal cord edge. Excessive tissue removal can result in incomplete closure and poor vocal fold vibration, a situation that is worse than the original disease.[24]

Prognosis

The prognosis for satisfactory voice should be excellent provided the aforementioned precautions to identify the cause of the disorder have been addressed.[25] Repeated surgical removal for recurrence can result in increased fibrosis. Whether surgery alone, surgery with speech therapy, or speech therapy alone is most efficient in the treatment of simple vocal cord nodules remains controversial.[26] It is the author's bias that therapy alone should be tried first in cases of vocal fold nodules, with surgery and therapy reserved for refractory cases. The prognosis for polyps should be excellent. Patients with Reinke's edema who undergo surgery followed by continued smoking may have a recurrence, although the duration and the likelihood of recurrence have not been studied.

Controversies

Considerable controversy exists as to whether CO_2 lasers should be used in the surgical management of benign vocal fold lesions, such as vocal cord polyps, nodules, and Reinke's edema.[27] Laser-tissue energy effects are complex, and unwanted collateral soft tissue injury may result in unintended complications. Advances in CO_2 laser instrumentation now allow for decreased laser spot size, superpulsed char-free cutting, and microsecond-pulsed duration.[28] When applied with care and in appropriate situations, CO_2 lasers, used in conjunction with traditional microsurgical instrumentation, should be complementary in performing highly precise microphonosurgery.

LARYNGOCELE

Clinical Presentation

Laryngoceles are outpouchings of the normal mucosa and air from the laryngeal ventricle and saccule. They may extend into the larynx and/or into the neck. Internal laryngoceles extend into the larynx by expansion and dilation of the false vocal fold, whereas external laryngoceles are outpouchings of mucosa through the thyrohyoid membrane and present as neck masses.[29] Internal laryngoceles present with airway-obstruction stridor or hoarse voice. Because laryngoceles may decompress spontaneously, they may cause variable symptoms. The laryngoceles may be a cause of congenital or neonatal stridor and should be differentiated from congenital cysts of the neck.[30] The acquired form of laryngocele is seen most frequently in patients, such as horn and wind instrumentalists, who are repeatedly subjected to excessive pharyngolaryngeal pressure. The pathophysiology of internal laryngoceles appears to involve either a congenital or an acquired weakness or dehiscence in the triangular membrane. External laryngoceles must be differentiated from pharyngoceles, whereas internal laryngoceles must be distinguished from epiglottic cysts, saccular cysts, and traumatic cysts of the vocal fold.

Symptoms and Signs

The chief symptom in patients with laryngocele is stridor and airway obstruction in children and hoarseness with airway obstruction in adults.[31] Infection of the laryngocele, with subsequent development of laryngopyocele, has been reported and may cause rapid deterioration in the airway.[32] Most laryngoceles are unilateral, and the most common type is internal.[33] In a review of 60 cases by Matino Soler,[33] the initial symptom in 56% was hoarseness, and acute respiratory distress subsequently developed in 20% of these patients.

Diagnosis

Evaluation of the patient with suspected laryngocele should include either plain x-ray films of the neck, ultrasonography, or CT scans of the neck.[30] A cystic mass, containing air and fluid, will be seen to be causing external compression of the airway. A CT scan will demonstrate the communication between the saccule and the neck mass, thereby differentiating the larygocele from other neck masses.

Treatment

Internal laryngoceles may be treated by endoscopic marsupialization using the CO_2 laser (Fig. 8–16). This involves a wide excision of the false vocal cord on the affected side. Laryngopyoceles may also be drained by this method to obviate the need for tracheotomy. If the laryngocele is inadequately marsupialized, it may recur, causing further obstruction of the airway. Mixed and external laryngoceles can be removed completely via an external cervical approach. If the laryngocele can be traced into the ventricle through the thyrohyoid membrane, there is no need to perform a thyrotomy. For complex internal and external laryngoceles, for which improved access to the supraglottic larynx and false vocal fold is desirable, a window of thyroid cartilage centered on the ipsilateral superior half of the thyroid ala may be removed to gain access and then replaced after laryngocele removal.

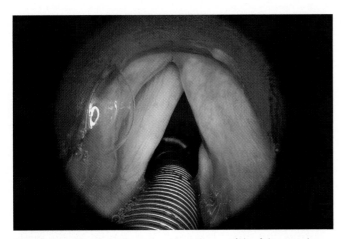

FIGURE 8–16 Saccular cyst with prolapse of the false vocal fold.

Prognosis

With adequate laryngocele removal, the prognosis for a full recovery is excellent. Patients who are at risk for recurrence, such as glass blowers and wind instrumentalists, should be monitored closely.

Controversies

There is a possibility of carcinoma arising from a laryngocele. Whether the laryngocele is a secondary or primary process has not been adequately resolved. In patients with suspected laryngocele, a CT scan of the neck and histologic examination of the tissue are warranted.

CONTACT ULCERS, INTUBATION GRANULOMA, AND CONTACT GRANULOMA

Contact granuloma is a clinical entity described by Jackson[34] as a contact ulcer resulting from epithelial thickening at or near the vocal process caused by excessive vocal process contact and reaction brought on by violent coughing, throat clearing, or voice abuse. This is an important clinical entity, as the underlying cause is often undetected, and treatment by surgery alone often fails. Injuries from intubation and granulation formation at the vocal process are termed intubation granulomas. In the patient with intubation granuloma, there is a clear, inciting injury from either acute or prolonged intubation. This is less true for contact granulomas. Contact ulcers and contact granulomas should be considered a phonologic disorder, and the treating physician should carefully consider the functional aspect of voice and laryngeal function in the pathophysiology of this disorder.

Clinical Presentation

Contact ulcers are primarily seen in adult men. The incidence of this disorder is thought to be greatest in highly stressed individuals with hard-driving, aggressive voice attacks. Contact granulomas have been seen in preachers, rabbis, singers, jailers, executives, and laborers. Many are in positions in which they must project authority through their voice. Some are imbued with inner tension and live highly charged lives. The speech pattern is characterized by abrupt breaks, and sentences are expelled in short, barking, staccato phrases. The voice is low-pitched and punctuated by vocal fry, and the voice resonance is far back, without a forward focus. The harsh, guttural voice with loud accents appears to be especially prone to producing harmful, harsh contact of the vocal processes. These patients speak with their chin tucked, and with great neck tension. Patients present with throat pain after short periods of phonation. Hoarse voice, chronic throat clearing, and habitual coughing are other characteristics that may prompt the patient to seek care. The voice abuse theory has been supported by von Leden[35] in a study involving high-speed motion pictures that document the aggressive closure of the vocal processes in voice abuse gestures, such as "coup de Glott." Further supporting evidence for vocal trauma contributing to contact ulcers is the development of contact granulomas in several patients with vocal cord paralysis who underwent voice therapy to close a large glottal chink.

Intubation granuloma is produced by a round endotracheal tube being placed into a triangular glottis. In the larynx, the point of maximal contact stress exerted by the circular tube is on the vocal process of the arytenoid cartilage. With the tube in place, the constant adduction of the vocal cords with swallow, cough, and other vegetative laryngeal movements facilitates injury of the mucosa overlying the vocal process. Ulceration of the mucosa, exposure of the raw surface to contaminated oral secretions, and possible contamination with acidic contents from the stomach contribute to an intense inflammatory reaction. When the tube is removed, the ulceration may heal with a scar or trough, or it may proceed to granulation formation. Intubation granuloma is directly related to tube injury. Therefore, avoidance of intubation trauma, selection of the appropriate endotracheal tube, and prevention of long-term endotracheal intubation all play a role in its prevention.

Symptoms and Signs

Patients present with hoarseness, throat pain, and chronic throat clearing. They complain of increased phlegm and foreign body sensation, which cause chronic throat clearing. Some patients can date the onset of the problem to a viral upper respiratory infection with spasms of coughing, in others, the onset of symptoms is insidious. Inquiries about

GERD symptoms may elicit reports of classic GERD symptoms, such as heartburn and belching, or they may reveal atypical symptoms such as (1) the taste of acid in the larynx, (2) laryngospasm, or (3) episodic, uncontrolled wheezing and coughing. These symptoms should alert the physician to search for GERD as a cofactor in patients with contact ulcer.

The physical findings of contact ulcers are limited to the posterior larynx. On laryngoscopy, the vocal process has a shaggy, superficially ulcerated lesion that, in the early stages, is hyperemic and may have superficial ulceration. The "hammer and anvil" analogy is apt, as the contact granulomas often have a prominent vocal process with heaped-up keratin and epithelial reaction on the contralateral vocal process (Fig. 8–17).[36] On the contralateral side, a prominent depression often develops over time. The projected arytenoid vocal process may be hypertrophied and hard, and it may fit into the contralateral bed with in such a way that it resembles a cup and saucer. Benjamin and others[37] have reported osteosclerosis of the arytenoid cartilage found on CT scan. It is not clear whether the osteosclerosis is a primary inciting factor for the development of contact granuloma or whether the osteosclerosis is a reaction to repeated trauma at the site.[37] In either case, osteosclerosis may result in an arytenoid process that is enlarged and anatomically difficult to correct.

Although the diagnosis may be suspected based on endoscopic criteria alone, the lesion may simulate an early vocal cord carcinoma of the posterior vocal fold, a granulomatous lesion, or ulceration from traumatic injury. Biopsy studies and operative endoscopy are indicated if atypical features are seen during endoscopic examination.

Patients with intubation granulomas present with a breathy, hoarse voice, the onset of which dates to the time of extubation. Although the voice usually improves after extubation, the improvement plateaus. The patient's voice is usually breathy, and great effort must be expended to produce audible sound. It is important to differentiate this group of patients from the group with contact ulcers, as the response to treatment is quite different. Intubation granulomas are solitary and mushroom-shaped and have exuberant granulation tissue. They arise from the medial surface of the vocal process. The lesions are often seen on a pedicle and may have a small site of origin despite their large size.

Diagnosis

Contact ulcers and intubation granulomas are easily identified by office laryngoscopy. Radiographic evaluation may not be necessary to establish the diagnosis. For patients with recurrent contact granulomas and those for whom osteosclerosis of the arytenoid cartilage is suspected, a CT scan should be performed to confirm the lesion.[37]

Treatment

Contact ulcers are more difficult to treat than intubation granulomas because of the mixed etiology of phonologic disorder and organic tissue change. A careful history should be helpful in differentiating the patient with intubation granuloma from one with contact ulcers. If the history of reflux laryngitis is suggestive, the work-up should include a 24-hour pH probe to document the presence or absence of reflux laryngitis. Evaluation of the patient's voice and therapy to correct voice and speech patterns are important considerations in all patients with contact ulcers.

Speech therapy consists of patient education about the underlying phonologic aspects contributing to the disorder, corrective retraining of voice to reduce contact stress on the ulcers, and substitution of less traumatic vegetative laryngeal gestures for cough and throat clearing. Voice retraining involves (1) reducing the harsh glottal attack; (2) changing the tone focus to a more resonant, tone-forward voice; (3) using soft glottal attacks; and (4) teaching proper respiratory support for the voice. Using such an approach, many patients will experience symptomatic improvement with only a few sessions. Medical therapy consists of antacid therapy, mucolytic therapy, and occasionally, inhaled topical steroids. The patient is re-evaluated in 4 to 6 weeks. If the granuloma is not improved, combined surgical and conservative therapy (voice therapy and treatment of infections, allergy, esophageal reflux, and psychogenic stress) is instituted in the treatment of vocal cord granuloma.[38]

Surgery for contact ulcer is indicated for large lesions, and this must be followed by immediate voice therapy. The removal of the granuloma should be done as atraumatically as possible, with care taken to avoid heat injury to the perichondrium or to the

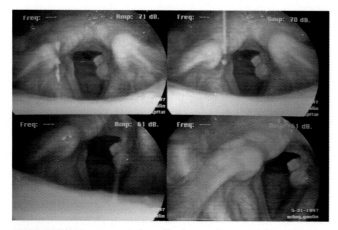

FIGURE 8–17 Contact ulcer. The lesion shows granulation tissue above and below the vocal process. The bed of the ulcer is keratinized and has a shaggy ulcer.

arytenoid cartilage. The excised bed is injected with the long-acting anti-inflammatory steroid methyl prednisolone acetate (Depo-Medrol) to prevent granulation production while allowing the new epithelium to form. The tendency for recurrence after excision alone has been well documented, so treatment should include proper medical and phoniatric therapy.[39] In patients with recalcitrant contact granulomas due to voice abuse, botulism toxin type A has been used to treat vocal fold granuloma.[40] The rationale for its use is to reduce contact stress and allow the vocal process to heal.

Treatment of intubation granulomas (Fig. 8–18) is comparatively easy. Voice retraining is not necessary. The management is primarily medical or surgical. The patient is begun on a course of gastric acid secretion inhibitor; an inhaled steroid spray (beclomethasone dipropionate/Vanceril) is used for 4 weeks. If the lesion is small, continued treatment for 8 weeks is usually adequate. Large intubation granulomas (Fig. 8–19) and those causing stridor are best treated by microsuspension laryngoscopy and surgical removal with scissors. After debridment, careful cautery of the remnant by CO_2 laser or electrocautery may be done. Antireflux medications, antibiotics, and voice rest are prescribed postoperatively to ensure mucosal healing.

Prognosis

The prognosis for intubation granulomas is excellent, although the voice may not return to normal due to intubation trauma and may need adjunctive phonosurgical procedures. The prognosis for contact granulomas depends on the ability of the affected individual to alter injurious behavioral patterns and to allow healing of the contact ulcer area. Patients undergoing repeated removal of contact ulcers with osteosclerosis of the arytenoid joint may show full healing yet complain of easy fatigue of the voice. These patients may need long-term phonologic care and retraining.

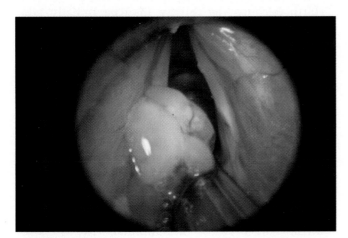

FIGURE 8–18 Intubation granuloma. The lesion is friable and exuberant granulation is present.

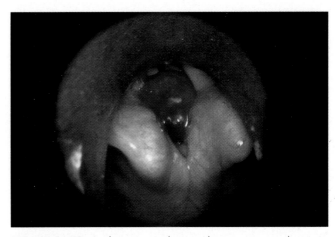

FIGURE 8–19 Intubation granuloma with acute airway obstruction after coughing and hemorrhage.

Controversies

The controversies surrounding contact granuloma involve the timing of surgical removal and whether the laser should be used in granuloma removal. The exact role of GERD in contributing to the contact ulcer is also uncertain, although most agree GERD is an important cofactor in development of posterior laryngitis.[41] Patients with contact granulomas secondary to voice abuse should be considered to have a phonologic disorder for which voice therapy and medical therapy are appropriate as the first line of treatment. Without appropriate phonologic retraining, recurrence after surgical excision may be expected. Treating physicians should avoid this scenario by carefully differentiating between the various forms of posterior vocal process granulomas.

AMYLOIDOSIS

Localized laryngeal amyloidosis is a rare and benign process affecting the larynx. The etiology for this disorder is obscure. Amyloid deposits of the upper airway may be seen as part of generalized amyloidosis with infiltration of the soft tissue of the upper aerodigestive tract. Isolated laryngeal amyloidosis is a subset of localized amyloid deposits and may commonly involve the larynx.[13] Amyloid deposits are routinely found in the aged population, as the process is a natural consequence of aging.[42] Localized laryngeal amyloid deposits affect mainly adults in middle age, although they have also been reported in the pediatric population.

Clinical Presentation

Localized amyloidosis of the larynx is usually asymptomatic until local infiltration results in airway obstruction or hoarse voice. The focal infiltration may cause stridor or obstructive apnea if there is local infiltration of the supraglottic larynx. Amyloid infiltration causes vascular wall fragility due to amyloid deposits, and they may cause hemoptysis or hematemesis.[43]

Symptoms and Signs

Amyloidosis of the larynx and upper aerodigestive tract presents with dyspnea, hoarseness, and symptoms of upper airway obstruction. The amyloid deposits may be nodular or diffuse in soft-tissue infiltration.[44,45] In the larynx, the supraglottic laryngeal infiltration of the false vocal folds may be extensive, yet the true vocal folds may be spared. Endoscopic examination shows the tumor to be a submucosal mass with the mucosa of the larynx remaining intact. The deposits may be nodular and irregular in appearance, with a yellowish to brownish color. On microlaryngoscopy, the nodular masses are firm and friable. Bleeding may be difficult to control owing to capillary fragility.

Diagnosis

A CT scan of the larynx is indicated to delineate the extent of the soft tissue infiltration. Histologic confirmation is made by biopsy. If there is extensive calcification present in the larynx and trachea, the differential diagnosis of tracheopathia osteoplastica should be considered.

Treatment

The histologic finding of amyloidosis of the larynx usually prompts a work-up for primary and secondary generalized amyloidosis. In the work-up, chest x-ray studies, renal function testing, urine protein electrophoresis, and bone marrow biopsy may be performed to rule out multiple myeloma. If the results of the work-up are negative, isolated laryngeal amyloidosis is diagnosed.

Laryngeal amyloidosis may be removed with minimal trauma and functional impairment using the CO_2 laser. If the infiltration is extensive, the laser is used as a tool to debulk and create an airway.[46] Staged endoscopic treatment of laryngeal amyloidosis may be necessary to prevent laryngeal stenosis. Laryngeal amyloidosis often has an indolent course of several years' duration. Aggressive surgical removal and tracheotomy is not usually necessary.

Prognosis

Isolated laryngeal amyloidosis may be an indolent disease that lasts for decades. The patients in the author's small series all had symptoms for many years prior to presentation and were managed with intermittent CO_2 laser treatment for airway clearance. Tracheobronchial involvement with amyloidosis may carry a worse prognosis owing to the long segmental involvement and the risk of upper airway hemorrhage.[44]

Controversies

Further research into the biochemistry of the amyloid protein and its categorization will help to delineate the pathogenesis and diagnosis of this disease.

IDIOPATHIC AND ACQUIRED SUBGLOTTIC STENOSIS

Clinical Presentation

Subglottic stenosis is a common problem. Subglottic stenosis can take three forms: acquired, congenital, and idiopathic. Acquired subglottic stenosis is by far the most common type seen in practice. It is caused by complications relating to endotracheal anesthesia, prolonged intubation, or smoke inhalation or burn injury. The acquired form of stenosis starts with mucosal injury and complications of infection and trauma. Children are at especially high risk owing to the small caliber of the airway at the cricoid and the occasional need for long-term intubation. Injury from the endotracheal tube may be due to cuff injury or mucosal erosion at the vocal process and erosion of the posterior cricoid mucosa. Pressure necrosis is commonly caused by the cuff used to create a seal between the trachea and subglottis for artificial ventilation. Factors that contribute to exacerbation of the mucosal injury include hypotension, sepsis, bacterial contamination, and reduced host defenses, as in patients with diabetes and renal failure. If the injury is severe, there is tissue loss resulting in tracheomalacia or laryngomalacia. Transmural injury by cuff injury can result in catastrophic events, such as tracheal-innominate artery erosion, tracheoesophageal fistula, and large, segmental, laryngotracheomalacia.

Congenital subglottic stenosis may not be detected at birth because the airway may be initially adequate. However, the airway becomes inadequate as the patient gains weight and the increased demand for air exchange is not met.

Idiopathic subglottic stenosis is a rare form of the disorder, occurring in patients identified as having subglottic stenosis but without an identified source of laryngotracheal intubation or injury. Inflammatory or systemic illness that may contribute to subglottic stenosis is also ruled out in these patients. Thus, the diagnosis of idiopathic subglottic stenosis is a diagnosis of exclusion. It is an affliction of adults in the latter part of life and is differentiated from the congenital form by its late presentation.

Obstruction of the airway may be classified as extrinsic, intrinsic, or intraluminal. The stenoses have further been classified as segmental or circumferential. The thickness of the stenosis is a critical factor in endoscopic staging and treatment selection.[47] There are many classification schemes for pediatric and adult subglottic stenosis. The usefulness of the various classification systems is primarily for clinical decision making.

Symptoms and Signs

Patients with subglottic stenosis and other benign strictures of the upper airway present with symptoms of increasing dyspnea on exertion, audible wheezing with exercise, and tachypnea. Cough and hoarse voice may accompany these symptoms. There may be positional variations in the severity of the dyspnea if the stenosis is supraglottic or if the site of stenosis is also marked by tracheobronchomalacia. Often, the patients have worse dyspnea in the supine position. This may prompt patients to sleep in an upright position. Audible sounds may be heard with slight exertion, such as with climbing stairs or walking. The stridor of subglottic stenosis is heard best either during inspiration or during both inspiration and expiration. The physical findings on auscultation show turbulent airway sounds heard loudest over the trachea with transmitted upper airway sounds distally. The patient may use intercostal breathing, chest breathing, or accessory muscles of respiration to assist in air exchange. The history of recent intubation followed by recent worsening of dyspnea should prompt a referral for airway evaluation.

The use of pulmonary function testing is helpful in the diagnosis of upper airway obstruction and in differentiating fixed versus variable upper airway obstruction. It has also been used to diagnose intrathoracic or extrathoracic airway involvement.[48] Decreased maximum voluntary ventilation and reduced forced expiratory volume in one second (FEV_1) are suggestive and may be used as objective

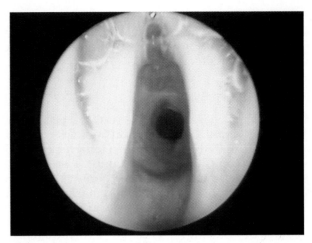

FIGURE 8–21 Circumferential subglottic stenosis. The injury is caused by intubation.

parameters to indicate severity. Unfortunately, flow loop studies are not useful for subtle differentiation of mild obstruction, and patients with obvious airway narrowing in the bronchus or upper airway cannot be distinguished from those with normal airways.

Examination of the airway by fiberoptic or rigid bronchoscopy is the main tool for evaluation of airway obstruction. With today's smaller diagnostic scopes, this examination can often be performed in the office setting with appropriate topical anesthesia of the upper airways. A more formal bronchoscopy with fiberoptic or rigid bronchoscopy and biopsy may be done if a pathologic specimen or diagnostic staging is necessary. The importance of examination of the larynx and trachea under local anesthesia is underscored by the need to evaluate the mobility and excursion of the vocal folds and the need to evaluate the airway for acquired laryngomalacia.

The endoscopic findings of benign strictures may be quite variable. Thin, web-like stenoses and those with subglottic synechia or bridge offer the best prognosis (Fig. 8–20). These may cause interarytenoid tethering and cause a pseudo–vocal cord palsy. The posterior glottic and subglottic web is often associated with arytenoid fixation.

Circumferential stenosis is a common form of subglottic stenosis (Fig. 8–21). The stenosis is usually fixed in diameter and should be measured as to the site, percent of luminal compromise, and the length of stenosis. Staging of the extent of stenosis has been proposed in the pediatric population by Cotton.[49] A proposed grading system for subglottic stenosis based on endotracheal tube sizes appears to be useful in predicting surgical results.[49] Stenosis resulting from granulation tissue that has mucosal inflammation should be differentiated from the white mature stricture, as should the benign subglottic stricture that causes complete obliteration of the airway. Strictures secondary to suspected sarcoidosis, histo-

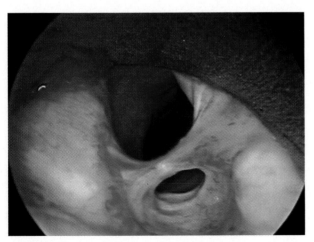

FIGURE 8–20 Interarytenoid synechia. This patient sustained a head injury and had stridor after decannulation. Laryngoscopy showed bilateral vocal fold immobility. A single treatment with CO_2 laser excision resulted in restoration of vocal fold motion.

plasmosis, tuberculosis, Wegener's granulomatosis, or acid reflux laryngitis have chronic inflammation and should undergo biopsy study and be cultured for the appropriate organisms.

Radiologic Evaluation

Radiographic evaluation of the airway starts with a chest x-ray study and a cervical radiograph of the lateral neck soft tissue, and then progresses to airway fluoroscopy, tomography, and CT scanning of the larynx and trachea. The chest x-ray is often normal, but may show tracheal airway narrowing in the upper trachea. Special attention should be paid to the airway when reviewing chest radiographs of patients with a history of prolonged dyspnea and wheezing. Lateral neck films with high kV views are used in the evaluation of adult and pediatric airways. The steeple sign and an irregular airway that does not fully open during inspiration may be seen on the anteroposterior and lateral neck films. This may indicate airway compromise when flexible endoscopy cannot easily be performed. The usefulness of radiographic evaluation of pediatric patients with stridor has been questioned in some studies.[50] Tostevin et al[50] reviewed their series of pediatric patients presenting with stridor and concluded that radiology had a limited screening role and that, in a child presenting with stridor, the initial radiologic assessment should be a chest radiograph, with further imaging and a barium swallow only if an abnormality is found at microlaryngoscopy. Radiographic examination cannot differentiate acquired stenosis from idiopathic or congenital stenosis. Idiopathic laryngotracheal stenosis produces focal stenosis of the cervical part of the trachea. The lumen is severely compromised, measuring no more than 5 mm in diameter at its narrowest portion. The stenosis can be concentric or eccentric and can have either smooth or lobulated margins.[51] Fluoroscopic examination of the upper airway is indicated to evaluate the presence of extrinsic compression, tracheobronchomalacia, and the collapsible airway. The use of tomograms has become less popular since the advent of CT scanning, but this modality remains useful in selected centers as it provides a coronal view of the thickness and caliber of the airway. CT scanning is used to evaluate the thickness of the stenosis and also the degree of involvement of the tracheal and cricoid cartilage. Loss of the cricoid cartilage ring and trachea and aberrant dystrophic calcifications are easily detected with thin-slice CT scans through the trachea and larynx. The scans should be used to help differentiate those patients requiring treatment by endoscopic laser technique or by open resection.

Treatment

The treatment of subglottic stenosis can be divided into endoscopic and open approaches. The endo-

scopic approaches include radial excision and dilation, endoscopic stenting, laser resection, balloon dilation, and a combination of these. Open surgical treatment of subglottic and tracheal stenosis consists of tracheal resection, laryngotracheal grafting, and single or multistage laryngotracheoplasty. Augmentation with soft and hard tissue may be necessary. Dilation has been used for many decades. Repeated dilation is often necessary to keep the airway patent. The recent application of radial dilation with balloon catheters may offer another alternative.[52]

At the outset, it should be clear that treatment of subglottic stenosis with glottic fixation is different than treatment of subglottic stenosis alone. For patients with impairment of vocal fold motion, laryngeal electromyography provides additional information as to the innervation pattern of the intrinsic laryngeal muscles (Fig. 8–22).

There have been innumerable approaches to the management of subglottic stenosis, bearing testimony to the difficulty in obtaining predictably satisfactory results.[53] Isolated, short, segmental, tracheal stenosis or subglottic stenosis may be treated by endoscopic laser radial incision and dilation.[54] Surgical intervention is indicated in patients with exertion dyspnea. Endoscopic laser incision and dilation can achieve excellent short-term results. Multiple serial dilations may be necessary, although in some patients palliation may be achieved with a single dilation. Restenosis is a problem with longer and more complex stenoses. These may require laryngotracheal resection and reconstruction.[55] Review of large series of pediatric patients undergoing single-stage laryngotracheoplasty for subglottic stenosis has shown a high success rate. The success rate (without further laryngotracheoplasty) for all patients in expert hands was 86% (89 of 104).[56] Segmental subglottic resection and primary thyrotracheal anastomosis have also been reported to show excellent re-

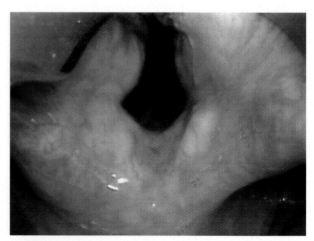

FIGURE 8–22 Bilateral cricoarytenoid joint ankylosis with intubation defect. The keyhole defect in the posterior cartlaginous glottis was associated with bilateral vocal fold fixation. Laryngeal electromyography was normal.

sults in the adult and pediatric populations.[47,57] Cricotracheal resection should be considered to be an important treatment option for severe subglottic stenosis in infants and children.[58]

Prognosis

Short, segmental stenoses may be treated by endoscopic resection with the CO_2 laser bronchoscope, followed by bronchoscopic dilation. This approach has an excellent palliative potential and the endoscopic approach allows patients to be discharged home after surgery with little hospitalization. The endoscopic CO_2 laser has also been used to excise posterior subglottic stenosis. Serial micro-trapdoor flap elevation and excision have been reported[59] without tracheotomy. Usually, the patients are immediately relieved of objective dyspnea. The procedure is safe in the hands of the experienced endoscopist. The problem is restenosis. This is especially a problem for patients with circumferential stenosis, stenosis greater than 1.5 cm, and in stenosis associated with loss of cartilaginous support. Restenosis usually occurs 6 months to 1 year after resection in these patients. Open surgery with tracheal resection and cricoid resection with excellent results have been reported by Grillo,[60] Pearson,[53] and others.

External trauma was found to have the best outcome when compared to other etiologies. The anatomic site of stenosis and its length were independent determinants of outcome, whereas its diameter was not. Involvement of the glottis in subglottic stenosis led to a significantly poorer outcome. The author recommends use of the length and site of stenosis as primary prognostic factors in the assessment of acquired laryngeal stenosis in the adult population.[61] Voice quality after surgery has been evaluated. Children with high-grade subglottic stenosis and multiple prior surgeries are at high risk for poor voice outcome after laryngotracheal reconstruction.[62]

Controversies

Open treatment by laryngoplasty, anterior and posterior split, and cartilage grafting has yielded excellent success rates in the pediatric population. In adults, the success rate is lower. One controversial point is whether one-stage laryngeal resection should be considered instead of the staged laryngotracheal reconstruction with stenting and grafting. Because no single technique offers completely successful surgery in patients with complex stenotic segments, staged laryngotracheal reconstruction should be considered in patients who have long segmental defects, those who are poor risks for hyoid release and thoracic tracheal release, those who have combined laryngeal and tracheal stenosis, and those who have failed previous open surgery. Previous open-heart surgery and poor medical condition are relative but not absolute contraindications to laryn-gotracheal resection. Although long-term stenting is a viable alternative, the need for a permanent tracheotomy and care usually makes this method of treatment a last resort and one that is reserved for those in whom more aggressive surgical alternatives have failed.

TEFLON GRANULOMAS, FOREIGN-BODY REACTIONS, AND METABOLIC DEPOSITS

The use of Teflon for vocal fold augmentation in the treatment of vocal cord paralysis was popularized by Arnold[63] and Dedo.[64] Complications of Teflon injection can occur and are related to overinjection, foreign-body giant cell reaction, and foreign-body granuloma. When injected into the mobile vocal fold or into the subglottis, Teflon can migrate from the larynx and present as a neck mass.[65] Recently, thyroplasty phonosurgical techniques have been developed to address the potential problems related to Teflon.

Symptoms and Signs

The most common problems related to the use of Teflon do not involve granuloma formation, but rather overinjection or a wrong site of injection. Teflon must be placed lateral to the vocal ligament and deep to the vocalis so as to be far away from the vocal fold edge. The injection sites available for vocal fold augmentation are limited to the membranous vocal fold. Thus, if the vocal fold defect is posterior and the Teflon is erroneously being used to augment a larger posterior chink, the Teflon may be overinjected into the membranous cord. This will result in a poor outcome, and will appear as a medial bowing of the true vocal folds. It will not effectively bridge the posterior chink, and patients will be left with a strained, breathy quality of voice. If Teflon is to be used, it should be used with appropriate caution, especially with regard to technique and site of injection.

If the voice is initially of good quality after Teflon injection but deteriorates over a period of many years, the diagnosis may be tissue reaction and granuloma formation. An unsatisfactory voice or a voice that is steadily deteriorating should alert the surgeon to the possibility of Teflon reaction. The biomechanical properties of the vocal cord seen after Teflon injection are often stiffness and nonpliability. These are consistent with the intraoperative finding of a scarred and stiff vocal fold at the time of Teflon granuloma removal. The vocal fold is red and hard. There may be thickening and bulging of the injected vocal fold. Stroboscopic examination reveals a stiff, nonvibrating vocal fold. If the airway is compromised, there is often a characteristic turbulent-sounding stridor upon inspiration. Biphasic stridor and dysphagia can also develop if the reaction to the Teflon injection is severe and the amount of tissue hyperemia is extensive. Subglottic overfilling is the most common condition.[66]

Radiologic Evaluation

A CT scan is indicated to assess the extent of the granuloma and the degree of airway compromise. A CT scan of the larynx is also indicated to rule out the possibility that the submucosal mass is a submucosal tumor. The CT scan of the larynx shows the Teflon to be calcified, and infiltration of the true vocal fold by Teflon is typical. The characteristic changes of dystrophic calcification in the larynx after Teflon injection make the differential diagnosis easy, especially when there is an antecedent history of Teflon injection.

Treatment

Dysphonia, secondary to Teflon injection, can result either from overinjection of Teflon or inappropriate injection, or from the proliferate granulomatous response of the larynx to the Teflon. The technique of laser incision into the superior aspect of the Teflon implant, followed by vaporization and preservation of a margin of mucosa of the cord medially, has been reported to have improved voice in 8 of 11 patients treated in this manner.[67]

Lasers in adult laryngeal surgery remain a valuable tool for the treatment of specific laryngeal diseases, such as Teflon granulomas. The laser is used to debulk excessive Teflon granuloma and to sculpt the remaining granuloma to produce a straighter edge of vocal fold.[68] When excising the Teflon, care must be taken to use low oxygen flows through the anesthesia circuit, as the Teflon particles cause a bright flare when struck by the CO_2 laser. The potential for airway fire is increased when high O_2 flows are used. Laryngotomy and removal of the Teflon have also been performed, but this approach may require airway control by tracheotomy.

Prognosis

Difficulties in the endoscopic removal of Teflon granulomas of the vocal fold have been reviewed.[69] Endoscopic removal of Teflon to create a linear vocal fold promotes vocal fold closure. Although the voice can be improved, the harsh quality related to the stiffness of the vocal cord will persist.

Controversies

The permanency of the poor voice quality resulting from complications of Teflon injection has prompted the search for alternatives to Teflon, such as fat,[70] and open techniques, such as medialization laryngoplasty[71] and arytenoid adduction. Until a prospec-

tive randomized study is conducted to study the effects of each procedure in functionally matched patients, controversy persists.

INFLAMMATORY MYOFIBROBLASTIC TUMOR (PLASMA CELL GRANULOMA)

Symptoms and Signs

Inflammatory myofibroblastic tumors of the larynx are uncommon lesions that easily may be misinterpreted as malignant epithelial or mesenchymal spindle cell neoplasms.[72] Although the lung is the best known and most common site, inflammatory myofibroblastic tumors occur in diverse extrapulmonary locations.[73] A mass, fever, weight loss, pain, and site-specific symptoms are the presenting complaints. Laboratory abnormalities may include anemia, thrombocytosis, polyclonal hypergammaglobulinemia, and elevated erythrocyte sedimentation rate. In a study of 84 cases, Coffin et al[73] reviewed the sites of involvement of extrapulmonary plasma cell granuloma. The most common sites included the abdomen, retroperitoneum, and pelvis (61 cases); head and neck, including the upper respiratory tract (12 cases); trunk (8 cases); and the extremities (3 cases).[73] The presentation and upper airway findings of plasma cell granuloma may mimic endobronchial malignant disease or asthma. This condition has also been reported to cause sudden asphyxia.[74] It can present as a variety of nonspecific symptoms which may delay diagnosis. It usually occupies a peripheral pulmonary location and gives rise to symptoms because of its local mass effect and destructive invasion.[75]

Radiologic Evaluation

Inflammatory myofibroblastic tumor presents as a mass lesion that may be difficult to differentiate from a malignant tumor. Mass lesions of the upper airway and trachea may present with obstruction of the endobronchial tree or as a mass in the larynx. A contrast enhanced CT scan of the trachea and larynx is indicated.

Treatment

Frequently misdiagnosed as malignant tumors, inflammatory myofibroblastic tumors cause localized morbidity by obstruction, erosion, and mass compression. The lesion is responsive to low-dose radiation therapy, excision, and steroid and antibiotic therapy.[73,76,77]

Prognosis

The prognosis for inflammatory myofibroblastic tumors is good. Complications are related to localized obstruction and invasion.

INFECTIOUS AND INFLAMMATORY DISORDERS

Acute inflammation of the upper airways is one of the most common causes of organic voice disorders. The effects of the common cold and other viruses result in temporary but troublesome dysphonia. Such afflictions are usually a transient annoyance unless the one affected is a voice professional or singer. If the problem fails to resolve over a period of weeks to months, a chronic problem may be present. This may progress to disabling and permanent dysphonia. When a condition results in painful, difficult effort during communication, it brings even the most recalcitrant patient to seek care.

The term laryngitis is a clinically descriptive term that covers the entire spectrum of disorders of the larynx that involve the process of inflammation. Laryngitis loosely encompasses a spectrum of disorders from acute inflammatory edema to scar formation, with scar being the sequel to tissue inflammation and repair. Because inflammatory response is a physiologic process of tissue, laryngitis is often classified clinically as acute, subacute, chronic, or recurrent. This helps to describe the clinical course and prognosis of these disorders, but does not specify their etiology. The pathogenesis of laryngitis may be attributable to a long list of pathologic processes, some of which are listed in Table 8–1. Unfortunately, the clinical examination may not differentiate between the various forms. Therefore, the laryngologist must distinguish between those disorders that result from pathogenic organisms (bacterial, fungus, viral) and laryngeal inflammation that arises as a result of systemic disease, trauma, or allergies.

Common to all forms of laryngitis is the basic process of inflammation and repair. With acute inflammation and repair, fluid and hemodynamic changes occur in the vocal folds, altering their mass and vibratory characteristics and producing dysphonia. Pharmacologic treatment and speech therapy can be used to blunt the severity of the response. Speech therapy may be used to decrease the inciting injury from vocal fold trauma due to voice abuse. Steroids may be used to reduce the severity of the body's response to injury. Inflammation, when it is persistent, may progress to chronic inflammation, resulting in permanent tissue changes and permanent dysphonia. Because vocal fold vibration depends on oscillation of delicate vocal folds, even small alterations in local tissue homeostasis can result in changes in the perceived voice result.

Laryngitis is defined as inflammation and reaction of the tissue of the larynx to injury. The tissue response sets in motion a complex sequence of events involving tissue defense and cellular repair. The inflammatory response is a highly organized series of steps designed to destroy, wall off, and repair the damage. In the process of repairing injury, an often undesirable functional side effect on the larynx is

TABLE 8–1   LARYNGITIS AND ITS VARIANTS

Acute Laryngitis

Viral laryngitis
Bacterial laryngitis
Allergic laryngitis
Traumatic laryngitis associated with voice abuse
Acute laryngitis associated with smoke inhalation, fumes, or toxins

Chronic Laryngitis

Fungal laryngitis
    Candida, blastomycosis, histoplasmosis
Tuberculosis laryngitis
Bacterial laryngitis—staphylococcal
Acid reflux laryngitis
Laryngitis with systemic diseases
    Wegener's granulomatosis
    Sjögren's syndrome
    Sarcoidosis
Atrophic laryngitis of aging
Nonspecific laryngitis
Polypoid corditis and Reinke's edema
Postradiation laryngitis

Endocrine and Metabolic Factors

Hypothyroidism
Use of virilization drugs
Postmenopausal voice changes

scar formation. It is because of attempts at inflammation and repair that common laryngeal disorders, such as laryngeal edema, acute and chronic laryngitis, and vocal fold scarring, result. These processes cause dysphonia. Although it is common to think of bacterial or viral diseases as causes for acute laryngitis, many forms of injury to the larynx may exist. These include thermal injury, radiation injury, chemical injury, and impact trauma of voice abuse. The larynx, by virtue of its anatomy, sits at the crossroads of the aerodigestive tract. Therefore, acute and chronic inflammation of these sites may also affect the larynx by local contamination. Examples of these problems include: (1) sinobronchial infection causing laryngitis (bacterial and viral); (2) reflux laryngitis (chemical and acid); (3) traumatic laryngitis (voice abuse); and (4) inhalation laryngitis (thermal).

It is useful, for prognosis and treatment purposes, to classify inflammatory disorders of the larynx into acute and chronic inflammatory patterns. The differential diagnoses for patients presenting with acute versus chronic laryngitis are different, as are the extent of work-up and treatment.

Acute Laryngitis

Acute laryngitis applies to an inflammatory disorder of the larynx that is usually of short duration, lasting hours to days, and that affects an otherwise healthy patient. The cause is usually identifiable as trauma or viral illness. During the early phase, the normal laryngeal mucosa experiences vascular dilation, increased blood flow, and vascular stasis. The tissue of the vocal folds undergoes increased vascular permeability with exudate of protein-rich fluid entering the extravascular space. The increased vascular permeability results in laryngeal edema. Permeability changes in the tissue are then followed by infiltration of white blood cells into the extravascular space. This corresponds to the classic observations of erythema (rubor), pain (dolor), and heat (calor) (Fig. 8–23).

Acute laryngitis and laryngeal edema may be seen following upper respiratory infection; intubation, prolonged shouting, as at rock concerts; and severe coughing.[78] Such acute inflammation may result in one of the following outcomes:

1. The laryngitis may completely resolve, with restoration of the site of injury to normal. This may occur when there has been limited injury and little tissue destruction.
2. Healing may occur by scar formation. When mucosal injury is extensive, or if an exudative process results, the healing process often involves fibrosis and scarring, with collagen deposition. In the delicate vocal folds, especially in the superficial layer of the lamina propria, dense collagen fibers are noticeably absent. When unwanted collagen is deposited as a result of the inflammatory response, it may interfere with the normal vibration of the vocal folds during phonation.

Chronic inflammation may be attributable to an ongoing stimulus that promotes laryngeal tissue reaction and repair or to a repair process that persists after the initial causative agent has been removed.

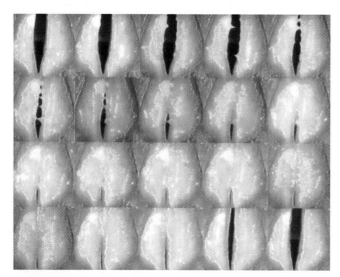

FIGURE 8–23 Acute suppurative laryngitis. Stroboscopic examination shows excessive phlegm on the vocal folds with the glistening surface of the vocal folds having a "salt and pepper" appearance.

Such a stimulus may be an irritant, such as smoke or alcohol, resulting in pachydermia laryngica, or it may be a condition, such as acid reflux, that results in chronic reflux laryngitis. It may be attributable to an autoimmune response resulting in rheumatoid arthritis, or it may be due to a host of bacterial and fungal agents that promote a chronic inflammatory response. Tuberculosis,[79] fungi, and other agents producing granulomatous laryngitis are examples of bacterial and fungal agents that produce chronic laryngitis. Figure 8–24 presents a schematic chart of the pathophysiologic response of the larynx that occurs with laryngitis, as well as its sequelae.

Acute Viral Laryngitis

Acute viral laryngitis is usually a consequence of viral inflammation of the upper respiratory tract. Rhinovirus and influenza virus are common pathogens, yet multiple other viral agents have also been implicated as causes of viral laryngitis.

The incidence of acute laryngitis is difficult to estimate. This is because most patients with acute laryngitis do not usually present for evaluation because it is a disease of limited duration. The affected individual often will embark on a course of expectant treatment while "waiting out" a cold or laryngitis. The same can be said for patients with acute laryngitis that arises after overexuberant voice use during a ball game or rock concert. Traumatically induced edema of the larynx lasts up to 2 to 3 days and gradually returns to normal with voice rest. Two exceptions to this scenario are (1) patients with bacterial suppurative laryngitis that results in fever and epiglottitis; and (2) patients with special voice needs. Patients with epiglottitis may progress to airway compromise and require emergency airway management. Voice professionals seek out care and treatment because of professional and vocational concerns related to special voice needs.

Symptoms and Signs

When a patient presents for evaluation of acute voice loss and suspected acute viral laryngitis, the chronologic history and identification of the inciting agent are most important in determining the appropriate diagnosis and treatment. Because acute laryngitis is a nonspecific inflammatory response, a careful history should help the clinician to differentiate between the various possibilities, which include voice abuse, nonspecific laryngitis, and bacterial or viral laryngitis.

Complaints of vocal dysfunction in laryngitis focus on limitation of vocal range and phonatory function. Pain or discomfort associated with voice production may also bring the patient in for evaluation. Cough and a painful, irritated larynx are symptoms that most commonly bring the patient in for evaluation.

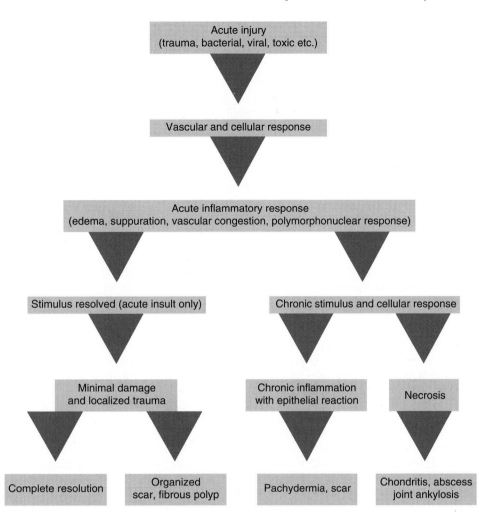

FIGURE 8–24 Schematic outline of the pathophysiology of acute and chronic laryngitis.

The well-trained voice professional usually considers a medical or organic condition to be the source of their vocal complaints. Although vocal fold hemorrhage, nodules, and acute inflammation do occur, in the author's experience, the finding of hyperfunction or functional voice abuse leading to an organic laryngeal finding is very common. Acute viral or bacterial laryngitis may be the suspected diagnosis made by the voice professional, but the cause is often due to voice misuse and other nonspecific inflammation.

Acute viral laryngitis is usually associated with other respiratory symptoms, such as coryza, rhinorrhea, and cough. A sore throat may herald the presence of pharyngitis prior to laryngitis. Fever, pain upon swallowing, and generalized throat irritation often accompany voice changes. Interestingly, the onset of voice changes is often delayed, and voice quality is often worse during the resolution stages of an acute upper respiratory infection. Occasionally, the tracheobronchial tree is spared and the patient may present with only pain and sore throat, followed by a husky, poor voice quality. A low-grade

fever is common, but a high fever with dysphagia should lead the clinician to suspect bacterial laryngitis or bacterial supraglottitis. If the infectious etiology is viral, the vocal symptoms rapidly clear within 4 to 6 days. During the resolution stage of acute laryngitis, the patient often complains of increased phlegm. Throat clearing and irritated throat symptoms lasting up to 2 weeks are not uncommon.

One exception to the rapid clearance of viral laryngitis is in the immunocompromised host. In a patient who tests positive for human immunodeficiency virus (HIV), acute laryngitis may persist so long that it becomes chronic laryngitis. Herpes simplex–induced chronic laryngitis and vocal cord lesions also have been reported.[80]

Bacterial infections, such as those caused by β-streptococcus, *Hemophilus influenzae,* and pneumococcus, may complicate the course of viral laryngitis and prolong the course of illness. Figure 8–23 shows an example of stroboscopic findings in a patient with acute laryngitis. Note the increased edema with thick mucus. The vocal folds show hyperemia and edema. These laryngeal findings may be associated with rigor, fever, and chills. Tenacious, thick phlegm with cough often prevents a good night's sleep and brings the patient to the physician's office after several days of home treatment. Such a history is easily differentiated from laryngitis due to other causes.

The medical history of patients with acute and chronic hoarseness should include a thorough review of prescription and nonprescription medications. Some medications (e.g., diuretics, antihypertensive medications, psychotropic drugs) may promote mucosal drying and mucositis. Over-the-counter medications (e.g., antihistamines, decongestants) may also cause local drying and mucosal injury.

A workplace history should also be obtained, including inquiries as to smoking and second-hand smoke; exposure to fumes, dyes, petrochemical distillates, and photochemical acids and bases; and rapid changes in cold and warm environments. Nonspecific allergies to environmental irritants are a common source of throat irritation and hoarseness.

From the patient's perspective, the symptoms of acute laryngitis may be trivial to catastrophic. For the average patient, the symptoms of dysphonia and throat pain are merely nuisances associated with an acute viral illness; however, if the patient is a singer, the implications may be severe. Singers with mild laryngeal edema may have a normal speaking voice but may lose their singing voice. The high vocal range is especially affected by mild laryngitis. Difficulty with control of the passages and a loss of brilliant tone in the midrange are other common complaints. For patients with extraordinary voice needs, a thorough search for factors that may contribute to laryngeal irritation is indicated. This may take the form of a questionnaire or directed questions. The interaction between organic illness and hyperfunctional disorder in voice professionals often warrants a multidisciplinary diagnosis and treatment approach involving speech pathologists, vocal coaches, and physicians. Such an approach is often useful in the more difficult cases in reducing the interval between onset and diagnosis and treatment.

The emotional and psychosocial adjustments caused by acute inflammation in the singer should not be trivialized. For the singer, voice restoration within a limited time frame is critical to reputation and livelihood. Distress is often attributable to either voice qualities that conflict with the singer's schedule or the fear of irreversible voice damage secondary to laryngeal trauma or hemorrhage. Such heightened fear of vocal fold injury may prompt a demand for a quick cure. This psychological aspect of voice should be recognized and understood.[81]

Acute laryngitis is usually preceded by symptoms of chills and malaise. The throat is dry and irritated. Because of the interstitial edema, the fundamental frequency often drops, and sustained phonation may become unreliable. Unreliability of the voice is present as the speaker attempts pitch changes resulting in voice breaks. There is often a husky, brassy voice characteristic that is recognizable to the public as "laryngitis." Progression of laryngeal inflammation results in severe dysphonia. Speaking is accomplished only with great effort, resulting in short bursts that sound much like a croak. Speaking becomes painful. Voice may cease. Despite voice cessation, the throat remains red and irritated, with the irritation causing the patient to clear the throat frequently.

During acute laryngitis, the vocal folds have a pink color and resemble fine velvet in appearance. The fine capillaries on the vocal fold surface are dilated as a result of increased blood flow. As the infection progresses, the stages of inflammation result in copious secretions that cause frequent expectoration and cough. Often, the patient cannot sleep at night due to excessive secretion and expectoration. Coughing and throat clearing become painful and sleep becomes impossible. The suppurative stage is usually limited to 48 to 72 hours and is followed by gradual resolution. During the resolution stage, the secretions become less viscous although they are still copious. Voice function returns, but still retains a veiled quality. Throat irritation lessens, but a scratchy, irritated throat is often present for many weeks after the acute inflammation has subsided. Full restitution of vocal function usually occurs within 7 to 10 days.

Examination of the vocal folds during laryngitis shows some typical findings. During the early hyperemic stage, the vocal folds may look quite normal except for their pink/rose color. However, attempts at phonation will often result in vocal folds that fail to oscillate. During the suppurative stage of inflammation, copious, thick secretions are present throughout the larynx and at the vocal fold contact area. Thickened strands of mucus between the vocal folds are often noted (see Fig. 8–23). If coughing is severe, the arytenoid and interarytenoid areas may be red and swollen. It is during the height of inflammation when singers and other voice users are most susceptible to vocal fold hemorrhage. Vocal fold hemorrhages are usually a result of mechanical trauma to the dilated vascular bed of the vocal folds. This can result in submucosal hemorrhage. Such mechanical trauma may be attributable to excessive voice use or harsh throat clearing.

Stroboscopic examination reveals changes in vocal fold oscillation. Although not diagnostic for acute inflammatory laryngitis, stroboscopic examination helps to stage the course of the disease, as well as to offer some prognostic signs as to return of vibratory function. Typical stroboscopic features associated with the various stages of laryngitis and its sequelae include symmetric loss in vibratory amplitude and mucosal wave; vocal fold edema and puffy, swollen vocal folds; rocking movement of the vocal cover; incomplete closure with glottal gap; and aperiodicity with pressed phonation.

Treatment

Most patients with viral laryngitis have a self-limited course. Voice rest and supportive measures are all that are necessary. To soothe the irritated dry throat, steam inhalation in moderate amounts may be useful. This may be accomplished using commercially available units or by home remedies, such as inhaling through a hot, wet towel.

To increase thin secretions and reduce irritation, many popular remedies exist. Herbal tea, lemon flavoring, and honey are favorites among many singers. Strong antiseptic mouthwash is to be avoided due to its irritative properties. Warm saltwater gargles, used frequently, can help to remove thick viscous secretions mechanically and reduce pharyngeal irritation. Inhalers and nebulizers may be used to instill moisture directly onto irritated, dry membranes. Saline nebulizers should be 7 to 20 μm in size and should use large-particle nebulizers for deposit in the upper airway.

Hydration is one of the best remedies for acute laryngitis. If a singer must perform with a minor ailment, it is wise to first document the underlying pathologic process to ensure that it is safe. During a bout of laryngitis, the efficiency of the vocal system in voice production is poor. This is due to the increased subglottic pressure and airflow necessary to produce vocal fold oscillation.[82] A few emergency training sessions with a voice coach or speech pathologist with training and experience in such treatments may be useful. The purpose of these sessions is not to teach the patient proper voice use but rather to provide the voice professional with performance techniques and insights for (1) avoiding vocal injury; (2) producing the least effortful voice with acceptable sound, and (3) addressing the special needs of the performer as they relate to performance.

Pharmacologic treatment of acute laryngitis is occasionally necessary. In patients with simple viral laryngitis, no pharmacologic intervention is necessary for a limited illness. In patients with significant symptoms, several drugs may be used.

To decrease the heavy cough and throat clearing, a combination of a cough suppressant and mucolytic is useful. Organidin and codeine, used in combination, hydrate the airway and reduce the cough reflex. If there is an associated hypersecretory state, such as in viral rhinitis, a decongestant may also be added to the regimen. Antihistamines should be used with caution because of their drying effect. High-dose guaifensin (1200 mg twice a day) is useful in reducing the viscosity of the mucus and the severity and frequency of dry throat and cough.

Mouthwash and sprays have been used by physicians over the centuries to reduce inflammation and edema. Afrin or epinephrine can be sprayed on the vocal folds to achieve temporary mucosal vasoconstriction and transient relief from dysphonia. This may be used by performers to provide a brief, symptomatic respite for a critical song or act. However, regular applications of systemic α-adrenergic medications carry the risk of medication rebound and the side effects of adrenergic stimulation, which may manifest as vocal tremor.

Atropine and its derivatives are occasionally used to dry excessive nasal secretions. Ipatropium (Atrovent), a new anticholinergic nasal spray, may be used with good effect to dry excessive secretions due to viral rhinitis and allergic rhinitis associated with copious rhinorrhea. Systemic or inhaled corticosteroids are occasionally used to blunt the physiologic effects of inflammation. Drugs such as these should always be monitored by the treating physician. If a systemic steroid is used in preparation for a performance, it should only be used for critical performances. Antibiotic coverage and antifungal prophylactic coverage during the acute and resolution phases of an acute illness is usually indicated if the patient has been receiving systemic steroids.

Antibiotics have been used with increasing frequency for acute viral and bacterial laryngitis, despite the lack of efficacy of antibiotics against vital pharyngitis or laryngitis. When laryngitis is associated with bacterial tonsillitis, sinusitis, or bronchitis, antibiotic therapy is justified. In laryngitis associated with high fever, suppuration, and toxemia, bacterial etiologies must be considered. There is an increasing incidence of drug resistance to traditional antibiotics, such as ampicillin and penicillin. *Branhamella catarrhalis*, β-streptococcus, pneumococcus, *Haemophilus influenzae,* and staphylococcus are common pathogens that have increasing resistance to antibiotics. Throat and nasal sinus cultures, followed by close monitoring, is necessary. In cases in which antibiotic resistance is suspected, sputum examination, direct laryngeal swab, and cultures may be done.

Prognosis

The prognosis for return of voice in acute laryngitis is excellent. Although a small group of patients have episodes of recurrent symptoms or prolonged symptoms, most regain normal vocal function 7 to 10 days after the initial onset of symptoms.

Noninfective or Nonspecific Laryngitis

Acute inflammation of the larynx that is not attributable to viral, fungal, or bacterial etiologies has been termed noninfective laryngitis. This includes allergic laryngitis; traumatic laryngitis of vocal abuse; and thermal, chemical, or caustic irritation of the larynx. Although the presentation and clinical course of this spectrum of disorders is variable, the pathogenesis, tissue response, and treatment are sufficiently similar to be considered together.

Mild traumatic laryngitis often occurs after exhaustive voice use. Teachers who spend their day lecturing often have mild, transient, mucosal edema with voice loss. Nonspecific irritants, such as second-hand smoke, hair spray, dry air, and sudden temperature changes, may also result in mild laryngeal edema with irritation. Medications that have drying effects on mucus include diuretics, antihypertensive medications, antihistamines, and psychotropic drugs with anticholinergic side effects.

Nonspecific laryngitis is suspected when voice loss and laryngeal irritation are present without the usual symptoms of upper respiratory infection. The clinical course of nonspecific laryngitis is variable and may be brief to prolonged. The causative agent of nonspecific laryngitis is usually a laryngeal irritant. Appropriate identification and avoidance of the inciting agent is the best course of treatment. For the patient with a habitual, loud voice and traumatic laryngitis, vocal re-education by a speech pathologist is the best approach. Patients with dry throats secondary to medication side effects are best treated by aggressive vocal hygiene, hydration, and changes in medication regimen.

Nonspecific laryngitis is often a difficult problem to manage, and a specific inciting agent may be difficult to identify. In its subacute form, frequent exacerbation of voice difficulties may occur at the most injudicious times. Drugs, such as corticosteroids, may be useful in temporizing symptoms. Definitive treatment depends on a successful search for the inciting agent. Such patients, because of their intermittent complaints and paucity of physical findings, may be labeled as having functional or psychogenic dysphonia. In such cases, interdisciplinary evaluations by otolaryngologists and speech pathologists can be most useful.

The vocal characteristics of nonspecific laryngitis are indistinguishable from those associated with acute laryngitis. Voice loss in nonspecific laryngitis follows a more variable clinical course than acute laryngitis. Vocal symptoms often have an indolent, subacute form which neither progresses to aphonia nor resolves to total restitution of voice. These patients often go from physician to therapist with a variety of diagnoses that are far from definitive and often are treated empirically with a host of medications and therapies.

Endoscopic examination can differentiate between acute laryngitis and nonspecific laryngitis. Allergic laryngitis is characterized by laryngeal findings that resemble those of the normal larynx. There is little erythema or increased production of mucus. The only hint of abnormality is the pale bluish color to the vocal fold edge with a hint of vocal fold edema. Erythema located over the posterior interarytenoid area may be present in patients with acid reflux laryngitis and in patients with habitual chronic throat clearing.

Stroboscopic examination helps to differentiate between acute and chronic laryngeal irritation. With prolonged irritation, the superior surface of the vocal fold loses its glistening, smooth appearance. The

smooth, glossy surface is replaced by a stippled surface that can easily be detected by stroboscopy. This has the appearance of salt and pepper speckled on the surface. Figure 8-25 shows an example of such a "salt and pepper" larynx in a patient with chronic laryngeal inflammation. In patients with mild inflammation, the mucosal vibratory amplitude remains good despite excessive secretion and color change. Mucosal wave propagation may be delayed relative to the vocal fold opening, and it may be erratic and jerky, imparting a sensation that there is increased inertia to movement. In patients with severe mucosal inflammation, the mucosal amplitude becomes progressively diminished. The mucosal wave is absent. When there is severe stiffness of the vocal folds, vibration of the vocal folds ceases. In severe laryngitis, the vocal folds fail to vibrate during phonation, showing absence of vibratory amplitude and mucosal wave.

Treatment

The primary treatment of nonspecific laryngitis lies in a careful search for and identification of the inciting agent. After correct identification, a plan to decrease or eliminate exposure is the best treatment. Voice rest, hydration, and mucolytics are useful adjuncts in the treatment of nonspecific laryngitis. Inhaled steroid spray or systemic steroid use may be indicated to bring about rapid symptomatic improvement.

Patients with throat pain and irritation often develop harmful voicing gestures. These include development of organic processes, such as contact ulcers, polyps, and nodules. Chronic hypophonia with bowed, incompletely closed, vocal folds are often

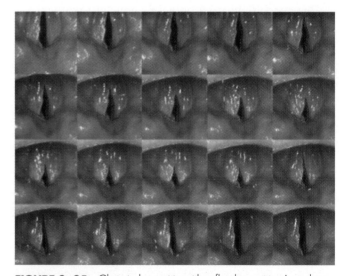

FIGURE 8-25 Chronic laryngitis with reflux laryngitis. A stroboscopic view shows the chronic vocal fold edema with reduced vibratory amplitude, incomplete closure, and reduced fundamental frequency of vibration.

seen in patients with contact granuloma. Ventricular phonation is often a compensatory gesture for immobile or nonpliable true vocal folds. In patients with these harmful voicing gestures, behavioral speech therapy, used in conjunction with appropriate medical supportive measures, should be initiated to speed recovery.

Vocal Fold Tear and Hemorrhage

Mucosal tear and submucosal hemorrhage are two feared complications of acute laryngeal inflammation and may result in permanently altered voice. Mucosal tear results from microtrauma when patients aggressively phonate or cough. The consequence of such a tear is often healing by secondary intention and vocal fold scarring. Unlike soft vocal fold nodules, which are reversible, microtears may result in residual scar and a nonvibratory segment. Such an adynamic segment of the vocal folds results in a further decrement in voice elasticity and may be permanent.

Vocal fold hemorrhage secondary to vascular leakage may result in normal healing without damage. Extensive macrophage and fibroblast stimulation followed by healing may change the layered viscoelastic properties of the vocal folds and reduce vocal fold pliability. Submucosal fibrosis will result in a nonvibratory segment. With stroboscopic light examination, the vocal fold hemorrhage is seen to cause localized stiffness of the affected fold, resulting in a unilateral reduction in amplitude and mucosal wave. Because of the asymmetric tension, vocal fold vibration may be associated with phase shift as one vocal fold opens and closes before the other. Phase shifts result in a vocal fold vibratory pattern that resembles a snake dance.

Treatment

Mucosal tears and submucosal hemorrhages are absolute indications for voice rest. It is critical that further injury to the delicate vocal folds be avoided. Therefore, performances may need to be canceled and lectures may need to be rescheduled. Voice rest, along with medical treatment to reduce cough and throat irritation, is used to allow uneventful healing and avoid further mucosal damage.

Chronic Laryngitis

Chronic laryngitis is a nonspecific, clinical term that describes multiple inflammatory processes and disorders of the larynx. This condition is distinguishable by the presence of chronic, inflammatory, cellular infiltration with a typical clinical pattern and presentation. Histologic examination may not distinguish the various possibilities. For example, reflux laryngitis and pachydermia associated with long-term smoking look similar. Both are characterized by acute and chronic inflammatory cellular infiltrate, with or without epithelial hyperplasia. Chronic laryngitis refers to a broad category of disorders resulting in a chronic inflammatory response. Patterns of chronic tissue response can take one of several forms, including (1) infiltrative disorders, such as amyloidosis; (2) chronic granulomatous diseases affecting the larynx (e.g., sarcoidosis, tuberculosis, fungal laryngitis); (3) chronic, nonspecific inflammation (e.g., bacterial laryngitis, laryngitis sicca); and (4) proliferative processes involving the epithelial layer (e.g., hyperplastic laryngitis, keratosis, sulcus vocalis).

Factors contributing to chronic laryngitis that are not of bacterial, viral, fungal, or systemic origin may include irritants that are inhaled or local contamination from adjacent structures. Some of these include: (1) environmental exposures to dust, chemicals, or toxins; (2) allergic response of the immediate or delayed-hypersensitivity type; and (3) chronic infection in organs contiguous with the larynx (e.g., chronic reflux laryngitis, chronic sinobronchial infections).

Chronic inflammation of the larynx appears to produce changes primarily at two sites. These changes occur in the epithelial and subepithelial layers of the vocal folds. Benign mucosal disorders may result in changes in normal epithelial proliferation and maturation. These proliferative epithelial disorders include hyperkeratosis, dyskeratosis, parakeratosis, acanthosis, and cellular atypia. Figure 8–26 is an example of benign keratosis in a chronic heavy smoker. Figure 8–25 is an example of chronic laryngitis with interarytenoid mucosal hyperplasia due to reflux laryngitis.

Besides the local tissue response to chronic irritation, systemic chronic inflammatory disorders may cause chronic laryngitis. Rheumatoid arthritis, systemic lupus erythematosus, and mucosal ulcerative

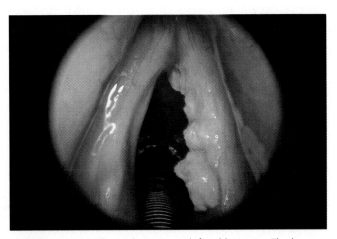

FIGURE 8-26 Chronic laryngitis with focal keratosis. The lesion is unusual in that it is limited to one vocal fold. The contralateral vocal fold has a sulcus vocalis.

disorders, such as pemphigus and Behçets syndrome,[83] may affect the laryngeal mucous membrane and joints. Airway and voice compromise occasionally complicate these systemic inflammatory disorders. To diagnose these disorders, there must be a high level of clinical suspicion, and biopsy studies, cultures, and special histopathologic studies may be necessary.

Chronic, Nonspecific Laryngitis

Chronic, nonspecific laryngitis is a disease affecting adult males in their fifth to seventh decades. Men appear to be more commonly afflicted than women due to a higher incidence of smoking and environmental exposure to fumes and work-related irritants.

Chronic, nonspecific laryngitis is found in heavy smokers and drinkers.[84] These patients rarely complain of dysphonia despite their severe symptoms. Occupational factors may play a role in the pathogenesis of chronic, nonspecific laryngitis. Patients who work in foundries, beauty shops, paper mills, printing shops, and other sites where chemical, thermal, and foreign bodies may be inhaled are at increased risk.

Medication side effects often contribute to this condition. Patients taking psychotropic drugs with anticholinergic side effects have a dry throat and a hoarse, rough voice sound. Medication side effects have been found to contribute to dysphonia and chronic laryngitis symptoms in the elderly.[85] Allergic and bacterial rhinosinusitis with laryngeal involvement may progress to chronic, nonspecific laryngitis if such antigen exposure is prolonged.

Physical Findings

The history of chronic laryngitis is one of recurrent episodes of dysphonia with progressive inability to return to normal voice. The severity of vocal difficulties may fluctuate, but voice quality does not return to normal. The voice gradually deteriorates over a period of weeks to many months. In most patients, pain and dysphonia are not prominent features. The patient may exhibit chronic throat clearing, but rarely will there be pain or discomfort. When the patient coughs, thick, tenacious fluid is often present. The thick mucus is a sign of infection or inflammation. In some patients, this is accompanied by a sensation of a lump in the throat. The voice in these patients is often poor, and ventricular phonation is a common finding.

A bacterial etiology for chronic laryngitis is to be suspected if there is transient improvement during a course of antibiotics, followed by recurrent relapses. Chronic bacterial laryngitis is also suggested by findings of diffuse inflammation with suppuration. The larynx is swollen and dry. Pachydermia of the interarytenoid area is often present. Tissue response to infection of the false vocal folds, arytenoid, and interarytenoid areas may be so intense that a mass lesion is suspected. Patients may be advised to undergo microlaryngeal examination to rule out neoplasia. Erythema of the aerodigestive tract is rarely limited to the larynx. Pharyngeal inflammation is often obvious. Thick mucus collects in the posterior pharynx. The posterior pharyngeal wall appears thickened and has an uneven, pebble-stone appearance due to areas of lymphoid hypertrophy.

The otolaryngologist will look for infections of the tonsil, nasopharynx, and sinus areas as primary sites of infection. The lung and tracheobronchial tree should also be considered as potential sites of infection. Sputum samples should be sent for culture for bacteria, fungus, and tuberculosis. When inhaled steroids have been used for a prolonged period, or when the patient is immunocompromised due to HIV infection, Candidal laryngitis should be suspected. If this is the case, endoscopic examination, biopsy, and culture should be considered.

The bacteriologic findings of chronic infectious laryngitis are different than those of acute laryngitis. The most common pathogenic organism isolated in chronic laryngitis is *Staphylococcus aureus*. Appropriate antibiotic coverage should include coverage for common gram-positive and gram-negative pathogens. If tuberculosis or fungal laryngitis is suspected, treatment should be guided by endoscopic biopsy and culture results.

Stroboscopic examination is also useful for differentiating mucosal stiffness secondary to epithelial hyperplasia and that caused by chronic inflammation. In patients with epithelial thickening, mucosal wave propagation is disturbed, but the folds continue to oscillate. The thickened epithelial layer will exhibit a rocking motion on an otherwise normal Reinke's layer. Like a boat riding the crest of a wave in a storm, the vocal fold will still oscillate. When there has been extensive epithelial and subepithelial involvement by inflammation, such rocking motion subsides and the vocal folds become stiff and immobile.

Treatment

Endoscopic evaluation and treatment may be necessary to establish the diagnosis. Biopsy studies and culture may be necessary to guide the management of chronic laryngitis. Histoplasmosis, tuberculosis, and sarcoidosis are causes of granulomatous laryngitis that should be diagnosed by tissue biopsy and culture. Autoimmune disorders, such as amyloidosis, Wegener's granulomatosis, lupus erythematosus, and rheumatoid arthritis with laryngeal involvement, should be suspected in patients with laryngeal findings consistent with chronic laryngitis but refractory to antibiotic and medical treatment. Early diagnosis and treatment may help prevent complications that can cause permanent damage to the larynx.

Besides medical and surgical treatment, supportive measures for patients with chronic laryngitis should include hydration, inhalation therapy, and awareness of mucosal hygiene. Hydration may be accomplished by a systemic fluid intake of 2 L per day. Hydration with steam inhalation or room humidifiers is helpful as a demulcent to thin thick mucus. Local rheologic factors contributing to mucosal stiffness and dryness should be reversed. A vocal hygiene program begins with identification of the local irritants to the larynx and planning for their reduced exposure. Simply wearing a filtered mask during work and performing saline nasal douching after work often helps patients exposed to particulate irritants. A reduction in local irritation will mean less coughing and trauma to the larynx. The treatment of allergy or irritation caused by noxious fumes and organic solvents is more complicated. In managing these patients, limitation of exposure and a change in work environment may be necessary. Second-hand smoke in the home and workplace is increasingly being implicated as a nonspecific laryngeal irritant, and should be addressed as part of the environmental assessment.

Speech pathologists are often called upon to assist with the care of patients with nonspecific laryngitis. Although hyperfunctional voice disorders are rarely a cause of chronic laryngitis, continued chronic laryngitis often promotes hyperfunctional voice disorder. Compensatory mechanisms during voicing often become necessary for the patient to talk. The endoscopic findings include ventricular phonation; short anterior to posterior laryngeal squeezing, and inappropriate laryngeal height during phonation. Fiberoptic videolaryngoscopy, performed with a speech pathologist in attendance, will help to identify these compensatory mechanisms. Rehabilitation of patients with chronic, nonspecific laryngitis often includes treatment by a speech pathologist to re-educate the patient as to appropriate voice production. Table 8–2 summarizes the speech pathologist's role in nonmedical management of chronic laryngitis. When the medical aspects of chronic organic voice disorder have been reversed, reversal of habitual hyperfunction with the aid of a speech pathologist can improve function.

Prognosis

Chronic laryngitis is a difficult problem to treat. Unless a specific etiology is identified and addressed, the disorder may be indolent and may cause ongoing morbidity characterized by voice loss, chronic cough, and occasionally, airway obstruction. The possibility of malignant degeneration is debated, but may be a contributing cofactor to laryngeal carcinoma. The clinical diagnosis of chronic laryngitis should be the beginning of a search for specific inciting factors. By process of elimination, via testing, endoscopy, biopsy, culture, and histologic examina-

TABLE 8 – 2	THE ROLE OF THE SPEECH–LANGUAGE PATHOLOGIST IN THE NONMEDICAL EVALUATION AND MANAGEMENT OF LARYNGITIS

1. Improve vocal hygiene.
2. Assess respiration and phonatory breath support.
3. Improve phonation range and loudness with better resonance.
4. Explore coping strategies with amplification and problem solving.
5. Reduce compensatory hyperfunction.
6. Monitor compliance with medical and nonmedical treatment.

tion, the differential diagnosis should be narrowed sufficiently to establish a working diagnosis of possible etiologies. Local and systemic medications, speech therapy evaluation, and surgery have important roles in disease reversal and symptomatic relief.

In patients with chronic laryngitis and epithelial reaction, the differentiation of benign versus malignant vocal fold lesions cannot be accomplished definitively by clinical methods alone. In some patients with risk factors for neoplasm, biopsy study and operative treatment are the logical treatment choices. Although low in incidence, the possibility of cancer should be discussed during preoperative counseling. Furthermore, the necessity of tissue examination may need to supersede other voice considerations. In most vocal folds showing cellular changes, the malignant potential of these lesions is low. Appropriate treatment should strike a balance between factors such as the malignant potential of the lesion and the voice needs of the patient.

Fungal Laryngitis and Laryngeal Infiltration

Clinical Presentation

Fungal laryngitis is a specific form of chronic laryngitis due to upper airway involvement with fungi. The organisms may be the result of superficial overgrowth of fungi in a host, or they may be invasive fungi. Immunocompromised patients are especially at risk. Such patients include those receiving high-dose steroids for asthma, insulin-dependent diabetics, transplant patients, dialysis patients, patients with acquired immunodeficiency syndrome (AIDS), and others. Medications and treatments may also place patients at risk for fungal laryngeal involvement. Examples include radiation therapy, long-term antibiotic use, steroid use, and chemotherapeutic agents. Alternatively, fungal laryngitis may arise secondary to laryngeal invasion by a fungus that is endemic to the home, as in histoblastosis, coccidiomycosis, and blastomycosis. Patients with compromised immunity are especially susceptible to unusual bacterial (*Mycobacterium tuberculosis*),[79] viral (e.g., herpes simplex),[80] and fungal (Candida) infections of the larynx.

Symptoms and Signs

Candidal Laryngitis and Pharyngitis

Superficial involvement of the larynx and pharynx with *Candida albicans* is not uncommon. This opportunistic infection is seen in patients receiving long-term inhaled steroid therapy, in patients taking cytotoxic drugs, and in patients with AIDS. Involvement of the larynx and pharynx, as well as the oral cavity, is typical.

The disease may present with local signs only or with systemic fever and rigor. The focal involvement starts with a hoarse voice, dysphagia, and throat pain. The larynx may be the only site of involvement in patients taking inhaled steroids, and patients may present with an unexplained hoarse voice of many months' duration. Immunocompromised hosts present with more diffuse involvement. The patients may complain bitterly of throat pain or ear pain. The severity of dysphonia and dysphagia may be out of proportion to the physical findings of red throat. The mucosa is violet-red and spotted with punctate white areas of exudate. The mucosa is rough, dry, and without its gleaming coat of mucus. Occasionally, microabscesses with ulcerations may be seen. Dysphagia may promote dehydration and further drying of the mucous membranes. Crusting and inspissated mucus may involve the larynx, mimicking chronic staphylococcal laryngitis or infiltrative diseases of the larynx. In these patients, the site of involvement is always diffuse, and some differentiation of the suspected organism may be possible on the basis of the history and the clinical sites of involvement.

Histoplasmosis and Blastomycosis

Invasive fungal laryngitis, such as blastomycosis and histoplasmosis, is a disease affecting populations in certain areas of the United States and the world where the infections are endemic. In the United States, the organisms *Histoplasma capsulatum* and *Blastomyces dermatitidis* are prevalent in the Ohio River area (histoplasmosis) and in the southwestern United States (blastomycosis). The route of infection is via an airborne vector by inhalation. Laryngeal involvement is rare. The disease is often confused with tuberculosis of the larynx and may mimic squamous cell carcinoma of the larynx. Fungal laryngitis may present as a supraglottic mass with exophytic or submucosal masses. Ulceration and necro-sis may be present, with extensive hyperemia of the surrounding ulcers.

Radiologic Evaluation

A barium swallow may show nonspecific esophagitis in patients with candidal pharyngitis. Patients with invasive fungal laryngitis may present with a laryngeal mass of the supraglottic or glottic larynx. There is no specific feature recognizable on CT scan of the larynx that would differentiate fungal laryngitis due to granulomatous involvement of the larynx with fungus from tuberculosis, except for the likelihood of posterior laryngeal involvement in the latter.

Treatment

Systemic and topical antifungal treatments have been used. Systemic treatment is appropriate in patients who are immunocompromised. Oral antifungal lozenges, combined with withdrawal of inhaled or systemic steroids or antibiotics, are effective in patients with candidal laryngitis who do not have a compromised immune status. Clinical suspicion and a differential diagnosis of squamous cell carcinoma, tuberculosis, blastomycosis, and histoplasmosis will help to alert the pathologist to the possibilities of invasive fungal laryngitis. Multiple biopsy studies and cultures may be necessary to establish the diagnosis of fungal laryngeal invasion. Systemic treatment with amphotericin B is indicated in laryngeal invasion with blastomycosis and histoplasmosis.

Prognosis

Candida rarely causes invasive tissue destruction; however, systemic and hematologic dissemination of *C. albicans* originating in the oral pharynx and larynx may cause life-threatening illness, especially in immunocompromised hosts. It can be a cause of multiorgan failure, sepsis, and death.

Invasive fungal laryngeal involvement responds to systemic antifungal treatment. However, the extent of laryngeal involvement may require tracheotomy. Subglottic stenosis and tracheal dependence may be a sequel of advanced laryngeal involvement.

Gastroesophageal Reflux Disease and the Larynx

Sufficient new interest has arisen recently regarding the importance of extraesophageal manifestations of GERD in a variety of laryngeal disorders to warrant a discussion of this disease. GERD is a ubiquitous disorder that affects 25% of the adult U.S. population. The two major clinical forms of this disease have been categorized as esophageal and extraesophageal. GERD involves refluxate of acid and pepsin outside the stomach into the esophagus, larynx, pharynx, and lungs. Whether the problem is primarily one of acid production or a motility disorder is still debated in the gastroenterologic literature. What is not controversial is the effect of mucosal injury caused by prolonged exposure to acid. It is of interest to laryngologists because of the variety of extraesophageal manifestations of GERD, which may present as GERD-related laryngeal symptoms and disorders.

Patients with hoarseness, dysphagia, globus sensation, laryngeal granulomas, and subglottic stenosis may have GERD as the primary cause of their disorder and should be evaluated for GERD.[41] As stated by Olson,[86] there is a large variety of symptoms presenting to the otolaryngologist that result from gastroesophageal reflux; some are merely nuisances, whereas others are life-threatening. The variety of GERD-related complications involving the laryngopharynx may vary from thick phlegm to mild, chronic, throat clearing to life-threatening subglottic stenosis.

Laryngotracheal Manifestations of GERD

Clinical Presentation, Symptoms, and Signs

An association between gastroesophageal reflux and vocal cord contact ulcer was first reported by Cherry and Margulies.[41] Since then, nonspecific laryngitis attributable to acid reflux has been reported by Delahunty[87] and Ward and Berci.[88] Head and neck manifestations of gastroesophageal reflux have been reviewed by others.[89] In an important contribution, Koufman carefully studied symptoms of extraesophageal manifestations of GERD and delineated the role of acid in the larynx in the animal model. Since then, various authors have further delineated the role of acid in the pharynx in the pathogenesis of chronic posterior laryngitis.[90,91] Hanson and colleagues[92] studied the response of chronic laryngitis attributable to acid reflux using endoscopic documentation and questionnaires and reported improvements in laryngeal indices. The laryngoscopic findings of acid laryngitis may be characteristic but subtle, spanning a spectrum from normal to severe laryngitis with stenosis. In a study of endoscopic findings, pH findings, and response to empirical antireflux therapy in patients with globus symptoms, pH abnormalities were not found to correlate directly with laryngeal findings of laryngeal edema, hyperemia, or posterior laryngitis.[93] The causes of posterior laryngitis were identified as a result of gastroesophageal reflux, with friction of both vocal processes during phonation and vocal abuse.

The role of acid reflux in the genesis of symptoms of hoarseness and cough has been reviewed, but large clinical trials remain to be done.[94,95] McNally and co-workers[95] evaluated a small series of patients and found that GERD was frequently seen in patients with idiopathic hoarseness (55%) and that patients with both throat pain and nocturnal heartburn were likely to have esophagitis. There is, however, conflicting evidence as to the prevalence of GERD in the genesis of cough and hoarseness in the general population. A review by Fraser[96] indicated that patient selection may be a factor in studies suggesting a major role of GERD in the symptoms of cough and hoarseness. It is possible that patients with cough and hoarseness present to an otolaryngologist because of low esophageal reflux exposure despite abnormal pharyngeal exposure. Other plausible explanations include: insensitivity of the esophageal mucosa to acid exposure or increased pharyngeal and laryngeal sensitivity to episodic pharyngeal reflux. Thus, although it is recognized that GERD is an important differential in patients presenting with cough and hoarseness, controversy exists as to its prevalence. Most authors agree that the selected use of certain diagnostic tests (biopsy, endoscopy, and 24-hour pH analysis) is indicated.

Radiologic Evaluation

A careful history and physical examination with a high index of suspicion is the first step in the workup of a patient presenting with suspected GERD or extraesophageal GERD symptoms. Esophagoscopy is commonly used to diagnose and to stage esophagitis,[97] however, normal findings on endoscopy cannot exclude reflux disease. Endoscopy is used to establish a diagnosis of reflux esophagitis, to exclude other esophageal disease, and to permit directed biopsy if columnar metaplasia, dysplasia, or carcinoma is suspected. The lesions of reflux esophagitis—erosions, ulceration, stricture, and metaplasia—should be identified and graded independently.

Twenty-four-hour pH analysis has recently become the "gold standard" for detection of gastroesophageal reflux.[98] In many patients, the reflux correlates with the GERD event. Technologic advancement has considerably simplified both the procedure and the interpretation of the data obtained, and there is currently reasonable consensus as to the parameters that best discriminate between physiologic and pathologic gastroesophageal reflux. There remains a need for internationally agreed upon definitions and standards, particularly with regard to the calculation of these parameters. Despite these considerations, the use of double-probe 24-hour pH monitoring in the diagnosis of otolaryngoloic manifestations of GERD has become the standard within the last 10 years. A pH exposure of less than 4 is considered to indicate a positive reflux episode. From the 24-hour tracing, a computer printout of the total acid exposure time, number of reflux events, and correlation with symptoms is generated. The percentage of time that the pH is less than 4 provides as much information as any other scheme of quantifying esophageal acid exposure, but symptom association is essential when evaluating atypical or sporadic symptoms. The enthusiasm for 24-hour pH monitoring must, however, be tempered with an analysis of its proven clinical utility in determining patient management, and this utility must rightfully be compared with that of an empirical trial of antireflux therapy. Ambulatory pH monitoring is probably most useful in examining patients without typical reflux symptoms or patients who have either partially or completely failed a trial of antireflux therapy. To date, there have not been any prospective, controlled clinical trials evaluating these uses. Suggested clinical indications for ambulatory pH monitoring include (1) documented abnormal esophageal acid exposure in endoscopy-negative patients being considered for surgical antireflux repair; (2) either normal or equivocal endoscopic findings and reflux symptoms that are refractory to proton pump inhibitor therapy; (3) suspected otolaryngologic manifestations of GERD after symptoms have failed to respond to at least 4 weeks of proton pump inhibitor therapy.[99]

The radiographic evaluation of patients with otolaryngologic manifestations of GERD has traditionally included a barium swallow study. A double-contrast upper gastrointestinal (GI) series is a medically and economically sound alternative to endoscopy for evaluating patients with dyspepsia or other upper GI symptoms who fail to respond to an empirical trial of medical therapy. The barium esophagram is used primarily for detecting the gross morphologic changes of reflux esophagitis, and it is a reliable screening method for diagnosing the more severe grades of disease. Its utility in the evaluation of gastroesophageal reflux by barium examination in patients without esophageal symptoms is less certain. The presence of hiatal hernia and the demonstration of reflux by provocative testing as evidence of GERD has been replaced by 24-hour pH analysis, endoscopy, and manometry.

Treatment

The goals of management of GERD are relief of symptoms, healing of esophagitis, prevention of complications, and maintenance of remission. Simple lifestyle changes may control GERD in up to 20% of patients. Promotility therapy addresses the pathophysiology of this disorder, but even the best results achieved, using Cisapride, have yielded only a 50% to 60% control rate. The more traditional agents (metoclopramide and bethanechol) are limited by side effects. Acid suppression using histamine receptor antagonists controls GERD in 50% to 60% of patients, whereas proton pump inhibitors offer the most effective control (80% to 100%). A surgical approach (especially using newly developed laparoscopic techniques) provides effective therapy for GERD in a high percentage of patients, but further comparisons are needed to define the long-term efficacy and cost-effectiveness associated with both surgical and chronic medical therapy of GERD.

Simple lifestyle and dietary modifications and reflux precautions are effective in the management of a percentage of reflux patients. Nonmedical treatment of GERD symptoms should be used first, or may be combined with medical therapy. Dietary restriction of fat, alcohol, and caffeine should be practiced. The maintenance of a height gradient between the upper and lower esophageal sphincters by bed elevation and upright posture after meals are simple yet effective methods of nonmedical reflux management.

The keystone of medical management of GERD is acid suppression. Two classes of drugs that have shown effectiveness in acid suppression are the H_2 histamine receptor antagonists (cimetidine, ranitidine, famotidine, nizatidine) and the newer proton pump inhibitors (Omeprazole, Lansoprazole). A combination of antacids and prokinetic agents (Cisapride, bethanechol, and metaclopramide hydrochloride) has also been used to effect acid suppression in the management of GERD.

In the 1980s, antihistamine H_2 antagonists were the traditional first line of medical therapy for acid suppression in the management of GERD. However, with the recent approval by the FDA of long-term therapy with proton pump inhibitors for acid suppression, the use of proton pump inhibitors in GERD management has increased. The proton pump inhibitor is more effective than H_2 blockers in total acid suppression. Given the wide variety of effective agents available, a stepwise approach to therapy, utilizing a number of drug classes, may be possible.[100]

The addition of prokinetic drugs in combination therapy with H_2 histamine receptor antagonists makes theoretical sense, but has been shown to be of modest healing benefit, especially when compared to the effectiveness of H_2 histamine receptor antagonists alone.

Several different antireflux procedures yield good to excellent results when performed by skilled and experienced practitioners.[101] Laparoscopic antireflux surgery using the Nissen fundoplication technique has been shown to result in excellent long-term success. Antireflux surgery is designed to correct a mechanically defective sphincter, defined as a sphincter with a mean pressure of less than 6 mm Hg, a mean length exposed to the positive pressure environment of the abdomen of less than 1 cm, or a mean overall length of less than 2 cm. However, the incidence of associated complications and poor operative results needs to be compared to the results achieved with long-term acid suppression. With the recent developments in both surgical and medical therapies, a comparison of therapeutic results between surgery and medical management has become difficult. Surgery is a reasonable alternative in the following cases: (1) in patients who have failed medical therapy; (2) in healthy patients who prefer surgery; (3) in refractory extraesophageal manifestations, such as reflux laryngitis and asthma; and (4) in patients with bleeding from refractory esophagitis.

Relapsing Polychondritis

Relapsing polychondritis is an unusual disease of the upper airway. The primary sites of involvement in the ear, nose, and throat are the cartilaginous structures of the outer ear, the cartilaginous nasal skeleton, and the laryngeal and tracheal cartilages. Other sites of involvement include the cartilages of the joints and heart valves. Systemic involvement of the skin, kidney, and central nervous system has been reported and is characterized by repeated inflammation followed by destruction of the cartilages. The cause is unknown, but an immune system etiology is suspected.[102]

Clinical Presentation

The disease occurs in adults in the fifth decade. The laryngeal involvement may present as unexplained hoarse voice, airway obstruction, or pain.[103] The localized laryngeal pain on palpation may be accompanied by dysphagia, choking, and stridor. Airway obstruction may occur during the acute exacerbation of the disease or during the convalescent phase. The most common cause of upper airway obstruction is glottic and subglottic edema and narrowing due to inflammation and swelling of the subglottic area. With healing and repair of the inflammatory chondritis, there may be scarring and stenosis that encroach on the airway. Finally, loss of the cartilaginous support with repeated inflammation may result in tracheomalacia and flow-related collapse of the upper airways.[104]

Symptoms and Signs

Patients present during the acute phase with swelling of the ear cartilage and chondritic changes of the auricular cartilage. The ear may be exquisitely tender with erythema and edema. The auricular landmarks are obscured. Involvement of the nasal cartilage may include nasal obstruction and thickening of the septum. Laryngeal involvement is less likely than involvement of the other cartilage sites, but it may occur in isolation. Nonspecific complaints, such as dysphagia, stridor, and wheezing, may be the only symptoms. Severe endobronchial obstruction with relapsing polychondritis has been reported.[105]

Diagnosis

The work-up of a patient suspected of having endobronchial involvement related to relapsing polychondritis should include radiographic examination, endoscopic evaluation, and pulmonary function testing. A flexible bronchoscopic examination of the airway correlates well to tracheal involvement and may help to document stenosis or malacia, or both. Segmental involvement should be differentiated from more diffuse involvement because the treatment differs (tracheotomy versus reconstruction, respectively). The radiographic work-up involves airway fluoroscopy, radiographic evaluation of the airway soft tissues, and CT scans. The soft-tissue x-ray films are useful as a screening tool for upper airway obstruction. Airway fluoroscopy in the anteroposterior and lateral views is helpful to rule out flow-related collapse of the upper airway. CT scans are helpful in documenting the presence of stenosis, but they may underestimate the degree of stenosis if there is significant airway collapse. The use of pulmonary function testing with volume flow loops is especially useful in evaluating flow during inspiratory and expiratory phases of respiration.

Treatment

Correct diagnosis of this immune-mediated disease by radiologic study, clinical examination, and histologic examination is mandatory. The treatment of recurrent episodic inflammatory lapses is primarily medical and involves the use of systemic anti-inflammatory, antimetabolite, and immunosuppressive medications. High-dose oral steroids (e.g., 60 mg of prednisone/day) are used in the acute stages for management of pain and swelling. Immunuosupressive drugs used to treat this disorder include cyclophosphamide, azathioprine, and 6-mercaptopurine.[106]

Surgical intervention is indicated in patients with airway obstruction. Airway obstruction may require tracheotomy to bypass and stent the trachea, but this approach may be inadequate in diffuse tracheobronchial involvement. Use of endobronchial stents has been reported in relapsing polychondritis.

Airway collapse from relapsing polychondritis may be a cause of death from asphyxiation.[107] Laryngotracheal reconstruction for discrete segmental stenosis may be performed using traditional methods of segmental resection or cartilaginous grafting. If the disease is diffuse, surgical treatment may not be feasible.

Prognosis

Involvement of the tracheobronchial tree may be a late manifestation of relapsing polychondritis, or it may be present at initial presentation. Patients with initial involvement of the tracheobronchial tree have a worse prognosis, with higher rates of upper airway involvement, than do those with later onset. Airway compromise as a cause of death is a pulmonary complication of relapsing polychondritis, which may be the cause of death in a significant percentage of patients with this unusual disease.

Wegener's Granulomatosis

Wegener's granulomatosis is a systemic autoimmune disorder which, in its full-blown form, involves multiple organs and sites. However, localized involvement of upper airway structures, such as the nose, sinus, larynx, and trachea, is common, and these may be the presenting sites prior to pulmonary, renal, or other organ involvement. In the localized form, Wegener's granulomatosis is often confused with other inflammatory or granulomatous diseases of the upper airway, including laryngeal tuberculosis, fungal laryngotracheitis, sarcoidosis, actinomycosis, idiopathic subglottic stenosis, and others. This is because the biopsy may be nondiagnostic, and multinucleated giant cells seen on biopsy are not pathognomonic of Wegener's granulomatosis. Vasculitis with small vessel involvement by fibrinoid necrosis is more diagnostic, but this cannot always be confirmed by biopsy of the airway lesion.

Clinical Presentation

Affected patients may present with stridor and upper airway stenosis of unexplained etiology. Early in the process, a fresh, friable, or red lesion may be identified by biopsy study. The biopsy may reveal granulation tissue and chronic inflammation.[108]

Total obstruction of the subglottic larynx and upper trachea by stenosis and granuloma has been reported.[109] Wegener's granulomatosis can lead to proliferative tissue growth with acute airway obstruction in the larynx and trachea.

Symptoms and Signs

Subglottic stenosis, ulcerating tracheobronchitis with or without inflammatory pseudotumors, and tracheal or bronchial stenosis without inflammation are the most common presentations (59%).[110] Endobronchial abnormalities secondary to Wegener's granulomatosis should be suspected in any patients without a previous history of surgery or trauma. Hemoptysis may be an initial presentation of Wegener's granulomatosis.

Radiologic and Serologic Evaluation

Radiographic examination of the soft tissues of the larynx may be done by CT or by soft tissue tomography. It shows nonspecific involvement of the larynx and trachea with a mass or narrowing. Chest x-ray films may document pulmonary involvement. CT scans and a sinus series should be performed in patients with laryngotracheal involvement to evaluate the upper airway and rule out sinonasal involvement.

Antineutrophil cytoplasmic antibody (ANCA) is now regarded as a serologic marker for glomerulonephritis, either in its renal-limited form or associated with systemic vasculitis, such as Wegener's granulomatosis.[111] The usefulness of ANCA detection for the diagnosis of these forms of vasculitis has now been established. ANCA serologic markers should be part of the work-up for unexplained laryngeal and subglottic stenosis. Antinuclear antibodies and other rheumatologic serologic markers may yield positive results.

Treatment

Focal Wegener's granulomatosis responds well to cytotoxic agents, such as cyclophosphamide, and systemic steroids. The mainstay of therapeutic intervention is early identification and long-term medical management using those classes of drugs. More recent modalities include plasmapheresis, folate antagonists, oral trimethoprim-sulfamethoxazole, and local radiotherapy.[108,111] Subglottic stenosis may be an especially difficult problem because it may occur independent of other features of active Wegener's granulomatosis. It is frequently unresponsive to systemic immunosuppressive therapy.[112] Tracheal dilation and steroid injection therapy are safe and effective for the treatment of subglottic stenosis associated with Wegener's granulomatosis, and may be used for involvement of the subglottis and trachea, often leading to compromise of the upper airway. Moreover, the stenotic segments may persist or progress despite control of the disease elsewhere in the body.[113]

Prognosis

The likelihood that localized Wegener's granulomatosis will be able to be controlled by medical treatment is excellent. Incorrect diagnosis may lead to prolonged morbidity and delayed treatment. Subglottic involvement with Wegener's granulomatosis was reviewed by McDonald et al,[112] who found that it responded to cyclophosphamide combined with steroids. Treatment of subglottic stenosis after adequate medical management may require endoscopic or open surgery for re-establishment of a patent airway.

LARYNGEAL MANIFESTATIONS OF CUTANEOUS DISEASE

Epidermolysis bullosa is a rare inherited skin disease that generally presents in the neonatal period. It is characterized by noninflammatory bullous lesions that can involve the mucous membranes of the oral cavity and oropharynx.[108] Mucous membrane involvement may be extensive. Tracheal and laryngeal involvement has been reported.

Pemphigus is an autoimmune disorder that involves the cutaneous and mucous membranes. It

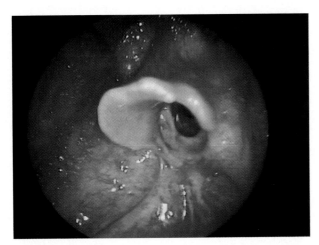

FIGURE 8–27   Cicatricial pemphigoid with supraglottic stenosis.

may occasionally affect the larynx, but is usually associated with oropharyngeal involvement.[115] The supraglottic larynx and the loose mucosal membranes around the larynx are most commonly involved. Bullae, ulceration, and stenosis are most commonly seen on the epiglottis and the aryepiglottic folds. Cicatricial pemphigoid may cause supraglottic stenosis (Fig. 8–27). This responds well to laryngoscopic dilation by laser and systemic medical treatment.

Hamartoma and Choristomas

Clinical Presentation

Laryngeal hamartoma is a rare, benign, congenital disorder of infancy.[116] It may be a cause of airway obstruction and should be considered in the differential diagnosis of neonatal stridor.

Symptoms and Signs

Hamartoma is a rare congenital abnormality of the larynx that must be considered in the differential diagnosis of benign lesions of the larynx. Presenting symptoms may include changes in voice, eating, and activity levels, and respiratory complaints.[117]

Radiologic Evaluation

Radiographic examination shows nonspecific mass lesions of the larynx. The differential diagnosis includes neoplasm and pseudotomor of inflammatory etiology.

Treatment

Endoscopic management by localized surgical resection using the CO_2 laser is the preferred method of management. Tracheotomy may be necessary.[118]

Prognosis

The outcome and prognosis after treatment is excellent.

Tracheopathia Osteoplastica

Clinical Presentation

Tracheopathia osteoplastica is a segmental degenerative disorder of the tracheobronchial tree that results in a narrowing of the major airways. It is a disorder affecting elderly men. The hallmark of this disorder is involvement of the submucosal tracheal lumen by multiple deposits of calcified nodules; a hard, calcified trachea that is rigid and narrowed is a finding on endoscopy and radiographic evaluation. Affected patients may present with stridor and progressive dyspnea, but this disorder may also present as a incidental finding of narrowed trachea on radiographic study. The narrowed, rigid trachea may preclude successful intubation during surgery, which may then prompt medical attention.

Symptoms and Signs

Tracheopathia osteoplastica is a relatively rare, benign disease of the trachea and major bronchi, characterized by cartilaginous and bony submucosal nodules covered by intact mucosa, which may cause narrowing and rigidity of the upper airways. The cause of tracheopathia osteoplastica is unknown, but is believed to be degenerative or due to chronic inflammation or irritation. The diagnosis of tracheopathia osteoplastica is rarely entertained because the condition is rare.[119] Patients present with a history of slow, indolent onset of dyspnea and hoarse voice, which is often progressive over many years.

Radiologic Evaluation

The radiographic findings show multiple submucosal nodules that are calcified. The cartilaginous rings are calcified and thickened. Individual nodules often have a rim of calcification on the surface of the nodule, covered by a thin rim of mucosa. The site of involvement usually involves a long segment of the trachea. The upper trachea and primary bronchi appear to be more involved than the lower airways. The multiple submucosal nodules narrow the lumen of the airway with irregular bumps, which are limited to the tracheal rings, sparing the posterior membranous wall of the trachea.

Treatment

Tracheopathia osteoplastica should be considered to be a benign dysplasia of the tracheobronchial tree. Localized involvement with minimal restriction of the airway may not require treatment or surgical intervention. Cases in which there is significant narrowing may need to be addressed by endoscopy, bronchoscopic removal by laser, and dilation.[120,121]

Prognosis

Relief of the airway by CO_2 laser excision or holmium laser excision of the nodules usually results in palliation of the disorder. The patient should be advised to reduce environmental irritants and to institute careful tracheobronchial hygiene to improve ciliary flow and pulmonary toilet.

REFERENCES

1. Bouchayer MCG, Witzig E, Loire R, Roch J. Epidermoid cysts, sulci, and mucosal bridges of the true vocal cord. *Laryngoscope.* 1985; 95:1087–1094.
2. Ford CN, Inagi K, Khidr A, Bless DM, Gilchrist KW. Sulcus vocalis: A rational analytical approach to diagnosis and management. *Ann Otol Rhinol Laryngol.* 1996; 105(3):189–200.
3. Tanaka S, Hirano M. Fiberscopic estimation of vocal fold stiffness in vivo using the sucking method. *Arch Otolaryngol Head Neck Surg.* 1990; 116(6):721–724.
4. Remacle M. The contribution of videostroboscopy in daily ENT practice. *Acta Otorhinolaryngol Belg.* 1996; 50(4):265–281.
5. Hirano M, Yoshida T, Tanaka S, Hibi S. Sulcus vocalis: Functional aspects. *Ann Otol Rhinol Laryngol.* 1990; 99(9 pt 1):679–683.
6. Belisle GM, Morrison MD. Anatomic correlation for muscle tension dysphonia. *J Otolaryngol.* 1983; 12(5):319–321.
7. Feder R. Varix of the vocal cord in the professional voice user. *Otolaryngol Head Neck Surg.* 1983; 91:435–440.
8. Glanz HK, Kleinsasser O. Chronische Laryngitis und Carcinom. *Arch Otorhinolaryngol.* 1976; 212:57–75.
9. Pontes P, Behlau M. Treatment of sulcus vocalis: Auditory perceptual and acoustical analysis of the slicing mucosa surgical technique. *J Voice.* 1993; 7(4):365–376.
10. Kass ES, Hillman RE, Zeitels SM. Vocal fold submucosal infusion technique in phonomicrosurgery. *Ann Otol Rhinol Laryngol.* 1996; 105(5):341–347.
11. Woo P, Casper J, Griffin B, Colton R, Brewer D. Endoscopic microsuture repair of vocal fold defects. *J Voice.* 1995; 9(3):332–339.
12. Courey MS, Garrett CG, Ossoff RH. Medial microflap for excision of benign vocal fold lesions. *Laryngoscope.* 1997; 107:340–344.
13. Kleinsasser O. *Microlaryngoscopy and Endolaryngeal Microsurgery.* St. Louis: Mosby; 1990.
14. Kumazawa H, Asako M, Yamashita T, Ha-Kawa SK. An increase in laryngeal aerosol deposition by ultrasonic nebulizer therapy with intermittent vocalization. *Laryngoscope.* 1997; 107(5):671–674.
15. Yanagisawa E, Hausfeld JN, Pensak ML. Sudden airway obstruction due to pedunculated laryngeal polyps. *Ann Otol Rhinol Laryngol.* 1983; 92(4 pt 1):340–343.
16. Gray SD, Hammond E, Hanson DF. Benign pathologic responses of the larynx. *Ann Otol Rhinol Laryngol.* 1995; 104(1):13–18.
17. Benninger MS, Jacobson B. Vocal nodules, microwebs, and surgery. *J Voice.* 1995; 9(3):326–331.
18. Ford CN, Bless DM, Campos G, Leddy M. Anterior commissure microwebs associated with vocal nodules: Detection, prevalence, and significance. *Laryngoscope.* 1994; 104(11 pt 1):1369–1375.
19. Morrison MD, Nichol H, Rammage LA. Diagnostic criteria in functional dysphonia. *Laryngoscope.* 1986; 96(1):1–8.
20. Benjamin B. Technique of laryngoscopy. *Int J Pediatr Otorhinolaryngol.* 1987; 13(3):299–313.
21. Strong MS, Vaughn VC. Vocal cord nodules and polyps—The role of surgical treatment. *Laryngoscope.* 1976; 81:911–923.
22. Woo P, Casper J, Colton R, Brewer D. Aerodynamic and stroboscopic findings before and after microlaryngeal phonosurgery. *J Voice.* 1994; 8(2):186–194.
23. Mahieu HF, Dikkers FG. Indirect microlaryngostroboscopic surgery. *Arch Otolaryngol Head Neck Surg.* 1992; 118(1):21–24.
24. Leonard RJ, Kiener D, Charpied G, Kelly A. Effects of repeated stripping on vocal fold mucosa in cats. *Ann Otol Rhinol Laryngol.* 1985; 94(3):258–262.
25. Benjamin B, Croxson G. Vocal nodules in children. *Ann Otol Rhinol Laryngol.* 1987; 96(5):530–533.
26. Lancer JM, Syder D, Jones AS, Le Boutillier A. The outcome of different management patterns for vocal cord nodules. *J Laryngol Otol.* 1988; 102(5):423–427.
27. Motta G, Villari G, Molta G Jr, Ripa G, Solerno G. The CO2 laser in the laryngeal microsurgery. *Acta Otolaryngol (Stockh).* 1986; 433(suppl):1–30.
28. Ossoff RH, Duncavage JA. The use of laser in head and neck surgery. In: Myers BC, Brackman DE, Krause CJ, eds. *Advances in Otolaryngology—Head and Neck Surgery.* Vol 1. Chicago: Year Book Medical Publishers; 1987:217–240.
29. Stell PMA. Laryngocoele. *J Laryngol Otol.* 1975; 89:915–924.
30. Chu L, Gussak GB, Orr JB, Hood D. Neonatal laryngoceles. A cause for airway obstruction. *Arch Otolaryngol Head Neck Surg.* 1994; 120(4):454–458.
31. Griffin JL, Ramadan HH, Wetmore SJ. Laryngocele: A cause of stridor and airway obstruction. *Otolaryngol Head Neck Surg.* 1993; 108(6):760–762.
32. Illum PNA. Laryngopyocele with a report of three cases. *J Laryngol Otol.* 1980; 94:211–218.
33. Matino Soler E, Martinez Vecina V, Leon Vintro X, Quer Agusti M, Burgues Vila J, Rel de Juan M. Laryngocele: Clinical and therapeutic study of 60 cases. *Acta Otorrinolaringol Esp.* 1995; 46(4):279–286.
34. Jackson C. Contact ulcer of the larynx. *Ann Otol Rhinol Laryngol.* 1928; 37:227–233.
35. von Leden HMP. Contact ulcer of the larynx: Experimental observations. *Arch Otolaryngol.* 1960; 72:746.
36. Svensson G, Schalen L, Fex S. Pathogenesis of idiopathic contact granuloma of the larynx. Results of a prospective clinical study. *Acta Otolaryngol [Suppl] (Stockh).* 1988; 449:123–125.
37. Benjamin B, Roche J. Vocal granuloma, including sclerosis of the arytenoid cartilage: Radiographic findings. *Ann Otol Rhinol Laryngol.* 1993; 102(10):756–760.
38. Jaroma M, Pakarinen L, Nuutinen J. Treatment of vocal cord granuloma. *Acta Otolaryngol(Stockh).* 1989; 107:296–299.
39. Cherry JMS. Contact ulcers of the larynx. *Laryngoscope.* 1968; 73:1937.
40. Nasri S, Sercarz JA, McAlpin T, Berke GS. Treatment of vocal fold granuloma using botulinum toxin type A. *Laryngoscope.* 1995; 105(6):585–588.
41. Cherry J, Margulies SI. Head and neck manifestations of gastroesophageal reflux. *Laryngoscope.* 1968; 78(11):1937–1940.
42. Friedman IF. *Granulomas and Neoplasms of the Larynx.* Edinburgh: Churchill Livingstone, 1988:357.
43. Chow LT, Chow WH, Shum BS. Fatal massive upper respiratory tract haemorrhage: An unusual complication of localized amyloidosis of the larynx. *J Laryngol Otol.* 1993; 107(1):51–53.
44. Simpson GSM, Skinner M, Cohen AS. Localized amyloidosis of the head and neck and upper aerodigestive and lower respiratory tracts. *Ann Otol Rhinol Laryrngol.* 1984; 93:374–379.
45. Ferrara G, Boscaino A. Nodular amyloidosis of the larynx. *Pathologica.* 1995; 87:94–96.
46. Walker PA, Courey MS, Ossoff RH. Staged endoscopic treatment of laryngeal amyloidosis. *Otolaryngol Head Neck Surg.* 1996; 114(6):801–805.
47. Grillo H. Congenital lesions, neoplasms, and injuries of the trachea. In: Sabiston DSF, ed. *Surgery of the Chest.* Philadelphia: WB Saunders; 1990:335–371.
48. Miller RHR. Evaluation of obstructing lesions of the trachea and larynx by flow-volume loops. *Am Rev Resp Dis.* 1973; 108:475–481.
49. Myer CM III, O'Connor DM, Cotton RT. Proposed grading system for subglottic stenosis based on endotracheal tube sizes. *Ann Otol Rhinol Laryngol.* 1994; 103(4 pt 1):319–23.
50. Tostevin PM, de Bruyn R, Hosni A, Evans JN. The value of radiological investigations in pre-endoscopic assessment of children with stridor. *J Laryngol Otol.* 1995; 109(9):844–848.
51. Bhalla M, Grillo HC, McLoud TC, Shepard JO, Weber AL,

Mark EJ. Idiopathic laryngotracheal stenosis: Radiologic findings. *AJR.* 1993; 161(3):515–517.

52. Axon PR, Hartley C, Rothera MP. Endoscopic balloon dilatation of subglottic stenosis. *J Laryngol Otol.* 1995; 109(9):876–879.

53. Pearson FG. Technique of management of subglottic stenosis. *Chest Surg Clin North Am.* 1996; 6(4):683–692.

54. Shapshay S. Laser application in the trachea and bronchi: A comparative study of soft tissue effects using contact and non-contact delivery system. *Laryngoscope.* 1987; 97(suppl 41):1–26.

55. Park SS, Streitz JM Jr, Rebeiz EE, Shapshay SM. Idiopathic subglottic stenosis. *Arch Otolaryngol Head Neck Surg.* 1995; 121(8):894–897.

56. Rothschild MA, Cotcamp D, Cotton RT. Postoperative medical management in single-stage laryngotracheoplasty. *Arch Otolaryngol Head Neck Surg.* 1995; 121(10):1175–1179.

57. Pearson FG, Gullane P. Subglottic resection with primary tracheal anastomosis: Including synchronous laryngotracheal reconstructions. *Semin Thorac Cardiovasc Surg.* 1996; 8(4):381–391.

58. Monnier P, Savary M, Chapuis G. Cricotracheal resection for pediatric subglottic stenosis: Update of the Lausanne experience. *Acta Otorhinolaryngol Belg.* 1995; 49(4):373–382.

59. Werkhaven JA, Weed DT, Ossoff RH. Carbon dioxide laser serial microtrapdoor flap excision of subglottic stenosis. *Arch Otolaryngol Head Neck Surg.* 1993; 119(6):676–679.

60. Grillo H. Surgical treatment of postintubation tracheal injuries. *J Thorac Cardiovasc Surg.* 1979; 78:860.

61. Massoud EA, McCullough DW. Adult-acquired laryngeal stenosis: A study of prognostic factors. *J Otolaryngol.* 1995; 24(4):234–237.

62. MacArthur CJ, Kearns GH, Healy GB. Voice quality after laryngotracheal reconstruction. *Arch Otolaryngol Head Neck Surg.* 1994; 120(6):641–647.

63. Arnold G. Vocal rehabilitation of paralytic dysphonia IX. Technique of intracordal injection. *Arch Otolaryngol.* 1962; 76:358–369.

64. Dedo HH, Urrea RD, Lawson L. Intracordal injection of Teflon in the treatment of 135 patients with dysphonia. *Ann Otol Rhinol Laryngol.* 1973; 82:661–667.

65. Walsh FM, Castelli JB. Polytef granuloma clinically simulating carcinoma of the thyroid. *Arch Otolaryngol.* 1975; 101:262–263.

66. Nakayama M, Ford CN, Bless DM. Teflon vocal fold augmentation: Failures and management in 28 cases. *Otolaryngol Head Neck Surg.* 1993; 109(3 pt 1):493–498.

67. Varvares MA, Montgomery WW, Hillman RE. Teflon granuloma of the larynx: Etiology, pathophysiology, and management. *Ann Otol Rhinol Laryngol.* 1995; 104(7):511–515.

68. Courey MS, Ossoff RH. Laser applications in adult laryngeal surgery. *Otolaryngol Clin North Am.* 1996; 29(6):973–986.

69. Ossoff RH, Koriwchak MJ, Netterville JL, Duncavage JA. Difficulties in endoscopic removal of Teflon granulomas of the vocal fold. *Ann Otol Rhinol Laryngol.* 1993; 102(6):405–412.

70. Zaretsky LS, Shindo ML, Detar M, Rice DH. Autologous fat injection for vocal fold paralysis: Long-term histologic evaluation. *Ann Otol Rhinol Laryngol.* 1995; 104(1):1–4.

71. Ishiki N, Morita H, Okamura H, Hiramoto M. Thyroplasty as a new phonosurgical technique. *Acta Otolaryngol (Stockh).* 1974; 78:451–457.

72. Wenig BM, Devaney K, Bisceglia M. Inflammatory myofibroblastic tumor of the larynx. A clinicopathologic study of eight cases simulating a malignant spindle cell neoplasm. *Cancer.* 1995; 76(11):2217–2229.

73. Coffin CM, Watterson J, Priest JR, Dehner LP. Extrapulmonary inflammatory myofibroblastic tumor (inflammatory pseudotumor). A clinicopathologic and immunohistochemical study of 84 cases [see comments]. *Am J Surg Pathol.* 1995; 19(8):859–872.

74. Fonseca CA, Suarez RV. Plasma cell granuloma of the larynx as a cause of sudden asphyxial death. *Am J Forensic Med Pathol.* 1995; 16(3):243–245.

75. Jayne D, Bridgewater B, Lawson RA. Endobronchial inflammatory pseudotumour exacerbating asthma. *Postgrad Med J.* 1997; 73:98–99.

76. Albizzati C, Ramesar KC, Davis BC. Plasma cell granuloma of the larynx (case report and review of the literature). *J Laryngol Otol.* 1988; 102(2):187–189.

77. Zbaren P, Lang H, Beer K, Becker M. Plasma cell granuloma of the supraglottic larynx. *J Laryngol Otol.* 1995; 109(9):895–898.

78. Baker DJ. Laryngeal problems in singers. *Laryngoscope.* 1962; 72:902.

79. Soda A, Rubio H, Salazar M, Ganem J, Berlanga D, Sanchez A. Tuberculosis of the larynx: Clinical aspects in 19 patients. *Laryngoscope.* 1989; 99(11):1147–1150.

80. Yeh V, Hopp ML, Goldstein NS, Meyer RD. Herpes simplex chronic laryngitis and vocal cord lesions in a patient with acquired immunodeficiency syndrome. *Ann Otol Rhinol Laryngol.* 1994; 103(9):726–731.

81. Punt N. *The Singer and Actor's Throat.* 3rd ed. London: William Heinemann Medical Books; 1979.

82. Rubin H. Vocal intensity, subglottic pressure and airflow in relationship to singers. *Folia Phoniatr (Basel).* 1967; 19:393.

83. Charrow A, Pass F, Ruken R. Pemphigus of the upper respiratory tract. *Arch Otol.* 1971; 93:209–210.

84. McGavran M, Bauer WC, Ogura JH. Isolated laryngeal keratosis: Its relation to Ca of the larynx based on clinical pathologic study of 87 consecutive cases with long-term follow-up. *Laryngoscope.* 1960; 70:932.

85. Woo P, Casper J, Colton R, Brewer D. Dysphonia in the aging: Physiology versus disease. *Laryngoscope.* 1992; 102(2):139–144.

86. Olson NR. The problem of gastroesophageal reflux. *Otolaryngol Clin North Am.* 1986; 19(1):119–133.

87. Delahunty JE. Acid laryngitis. *J Laryngol Otol.* 1972; 86(4):335–342.

88. Ward PH, Berci G. Observations on the pathogenesis of chronic non-specific pharyngitis and laryngitis. *Laryngoscope.* 1982; 92(12):1377–1382.

89. Bain WM, et al. Head and neck manifestations of gastroesophageal reflux. *Laryngoscope.* 1983; 93(2):175–179.

90. Contencin P, et al. Long-term esophageal and oropharyngeal pH-metry in ORL manifestations of gastroesophageal reflux in children. *Ann Otolaryngol Chir Cervicofac.* 1992; 109(3):129–133.

91. Sataloff RT, Spiegel JR, Hawkshaw M, Rosen DC. Gastroesophageal reflux laryngitis. *Ear Nose Throat J.* 1993; 72(2):113–114.

92. Hanson DG, Kamel PL, Kahrilas PJ. Outcomes of antireflux therapy for the treatment of chronic laryngitis. *Ann Otol Rhinol Laryngol.* 1995; 104(7):550–555.

93. Woo P, Nordij P, Ross JA. The association of gastroesophageal reflux and globus. *Otolaryngol Head Neck Surgery.* 1996; 115:502–507.

94. Thompson AR. Pharmacological agents with effects on voice. *Am J Otolaryngol.* 1995; 16(1):12–18.

95. McNally PR, Maydonovitch CL, Prosek RA, Colton RP, Wong RK. Evaluation of gastroesophageal reflux as a cause of idiopathic hoarseness. *Dig Dis Sci.* 1989; 34(12):1900–1904.

96. Fraser AG. Review article: Gastro-oesophageal reflux and laryngeal symptoms. *Aliment Pharmacol Ther.* 1994; 8(3):265–272.

97. Lorenz R, Jorysz G, Classen M. The value of endoscopy and endosonography in the diagnosis of the dysphagic patient. *Dysphagia.* 1993; 8(2):91–97.

98. Bollschweiler E, Feussner H, Holscher AH, Siewert JR. pH monitoring: The gold standard in detection of gastrointestinal reflux disease? *Dysphagia.* 1993; 8(2):118–121.

99. Kahrilas PJ, Quigley EMM. American Gastroenterological Association medical position statement: Guidelines on the use of esophageal pH recording. *Gastroenterology.* 1996; 110:1981–1996.

100. Reynolds JC. Individualized acute treatment strategies for gastroesophageal reflux disease. *Scand J Gastroenterol [Suppl].* 1995; 213:17–24.

101. Naunheim KS. Medical and surgical treatment of uncomplicated gastroesophageal reflux. *Chest Surg Clin North Am.* 1994; 4(4):653–671.

102. Zeuner M, Straub RH, Rauh G, Albert ED, Scholmerich J, Lang B. Relapsing polychondritis: Clinical and immunogenetic analysis of 62 patients. *J Rheumatol.* 1997; 24(1):96–101.

103. Wenig BM. Necrotizing sialometaplasia of the larynx. A report of two cases and a review of the literature [see comments]. *Am J Clin Pathol.* 1995; 103(5):609–613.

104. Mohsenifar Z. Pulmonary function in patients with relapsing polychondritis. *Chest.* 1982; 81:711–717.

105. Sacco O, Fregonese B, Oddone M, et al. Severe endobronchial obstruction in a girl with relapsing polychondritis: Treatment

with Nd YAG laser and endobronchial silicon stent. *Eur Respir J.* 1997; 10(2):494–496.

106. Kovarsky J. Otorhinolaryngologic complications of rheumatic diseases. *Semin Arthritis Rheum.* 1984; 14:141–150.

107. Shah R, Sabanthan S, Mearns HJ, Featherstone H. Self-expanding tracheobronchial stents in the management of major airway problems. *J Cardiovasc Surg (Torino).* 1995; 36(4):343–348.

108. Thompson JW, Ahmed AR. Dudley JP. Epidermolysis bullosa dystrophica of the larynx and trachea. Acute airway obstruction. *Ann Otol Rhinol Laryngol.* 89(5 pt 1):428–429.

109. Matt BH. Wegener's granulomatosis, acute laryngotracheal airway obstruction and death in a 17-year-old female: Case report and review of the literature. *Int J Pediatr Otorhinolaryngol.* 1996; 37(2):163–172.

110. Daum TE, Specks U, Colby TV, et al. Tracheobronchial involvement in Wegener's granulomatosis. *Am J Respir Crit Care Med.* 1995; 151(2 pt 1):522–526.

111. Lesavre P. The diagnostic and prognostic significance of ANCA. *Renal Fail.* 1996; 18(5): 803–812.

112. Langford CA, Sneller MC, Hallahan CW, et al. Clinical features and therapeutic management of subglottic stenosis in patients with Wegener's granulomatosis. *Arthritis Rheum.* 1996; 39(10):1754–1760.

113. Herridge MS, Pearson FG, Downey GP. Subglottic stenosis complicating Wegener's granulomatosis: Surgical repair as a viable treatment option. *J Thorac Cardiovasc Surg.* 1996; 111(5): 961–966.

114. Govender D, Chetty R. Inflammatory pseudotumour and Rosai-Dorfman disease of soft tissue: A histological continuum? *J Clin Pathol.* 1997; 50(1):79–81.

115. Wallner L, Alexander RW. Pemphigus of the larynx. *Laryngoscope.* 1964; 74:575–586.

116. Cenik Z, Uyar Y, Ozer B, Gungor S, Bulun E. An unusual laryngeal hamartoma: Lipofibroleiomyoma. *J Otolaryngol.* 1993; 22(2):136–137.

117. Fine ED, Dahmas B, Arnold JE. Laryngeal hamartoma: A rare congenital abnormality. *Ann Otol Rhinol Laryngol.* 1995; 104(2): 87–89.

118. Linder A. Hamartoma of the larynx causing neonatal respiratory distress. *J Laryngol Otol.* 1997; 111(2):166–168.

119. Park SS, Shin DH, Lee DH, Jeon SC, Lee JH, Lee JD. Tracheopathia osteoplastica simulating asthmatic symptoms. Diagnosis by bronchoscopy and computerized tomography. *Respiration.* 1995; 62:43–45.

120. Birzgalis AR, Farrington WT, O'Keefe L, Shaw J. Localized tracheopathia osteoplastica of the subglottis. *J Laryngol Otol.* 1993; 107(4):352–353.

121. Gleich LL, Rebeiz EE, Pankratov MM, Shapshay SM. The holmium:YAG laser-assisted otolaryngologic procedures. *Arch Otolaryngol Head Neck Surg.* 1995; 121(10):1162–1166.

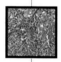

II. CLINICAL CONSIDERATIONS FOR NEOPLASMS OF THE LARYNX

■ GLENN J. SCHWARTZ

■ BARRY L. WENIG

INCIDENCE/EPIDEMIOLOGY

Carcinoma of the larynx comprises 2% to 5% of all malignant diseases diagnosed worldwide.[1] It is the second most common malignant lesion of the upper aerodigestive tract, exceeded only by carcinoma of the oral cavity.[2] In the United States, 12,500 new cases are diagnosed annually,[2] yielding an annual incidence of 5.6 per 100,000.[3] Approximately 4000 deaths occur each year as a result of laryngeal cancer, representing nearly 1% of all cancer-related deaths. Because squamous cell carcinoma accounts for greater than 95% of all laryngeal malignant diseases,[4] it is the focus of this chapter.

Laryngeal cancer is a disease of midlife. More than 80% of tumors are diagnosed in patients 50 to 75 years of age, with a peak incidence between the ages of 59 and 65.5 years. For both men and women, this trend has remained constant over several decades.[5–10] Although there is a male predominance for laryngeal carcinoma, the male:female ratio has been decreasing. A comparison of the 15-year periods from 1959 to 1973 and 1974 to 1988 reveals a drop in the male:female ratio from 5.6:1 to 4.5:1. This can be ascribed to the increasing number of women who smoke.[3,11] Despite improvements in diagnosis and new modalities of treatment, mortality has remained relatively stable over the last 20 years.[2] The estimated 5-year survival across all stages is 68%, making laryngeal carcinoma one of the more curable head and neck cancers.

ETIOLOGY

Multiple factors have been identified as having a role in the development of carcinoma of the larynx. Foremost among these etiologic agents is tobacco smoke. Although nicotine has not been implicated, the tars in tobacco smoke, which contain polycyclic aromatic hydrocarbons, have been shown to be carcinogenic.[12] The risk of carcinoma related to cigarette smoking appears to be dose-dependent.[13,14] In a large, case-controlled study, Falk et al[15] reported the risk for individuals who smoke one-half pack of cigarettes per day to be 4.4 times greater than that for nonsmokers; for those who smoke two packs per day, the risk was 10.4 times greater. Similarly, Hiranandani[16] found that 70% of a large cohort of heavy smokers developed keratotic changes of the laryngeal mucosa, and 20% of those determined to be at risk eventually developed cancer. Conversely, only 0.3% of the nonsmoking cohort developed cancer.[16] Mucosal changes induced by tobacco smoke are reversible if the individual stops smoking prior to the development of cancer.[17] In addition, it appears that cessation of smoking ameliorates the risk of developing laryngeal cancer,[18] with risk returning to that of a nonsmoker after 15 years of abstinence.[19]

The relationship of alcohol to the development of laryngeal carcinoma is less well defined. Some investigators believe alcohol is an independent risk factor for supraglottic carcinoma,[15,20] whereas others do not believe alcohol has an independent etiologic role.[19,21] Most individuals who consume large amounts of alcohol are also heavy smokers, making it difficult to conduct studies on the effects of alcohol as a single etiologic agent. Alcohol and tobacco appear to have a synergistic effect on the development of laryngeal cancer.[15,22,23] Individuals who abuse both alcohol and tobacco have a 25% to 50% increased risk of developing laryngeal cancer over the expected additive rate.[12,24] Most likely, alcohol is a cocarcinogen, but exactly how it potentiates the development of laryngeal cancer is still unclear.

Radiation exposure has also been identified as a risk factor for the development of laryngeal carcinoma.[25,26] External beam radiation, which historically has been used for a multitude of benign diseases, including adenotonsillar hypertrophy, thyrotoxicosis, and laryngeal papillomatosis,[25] may be responsible for the development of laryngeal carcinoma years later. Metachronous carcinomas in patients who were treated with radiation therapy for squamous cell carcinoma of the head and neck years earlier may be radiation-induced.[27,28]

Other occupational exposures have been associated with an increased risk for laryngeal cancer. These include steam and heat inhalation; thermal burns; organic chemical compounds, such as polycyclic aromatic hydrocarbons and nitrosamines that are produced in the iron, rubber, and coal industries; alkylating agents produced in mustard gas factories;[29] fumes from diesel and gasoline;[29,30] formaldehyde and vinyl chloride; benzopyrenes in insecticides; chronic exposure to wood dust;[29,31] asbestos;[29,32,33] nickel and chromate mining; and fibers found in textile manufacturing and the leather industry.[34–40]

The observation of clusters of relatives with squamous cell carcinoma of the upper aerodigestive tract suggests a hereditary predisposition, although no specific genetic factor has been identified. One study reported a 30% incidence of nonsmokers in a large cohort of patients diagnosed with head and neck cancer before the age of 40 years, compared to only 9% of nonsmokers in the control group. In the absence of this major risk factor, a hereditary predisposition to head and neck cancer is suspect. In addition, a significant family history of squamous cell carcinoma of the upper aerodigestive tract was identified in the nonsmoker group. The mortality rate was higher in the nonsmoking cohort as well, suggesting that these patients may develop tumors that are more biologically aggressive.[12]

Because of the long acknowledged association between the human papillomavirus (HPV) and squamous cell carcinoma of the genitourinary tract in women, attention has been given to this virus as a possible causative agent in carcinoma of the upper aerodigestive tract. Studies using the polymerase chain reaction to detect HPV DNA have revealed evidence of viral infection in malignant neoplasms of the tonsil and oral cavity, but no viral DNA has been identified in normal tonsils or healthy oral mucosal tissue.[41–43] In addition, a preponderance of HPV strains, (16, 18, and 33) all previously linked to carcinogenesis in the female genitourinary tract, has been detected. Kashima and co-workers[44] found HPV capsid antigen in 14 of 20 tumor specimens removed from individuals with laryngeal cancer. Portugal and associates[43] correlated HPV infection in squamous cell carcinoma of the head and neck with a lower rate of alcohol consumption, suggesting a role in cancer induction, independent of alcohol intake.

Extensive work has been done on the tumor marker p53 in order to characterize its role in carcinogenesis. Located on the short arm of chromosome 17, mutation of the *p53* gene has been observed in both premalignant lesions and malignant neoplasms.

Mutations of the *p53* gene are the most common genomic aberrations found in human cancers.[45,46] Overexpression of the p53 tumor suppressor protein has been identified in colorectal carcinoma,[47,48] lung cancer,[49] breast cancer,[50,51] leukemia, ovarian cancer,[52] and squamous cell carcinoma of the head and neck. The incidence of the p53 mutation in laryngeal carcinoma specimens has been reported to be about 60%.[53–55] Although this mutation may represent an early change in the process of tumorigenesis, p53 overexpression has not been correlated with tumor grade; stage; tumor-node-metastasis (TNM) classification; recurrence; or survival rates.[43] The development of laryngeal carcinoma is clearly a complex process that involves interaction between the host and various environmental factors.

EMBRYOLOGY

The larynx is derived from ectodermal, endodermal, and mesodermal tissues from the third, fourth, and sixth branchial arches and pharyngeal pouches. The supraglottic larynx develops from the buccopharyngeal anlage (third and fourth arches), whereas the glottis and subglottis arise from the tracheobronchial anlage (fourth and sixth arches).[56] This embryologic separation provides an oncologic basis for performing a supraglottic laryngectomy. The embryonic period comprises the first 8 weeks of gestation, and laryngeal development begins during the fourth week.[57] Initially, a ventral midline diverticulum referred to as the respiratory primordium arises in the caudal end of the primitive pharynx. As this structure deepens, it becomes the laryngotracheal groove, which has the appearance of a ridge on the external surface of the primitive pharynx. The endoderm lining the laryngotracheal groove gives rise to the epithelium and glands of the larynx, trachea, bronchi, and lungs. As the embryo further develops, the laryngotracheal groove evaginates to form a respiratory diverticulum on the ventral surface of the primitive pharynx. This diverticulum develops bilateral projections called bronchopulmonary buds, which progress to form the lower respiratory tract. The respiratory diverticulum becomes separated from the primitive pharynx through fusion of longitudinal tracheoesophageal folds, resulting in a partition known as the tracheoesophageal septum. This septum divides the foregut into the ventral laryngotracheal tube and the dorsal esophagus. The laryngotracheal tube gives rise to the larynx, trachea, bronchi, and lungs.[58]

During the fifth to sixth weeks of embryologic development, three tissue masses appear around the primordial laryngeal slit at the bases of the third and fourth branchial arches. The most anterior mass is the primitive epiglottis. The epiglottis arises from the caudal aspect of the hypobranchial eminence, a mesenchymal proliferation from the third and fourth branchial arches. Posteriorly, two paired arytenoid swellings develop from the sixth branchial arch, converting the previously slit-like laryngeal aperture into a T-shaped opening. Rapid growth of the laryngeal epithelium at this level temporarily occludes the lumen, which recanalizes by the end of the eighth week of embryonic life.

In the second month of laryngeal embryogenesis, the thyroid cartilage anlage begins to develop from the cartilage of the fourth branchial arch; at the same time, the cricoid cartilage arises from the sixth branchial arch. As the thyroid cartilage develops, the mucosal anlage of the vocal folds extends from the arytenoids to the inner surface of the thyroid lamina. Concurrently, the vestibular sinuses develop, eventually becoming the laryngeal ventricles and saccules. The intrinsic laryngeal muscles arise from myoblasts in the fourth and sixth branchial arches and migrate to their appropriate points in the larynx. The recurrent laryngeal nerves are also derived from the sixth branchial apparatus; they migrate cephalad with the muscle masses to insert into the larynx. The ligamentum arteriosum, a sixth aortic arch remnant, tethers the left recurrent laryngeal nerve in the chest during its embryologic ascent. The right recurrent laryngeal nerve migrates until it reaches the subclavian artery, a remnant of the fourth branchial arch that remains postnatally.

ANATOMY

A complete description of the laryngeal framework, including origins and insertions of the intrinsic musculature of the larynx, is beyond the scope of this chapter. This information has been extensively detailed in numerous anatomy texts. This section provides an overview of anatomy as it pertains to the spread of laryngeal cancer. This will help in providing a basis for the oncologic procedures that have developed in the management of laryngeal cancer.

Skeletal support for the larynx is provided by the hyoid bone and six cartilages, which are bridged to each other by joints and membranes. The cartilages include the epiglottis, thyroid, cricoid, and paired arytenoid, corniculate, and cuneiform cartilages. Histologic studies have confirmed that the cartilages and membranes of the larynx provide natural barriers to the spread of endolaryngeal tumors.[59,60] The most superior support structure of the larynx is the hyoid bone. Although this sesamoid bone is not uniformly considered to be part of the larynx, it serves as the point of attachment for various muscles and ligaments that are critical to laryngeal function. Additionally, the hyoid bone contributes to the anterior boundary of the pre-epiglotic space, which has oncologic significance. The thyrohyoid membrane stretches from the upper border of the thyroid cartilage to insert onto the hyoid bone. This membrane is perforated bilaterally by the superior neurovascu-

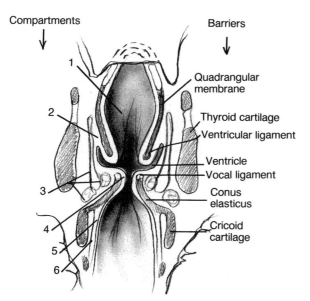

FIGURE 8-28 Coronal view of the larynx at the midcord level demonstrating barriers to tumor spread, as well as spaces through which tumor may spread easily. Compartments: *1,* supraglottic area; *2,* portion of paraglottic space continuous with pre-epiglottic space; *3,* paraglottic space; *4,* Reinke's space; *5,* subglottic space; *6,* cricoid area. From Fried MP, Girdhar-Gopal HV. *Advanced cancer of the larynx.* In: Bailey BJ, ed. *Head and Neck Surgery—Otolaryngology.* Philadelphia: JB Lippincott; 1993:1348, with permission.

lar bundle, consisting of the superior laryngeal artery and vein and the internal laryngeal nerve. This dehiscence allows for tumor involving the pre-epiglottic space to extend to adjacent structures outside the larynx.[59,61] The greater cornua of the thyroid car-

tilage articulate with the greater cornua of the hyoid bone superiorly, whereas the lesser cornua of the thyroid cartilage articulate with the cricoid cartilage inferiorly. The cricothyroid membrane bridges the gap anteriorly and laterally between the cricoid and thyroid cartilages.

Internal support for the supraglottic larynx comes from the quadrangular membrane, which arises from the edges of the epiglottis and attaches posteriorly to the arytenoid cartilages and inferiorly to the false cords. The mucosa-covered free edges of the quadrangular membrane form the aryepiglottic folds. The vocal ligaments provide structure to the free margin of the vocal folds, traversing from the vocal processes of the arytenoid cartilages to insert onto the midline inner surface of the thyroid cartilage. The fibrous attachment of the vocal ligaments to the thyroid cartilage is referred to as Broyles' ligament.[62] This ligament contains blood vessels and lymphatics that actually penetrate the inner perichondrium and thyroid cartilage to contact the outer perichondrium. Thus, carcinoma involving the anterior commissure may utilize Broyles' ligament as an avenue for extralaryngeal spread.[59,62–64] The conus elasticus, which provides structural support for the vocal folds, extends from the inner lower surface of the cricoid cartilage to insert onto the vocal ligaments, thyroid cartilage, and arytenoids. This membrane acts as a barrier to the spread of tumor to the subglottis.[65]

The various membranes, cartilages, and ligaments of the larynx create potential spaces that have oncologic significance (Fig. 8–28). These include the pre-epiglottic and paraglottic spaces (Fig. 8–29). The pre-epiglottic space, which contains fat and loose

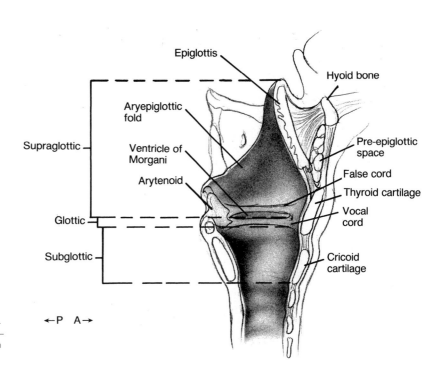

FIGURE 8-29 Midline sagittal section of larynx demonstrating the supraglottic and glottic regions, as well as the pre-epiglottic space. *P,* posterior; *A,* anterior. From Fried MP, Girdhar-Gopal HV. *Advanced cancer of the larynx.* In: Bailey BJ, ed. *Head and Neck Surgery—Otolaryngology.* Philadelphia: JB Lippincott; 1993:1348, with permission.

areolar tissue, is contiguous with the paraglottic space laterally. It is bounded superiorly by vallecular mucosa and the hyoepiglottic ligament. The hyoepiglottic ligament bridges the hyoid bone to the lingual surface of the epiglottis. This ligament has been shown to prevent the spread of tumor from the pre-epiglottic space to the oropharynx, providing oncologic justification as the superior margin in a supraglottic laryngectomy.[66] The anterior border of the pre-epiglottic space consists of the hyoid bone, thyrohyoid membrane, and the superior portion of the thyroid cartilage. Posteriorly, the border is defined by the anterior surface of the epiglottis and thyroepiglottic ligament. The elastic cartilage of the epiglottis has multiple perforations for tiny blood vessels throughout its surface, which may allow for carcinoma on the laryngeal surface of the epiglottis to extend into the pre-epiglottic space.[59,61,67–71]

The paraglottic space, external to the endolarynx, is similarly filled with fat and loose areolar tissue. It is bound laterally by the thyroid alae, superomedially by the quadrangular membrane, medially by the ventricle, inferomedially by the conus elasticus, and posteriorly by the pyriform sinus mucosa. Once a tumor enters the paraglottic space, it has a high propensity for thyroid cartilage invasion. The paraglottic space also allows deeply infiltrative tumors to pass from the true vocal cord to the false cord, and vice versa. Tumors that involve both the supraglottic and glottic larynx or glottic and subglottic larynx are called transglottic tumors. Extralaryngeal tumor spread from the paraglottic space may occur superiorly through dehiscences in the thyrohyoid membrane, anteriorly through direct communication with the pre-epiglottic space, or anteroinferiorly between the thyroid and cricoid cartilages.

For staging purposes, the larynx is divided into the supraglottis, glottis, and subglottis. This anatomic distinction is based on the embryologic development of the larynx above and below the level of the true vocal cords. Dye studies have confirmed this compartmentalization of lymphatics and blood supply.[72,73] The supraglottic larynx includes the lingual and laryngeal aspects of the epiglottis, the laryngeal apsect of the aryepiglottic folds, the arytenoids, and the ventricular bands (false cords). The inferior extent of the supraglottic larynx is defined by a horizontal plane passing through the apex of the ventricle.[74] Although this is the accepted clinical landmark, the true anatomic separation between the supraglottis and glottis is at the arcuate line, where the mucosa transitions from pseudostratified ciliated columnar epithelium to stratified squamous epithelium; this line is not reliably located at the apex of the ventricle.[75] Tumors located on the aryepiglottic fold and suprahyoid epiglottis, both subsites of the supraglottic larynx, exhibit biologic behavior similar to that of more aggressive tumors of the pyriform sinus and are, therefore, classified as marginal lesions.[12,59,75–77] The supraglottis is richly supplied with lymphatics that freely cross the midline and

drain into the superior and middle group of jugular nodes. Therefore, supraglottic carcinomas often present with ipsilateral, contralateral, or bilateral regional metastases.[78–82]

The glottic larynx includes the true vocal cords, the anterior commissure, and the interarytenoid region. The inferior limit of the glottis is defined by a horizontal plane passing 5 mm below the level of the free margin of the vocal fold. The vocal cord mucosa is nonkeratinizing, stratified, squamous epithelium on the free edges, transitioning to pseudostratified, ciliated epithelium at the superior and inferior aspects where it merges with the mucosa of the supraglottis and subglottis, respectively. The specialized lamina propria of the glottis, called Reinke's space, is not a true potential space (Fig. 8–30). It contains superficial, intermediate, and deep layers that possess varying amounts of elastic and collagenous fibers. A paucity of blood vessels and lymphatics exists within Reinke's space, conferring a resistance to the direct spread of tumor at the level of the glottis. For this reason, regional metastasis is a late event in glottic carcinoma, often occurring after disease has extended to other laryngeal sites. As previously mentioned, the conus elasticus provides additional resistance to the spread of cancer to the subglottis.

The subglottic larynx extends from 5 mm below the free edge of the vocal folds to the lower border of the cricoid cartilage. Subglottic primary carcinomas are rare, constituting less than 5% of laryngeal malignant lesions;[83] however, advanced glottic le-

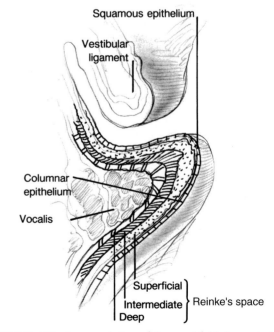

FIGURE 8–30 A coronal view of the vocal fold demonstrates the three layers of the lamina propria comprising Reinke's space.
Adapted from Woodson GE. Upper airway anatomy and function. In: Bailey BJ, ed. *Head and Neck Surgery—Otolaryngology.* Philadelphia: JB Lippincott; 1993:496, with permission.

sions frequently extend to involve this site. Tumors of the subglottis have an increased incidence of extralaryngeal spread, gaining access through the cricothyroid membrane. Like the supraglottic larynx, lymphatics are richly supplied in the subglottic larynx, but drainage tends to be ipsilateral. Lymphatic drainage occurs through the cricothyroid membrane to the prelaryngeal (Delphian) node, the middle and inferior jugular nodes, and the paratracheal lymph nodes.[61]

The intrinsic muscles of the larynx include the posterior cricoarytenoid (the only abductor of the vocal folds), lateral cricoarytenoid, transverse arytenoid, oblique arytenoid, aryepiglottic, thyroepiglottic, cricothyroid, and thyroarytenoid muscles. All intrinsic muscles of the larynx, with the exception of the cricothyroid, are innervated by the recurrent laryngeal nerve. The cricothyroid muscle is supplied by the external branch of the superior laryngeal nerve. Both the recurrent laryngeal and superior laryngeal nerves arise from the vagus nerve. The thyroarytenoid muscle, which runs just lateral to the vocal ligament and sometimes surrounds it, may become invaded by carcinoma of the glottis. Studies have shown that a deep invasion of the thyroarytenoid muscle is associated with fixation of the vocal cord.[84-86]

The extrinsic muscles of the larynx comprise the suprahyoid and infrahyoid musculature. The suprahyoid muscles include the digastric, stylohyoid, geniohyoid, mylohyoid, stylopharyngeus, and thyrohyoid muscles, all of which are elevators of the larynx. The infrahyoid (strap) muscles include the sternohyoid, omohyoid, sternothyroid, and thyrohyoid muscles. This group of muscles is involved in gross movement of the laryngotracheal complex and also aids in tensing the vocal folds. The middle and inferior constrictor muscles are also extrinsic muscles of the larynx, but their role is predominantly in swallowing.

TUMOR STAGING

An ideal staging system is one that provides prognostic information, aids the clinician in planning treatment, and allows for comparison of results. The two major staging systems are the Union Internationale Contre Cancer (UICC) and the American Joint Committee on Cancer (AJCC), developed in Copenhagen and the United Stages, respectively. After revisions in 1987, both systems are now identical for staging laryngeal carcinoma. The AJCC system, more commonly employed in the United States, utilizes the TNM classification for the staging of laryngeal tumors. This classification categorizes tumors based on their location and local extent (T stage); the presence, site, and size of cervical lymph node metastasis (N stage); and the presence or absence of distant metastatic disease (M stage) (Fig. 8–31). De-

pending on this information, the tumor is assigned a stage of I to IV. The TNM classification is useful for describing the anatomic extent of a tumor, but it does not take into account patient comorbidity or the biological behavior of the malignant lesion. Thus, it has shortcomings in accurately and consistently predicting survival. A staging system developed by Piccirillo and associates[87] includes both TNM data and clinical information related to the patient. This system has been shown to predict survival more accurately than does the TNM system alone. Attention to the entire patient represents important progress, and consideration should be given to application of this staging system on a more widespread level.

DIAGNOSIS

A systematic approach to the patient with a suspected laryngeal malignant lesion is critical. The elements of a proper assessment include: (1) history, (2) physical examination, (3) radiologic evaluation, (4) endoscopic evaluation with biopsy, and (5) medical and laboratory evaluation.

History

During the history taking, information should be elicited regarding the abuse of tobacco and alcohol, as well as contact with any of the multitude of occupational exposures that may play a role in carcinogenesis (see the previous section on etiology). The duration of symptoms may provide insights as to the extent of the tumor. Any associated past medical history is important in planning treatment so that appropriate medical consultation may be sought if necessary. This is especially critical if major surgery is anticipated. Signs and symptoms of laryngeal carcinoma vary depending on the location of the primary tumor, how locally advanced the tumor is, and the presence or absence of regional or distant metastatic disease.

Hoarseness, the cardinal symptom of laryngeal cancer, is caused by impairment of vocal cord function. Normal phonatory function depends on the ability of the vocal folds to freely vibrate in response to airflow through the glottis. Although a myriad of benign conditions may cause dysphonia, any patient with persistent hoarseness for more than 2 weeks should undergo a thorough evaluation of the larynx, particularly if the patient has risk factors for laryngeal cancer. Carcinoma of the larynx disrupts phonatory function by causing mucosal irregularities on the vocal folds, obstructing airflow through a narrowed glottic aperture, tethering the vocal fold mucosa too tightly to the submucosa, or fixation of the vocal cord. Hoarseness is an early symptom in carcinoma arising in the glottis; however, in tumors originating in the supraglottic or

Primary tumor (T)

TX   Primary tumor cannot be assessed
T0   No evidence of primary tumor
Tis   Carcinoma in situ

Supraglottis

T1   Tumor limited to one subsite of supraglottis, with normal vocal cord mobility
T2   Tumor invades more than one subsite of supraglottis or glottis, with normal vocal cord mobility
T3   Tumor limited to larynx with vocal cord fixation and/or invades postcricoid area, medial wall of piriform sinus, or pre-epiglottic tissues
T4   Tumor invades through thyroid cartilage and/or extends to other tissues beyond the larynx (e.g., to oropharynx, soft tissues of neck)

Glottis

T1   Tumor limited to vocal cord(s) (may involve anterior or posterior commissures) with normal mobility
      T1a Tumor limited to one vocal cord
      T1b Tumor involves both vocal cords
T2   Tumor extends to supraglottis and/or subglottis, and/or with impaired vocal cord mobility
T3   Tumor limited to the larynx with vocal cord fixation
T4   Tumor invades through thyroid cartilage and/or extends to other tissues beyond the larynx (e.g., to oropharynx, soft tissues of the neck)

Subglottis

T1   Tumor limited to the subglottis
T2   Tumor extends to vocal cord(s) with normal or impaired mobility
T3   Tumor limited to the larynx with vocal cord fixation
T4   Tumor invades through cricoid or thyroid cartilage and/or extends to other tissues beyond the larynx (e.g., to oropharynx, soft tissues of the neck)

A

Regional lymph nodes (N)

NX   Regional lymph nodes cannot be assessed
N0   No regional lymph node metastasis
N1   Metastasis in a single ipsilateral lymph node, 3 cm or less in greatest dimension
N2   Metastasis in a single ipsilateral lymph node, more than 3 cm but not more than 6 cm in greatest dimension; or in multiple ipsilateral lymph nodes, none more than 6 cm in greatest dimension; or in bilateral or contralateral lymph nodes, none more than 6 cm in greatest dimension
      N2a   Metastasis in a single ipsilateral lymph node, more than 3 cm but not more than 6 cm in greatest dimension
      N2b   Metastasis in multiple ipsilateral lymph nodes, none more than 6 cm in greatest dimension
      N2c   Metastasis in bilateral or contralateral lymph nodes, none more than 6 cm in greatest dimension
N3   Metastasis in a lymph node more than 6 cm in greatest dimension

B

Distant metastases (M)

MX   Presence of distant metastasis cannot be assessed
M0   No distant metastasis
M1   Distant metastasis

C

Stage grouping

Stage		T	N	M
Stage	0	Tis	N0	M0
Stage	I	T1	N0	M0
Stage	II	T2	N0	M0
Stage	III	T3	N0	N0
		T1	N1	M0
		T2	N1	M0
		T3	N1	M0
Stage	IV	T4	N0, N1	M0
		Any T	N2, N3	M0
		Any T	Any N	M1

D

FIGURE 8–31   *A,* Classification system of primary tumor (T) for carcinoma of the larynx according to the American Joint Committee on Cancer. *B,* Classification system of regional lymph nodes (N) according to the American Joint Committee on Cancer. *C,* Classification of distant metastases (M). *D,* Stage grouping. From *AJCC Cancer Staging Manual.* 5th ed. Philadelphia: Lippincott Williams & Wilkins; 1997: 427, with permission.

subglottic larynx, hoarseness occurs as a late symptom, indicating spread from these sites to the vocal cord, arytenoid, or cricoarytenoid joint.

As the laryngeal tumor enlarges and progressively obstructs the airway, dyspnea and stridor may ensue. Airway compromise occurs as a result of tumor bulk, accumulation of secretions, or vocal cord fixation. Lesions at any site in the larynx can cause airway obstruction, and stridor varies in relation to the site of the lesion. Exophytic supraglottic tumors cause inspiratory stridor by "ball valving" into the laryngeal inlet on inspiration. Patients with subglottic tumors present with expiratory stridor, whereas those with glottic or transglottic tumors have biphasic stridor. In general, laryngeal lesions are slow growing, so patients often complain of progressively worsening shortness of breath. However, the edema associated with a recent upper respiratory infection or sudden hemorrhage into the tumor can precipitate acute respiratory embarrassment, which requires emergency intubation or an awake tracheostomy to control the airway. If possible, it is worthwhile to proceed with a staging panendoscopy and biopsy at this time to avoid an additional visit to the operating room.

Lesions of the supraglottis may exist silently for

long periods of time and are often large when diagnosed. Presenting symptoms include chronic cough, throat irritation or pain, and a muffled "hot potato" voice.[83] Dysphagia, or difficulty swallowing, is another common symptom caused by tumors involving the supraglottis. Odynophagia, or pain induced by swallowing, often indicates spread of a laryngeal tumor to the tongue base, postcricoid space, or the esophageal inlet, sites that are important in deglutition.[12] Patients with dysphagia and/or odynophagia have usually curtailed their oral intake greatly and are, therefore, very malnourished. Weight loss may be related to their decreased oral consumption, but is also a symptom associated with the presence of distant metastasis. Hemoptysis, referred otalgia to the ipsilateral ear, and aspiration pneumonia are other less common presentations of laryngeal carcinoma. Subglottic tumors often present insidiously, initially manifesting as a lump in the throat or a vague tickling sensation.

Occasionally, the presenting symptom is a neck mass, which indicates regional metastasis or direct tumor extension into the neck. Cervical nodal metastasis in purely glottic tumors is fairly uncommon, occuring with an incidence of 5% for T1 tumors, 5% to 10% for T2 lesions, 10% to 20% for T3 tumors, and 25% to 40% for T4 lesions.[88-90] The incidence rate of regional metastases for supraglottic neoplasms is much higher, occurring in 60% to 80% of cases, depending on the T stage.[88,91-93] Subglottic tumors more commonly metastasize to the paratracheal region,[12,93] which is often not palpable, but cervical metastasis does occur 20% to 25% of the time.[12,83,93] Although a neck mass may be what brings the patient to the otolaryngologist's office, probing questions will usually identify symptoms referable to the larynx, as the presence of clinically palpable nodes generally indicates an advanced laryngeal carcinoma. A laryngocele, which may also be palpable in the neck, should raise the index of suspicion for a laryngeal cancer, given the association between these two entities, which occurs in 4.9% to 28.8% of cases.[94]

Physical Examination

A complete otolaryngologic examination includes careful inspection of the larynx. A large-diameter laryngeal mirror provides an adequate view of the tongue base and larynx, but often, visualization of the anterior commissure is insufficient. Flexible or rigid fiberoptic examination performed in the office is well tolerated, and provides optimal lighting and exposure. An additional advantage of the flexible fiberoptic laryngoscope is that it allows for examination of the nasopharynx. During laryngoscopy, attention should be directed toward the mucosa of the tongue base, epiglottis, aryepiglottic folds, arytenoids, false cords, true vocal cords, pyriform sinuses, and the upper portion of the postcricoid space. Any impairment of vocal fold mobility

should be noted and documented. In addition, the status of the airway should be assessed. Digital palpation of the tongue base and vallecula is important in the assessment of supraglottic tumors, as induration indicates the presence of submucosal spread to the oropharynx. Videostroboscopy may also serve as an adjunct in diagnosing laryngeal cancer. By detecting subtle abnormalities in the mucosal wave, videostroboscopy has successfully identified early invasive primary and recurrent carcinoma of the glottis.[95]

During examination of the neck, the larynx should be palpated externally. Splaying of the thyroid cartilage signifies an advanced laryngeal tumor with probable cartilaginous invasion, whereas fullness of the thyrohyoid or cricothyroid membranes implies extralaryngeal spread of tumor. Loss of laryngeal crepitus, the "click" that is palpated with sideways movement of the larynx against the vertebral bodies, indicates cancerous invasion of the postcricoid space or esophagus. A careful and systematic examination of the neck is also necessary to identify cervical lymphadenopathy, as the presence of regional metastasis significantly worsens the prognosis.[96,97] Metastatic lymph nodes may be located within the jugular chain, be prelaryngeal (Delphian), or, less commonly, may be situated in the submandibular or posterior triangles.[98,99] If lymph nodes are palpable, they must be characterized in terms of size, location, tenderness, and mobility. Immobility of a jugular chain lymph node in the cephalocaudad direction is suggestive of fixation of the node to the carotid artery, which some surgeons consider unresectable. Despite the most diligent physical examination, the overall error in clinically assessing the presence or absence of cervical lymph node metastasis is between 20% and 40%. The addition of either CT scanning or magnetic resonance imaging (MRI) of the neck has improved accuracy in diagnosing nodal disease.[12] After completion of the head and neck examination, patients with suspected laryngeal cancer should undergo a complete general physical examination, as these patients frequently have associated comorbidities. The assistance of an experienced internist in managing medical problems can be invaluable. Additionally, it is prudent to address medical issues prior to the administration of general anesthesia, which is required for panendoscopy and biopsy.

Radiologic Evaluation

Radiographic imaging should be performed prior to proceeding with triple endoscopy because of the tissue trauma produced at the biopsy site. This trauma leads to inflammation and, potentially, lymphadenopathy, which may be misinterpreted as tumor or regional metastasis on a subsequent imaging study. All patients should have a routine preoperative chest x-ray film, as 7% to 12% of patients with laryngeal carcinoma have distant metastasis at presentation.[100–103] A barium esophagram is an effective tool for detecting synchronous lesions of the hypopharynx and esophagus; indeed, some surgeons favor this noninvasive test over routine esophagoscopy.[104]

Certain radiologic techniques, such as laryngography, xeroradiography, and tomography, are only of historical interest since the advent of CT and MRI. Both of these modalities have greatly improved pretreatment staging by more accurately evaluating the full extent of the primary tumor. This includes determining the degree of involvement of adjacent laryngeal sites as well as the presence of extralaryngeal cancer. CT scanning offers the advantage of rapid imaging, which cuts down on movement artifact.[78] The soft tissues and structural framework of the larynx have a characteristic appearance on CT, enabling easy identification of pathologic processes. CT scans are also able to identify subclinical lymphadenopathy; nodes as small as 3 to 5 mm are usually detectable. This is particularly useful for nodes deep to the sternocleidomastoid muscle, within the retropharyngeal space, and along the tracheoesophageal groove, as these are regions that often elude the physical examiner.[105] The size and shape of a lymph node, its relationship to adjacent structures, and the presence of either central necrosis or extracapsular spread may readily be assessed by CT scanning.[105] One of the problems with CT scans is the difficulty in determining cancerous invasion of the cartilaginous laryngeal framework. The degree of cartilaginous ossification varies with age,[78,106–108] and nonossified cartilage and tumor-invaded cartilage have the same radiographic appearance on CT scan.[109–111] Although some authors have suggested that MRI may be a superior modality for assessing cartilaginous invasion,[112] others have not found MRI to be of benefit in this regard.[113] An additional disadvantage of CT scanning is that imaging is limited to the axial plane.

Three types of MR images are routinely obtained, determined by the time to repetition (TR) and the time to echo (TE). Short TR/short TE scans result in T1-weighted (T1W) images, which most clearly display anatomy. Long TR/long TE scans produce T2-weighted (T2W) images, which offer the best distinction between pathologic and normal tissues. Proton density images are scanned with a long TR/short TE mode; these sequences provide both T1W and T2W information. The ability of MRI to differentiate various soft tissues is useful in assessing the possibility of cancer invading the laryngeal framework.[114,115] Tumor and nonossified cartilage have the same appearance on T1W scans, but tumor appears brighter than nonossified cartilage with T2W sequences, allowing radiologists to make a distinction.[78,112] MRI also enables imaging in the axial, coronal, and sagittal planes; coronal images are helpful in delineating the false cord–ventricle–true cord complex. Caution must be exercised when interpret-

ing the presence of metastatic lymph nodes, as their appearance may vary with MRI. Lymph nodes that are heavily infiltrated with tumor cells appear as an area of low to intermediate signal intensity on all imaging sequences, whereas necrotic lymph nodes produce low to intermediate T1W signal intensity and high (bright) T2W signal intensity. Finally, lymph nodes that have tumor infiltration admixed with necrosis appear to have intermediate signal intensity on all imaging sequences.[105] Another disadvantage with MRI is the length of time required for examination. Depending on how many sequences and views are requested, scanning may take from ½ hour to 2 hours. MRI is also more sensitive to small movements than CT, and with prolonged time on the scanning table, patients are more likely to move and create image deterioration.[78,105] Cost is also a significant factor, as MRI is often twice as expensive as CT.

Detection of cartilaginous invasion is a critical oncologic issue, as this occurrence has traditionally been considered a contraindication to both radiotherapy and conservation surgery.[78,116–118] Despite the ability of MRI to delineate normal and pathologic tissues accurately, controversy still exists as to which imaging modality is superior in detecting cartilaginous invasion. Studies have shown that invasion of laryngeal cartilage occurs significantly more frequently than what is predicted by pretreatment CT.[119,120] Munoz and colleagues[121] determined that CT had a 46% positive predictive value in identifying cartilaginous invasion. Several other investigators have claimed that MRI is more suitable than CT for predicting neoplastic cartilaginous invasion.[108,115,122] In a prospective study of 40 patients with laryngeal cancer, Zbaren and associates[109] found that MRI was more sensitive than CT scanning in predicting cartilaginous invasion, but that CT scanning was more specific than MRI in this capacity. Moreover, both modalities were found to be more accurate in predicting cartilaginous invasion than clinical examination alone. There was no significant difference between the two modalities in overall accuracy, which was approximately 80%.[109] Nakayama and Brandenberg[123] established five criteria for increased risk of cartilaginous invasion in laryngeal cancer: (1) paraglottic spread (74%); (2) extensive cartilaginous ossification (73%); (3) a tumor diameter greater than 2 cm (66%); (4) extensive involvement of the anterior commissure (67%); and (5) vocal cord fixation. Note that both CT and MRI are adequate for determining the first three parameters.

It is particularly challenging to determine the full extent of supraglottic tumors because of their tendency to spread submucosally and invade potential spaces. Sites, such as the pre-epiglottic and paraglottic spaces, cannot be examined endoscopically, which can lead to understaging of these tumors.[109,124,125] Zeitels and Vaughan[71] conducted a retrospective review of 36 supraglottic lesions staged as T1 or T2, and identified 24 tumors that had invaded the pre-epiglottic space, indicating actual T3 staging. Both CT scanning and MRI are excellent modalities for differentiating between normal fat density in these sites and malignant lesions.[78,109] An accurate knowledge of tumor boundaries, often supplemented by the information CT and MRI can provide, ultimately dictates surgical treatment. For example, extension of a supraglottic tumor to the ipsilateral thyroarytenoid muscle renders a supraglottic laryngectomy unfeasible.[78] Likewise, superior extension of a supraglottic tumor into the vallecula necessitates resection of a portion of the base of tongue in order to achieve an adequate margin. This may significantly alter the rehabilitative process with respect to deglutition, and should be anticipated prior to surgery.

Determination of the full extent of glottic tumors is usually less of a challenge. The major contribution of radiography here is in determining subglottic extension and the status of the laryngeal ventricle. Both CT scans and MRI are useful in assessing subglottic extension, a condition that usually mandates total laryngectomy.[78,109] Because detailed coronal images can be obtained with MRI, it may be more useful than CT in detecting involvement of the laryngeal ventricle.[78,126] The anterior commissure is a well-established pathway for cartilaginous invasion and extralaryngeal spread of tumor through Broyles' ligament.[59,62–64,109,118] Bulky tumors can often obscure the anterior commissure during endoscopy. Radiographic imaging has been shown to increase the sensitivity in determining involvement of the anterior commissure.[78,109,112] Clearly, CT scanning and MRI have their strengths and weaknesses; however, both modalities improve the staging accuracy achieved with clinical examination alone. Because of the significant difference in cost, CT scanning is usually the preferred modality in the initial evaluation of the neck. At least one imaging modality is essential in the work-up of most laryngeal malignant lesions in order to optimize pretreatment staging.

Endoscopic Evaluation

After a thorough history and physical examination and a review of appropriate radiographs, the patient is taken to the operating room for triple endoscopy with biopsy. The triple endoscopy, which includes direct laryngoscopy, bronchoscopy, and esophagoscopy, is really an extension of the physical examination. The purpose of this evaluation is threefold: (1) to assess the full extent of the tumor for mapping and staging; (2) to obtain biopsy specimens of the lesion for histopathologic confirmation of the disease and histologic grading; and (3) to rule out a second primary malignant lesion of the upper aerodigestive tract. The incidence of multiple primary carcinomas

of the upper aerodigestive tract ranges from 5% to 16%, and the presence of a synchronous malignant lesion in the head and neck significantly worsens the prognosis.[12,104,127,128] Five-year survival rates for synchronous lesions are reported to be as low as 18%.[128] Common locations for second primary carcinomas in association with laryngeal cancer include the oropharynx, oral cavity,[128] lung, and esophagus. The mucosa of the tracheobronchial tree and esophagus should be inspected carefully, and a biopsy sample of any suspicious lesions should be obtained. Although rigid endoscopy has been the technique utilized by otolaryngologists for more than 100 years, some surgeons now favor flexible fiberoptic endoscopy to evaluate both the esophagus and tracheobronchial tree. A recent study comparing the results of rigid and flexible esophagoscopy in 195 patients with head and neck cancer reported a discrepancy in 10 patients. Five (50%) of the 10 patients had esophageal carcinoma that was not detected by rigid esophagoscopy. Based on the improved diagnostic accuracy and lower cost of flexible fiberoptic endoscopy, the authors recommended that this modality replace rigid endoscopy for the evaluation of esophageal disease.[129]

In order to prevent blood from obscuring the tissues during endoscopic examination, biopsy samples should be taken at the conclusion of the triple endoscopy. A systematic approach during direct laryngoscopy ensures that all anatomic areas of the oropharynx, hypopharynx, larynx, and esophageal inlet are examined. The surgeon should be as precise as possible in defining the anatomic extent of the tumor. Generous biopsy specimens should be obtained from areas that straddle a margin between tumor and apparently normal mucosa. Although not essential, frozen sections are helpful in guaranteeing the adequacy of the biopsy specimen, thus avoiding a repeat visit to the operating room owing to sampling error. Directed biopsy sampling in sites that appear to have normal mucosa may be helpful in determining the appropriateness of conservation versus radical surgery.[61] For example, a biopsy of the interarytenoid space could rule out extension of a glottic tumor to this region in order to ensure the suitability of a vertical hemilaryngectomy. If a tumor is bulky and there is substantial airway compromise, debulking with a forceps or the CO_2 laser may obviate the need for a tracheostomy.[61]

At the completion of the endoscopic examination, with the information still fresh in the surgeon's mind, the tumor is mapped on a standardized tumor diagram. Any cervical lymphadenopathy, whether noted clinically or radiographically, is also documented. Based on this information, the patient is then appropriately staged. This tumor map serves as an excellent reference during consultations between the otolaryngologist, oncologist, radiation therapist, and all other members of the treatment team.

Medical and Laboratory Evaluation

In addition to a general medical examination, a preoperative pulmonary evaluation may also be helpful in determining the risk of general anesthesia to the patient. Patients with laryngeal cancer are, almost without exception, long-time smokers, and they frequently suffer from chronic obstructive pulmonary disease. Pulmonary function tests are mandatory if any type of conservation laryngeal surgery is planned. Invariably, patients will have some degree of aspiration after partial laryngectomy, and sufficient pulmonary reserve is necessary to compensate adequately for this. Most individuals with laryngeal cancer are older than 40 years of age, so a preoperative electrocardiogram is warranted. If any abnormalities are detected, a cardiology consultation is requested and additional tests are ordered as necessary. Routine preoperative laboratory tests include a complete blood count, chemistry panel, prothrombin time, and partial thromboplastin time. Liver function tests are also obtained as a screen for liver metastasis.

Nutritional status is another important component in the assessment of a patient with laryngeal carcinoma. This can be ascertained using laboratory indices, such as albumin and transferrin levels, as well as through consultation with an experienced nutritionist. Patients with laryngeal cancer are often heavy drinkers who consume little each day except for alcohol. Malnutrition is, therefore, a common finding, and patients generally benefit greatly from enteral or parenteral alimentation. If prolonged nothing by mouth (NPO) status is anticipated, placement of a feeding nasogastric tube or percutaneous gastrostomy tube can be helpful. Patients should be asked about withdrawal symptoms when they refrain from drinking alcohol. The abrupt removal of alcohol may precipitate symptoms ranging from mild tremors to hallucinations associated with delirium tremens (DTs). This latter condition is usually self-limiting, lasting for 2 to 10 days. However, death has occurred secondary to DTs, so this condition should not be taken lightly. Consultation with an addictions specialist can be life-saving.

PATTERNS OF SPREAD

Much of the current information available about the patterns of spread for laryngeal carcinoma comes from Kirchner's studies involving whole organ sections of the larynx and Pressman's dye injection studies. These investigations revealed several natural barriers to the spread of early cancer and demonstrated variations in tumor spread, depending on the site within the larynx. This knowledge was instrumental in the development of conservation laryngeal surgery. A thorough understanding is essential to the management of laryngeal carcinoma.

Supraglottis

In the 1950s, Pressman[130] performed studies that involved injecting dye and radioisotopes into the submucosa of the supraglottis. He observed that spread tended to be limited to the tissues above the ventricle.[130] Indeed, only after massive infusions into the false vocal fold was spread to the glottis observed, by way of the paraglottic space.[131] These studies implied the presence of an anatomic barrier within the ventricle; however, whole organ sections failed to demonstrate a structure to account for this phenomenon.[132,133] Nevertheless, cancer that grossly remained confined to the supraglottic larynx was usually found to spare the ventricle in whole organ sections. This has provided an oncologic basis for performing a horizontal supraglottic laryngectomy with an inferior margin of only a few millimeters through the ventricle. Further support for this approach comes from the fact that recurrences after supraglottic laryngectomy are almost always in the area of the tongue base, not the glottis.[134] The separate embryologic anlagen of the supraglottis and glottis has been proposed as an explanation for this oncologic independence.[135,136] In the absence of a physical barrier, however, this phenomenon is not completely understood.

Cancer originating on the infrahyoid epiglottis may spread anteriorly to the pre-epiglottic space, passing through natural fenestrations in the epiglottic cartilage. Characteristically, tumors within the pre-epiglottic space have a pseudocapsule, which is thought to arise from the perichondrium of the epiglottis.[66] Rather than spreading with an infiltrative margin, the pseudocapsule leads to invasion with a broad pushing margin, which makes involvement of the hyoid bone and thyroid cartilage rare events.[71,132,137] In Kirchner's series only 2 of 112 supraglottic lesions invaded the hyoid bone. This fact allows for preservation of the hyoid bone in supraglottic laryngectomy, which may lead to earlier rehabilitation of deglutition. Additionally, none of the 112 supraglottic lesions had invaded the thyroid cartilage, which oncologically supports preservation of the outer perichondrium of the thyroid cartilage in a horizontal supraglottic laryngectomy.[132,133] The roof of the pre-epiglottic space is the hyoepiglottic ligament, a connective tissue structure that bridges the hyoid bone to the epiglottis. This ligament separates the supraglottic larynx from the tongue base[67,138,139] and serves to prevent occult invasion of the tongue base by tumors arising on the infrahyoid epiglottis. This may eliminate the need for resection of a portion of the tongue base as a cephalic margin in a supraglottic laryngectomy,[66] which can have a significant impact on rehabilitation. The floor of the pre-epiglottic space is the thyroepiglottic ligament, which attaches the epiglottis to the thyroid cartilage. The anterior commissure tendon, which is the confluence of the thyrogepiglottic ligament, vocal ligaments, conus elasticus, and the inner thyroid cartilage perichondrium, is an avascular fibroelastic mass that prevents inferior spread of cancer within the larynx.

Marginal zone tumors, which occur on the aryepiglottic fold and suprahyoid epiglottis, behave much more aggressively than other supraglottic neoplasms.[140] The aryepiglottic fold serves as the medial border of the pyriform sinus, allowing for early spread of these lesions into the hypopharnx. Tumors on the suprahyoid epiglottis are very likely to destroy the hyoepiglottic ligament, providing a gateway to the tongue base and oropharynx.[66] In a histologic study conducted by Zeitels and Kirchner,[66] four of six aryepiglottic fold lesions had invaded through the pharyngoepiglottic fold into the oropharynx, and all six tumors had invaded the pre-epiglottic space, paraglottic space, or both sites. All 16 lesions arising on the suprahyoid epiglottis had spread to the tongue base, and 9 of 16 had invaded both the pre-epiglottic and paraglottic spaces.[66] The rich lymphatic supply in the oropharynx and hypopharynx contributes to an increased incidence of regional metastasis with marginal tumors compared to other supraglottic subsites.[12,132,141,142]

Glottis

The four major barriers to the spread of cancer in the glottis are the anterior commissure, the conus elasticus, the vocal ligament, and the thyroglottic ligament, which is an extension of the vocal ligament along the floor of the ventricle. Tumors arising on the free margin of the vocal fold are initially confined to Reinke's space. Often, these lesions spread along the mucosa of the vocal cord and cross the anterior commissure before infiltrating deeply to involve the thyroarytenoid muscle and impair vocal cord motion.[133] There is controversy concerning tumors that involve the anterior commissure. The dense fibroelastic tissue that comprises the anterior commissure tendon is believed to act as a barrier to the spread of early glottic cancer.[64,143] However, the thyroid cartilage is devoid of perichondrium at the point of insertion of the anterior commissure tendon, theoretically making this site vulnerable to subclinical cartilaginous invasion and eventual extralaryngeal spread of tumor.[144,145] Yeager and Archer[146] detected cancer cells growing along the collagen bundles that make up the anterior commissure tendon, providing a passageway for cartilaginous invasion. On the other hand, Kirchner and Carter[132] reported that, when vocal cord motion was unimpaired, cartilaginous invasion did not occur in glottic lesions involving the anterior commissure. They observed that only anterior glottic lesions that extended upward along the base of the epiglottis invaded the thyroid cartilage.[132] The anterior commissure is likely a barrier to the early spread of cancer, but the potential for subclinical cartilaginous inva-

sion exists, and it is impossible to determine exactly when microscopic invasion has occurred. Thus, extreme vigilance and caution are warranted when managing tumors that involve the anterior commissure.

Dye studies conducted by Welsh and Welsh[131] have delineated the pattern of spread of glottic carcinoma once Reinke's space is violated. Initially, dye injected into the loose connective tissue within Reinke's space flows laterally into the thyroarytenoid muscle. It then travels inferiorly, where it is temporarily inhibited by the conus elasticus, a known barrier to tumor spread. Increased volume of instillate, however, overwhelms this fibrous barrier, and eventually, penetration occurs, allowing the dye to pass through the cricothyroid membrane and outside the larynx.[131] Invasion of the thyroarytenoid muscle is clinically manifested as vocal cord fixation. This muscle is located within the paraglottic space, which is bounded medially by the conus elasticus, superiorly by the thyroglottic ligament, and laterally by the thyroid cartilage and perichondrium. Two routes of tumor invasion into the paraglottic space have been demonstrated in whole organ sections of the larynx. The first route is along the superior surface of the vocal cord beyond the lateral extent of the thyroglottic ligament; the tumor thus enters the paraglottic space from above. The second pathway into this compartment is by direct invasion through the conus elasticus.[133] Once the lesion occupies the paraglottic space, it is considered to be transglottic, and it may spread laterally toward the thyroid cartilage and/or downward toward the cricothyroid membrane. Invasion of the laryngeal framework often occurs in glottic lesions with more than 1 cm of subglottic extension and in transglottic tumors that are 3 cm or larger.[147] Both the thyroid cartilage and its perichondrium appear to be effective barriers to the spread of cancer.[148] This concept is supported by the fact that tumor invades ossified portions of the laryngeal skeleton preferentially over cartilaginous portions.[133] Two common sites of early ossification are the superior rim of the cricoid cartilage and the inferior rim of the thyroid cartilage.[149] Consequently, these sites are frequently invaded by cancer within the paraglottic space as it transgresses the cricothyroid membrane.

Subglottis

Only 5% of laryngeal malignant lesions arise within the subglottis. Because of the scant submucosa in this region, dye injection studies reveal rapid permeation of the entire subglottic circumference. Penetration of the conus elasticus quickly occurs, with subsequent invasion of the thyroarytenoid muscle. Once into the paraglottic space, the injected dye readily spreads extralaryngeally through the cricothyroid membrane.[131] Clinically, tumors may invade the thyroarytenoid muscle and cause vocal cord fixation without causing any mucosal abnormality.[150] The presence of mucous glands within the subglottis allows for direct penetration of the cricoid cartilage and cricothyroid membrane.[151] Posterointerior extension leads to involvement of the hypopharynx and cervical esophagus.[93]

Lymphatic Metastasis

The likelihood of cervical lymph node metastasis varies with the location and size of the primary laryngeal tumor. Although tumors of the glottis rarely present with nodal disease, lesions located in the supraglottic and subglottic larynx very commonly involve regional lymph nodes. The presence of cervical lymph node metastasis is important to the patient with laryngeal carcinoma, as this event significantly decreases survival.[12,88,152–155] Many investigators have shown that the presence of nodal disease has a greater impact on prognosis than does the primary tumor itself.[96,97] Across all disease stages, it is estimated that the presence of clinically palpable lymph nodes decreases survival by one third;[12] extracapsular spread of tumor has been reported to reduce survival by 50%.[88]

At this time, our ability to assess the presence of nodal disease is limited. Both the deep location of the jugular nodes beneath the sternocleidomastoid muscle and the significant incidence of occult metastasis contribute to this difficulty.[156] Bocca and colleagues[92] reported a 12% rate of cervical metastasis in a cohort of patients staged as N0 who underwent elective neck dissection. In the same study, 34% of 62 patients who were found to have clinically suspicious nodes by physical examination had no evidence of disease after therapeutic neck dissection. Snyderman and associates[157] reported a 20% incidence of cervical nodal metastasis in a group of patients with clinically staged N0 disease; 50% of these patients had extracapsular spread. Even in the most experienced hands, there is an estimated 20% to 40% margin of error in detecting nodal disease by physical examination alone.[12,152] Although the addition of imaging modalities, such as CT scanning and MRI, have significantly improved the sensitivity in detecting regional lymphadenopathy, the rate of occult metastasis is still reported to be as high as 12%.[156]

Carcinoma of the supraglottic larynx has the highest propensity for regional metastasis of any laryngeal subsite. This is because of the rich lymphatic supply to the supraglottis, which allows for free lymphatic flow to both sides of the neck.[150] The bilateral regional spread of supraglottic carcinoma has been confirmed in numerous studies. Lutz and associates,[158] from the University of Pittsburgh, reviewed more than 200 patients with supraglottic carcinoma treated with surgery and unilateral neck dissection. Recurrent neck disease was observed in 20% of these patients, and 75% of these failures were in the

contralateral or undissected side of the neck. In a follow-up study conducted at the same institution, the neck relapse rate was reduced to 9% after instituting a policy of bilateral neck dissections for supraglottic carcinoma.[79] Levendag and coauthors[159] reviewed 104 patients with supraglottic carcinoma who were treated surgically. Of the neck relapses, 78% occurred in the contralateral neck. The authors concluded that both sides of the neck should be operated on in patients with supraglottic carcinoma.[159]

The incidence of cervical metastasis is strongly related to the size of the primary tumor. In a series of 267 patients with supraglottic carcinoma, Lindberg[160] reported 147 (55%) patients to have cervical metastatic disease. Thirty-nine percent of the patients with T1 disease presented with nodal metastasis, whereas 65% of the individuals with T3 and T4 lesions had regional disease. Several other investigators have reported the regional metastatic rate for supraglottic carcinoma according to T stage.[81,91,92] For T1 lesions, the metastatic rate ranges from 6% to 25%; for T2 lesions, the rate is 30% to 70%; and for T3 and T4 disease, the rate is 65% to 80%. The rate of occult metastasis varies from 20% to 50%, also increasing with T stage.[150]

Supraglottic lesions occupying the so-called marginal zone have been observed to metastasize to the cervical lymph nodes more frequently than other supraglottic subsites. Marks and associates[142] reviewed 540 patients and noted a 57% incidence of palpable lymphadenopathy when tumors involved the suprahyoid epiglottis, vallecula, or base of the tongue. Likewise, tumors arising on the aryepiglottic fold, arytenoid, or the free margin of the epiglottis were associated with palpable lymph nodes in 48% of cases. Although still quite significant, only 32% of patients with tumors arising on the infrahyoid epiglottis presented with palpable lymphadenopathy. Further analysis of this patient population revealed that the primary tumor subsite did not correlate with the incidence of cervical metastasis that developed subsequent to presentation.[142] Jorgensen and colleagues[141] also separated the supraglottic larynx into suprahyoid and infrahyoid epiglottis and noted a similar difference in the rates of cervical metastasis. Forty percent of the patients with tumors of the suprahyoid epiglottis and aryepiglottic fold had clinical evidence of regional disease, whereas only 15% of the patients with tumors of the false cord, and 25% of patients with lesions arising on the infrahyoid epiglottis, had palpable lymphadenopathy.

Cervical lymph node metastasis in supraglottic carcinoma usually involves lymph nodes in levels II, III, and IV (Fig. 8–32). Wenig and Applebaum[98] reviewed 239 patients with carcinoma of the larynx and hypopharynx, identifying 90 patients (40%) who developed cervical metastasis. Seventy percent of the metastatic disease was concentrated within levels II and III, and only 2% of the patients who developed

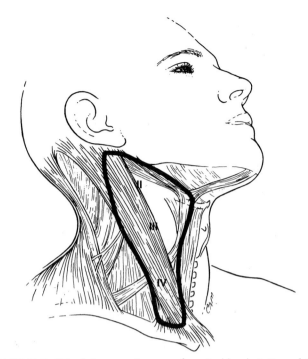

FIGURE 8-32 Schematic diagram of cervical levels II, III, and IV. This lymphatic bed is most likely to be involved in metastatic laryngeal cancer. From Suen JY, Stern SJ. *Cancer of the neck.* In: Myers EN, Suen JY, eds. *Cancer of the Head and Neck.* 3rd ed. Philadelphia: WB Saunders; 1996:475, with permission.

nodal disease had involvement of the submandibular triangle (level I). Similarly, Shah[99] reported on 119 patients with supraglottic carcinoma associated with palpable lymphadenopathy, and identified only 5% of the patients as having involvement of level I; 50% of these patients also had palpable nodes in levels II, III, or IV. Furthermore, a histopathologic analysis of radical neck dissection specimens obtained from patients with supraglottic carcinoma with clinical stage N0 necks detected only 1% and 6% with metastasis to levels I and V, respectively.[99] Based on these findings, Shah[99] recommends a selective neck dissection to include levels II, III, and IV for stage N0 and N1 necks, and a classic radical neck dissection for patients with either stage N2 or stage N3 necks, or T4 primary tumors.

The incidence of cervical metastasis with purely glottic lesions is very low owing to the paucity of lymphatics in this region. Electron microscopic studies have revealed that the lymphatics within the glottis are most dense at the arytenoid, and progressively decrease in density as one moves anteriorly along the vocal fold. Lymphatics are most sparse on the anterior vocal cord, where most glottic lesions originate.[161] In general, the risk for cervical metastasis increases with the size of the tumor and degree of infiltration. In a series of 620 patients with carcinoma of the glottis, Leroux-Robert[162] reported a 2.5% incidence of cervical metastasis, and 93% of

these patients had T3 or T4 lesions. Hawkins[163] similarly noted a 7% metastasis rate in 800 patients and glottic carcinoma, and most patients had T3 or T4 neoplasms. Other investigators have reported the risk of nodal metastasis of the glottis to be less than 5% for T1 lesions; 5% to 10% for T2 lesions; 10% to 20% for T3 tumors; and 25% to 40% for T4 neoplasms.[88-90] Like supraglottic tumors, glottic lesions typically metastasize to the jugular chain lymph nodes in levels II, III, and IV.[99,164] Bilateral and contralateral disease are uncommon with glottic lesions unless the tumor has invaded the laryngeal cartilage or extended to other sites; in this event, a comparable nodal distribution is observed on the contralateral side of the neck.[164]

Glottic neoplasms with subglottic extension have an increased risk for the development of cervical metastasis, in close relation to the size of the tumor. When there was less than 10 mm of subglottic extension, Castellanos and associates[12] observed only 5 (3.8%) patients, in a series of 132 with glottic lesions extending to the subglottis, to have clinically palpable nodes. To the contrary, Fleischer[165] reported regional metastasis in 30% to 40% of patients who presented with glottic tumors that extended more than 20 mm into the subglottis. Purely subglottic carcinomas are uncommon; however, these lesions metastasize to the cervical lymph nodes somewhat more frequently than tumors of the glottic larynx. Lederman[166] reported a 4.3% incidence of cervical metastasis in 140 patients with subglottic tumors, whereas Pietrantoni and colleagues[167] identified five patients (9.2%) with regional metastasis in a series of 54 individuals with subglottic cancer. The cervical metastasis rate is generally reported to be less than 20% when all stages are included.[150] Although the jugular chain lymph nodes are often spared, carcinoma of the subglottis commonly metastasizes to the paratracheal lymph nodes;[168] Harrison[93] reported a 65% incidence of paratracheal node involvement.

PREMALIGNANT LESIONS

Histologic abnormalities of the laryngeal mucosa include hyperplasia, keratosis, atypia (dysplasia), and carcinoma in situ (Table 8-3). Each of these processes may occur alone or in combination with one another. Risk factors for precancerous lesions of the larynx are the same as for invasive squamous cell carcinoma, with tobacco and its synergistic activity with alcohol being the main culprits. Also, like laryngeal cancer, premalignant lesions are far more common in men than women, with a sex ratio of 9:1.[169] The most frequent location within the larynx is on the anterior portion of the vocal fold. Clinically, these lesions appear as diffuse, white plaques (leukoplakia); red, nonkeratinizing, epithelial changes (erythroplakia); or complete epithelial thickening

T A B L E 8 – 3	HISTOPATHOLOGIC CLASSIFICATION OF PREMALIGNANT LARYNGEAL LESIONS

GROUP	DEFINITION
I	Squamous cell hyperplasia with or without keratosis and/or mild dysplasia
II	Squamous cell hyperplasia with moderate dysplasia
III	Squamous cell hyperplasia with severe dysplasia or classic carcinoma in situ with full-thickness atypia

From Hellquist H, Lundgren J, Olofsson J. Hyperplasia, keratosis, dysplasia, and carcinoma in situ of the vocal cords—a follow-up study. *Clin Otolaryngol.* 1982; 7:13, with permission.

(pachydermia).[169] Although not all lesions progress to invasive squamous cell carcinoma, some have clearly demonstrated malignant potential.

Hyperplasia refers to uniform thickening of the vocal cord epithelium. It may be associated with both keratosis and cellular atypia; when extensive, it is referred to as acanthosis. Regions of hyperplastic epithelium with atypia may protrude deeper than the surrounding epithelium, and may occasionally be misdiagnosed as invasive squamous carcinoma. Surface keratosis results from deposition of keratin on the mucosa of the vocal cords. Initially, epithelial cells within the prickle cell layer form keratohyalin granules. As these cells migrate superficially to the mucosal surface and die, the granules release their keratin, which persists as a layer on the vocal cords. Keratinization may also occur within individual cells in the prickle cell layer; this process is called dyskeratosis. Crissman[170] reported 94 cases of laryngeal keratosis, with or without cellular atypia, and observed that only four patients developed invasive laryngeal carcinoma. All four patients had severe atypia. McGavran and colleagues[171] published similar findings in a review of 87 cases of laryngeal keratosis. It seems justifiable to conclude that this lesion is not a predictor of progression to invasive squamous cell carcinoma; however, the presence of a suspicious lesion on the surface of the vocal cords warrants biopsy study in almost all circumstances.

Cellular atypia, or dysplasia, is a histopathologic term that refers to the presence of nuclear aberrations within cells. These include excessive nuclear enlargement, irregular chromatin clumping, nuclear pleomorphism, and/or abnormally dense nuclear staining. Owing to disorganized maturation of cells, mitoses are often seen in the midepithelium rather than in their normal location along the basal layer. Cellular atypia occurs with a severity that ranges from mild to severe, depending on the amount of epithelium replaced by abnormal cells. When malignant-appearing cells have effaced the entire epithelium but not violated the basement membrane, carcinoma in situ has ensued.[169,172] Once

discrete malignant cells are observed deep to the basement membrane, a diagnosis of microinvasive squamous cell carcinoma is made.[173] Although it is generally accepted that greater levels of cellular atypia increase the likelihood of progression to malignant invasion, no universal grading system to differentiate the varying levels of atypia from carcinoma in situ has been implemented.[169,174–176] This has led to wide variations in the reported incidence of carcinoma in situ, which ranges from 1.3% to 16% in the literature.[177–180] Grading classification systems have been proposed by Kleinsasser,[169] Hellquist and colleagues,[174] and others.[176,181] A simple, standardized grading system would consistently identify lesions that are likely to progress to invasive carcinoma, and would also facilitate a comparison of outcomes with various treatment regimens.

Clinically, the difference between severe atypia and carcinoma in situ is not critical, as both lesions are considered to be significant risk factors for the development of invasive laryngeal carcinoma.[150] Thus, in some grading systems, both severe atypia and carcinoma in situ are classified as grade III lesions.[169,174] In Kleinsasser's[182] series of 20 patients with grade III disease, 19 (95%) patients progressed to invasive carcinoma over an average period of 5 to 7 years. Stenersen and associates[183] reported the development of invasive cancer in 19 (46%) of 41 patients with biopsy-proven carcinoma in situ, whereas in a series reported by Hintz,[184] 18 (66%) of 27 patients went on to develop invasive carcinoma. Although it is clear that cellular atypia and carcinoma in situ are premalignant lesions, their variable biological behavior remains a mystery. There are several explanations why carcinoma in situ and severe atypia lead to invasive carcinoma in some, but not all, patients. One possibility is that the entire lesion may be excised during the initial biopsy, making it a curative procedure in some patients. Another possibility is that small foci of invasive carcinoma may already exist in sites adjacent to the carcinoma in situ, but may not be detected during biopsy. Clearly, these patients would have an increased propensity for developing invasive carcinoma. Finally, studies have suggested that, with cessation of smoking, carcinoma in situ and cellular atypia may be reversible lesions. In a cohort of 644 smokers, Auerbach and associates[185] observed a 16% incidence of laryngeal carcinoma in situ at autopsy; this finding was absent in 116 former smokers. Twenty-five percent of the ex-smoker group had milder degrees of atypia, and 75% had normal epithelium. The findings in the ex-smoker cohort were identical to the percentages reported for a group of 88 individuals who never smoked. Although impossible to prove, it is reasonable to assume that during the time the ex-smokers were actively smoking, the incidence of severe atypia and carcinoma in situ was similar to that observed in the smoking group, but that upon removal of the tobacco, these laryngeal changes regressed.[185]

TREATMENT

Carcinoma In Situ

Treatment modalities for carcinoma in situ and microinvasive carcinoma include primary radiation therapy, vocal cord stripping, and excisional laser surgery. The optimal treatment for carcinoma in situ is a subject of considerable controversy, as each modality has its advantages and disadvantages. Mendenhall and associates[186] have recommended radiation therapy for carcinoma in situ, stating that postirradiation voice quality is superior to that obtained after surgical management. This is particularly important for individuals whose careers depend on a strong, functional voice. Patients with carcinoma in situ along with multiple other medical problems are usually poor candidates for general anesthesia and are, therefore, better served by radiation therapy, especially because multiple vocal cord strippings are often required to control the disease.[187,188] Carcinoma in situ that involves the anterior commissure, a region that is difficult to assess endoscopically, may also be a suitable candidate for radiation therapy.[189] Other lesions for which radiation therapy has been recommended include those that have either rapidly recurred or have recurred multiple times after vocal cord stripping.[190] Finally, proponents of radiation therapy point out that it provides definitive therapy for patients who cannot be monitored closely in follow-up, either because of excessive travel distances or unreliability.[186,190]

Those in favor of surgical treatment for carcinoma in situ argue that close follow-up monitoring is necessary, regardless of the initial treatment, as local recurrence rates are reported to be as high as 50% and 60% after radiation therapy and surgery, respectively.[180,184] More often than not, these treatment failures represent invasive squamous cell carcinoma, further underscoring the importance of close follow-up monitoring. Stenersen and co-workers[191] identified 19 recurrences in a series of 41 patients with carcinoma in situ treated with vocal cord stripping; all 19 patients had invasive carcinoma. Similarly, Miller and Fisher[180] reported recurrent disease in 22 of 41 patients with carcinoma in situ treated with radiation therapy; 18 of the 22 individuals had invasive cancer. Other authors have reported similar recurrence patterns after both surgical treatment and irradiation.[192–195] The use of radiation therapy in the initial treatment of carcinoma in situ eliminates the possibility of this important modality in the future. On the contrary, both vocal cord stripping and laser surgery may be repeated without significant untoward complications, while reserving salvage surgery and radiation therapy for invasive disease.

Both radiation therapy and surgery have comparable success rates in terms of local control, ultimate control, and laryngeal preservation. In a study comparing the two treatment modalities, Murty et al[196] reported local and ultimate control rates of 85% and 95% in the 20 patients treated with radiation therapy, and rates of 75% and 88%, respectively, in the 17 patients treated with excisional biopsy. The laryngeal preservation rates for the radiation and surgery cohorts were 85% and 94%, respectively.[196] Mendenhall and colleagues[186] reviewed 17 series, including one in which 235 patients were treated with vocal cord stripping and 481 patients were treated with primary radiotherapy. The local control, ultimate control, and laryngeal preservation rates were 66%, 92%, and 88%, respectively, for the vocal cord stripping group and 84%, 98%, and 93%, respectively, for the radiation therapy group.[186] With such comparable outcomes, the ultimate decision as to treatment modality should be individualized to each patient. Carcinoma in situ that can be completely visualized during suspension microlaryngoscopy is amenable to either laser surgery or vocal cord stripping with micro-cup forceps. Patients with biopsy specimens that demonstrate microinvasion can be further ablated with the CO_2 laser. Radiation therapy, on the other hand, is best suited for lesions that are difficult to visualize endoscopically, for recurrent disease (either carcinoma in situ or invasive carcinoma), for patients who are very concerned about voice quality (e.g., singers), and for debilitated patients who are not candidates for surgery.

Supraglottic Carcinoma

EARLY-STAGE CANCER

Carcinoma of the supraglottic larynx can be difficult to diagnose because symptoms are often mild. With early-stage lesions (T1 to T2), patients may only complain of otalgia or vague throat discomfort, or they may even be asymptomatic. Thus, supraglottic carcinoma frequently presents at an advanced stage (T3 to T4). For early-stage lesions, there are two available treatments: surgery and radiation therapy, both used as a single modality. The addition of radiation therapy after surgery has not been shown to improve local control for early lesions arising in the supraglottic larynx.[92,158,197–199] Local control rates are comparable for both surgery and primary radiotherapy. Surgery is able to achieve a 90% to 95% local control rate for T1 lesions, and an 80% to 90% rate for T2 neoplasms.[92,158,200–203] On the other hand, primary radiotherapy without surgical salvage is able to control T1 tumors in 80% to 90% of cases, and T2 tumors in 70% to 80% of cases.[204–209] With the addition of salvage surgery for radiation failures, the local control rates between the two methods are equal.

Proponents of radiation therapy for early supraglottic carcinoma state that this approach provides the best opportunity to preserve the larynx. Irradiation is particularly attractive for T1 and T2 primary tumors without evidence of regional metastasis. In this scenario, the clinically negative neck is electively radiated bilaterally, covering levels II, III, and IV. The surgical alternative is a supraglottic laryngectomy with bilateral staging neck dissections. Although some authors advocate the use of radiation therapy alone for treatment of metatstatic nodes that are less than 3 cm in diameter,[210] others believe that a neck dissection is warranted in the presence of palpable lymphadenopathy.[211] Radiation therapy may be used in combination with surgery for patients with early-stage primary lesions and advanced neck disease. In this situation, the primary tumor is usually effectively controlled with irradiation; however, a neck dissection is necessary to adequately address the nodal disease. Because of the propensity for supraglottic tumors to metastasize bilaterally, the contralateral neck should also be addressed,[79] especially in the setting of advanced regional disease. The routine use of postoperative radiation therapy after supraglottic laryngectomy is avoided, as this may result in marked laryngeal edema and potential airway obstruction.[210] Postoperative radiotherapy is reserved for specific indications, including positive surgical margins, involvement of multiple nodes, or extracapsular spread of disease.[210]

Radiation therapy is associated with both early and late complications. During the course of treatment, patients experience skin desquamation, loss of taste, a sore throat, and xerostomia. Approximately 10% of patients will require a feeding tube for nutritional support during therapy.[210] Mild late side effects include xerostomia and a concomitant increased risk for dental caries. After radiation therapy, patients are also at increased risk for fistula formation if salvage laryngectomy becomes necessary.[212,213] Severe late complications include laryngopharyngeal edema requiring tracheotomy, osteoradionecrosis of the mandible, radiation-induced myelitis, and chondroradionecrosis potentially requiring permanent tracheotomy or laryngectomy in approximately 2% of cases.[214–216] Although the risk of radiation inducing a second malignant lesion is negligible,[217,218] consideration must be given to such morbidities when deciding on appropriate therapy.

Surgical options for treating early-stage supraglottic neoplasms include: (1) horizontal supraglottic laryngectomy; (2) endoscopic excision; (3) near-total laryngectomy; and (4) total laryngectomy. Whole organ sections of the larynx have demonstrated that a supraglottic laryngectomy is an oncologically safe operation. Local control rates with supraglottic laryngectomy are equal to those obtained with a total laryngectomy,[158,198,202,219] although the former operation results in considerably less morbidity than the latter. Herranz-Gonzalez and associates[220] reviewed 110 patients who underwent supraglottic laryngectomy, reporting a 94.5% decannulation rate. Moreover, most of these patients were able to eat within 2 to 3 weeks of surgery. Supraglottic laryngectomy is generally considered to be appropriate for T1 and T2 neoplasms arising in the supraglottis, as well as selected T3 lesions that involve a portion of the tongue base. However, with T3 lesions, closure is done under increased tension, and the risk of aspiration increases when a portion of the base of tongue is removed. Prior to surgery, one must rule out involvement of the anterior commissure and ensure that the vocal cords have normal mobility; cord fixation implies involvement of the cricoarytenoid joint or the thyroarytenoid muscle.[221] Other tumors that preclude a supraglottic laryngectomy are those that invade the thyroid or arytenoid cartilage, or extend posterolaterally to the apex of the pyriform sinus. Frozen sections should be used to control the tumor margins, and biopsy specimens should be taken from the patient rather than from surgical specimens. When positive margins are identified, a total or near-total laryngectomy should be performed. It is a risky oncologic policy to depend on postoperative radiation therapy to deal with inappropriately excised tumor.[220,222,223]

A standard horizontal supraglottic laryngectomy involves removal of the epiglottis, aryepiglottic folds, false vocal cords, pre-epiglottic space, superior half of the thyroid cartilage, and the hyoid bone, with preservation of the arytenoids and vocal cords to allow for phonation (Figure 8–33). Upon removal of these structures, patients lose the ability to protect the airway during deglutition and, consequently, experience postoperative aspiration to varying degrees. Thus, not all patients are able to tolerate a supraglottic laryngectomy; appropriate patient selection is a critical responsibility of the head and neck surgeon. Chronologic age alone should not prevent a patient from undergoing a supraglottic laryngectomy. A robust 75-year-old patient is a better candidate than a frail 50-year-old with multiple medical problems. Individuals who are relatively healthy with good pulmonary reserve are ideal candidates for a supraglottic laryngectomy. On the contrary, debilitated patients with either congestive heart failure or chronic obstructive pulmonary disease are unable to tolerate even small amounts of aspiration and are, therefore, poor candidates. Such individuals should be considered for either primary radiation therapy or a total laryngectomy. Studies have been conducted to elucidate parameters related to cardiopulmonary status that will predict a successful outcome after supraglottic laryngectomy. Beckhart and associates[224] studied patients preoperatively and postoperatively and found that a FEV_1/FVC (ratio of forced expiratory volume in 1 second to forced vital capacity) of less than 50% was associated with an increased risk of complications secondary to aspiration. Thus far, no criteria have been able to predict reliably the likelihood of postoperative complications. Ultimately, the clinical judgment and experience of the surgeon must prevail in deciding whether a patient is a suitable candidate for a supraglottic laryngectomy.

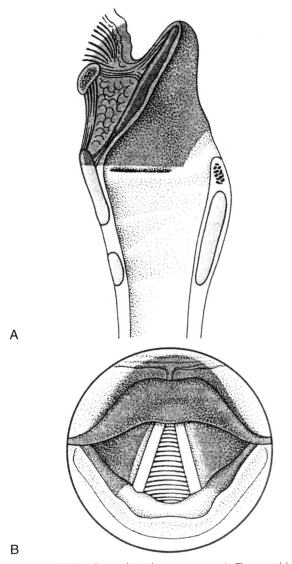

A

B

FIGURE 8-33 Supraglottic laryngectomy. *A,* The possible maximal extent of the supraglottal resection. *B,* Both arytenoid cartilages should be preserved to maintain a functioning laryngeal stump. Extension of the resection into the base of the tongue should be limited. From Squamous cell carcinomas. In: Kleinsasser O, ed. *Tumors of the Larynx and Hypopharynx.* New York: Thieme Medical Publishers; 1988:184, with permission.

Those in favor of surgery for early-stage supraglottic lesions point out that recurrences are difficult to detect in the irradiated larynx. This is particularly true with supraglottic tumors because they are often submucosal or involve the pre-epiglottic space, which cannot be visualized endoscopically. Recurrent carcinoma may go unnoticed until the patient presents with vocal cord fixation or airway obstruction.[225] At this point, the only acceptable operation for salvage is a total laryngectomy. DeSanto and co-workers[226] have estimated that as many as two thirds of the patients with early lesions treated with primary radiation eventually lose their larynx be-

cause of inadequate local control.[226] Most authors would agree that, after radiation failure, total laryngectomy provides the highest salvage cure rate with the lowest complication rate.[226,227] Although most patients at the authors' institution who fail primary radiation therapy are salvaged with a total laryngectomy, numerous patients have been salvaged with supraglottic laryngectomy, with an acceptable complication rate.[228] However, the authors' criteria for performing a salvage supraglottic laryngectomy are stringent. Patients must be young, healthy, and have good pulmonary reserve. Additionally, the recurrent tumor must be detected early and be completely visualized endoscopically.

Recently, endoscopic surgery has been used to resect early-stage cancers of the supraglottic larynx. Zeitels and associates[229] reported their experience in resecting supraglottic lesions with the CO_2 laser, either with or without postoperative radiation therapy. They emphasized that lesions arising on the suprahyoid epiglottis, aryepiglottic fold, and vestibular fold were well suited for endoscopic excision because of their perpendicular orientation with the lumen of the laryngoscope. Conversely, tumors of the infrahyoid epiglottis and upper false vocal fold were more difficult to resect transorally owing to their tangential alignment with the laryngoscope. In Zeitels et al's[229] series, 19 patients with T1 to T2 lesions underwent transoral resection without adjuvant radiotherapy; of these, 13 patients were monitored for a minimum of 2 years. None of these patients experienced failure of therapy in the larynx, and one developed nodal disease that was successfully managed with a salvage neck dissection. Six patients had only a short follow-up period owing to the development of an incurable second primary tumor, yet none had recurrences in the head and neck. Twenty-three patients with stage T2 to T3N0 lesions were treated with endoscopic resection followed by radiation therapy. Sixteen of these patients had histologically negative margins, with 100% local control in this group. Two patients had tumor recurrences in the neck and died despite salvage neck dissection. Of the seven patients with positive margins, four recurred in the larynx after radiation therapy and required a salvage total laryngectomy. Although endoscopic laser excision appears to be an effective modality for controlling T1 and early T2 lesions, it is difficult to draw conclusions about more advanced tumors because postoperative radiation therapy is utilized. Other authors have also reported encouraging results;[230-233] however, studies with increased numbers of patients and long-term follow-up evaluation are necessary in order to establish the efficacy of endoscopic laser surgery for managing early-stage supraglottic carcinoma.

Treatment for early supraglottic carcinoma can be simplified by choosing a single modality rather than a combination. For T1 and T2 supraglottic lesions with a clinically negative neck, both radiation and surgery are effective modalities; whichever treatment is chosen, the neck should be addressed prophylactically. For early tumors associated with palpable lymphadenopathy, the authors' approach is a supraglottic laryngectomy with bilateral selective neck dissections. Patients who are medically unsuitable for a supraglottic laryngectomy, or who refuse surgery, may be treated with primary radiation therapy with surgical salvage in the form of a total laryngectomy or neck dissection. Selected T1 and T2 supraglottic lesions may be managed with endoscopic resection using the CO_2 laser as an alternative to supraglottic laryngectomy.

ADVANCED-STAGE CANCER

There is a significantly increased likelihood of cervical metastasis with advanced tumors of the supraglottic larynx. Shah and Tollefesen[234] observed this trend in 352 patients with supraglottic carcinoma, reporting regional metastasis in 40%, 42%, 55%, and 65% of patients with T1, T2, T3, and T4 disease, respectively. Because it is generally agreed upon that the N stage is more predictive of survival than the T stage,[235,236] it is not surprising that survival rates significantly worsen with T3 and T4 neoplasms of the supraglottic larynx. Myers and Alvi[159] reported an 84% 2-year survival rate in 49 patients without nodal disease, and a 46% 2-year survival in 50 patients with regional disease. Similarly, Castellanos and co-workers[12] observed a decline in 3-year determinate survival from 82% for stage I disease to 50% for stage IV cancer. Others have reported cure rates for stage III and IV supraglottic lesions to range from 20% to 40%.[237,238]

Treatment options for advanced supraglottic carcinoma include primary radiation therapy with surgical salvage, horizontal supraglottic laryngectomy, and total laryngectomy. The benefit of postoperative irradiation still remains unclear; however, several authors support the use of combination therapy.[56,239] Supraglottic laryngectomy has its greatest potential when used for early to moderately advanced supraglottic carcinoma. Cancers that are staged as T3 lesions because of invasion of the pre-epiglottic space are suitable for supraglottic laryngectomy, as the operation removes the entire pre-epiglottic space. Bocca and associates[92] have described three indications for an extended supraglottic laryngectomy: (1) lateral and posterior extension of the tumor involving the aryepiglottic fold, arytenoid, and medial wall of the pyriform sinus; (2) anterior extension of the lesion to the base of tongue; and (3) combined anterior and posterolateral tumor extension involving the base of tongue plus one arytenoid and the adjacent medial wall of the pyriform sinus.[92] Anterior resection of the tongue base can usually be extended up to the circumvallate papillae with maintenance of adequate deglutition,[150] although the surgeon should anticipate a prolonged recovery. Tumors associated with vocal cord fixation, invasion of

the laryngeal framework, involvement of the postcricoid space, or extension beyond the medial wall of the pyriform sinus require a total laryngectomy.

Overall, local control rates with primary radiation therapy are approximately 60% for T3 lesions, and 40% to 50% for T4 lesions.[204,205,208,209,240] Much of the experience with primary radiation therapy for advanced supraglottic carcinoma comes from Mendenhall's group[240] at the University of Florida, and from the work of Harwood and associates[241] at the Princess Margaret Hospital in Toronto. Mendenhall and co-workers[240] published the results of 129 patients with supraglottic carcinoma, of whom 50 had T3 to T4 primary tumors. In this retrospective review, local control was achieved in 61% and 33% of individuals with T3 and T4 lesions, respectively. After surgical salvage, ultimate control in these two groups was 83% and 67%, respectively. More importantly, ultimate local control with voice preservation was achieved in 69% and 57% of patients with T3 and T4 tumors, respectively. The high complication rate that was observed with primary irradiation for T4 lesions led the authors to favor total laryngectomy for these patients, with or without postoperative radiation therapy. Harwood and associates[205] reported the 20-year experience at the Princess Margaret Hospital with primary irradiation for advanced supraglottic carcinoma. Local control rates for T3N0 and T4N0 tumors at 5 years were 56% and 52%, respectively; among survivors, 64% retained their larynx. Similarly, Robson and co-authors[206] reviewed their 20-year experience with primary radiotherapy and surgical salvage for laryngeal carcinoma. Their study included 84 patients with supraglottic carcinoma, of whom 52% had T3 or T4 lesions. The 5-year cure rate with radiation therapy alone was 55% and 59% for T3 and T4 tumors, respectively, resulting in an overall cure rate of 57%. With the addition of salvage surgery, the 5-year cure rate improved to 67%. Radical radiation therapy with surgical salvage results in ultimate local control rates that are similar to those achieved with surgical therapy, and a significant number of patients will retain their larynx, which may lead to improved quality of life for the patient.[241]

Local control rates are generally better with surgical treatment than with primary irradiation for advanced supraglottic carcinoma, ranging from 70% to 90%. Ogura and co-workers[144] reported results in 22 patients with T3 and T4 supraglottic carcinoma treated with supraglottic laryngectomy, with or without preoperative radiation therapy. The 3-year cure rate for T3N0M0 and T4N0M0 lesions was 70% and 75%, respectively. An additional 35 patients had advanced tumors that were deemed unsuitable for supraglottic laryngectomy; these patients consequently underwent preoperative radiation therapy followed by total laryngectomy. The 3-year determinate survival in this cohort was 66%. Based on the improved survival rates with supraglottic laryngectomy compared to primary irradiation across all T stages, the authors stated that, when anatomically suitable, conservation surgery should be the treatment of choice for supraglottic carcinoma.[140] Bocca and colleagues[92] published their 30-year experience with conservation surgery for supraglottic carcinoma, including 467 patients across all stages. The overall 5-year survival rate was 75%, and for the 52 patients with T4 lesions, local control was achieved with extended supraglottic laryngectomy in 77%. The addition of radiotherapy for advanced tumors did not improve the prognosis.[92] Desanto[202] reported a 97% local control rate in 65 patients with T3 lesions treated with surgery alone, and 75% were either alive or had died of something other than laryngeal cancer after a minimum follow-up of 2½ years. In the 21 patients with T4 cancers, the local control rate was 90%, and 52% of the patients were either alive or had died of another cause.

Difficulty arises when comparing results after primary radiation therapy to those obtained with supraglottic laryngectomy. This is because series of patients treated with irradiation include individuals with lesions that are unsuitable for supraglottic laryngectomy, as well as patients whose medical condition precludes this operation. These factors create an unfavorable bias against the radiation therapy series. Additional bias to comparison is created by the frequent addition of postoperative radiation therapy following partial or total laryngectomy. Although postoperative radiotherapy has not conclusively been shown to be more effective than single-modality therapy for supraglottic carcinoma, some nonrandomized studies have suggested that combined therapy may be associated with higher local control rates, particularly with advanced-stage supraglottic cancer.[56] Support for combination therapy comes from the experience at the M.D. Anderson Cancer Center.[242] Sixty patients with supraglottic carcinoma were treated with supraglottic laryngectomy, and 50 of these patients received postoperative radiation therapy. There were no local recurrences, four regional recurrences, and three distant failures; disease-free survival was 96% at 2 years and 91% at 5 years. Although these researchers reported excellent local-regional control rates, 53 of the 60 patients had stage T2 or T3 tumors, leaving unanswered the question as to the impact combination therapy has on T4 tumors of the supraglottis.[242] Furthermore, other authors have not been able to show improved survival with the addition of radiotherapy to surgery.[92,199] In view of the conflicting support for combined therapy, the head and neck oncologist must utilize postoperative radiation therapy very judiciously, as it may introduce additional morbidity following conservation laryngeal surgery. Such complications include persistent laryngeal edema that may require prolonged or permanent tracheostomy and intractable aspiration, ultimately necessitating a completion laryngectomy.

THE NECK

The presence of nodal disease has consistently been reported as the most significant predictor of survival for patients with supraglottic carcinoma.[150,159,189] The incidence of regional metastasis ranges from 25% to 50%, with 30% to 50% of these patients presenting with clinically palpable nodes.[56] Those individuals without palpable lymphadenopathy are reported to have histologic evidence of nodal disease in about 20% to 40% of cases.[56,81,159,242–244] The presence of extracapsular spread is a particularly ominous occurrence. Meyers and Alvi[243] reported nodal metastasis in 50 of 99 patients with supraglottic carcinoma, and 32 patients had extracapsular spread. Of the patients without extracapsular spread, 72% were alive at 2 years, whereas only 31% of the patients with extracapsular spread survived for this time period. Snyderman and colleagues[157] have also reported the presence of extracapsular spread to be a poor prognostic sign for patients with supraglottic cancer. Extracapsular spread may also predict subsequent development of distant metastasis.[243]

Although some authors advocate the use of radiation therapy for the clinically N0 neck,[210] others recommend that bilateral neck dissections be performed.[92,158,242,243,245–247] Approximately 40% to 50% of regional failures occur in nondissected N0 necks, despite the use of radiation therapy.[158,242] Ramadan and Allen[248] reported a 40.5% neck relapse rate in 63 patients with N0 supraglottic carcinoma; the relapse rate was only 14.3% in the group of patients treated with neck dissection. Likewise, Lutz and associates[158] reviewed 202 patients with supraglottic carcinoma of all stages and reported a regional recurrence rate of 21% for patients who underwent a unilateral neck dissection, this rate was only 7% for those treated with bilateral neck dissections. Furthermore, radiation therapy was ineffective in preventing metastasis in the contralateral neck.[158] These findings prompted the authors to adopt a strategy that included bilateral neck dissections. In a follow-up study of 76 patients whose treatment included bilateral neck dissections, only seven patients relapsed in the neck. Thus, their regional failure rate decreased from 20% to 9% without increasing morbidity.[79] Levendag and associates[159] reviewed 104 patients with supraglottic carcinoma treated with primary surgery, with or without a unilateral neck dissection. Of the patients who developed neck relapses, 78% involved the contralateral, nondissected neck. Bilateral neck dissections have been shown to reduce the regional recurrence rate to between 3% and 6%. This approach is currently used at the authors' institution for patients with supraglottic carcinoma. Radiation therapy is reserved for patients with multiple positive lymph nodes, extracapsular spread, or those with a stage N0 neck whose primary tumor is being treated with radiation therapy.

Glottic Carcinoma

EARLY-STAGE CANCER

In contrast to supraglottic carcinoma, which may exist silently for long periods of time, cancer of the glottis causes symptoms, such as hoarseness, early in the course of disease. Fortunately, this often prompts the patient to seek medical attention. The sparse lymphatics within the glottic larynx diminish the likelihood of cervical metastasis until the tumor has become quite advanced. Thus, control of the primary lesion is often equivalent to cure. In addition to the obvious goal of cure, other objectives of treatment include minimizing the recurrence rate and preserving good voice quality.

Early-stage glottic carcinoma can be managed successfully with single-modality therapy, utilizing either primary radiation therapy or surgery. The major advantage of radiotherapy, as asserted by its proponents, is that voice quality is generally better after irradiation than after surgery, although this has been the subject of debate in the literature. Controversy stems from the lack of objective, measurable criteria concerning what constitutes a good voice. Rydell and associates[249] reported the results of 36 patients with stage T1a glottic carcinoma, 18 of whom were treated with radiation therapy and 18 of whom were treated with CO_2 laser cordectomy. Based on acoustic and perceptual variables applied at both 3 months and 2 years, the authors concluded that voice quality was superior in patients who received radiation therapy. Other investigations have supported these findings.[250,251] On the other hand, Cragle and Brandenburg[252] studied 11 patients treated endoscopically for T1 glottic cancer and 20 patients treated with radiotherapy for similarly staged lesions. They found the two groups to have similar outcomes when comparing acoustic variables, such as maximum phonation time, frequency range, intensity range, jitter, shimmer, and signal-to-noise ratio.

Although some institutions employ primary irradiation with surgical salvage for laryngeal lesions of all stages, most authors agree that radiation therapy is best utilized for T1 and T2 tumors. Local control rates for radiation therapy range from 85% to 95% for T1 lesions, and 65% to 75% for T2 lesions.[253–261] One half to two thirds of radiation failures are amenable to salvage surgery,[150] resulting in ultimate control rates that are comparable to that obtained with surgery alone. Because 80% to 100% of recurrences will present in the first 36 months after radiation therapy, close monitoring is essential during this time period.[262,263] Early recurrences can often be managed with conservation procedures, such as CO_2 laser surgery or vertical partial laryngectomy. If conservation techniques fail, total laryngectomy is still a viable option. Outzen and Illum[262] cured 17 patients with recurrent supraglottic and glottic carcinoma us-ing the CO_2 laser, and reported no additional recurrences in 13 patients who were followed over a period of 2 months to 5 years.[262] These authors concluded that small recurrences could be managed adequately with the CO_2 laser, and cited the following advantages compared to conventional partial laryngectomy: (1) minimal bleeding and increased precision; (2) a lessor degree of trauma; (3) shorter operating time; (4) shorter hospitalization time; and (5) the avoidance of tracheostomy. Kooper and co-workers[263] published the results achieved in a series of 61 patients with recurrent carcinoma of the glottis who underwent salvage operation with a vertical partial laryngectomy. They reported a local control rate of 85%, and an actuarial overall survival of 88% at 5 years. The authors stressed that a prerequisite to salvage partial laryngectomy was that the recurrence, as well as the initial tumor before irradiation, must be amenable to conservation surgery. If the original tumor could not be managed by a vertical partial laryngectomy, then its recurrence after radiotherapy should not be treated with conservation surgery either.[263]

Several studies have attempted to elucidate factors associated with T1 and T2 lesions that make them more likely to recur after radiation therapy. The four criteria that have received the most attention are the presence of vocal cord motion impairment, anterior commissure involvement, the absolute size of the tumor, and the degree of subglottic extension. Vocal cord motion impairment implies a greater depth of tumor invasion, and has most consistently been associated with an increased likelihood of recurrence after radiotherapy.[264–266] This was the experience at the Princess Margaret Hospital in Toronto. Harwood and colleagues[266] reported a series of 154 patients with T2N0 glottic carcinoma treated with primary irradiation. They observed local control rates of 77% for patients with normal vocal cord mobility, but only a 51% local control rate when cord motion was impaired. A subsequent study from the University of Florida, conducted by Fein and associates,[261] further demonstrated the significance of vocal cord motion impairment for prognosis. In 115 patients who received radiation therapy for T2 glottic carcinoma, local control rates of 87% for patients with normal vocal cord motion and 76% for those with motion impairment were reported. The relationship of cord motion to prognosis has led several authors to support the subclassification of T2 tumors of the glottis as either T2a lesions (normal cord mobility) or T2b lesions (impaired cord mobility).

The influence that anterior commissure involvement has on the efficacy of radiation therapy is less clear. Concern stems from the fact that there is no perichondrium on the inner surface of the thyroid cartilage at the anterior commissure, which renders it vulnerable to cancerous invasion into the laryngeal framework. Tumor cells within the thyroid cartilage may be protected from exposure to the therapeutic radiation beam, which explain would an increase in recurrence rate when the anterior commissure is involved. Although some authors have reported recurrence rates as high as 61% to 88% with anterior commissure involvement,[267,268] others have stated that local control rates are comparable to those achieved when the anterior commissure is spared.[144,269] Large, bulky tumors with significant subglottic extension have also been identified as glottic lesions that are unlikely to respond to radiation therapy. Dickens and associates[265] reported a 26% recurrence rate for tumors greater than 15 mm in diameter, in contrast to a recurrence rate of only 4% for tumors that were 5 to 15 mm in diameter. Furthermore, in 49 patients with T2 carcinoma of the glottis, the authors reported a recurrence rate of 25% when there was no subglottic extension, 38% when there was less than 5 mm of subglottic extension, and 50% when subglottic extension exceeded 5 mm.[265]

Surgical options for early-stage glottic carcinoma include endoscopic excision (with or without use of the CO_2 laser), laryngofissure with cordectomy, and vertical partial laryngectomy. Since the first report of the use of the CO_2 laser for treatment of laryngeal malignant lesions by Strong and Jako[270] in 1972, the CO_2 laser has gained increased acceptance as a treatment for this condition. Eckel and Thumfart[230] reported achieving local control in 52 of 58 patients with T1 to T2 glottic carcinoma treated with endoscopic CO_2 laser treatment, based on an average follow-up period of 22 months. Similarly, Mahieu and associates[271] achieved endoscopic local control in 29 of 31 (94%) patients with carcinoma in situ or T1a carcinoma of the glottis. Although endoscopic excision appears to be very effective for treating early glottic lesions, its role in controlling more advanced tumors is less well defined. Eckel and Thumfart[230] were unable to excise 9 of 10 lesions endoscopically that were preoperatively staged as T3 lesions. Thus, they believe that this modality is inappropriate for advanced cancer of the larynx. Tumors that involve the anterior commissure should also be addressed with caution, particularly when planning an endoscopic excision. Krespi and Meltzer[145] treated five patients with carcinoma involving the anterior commissure with endoscopic laser surgery; in all five patients, recurrent disease developed within 12 months of initial treatment. The authors pointed out that only 2 to 3 mm of space exists between the anterior commissure ligament and the thyroid cartilage; consequently, a T1 lesion may actually be a T4 lesion if the thyroid cartilage is invaded.[145] In this instance, endoscopic laser surgery is clearly undertreatment. In order to avoid this problem, Zeitels has recommended raising a mucosal flap at the anterior commissure to visualize the extent of tumor in this region directly, proceeding with laser excision only if the thyroid cartilage has not been invaded (personal communication, 1999). Although some authors have achieved good results treating carcinoma

of the anterior commissure endoscopically, most agree that extra precautions are warranted for tumors involving this site.

Laryngofissure with cordectomy is another suitable operation for early-stage cancer of the glottis when vocal cord motion is unimpaired. It is ideal for lesions that cannot be completely visualized endoscopically. It can also be utilized for tumors that involve the anterior commissure or the vocal process of the arytenoid. Although this procedure is appropriate after failure of radiation therapy, it should not be applied to lesions that would not have been deemed suitable prior to irradiation.[272] The laryngofissure operation involves a vertical thyrotomy through the thyroid cartilage on the side opposite the tumor, with entrance to the larynx through an incision placed in the cricothyroid membrane. The resection margins are as follows: superiorly, above the false vocal cord; inferiorly, at the lower border of the thyroid cartilage; and posteriorly, immediately anterior to the vocal process of the arytenoid. The deep margin is the inner aspect of the thyroid cartilage. When the anterior commissure is involved, a small vertical strip of thyroid cartilage is also resected. The mucosal defect heals by granulation and re-epithelialization, creating a neocord of scar tissue that the normal vocal cord bulk can oppose. Various reconstructive techniques to improve voice quality after laryngofissure and cordectomy have been described.[273] With proper patient selection, cure rates after laryngofissure and cordectomy approach 90%. In a series of 188 patients treated with laryngofissure and cordectomy, Neel and associates[274] reported only four local recurrences, and only two deaths were caused by cancer.[274]

Vertical partial laryngectomy has also been termed vertical hemilaryngectomy,[275] verticofrontolateral laryngectomy,[276] and extended verticofrontolateral laryngectomy.[277] This operation is appropriate for T1 to T3 lesions of the glottic larynx, and can be used both for primary tumors and for surgical salvage after radiation failure.[263] Mohr and colleagues[276] defined their criteria for performing a vertical hemilaryngectomy as follows:

1. T1 lesions of the glottis that do not
   a. involve more than one third of the opposite vocal cord,
   b. extend more than 10 mm into the subglottis at the anterior or mid-cord level, or 5 mm posteriorly, or
   c. extend beyond the mid-ventricle;
2. T2 carcinoma of the glottis associated with vocal fold motion impairment;
3. T3 glottic carcinoma with vocal cord fixation caused primarily by tumor bulk, and minimally by invasion of the vocalis muscle.

Consent for a possible total laryngectomy should be obtained from all patients prior to performing a vertical hemilaryngectomy.

Resection margins in vertical hemilaryngectomy are depicted in Figure 8–34. The classical vertical hemilaryngectomy involves removal of the involved vocal cord (with or without the arytenoid) and the ipsilateral thyroid ala, along with 1 cm of thyroid cartilage on the contralateral side. The outer peri-

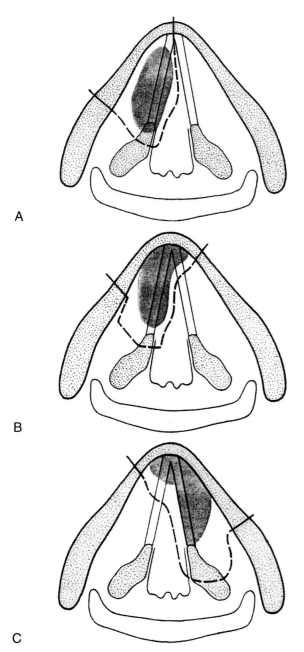

A

B

C

FIGURE 8–34   *A,* Vertical hemilaryngectomy with cartilage and soft-tissue resection. *B,* Extended partial laryngectomy, with cartilage and soft-tissue resection, when tumor involves the anterior commissure. *C,* Frontolateral partial laryngectomy, with cartilage and soft-tissue resection, when tumor involves the anterior commissure and extends up to the arytenoid cartilage. From Kleinsasser O. Surgical treatment of carcinoma of the larynx and hypopharynx and squamous cell carcinoma. In: Kleinsasser O, ed. *Tumors of the Larynx and Hypopharynx.* New York: Thieme Medical Publishers; 1988:173,176, with permission.

chondrium of the ipsilateral thyroid ala is preserved, and is used to resurface the neocord, which derives its bulk from the strap muscles.[277–279] Advancement of the pyriform sinus mucosa can also be utilized to epithelialize the reconstructed hemilarynx. The inferior margin of resection is the upper border of the cricoid cartilage but, if necessary, the mucosa overlying the cricoid may be incised and elevated off the cricoid cartilage to extend the subglottic margin.[280] Biller and Som[281] have described an extended hemilaryngectomy, which involves resection of up to 75% of the lateral and posterior portions of the cricoid cartilage, with reconstruction using a pedicled thyroid cartilage graft. Reconstruction after hemilaryngectomy should allow for adequate visualization of the larynx. An excessively bulky neocord for improved vocalization should not be created at the expense of lesser laryngeal visualization, as this may prevent detection of tumor recurrence. The epiglottis should be suspended at the conclusion of the procedure in order to improve endolaryngeal visualization further.

Surgical resection margins are very close in vertical hemilaryngectomy, with margins of 1 mm considered acceptable.[282] Intuitively, the closer one cuts to the tumor, the greater the possibility of leaving residual tumor within the patient. Close margins additionally increase the likelihood of erroneous pathologic interpretation. Analysis of frozen sections obtained from tissue in situ helps to avoid this unfortunate circumstance; however, situations will arise in which frozen section studies yield negative results and permanent sections reveal tumor-positive margins. Bauer and co-workers[283] reviewed 111 patients who underwent hemilaryngectomy. They found that patients with tumor-positive margins had a threefold increase in recurrence compared to those with negative margins, but that survival was not adversely affected.[283] Similarly, Wenig and Berry[284] identified 11 of 39 patients who underwent vertical hemilaryngectomy for T1 to T3 glottic carcinoma who had at least one positive surgical margin. Although the recurrence rate was seven times greater for this group of patients compared to the rate in those who had clear margins, there was no adverse effect on overall survival when salvage surgery was included. The authors concluded that completion laryngectomy need not be performed in the face of positive surgical margins, but rather that a policy of watchful waiting is acceptable. Other investigators have supported this contention.[263] Although data are limited on the effect radiation therapy has on positive margins, other authors have recommended the use of postoperative irradiation in this setting.[282]

ADVANCED-STAGE CANCER

Management of advanced carcinoma of the glottis is a topic that has generated much controversy and debate. Historically, radical radiation therapy as a single modality for T3 and T4 lesions has only been able to achieve cure rates of 20% to 30%.[166,285] For this reason, advanced laryngeal cancer was considered to be a surgical disease that necessitated a total laryngectomy. The addition of radiation therapy following total laryngectomy was later observed to improve local-regional control without significantly increasing complications,[286] and this then became the standard of care for advanced laryngeal carcinoma. The use of definitive radiation therapy for advanced laryngeal cancer was reserved for patients with unresectable tumors, those who were not surgical candidates because of associated medical conditions, or those who refused surgery. The recent success with "organ-sparing" chemotherapy and radiation therapy trials has further stirred the controversy over the appropriate initial treatment for advanced laryngeal cancer. Protocols utilizing a combination of chemotherapy and irradiation have reported survival rates that are comparable to those achieved with surgery and radiation therapy, and in a significant number of patients, the larynx has been preserved. This subject is addressed in further detail in a subsequent section of the chapter. At present, the three acceptable therapeutic approaches to advanced laryngeal carcinoma are: (1) radical radiation therapy with surgical salvage; (2) surgery combined with postoperative radiation therapy; and (3) combined chemotherapy and radiation therapy with surgical salvage. At the authors' institution, the latter two are most commonly employed.

Over the last 2 decades, improved techniques for delivering definitive radiation therapy, as well as higher therapeutic doses, have resulted in local control rates of 40% to 60%. Actuarial survival rates after surgical salvage range from 50% to 70%, depending on how many T4 cancers are included in the patient population and whether or not patients with cervical metastasis are included in the particular study.[209,287-293] Some of the most impressive results have been reported by the group from the Princess Margaret Hospital in Toronto. Harwood and associates[290] reported on 112 patients with T3N0M0 glottic carcinoma treated with radical radiation therapy. Of the 55 (49%) patients who developed recurrence, 48 underwent a partial or total laryngectomy, and 65% of these patients were cured with salvage surgery. The overall local control and 3-year survival rates were 76% and 68%, respectively.[290] The same authors also reported the results of treatment with radical radiation in 43 patients with T4 cancer. Local control was achieved in 53% of the patients with radiation alone. Three local recurrences were salvaged with surgery, resulting in an overall 60% local control rate.[294] Karim and co-workers[287] published the Amsterdam experience with definitive radiation therapy for advanced laryngeal carcinoma. In a series of 137 patients, radiation therapy with surgical salvage achieved a 3-year local control rate of 85%. Moderate to severe complications were observed in 14 of 38 patients in this series who underwent salvage surgery after radiation failure. This complication rate is higher than the "acceptable morbidity" rate reported by Harwood and associates[294] following salvage surgery, possibly owing to the higher radiation doses delivered in the Amsterdam study. Definitive radiation therapy is a viable option for patients with advanced laryngeal carcinoma who cannot or will not undergo surgery, either for medical or personal reasons. With this approach, a significant number of patients may be cured, some of whom may potentially retain a functional larynx.

For most T3 and T4 glottic cancers, the surgical procedure that offers the greatest likelihood of cure is total laryngectomy. In selected patients, a less aggressive operation may be performed and still effect cure. It must be emphasized, however, that the potential for cure should not be jeopardized in a vain attempt at vocal salvage. The primary goal in the treatment of advanced laryngeal carcinoma is cure, with preservation of function an important secondary objective. Conservation surgical procedures include the near-total laryngectomy described by Pearson[295] and the supracricoid partial laryngectomy championed by Laccourreye and co-workers.[296] Near-total laryngectomy involves ablation of one entire hemilarynx while creating a dynamic tracheoesophageal shunt to allow for the preservation of lung-powered voice. Breathing is maintained through a permanent tracheostomy, which must be occluded during phonation. Tumors that are oncologically encompassed by the near-total laryngectomy include unilateral T3 and T4 lesions, transglottic tumors, and pyriform sinus carcinomas. Because one arytenoid and at least two thirds of the uninvolved vocal cord must be preserved in order to create the vocal shunt, tumor involvement of the interarytenoid and postcricoid spaces are contraindications to near-total laryngectomy. The role of near-total laryngectomy for recurrent cancer after radiation therapy is unclear. Some authors advocate a total laryngectomy for recurrences on the basis that radiation therapy obscures tumor margins, thereby making preservation of the contralateral arytenoid an oncologically questionable approach.[297,298] Others have utilized the operation for T1 lesions that failed to respond to primary radiotherapy and were restaged as T3 cancers.[298]

In appropriately selected patients, the local control rate with near-total laryngectomy matches that of total laryngectomy.[298] Pearson and Keith[298] published the Mayo Clinic's experience with near-total laryngectomy. This study of 66 patients with tumors in all laryngeal sites represents the largest series to date. For all laryngeal sites, the authors reported a 53% 3-year cure rate; 20 of 29 (69%) patients with glottic, subglottic, or transglottic lesions achieved a 3-year cure.[298] Chandrachud and co-workers[299] reported an impressive 100% cure rate in 11 patients treated with near-total laryngectomy. Their patient population consisted of three patients with glottic tumors, five with transglottic tumors, and three with supraglottic carcinomas.

Supracricoid partial laryngectomy involves resection of the entire thyroid cartilage, epiglottis, and paraglottic and pre-epiglottic spaces, while preserving the cricoid cartilage, hyoid bone, and at least one arytenoid cartilage. Originally, reconstruction was done with a cricohyoidopexy (CHP), but extended operations have been described that entail either a cricohyoidoepiglottopexy (CHEP) or a tracheocricohyoidoepiglottopexy (TCHEP). The indications for a supracricoid laryngectomy, as defined by Laccourreye and associates,[300] are as follows: (1) T1 and T2 supraglottic lesions extending to the ventricle, infrahyoid epiglottis, and the posterior third of the false vocal cord; (2) T1 and T2 supraglottic lesions extending to the glottis and the anterior commissure with or without impaired mobility of the true vocal cord; (3) T3 transglottic carcinomas with marked limitation of the true vocal cord; and (4) selected cases of T4 supraglottic and transglottic cancers invading the thyroid cartilage. Based on the experience of Laccourreye and co-workers at the Laennec Hospital, University of Paris, local control and survival rates appear to be commensurate with those obtained with total laryngectomy, yet with considerably less morbidity. In their review of 68 patients, the local control rate was 100%, with a 3-year actuarial survival rate of 71%.[300] More importantly, 95% of the patients recovered physiologic deglutition and none required permanent tracheostomy. Although the postoperative voice was regarded as harsh, it provided for normal social interaction.

Encouraged by the long-term oncologic and functional results achieved with this operation, Laccourreye and co-workers[301] extended the supracricoid laryngectomy to include resection of the anterior subglottis. This extended operation was designed for patients with 10 to 15 mm of subglottic involvement, and reconstruction involved TCHEP. The authors published preliminary results for 16 patients with glottic carcinoma who would have required a total laryngectomy, reporting an overall 3-year survival rate of 68%. Laryngeal preservation and local control rates were 87% and 94%, respectively. Although numbers were small in this study, the authors concluded that the TCHEP procedure may be a valid alternative to total laryngectomy in controlling glottic carcinoma that presents with 10 to 15 mm of subglottic extension.[301]

In a subsequent study, the same authors investigated the safety and efficacy of the supracricoid laryngectomy to manage recurrence after failed radiation therapy.[302] Their patient population consisted of 12 patients with recurrent carcinoma after primary radiotherapy that would have required salvage total laryngectomy. After supracricoid partial laryngectomy, local recurrence was reported in 2 of 12 patients, resulting in a 3-year actuarial local control rate of 83%. With salvage total laryngectomy included, the overall local control and laryngeal preservation rates were 100% and 75%, respectively.[302] Postoperative complications included laryngeal perichondritis, anterior neck abscess, and persistent arytenoid edema resulting in prolonged tracheostomy. The incidence of complications in this study was not higher than that in previously reported series using vertical partial laryngectomy[303–305] or horizontal supraglottic laryngectomy[306–308] after failed radiation therapy. However, when compared to the typical postoperative course in nonirradiated patients undergoing supracricoid partial laryngectomy, there were significant differences. Most notably, the duration of tracheostomy was twice as long in irradiated patients.[302] Although extensive data from multiple institutions are lacking in the literature, the supracricoid partial laryngectomy appears to be a viable alternative to total laryngectomy for selected patients with supraglottic carcinoma that is not amenable to horizontal supraglottic laryngectomy. Preliminary data suggest that it may also be an appropriate salvage operation after radiation failure, but one should anticipate an increased risk of complications in this instance.

Total laryngectomy is the time-tested surgical procedure for laryngeal carcinoma. It is indicated for T3 and T4 lesions, either as primary treatment or as a surgical salvage procedure after failed radiotherapy (with or without induction chemotherapy). Completion laryngectomy is the procedure of choice for recurrent or persistent tumor after previously performed conservation surgery.[309] For rare tumors of the larynx, total laryngectomy is also the procedure of choice. These lesions include adenocarcinoma,[310] salivary gland malignant lesions,[311] fibrosarcoma,[312] melanoma,[313] chondrosarcoma,[314] paraganglioma,[315] and verrucous carcinoma.[316] Although disputed in the literature, some surgeons advocate emergency laryngectomy for obstructing carcinoma of the larynx in order to avoid the theoretical risk of stomal recurrence associated with a tracheostomy, particularly in the presence of subglottic extension. Finally, total laryngectomy is the treatment of choice for chondroradionecrosis, a rare, but devastating sequela of primary radiotherapy for laryngeal carcinoma.

The local-regional control rates after primary laryngectomy are best demonstrated by the experience of institutions where this procedure is routinely performed for T3 and T4 cancer. DeSanto[317] achieved local control in 68 of 69 previously untreated patients with T3N0 glottic carcinoma who underwent primary laryngectomy alone. Seven patients had recurrences in the neck, and one patient had a distant tumor, resulting in a 5-year actuarial survival of 80%.[318] In a similar study, Razack and associates[318] treated 128 patients with T3 and T4 glottic carcinoma with total laryngectomy, with or without neck dissection. They reported a 95% local control rate.

Despite the impressive control at the primary site, 5-year survival was only 53% after surgery alone, and 63% after salvage radiation therapy, owing to the development of regional and distant metastasis. Finally, Johnson and colleagues[319] published a report of a series of patients with 144 T3 and 34 T4 lesions treated with total laryngectomy, with or without neck dissection. Thirty-five patients in the study received postoperative radiation therapy. The local control rate was 94% for patients with T3 lesions and 86% for those with T4 cancers; 2-year disease-free survival was 79% and 58%, respectively.[319]

The benefit of postoperative radiation therapy following partial or total laryngectomy is not clear, particularly because surgery alone is able to achieve good local control rates, even with advanced glottic tumors. The advantages of postoperative radiation therapy must be weighed against the morbidity associated with irradiation. Short-term side effects include mucositis and odynophagia; long-term sequelae include xerostomia, persistent laryngeal edema, and radiation-induced necrosis. The latter two complications are of special concern following conservation laryngeal surgery. Persistent laryngeal edema may impede phonation and necessitate tracheostomy, whereas radiochondronecrosis, although uncommon, is usually an indication for a complete laryngectomy. The following criteria have been established by numerous authors for the use of postoperative radiation therapy following partial or total laryngectomy:[150,320–322]

1. Significant subglottic extension
2. Extension to the adjacent hypopharynx or tongue base
3. Invasion through the laryngeal framework to the neck soft tissues
4. Unsatisfactory surgical margins
5. Undifferentiated cancer
6. Presence of perineural or vascular invasion or
7. Concomitant regional metastatic disease requiring radiation therapy.

Several studies have demonstrated the effectiveness of postoperative radiation therapy in preventing locoregional recurrence following partial or total laryngectomy, with or without neck dissection. Vikram and co-workers,[323] from the Memorial Sloan-Kettering Cancer Center, treated 114 patients with head and neck cancer of all sites with a combination of surgery and postoperative radiation therapy; local recurrences were reported in only 6 (5%) patients. In a stage-matched cohort of historical controls who were treated with surgery alone, 39% developed local recurrences, resulting in statistically significant improvement with the addition of postoperative radiation therapy.[239] An additional study by this group demonstrated a significant decrease in the number of failures in the neck after the initiation of postoperative radiation therapy. Moreover, for the

53 patients who were treated with radiotherapy within 6 weeks of surgery, only 2% experienced relapses in the neck, whereas 29% of the 41 patients who received radiation therapy more than 6 weeks after surgery developed nodal recurrences. Based on these findings, the authors recommended the routine use of postoperative radiation therapy for advanced head and neck cancer, and further recommended that it be administered within 6 weeks of surgery to obtain the best results.[323] Other authors have reported similarly improved results with postoperative radiotherapy for advanced laryngopharyngeal cancers.[320,324,325] At the authors' institution, patients with T3 and T4 glottic tumors are routinely treated with postoperative radiation therapy. Additionally, those with multiple metastatic lymph nodes or extracapsular spread are also treated with irradiation of the neck and the primary site.

THE NECK

In contrast to other laryngeal sites, true glottic carcinoma rarely metastasizes to the cervical lymph nodes until there is invasion of the laryngeal framework or extension into adjacent sites, such as the supraglottic or subglottic larynx or the pyriform sinus.[88,164] A review of 800 patients with glottic carcinoma conducted by Hawkins[163] revealed nodal metastasis in only 7% of patients, and most of these had T3 and T4 lesions. Similarly, Leroux-Robert[162] observed metastasis in only 15 of 620 patients with carcinoma of the glottis; 14 of these 15 patients had T3 and T4 tumors. All told, the risk of cervical metastasis for patients with T1 to T2 lesions is approximately 5% to 8%; for those with T3 to T4 lesions, the risk ranges from 15% to 40%.[162]

For patients with palpable cervical lymphadenopathy, management of the neck is fairly straightforward. For patients with N1 disease, the authors advocate either a selective or modified radical neck dissection; for those with N2 to N3 stage neck disease, a modified radical or classical radical neck dissection is recommended. If pathologic analysis reveals multiple positive lymph nodes or extracapsular spread, postoperative radiation therapy is administered. In the absence of clinically or radiographically detectable lymph nodes, the head and neck oncologist has three reasonable options: (1) no immediate therapy with close follow-up monitoring and therapeutic neck dissection if regional metastasis occurs; (2) elective neck dissection; or (3) elective radiation therapy. Some authors contend that close follow-up evaluation is acceptable for stage N0 neck disease in patients with early-stage squamous cell carcinoma that is confined to the true vocal cords.[162] Wing Yuen and colleagues[326] conducted a study to determine the efficacy of a watchful waiting policy for N0 neck disease. Their study consisted of 130 patients with advanced laryngeal carcinoma of all sites, including 80 transglottic tumors, 21 supraglottic tumors, and 21 infraglottic tumors (involving the glottis and subglottis). None of the 11 patients who underwent an elective neck dissection developed nodal recurrence, whereas 19 of 122 patients who did not initially undergo neck dissection ultimately developed cervical metastasis. After salvage neck dissection, only 10% of the 122 patients whose necks were not electively dissected died of nodal recurrence. The authors concluded that a watchful waiting policy is a satisfactory option for N0 stage neck disease.[326]

Other investigators believe that elective treatment of a stage N0 neck lesion is indicated for advanced glottic carcinoma when the primary tumor is treated with an open surgical procedure.[318] An ipsilateral selective neck dissection with attention to levels II, III, and IV introduces little morbidity and offers useful prognostic information. Transglottic cancers, which involve the paraglottic space and supraglottic larynx, have a significantly higher propensity for metastasizing to the cervical lymph nodes than do purely glottic tumors. Ogura and associates[327] described 63 patients with T3 transglottic cancer in whom the overall metastatic rate was 26% (and the occult metastatic rate was 11%), compared to a metastatic rate of only 13% in patients with pure T3 glottic carcinoma.[327,328] Similarly, Hao and coauthors[329] retrospectively compared 79 patients with T3 transglottic carcinoma to 65 patients with pure T3 glottic carcinoma. Twenty-one (27%) patients with transglottic carcinoma developed regional metastasis, compared to only 11 (17%) patients with glottic carcinoma. In addition, the group of patients with transglottic tumors had an increased likelihood of having extracapsular nodal spread, which has been shown to decrease survival significantly.[157,329] Based on their findings, the authors recommend that patients with T3 transglottic tumors routinely undergo elective neck dissection.[328]

When radical radiation therapy with surgical salvage is used for advanced glottic carcinoma, radiation therapy is routinely delivered to both sides of the neck. This is an effective modality for preventing nodal recurrence, provided the primary site is controlled; however, relapse in the neck is associated with recurrence at the primary site.[216,287] Mendenhall and associates[330] found that 22% of patients with T2N0 carcinoma of the glottis that recurred or persisted after radiation therapy eventually developed nodal metastasis. This observation prompted these authors to recommend an ipsilateral elective neck dissection for patients in whom primary radiation therapy fails. There is no single answer as to the appropriate management of the N0 stage neck lesion in advanced laryngeal cancer. The ultimate decision depends on several variables, and can only be made after carefully mapping out the extent of the primary tumor and then discussing with the patient all treatment options for both the primary tumor and the neck.

Subglottic Carcinoma

Primary subglottic carcinoma accounts for only 5% to 8% of laryngeal cancers,[83] resulting in a relative paucity of studies pertaining to the appropriate treatment of this lesion. Both radical radiation therapy and primary surgery have been utilized for subglottic lesions with varying degrees of success. Chemoradiotherapeutic protocols are being tested for their effectiveness in controlling tumors in this site. Because subglottic carcinomas are often silent until they produce obstructive symptoms, they are usually in an advanced stage at presentation. For this reason, surgical management usually involves total laryngectomy. Several authors have reported results with total laryngectomy, either with or without postoperative radiation therapy, to control primary subglottic carcinoma. Shaha and Shah[331] published their 25-year experience at the Memorial Sloan-Kettering Cancer Center with primary subglottic carcinoma in a series of 16 patients. Local control was achieved in all 3 patients treated with partial laryngectomy for stage I to II disease and in 10 of 13 patients treated with wide-field laryngectomy. Based on their findings, the authors recommended laryngectomy with thyroidectomy and paratracheal node dissection, in combination with postoperative radiation therapy, for advanced tumors.[331] In another review of primary subglottic carcinoma, local control was achieved in 24 (53%) of 45 patients treated with wide-field laryngectomy.[332]

Radical radiation therapy for subglottic carcinoma has yielded similar poor results. Vermund[333] reviewed 20 articles on the treatment of subglottic carcinoma, compiling data on 185 patients. Primary radiotherapy was utilized in 127 patients, resulting in a 36% 5-year survival rate. Conversely, 58 patients underwent primary surgery, resulting in a 42% 5-year survival.[333] Warde and associates[334] published the Toronto experience with primary subglottic carcinoma, reporting on 23 patients treated with primary radiotherapy. Local control was achieved in 70% of the patients, which included all T1 to T3 cancers. On the other hand, recurrences were noted in 7 of the 11 patients with T4 carcimomas.[334] At the University of Florida, six patients with subglottic carcinoma were treated over a 21-year period. Local control was achieved with primary irradiation in one patient with carcinoma in situ, in one of two patients with T2N0 stage cancer, and in two of three patients with T4N0 cancer.[335]

The incidence of cervical metastasis with purely subglottic carcinomas is less than 20% across all disease stages;[166,167] however, involvement of the paratracheal lymph nodes has been reported to be as high as 65%.[93] Therefore, in the absence of clinical or radiographic lymphadenopathy, neck dissection is not routinely performed. The paratracheal lymph nodes are either dissected or irradiated, depending on which modality is used for the primary tumor. If this lymphatic bed is dissected and found to have histopathologic evidence of disease, postoperative radiation therapy is recommended.

Chemotherapy in Advanced Laryngeal Cancer

Traditionally, total laryngectomy with postoperative radiation therapy has been the standard of care for advanced laryngeal cancer,[336–338] and chemotherapy has primarily played a palliative role.[12] However, over the past decade, experience has accumulated with the use of chemotherapy in the initial management of squamous cell carcinoma of the head and neck, particularly in cases of advanced carcinoma of the larynx. Several clinical trials have demonstrated tumor regression with the use of induction chemotherapy.[339–342] As a result of this, recent protocols have been designed as alternatives to ablative surgery, placing emphasis on the concept of "organ preservation" (Fig. 8–35). Although numerous trials have demonstrated the ability of salvage surgery with postoperative radiation therapy to preserve the larynx without compromising overall survival,[336,342–345] no study has been able to show an improvement in survival compared to surgery with radiation therapy.[340–342,346–348]

The most significant clinical trial was reported by the Department of Veterans Affairs (VA) Laryngeal Cancer Study Group.[346] This was a multi-institu-tional study that included 332 patients with stage III and IV squamous cell carcinomas of the larynx. In this study, patients were randomly assigned to one of two treatments. The first group of patients received three cycles of chemotherapy consisting of cisplatin and fluorouracil, followed by definitive radiation therapy. The second group was treated with wide-field total laryngectomy, with or without neck dissection, followed by postoperative radiation therapy. Patients who received the first treatment regimen were evaluated at the end of the second cycle to determine the tumor's clinical response to chemotherapy. Those with at least a partial response, defined as a reduction in tumor volume by 50% without progression of neck disease, were given a third cycle of chemotherapy and subsequent irradiation. Patients who did not achieve an adequate tumor response, or who developed regional metastasis, were treated with salvage laryngectomy and postoperative radiation therapy; a neck dissection was also performed if necessary. After a median follow-up of 33 months, the 2-year survival was 68% in both treatment groups. In the group receiving chemotherapy, the estimated laryngeal preservation rate at 2 years was 66%, but only 39% of the patients retained a "functional larynx."[346] The morbidity associated with a nonfunctional larynx includes the inability to phonate, the loss of airway protection, and chronic pain related to speaking or swallowing. These symptoms often form the basis for performing a laryngectomy; the number of patients who underwent a laryngectomy to address these issues was not mentioned in the publication.[12] Nonetheless, the importance of this study is that a significant number of patients with advanced laryngeal carcinoma treated with induction chemotherapy and radiation therapy can achieve laryngeal preservation without compromising survival.

One of the most common criticisms of the VA study is that it did not include a third treatment group of patients who received only radiation therapy. The rationale provided by the project's chiefs was that it would have been unethical to so design the study, as radiation therapy is already known to be less effective than surgery plus radiotherapy.[317,318,349,350] However, studies in Canada and Europe have reported results comparable to those cited in the VA study. Harwood and associates[205] published a series of 265 patients with T3N0 and T4N0 supraglottic tumors treated with primary radiation therapy and surgical salvage. They reported a 5-year survival rate of 51% with a laryngeal preservation rate of 64% in the survivors. Similarly, Croll and co-workers[351] reported results in 55 patients with T3N0 and T4N0 tumors without invasion of the laryngeal framework, noting a 52% cure rate with preservation of the larynx in 73% of the survivors. Thus, it is difficult to determine whether induction chemotherapy actually had a therapeutic role in those patients with good outcomes. Based on variations in tumor

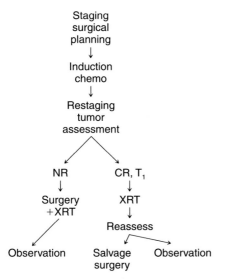

FIGURE 8–35 General schema of organ preservation treatment strategies incorporating chemotherapy (chemo) to select patients for definitive radiation therapy. CR, complete response; NR, no response; XRT, radiation therapy. From Wolf GT, Hong WK. Induction chemotherapy for organ preservation in advanced laryngeal cancer: Is there a role? *Head Neck.* 1995; 17(4):280.

biology, it is possible that a good clinical response to chemotherapy identified the patients who would have responded well to radiation therapy alone.

Subsequent to the VA study, additional investigations using induction chemotherapy have been published with equally encouraging results, although with smaller numbers. De Andres and associates[352] reported results in 46 patients with stage III laryngeal carcinoma who received induction chemotherapy (cisplatin and fluorouracil) followed by either radiation therapy or surgical salvage. They reported preservation of a functional larynx in 57% of all patients included in the study, and in 64% of 3-year survivors. As in the VA study, the term "functional larynx" was not defined. A noteworthy factor in this study was that 6 of the 14 patients who had an insufficient response to chemotherapy were able to be salvaged with conservation laryngeal surgery followed by radiation therapy. However, details of the operations were not provided. The remaining eight patients underwent salvage total laryngectomy.[352] Shirinian and colleagues[353] recently reported the M.D. Anderson Cancer Center's experience with the use of induction chemotherapy in the treatment of advanced carcinoma of the larynx, hypopharynx, and oropharynx. This was considered to be an organ-preservation study, as all 64 subjects were judged to have tumors that would have necessitated total laryngectomy in order to achieve adequate local control. One half of the patients in this study received a chemotherapeutic regimen consisting of cisplatin and fluorouracil, whereas the remaining patients received cisplatin, bleomycin, and fluorouracil. Partial plus complete response rates between the two cohorts were comparable at 79% and 73% for PF and PBF, respectively. With follow-up ranging from 15+ to 54+ months, the laryngeal preservation rates were 44%, 28%, and 22%, and the overall 2-year survival rates were 71%, 46%, and 38% for lesions of the larynx, hypopharynx, and oropharynx, respectively. The lower rates of laryngeal preservation achieved in patients with tumors of the hypopharynx and oropharynx reflect the more aggressive biologic behavior of these tumors compared to laryngeal carcinoma.[353] A similarly designed study was recently conducted at the Memorial Sloan-Kettering Cancer Center.[354] Forty patients with advanced but resectable carcinoma of the larynx, hypopharynx, and oropharynx were treated with cisplatin and either bleomycin or vinblastine in one to three cycles, followed by radiation therapy. After surgical salvage, the 5-year disease-free survival rate was 33%, and 68% of the patients were able to retain their larynx.[354] Recently, Vokes and colleagues[355] at the University of Chicago published data on a series of 71 patients with advanced head and neck cancer of all sites. These patients were treated with an aggressive regimen of induction chemotherapy (cisplatin, fluorouracil, leucovorin, and interferon α-2b), followed by optional organ-sparing surgery and seven or eight cycles of fluorouracil, hydroxy-

urea, and concurrent radiation for 5 days (to a total dose of 65 to 75 Gy). The 3-year survival rate was 60%; however, toxicity was quite significant with this chemoradiotherapeutic regimen. Severe or life-threatening mucositis occurred in 54% of patients, and myelosuppression was reported in 60%; five patients died from toxicity.[355] A follow-up study by the same authors included 93 patients with head and neck cancer of all sites.[356] The 5-year survival rate was reported to be 62%, again with very significant toxicity. Of the 34 patients who underwent chemoradiotherapy, only one laryngectomy and no glossectomies were performed, confirming the organ-preserving nature of this approach.

Chemoradiotherapeutic protocols that attempt to preserve the larynx and improve survival are important in the quest for improved management of laryngeal cancer. Studies have shown that induction chemotherapy, followed by radiation therapy, does provide a chance for cure with laryngeal preservation in a significant number of individuals. However, few studies have been conducted in a randomized prospective manner, limiting comparisons to historical controls that inevitably introduce bias. Additionally, chemotherapeutic regimens and dosing schedules differ between various trials, making it difficult to draw reasonable conclusions about the benefits of these agents. Finally, studies to date have not been able to demonstrate an appreciable increase in survival when compared to surgery plus radiation therapy. At this point, chemoradiotherapeutic protocols are still merely investigational alternatives for individuals who refuse total laryngectomy. Protocols should be conducted at an institution where multispecialty support is available for the close monitoring of patients and surgical management of treatment failures. The standard of care for resectable advanced laryngeal cancer at this time is still surgical resection with postoperative radiation therapy.

PERISTOMAL RECURRENCE

Peristomal recurrence refers to carcinoma arising from the tracheal or pharyngeal resection margins, or from the lymph nodes or adjacent soft tissues in the peristomal area. It is one of the most dreaded and fatal complications following total laryngectomy for squamous cell carcinoma.[357] The incidence of stomal recurrence reported in the literature varies from 2.5% to 15%, with a mean of 5.8%.[358–361] Most often, recurrence appears within 1 to 2 years following total laryngectomy, but in some cases, it can present within a few months after surgery.[358,362,363] Inadequate tumor resection at the inferior margin probably contributes to early recurrence in these cases.[169] The clinical presentation of stomal recurrence varies. In some instances, the tumor resembles granulation tissue at the mucocutaneous junction of the tracheostoma, but more commonly, a subcutaneous nodule develops adjacent to the stoma. The tumor then grows concentrically, narrowing the tracheal lumen and eventually ulcerating through the mucosa. Massive bleeding and airway obstruction ultimately lead to the patient's death.

The system utilized for classifying stomal recurrences was developed by Sisson and co-workers.[364,365] Stomal recurrences are categorized into four types, based on their location with respect to the stoma and their local extent.

Type I—Tumor involves the superior one half of the stoma without esophageal involvement.

Type II—Tumor involves the superior one half of the stoma with esophageal involvement.

Type III—Tumor involves the inferior one half of the stoma and extends into the superior mediastinum.

Type IV—Tumor extends laterally underneath both clavicles and into the superior mediastinum.

Multiple risk factors have been implicated in the development of peristomal recurrence. Most prominent among these is the presence of tumor in the subglottis, either as a primary lesion or a transglottic lesion.[150,359,362,366] In Kleinsasser's series,[169] 80% of the cases of stomal recurrence had subglottic involvement. The increased stomal recurrence rate with tumors involving the subglottis may be explained by looking at the pattern by which these lesions spread. Carcinoma of the subglottis penetrates the cricothyroid membrane, spreading to adjacent structures, such as the thyroid gland, trachea, and hypopharynx.[93,367,368] Furthermore, subglottic tumors metastasize to the paratracheal lymph nodes in up to 65% of cases.[93] These nodes are seldom palpable on physical examination and are not routinely included in neck dissection. Thus, residual disease left in the adjacent peristomal tissue, and occult cancer within the paratracheal lymph nodes, both contribute to an increased risk for stomal recurrence. Hosal and co-workers[357] reported a decrease in the incidence of peristomal recurrence from 11.5% to 2.7% after the paratracheal lymph nodes were addressed. They currently recommend dissecting out the paratracheal, pretracheal, and retrosternal lymph nodes in all patients with laryngeal tumors with subglottic involvement. Furthermore, if any nodes are found to be histologically positive, these researchers advise that postoperative radiation therapy be administered.[357] Histologic evidence of disease in the paratracheal lymph nodes, however, is an ominous finding. Weber and associates[369] reported a 0% survival rate beyond 42 months in 645 patients with metastasis to this lymphatic bed.

Prior tracheotomy is the most controversial risk factor for stomal recurrence. Patients with large, bulky tumors frequently present with airway ob-struction requiring urgent or emergent tracheotomy. It has been hypothesized that, during the procedure, dislodged tumor cells may become implanted in the fresh granulation tissue of the tracheostoma wound. Support for this concept comes from case reports of tumor recurrence at a recent gastrostomy site in a patient with tongue carcinoma,[370] and along the donor site of a pectoralis major myocutaneous flap that was used to close a retromolar trigone defect.[371,372] The increased incidence of stomal recurrence in patients who receive prior tracheotomy has been observed by many investigators,[373–375] and this has led authors to advocate "emergency laryngectomy" rather than tracheotomy.[376–378] Recent studies, however, have failed to demonstrate a relationship between preoperative tracheotomy and an increased stomal recurrence rate.[357,367,379–381] Rubin and associates[367] published the results of a series of 444 patients with laryngeal carcinoma who underwent total laryngectomy, reporting no difference in the stomal recurrence rate in patients with subglottic involvement who required preoperative tracheotomy. Differences reported in the literature likely reflect the location and size of the lesion in the subglottis. Patients who present with airway obstruction requiring tracheotomy usually have extensive disease, which increases their risk for stomal recurrence. Preoperative tracheotomy, in and of itself, does not appear to be an independent risk factor.[357,367] Thus, at the authors' institution, emergency laryngectomy is not performed; however, definitive surgery is scheduled at the earliest possible interval after emergent tracheostomy.

Some debate exists regarding the impact preoperative tumor extent (T stage) has on the stomal recurrence rate. A multivariate analysis of risk factors conducted by Rubin and colleagues[367] revealed that only subglottic involvement and T stage were significant predictors of peristomal recurrence. This has been corroborated by some studies,[362,379,382] whereas others have failed to show a relationship between the initial tumor stage and stomal recurrence.[359,360,383]

Treatment options for managing stomal recurrences include surgery, radiation therapy, surgery with radiation therapy, and chemotherapy with radiation therapy. As a single technique, radiation therapy may provide patients with some palliation, but it is ineffective in controlling stomal disease. Furthermore, radiation therapy is not always a viable option, as many patients have already received radiation therapy after their initial surgery. A combined regimen of chemotherapy and irradiation has shown promising results in a small group of patients; however, additional studies are necessary before conclusions about improved survival can be made. Thus, the primary treatment for stomal recurrence is radical surgery, largely based on the research of Sisson and colleagues.[364,365] Surgical resection involves removal of the tracheostoma with a margin of 3 cm of surrounding skin, resection of the upper portion of the manubrium (with or without the sternal ends of the clavicles), removal of any involved pharyngoesophageal tissue, and excision of any remaining thyroid gland. Additionally, lymph nodes in the superior mediastinal, paratracheal, and tracheoesophageal regions are included with the specimen. Reconstruction and obliteration of the dead space are usually accomplished with a pectoralis major myocutaneous flap.

Survival rates after stomal recurrence surgery have been very poor, prompting some authors to suggest that increased emphasis be placed on prevention rather than treatment. Sisson and co-workers[384] performed transsternal radical neck dissections on 28 patients with peristomal recurrence, reporting 3- and 5-year survival rates of 29% and 17%, respectively. In a cohort of 41 patients with all types of stomal recurrences, Gluckman and associates[385] reported a 16% overall survival rate, with a 24% determinate survival rate. After stratifying the patient population by the type of lesion, however, a 45% survival rate was noted in those individuals with type I or II stomal recurrences; the survival for patients with type III or IV lesions was only 9%. Adequate palliation of pain and airway obstruction was obtained in the nonsurvivors.[385] Currently, mediastinal dissection with postoperative radiation therapy (if this modality has not already been used) is recommended for patients with type I or II stomal recurrences. Mediastinal dissection may be attempted in selected patients with type III or IV stomal recurrences who are medically fit to tolerate the operation; however, the morbidity and mortality rates may be unacceptably high considering the dismal survival rates reported.

Stomal recurrence surgery is fraught with a multitude of complications, many of which are fatal. The perioperative mortality rate approaches 15%.[150] Complications may be divided into three categories: intraoperative, immediate postoperative, and late complications.[386] Injury to one of the great vessels represents the most devastating intraoperative complication. The aorta, innominate artery and vein, and carotid arteries are immediately within the operating field. Damage to any of these vascular structures results in profuse hemorrhage, which is often difficult to control, leading to exsanguination. Other serious intraoperative complications include air embolism, pneumothorax, and chyle leak. Immediate postoperative complications are those that occur within the first 5 days after surgery. The most severe and potentially fatal complication is mediastinitis, which may arise from an infected hematoma, seroma, or an anastomotic leak. Once diagnosed, mediastinitis requires immediate thoracotomy and drainage, as well as intravenous antibiotic therapy and wound care. Local wound infection, a seemingly benign postoperative complication, can progress to sepsis, shock, and death if not diagnosed early and treated aggressively. Late postoperative events, which occur more than 5 days after surgery, may be just as catastrophic as early complications. Vascular rupture is the most life-threatening delayed complication. With the lower position of the tracheostoma and the intimate relationship of the trachea to the great vessels, the potential exists for erosion of either the innominate artery or aorta into the tracheal lumen. The continuous trauma that mechanical ventilation imparts to the trachea increases the possibility of this devastating event. Other delayed complications include flap necrosis, hypothyroidism, hypoparathyroidism, and aspiration pneumonia.

SUMMARY

As a prerequisite to the treatment of laryngeal carcinoma, one must have a thorough knowledge of the anatomy and physiology of the larynx. Additionally, an understanding of the typical patterns of tumor spread for lesions arising from the various sites within the larynx is essential. Surgical treatment for laryngeal carcinoma has changed over the last several decades, evolving from radical ablative surgery to various conservation techniques that preserve phonation and deglutition. The oncologic basis for conservation laryngeal surgery has been established through extensive laboratory and clinical studies, and in properly selected patients, it is as effective as total laryngectomy. Newer techniques for delivering radiation therapy, as well as higher therapeutic doses, have led to improved local-regional control of laryngeal tumors. In addition, various protocols using induction chemotherapy prior to irradiation have, in many instances, allowed laryngeal preservation. At this time, however, chemoradiotherapeutic protocols have not been able to achieve improved survival compared to standard therapy. Future directions in the management of laryngeal cancer will include a better understanding of tumor biology, as well as the development of biologic response modifiers and newer chemotherapeutic agents for preventing the growth and spread of laryngeal cancer.

REFERENCES

1. Brockmuehl F. *Die Behandlung und Prognose des Kehlkopfkrebses in der DDR von 1956–1966 und epidemiologisch Gesichtspunken.* Berlin: Habel; 1977.
2. DeRienzo DP, Grennberg SD, Fraire AE. Carcinoma of the larynx. Changing incidence in women. *Arch Otolaryngol Head Neck Surg.* 1991; 117:681.
3. Young JL Jr, Percy CL, Asire AJ, eds. *Surveillance, Epidemiology, and End Results: Incidence and Mortality Data, 1973–1977.* NCI Monograph 57. NIH, PHS, DHEW Publication (NIH) 81-2330, 1981.
4. Roels H. Histopathology of laryngeal tumours. *Acta Otorhinolaryngol (Belg).* 1992; 46:127.
5. Ringertz N. Cancer incidence in Finland, Norway, Iceland, and Sweden. *Acta Pathol Microbiol Immunol Scand.* 1971; 224 (suppl):1.

6. Doll R, Payne P, Waterhouse J. *Cancer Incidence in Five Continents*. Vol 1. Geneva: UICC; 1966.

7. Doll R, Payne P, Waterhouse J. *Cancer Incidence in Five Continents*. Vol 2. Geneva: UICC; 1970.

8. Muir C, Waterhouse J, Mack T, et al. *Cancer Incidence in Five Continents*. vol 5. Lyon: International Agency for Research on Cancer (IARC); 1987.

9. Waterhouse J, Muir CS, Correa P, et al. *Cancer Incidence in Five Continents*. vol 3. Lyon: IARC; 1976.

10. Waterhouse J, Muir C, Shanmugaratnam K, et al. *Cancer Incidence in Five Continents*, vol 4. Lyon: IARC; 1982.

11. Silverberg E. Cancer statistics, 1983. *CA*. 1983; 33:9–25.

12. Castellanos PF, Spector JG, Kaiser TN. Tumors of the larynx and laryngopharynx. In: Ballenger JJ, Snow JJ Jr, eds. *Otorhinolaryngology Head and Neck Surgery*. Philadelphia: Williams & Wilkins; 1996.

13. Breslow NE, Eustrom JE. Geographic correlations between cancer mortality rates and alcohol-tobacco consumption in the U.S. *J Natl Cancer Inst*. 1974; 53:631.

14. Wynder EL, Stillman SD. Comparative epidemiology of tobacco related cancers. *Cancer Res*. 1977; 37:4608.

15. Falk RT, Pickle LW, Brown LM, et al. Effect of smoking and alcohol consumption on laryngeal cancer risk in coastal Texas. *Cancer Res*. 1989; 49:4024.

16. Hiranandani LH. Panel on epidemiology and etiology of laryngeal carcinoma. *Laryngoscope*. 1975; 85:1197.

17. Moore C. Cigarette smoking and cancer of the mouth, pharynx, and larynx: A continuous study. *JAMA*. 1971; 218:553.

18. Wynder EL, Stillman SD. Impact of long-term filter cigarette usage on lung and larynx cancer risk: A case control study. *J Natl Cancer Inst*. 1979; 62:471.

19. Spitz MR, Fueger JJ, Goepfert H, et al. Squamous cell carcinoma of the upper aerodigestive tract. A case comparison analysis. *Cancer*. 1988; 61:203.

20. Brugers J, Guenel P, Leclerc A, et al. Differential effects of tobacco and alcohol in cancer of the larynx, pharynx, and mouth. *Cancer*. 1986; 57:391.

21. Zheng W, Blot WJ, Shu XO, et al. Diet and other risk factors for laryngeal cancer in Shanghai, China. *AJ Epidemiol*. 1992; 136:178.

22. Hedberg K, Vaughan TL, White E, et al. Alcoholism and cancer of the larynx: A case-control study in western Washington. *Cancer Causes Control*. 1994; 5:3.

23. Flanders WD, Rothman KJ. Interaction of alcohol and tobacco in laryngeal cancer. *Am J Epidemiol*. 1982; 115:371.

24. Wynder EL, Bross JJ, Day E. Epidemiological approach to the etiology of cancer of the larynx. *JAMA*. 1956; 160:1384.

25. Brandwein MS, Nuovo GJ, Biller H. Analysis of prevalence of human papillomavirus in laryngeal carcinoma. Study of 40 cases using polymerase-chain reaction and consensus primers. *Ann Otol Rhinol Laryngol*. 1993; 102:309.

26. Amendola BE, Amendola MA, McClatchey KD. Radiation induced carcinoma of the larynx. *Surg Gynecol Obstet*. 1985; 161:30.

27. Aaronsen JP, Olofsson J. Irradiation-induced tumours of the head and neck. *Acta Otolaryngol (Stockh)*. 1979; 360(suppl): 178.

28. Lawon S, Som M. Second primary cancer after irradiation of laryngeal cancer. *Ann Otol Rhinol Laryngol*. 1975; 84:771.

29. Wortley P, Vaughan TL, Davis S, et al. A case-control study of occupational risk factors for laryngeal cancer. *Br J Indust Med*. 1992; 49:837.

30. Brown LM, Mason TJ, Pickle LW, et al. Occupational risk factors for laryngeal cancer on the Texas Gulf Coast. *Cancer Res*. 1988; 48:1960.

31. Muscat JE, Wynder EL. Tobacco, alcohol, asbestos, and occupational risk factors for laryngeal cancer. *Cancer*. 1992; 69: 2244.

32. Smith AH, Handley MA, Wood R. Epidemiological evidence indicates asbestos causes laryngeal cancer. *J Occup Med*. 1990; 32:499.

33. Chan CK, Gee JB. Asbestos exposure and laryngeal cancer: An analysis of the epidemiologic evidence. *J Occup Med*. 1988; 30:23.

34. Flanders WD, Rothman KJ. Occupational risk for laryngeal cancer. *Am J Public Health*. 1982; 72:369.

35. Klayman MB. Exposure to insecticides. *Arch Otolaryngol Head Neck Surg*. 1968; 88:116.

36. Manning KP, Skegg DC, Stell PM, et al. Cancer of the larynx and other occupational hazards of mustard gas workers. *Clin Otolaryngol*. 1981; 6:165.

37. Moss E. Oral and pharyngeal cancer in textile workers. *Ann NY Acad Sci*. 1976; 271:301.

38. Stell PM, McGill T. Exposure to asbestos and laryngeal carcinoma. *J Laryngol Otol*. 1971; 89:513.

39. Liddell FDK. Laryngeal cancer and asbestos. *Br J Ind Med*. 1990; 47:289.

40. Parnes SM. Asbestos and cancer of the larynx: Is there a relationship? *Laryngoscope*. 1990; 100:254.

41. Snijders PJF, Cromme FV, Van Den Brule AJC, et al. Prevalence and expression of human papillomavirus in tonsillar carcinomas, indicating a possible viral etiology. *Int J Cancer*. 1992; 51:845.

42. Bercovich JA, Centeno CR, Aguilar OG, et al. Presence and integration of human papillomavirus type 6 in a tonsillar carcinoma. *J Gen Virol*. 1991; 72:2569.

43. Portugal LG, Goldenberg JD, Wenig BL, et al. Human papillomavirus expression and p53 mutations in squamous cell carcinoma of the oral cavity and tonsil. *Arch Otolaryngol Head Neck Surg*. 1997; 123:1230.

44. Kashima H, Mounts P, Kuhajda F, et al. Demonstration of human papilloma virus capsid antigen in carcinoma in situ of the larynx. *Ann Otol Rhinol Laryngol*. 1986; 95:603.

45. Levine AF, Momand J, Finlay CA. The p53 tumor suppressor gene. *Nature*. 1991; 351:453.

46. Hollstein M, Sidransky D, Vogelstein B, et al. p53 mutations in human cancers. *Science*. 1991; 253:49.

47. Rodriguez NR, et al. p53 mutations in colorectal carcinoma. *Proc Natl Acad Sci USA*. 1990; 87:7555.

48. Purdic CA, O'Grady J, Piris J, et al. p53 expression in colorectal tumors. *Am J Pathol*. 1991; 138(4):807.

49. Takahashi T, Nau MM, Chiba I, et al. p53: A frequent target for genetic abnormalities in lung cancer. *Science*. 1989; 246:491.

50. Davidoff AM, Kerns BJ, Iglehart JD, et al. Maintenance of p53 alterations throughout stages of breast cancer progression. *Cancer Res*. 1991; 51:2605.

51. Bartek J, Bartkova J, Vojtesek B, et al. Patterns of expression of the p53 tumor suppressor in human breast tissues and tumors in situ and vivo. *Int J Cancer*. 1990; 46:839.

52. Marks JR, Davidoff AM, Kerns BJ, et al. Over-expression and mutation of p53 in epithelial ovarian cancer. *Cancer Res*. 1991; 51(11):2979.

53. Schantz SP. Carcinogenesis, markets, staging and prognosis of head and neck cancer. *Curr Opin Oncol*. 1993; 5:483.

54. Carter RL. Pathology of squamous carcinomas of the head and neck. *Curr Opin Oncol*. 1993; 5:491.

55. Dolcetti R, Doglioni C, Maestro R, et al. p53 over-expression is an early event in the development of human squamous-cell carcinoma of the larynx: Genetic and prognostic implications. *Int J Cancer*. 1992; 52:178.

56. Frazer EJ. The development of the larynx. *J Anat Physiol*. 1909; 44:156.

57. Henick DH. Three-dimensional analysis of murine laryngeal development. *Ann Otol Rhinol Laryngol*. 1993; 102(suppl 159): 1.

58. Moore KL. The respiratory system. In: *The Developing Human: Clinically Oriented Embryology*. Philadelphia: WB Saunders; 1998.

59. Ogura JH. Surgical pathology of cancer of the larynx. *Laryngoscope*. 1955; 65:867.

60. Tucker GF, Smith HR. A histopathological demonstration of the development of laryngeal connective tissue compartments. *Trans Am Acad Ophthalmol Otolaryngol*. 1962; 66:308.

61. Tucker HM. *The Larynx*. New York: Thieme Medical Publishers; 1987.

62. Broyles EN. The anterior commissure tendon. *Ann Otol Rhinol Laryngol*. 1943; 52:341.

63. Kirchner JA. Anterior commissure cancer. *Can J Otolaryngol.* 1975; 4:671.

64. Bagatella F, Bignardi L. Behavior of cancer at the anterior commissure of the larynx. *Laryngoscope.* 1983; 93:353.

65. Kirchner JA. *Vocal Fold Histopathology.* San Diego: College Hill Press; 1986.

66. Zeitels SM, Kirchner JA. Hyoepiglottic ligament in supraglottic cancer. *Ann Otol Rhinol Laryngol.* 1995; 104:770.

67. Clerf LH. The preepiglottic space. Its relation to carcinoma of the epiglottis. *Arch Otolaryngol.* 1944; 40:177.

68. Kirchner JA. One hundred laryngeal cancers studied by serial section. *Ann Otol Rhinol Laryngol.* 1969; 78:689.

69. Bocca E, Pignataro O, Mosciaro O. Supraglottic surgery of the larynx. *Ann Otol Rhinol Laryngol.* 1968; 77:1005.

70. Gregor RT. The preepiglottic space revisited: Is it significant? *Am J Otolaryngol.* 1990; 11:161.

71. Zeitels SM, Vaughan CW. Preepiglottic space invasion in "early" epiglottic cancer. *Ann Otol Rhinol Laryngol.* 1991; 100: 789.

72. Pressman JJ, Dowdy A, Libby R, et al. Further studies upon the submucosal compartments and lymphatics of the larynx by injections of dyes and radioisotopes. *Ann Otol Rhinol Laryngol.* 1956; 65:963.

73. Pearson BW. Laryngeal microcirculation and pathways of cancer spread. *Laryngoscope.* 1975; 85:700.

74. American Joint Committee on Cancer, 1997.

75. Nassar VH, Bridger GP. Topography of the laryngeal mucous glands. *Arch Otolaryngol.* 1971; 94:490.

76. Ogura JH, Spector GJ, Sessions DG. Conservation surgery for epidermoid carcinoma of the marginal area (aryepiglottic fold extension). *Laryngoscope.* 1975; 85:1801.

77. Sessions DG, Ogura JH. Classification of laryngeal cancer. In: Alberti PW, Bryce DB, eds. *Workshops from the Centennial Conference on Laryngeal Cancer.* New York: Appleton-Century-Crofts; 1976:83.

78. Valvassori GE, Mafee MF, Carter BL. *Imaging of the Head and Neck.* New York: Thieme Medical Publishers; 1995.

79. Weber PC, Johnson JT, Myers EN. The impact of bilateral neck dissection on pattern of recurrence and survival in supraglottic carcinoma. *Arch Otolaryngol Head Neck Surg.* 1994; 120:703.

80. Bocca E. Surgical management of supraglottic cancer and its lymph node metastases in conservative perspective. *Ann Otol Rhinol Laryngol.* 1991; 100:261.

81. Bocca E, Calearo C, De Vincentiis I, et al. Occult metastases in cancer of the larynx and their relationship to clinical and histological aspects of the primary tumor: A four-year multicentric research. *Laryngoscope.* 1984; 94:1086.

82. Razack MS, Baffi R, Sako K. Bilateral radical neck dissection. *Cancer.* 1981; 47:197.

83. Olofsson J. Clinical manifestations and diagnostic procedures. In: Ferlito, ed. *Neoplasms of the Larynx.* New York: Churchill Livingstone; 1993:361.

84. Kirchner JA, Som ML. Clinical significance of the fixed vocal cord. *Laryngoscope.* 1971; 81:1029.

85. Mittal B, Marks JE, Ogura JH. Transglottic carcinoma. *Cancer.* 1984; 53:151

86. Olofsson J, Lord IJ, van Nostrand AWP. Vocal cord fixation in laryngeal carcinoma. *Acta Otolaryngol (Stockh).* 1973; 75: 496.

87. Piccirillo JF, Wells CK, Sasaki CT, et al. New clinical severity staging system for cancer of the larynx. *Ann Otol Rhino Laryngol.* 1994; 103:83.

88. Johnson JT, Myers EN. Cervical lymph node disease in laryngeal cancer. In: Silver CE, ed. *Laryngeal Cancer.* New York: Thieme Medical Publishers; 1991.

89. Daly CJ, Strong EW. Carcinoma of the glottic larynx. *Am J Surg.* 1975; 130:489.

90. Jesse RH. The evaluation and treatment of patients with extensive squamous cancer of the vocal cords. *Laryngoscope.* 1975; 85:1424.

91. Redaelli de Zinis LO, Nicolai P, Barezzani MG, et al. Incidence and distribution of lymph node metastases in supra-

glottic squamous cell carcinoma: Therapeutic implications. *Acta Otorhinolaryngol Ital.* 1994; 14:19.

92. Bocca E, Pignataro O, Oldini C. Supraglottic laryngectomy: 30 years of experience. *Ann Otol Rhinol Laryngol.* 1983; 92:14.

93. Harrison DF. The pathology and management of subglottic cancer. *Ann Otol Rhinol Laryngol.* 1971; 80:6.

94. Celin SE, Johnson J, Curtin H, Barnes L. The association of laryngoceles with squamous cell carcinoma of the larynx. *Laryngoscope.* 1991; 101:529.

95. Sataloff RT, Spiegel JR, Hawshaw MJ. Strobovideolaryngoscopy: Results and clinical value. *Ann Otol Rhinol Laryngol.* 1991; 100:725.

96. Zamora RL, Harvey JE, Sessions DG, et al. Clinical staging for primary malignancies of the supraglottic larynx. *Laryngoscope.* 1993; 103:69.

97. Patel P, Snow GB. Metastases of carcinoma of the larynx. *Acta Otorhinolaryngol (Belg).* 1992; 46:141.

98. Wenig BL, Applebaum EL. The submandibular triangle in squamous cell carcinoma of the larynx and hypopharynx. *Laryngoscope.* 1991; 101:516.

99. Shah JP. Patterns of cervical lymph node metastasis from squamous carcinoma of the upper aerodigestive tract. *Am J Surg.* 1990; 160:405.

100. Papae RJ. Distant metastases from head and neck cancer. *Cancer.* 1984; 53:342.

101. Alonso JM. Metastasis of laryngeal and hypopharyngeal carcinoma. *Acta Otolaryngol (Stockh).* 1967; 64:353.

102. Abramson A, Pansier SC, Zamansky MJ, et al. Distant metastasis from carcinoma of the larynx. *Laryngoscope.* 1971; 81: 1503.

103. Mummer CS, Chusid CA. Distant metastases from primary malignancies of the endolarynx. *Laryngoscope.* 1961; 71:524.

104. Shaha A, Hoover E, Marti J, et al. Is routine triple endoscopy cost-effective in head and neck cancer? *Am J Surg.* 1988; 155: 750.

105. Som PM. Evaluation of cervical nodes by computed tomography and magnetic resonance imaging. In: Silver CE, ed. *Laryngeal Cancer.* New York: Thieme Medical Publishers; 1991.

106. Isaacs JH, Mancuso AA, Mendenhall WM, et al. Deep spread patterns in CT staging of T2–4 squamous cell carcinoma. *Otolaryngol Head Neck Surg.* 1988; 99:455.

107. Yeager VL, Lawson C, Archer CR. Ossification of the laryngeal cartilages as it relates to computed tomography. *Invest Radiol.* 1982; 17:11.

108. Curtin HD. Imaging of the larynx: Current concepts. *Radiology.* 1989; 173:1.

109. Zbaren P, Becker M, Lang H. Pretherapeutic staging of laryngeal carcinoma: Clinical findings, computed tomography, and magnetic resonance imaging compared with histopathology. *Cancer.* 1996; 77:1263.

110. Hoover LA, Calcaterra TC, Walter GA, et al. Preoperative CT scan evaluation for laryngeal carcinoma: Correlation with pathological finding. *Laryngoscope.* 1984; 94:310.

111. Archer CR, Yeager VL. Evaluation of laryngeal cartilages by computed tomography. *J Comput Assist Tomogr.* 1979; 35:604.

112. Castelijns JA, van den Brekel MW, Tobi H, et al. Laryngeal carcinoma after radiation therapy: Correlation of abnormal MR imaging signal patterns of laryngeal cartilage with risk of recurrence. *Radiology.* 1996; 198:151.

113. Wenig BL, Ziffra K, Mafee MF, et al. Magnetic imaging of squamous cell carcinoma of the larynx and hypopharynx. *Otolaryngol Clin North Am.* 1995; 28:609.

114. Castelijns JA, Doornbos J, Verbeeten F Jr, et al. Magnetic resonance imaging of the normal larynx. 1985; 9:919.

115. Becker M, Zbaeren P, Laeng H, et al. Neoplastic invasion of the laryngeal cartilage: Comparison of MR imaging and CT with histopathologic correlation. *Radiology.* 1995; 194:661.

116. Castelijns JA, Golding RP, van Schaik C, et al. MR findings of cartilage invasion by laryngeal cancer: Value in predicting outcome of radiation therapy. *Radiology.* 1990; 174:669.

117. Kirchner JA, Owen JR. Five hundred cancers of the larynx

and piriform sinus: Results of treatment by radiation and surgery. *Laryngoscope.* 1977; 87:1288.

118. Giron J, Joffre P, Serres-Cousine O, et al. CT and MR evaluation of laryngeal carcinomas. *J Otolaryngol.* 1993; 22:4.

119. Million RR. The larynx . . . so to speak: Everything I wanted to know about laryngeal cancer I learned in the last 32 years. *Int J Radiat Oncol Biol Phys.* 1992; 23:691.

120. Lam KH. Extralaryngeal spread of cancer of the larynx: A study with whole organ sections. *Head Neck Surg.* 1983; 5: 410.

121. Munoz A, Ramos A, Ferrando J, et al. Laryngeal carcinoma: Sclerotic appearance of the cricoid and arytenoid cartilage–CT pathologic correlation. *Radiology.* 1993; 189.

122. Adlington P, Woodhouse MA. The ultrastructure of chemodectoma of the larynx. *J Laryngol Otol.* 1972; 86:1219.

123. Nakayama M, Brandenburg JH. Clinical underestimation of laryngeal cancer. Predictive indicators. *Arch Otolaryngol Head Neck Surg.* 1993; 119:950.

124. Pillsbury HRC, Kirchner JA. Clinical versus histopathologic staging in laryngeal cancer. *Arch Otolarnygol Head Neck Surg.* 1979; 105;157.

125. Sulfaro S, Barzan L, Qurein F, et al. T staging of the laryngohypopharyngeal carcinoma. *Arch Otolaryngol Head Neck Surg.* 1989; 115:613.

126. Mancuso AA. Evaluation and staging of laryngeal and hypopharyngeal cancer by computed tomography and magnetic resonance imaging. In: Silver CE, ed. *Laryngeal Cancer.* New York: Thieme Medical Publishers; 1991.

127. Gluckman JL, Crissman JD. Survival rates in 548 patients with multiple neoplasms of the upper aerodigestive tract. *Laryngoscope.* 1983; 33:71.

128. Panosetti E, Luboinski B, Mamelle G, et al. Multiple synchronous and metachronous cancers of the upper aerodigestive tract: A nine-year study. *Laryngoscope.* 1989; 99:1267.

129. Glaws WR, Etzkorn KP, Wenig BL, et al. Comparison of rigid and flexible esophagoscopy in the diagnosis of esophageal disease: Diagnostic accuracy, complications, and cost. *Ann Otol Rhinol Laryngol.* 1996; 105:262.

130. Pressman JJ. Submucosal compartmentalization of the larynx. *Ann Otol Rhinol Laryngol.* 1956; 65:766.

131. Welsh LW, Welsh JJ, Rizzo TA. Internal anatomy of the larynx and the spread of cancer. *Ann Otol Rhinol Laryngol.* 1989; 98:228.

132. Kirchner JA, Carter D. Intralaryngeal barriers to the spread of cancer. *Acta Otolaryngol (Stockh).* 1987; 103:503.

133. Kirchner JA. Spread and barriers to spread of cancer within the larynx. In: Silver CE, ed. *Laryngeal Cancer.* New York: Thieme Medical Publishers; 1991.

134. Som ML. Conservation surgery for carcinoma of supraglottis. *J Laryngol Otol.* 1970; 84:655.

135. Ogura JH. Supraglottic subtotal laryngectomy and radical neck dissection for carcinoma of the epiglottis. *Laryngoscope.* 1958; 48:983.

136. Bocca E. Supraglottic cancer. *Laryngoscope.* 1975; 85:1318.

137. Kirchner JA. What have whole organ sections contributed to the treatment of laryngeal cancer? *Ann Otol Rhinol Laryngol.* 1989; 98:661.

138. Pernkopf E. Head and neck. In: *Atlas of Topographical and Applied Human Anatomy.* Vol 1. Philadelphia: WB Saunders; 1963:330.

139. Tucker GF. *Human Larynx Coronal Section Atlas.* Washington, DC: Armed Forces Institute of Pathology; 1971:12.

140. Ogura JH, Sessions DG, Spector GJ. Conservation surgery for epidermoid carcinoma of the supraglottic larynx. *Laryngoscope.* 1975; 85:1808.

141. Jorgensen K, Munk J, Anderson JE, et al. Carcinoma of the larynx. Series of 410 patients treated primarily with Co irradiation. *Acta Radiol Oncol.* 1984; 23:321.

142. Marks JE, Breaux S, Smith PG, et al. The need for elective irradiation of occult lymphatic metastases from cancers of the larynx and pyriform sinus. *Head Neck* 1985; 8:3.

143. Kirchner JA, Fischer J. Anterior commissure cancer—A clinical and laboratory study of 39 cases. *Can J Otolaryngol.* 1975; 4:637.

144. Olofsson J, Williams GT, Rider WD, et al. Anterior commissure carcinoma. Primary treatment with radiotherapy in 57 patients. *Arch Otolaryngol.* 1972; 95:230.

145. Krespi YP, Meltzer CJ. Laser surgery for vocal cord carcinoma involving the anterior commissure. *Ann Otol Rhinol Laryngol.* 1989; 98:105.

146. Yeager VL, Archer CR. Anatomical routes for cancer invasion of laryngeal cartilages. *Laryngoscope.* 1982; 92:449.

147. Kirchner JA, Cornog JL, Holmes RE. Transglottic cancer. *Arch Otolaryngol.* 1974; 99:247.

148. Langer R, Brem H, Falterman K, et al. Isolation of a cartilage factor that inhibits tumor neovascularization. *Science.* 1976; 201:70.

149. Gregor RT. Framework invasion in laryngeal carcinoma. In: Silver CE, ed. *Laryngeal Cancer.* New York: Thieme Medical Publishers; 1991.

150. Sinard RJ, Netterville JL, Garrett CG, et al. Cancer of the larynx. In: Myers EN, Suen JY, eds. *Cancer of the Head and Neck.* 3rd ed. Philadelphia: WB Saunders; 1996:381.

151. Bridger GP, Nassar VH. Carcinoma in situ involving the laryngeal mucus glands. *Arch Otolaryngol.* 1971; 94:389.

152. Ali S, Tiwari RM, Snow GB. False-positive and false-negative neck nodes. *Head Neck Surg.* 1985; 8:78.

153. Candela FC, Shah J, Jaques DP, et al. Patterns of cervical node metastases from squamous carcinoma of the larynx. *Arch Otolaryngol Head Neck Surg.* 1990; 116:432.

154. Grandi C, Alloiso M, Moglia D, et al. Prognostic significance of lymphatic spread in head and neck carcinomas: Therapeutic implications. *Head Neck Surg.* 1985; 8:67.

155. Yuen A, Medina JE, Goepfert H, et al. Management of stages T3 and T4 glottic carcinomas. *Am J Surg.* 1984; 148:467.

156. Friedman M, Mafee MF, Pacella BL Jr, et al. Rationale for elective neck dissection in 1990. *Laryngoscope.* 1990; 100:65.

157. Snyderman NL, Johnson JT, Schramm VL Jr, et al. Extracapsular spread of carcinoma in cervical lymph nodes: Impact upon survival in patients with carcinoma of the supraglottic larynx. *Cancer.* 1985; 56:1597.

158. Lutz CK, Johnson JT, Wagner RL, et al. Supraglottic carcinoma: Patterns of recurrence. *Ann Otol Rhinol Laryngol.* 1990; 99:12.

159. Levendag P, Sessions R, Vikram B, et al. The problem of neck relapse in early stage supraglottic larynx cancer. *Cancer.* 1989; 63:345.

160. Lindberg RD. Sites of first failure in head and neck cancer. *Cancer Treat Symp.* 1983; 2:21.

161. Werner JA, Schunke M, Rudert H, et al. Description and clinical importance of the lymphatics of the vocal fold. *Otolaryngol Head Neck Surg.* 1990; 102:13.

162. Leroux-Robert J. A statistical study of 620 laryngeal carcinomas of the glottic region personally operated upon more than five years ago. *Laryngoscope.* 1975; 85:1440.

163. Hawkins NV. The treatment of glottic carinoma: An analysis of 800 cases. *Laryngoscope.* 1975; 85:1485.

164. Kowalski, LP, Franco EL, Sobrinho JA. Factors influencing regional lymph node metastasis from laryngeal carcinoma. *Ann Otol Rhinol Laryngol.* 1995; 104:442.

165. Fleischer I. Morphologische untersuchungen an sublottischen kehikopfcarcinomen. Dis., Marburg 1977.

166. Lederman M. Radiotherapy of cancer of the larynx. *J Laryngol Otol.* 1970; 84:867.

167. Pietrantoni L, Agazzi C, Fior R. Indications for surgical treatment of cervical lymph nodes in cancer of the larynx and hypopharynx. *Laryngoscope.* 1962; 72:1511.

168. Harris HH, Butler E. Surgical limits in cancer of the subglottic area. *Arch Otolaryngol.* 1968; 87:64.

169. Kleinsasser O. Special morphology. In: *Tumors of the Larynx and Hypopharynx.* New York: Thieme Medical Publishers; 1988.

170. Crissman JD. Laryngeal keratosis preceding laryngeal carcinoma: A report of four cases. *Arch Otolaryngol Head Neck Surg.* 1982; 108:445.

171. McGavran MH, Bauer WC, Ogura JH. Isolated laryngeal keratosis. Its relation to carcinoma of the larynx based on a

clinicopathologic study of 87 consecutive cases with long-term follow-up. *Laryngoscope.* 1960; 70:932.

172. Broders AC. Carcinoma in situ contrasted with benign penetrating epithelium. *JAMA.* 1932; 99:1670.

173. Barnes L, Gnepp D. Diseases of the larynx, hypopharynx, and esophagus. In: Barnes L, ed. *Surgical Pathology of the Head and Neck.* New York: Marcel Dekker; 1985:141.

174. Hellquist H, Lundgren J, Olofsson J. Hyperplasia keratosis, dysplasia and carcinoma in situ of the vocal cords—A follow-up study. *Clin Otolaryngol.* 1982; 7:11.

175. Crissman JG, Gnepp DR, Goodman ML, et al. Preinvasive lesions of the upper aerodigestive tract: Histologic definitions and clinical complications (a symposium). *Pathol Annu.* 1987; 22:311.

176. Kleinsasser O. Die Klassifikation und differentialdiagnose der epistelhyperpllasien der kelkopfschleimhaut auf grund histomorphologischar merkmale. *Z Laryngol Rhinol Otol Ihre Grenzgeb.* 1963; 42:339.

177. Bauer WC, McGavran MH. Carcinoma in situ and evaluation of epithelial changes in laryngopharyngeal biopsies. *JAMA.* 1972; 221:72.

178. Fisher HR. The delineation of carcinoma in situ of the larynx. In: Alberti PW, Bryce DP, eds. *Centennial Conference on Laryngeal Cancer.* New York: Appleton-Century-Crofts; 1974; 116.

179. Ferlito A, Polidoro F, Rossi M. Pathological basis and clinical aspects of treatment policy in carcinoma-in-situ of the larynx. *J Laryngol Otol.* 1981; 95:141.

180. Miller AH, Fisher HR. Clues to the life history of carcinoma in situ of the larynx. *Trans Am Laryngol Rhinol Otol Soc.* 1971; 1475.

181. Miller AH, Batsakis JG. Premalignant laryngeal lesions, carcinoma in situ, superficial carcinoma—definition and management. *Can J Otolaryngol.* 1974; 3:573.

182. Kleinsasser O. Ubr den krankheitsverlauf bci epithelhyperlasein der kehlkopfschleimhaut und die entstehung von karzinomen. *Laryngol Rhinol Otol (Stuttg).* 1963; 42:541.

183. Stenersen TC, Hoel PS, Boysen M. Carcinoma in situ of the larynx: An evaluation of its natural clinical course. *Clin Otolaryngol.* 1991; 16:358.

184. Hintz BL, Kagan AR, Nussbaum H, et al. A "watchful waiting" policy for in situ carcinoma of the vocal cords. *Arch Otolaryngol.* 1981; 107:746.

185. Auerbach O, Hammond EC, Garfinkel L. Histologic changes in larynx in relation to smoking habits. *Cancer.* 1970; 25:92.

186. Mendenhall WM, Parsons JT, Stringer SP, et al. Management of Tis, T1, and T2 squamous cell carcinoma of the glottic larynx. *Am J Otolaryngol.* 1994; 15:250.

187. Small W Jr, Mittal BB, Brand WN, et al. Role of radiation therapy in the management of carcinoma in situ of the larynx. *Laryngoscope.* 1993; 103:663.

188. Rothfield RE, Myers EN, Johnson JT. Carcinoma in situ and microinvasive squamous cell carcinoma of the vocal cords. *Ann Otol Rhinol Laryngol.* 1991; 100:793.

189. Myssiorek D, Vambutas A, Abramson AL. Carcinoma in situ of the glottic larynx. *Laryngoscope.* 1994; 104:463.

190. Fein DA, Mendenhall WM, Parsons JT, et al. Carcinoma in situ of the larynx: The role of radiotherapy. *Int J Radiat Oncol Biol Phys.* 1993; 27:379.

191. Stenersen TC, Hoel PS, Boysen M. Carcinoma in situ of the larynx. Results with different methods of treatment. *Acta Otolaryngol (Stockh).* 1988; 449(suppl):131.

192. Doyle PJ, Flores A, Douglas GS. Carcinoma in situ of the larynx. *Laryngoscope.* 1977; 87:310.

193. Elman AJ, Goodman M, Wang CC, et al. In situ carcinoma of the vocal cords. *Cancer.* 1979; 43:2422.

194. Maran AGD, Mackenzie IJ, Stanley RE. Carcinoma in situ of the larynx. *Head Neck Surg.* 1984; 7:28.

195. Crissman JD, Zarbo RJ, Drozdowicz S, et al. Carcinoma in situ and microinvasive squamous carcinoma of the laryngeal glottis. *Arch Otolaryngol Head Neck Surg.* 1988; 114:299.

196. Murty GE, Diver JP, Bradley PJ. Carcinoma in situ of the glottis: Radiotherapy or excision biopsy? *Ann Otol Rhinol Laryngol.* 1993; 102:592.

197. DeSanto L. Early supraglottic cancer. *Ann Otol Rhinol Laryngol.* 1990; 99:593.

198. Suarez C, Rodrigo JP, Herranz J, et al. Supraglottic laryngectomy with or without postoperative radiotherapy in supraglottic carcinomas. *Ann Otol Rhinol Laryngol.* 1995; 104:358.

199. Schuller DE, McGuirt WF, Krause CJ, et al. Increased survival with surgery alone vs. combined therapy. *Laryngoscope.* 1979; 89:582.

200. Tabb HG, Druck NS, Thornton RS, et al. Supraglottic laryngectomy. *South Med J.* 1978; 71:114.

201. Ogura JH, Marks JE, Freeman RB. Results of conservation surgery for cancers of the supraglottis and pyriform sinus. *Laryngoscope.* 1980; 90:591.

202. DeSanto LW. Cancer of the supraglottic larynx: A review of 260 patients. *Otolaryngol Head Neck Surg.* 1985; 93:705.

203. Soo KC, Shah JP, Gopinath KS, et al. Analysis of prognostic variables and results after supraglottic partial laryngectomy. *Am J Surg.* 1988; 156:301.

204. Fletcher GH, Jesse RH, Lindber RD, et al. The place of radiotherapy in the management of squamous cell carcinoma of the supraglottic larynx. *AJR.* 1970; 108:19.

205. Harwood AR, Beale FA, Cummings BJ, et al. Supraglottic laryngeal carcinoma: An analysis of dose-time-volume factors in 410 patients. *Int J Radiat Oncol Biol Phys.* 1983; 9:311.

206. Harwood AR, Beale FA, Cummings BJ, et al. Management of early supraglottic laryngeal carcinoma by irradiation with surgery in reserve. *Arch Otolaryngol.* 1983; 109:583.

207. Spaulding CA, Krochak RJ, Hahn SS, et al. Radiotherapeutic management of cancer of the supraglottis. *Cancer.* 1986; 57: 1292.

208. Weems DH, Mendenhall WM, Parsons JT, et al. Squamous cell carcinoma of the supraglottic larynx treated with surgery and/or radiation therapy. *Int J Radiat Oncol Biol Phys.* 1987; 13:1483.

209. Robson NL, Oswal VH, Flood LM. Radiation therapy of laryngeal cancer: A twenty year experience. *J Laryngol Otol.* 1990; 104:699.

210. Mendenhall WM, Parsons JT, Cassisi NJ, et al. Radiation therapy in the management of early laryngeal and pyriform sinus cancer. In: Silver CE, ed. *Laryngeal Cancer.* New York: Thieme Medical Publishers; 1991:1347.

211. Fried MP, Girdhar-Gopal HV. Advanced cancer of the larynx. In: Bailey BJ, Johnson JT, Kohut RI, Pillsbury HC, Tardy ME, eds. *Head and Neck Surgery—Otolaryngology.* Philadelphia: JB Lippincott; 1993.

212. McCombe AW, Jones AS. Radiotherapy and complications of laryngectomy. *J Laryngol Otol* 1993; 107:130.

213. Natvig K, Boysen M, Tausjo J. Fistulae following laryngectomy in patients treated with irradiation. *J Laryngol Otol.* 1993; 107:1136.

214. Keene M, Harwood AR, Bryce DP, et al. Histopathological study of radionecrosis in laryngeal carcinoma. *Laryngoscope.* 1982; 92:173.

215. Slevin NJ, Vasanthan S, Dougal M. Relative clinical influence of tumor dose versus dose per fraction on the occurrence of late normal tissue morbidity following radiotherapy. *Int J Radiat Oncol Biol Phys.* 1993; 25:23.

216. Viani L, Stell PM, Dalby JE. Recurrence after radiotherapy for glottic carcinoma. *Cancer.* 1991; 67:577.

217. Seydel HG. The risk of tumor induction in man following medical irradiation for malignant neoplasm. *Cancer.* 1975; 35: 1641.

218. Parker RG, Enstrom JE. Second primary cancers of the head and neck following treatment of initial primary head and neck cancers. *Int J Radiat Oncol Biol Phys.* 1988; 14:561.

219. Robbins KT, Davidson W, Peters LJ, et al. Conservation surgery for T2 and T3 carcinoma of the supraglottic larynx. *Arch Otolaryngol Head Neck Surg.* 1988; 114:421.

220. Herranz-Gonzales J, Gavilan J, Martinez-Vidal J, et al. Supraglottic laryngectomy: Functional and oncologic results. *Ann Otol Rhinol Laryngol.* 1996; 105:18.

221. Ogura JH. Selection of patients for conservation surgery of the larynx and pharynx. *Trans Am Acad Ophthalmol Otolaryngol.* 1972; 76:741.

222. Amdur RJ, Parsons JT, Mendenhall WM, et al. Postoperative irradiation for squamous cell carcinoma of the head and neck: An analysis of treatment results and complications. *Int J Radiat Oncol Biol Phys.* 1989; 16:25.

223. Mantravadi RVP, Haas RE, Liebner EJ. Postoperative radiotherapy for persistent tumor at the surgical margin in head and neck cancers. *Laryngoscope.* 1983; 93:1337.

224. Beckhart RN, Murray JG, Ford CN, et al. Factors influencing functional outcome in supraglottic laryngectomy. *Head Neck.* 1994; 16:232.

225. DeSanto LW, Vaughan CW. Early carcinoma of the larynx. In: Silver CE, ed. *Laryngeal Cancer.* New York: Thieme Medical Publishing; 1991.

226. De Santo LW. Supraglottic laryngectomy. In: Bailey BJ, Johnson JT, Kohut RI, Pillsbury HC, Tardy ME, eds. *Head and Neck Surgery—Otolaryngology.* Philadelphia: JB Lippincott; 1993:1334.

227. Shaw HJ. Surgical salvage for squamous cancer involving the supraglottic larynx. *J Laryngol Otol.* 1988; 102:704.

228. Wenig BL, Bussell GS, Portugal LG. The role of salvage supraglottic laryngectomy following radiation therapy. Presented at the American Laryngological Society; April 24, 1999; Palm Desert, CA.

229. Zeitels SM, Koufman JA, Davis RK, et al. Endoscopic treatment of supraglottic and hypopharynx cancer. *Laryngoscope.* 1994; 104:71.

230. Eckel HE, Thumfart WF. Laser surgery for the treatment of larynx carcinomas: Indications, techniques, and preliminary results. *Ann Otol Rhinol Laryngol.* 1992; 101:113.

231. Davis RK, Shapshay SM, Strong MS, et al. Transoral partial supraglottic resection using the CO_2 laser. *Laryngoscope.* 1983; 93:429.

232. Zeitels SM, Vaughan CW, Domanowski GF. Endoscopic management of early supraglottic cancer. *Ann Otol Rhinol Laryngol.* 1990; 99:951.

233. Davis RK, Kelly SM, Hayes J. Endoscopic CO_2 laser excisional biopsy of early supraglottic cancer. *Laryngoscope.* 1991; 101:680.

234. Shah JP, Tollefesen HR. Epidermoid carcinoma of the supraglottic larynx: Role of neck dissection in initial surgical treatment. *Am J Surg.* 1974; 128:494.

235. Shah JP. Cervical lymph node metastases—Diagnostic, therapeutic, and prognostic implications. *Oncology.* 1990; 4:61.

236. Reid AP, Robin PE, Powell J, et al. Staging carcinoma: Its value in cancer of the larynx. *J Laryngol Otol.* 1991; 105: 456.

237. Hansen HS. Supraglottic carcinoma of the aryepiglottic fold. *Laryngoscope.* 1975; 85:1667.

238. Sirrala U, Paavolainen M. The problem of advanced supraglottic carcinoma. *Laryngoscope.* 1975; 85:1633.

239. Vikram B, Strong EW, Shah JP, et al. Failure at the primary site following multimodality treatment in advanced head and neck cancer. *Head Neck Surg.* 1984; 6:720.

240. Mendenhall WM, Parsons JT, Stringer SP, et al. Carcinoma of the supraglottic larynx: A basis for comparing the results of radiotherapy and surgery. *Head Neck.* 1990; 12:204.

241. Harwood AR, Rawlinson E. The quality of life of patients following treatment for laryngeal cancer. *Int J Radiat Oncol Biol Phys.* 1983; 9:335.

242. Lee NK, Goepfert H, Wendt CD. Supraglottic laryngectomy for intermediate-stage cancer. UTMD Anderson Cancer Center experience with combined therapy. *Laryngoscope.* 1990; 100:831.

243. Myers EN, Alvi A. Management of carcinoma of the supraglottic larynx: Evolution, current concepts, and future trends. *Laryngoscope.* 1996; 106:559.

244. Gavilan C, Gavilan J. Five-year results of functional neck dissection for cancer of the larynx. *Arch Otolaryngol Head Neck Surg.* 1989; 115:1193.

245. Burstein FD, Calcaterra TC. Supraglottic laryngectomy: Series report and analysis of results. *Laryngoscope.* 1985; 95:833.

246. Suarez C, Llorente JL, Nunez F, et al. Neck dissection with or without radiotherapy in supraglottic carcinomas. *Otolaryngol Head Neck Surg.* 1993; 109:3–9.

247. Weber PC, Johnson JT, Myers EN. Impact of bilateral neck dissection on recovery following supraglottic laryngectomy. *Arch Otolaryngol Head Neck Surg.* 1993; 119:61.

248. Ramadan HH, Allen GC. The influence of elective neck dissection on neck relapse in NO supraglottic carcinoma. *Am J Otolaryngol.* 1993; 14:278.

249. Rydell R, Schalen L, Fex S, et al: Voice evaluation before and after laser excision vs. radiotherapy of T1A glottic carcinoma. *Acta Otolaryngol (Stockh).* 1995; 115:560.

250. Hirano M, Hirade Y, Kawaski H. Vocal function following carbon dioxide laser surgery for glottic carcinoma. *Ann Otol Rhinol Laryngol.* 1985; 94:232.

251. Epstein BE, Lee D, Kashima H, et al. Stage T1 glottic carcinoma: Results of radiation therapy or laser excision. *Radiology.* 1990; 175:567.

252. Cragle SP, Brandenburg JH. Laser cordectomy or radiotherapy: Cure rates, communication, and cost. *Otolaryngol Head Neck Surg.* 1993; 108:648.

253. Harwood AR. Cancer of the larynx—the Toronto experience. *J Otolaryngol.* 1982; 11(suppl):1.

254. Mendenhall WM, Parsons JT, Stringer SP, et al. T1-T2 vocal cord carcinoma: A basis for comparing the results of radiotherapy and surgery. *Head Neck Surg.* 1988; 10:373.

255. Wang CC. Treatment of squamous cell carcinoma of the larynx by radiation. *Radiol Clin North Am.* 1978; 16:209.

256. Howell-Burke D, Peters LJ, Goepfert H, et al. T2 glottic cancer. *Arch Otolaryngol Head Neck Surg.* 1990; 116:830.

257. Kelly MD, Spaulding CA, Constable WC, et al. Definitive radiotherapy in the management of stage I and II carcinomas of the glottis. *Ann Otol Rhinol Laryngol.* 1989; 98:235.

258. Shimm DS. Early-stage glottic carcinomas: Effect of tumor location and full-length involvement on local recurrence after radiation therapy. *Radiology.* 1994; 192:873.

259. Small W Jr, Mittal BB, Brand WN, et al. Results of radiation therapy in early glottic carcinoma: Multivariate analysis of prognostic and radiation therapy variables. *Radiology.* 1992; 183:789.

260. Pellitteri PK, Kennedy TL, Vrabec DP, et al: Radiotherapy. The mainstay in the treatment of early glottic carcinoma. *Arch Otolaryngol Head Neck Surg.* 1991; 117:297.

261. Fein DA, Mendenhall WM, Parsons JT, et al. T1-T2 squamous cell carcinoma of the glottic larynx treated with radiotherapy: A multivariate analysis of variables potentially influencing local control. *Int J Radiat Oncol Biol Phys.* 1993; 25: 605.

262. Outzen KE, Illum P. CO_2-laser therapy for carcinoma of the larynx. *J Laryngol Otol.* 1995; 109:111.

263. Kooper DP, Van Den Broek P, Manni JJ, et al. Partial vertical laryngectomy for recurrent glottic carcinoma. *Clin Otolaryngol.* 1995; 20:167.

264. Chacko DC, Hendrickson F, Fisher A. Definitive irradiation of T1–T4 NO larynx cancer. *Cancer.* 1983; 51:994.

265. Dickens WJ, Cassisi NJ, Million RR, et al. Treatment of early vocal cord carcinoma: A comparison of apples and apples. *Laryngoscope.* 1983; 93:216.

266. Harwood AR, Deboer G. Prognostic factors in T2 glottic cancer. *Cancer.* 1980; 45:991.

267. Kirchner JA. Cancer at the anterior commissure of the larynx. Results with radiotherapy. *Arch Otolaryngol.* 1970; 91: 524.

268. Som ML, Silver CE. The anterior commissure technique of partial laryngectomy. *Arch Otolaryngol.* 1968; 87:138.

269. Jesse RH, Lindberg RD, Horiot JC. Vocal cord cancer with anterior commissure extension. Choice of treatment. *Am J Surg.* 1971; 122:437.

270. Strong MS, Jako GJ. Laser surgery in the larynx. Early clinical experience with continuous CO_2 laser. *Ann Otol Rhinol Laryngol.* 1972; 81:791.

271. Mahieu HF, Patel P, Annyas AA, et al. Carbon dioxide laser vaporization in early glottic carcinoma. *Arch Otolaryngol Head Neck Surg.* 1994; 120:383.

272. Silver CE. Technical aspects of conservation surgery. In: Sil-

ver CE, ed. *Laryngeal Cancer*. New York: Thieme Medical Publishers; 1991:960.

273. Bailey BJ. Glottic reconstruction after hemilaryngectomy: Bipedicle muscle flap laryngoplasty. *Laryngoscope*. 1975; 85:960.

274. Neel HB III, Devine KD, De Santo LW. Laryngofissure and cordectomy for early cordal carcinoma: Outcome in 182 patients. *Otolaryngol Head Neck Surg*. 1980; 88:79.

275. Norris CM. Role and limitations of vertical hemilaryngectomy. *Can J Otolaryngol*. 1975; 4:426.

276. Mohr RM, Quenelle DJ, Shumrick DA. Vertico-frontolateral laryngectomy (hemilaryngectomy). Indications, technique, and results. *Arch Otolaryngol*. 1983; 109:384.

277. Norris CM. Technique of extended fronto-lateral partial laryngectomy. *Laryngoscope*. 1958; 68:1240.

278. Stegnjajic A, Wenig BL, Guberina L, et al. Glottic reconstruction with investing cervical fascia following vertical partial laryngectomy. *Arch Otolaryngol Head Neck Surg*. 1985; 111: 472.

279. Wenig BL, Stegnjajic A, Abramson AL. Glottic reconstruction following conservation laryngeal surgery. *Laryngoscope*. 1989; 99:983.

280. Biller HF, Lawson W. Partial laryngectomy for vocal cord cancer with marked limitation or fixation of the vocal cord. *Laryngoscope*. 1986; 96:61.

281. Biller H, Som M. Vertical partial laryngectomy for glottic carcinoma with posterior subglottic extension. *Ann Otol Rhinol Laryngol*. 1977; 86:715.

282. Mohr RM. Vertical partial laryngectomy. In: Silver CE, ed. *Laryngeal Cancer*. New York: Thieme Medical Publishers; 1991.

283. Bauer WC, Lesinski SG, Ogura JH. The significance of positive margins in hemilaryngectomy specimens. *Laryngoscope*. 1975; 85:1.

284. Wenig BL, Berry BW Jr. Management of patients with positive surgical margins after vertical hemilaryngectomy. *Arch Otolaryngol Head Neck Surg*. 1995; 121:172.

285. Wang CC. Treatment of glottic carcinoma by megavoltage radiation therapy and results. *AJR*. 1974; 130:157.

286. Arriagada R, Eschwege F, Cachin Y, et al. The value of combining radiotherapy with surgery in the treatment of hypopharyngeal and laryngeal cancers. *Cancer*. 1983; 51:1819.

287. Karim BMF, Kralendonk JH, Njo KH, et al. Radiation therapy for advanced (T3-T4NO-N3M0) laryngeal carcinoma. The need for a change of strategy: A radiotherapeutic viewpoint. *Int J Radiat Oncol Biol Phys*. 1987; 13:1625.

288. Mendenhall WM, Parsons JT, Stringer SP, et al. Stage T3 squamous cell carcinoma of the glottic larynx: A comparison of laryngectomy and irradiation. *Int J Radiat Oncol Biol Phys*. 1992; 23:725.

289. Woodhouse RJ, Quivey JM, Fu KK, et al. Treatment of carcinoma of the vocal cord. A review of 20 years experience. *Laryngoscope*. 1981; 91:1155.

290. Harwood AR, Beale FA, Cummings BJ, et al. T3 glottic cancer: An analysis of dose time-volume factors. *Int J Radiat Oncol Biol Phys*. 1980; 6:675.

291. Terhaard CH, Wiggenraad RG, Hordijk GJ, et al. Regression after 50 Gy as a selection for therapy in advanced laryngeal cancer. *Int J Radiat Oncol Biol Phys*. 1988; 15(3):591.

292. Meredith AP, Randall CJ, Shaw HJ. Advanced laryngeal cancer: A management perspective. *J Laryngol Otol*. 1987; 101: 1046.

293. Terhaard CH, Karim AB, Hoogenraad WJ, et al. Local control in T3 laryngeal cancer treated with radical radiotherapy, time dose relationship. *Int J Radiat Oncol Biol Phys*. 1991; 20: 1207.

294. Harwood AR, Beale FA, Cummings BJ, et al. T4N0M0 glottic cancer—an analysis of dose-time volume factors. *Int J Radiat Oncol Biol Phys*. 1981; 7:1507.

295. Pearson BW. Management of the primary site: Larynx and hypopharynx. In: Pillsbury HC III, Goldsmith MM III, eds. *Operative Challenges in Otolaryngology and Head and Neck Surgery*. Chicago: Medical Yearbook; 1990:346.

296. Laccourreye H, Brasnu D, Lacau ST, et al. New concepts in

297. Donald PJ, Pearson BW. The larynx. In: Donald PJ, ed. *Head and Neck Cancer–Management of the Difficult Case*. Philadelphia: WB Saunders; 1984.

298. Pearson BW, Keith RL. Near-total laryngectomy. In: Johnson JJ, Biltzer A, Ossoff RH, Thomas JR, eds. *American Academy of Otolaryngology—Head and Neck Surgery, Instructional Courses*. vol 2. St. Louis: Mosby; 1989:309.

299. Chandrachud HR, Chaurasia MK, Sinha KP. Subtotal laryngectomy with myomucosal shunt. *J Laryngol Otol*. 1989; 103: 504.

300. Laccourreye H, Laccourreye O, Weinstein G, et al. Supracricoid laryngectomy with cricohypoidopexy: A partial laryngeal procedure for selected supraglottic and transglottic carcinomas. *Laryngoscope*. 1990; 100:735.

301. Laccourreye O, Ross J, Brasnu D, et al. Extended supracricoid partial laryngectomy with tracheocricohyoidoepiglottopexy. *Acta Otolaryngol (Stockh)*. 1994; 114J:669.

302. Laccourreye O, Weinstein G, Naudo P, et al. Supracricoid partial laryngectomy after failed laryngeal radiation therapy. *Laryngoscope*. 1996; 106:495.

303. Biller HF, Barnhill FR, Ogura JH, et al. Hemilaryngectomy following radiation failure for carcinoma of the vocal cords. *Laryngoscope*. 1970; 80:249.

304. Nichols RD, Mickelson S. Partial laryngectomy after irradiation failure. *Ann Otol Rhinol Laryngol*. 1991; 100:176.

305. Sorensen H, Hansen HS, Thomsen KA. Partial laryngectomy following irradiation. *Laryngoscope*. 1980; 90:1344.

306. Shaw HJ. Role of partial laryngectomy after irradiation in the treatment of laryngeal cancer: A view from the United Kingdom. *Ann Otol Rhinol Laryngol*. 1991; 100:268.

307. Burns H, Bryce DP, van Nostrand AWP. Conservation surgery in laryngeal cancer and its role following failed radiotherapy. *Arch Otolaryngol*. 1979; 105:234.

308. Eillis PDM. Conservation laryngectomy after radiotherapy. *J Laryngol Otol*. 1977; 91:209.

309. Myers EN, Ogura JH. Completion laryngectomy. *Ann Otol Rhinol Laryngol*. 1979; 88:172.

310. Whicker JH, Neel BH, Weiland LH, et al. Adenocarcinoma of the larynx. *Ann Otol Rhinol Laryngol*. 1974; 83:487.

311. Spiro RH, Lewis JS, Hajdu SI, et al. Mucus gland of the larynx and laryngopharynx. *Ann Otol Rhinol Laryngol*. 1976; 85:498.

312. Flanagan P, Cross RMP, Locke JH. Fibrosarcoma of the larynx. *J Laryngol Otol*. 1965; 79:1049.

313. Moore ES, Martin H. Melanoma of the upper respiratory tract and oral cavity. *Cancer*. 1955; 8:1167.

314. Swerdlow RS, Som ML, Biller HF. Cartilaginous tumors of the larynx. *Arch Otolaryngol*. 1974; 10:269.

315. Adlington P, Woodhouse MA. The ultrastructure of chemodectoma of the larynx. *J Laryngol Otol*. 1972; 86:1219.

316. Van Norstrand WP, Olofsson J. Verrucous carcinoma of the larynx. *Cancer*. 1972; 30:691.

317. DeSanto LW. T3 glottic cancer: Options and consequences of the options. *Laryngscope*. 1984; 94:1311.

318. Razack MS, Maipang T, Sako K, et al. Management of advanced glottic carcinomas. *Am J Surg*. 1989; 158:318.

319. Johnson JT, Myers EN, Hao SP, et al. Outcome of open surgical therapy for glottic carcinoma. *Ann Otol Rhinol Laryngol*. 1993; 102:752.

320. Byers RM. The use of postoperative irradiation—its goals and 1978 attainments. *Laryngoscope*. 1979; 89:567.

321. Chung CT, Sagerman RH, King GA, et al. Complications of high dose preoperative irradiation for advanced laryngeal-hypopharyngeal cancer. *Radiology*. 1978; 128:467.

322. Goepfert HH, Zaren HA, Jesse RH, et al. Treatment of laryngeal carcinoma with conservative surgery and postoperative radiation therapy. *Arch Otolaryngol*. 1978; 104:576.

323. Vikram B, Strong EW, Shah JP, et al. Failure in the neck following multimodality treatment for advanced head and neck cancer. *Head Neck Surg*. 1984; 6:724.

324. Byhardt RW, Cox JD. Patterns of failure and results of pre-

operative irradiation vs radiation therapy alone in carcinoma of the pyriform sinus. *Int J Radiat Oncol Biol Phys.* 1980; 6: 1135.

325. Goepfert HH, Jesse RH, Fletcher GH, et al. Optimal treatment for the technically resectable squamous cell carcinoma of the supraglottic larynx. *Laryngoscope.* 1975; 85:14.

326. Po Wing Yuen A, Wei WI, Hon Wai Wong S. Critical appraisal of watchful waiting policy in the management of N0 neck of advanced laryngeal carcinoma. *Arch Otolaryngol Head Neck Surg.* 1996; 122:752.

327. Ogura JH, Biller HF, Wette R. Elective neck dissection for pharyngeal and laryngeal cancers: An evaluation. *Ann Otol Rhinol Laryngol.* 1971; 80:646.

328. Leemans CF, Tiwari R, Nauta JJP, et al. Regional lymph node involvement and its significance in the development of distant metastasis in head and neck carcinoma. *Cancer.* 1993; 71:452.

329. Hao S, Myers EN, Johnson JT. T3 glottic carcinoma revisited: Transglottic vs pure glottic carcinoma. *Arch Otolaryngol Head Neck Surg.* 1995; 121:166.

330. Mendenhall WM, Parsons JT, Brant TA, et al. Is elective neck treatment indicated for T2N0 squamous cell carcinoma of the glottic larynx? *Radiother Oncol.* 1989; 14:199.

331. Shaha AR, Shah JP. Carcinoma of the subglottic larynx. *Am J Surg.* 1982; 144:456.

332. Stell PM, Tobin KE. The behavior of cancer affecting the subglottic space. *Can J Otolaryngol.* 1975; 4:612.

333. Vermund H. Role of radiotherapy in cancer of the larynx as related to the TNM system of staging: A review. *Cancer.* 1970; 25:485.

334. Warde P, Harwood A, Keane T. Carcinoma of the subglottis: Results of initial radical radiation. *Arch Otolaryngol Head Neck Surg.* 1987; 113:1228.

335. Guedea F, Parsons JF, Mendenhall WM, et al. Primary subglottic cancer: Results of radical radiation therapy. *Int J Radiat Oncol Biol Phys.* 1991; 21:1607.

336. Wolf G, Lippman SM, Laramore G, et al. Head and neck cancer. In: Holland JF, Frei E, Bast RC Jr, Dufe DW, Morton DL, Weichselbaum R, eds. *Cancer Medicine.* 3rd ed. Philadelphia: Lea and Febiger; 1992.

337. Hong WK, Bromer R. Chemotherapy in head and neck cancer. *N Engl J Med.* 1983; 308:75.

338. Vokes EE, Weichselbaum RR, Lippman SM, et al. Head and neck cancer. *N Engl J Med.* 1993; 328:184.

339. Head and Neck Contract Program. Adjuvant chemotherapy for advanced head and neck squamous carcinoma. *Cancer.* 1987; 60:301.

340. Holoye PY, Grossman TW, Toohill RJ, et al. Randomized study of adjuvant chemotherapy for head and neck cancer. *Otolaryngol Head Neck Surg.* 1985; 93:712.

341. Schuller DE, Metch B, Stein DW, et al. Preoperative chemotherapy in advanced resectable head and neck cancer—final report of the Southwest Oncology Group. *Laryngoscope.* 1988; 98:1205.

342. Taylor SG, Applebaum E, Showell JL, et al. A randomized trial of adjuvant chemotherapy in head and neck cancer. *J Clin Oncol.* 1985; 3:672.

343. Hong WK, Choksi A, Dimery IW. Sequential induction chemotherapy and radiotherapy for advanced head and neck cancer: Potential impact of treatment in advanced laryngeal and nasopharyngeal carcinomas. In: Fee WE Jr, ed. *Head and Neck Cancer.* Vol. 2. Philadelphia: BL Decker; 1990.

344. Choksi AJ, Dimery IW, Hong WK. Adjuvant chemotherapy of head and neck cancer: The past, the present, and the future. *Semin Oncol.* 1988; 15:45.

345. Karp D, Vaughan C, Carter R, et al. Larynx preservation using induction chemotheray plus radiation therapy as an alternative to laryngectomy in advanced head and neck cancer: A long-term follow-up. *Am J Clin Oncol.* 1991; 14:273.

346. The Department of Veterans Affairs Laryngeal Study Group. Induction chemotherapy plus radiation in patients with advanced laryngeal cancer. *N Engl J Med.* 1991; 324:1685.

347. Shirinian M, Zatopek N, Lippman SM, et al. Adjuvant therapy in head and neck cancer. In: Jones SE, Salmon SE, eds. *Adjuvant Therapy of Cancer VI.* New York: Grune and Stratton; 1990.

348. Laramore GE, Scott CB, Al-Sarraf M, et al. Adjuvant chemotherapy for resectable squamous cell carcinoma of the head and neck: Report on intergroup study 0034. *Int J Radiat Oncol Biol Phys.* 1992; 23:705.

349. Kazem I, van den Brock P. Planned preoperative radiation therapy vs. definitive radiotherapy for advanced laryngeal carcinoma. *Laryngoscope.* 1984; 94:1355.

350. Harwood AR, ENT Group. The management of advanced supraglottic carcinoma by delayed combined therapy. *Int J Radiat Oncol Biol Phys.* 1982; 8(suppl 1):101. Abstract.

351. Croll GA, Gerrisen GJ, Tiwari RM, et al. Primary radiotherapy with surgery in reserve for advanced laryngeal carcinoma: Results and complications. *Eur J Surg Oncol.* 1989; 15: 350.

352. De Andres L, Brunet J, Lopez-Pousa A, et al. Function preservation in stage III squamous laryngeal carcinoma: Results with an induction chemotherapy protocol. *Laryngoscope.* 1995; 105:822.

353. Shirinian MH, Weber RS, Lippman SM, et al. Laryngeal preservation by induction chemotherapy plus radiotherapy in locally advanced head and neck cancer: The M.D. Anderson Cancer Center experience. *Head Neck.* 1994; 16:39.

354. Pfister DG, Strong E, Harrison L, et al. Larynx preservation with combined chemotherapy and radiation therapy in advanced but resectable head and neck cancer. *J Clin Oncol.* 1991; 9:850.

355. Vokes EE, Kies M, Haraf DJ, et al. Induction chemotherapy followed by concomitant chemoradiotherapy for advanced head and neck cancer: Impact on the natural history of the disease. *J Clin Oncol.* 1995; 13:876.

356. Kies MS, Haraf DJ, Athanasiadis I, et al. Induction chemotherapy followed by concurrent chemoradiation for advanced head and neck cancer: Improved disease control and survival. *J Clin Oncol.* 1998; 16:2715.

357. Hosal N, Onerci M, Turan E. Peristomal recurrence. *Am J Otolaryngol.* 1993; 14:206.

358. Zbaren P, Greiner R, Kenglebacher M. Stoma recurrence after laryngectomy: An analysis of risk factors. *Otolaryngol Head Neck Surg.* 1996; 114:569.

359. Keim WF, Shaprio MJ, Rosin HD. Study of postlaryngectomy stomal recurrence. *Arch Otolaryngol.* 1965; 81:183.

360. Stell PM, Van Den Broek P. Stomal recurrence after laryngectomy: Aetiology and management. *J Laryngol Otol.* 1971; 850:131.

361. Kuehn PG, Teunant R. Surgical treatment of stomal recurrences in cancer of the larynx. *Am J Surg.* 1971; 122:445.

362. Bonneau RA, Lehmann RH. Stomal recurrence following laryngectomy. *Arch Otolaryngol.* 1975; 101:408.

363. Modlin B, Ogura JH. Post-laryngectomy tracheal stomal recurrences. *Laryngoscope.* 1969; 79:239.

364. Sisson GA, Strachley CJ Jr, Johnson NE. Mediastinal dissection for recurrent cancer after laryngectomy. *Laryngoscope.* 1962; 72:1064.

365. Sisson GA, Edison BP, Bytell DE. Transsternal neck dissection. *Arch Otolaryngol.* 1979; 101:46.

366. Norris CM. Causes of failure in surgical treatment of malignant tumors of the larynx. *Ann Otol Rhinol Laryngol.* 1959; 68: 487.

367. Rubin J, Johnson JT, Myers EN. Stomal recurrence ater laryngectomy: Interrelated risk factor study. *Otolaryngol Head Neck Surg.* 1990; 103:805.

368. Olofsson J. Specific features of laryngeal carcinoma involving the anterior commissure and the subglottic region. *Can J Otolaryngol.* 1975; 4:618.

369. Weber RS, Marvel J, Smith P, et al. Paratracheal lymph node dissection for carcinoma of the larynx, hypopharynx, and cervical esophagus. *Otolaryngol Head Neck.* 1993; 108:11.

370. Alagaratnam TT, Oug GB. Wound implantation—a surgical hazard. *Br J Surg.* 1977; 64:872.

371. Robbins KT, Woodson GE. Chest wall metastasis as a complication of myocutaneous flap reconstruction. *J Otolaryngol.* 1984; 13:13.

372. Carr RJ, Gilbert PM. Tumor implantation to a temporalis muscle flap donor site. *Br J Oral Maxillofac Surg.* 1989; 24:295.

373. Biguardi L, Vavioli L, Staffieri A. Tracheostomal recurrences after laryngectomy. *Arch Otorhinolaryngol.* 1983; 238:107.

374. Barr GD, Robertson AG. Stomal recurrence: A separate entity? *J Surg Oncol.* 1990; 44:176.

375. Rockley TJ, Powell J, Robin PE, et al. Post-laryngectomy stomal recurrence: Tumor implantation or paratracheal lymphatic metastasis? *Clin Otolaryngol.* 1991; 16:43.

376. Baluyot ST, Shumrick DA, Everts EC. Emergency laryngectomy. *Arch Otolaryngol.* 1971; 94:414.

377. Davis RK, Shapshay SM. Peristomal recurrence: Pathophysiology, prevention, treatment. *Otolaryngol. Clin North Am.* 1980; 13:499.

378. Hoover WB, King BD. Emergency laryngectomy. *Arch Otolaryngol.* 1954; 59:431.

379. Mantravadi R, Katz AM, Skolaik EM, et al. Stomal recurrence. A critical analysis of risk factors. *Arch Otolaryngol.* 1981; 107:735.

380. Coancon HA. Post-laryngectomy stomal recurrence: The influence of endotracheal anesthesia. *Br J Anaesth.* 1969; 41:531.

381. DeJong PC. Intubation and tumor implantation in laryngeal carcinoma. *Practica Otorhinolaryngol.* 1969; 31:119.

382. Schneider JJ, Lindberg RD, Jesse RH. Prevention of tracheal stomal recurrence after total laryngectomy by postoperative irradiation. *J Surg Oncol.* 1975; 7(3):187.

383. Hermanek P, Scheibe O, Spiessl B, et al. *TNM Classification of Malignant Tumors.* 4th ed. Berlin: Springer; 1987.

384. Sisson GA, Bytell DE, Edison BD, et al. Transsternal radical neck dissection for control of stomal recurrences—end results. *Laryngoscope.* 1975; 85:1504.

385. Gluckman JL, Hamaker RC, Weissler MC, et al. Surgical salvage for stomal recurrence: A multi-institutional experience. *Laryngoscope.* 1987; 97:1025.

386. Josephson JS, Krespi YP. Management of stomal recurrence. In: Silver CE, ed. *Laryngeal Cancer.* New York: Thieme Medical Publishing; 1991.

III. PATHOLOGY OF THE LARYNX, HYPOPHARYNX, AND TRACHEA

■ LESTER D. R. THOMPSON

GROSS AND FROZEN SECTION PROCEDURES FOR LARYNGEAL SPECIMENS

If a biopsy specimen is obtained from the larynx, the specimen should be fixed by washing the biopsy forceps with formaldehyde or formalin. In the alternative, the specimen may be sent fresh for frozen section or microbiologic cultures, wrapped in saline-infused gauze. A description should be given of the number, color, and size of the fragments of the biopsy, which should be completely embedded. The mucosal surface needs to be sectioned on edge. If the sample of tissue is greater than 4 mm in diameter, the specimen should be bisected. When the tissue is smaller than 4 mm, multiple serial cuts should be requested at the time of the initial sectioning to avoid loss of diagnostic material in subsequent recut requests. If needed, alternate levels may be stained with hematoxylin and eosin (H&E), with the unstained (or charged) slides held for additional studies as required.[1,2]

The specimen for frozen section should be chosen by the surgeon and pathologist to represent the diagnostic issue at hand. A variety of commercial preparations are available for preparing and cutting the specimens, and no one specific technique or product is better than another. Perpendicular sections to the surface epithelium are mandatory, especially when ascertaining margins of resection. A permanent record of the frozen section request and diagnosis should be maintained in the patient's record and in the pathology suite (electronically, as allowed by governing bodies). Although diagnoses may be deferred, there is a high degree of accuracy with frozen section techniques.[1,3-6] There are four areas in which errors can be committed: (1) inadequate sampling (by surgeon or pathologist); (2) incorrect interpretation; (3) inaccurate communication; and (4) technical difficulties. The most problematic area of histopathologic interpretation of frozen section samples involves epithelial lesions, especially epithelial hyperplasia, pseudoepitheliomatous hyperplasia, radiation changes, and squamous cell carcinoma (verrucous and spindle cell types). Insufficient sampling is a common problem with mesenchymal and inflammatory lesions, as the diagnostic material rests in the submucosal deep tissues of the larynx. Each of these topics is covered in greater detail in subsequent sections; however, it is probably advisable to err on the side of benignancy and to delay definitive therapy rather than perform radical surgery for a benign disease.

There are only a selected number of instances in which a biopsy of the larynx requires a frozen section diagnosis, as when:

1. Special procedures are required based on the diagnosis of the lesion, such as ultrastructural examination, cultures, immunophenotypic analysis, or flow cytometry (specimen adequacy).
2. A different definitive therapy would be instituted based upon the diagnosis.
3. Numerous previous attempts at diagnosis have been unsuccessful.
4. An assessment of adequate surgical margins of resection must be made.

When assessing margins of resection, specimens should be obtained (after appropriate inking and orientation) to include the closest margin, as well as other mucosal margins (proximal, distal, medial, and lateral, as indicated). Margins should be examined routinely on all head and neck carcinoma resections. A frozen section biopsy should never be performed just for academic curiosity, gamesmanship, financial gain, or rote examination, and should be discouraged when the tissue is heavily calcified, when the specimen is very small, and when the lesions to be studied are thought to be unique, requiring a number of additional studies (e.g., in the case of infectious agents, lymphomas, or neuroendocrine tumors).[1,3,4,7-10]

Resections

A *hemilaryngectomy* specimen includes the true and false vocal cords and the underlying soft tissue and cartilage. The procedure is generally performed for a localized glottic carcinoma. It is imperative to determine whether the tumor involves the anterior and posterior commissures, as well as the other mucosal and soft-tissue margins. This may be made easier with the use of India ink at the resection margins. The connective tissue at the anterior commissure and the conus elasticus are two barriers to cancer spread that need to be examined histologically to ascertain the extent of disease. After measuring the specimen (which should include a measurement of the tumor), the gross abnormalities are described before fixing the specimen in formalin for at least 2 to 4 hours. The gross description should include the tumor's exact location, size, extent, and depth of invasion, as well as the appearance of the uninvolved mucosa. The cartilage should be separated from the soft tissue of the vocal cord. Sections should be taken vertically, at 2- to 3-mm intervals, and sequentially from anterior to posterior (Fig. 8–36A). These slices are placed separately in labeled cassettes, in the same order as sectioned, to allow the best localization and determination of tumor extent. If a neck dissection has been performed, the lymph nodes should be retrieved from the upper, middle, and lower thirds of the specimen unless individual lymph nodes are submitted separately. It is important to state whether the specimen is from the right or left side.[2,10-13]

A *total laryngectomy* specimen is handled in a slightly different fashion. The larynx should be separated from the radical neck dissection sample (if present). It is important to preserve soft-tissue relationships if the tumor extends into the soft tissue from the larynx. If the thyroid gland is included, it is dissected away from the larynx and "breadloafed" at 3-mm intervals, with any abnormal areas being embedded. Alternatively, if there are no abnormalities, a section from each lobe may be submitted for testing. Parathyroid glands should be sought along the posterior surface of the thyroid and these, too, should be embedded.

The larynx should be opened posteriorly down the midline. A description of the tumor, including its color, growth pattern (endophytic, exophytic), and location (mucosal or submucosal), should be given, and the presence or absence of surface ulceration, tumor necrosis, hemorrhage, or degeneration should be noted. It should be determined whether there is involvement of the true or false vocal cords; whether the lesion is supraglottic, transglottic, or subglottic; and whether it is unilateral or extends across the midline. Distances from the tumor to the tracheal margin and the anterior mucosal margin (base of tongue, epiglottic fold, and aryepiglottic fold) should also be documented. The mucosal mar-

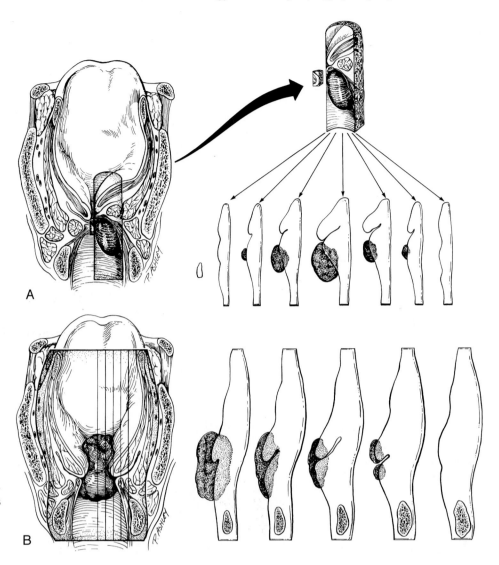

FIGURE 8–36 *A*, Hemilaryngectomy, including the type of sections to embed; *B*, Total laryngectomy, including the type of sections to embed.

gins (tracheal, pharyngeal, and lingual) can be inked with a permanent ink, and photographs may be taken if desired. The specimen must be fixed for several hours or, preferably, ovenight to obtain the best sections when cutting through the tumor. If the specimen cannot be properly oriented, clarification from the surgeon is imperative prior to fixation. There is no remedy for a poorly oriented specimen that has already been dissected.

Although whole-organ serial saggital sectioning has been advocated as a method of submitting sections, especially in light of the ease of comparison with similar computed tomography (CT) slices, the long period required for fixation and/or decalcification and the special equipment required make the method cumbersome.[1,14,15] A slightly easier, and less equipment-intensive method has been suggested (Fig. 8–36*B*). After cutting vertically through the tumor, the size, shape, color, and consistency of the tumor are described, noting specifically the depth of tumor invasion and extension to or through the laryngeal cartilages. At least two to three vertical sec-

tions through the tumor, at the deepest point of invasion and in an area which will demonstrate the tumor's relationship to surrounding structures, should be submitted, with division into several blocks, as necessary. If there is only scar tissue remaining after radiotherapy, an adequate number of sections is obtained from the abnormal areas. If the carcinoma involves only one side of the larynx, a section from the anterior commissure (to document bilateral or unilateral involvement) and the middle of the other vocal cord should be submitted. These samples should be taken vertically and should include the soft tissue up to, but not including, the cartilage. If the cartilage or bone is involved, these sections are submitted separately for decalcification. If the tumor does not involve the bone or cartilage, no sections of these structures are necessary. If the tumor is nonlaryngeal, a section of both cords, as described earlier, should be embedded. A section of the epiglottis, including the anterior mucosal margin, should also be included.[2,3]

LARYNGEAL HISTOLOGY

The larynx is a mucosa-covered package of intricately related cartilages, ligaments, and muscle. There are seven cartilages, composed of either elastic or hyaline-type cartilage, including the epiglottis (elastic), thyroid, cricoid, arytenoid, corniculate (elastic), cuneiform (elastic), and triticeous (the latter four of which are arranged in matching pairs). Each of the cartilages has a unique appearance and physiologic function in the passage of air and in phonation. Each is connected to other structures in the larynx, to the joints of the organ, or to the fibrous framework that comprises the connective tissue. The larynx is divided into the supraglottic, glottic, and subglottic regions. The supraglottic region contains the epiglottis, false cords, ventricular cavities, aryepiglottic folds, and arytenoid cartilages. The glottis is the region at the level of the true vocal cords and anterior commissure. The subglottis is found below the vocal cords, extending to the lower edge of the cricoid cartilage where the trachea begins. The epiglottis and true vocal cord are covered by nonkeratinizing, stratified, squamous epithelium, whereas the supraglottis and subglottis are covered with a pseudostratified, ciliated, respiratory epithelium (Fig. 8–37A). A transitional-type epithelium is interposed between these two epithelial types, frequently causing diagnostic problems with dysplasia or laryngeal intraepithelial neoplasia (Fig. 8–37B). Mucoserous glands can be found in the lower epiglottis and in the ventricular stromal connective tissue. A rich vascular and lymphatic investment is seen in the stroma of the larynx, although the free surfaces of the cords are considered to be devoid of these structures.

The epithelium of the hypopharynx is a stratified squamous epithelium that is rich with mucoserous glands. By contrast, the tracheal epithelium is a pseudostratified, ciliated, respiratory epithelium.

NON-NEOPLASTIC LESIONS

Reactive Epithelial Changes

Gross Pathology

The gross appearance of reactive epithelial lesions ranges from ulcerated to flat to polypoid, smooth or nodular, papillary or verrucoid. These lesions may be white (leukoplakic) or, less often, red (erythroplakic) and may involve a small area or expand to cover the entire larynx (pachyderma laryngis).[17,19–21,23–25]

Microscopic Pathology

The histologic appearance is variable and frequently reflects a combination of findings. Histologic changes may include *hyperplasia* (a thickening of the epithelium by an absolute increase in cell number) (Fig. 8–38A); *metaplasia* (changing from a specialized epithelium, such as respiratory, to a simpler epithelium, such as stratified squamous epithelium); *keratosis* (an accumulation of keratinized cells or material); *parakeratosis* (incomplete keratinization with cells retaining their nuclei); *koilocytosis* (a crenated nucleus surrounded by a clear cytoplasm with a prominent, thick cell border); *oncocytosis* (abundant, eosinophilic cytoplasm); dyskeratosis; or a vague cytologic atypia characterized by varying degrees of each of these changes. These changes may be focal or may be found throughout the specimen. The degree or the quantity of the change may also influence the diagnosis, especially as the assemblage of characteristics becomes more prominent or cytologically atypical.[16–22,25,26]

Special Studies

Immunohistochemical reactions for the subtypes of keratins have been proposed as a means of distinguishing between reactive epithelial changes and

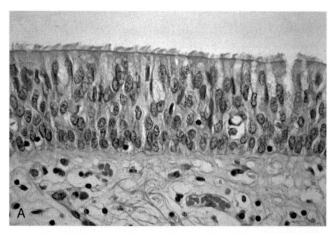
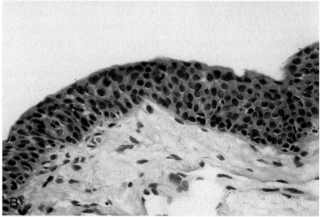

FIGURE 8–37   *A,* Pseudostratified, ciliated respiratory epithelium (H&E, × 300); *B,* Transitional or intermediate epithelium, often misdiagnosed as laryngeal intraepithelial neoplasia (H&E, × 300).

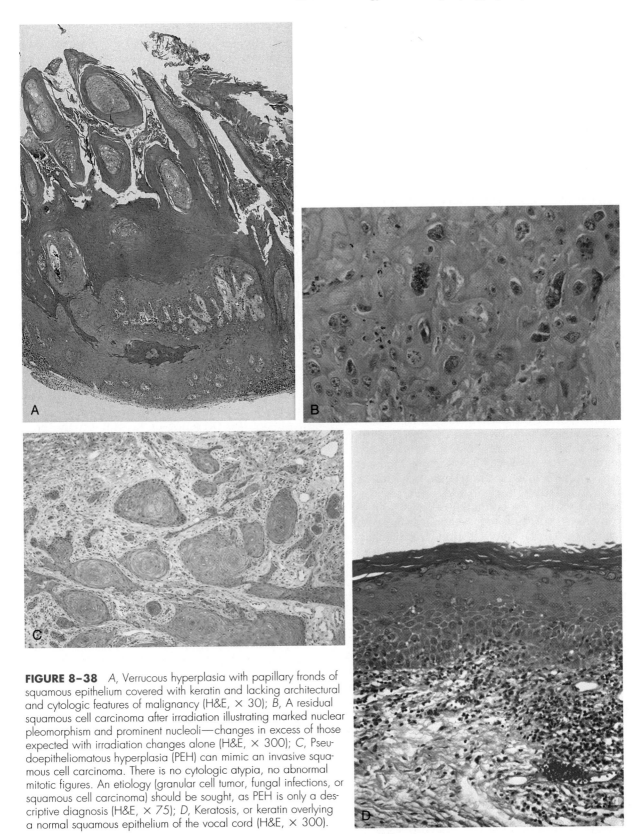

FIGURE 8-38 *A,* Verrucous hyperplasia with papillary fronds of squamous epithelium covered with keratin and lacking architectural and cytologic features of malignancy (H&E, × 30); *B,* A residual squamous cell carcinoma after irradiation illustrating marked nuclear pleomorphism and prominent nucleoli—changes in excess of those expected with irradiation changes alone (H&E, × 300); *C,* Pseudoepitheliomatous hyperplasia (PEH) can mimic an invasive squamous cell carcinoma. There is no cytologic atypia, no abnormal mitotic figures. An etiology (granular cell tumor, fungal infections, or squamous cell carcinoma) should be sought, as PEH is only a descriptive diagnosis (H&E, × 75); *D,* Keratosis, or keratin overlying a normal squamous epithelium of the vocal cord (H&E, × 300).

carcinoma. However, from a practical standpoint, these reactions are insufficiently reliable to be used in a clinical setting at this time.

Differential Diagnosis

The importance of reactive epithelial changes, especially in terms of the degree of change, rests on their association with squamous cell carcinoma, both verrucous and well differentiated. When keratosis is present, the underlying degree of nuclear atypicality seems to have a positive correlation with the later development of invasive carcinoma. A certain degree of judgment is often required to elucidate the true nature of the disease, often requiring expert consultation or multiple biopsies taken sequentially over a number of months. Although there is no proof of development of carcinoma in these laryngeal lesions, there is certainly a well-documented association with squamous cell carcinoma. The prescence of carcinoma may represent sampling at the time of biopsy, or may represent progression of the disease. In either case, careful monitoring of these patients is imperative, especially of those in high-risk groups.[16–20,23,25]

Reactive epithelial changes can also be associated with radiation-induced changes. Mucositis is the initial change, evidenced by inflammation of the mucosa and a lack of mucus-secreting cells, especially within the ciliated respiratory epithelium. Submucosal edema fluid is present, with hyalinization and disruption of the tissues. The reactive changes of nuclear enlargement—multinucleation within cells that have maintained nucleocytoplasmic ratio—can be identified within the epithelial cells, as well as in the stromal cells. Cytoplasmic vacuolization, cellular atrophy, and vascular proliferation are all changes attributable to radiation damage. The antecedent event is generally known; the difficulty lies in ruling out recurrent or residual disease (which can occur frequently) and distinguishing it from a benign reactive epithelial response, which frequently is associated with bacterial infection or cartilaginous degeneration. Careful examination for the features of malignancy will help to differentiate recurrent tumor from reactive changes (Fig. 8–38B).

Verruca vulgaris can occur in the larynx, although it is decidedly rare. When it does occur, there is marked acanthosis; papillomatosis; orthokeratosis; a prominent granular cell layer; irregular, coarsely aggregated, keratohyaline granules; koilocytes; and thin, penetrating rete pegs.[26] A contact ulcer, especially one of prolonged duration, will demonstrate re-epithelization of the denuded surface, resulting in epithelial hyperplasia. Upon biopsy examination, the underlying granulation-type tissue reaction, characterized by hemosiderin-laden macrophages, red blood cells, fibrin exudate, and inflammatory cells, will help to confirm the diagnosis.

Mucoserous or mucosal gland hyperplasia can be recognized by an increase in the absolute number of stromal glands and associated duct structures. An overall lobular architecture is maintained without a disordered growth pattern, and there is no evidence of infiltration, although fibrosis is noted when associated with inflammation.

A keratoma is a flat to warty or villous mass that can be seen along the anterior to middle third of the vocal cord; involvement of the entire length can occur. Keratoma includes an epithelial hyperlasia that produces verrucous or papillary growth with surface keratinization, but without loss of polarity and nuclear atypia.

Clinicopathologic Correlation

Hyperplasia is an absolute increase in the number of cell layers and is not considered to be a precancerous lesion. Pseudoepitheliomatous hyperplasia is a form of reactive hyperplasia of the squamous epithelium in which there may be an exuberant overgrowth displaying no cytologic evidence of malignancy. However, because this entity is characterized by an architectural growth pattern that is similar to that of invasive squamous cell carcinoma (Fig. 8–38C), it is often misdiagnosed. Squamous metaplasia of the respiratory epithelium can also occur, often as a result of trauma or in response to noxious stimuli. Keratosis, the presence of keratin on the epithelial surface, often presents in an exophytic or stalactitic pattern. The term has been used synonymously with hyperkeratosis (a redundant term since keratin is not a normal constituent of the epithelium of the larynx) (Fig. 8–38D), leukoplakia (a clinical term), and pachydermia (a diffuse layering of squames). Although any of these reactions can occur in the setting of injury or other provocation, they can also be seen in association with tumors, both benign and malignant. Their presence alone is just a morphologic diagnosis and may not indicate a specific pathologic condition. A certain degree of epithelial atypia can be seen in these conditions, but generally, the epithelial architecture is maintained in an orderly growth pattern with maturation toward the surface, no atypical mitotic figures, and without abnormal keratinization.[16–25]

Vocal Cord Polyps and Nodules

Gross Pathology

Vocal cord nodules and polyps are not clinically synonymous, but they frequently are interchangeable terms by pathologic standards. A nodule is a thickening on opposing surfaces of the vocal folds that is almost always bilateral and that typically involves the middle one third of the vocal cord. These lesions may be edematous, gelatinous, or hemorrhagic, firm or fixed, and usually measure a few millimeters in diameter.[27,28]

Polyps usually involve either Reinke's space or the ventricular space, appear on a single vocal cord (in more than 90% of the cases), and areas on the anterior to midpoint of the vocal cord. Polyps can range from sessile, raspberry-like to pedunculated, with a soft, rubbery, or firm consistency, and may range in color from translucent white to red (in the telangiectatic type). They may be as large as a few centimeters in maximum dimension, depending on their stage of development.[27–31]

Microscopic Pathology

During the early stages of nodule formation edema fluid collects, leading to a protein accumulation and the formation of a loose, myxoid matrix with early deposition of collagen fibers. An organizational process progresses with continued insult and the lesion becoming fibrotic with time. The surface epithelium may become keratotic and hyperplastic (Fig. 8–39A).

Vocal cord polyps are usually divided into four main histologic subtypes: edematous, vascular, hyaline, and fibrous. They frequently demonstrate a spectrum of changes within the same polyp in varying proportions, perhaps related to the progression of time or stages in the development of polyps. The edematous type also has a loose, myxoid, vascularized stroma admixed with a submucosal, pale blue to pink matrix material (Fig. 8–39B). Vascular polyps have many dilated vessels, infrequently demonstrating a more prominent central vessel, and they are often associated with hemorrhage. However, the complex arborization of the lymphatics in this region makes definitive determination of vascular type difficult.[32] Granulation tissue and/or dense, homogeneous, eosinophilic material may be present in association with fibrous organization and as a response to the hemorrhage. The hyaline type of polyp is characterized by a fibrin-like material that is closely juxtaposed to vascular spaces (Fig. 8–39C). The fibrous type of polyp shows spindle cells in a dense, fibrous stroma (Fig. 8–39D). The surface epithelium can be metaplastic, atrophic, keratotic, hyperplastic, or even malignant in rare instances (see Fig. 8–39A). A variable degree of inflammation may be evident, but it is generally scarce.[27,28,30,31]

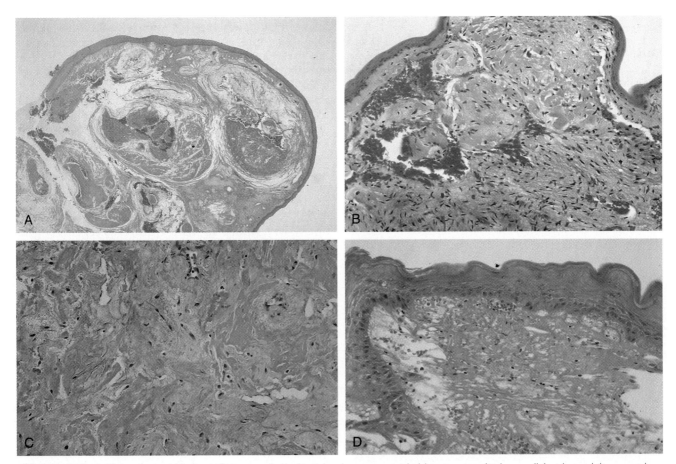

FIGURE 8–39 A, The surface epithelium of a myxoid vocal cord polyp is unremarkable, covering the hypocellular, basophilic myxoid stroma (H&E, × 7.5); B, A polypoid mass with dilated vessels and scant stroma can be seen in a vascular or edematous polyp (H&E, × 150); C, Degenerative changes can occur within polyps, such as the fibrinoid degeneration identified in this laryngeal polyp (H&E, × 150); D, A singer's vocal cord nodule shows a fibrous connective tissue deposition beneath an unremarkable epithelium. This diagnosis requires a clinical correlation (H&E, × 200).

Special Studies

Hyalin deposition may suggest the presence of amyloid, but special stains for amyloid (e.g., Congo red) yield negative results. Although seldom necessary for diagnostic purposes, fibrin deposits can be identified in vocal cord polyps by ultrastructural studies. The vessels demonstrate occasional gaps between the endothelial cells, which are incompletely surrounded by basement membrane material mixed with collagen fibers. Ultrastructural changes of the extracellular matrix proteins have also been reported.[33,57]

Differential Diagnosis

There is no evidence of amyloid deposition in these types of polyps. Myxoid vocal cord polyps are frequently misdiagnosed as laryngeal myxoma. Myxoma, however, is extraordinarily rare in the larynx, and will generally infiltrate the surrounding stroma with stellate cells with bland nuclei, a reticular fiber network, and mast cells within the viscid myxoid background material[22,34] (Fig. 8–40).

Contact Ulcer

Gross Pathology

Contact ulcer is usually an ulcerated, polypoid, or nodular mass involving the posterior vocal cord and arytenoid and, occasionally, the trachea. The lesion is beefy red to tan-white in appearance, measuring up to 3 cm in greatest dimension. A "kissing ulcer" may be present on the opposite side. Involvement of the cartilage may be seen on generous biopsy specimens.[35–40]

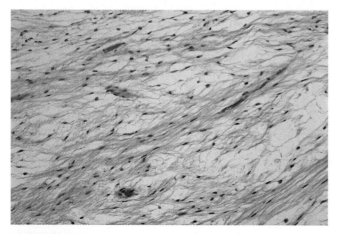

FIGURE 8–40. A myxoma is a rare lesion in the larynx, with scattered spindled to stellate cells, focal vascularity, and mast cells present. This lesion must be distinguished from a myxomatous polyp (H&E, × 150).

Microscopic Pathology

The ulcerated surface is covered by a layer of fibrin or fibrinoid necrosis. Exuberant granulation tissue is present below the fibrin layer (Fig. 8–41A). This marked vascular proliferation is characterized by plump endothelial cells within the vascular spaces and a haphazard architectural arrangement. There is a rich investment of inflammatory cells, including lymphocytes, plasma cells, neutrophils, and histiocytes (including giant cell forms) (Fig. 8–41B). A spindle cell proliferation often accompanies the granulation tissue reaction, frequently demonstrating atypical features. In the early stages, surface ulceration without granulation tissue may be identified. With the progression of time a chronic phase may develop, with an irregular hyperplastic epithelium arising as a result of the regenerative surface re-epithelization (Fig. 8–41C). Prominent fibrosis may also be present in the stroma with progression of the disease.[35,37,38,40,41]

Differential Diagnosis

The aggregate of histologic features is not specific for contact ulcer, but certainly should raise it as a diagnostic and etiologic possibility. Because some of the findings are nonspecific, the histologic differential diagnosis includes infectious processes (tuberculosis, fungal disease, bacterial infection, syphilis), inflammatory conditions (infections, Wegener's granulomatosis, Crohn's disease, and inflammatory pseudotumor), vascular lesions (bacillary angiomatosis, Kaposi's sarcoma, angiosarcoma, lobular capillary hemangioma, and epithelioid hemangioma), and neoplastic conditions. Infectious agents can be ruled out with special stains for specific organisms (Gomori methenamine silver [GMS], periodic acid–Schiff [PAS], Brown-Hopps [tissue gram stain], and Warthin-Starry stains) or with cultures. Wegener's granulomatosis also may be characterized by surface ulceration, but optimal biopsy samples will show ischemic or geographic-type necrosis combined with genuine vasculitis, mixed chronic inflammation, and scattered multinucleated giant cells. In addition, patients with active Wegener's granulomatosis generally have elevated serum titers of antineutrophil cytoplasmic antibodies (ANCA).

A diagnosis of squamous cell carcinoma—well-differentiated, verrucous, or spindle cell type—should be carefully excluded, but this lesion frequently demonstrates a distinctive infiltrative growth pattern and single cell immunoreactivity with keratin in the stroma.[35,36,39,40,42] A variety of vascular neoplasms should also be considered in the differential diagnosis. Lobular capillary hemangioma will have a similar granulation tissue-like appearance, although the lobular arrangement around a central vessel is generally absent in a contact ulcer.[43] Lobular capillary hemangioma (pyogenic granuloma) is also considered to be a benign neoplasm,

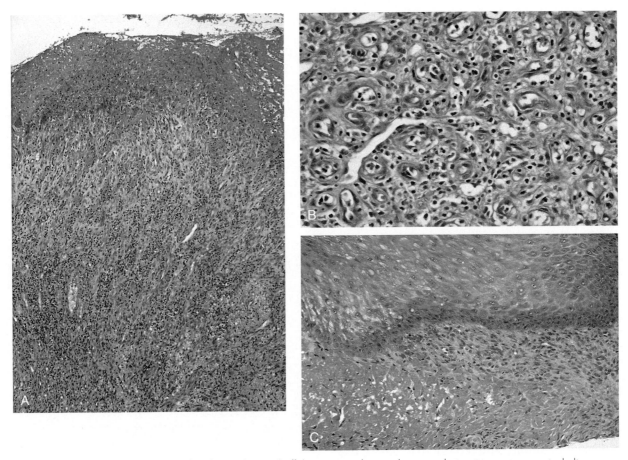

FIGURE 8–41. *A*, The surface epithelium has been ulcerated off this contact ulcer, with a granulation tissue response, including endothelial cell hyperplasia and mixed inflammation (H&E, × 75); *B*, The deeper portion of the contact ulcer contains a rich investment of vessels and inflammatory elements. These lesions can be confused with hemangiomas (H&E, × 300); *C*, The surface epithelium will eventually regenerate over the ulcerated area, but remnants of the fibrinoid necrosis are still present (H&E, × 150).

arising spontaneously and unassociated with an identifiable etiology. Thus treatment of an underlying cause of a contact ulcer may be overlooked if the incorrect diagnosis is rendered.[43] While not yet documented to occur in the larynx, bacillary angiomatosis may have plump epithelioid cells exhibiting nuclear atypia, neutrophils, and granular (bacterial) material.[44] Likewise, epithelioid hemangioma has not been described in the larynx.[45] Kaposi's sarcoma will invade the surrounding tissues, and the irregular and slit-like vascular spaces will be lined by spindled endothelial cells. The fascicular arrangement and spheroid hyaline globules of Kaposi's sarcoma are not seen in contact ulcer.[46] An atypical "hobnail" configuration, anastomosing vascular channels, invasive growth, and a lack of inflammatory elements will differentiate angiosarcoma from a contact ulcer.

Clinicopathologic Correlation

Specific causes for contact ulcer should be sought, including vocal abuse (shouting, persistent coughing or clearing of the throat, harsh or deep throaty voice); postintubational trauma (more common in female patients, who have a narrower glottis and a thinner mucoperichondrium, than in male patients), which may yield a hematoma and not a classic contact ulcer;[36,38–41,47] and gastric-laryngeal reflux, often associated with hiatal hernia. Gastric-laryngeal reflux or gastroesophageal reflux disease (GERD) is frequently missed, as the patient may be unaware of the underlying cause. A hiatal hernia, peptic esophagitis, or gastritis will cause acid reflux, usually during sleep, thereby causing a contact ulcer without the patient's knowledge. Pepsin, and not hydrochloric acid, is thought to be the injurious agent. In addition to the development of granulation tissue, stenosis of the trachea or larynx may result in contact ulcer formation.[39,48–50]

The ability to suggest a specific diagnosis with its causative factors is predicated on the correct morphologic interpretation. If the correct specific diagnosis of contact ulcer is made, appropriate therapy can be instituted early, decreasing the associated morbidity.

Necrotizing Sialometaplasia

Gross Pathology

Necrotizing sialometaplasia most commonly appears as an ulcerative, crater-like lesion, although it can also manifest as a submucosal nodular swelling. After sloughing, the nodule may form the deep crater-like ulceration, which generally does not exceed 3 cm in diameter. The lesion often appears over the tracheal rings first, resulting in a stratified squamous epithelium replacing a pseudostratified respiratory epithelium, although any location of the larynx or trachea can be involved.[35,51-54]

Microscopic Pathology

The marker for this disease is maintenance of the lobular architectural arrangement of the accessory salivary glands with necrosis of the mucoserous acinar cells. In an attempt at re-epithelization, squamous metaplasia of the residual glands and acini develops (Fig. 8–42A). In the immediate area, remnants of uninvolved acini and ducts can be seen, along with mucin-producing cells. Frequently, associated acute and chronic inflammation is evident, in addition to mucus extravasation related to the necrosis of the duct or acinar epithelium (see Fig. 8–42A). The lobules of the minor salivary gland ducts, which remain smooth in contour, are lined by a metaplastic squamous epithelium that has a bland appearance (Fig. 8–42B). However, as with any reparative or regenerative epithelium, enlarged nuclei, prominent nucleoli, apoptosis, and mitotic figures can be seen (see Fig. 8–42B, right). Frequently, the changes will extend along the ducts of the minor salivary glands to merge with the surface epithelium. Although common in other sites of necrotizing sialometaplasia, pseudoepitheliomatous hyperplasia is ordinarily not seen. However, the degree of hyperplasia in other sites has been so florid as to simulate squamous cell carcinoma.[35,51-56]

Special Studies

Mucicarmine or PAS with diastase may be helpful in identifying the contents of the necrotic acini and any residual mucocytes.

Differential Diagnosis

When there is a fair degree of nuclear atypia but no architectural disruption, the differential diagnosis should include a number of malignant epithelial tumors: squamous cell carcinoma, adenosquamous cell carcinoma, and mucoepidermoid carcinoma. Distinguishing between necrotizing sialometaplasia and carcinomas becomes increasingly difficult when the biopsy specimen is small and the bulk of it is composed of fibrous connective tissue and inflammatory elements, with only isolated epithelial islands. However, with deeper sections and/or a larger biopsy

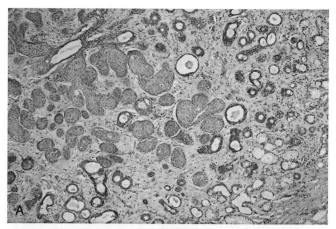

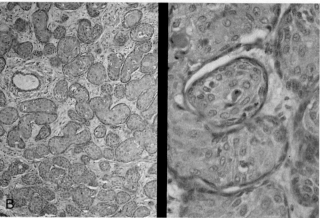

FIGURE 8–42. *A,* Necrotizing sialometaplasia is a lobular process, with areas of squamous metaplasia confined to the previous lobular architecture of a mucoserous gland. Uninvolved mucoserous glands can be identified at the periphery (H&E, × 75); *B,* The lobular architecture of necrotizing sialometaplasia (*left*) can demonstrate dyskeratosis and focal nuclear atypia (*right*). The distinction from squamous cell carcinoma requires an adequate biopsy size, careful clinical history, and recognition of the lobular architecture on low power (H&E, × 75 [*left*] and × 300 [*right*]).

sample, the true nature of the lesion will become apparent. The lobular architecture, smooth edges of the epithelial islands, and the uninvolved subtending salivary glands can help to differentiate between these diseases. One must hasten to add that necrotizing sialometaplasia is frequently associated with an underlying cause, and therefore, does not exclude the possibility of a squamous cell carcinoma (or other carcinoma) being present synchronously. The intermediate cells and mucocytes of the lower-grade mucoepidermoid carcinoma and the marked cytologic atypia of adenosquamous carcinoma may also help to identify these tumors. Often, the self-limiting nature of necrotizing sialometaplasia will help to define the true nature of the disease.[35,51-54]

Clinicopathologic Correlation

It is important to try to identify the etiologic agent of the necrotizing sialometaplasia, if possible, based on histologic preparations. For example, atheromatous emboli have been known to cause necrotizing sialometaplasia.[53] The finding of inclusion bodies on H&E–stained slides or immunohistochemical confirmation of herpes simplex virus may be helpful in establishing the cause of the disease, but usually, prolonged intubation is a factor.[57,58]

Amyloidosis

Gross Pathology

Isolated amyloidosis (without plasmacytoma) frequently occurs along the false vocal cord, although any portion of the larynx, hypopharynx, and trachea can be affected. When it involves the supraglottic or glottic region, the lesion most commonly presents as an elevated, smooth or bosselated, polypoid, mucosa-covered, firm mass. Subglottic amyloidosis presents as a more generalized, diffuse swelling. Multifocal deposits occur quite frequently. Surface ulceration has been identified in larger lesions. The mass is firm, with a waxy, translucent cut surface ranging in color from tan-yellow to red-grey.[35,59–69]

Microscopic Pathology

The histologic appearance of amyloid is identical whether it is isolated, secondary, associated with systemic disease, or part of a plasmacytoma. Histologic examination reveals an extracellular, acellular, eosinophilic matrix material dispersed randomly throughout the stroma or lamina propria, but sparing the overlying epithelium (Fig. 8–43A). The hyalin-like, homogeneous material may appear as flecks or large masses, and has a perivascular (or part of the vessel wall) and periglandular deposition, obliterating the seromucous glands through compression atrophy (Fig. 8–43B). An inflammatory infiltrate composed of mature lymphocytes, histiocytes, and occasional plasma cells is often identified. Depending upon the extent of the disease, a foreign-body giant cell reaction can also be seen (Fig. 8–43 A and C). Metaplastic bone has also been noted within the amyloid deposition.[35,59–64,66–68]

Special Techniques

When iodine and sulfuric acid are placed on the gross specimen, a blue reaction is most suggestive of amyloid. Staining with Congo red (apple-green birefringence under polarized light) (see Fig. 8–43C), crystal or methyl violet, or thioflavin-T stains can confirm the presence of amyloid, but will not help to rule out an associated lymphoproliferative disorder.

In order to diagnose amyloid tumor accurately and to exclude a plasmacytoma, careful immunohistochemical testing for immunoglobulin light chain restriction (whether performed by immunohistochemical reactions or molecular testing) and amyloid P com-

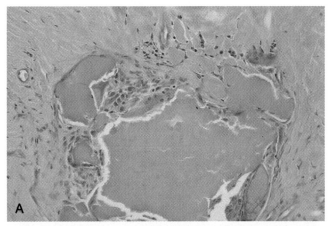

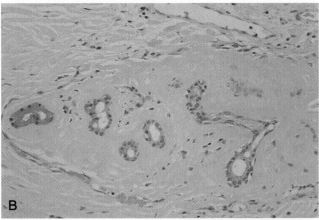

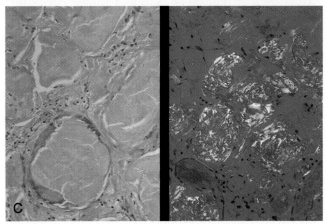

FIGURE 8–43. *A,* Fragments of amorphous, acellular, eosinophilic amyloid material is found in the stroma, with a foreign-body giant cell reaction (H&E, × 150); *B,* Periductal deposition with compression atrophy is characteristic for amyloid (H&E, × 150); *C,* The left of the split field demonstrates a fragment of amyloid, while the right demonstrates the "apple green" birefringence of amyloid when viewed under polarized light. The yellow splinter-like areas are collagen fibers (H&E, × 150).

ponent must be performed. P component is a glycoprotein present in most types of amyloid, and laryngeal amyloidosis is usually of the AL (light chain–derived) type, composed of κ or λ light chains. Protein sequencing suggests that laryngeal amyloid is of immunoglobulin origin. Amyloid tumor tests negative for amyloid A protein, prealbumin, and β_2-microglobulin.

Although electron microscopy can be utilized to document the characteristic presence of linear, non-branching fibrils of varying diameter in amyloid, it is seldom necessary to confirm the diagnosis. There are a number of different patterns of amyloid, identifiable both chemically and by electron microscopy, but this distinction is often unnecessary when the clinical presentation is taken into consideration.[35,60–62,65–68]

Differential Diagnosis

The most common amyloid lesion seen in the larynx is amyloid deposition alone, localized amyloid deposit, or amyloid tumor (without associated lymphoproliferative disorder). This lesion is generally unassociated with serum or urine electrophoretic abnormalities. However, careful studies must be performed to distinguish between tumor-forming amyloid, primary systemic amyloidosis (diagnosed by serum or urine immunoelectrophoresis or rectal biopsy), secondary amyloidosis (associated with some other predisposing disease), and plasmacytoma, whether it be solitary or part of multiple myeloma. Amyloid deposition in association with a plasmacytoma has a similar distribution, but does not have a predilection for the false cord and will be monoclonal.[22,35,60,63,66–68] However, amyloid tumor deposition as a mass has been shown to demonstrate monoclonal immunoglobulin A (IgA) proliferations that could possibly lead to amyloidosis, perhaps representing a solitary plasmacytoma arising in mucosa-associated lymphoid tissue.[63,70] Atypical carcinoid also may present with amyloid deposition. Ligneous conjunctivitis, a hereditary or familial disease, is characterized by pseudomembrane-covered, fibrous, woody, plaque-like deposits of accumulated acid mucopolysaccharides and hyaluronic acid surrounded by inflammatory cells and vessels. These deposits can be seen in the larynx or trachea, but test negative with amyloid stains, besides demonstrating a distinct clinical picture.[71] Lipoid proteinosis (hyalinosis cutis et mucosae) may have a similar clinical appearance to amyloidosis, but tends to have more widespread extracellular deposition of amorphous hyaline lipoproteins (both skin and mucous membranes), which are neutral and acid mucopolysaccharides that test negative with amyloid stains.[72] Hyalinized vocal cord nodules or polyps can also be included in the differential diagnosis, but these, too, test negative with amyloid stains.[66]

Clinicopathologic Correlation

A number of patients (up to 15%) with laryngeal amyloid may also manifest amyloid deposition in other head and neck sites. Clinical assessment is particularly important in such instances.

Subglottic Stenosis

Gross Pathology

Most cases of subglottic stenosis can be classified clinically as cartilaginous or soft-tissue stenosis ("hard" or "soft", respectively), although fibrosis of both categories can occur, depending upon maturity of the fibrous tissues. Abnormalities of the cricoid cartilage (absence, deformity, small for age), a trapped first tracheal ring, and fibrosis of the cartilage constitute the cartilaginous types, whereas granulation tissue, mucinous gland hyperplasia (usually on the posterior wall), and associated fibrosis constitute the soft-tissue types of stenosis. A large anterior or posterior lamina and generalized thickening resulting in circumferential narrowing, elliptical shape, or submucous cleft are the most frequent size and shape abnormalities affecting the cricoid cartilage. The cartilage may also be too small (hypoplastic) for the size of the larynx. Absence of the cricoid is also found in association with laryngotracheoesophageal cleft or atresia. It is uncommon to find only a single abnormality; instead, there are usually varying degrees of both "hard" and "soft" involvement in the same specimen.[35,73–80]

Microscopic Pathology

Although the histologic findings are nonspecific, careful documentation of the abnormalities of the gross specimen will allow appropriate clinical management. Histologic features include submucosal fibrosis with dense, eosinophilic collagen deposition intimately associated with fibroblasts. The fibroblasts are spindle-shaped and contain oval nuclei, inconspicuous nucleoli, and a variable amount of cytoplasm. The inflammatory infiltrate is variable, ranging from scant to heavy.[35,73,75,77–79]

Differential Diagnosis

Although there are a number of causes of subglottic stenosis, the differential diagnosis, based on histopathologic specimens, usually includes only a few entities, as clinicopathologic correlation is requisite. Infectious diseases, Wegener's granulomatosis, neurilemmoma, fibrous histiocytoma, and other nonspecific inflammatory conditions may be included in the histologic differential diagnosis, but each has specific, distinguishing clinical features. Among the congenital conditions (versus the acquired lesions), the symptom of stridor suggests a number of laryngeal abnormalities, including webs, stenosis, atresia, laryngomalacia, and idiopathic disease. Clinical examination of the larynx will help to distinguish between these entities. Membranous sheets occluding the lumen of the larynx can be seen in individuals with glottic webs, and no breath sounds will be appreciated at birth in cases of atresia or laryngeal dysgenesis.[77,80–86] Laryngomalacia (congenital laryngeal stridor) is a developmental anomaly associated with hypotonia or anatomic abnormalities, and may be the cause of stridor (with appropriate laryngoscopic findings) when other conditions have been excluded.[84,87,88] Other abnormalities of the epiglottis, aryepiglottic folds, and arytenoids can give a flaccid, tubular configuration to the supraglottic larynx. Biopsy study of such a lesion frequently contributes little to the clinical management, but may exclude other conditions.[89] Infections or inflammation must be excluded by appropriate cultures or histochemical staining, as these can complicate the picture, especially when superinfections produce nearly complete obstruction.[35,73,78,90] Acromegaly is also associated with deformity of the laryngeal cartilages, but is quite unique.[22]

Clinicopathologic Correlation

Subglottic stenosis involves the region extending from the insertion of the conus elasticus into the vocal cords to the inferior margin of the cricoid cartilage, not including the upper trachea. The histopathology of subglottic stenosis is the most definitive classification scheme, although etiology and clinical or anatomic appearance are important corroborating factors.

Teflonomas

Gross Pathology

Although paraffin, tantalum powder, silicone, and Gelfoam paste have been identified as laryngeal foreign substances in the past, Teflon (fluorocarbon, polytef) is the most frequently identified foreign substance in the larynx. The amount of Teflon paste used determines the size of the overall gross lesion. If too much has been used, the extruded material may create a larger nodule than normally encountered in the diffusely enlarged cord. The extravasated material yields a "teflonoma," or tumor-like accumulation of the Teflon. A teflonoma is a submucosal, polypoid, indurated mass, measuring 2 cm or less in diameter, and most often involving the subglottis.[35,91–96]

Microscopic Pathology

A foreign-body giant cell reaction or granulomatous response is most frequently identified in the arytenoid region, rather than in the mid–vocal cord itself, perhaps because of the volume of Teflon used or the vascular supply. The giant cell reaction is submucosal, with extension into the underlying muscle and cartilage (Fig. 8–44A). Depending on the exact chronologic point at which the biopsy specimen is obtained, the initial findings may include edema, inflammation, and a marked mononuclear histiocytic response. The irregular granules or

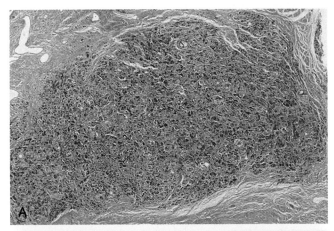

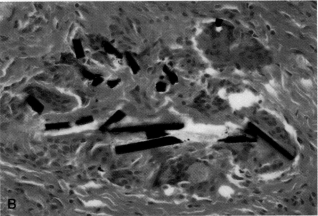

FIGURE 8–44. *A,* The particles of Teflon are aggregated in this circumscribed stromal nodule. Note the lack of significant inflammatory or foreign-body giant cell reaction (H&E, × 30); *B,* Carbon coating sometimes used on Teflon yields black rod-shaped particles, often identified within foreign-body giant cell macrophages (H&E, × 300); *C,* Polarization of the specimen will show the highly refractile particles of Teflon (H&E, polarized, × 150).

brownish fibers of Teflon appear as glassy crystals either within the giant cells or loose, within an extensive fibrous connective tissue. If carbon-coated, they will appear as black fibers (Fig. 8–44*B*). Long-standing lesions may only show a limited inflammatory reaction with dense, fibrous connective tissue "encapsulating" the lesion. Giant cells are only occasionally seen at this late stage of the disorder (see Fig. 8–44 A and B).

Special Studies

Teflon is birefringent under polarized light (Fig. 8–44C). Teflon particles may be positively identified by using infrared absorption spectrophotometry (IAS) after sodium hydroxide digestion or energy-dispersive x-ray analysis (EDXA).[96,97] There is a high content of C-F groups in Teflon (fluorocarbon derivation), which exhibits a pair of intense bands in the 8- to 9-μm region by IAS. Teflon can also be confirmed by EDXA, demonstrating a major peak for fluorine at 0.68 keV. Alternatively, numerous ovoid to spherical particles with a "flaky" appearance can be identified both intracellularly and extracellularly by scanning electron microscopy. It should be pointed out, however, that it is seldom necessary to go to this extent to document the nature of the polytef (Teflon), as there is usually a history of Teflon injection and the histologic appearance is characteristic.[35,96]

Differential Diagnosis

Silicone has been identified in the vocal cords, but usually occurs only in small quantities; moreover, soon after initial instillation (within a few months), it is resorbed by the body.[35,91,93,94,96,98] Silicone has a histologic response similar to that of Teflon, with an encapsulated mass of thin, fibrous connective tissue intersecting the clear, ghost-like spaces occupied by vulcanizing silicone, scattered foreign-body giant cells, and scant inflammatory cell infiltrate. The small amounts of silicone used in the larynx have not been associated with migration or systemic collagen vascular disorders.[95] Autogenous fat has also been used, but has not elicited a foreign-body response.[99]

Clinicopathologic Correlation

The proper technique and placement of the Teflon is the most important component of its beneficial result, to say nothing of appropriate patient selection for this type of therapy. Therefore, once the decision is made to use Teflon, critical attention must be paid to the exact location of injection and the amount injected at each session.

Foreign Bodies

Gross Pathology

The size and shape of foreign bodies are important in determining where they may lodge. Food is the most frequently identified foreign body in the larynx

and trachea, whereas coins are the foreign bodies most often found in the esophagus. Most of the food objects are irregular or pointed and small in size (usually nuts), characteristics that allow easier entry into the larynx compared to larger, rounded items. A very small "third" dimension may account for incomplete airway obstruction, thereby avoiding fatality. Objects such as balloons, however, conform to the larynx and can completely obstruct the airway. The age of the patient may also determine the type of object lodged in the upper airway, as nonfood items are more prevalent among individuals older than 5 years of age, whereas food items are more commonly ingested by those younger than 5 years. Prompt removal of the foreign body yields the best outcome, although fatalities have been reported, particularly by the Consumer Product Safety Commission.[100–103]

Microscopic Pathology

Microscopic analysis of the foreign body is generally not indicated, as its identity is usually apparent on gross examination. However, vegetable or plant material can be so identified if the material lodged in the larynx is a food substance. A laryngolith (calcified amorphous mass) or laryngeal stone may lodge in the larynx, but is extremely rare.[104] Further studies may be indicated if clinical, radiographic, or gross examination proves inconclusive.

Inflammatory Myofibroblastic Tumor (Inflammatory Pseudotumor or Plasma Cell Granuloma)

Gross Pathology

Inflammatory myofibroblastic tumors (IMT) can be polypoid, pedunculated, spherical, lobular, or nodular, with a smooth external appearance. They may be confined to the immediate submucosal region, and not truly invading. They are firm in consistency, fleshy, and gritty on cut surface, grey-yellow or tan-white, and may measure up to 3 cm in greatest dimension. These lesions are usually located on the true vocal cord, although the subglottis and trachea can be involved as well. The lesions may demonstrate a myxomatous appearance, but do not exhibit necrosis or hemorrhage.[105–116]

Microscopic Pathology

The characteristic finding in IMT, similar to that described in the lung and other locations, is an unencapsulated and nodular proliferation of spindle-shaped to stellate cells, arranged in a loosely organized growth pattern within a myxoid or fibrous background stroma (Fig. 8–45A). Some lesions may exhibit relatively compact growth, whereas others demonstrate dense, plate-like collagen deposition

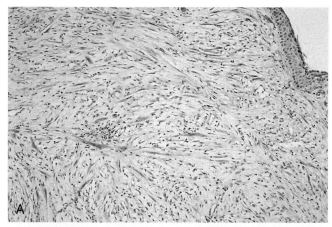

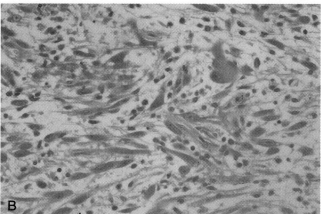

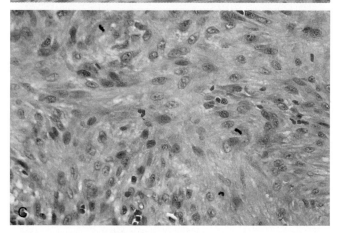

FIGURE 8–45. *A,* The surface epithelium is intact in this case of inflammatory myofibroblastic tumor (IMT). The myofibroblasts and inflammatory elements are easily identified in this specimen, with nuclear atypicality (H&E, × 100); *B,* A high-power view of IMT demonstrates the haphazard arrangement, the atypical spindle cell, and a mixed inflammatory response (H&E, × 300); *C,* The differential diagnosis occasionally includes nodular fasciitis, which may have a similar histologic appearance, but will contain no atypical cells, numerous mitotic figures (all normal), and extravasated erythrocytes (H&E, × 300).

and/or calcifications. The inflammatory infiltrate varies from sparse to abundant, and contains mature lymphocytes, histiocytes, plasma cells, neutrophils, and eosinophils. Russell bodies may be seen, but no

vascular compromise or thrombosis is evident. Cellularity is variable, with the myofibroblasts having round to oval nuclei with dense chromatin and an inapparent to prominent eosinophilic nucleolus, surrounded by adequate eosinophilic, fibrillar cytoplasm. These cells may be round to spindle-shaped, often creating long cytoplasmic extensions. A certain degree of nuclear atypicality, even remarkable atypia, may be seen, but generally, there is a normal nucleocytoplasmic ratio (Fig. 8–45 *A* and *B*). No cytoplasmic cross-striations or Z-bands are identified, nor is a "cambium" layer present in these proliferations. Anaplasia and necrosis are not usually seen. Mitotic figures may be identified and may be numerous, but atypical mitoses are not present. The proliferation is halted at the mucosal surface without invasion of the overlying surface mucosa or the surrounding mesenchymal tissues. The surface epithelium is generally unremarkable, although ulceration and reactive hyperplasia may be seen.[105–113,115–122] (see Fig. 8–45*A*).

Special Studies

Immunohistochemical studies show that myofibroblasts react with vimentin, muscle-specific actin, and smooth muscle actin, but have no immunoreactivity for S-100 protein. Cytokeratin reactivity may rarely be seen focally in the cytoplasm.

Ultrastructural analysis reveals lymphocytes, plasma cells, and histiocytes, in addition to spindle cells with irregular cellular outlines and cytoplasmic extensions, which are incompletely surrounded by fragmented basal lamina. Many of the cells have a blunt end. The nuclei are round, with deep indentations and nucleoli. Thin microfilaments, arranged parallel to the long axis, are seen beside intercalated dense bodies with rare junctional complexes.[106,107,111,113,114,119,120]

Differential Diagnosis

The chief differential diagnosis centers around spindle cell squamous carcinoma (SCSC), but inflammatory fibrosarcoma, nerve sheath tumors, nodular fasciitis, and nonspecific inflammation must also be excluded. SCSC will often demonstrate a surface component or an invasive squamous cell carcinoma in addition to the spindled component, in which case it is frequently mislabeled as pseudosarcoma. The atypical spindle cells in the underlying proliferation will demonstrate a degree of pleomorphism that is not seen in an inflammatory myofibroblastic tumor. Atypical mitotic figures may be identified in an SCSC, but they are generally not a feature of IMT. If needed, immunohistochemical evaluation with keratin and vimentin, along with the actins, should help to distinguish the two, although a number of SCSCs may only demonstrate focal keratin reactivity, or may not be reactive with keratin at all. A lack of nuclear pleomorphism without atypical mitotic figures distinguishes IMT from inflammatory fibrosarcoma, malignant peripheral nerve sheath tumor, leiomyosarcoma, and spindle cell rhabdomyosarcoma. These mesenchymal tumors are exceedingly rare in the larynx. However, when these mesenchymal tumors do exist as separate entities, they arise in the deep tissues of the larynx (rather than the submucosal region) and have malignant characteristics. A benign peripheral nerve sheath tumor (neurilemmoma) usually has whorled spindle cells, but palisading of the nuclei, along with a positive S-100 protein immunoreaction and neural features on electron microscopy, helps to distinguish it from inflammatory myofibroblastic tumor. Nodular fasciitis primarily affecting the larynx is exceedingly rare, even though it may have similar histologic features. Both lesions may have similar, widely separated, spindled cells, myxoid stroma, rich vascularity, and an occasional storiform pattern. However, nodular fasciitis usually has less inflammatory infiltrate, extravasated erythrocytes, more prominent collagen, and a greater number of mitotic figures (Fig. 8–45C). No single criterion is sufficient to distinguish these proliferations but, collectively, they may help to establish a diagnosis. Nonspecific inflammation may be the harbinger of an infectious agent, and cultures or special stains should be performed to exclude this possibility. Atypical cells in the stroma of a polyp or in a postirradiation reactive process can also be seen, but in such cases, the nucleocytoplasmic ratio is usually maintained and there is a corroborating clinical history of irradiation. Immunoreactivity will identify the myofibroblastic nature of these changes. If the plasma cells are predominant, they are polyclonal without κ or λ light chain restriction, underscoring the reactive nature of this lesion and also excluding an extramedullary plasmacytoma.[35,106–108,110,112,113,116,118,120,122–124] Non-neoplastic conditions, such as sarcoidosis, amyloidosis, Wegener's granulomatosis, relapsing polychondritis, syphilis (plasma cell–rich infiltrate), and malignant lymphoma usually do not have the atypical spindle cell component and can be excluded on the basis of clinical studies (cultures) and other histologic features.[111,118]

Although no specific etiologic agent has been identified for laryngeal IMT, Epstein-Barr virus (EBV) has been identified in similar lesions in other anatomic sites.[125] There seems to be a spectrum of growth from the "plasma cell granuloma" end of the spectrum to the IMT with phenotypic variability from one to the other. The lesions may present with a predominance of one of the histologic features, but generally, with adequate sampling, the spectrum of changes can be identified in most of the lesions.

Clinicopathologic Correlation

IMT may recur if incompletely excised, and in rare cases, metastasis has been reported. However, to date, no laryngeal lesions have metastasized or been identified as the direct cause of death in a patient.[107,113,121] Recent evidence has shown the presence of anaplastic lymphoma kinase (*ALK*) gene rearrangements in IMT. Oncogenic *ALK* expression may be an important mechanism in the pathogenesis of IMT and supports the concept that IMTs are neoplastic.[126,127]

Fibroma

Gross Pathology

Fibroma generally presents as a polyp or nodule, either sessile or pedunculated in attachment, soft or firm, and its size dependent on the duration of the lesion and intensity of the exposure to the irritating factors. Most of the lesions are covered by an intact epithelium, often exhibit keratosis, and measure up to 4 cm in maximum dimension. The cut surface is grey-white to pink. Many of these fibromas involve Reinke's space (the submucosal space of the vocal cord), arising from the anterior two thirds of the vocal cord, but a number have also been identified along the trachea.[22,128–130]

Microscopic Pathology

Initially, there is chronic edema, associated with inflammatory cells and variable vascularity. With time fibrous tissue develops, giving the lesion its name. Although neovascularization can be identified, the dominant histologic presentation is one of a fibrous connective stroma (Fig. 8–46). Inflammatory cells of all types can be identified in fibromas, and in cases of long duration, hyalinized collagen will be seen in the stroma. The overlying surface epithelium may be ulcerated or atrophic, or it may exhibit any of the other reactive epithelial changes described previously (see reactive epithelial changes). Special studies are generally neither helpful nor indicated.[128–130]

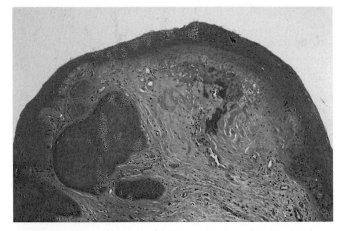

FIGURE 8–46. Fibroma or fibrous nodule, usually associated with smoking, displaying a dense fibrous connective tissue in a late stage of the process (H&E, × 75).

Differential Diagnosis

It is necessary to differentiate fibroma from fibromatosis, nodular fasciitis, fibrous histiocytoma, and nonspecific inflammatory or infectious disease. There is generally more of a clinically similar appearance than a histologic similarity for the inflammatory and infectious etiologies. Fibromatosis is a proliferative tumor, often associated with systemic disease, that appears grossly granular; contains slender, well-differentiated fibroblasts set in a prominent collagen matrix; and fibromatosis frequently encompasses muscle fibers. There is no associated inflammation, and these lesions are usually amitotic. The muscle fibers are usually atrophic. Nodular fasciitis is much more proliferative than fibroma and exhibits greater cellularity, mitotic activity, and extravasated erythrocytes. In fibrous histiocytoma, cells are arranged in a storiform growth pattern with plump cells, giant cells, and inflammatory elements. A number of infectious agents (specifically, tuberculosis) should be ruled out, especially ones of a long duration, as fibrous connective tissue may be all that remains of the granulomatous inflammation.[129–132]

Clinicopathologic Correlation

A fibroma probably represents a reactive change and is not a true neoplasm. With removal of the inciting condition, healing may occur after the mass has been surgically excised.

INFECTIOUS AND INFLAMMATORY DISEASES

Both infectious and inflammatory conditions can result in laryngitis, which is classified as acute or chronic. Often conditions occur more frequently in adults and others occur more frequently in children. Pharyngitis, laryngitis, "croup," epiglottitis, and laryngeotracheobronchitis, in either acute or chronic form, are all appellations applied to the various infections or inflammations of the larynx, trachea, and hypopharynx. Clearly, these terms have clinical implications based on anatomic location, but they can be caused by a variety of different etiologic agents.

The findings on histologic examination may be nonspecific, with edema and an inflammatory infiltrate being identified in cases of infectious disease, inflammatory disease, allergy, trauma, and environmental exposure to noxious substances, without a specific focal lesion. There may also be vocal cord compromise and ulceration. Therefore, close correlation with the clinical findings is imperative in order to clarify the disease process, as are serologic, cytologic, and microbiologic testing, and precipitant tests for fungi and other clinical studies (thyroid function tests, skin tests, etc.). Infections may be manifested in a variety of clinical diseases, depending upon the age of the patient, with a single organism causing bronchiolitis in an infant, croup in an older child, pharyngitis in another, and a subclinical syndrome in another individual.

Infectious Diseases

For purposes of classification, a brief discussion of viral, bacterial, fungal, and parasitic infections is presented, followed by an overview of inflammatory processes.

VIRAL

A full spectrum of viral infections can affect the larynx, trachea, and hypopharynx, including, but not limited to, Picornaviridae (rhinovirus and enterovirus); Paramyxoviridae, including parainfluenza viruses; mumps; measles (Morbillivirus); respiratory syncytial virus (RSV) (Pneumovirus); Orthomyxoviridae (influenza viruses); adenovirus; and Herpesviridae (cytomegalovirus [CMV], herpes simplex, varicella zoster, and EBV). With few exceptions, the histologic appearance is identical, as are the clinical manifestations, which are frequently dependent on the age, sex, nutritional, and immunity status of the individual. Extensive laboratory investigation to document the specific type of virus is probably not warranted except in extreme cases. The mucous membranes are erythematous and swollen on gross examination. The histologic findings include nonspecific inflammatory cells and edema fluid, occasionally coupled with specific inclusions (CMV, herpes simplex viruses, measles, RSV, etc.) (Fig. 8–47 A and B). Frequent secondary infections by bacterial agents can complicate the clinical and histologic appearance. Fibrinous laryngotracheobronchitis is believed to be caused by both a virus and secondary bacterial infection, with destruction of the ciliated epithelium.[133] Uremia can give rise to a similar histologic picture, but cultures will help identify the superinfecting bacteria so that additional, specific antibiotic therapy may be instituted. However, the appropriate clinical management of the patient prior to definitive laboratory results is imperative.[58,134–136]

Infectious mononucleosis is most often caused by EBV, although tissue confirmation of the diagnosis is generally not required. Marked swelling and erythema of the hypopharynx (or tonsils) are evident. Appropriate clinical laboratory findings are more helpful in confirming this diagnostic possibility than tissue biopsy and include an absolute lymphocytosis, prominent atypical lymphocytes (T lymphocytes) and a positive Monospot test. If necessary, EBV nuclear antigen antibodies or EBV capsid antigen antibodies (either IgM or IgG) may be useful in documenting an infection. The immunohistochemical markers for both B cells and T cells are positive, and there is no immunoreactivity for CD15. If these findings are equivocal, an absence of gene rearrangements or detection of the EBV-encoded polypeptide sequence will help to confirm the diagnosis. Large

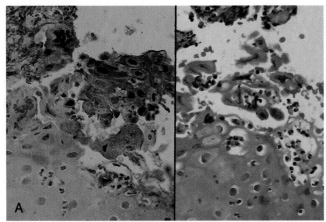

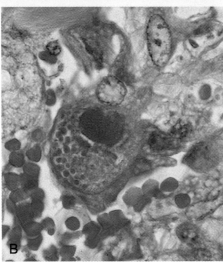

FIGURE 8–47. *A*, Herpes simplex virus (HSV) gives a characteristic "ground glass" appearance in the nuclei, especially in a multinucleated giant cell (*right*, IHC, × 300). Immunoreactivity for HSV (*left*, IHC, × 300) can confirm the hematoxylin and eosin stained impression; *B*, Cytomegalovirus infection produces a characteristic eosinophilic intranuclear "bulls-eye" type inclusion, with a more basophilic cytoplasmic inclusion (H&E, × 750).

cell or immunoblastic lymphoma and anaplastic large cell lymphomas can be difficult to distinguish on the basis of histologic features alone. Hodgkin's disease may also be considered, but it can generally be excluded on the basis of the aforementioned molecular or immunophenotypic studies. Changes associated with human immunodeficiency virus (HIV) can also mimic an EBV infection, but generally, vascular changes, relative lymphocytic depletion, and clinical assessment can help differentiate between these two infections.[46]

BACTERIAL

Bacterial infections may involve *Haemophilus influenzae* (type B, specifically, although all subtypes are involved), pneumococci, hemolytic streptococci or staphylococci (also including scarlet fever sequelae), Neisseria species, micrococci, Klebsiella species, *Bordetella pertussis* (whooping cough), *Corynebacterium diphtheriae* (diphtheria), *Salmonella typhi* (typhoid fever) and Rickettsia species (typhus). These bacteria may be associated with acute epiglottitis, acute laryngotracheobronchitis, and laryngeal diphtheria, usually resulting in a diffuse erythema of the laryngeal mucosa with exudate, which often extends into the subglottis or trachea. Mucopurulent discharge may be seen on gross examination. Histologic examination demonstrates microabscesses and mixed inflammation, often with surface ulceration. Clinical management is mandatory, often requiring emergent therapy without laboratory confirmation of the etiologic agent. Once the etiologic agent is determined, appropriate antibiotic therapy can be instituted.[137–146] Diphtheria still occurs, and antitoxin should be given as clinically indicated, not delayed by lack of laboratory confirmation or a Schick test. A diphtheritic, dirty-grey membrane will be evident, coupled with a foul odor.[138,147]

Retropharyngeal, peritonsillar, or laryngeal abscess may result in obstruction of the larynx. This is usually a consequence of a suppurative infection of a retropharyngeal lymph node or the posterior tonsillar pillar, or related to deep, penetrating trauma. Rather than waiting for culture results, the necessary surgical intervention should be undertaken promptly. *H. influenzae* is the most common infecting organism.[148–151]

Granulomatous inflammation can be identified in a variety of infections, including those of bacterial, mycobacterial, and fungal origin. Nodules are evident throughout the respiratory tract, as are the characteristic epithelioid histiocytes, giant cells, chronic inflammation, and variable necrosis or caseation, depending upon the infectious agent (Fig. 8–48*A*). The overlying epithelium may be atrophic, normal, or hyperplastic with pseudoepitheliomatous hyperplasia, demonstrating ulceration to nodularpapillary growth. The degree of granulomatous inflammation may be variable, depending on the host's immune response to the organism. This means that a nonspecific inflammation, rather than the characteristic caseating granulomas, may be encountered in a *Mycobacterium tuberculosis* infection in an immunocompromised patient. Therefore, careful histologic examination, often under oil immersion and frequently involving multiple slides, is necessary to identify the causative agent. Mycobacterial agents, including tuberculosis, avium complex, and leprosy, can be identified using acid-fast stains (Ziehl-Neelsen) or fluorochrome dyes (auramine and rhodamine).[42,59,142,152–158] Lupus vulgaris is a secondary form of tuberculosis that can present in the mucosa of the larynx, usually as a result of extension from cervical lymphadenitis. *Klebsiella rhinoscleromatis* can be documented by tissue gram stain, whereby the organisms fill the histiocytes (so-called Mikulicz's cells) identified within the rich inflamma-

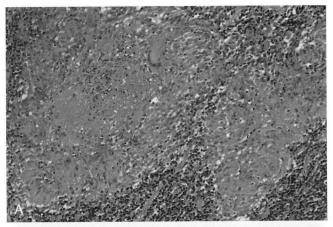

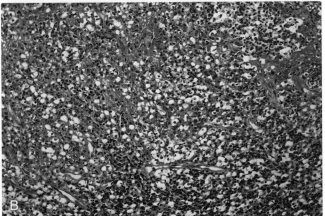

FIGURE 8–48. *A*, Granulomatous inflammation with caseation is characteristic for a tuberculosis infection, but other infectious agents should be excluded through culture or staining. Central necrosis, giant cells and inflammatory cells are found with epithelioid histiocytes. Granulomatous inflammation is a descriptive diagnosis, for which a cause should be actively sought (H&E, × 150); *B*, the bacteria *Klebsiella rhinoscleromatis* produced a histiocytic response in which the submucosa is filled with sheets of histiocytes and inflammatory elements. Tissue gram stain will demonstrate the organisms stuffed into the histiocytes (H&E, × 75).

tory infiltrate and granulomatous inflammation. The response is variable, though, depending upon the stage of the disease at the time of biopsy[59,142,159–162] (Fig. 8–48B). *Actinomyces israelii* (usually part of the oral flora), the most frequent clinical isolate of the Actinomycetales order, also yields a granulomatous inflammation, but usually with a greater degree of necrosis (abscess formation) and fibrosis. Actinmycoses often demonstrate spheres of organisms arranged in a radiating pattern (sulfer granules). Gram stains accentuate the fine filamentous organisms, which do not test positive with acid-fast stains.[59,163,164] Cat-scratch disease may extend into the larynx from the surrounding lymph nodes, in which case a palisaded granuloma with stellate necrosis is characteristic. A Warthin-Starry stain will help to identify the gram-negative bacillus.

FUNGAL

A variety of fungi can cause laryngitis, all with a similar histologic appearance of acute and chronic inflammation, usually granulomatous in nature. Fungal organisms (either yeast or mold forms) include the following:[46,59,142,145,156,164–176]

Candida albicans—oval, budding cells with long, tubular hyphae that can be seen on gram stain

Histoplasma capsulatum—small, variably shaped, intracytoplasmic organisms, often in regions of viable tissues

Coccidioides immitis—thick, double-walled spherules with endospores (Fig. 8–49A)

Cryptococcus neoformans—polysaccharide-encapsulated, variably sized, oval-shaped organisms

Blastomyces dermatitidis—thick, double-contoured "refractile" organisms with broad-based budding (Fig. 8–49B)

Paracoccidioides brasiliensis—circular organisms with "mariner's wheel" type multiple budding

Aspergillus species—narrow fungi with acute-angle branching and septations

Mucor species—broad, aseptate, ribbon-like mold forms

Sporothrix schenckii and rhinosporidiosis—free trophocytes or round sporangia filled with sporoblasts/endospores

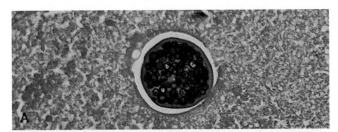

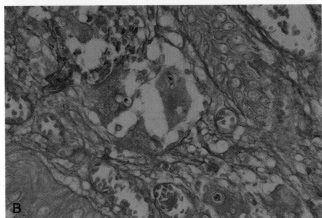

FIGURE 8–49. *A*, The spherule of *Coccidioides immitis*, accentuated with a Gomori methenamine silver stain, which also highlights the endospores (GMS, × 300); *B*, Broad-based budding can be seen in this example of blastomycosis, accentuated with a periodic acid-Schiff preparation (PAS, × 300).

Each of these organisms has a characteristic fungal or yeast form in tissue or in culture. Documentation of the organism in tissue can be facilitated by mucicarmine, PAS, calcafluor white, Warthin-Starry, GMS, and immunoperoxidase antibody studies. Confirmation by blood cultures, serologic titers (complement fixation, latex agglutination, or precipitant test), or cutaneous hypersensitivity testing (less specific), may also be performed. Although isolated disease can occur, fungal infections are most often part of systemic disease, and are particularly prevalent in immunocompromised patients. Laryngeal manifestations of acquired immunodeficiency syndrome (AIDS) may include a variety of infections, most frequently candidiasis or herpes simplex lesions.[46]

A modified Dieterle's stain will document the presence of spirochetes if syphilis or borreliosis is suspected. The presentation of syphilis will vary depending on primary (mucosal ulceration), secondary, or tertiary manifestations (perichondritis, gumma formation, and fibrosis). The tertiary stage is the most common laryngeal manifestation, associated with gumma, granuloma, and ulceration. The associated vasculitis, rich plasma cell infiltrate, and positive Venereal Disease Research Laboratory (VDRL) or fluorescent treponemal antibody absorption (FTA-ABS) test results should confirm the diagnosis.[59,145,177,178] In the setting of a granulomatous inflammation, malacoplakia must also be excluded. The demonstration of Michaelis-Gutmann bodies (round, target-like calcified structures) is sufficient to establish the diagnosis, although cultures will usually grow *Escherichia coli* or another bacterial organism.[179] Granulomatous inflammation is not a complete diagnosis, but requires clinicopathologic correlation. After infectious agents have been ruled out, other causes of granulomatous inflammation (e.g., sarcoid, carcinoma, Wegener's granulomatosis, foreign bodies, and Teflon) must also be excluded.[180]

Only rare case reports document laryngeal involvement by parasitic organisms. These organisms include Trichinella species, *Ascaris lumbricoides*, *Hirudinea genera* (leeches), *Limnatis maculosa*, and Leishmania species.[181–183]

Inflammatory Diseases

Gross Pathology

On gross examination, the biopsy specimen of inflammatory diseases is usually pale and edematous rather than erythematous, the latter being seen more frequently in bacterial or viral infections. The histologic examination usually only shows edema fluid and variable inflammation. Inflammatory conditions are usually abrupt in clinical onset and exhibit a rapid response to epinephrine, which is quite distinct from the nature of infectious agents. Previous

allergic sensitivity can help to differentiate these disorders.[138,142,145,184,185]

The gross appearance of perichondritis and chondronecrosis is variable, depending upon the degree of inflammation. Edema is evident in the initial stages, but extensive disease, especially of the cricoid, can result in complete destruction of the cartilaginous tissues, with subsequent frank collapse. This complication is infrequent and usually occurs late in the disease course.

Microscopic Pathology

On histologic examination, the perichondrium seems to be affected initially, with degeneration of the nuclei, vascular proliferation, and infiltration by inflammatory cells. With time, fibrosis and hyalinization of the perichondrium can be seen.

"Reinke's edema" generally involves the entire space of Reinke and is characterized by a smooth surface contour and gelatinous, greyish edema fluid. The histologic appearance is one of edema fluid without any fibrous connective tissue or myofibroblasts, which is different from the appearance of degenerative polyps. The overlying epithelium may be quite thinned, extending over the sharply delimited swelling. Hypothyroidism can result in edema of Reinke's space with progression to a floppy, polypoid appearance. The cordal tissues are filled with mucoproteinaceous ground substance. Replacement therapy may yield resolution of the edema.[156,186,187]

Differential Diagnosis

Supraglottic allergic edema (angioedema) and subglottic allergic edema (spasmodic croup or false croup) are not generally related to an infectious etiology, but are associated with allergic stimuli; sensitivity to food, animal dander, dust, feathers, pollens, or drugs; trauma; and environmental exposure to noxious, inhaled substances. Chronic, nonspecific inflammation with associated squamous metaplasia and epithelial thickening may result from repeated episodes of laryngitis, voice abuse, environmental exposure (chemicals, smoke, climatic extremes), acid reflux, and systemic diseases. Nodules, polyps, contact ulcers, and specific infections or inflammations must be excluded, as should a laryngeal intraepithelial neoplasia, before the diagnosis of chronic laryngitis can be definitively applied to these nonspecific changes.

Clinicopathologic Correlation

The antecedent events for inflammation may be related to infection (mycotic infections or mycobacteria), trauma, neoplasms, surgery (vascular compromise), iatrogenic causes (feeding tubes or tracheostomy tubes), foreign bodies, or irradiation. A number of etiologies may be present synchronously, as in an infection that develops in association with radiation therapy, so multiple etiologies must be addressed. The mucositis of early radiation changes is reversible, but generally, the chondronecrosis associated with irradiation is irreversible. The cartilages may be involved in isolation or in the aggregate.[142,188–191] Predisposing factors should be removed in an attempt to treat the underlying cause of the disease.[22,48,142,145,180]

Sarcoidosis

Gross Pathology

A pale-red, diffuse, symmetric, swollen, nodular, exophytic, or edematous lesion, most often of the supraglottic structures, is a common finding in sarcoidosis. Miliary, small, nodular lesions to larger, lobulated, submucosal masses have also been described. There is occasionally an associated epithelial hyperlasia or keratosis. Ulceration and scarring of the larynx are generally not identified.[35,59,90,159,192–198]

Microscopic Pathology

The microscopic diagnosis of sarcoidosis is generally one of exclusion, so clinical, radiographic, and laboratory correlations are needed to confirm the histologic diagnosis. Small to medium-sized, tightly clustered, noncaseating, epithelioid granulomas are present in the stroma, and a rich inflammatory infiltrate of plasma cells and lymphocytes is seen interspersed with occasional Langhans' and foreign-body giant cells. The epithelioid histiocytes are polyhedral cells with abundant cytoplasm and vesicular nuclei (Fig. 8–50). Bands of fibrous connective tissue septa separate the granulomas. Although not specific for sarcoid, asteroid bodies (stellate, intracytoplasmic inclusions in giant cells), Schaumann's bodies (concentrically laminated, calcified bodies), and Hamazaki-Wesenberg bodies (yellow-brown structures that resemble fungal organisms) may be identified. Although fibrinoid necrosis may be identified in sarcoidosis, it is an extraordinary finding, so an infectious etiology should be excluded first. With progression of the disease, fibrosis and hyalinization of the stroma occurs, possibly obscuring the granulomatous inflammation and leaving a fibrous scar in place of the granuloma.[35,192,194–196,198]

Differential Diagnosis

It is imperative that other infectious, inflammatory, or neoplastic conditions be ruled out, as the diagnosis of sarcoidosis is one of exclusion. Evidence of mycobacterial organisms (tuberculosis, avium complex, leprosy), cat-scratch disease, Haemophilus species, syphilis, tularemia, histoplasmosis, blastomycosis, actinomycosis, rhinosporidiosis, toxoplasmosis, and brucellosis should be sought through tissue staining or culture.[35,59,192,194–198] A foreign-body reaction can be excluded by polarization. Systemic diseases, such as beryliosis and Wegener's granulomatosis, can be ruled out with demonstration of foreign material and a true vasculitis, geographic-type necrosis, and appropriate serum titers (serum angiotensin-converting enzyme and ANCA, respectively).[193] Patients with malacoplakia will demonstrate Michaelis-Gutmann bodies as part of the granulomatous inflammation.[179] Granulomatous inflammation can also be seen in association with malignant tumors, especially as a reaction to the keratinous debris of a squamous cell carcinoma. Therefore, it is prudent to submit all of the tissue and examine the overlying surface epithelium closely for features of malignancy.

Clinicopathologic Correlation

Isolated laryngeal sarcoidosis has been described, but such a diagnosis must be supported by additional clinical, radiographic, or laboratory evidence. Involvement of the larynx as part of systemic disease is a much more likely scenario, and cutaneous manifestations, fevers, and adenopathy can usually be found on clinical evaluation.[35,192,194,198]

SYSTEMIC, AUTOIMMUNE, AND CONNECTIVE TISSUE DISEASES

Rheumatoid Nodules

Gross Pathology

Erythematous vocal cords with submucosal nodules, often bilateral, can be identified on laryngoscopy. The lesion can be found within the cords or involving the cricoarytenoid joint, frequently exhibiting ulceration. Upon cut section, the nodule is often yellow.[199,200]

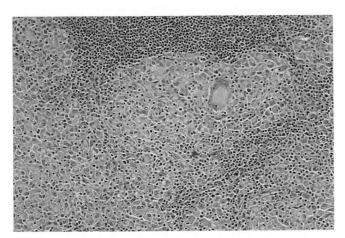

FIGURE 8–50. Epithelioid histiocytes are arranged in a granuloma, with a giant cell and chronic inflammatory cells (H&E, × 150).

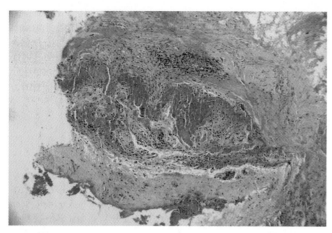

FIGURE 8–51. Rheumatoid arthritis of the larynx can be documented with the deposition of amorphous materials accompanied by an inflammatory and foreign-body giant cell reaction (H&E, × 75).

Microscopic Pathology

The joint manifestations in the acute phase include inflammation, joint effusion, and a synovial proliferation. In rheumatoid nodules, subepithelial areas of fibrinoid necrosis of the collagen are surrounded by palisading histiocytes with associated fibrosis and inflammatory cells (Fig. 8–51). More extensive inflammation with fibroblasts, edema, and endothelial proliferation in the fibrous connective tissue may be seen.[199,200]

Differential Diagnosis

The differential diagnosis includes other causes of arthritis in the laryngeal joints (systemic lupus erythematosis, gout, Reiter's disease) and other granulomatous-type inflammations (frequently infectious). The clinical setting of the disease is generally helpful in defining the sometimes nonspecific inflammatory findings.[199–202] Gout can present as arthritis of the intralaryngeal joints, while the classic submucosal tophus near the laryngeal joints has also been documented (amorphous mass of urate crystals, inflammatory cells, macrophages, and foreign-body giant cells). Cultures or tissue staining for infectious agents, birefringence to document the crystals of gout (if processed correctly), and the exclusion of Wegener's granulomatosis can be performed, depending upon the degree of necrosis and granulomatous-type inflammation.[203–205]

Relapsing Polychondritis

Gross Pathology

Although the gross findings are nonspecific, there is an overall thickening to the epiglottis and aryepiglottic folds, with softening and friability of the cricoid and tracheal rings (and tracheal wall), as well as an overall decrease in the size of the larynx and trachea or frank collapse in the later stages of the disease.[90,206–210] No specific mucosal lesion is generally present, although if a mucosal lesion is present it may be erythematous and swollen.[206–211]

Microscopic Pathology

The low-power view of relapsing polychondritis (polychondropathy) reflects a loss of cartilage basophilia, assuming an eosinophilic quality. There is fragmentation of the cartilage, with necrosis and lysis of the cartilaginous plates. The outer perichondrium is permeated by a spectrum of inflammatory cells, including neutrophils, eosinophils, lymphocytes, and plasma cells, frequently associated with edema or gelatinous cystic degeneration (Fig. 8–52). Rather than a well-defined perichondrium, there is an imperceptible blending of the degenerated fibrillar cartilage with the surrounding inflammatory cells (see Fig. 8–52). With progression of the disease, the dissolved lacunae are replaced with granulation-type tissue or fibrosis, which can completely replace the cartilage structure. Occasionally, a deranged architecture of the cartilage may be present, perhaps affiliated with regeneration, as the disease progresses.[206–216]

Special Techniques

Although electron microscopy is not performed routinely for this disease, many of the chondrocytes contain increased lysosomes and lipids in addition to electron-dense multivesicular bodies.[206,213]

Differential Diagnosis

Clinically, diffuse tracheal stenosis can be caused by a variety of disorders, including sarcoid, infectious

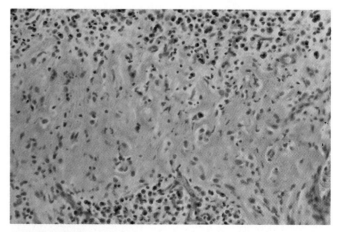

FIGURE 8–52. Relapsing polychondritis shows characteristic loss of cartilage basophilia with acute and chronic inflammatory cells destroying the cartilage from the perichondrium in toward the center. This is a systemic autoimmune disorder, frequently presenting with otic or nasal manifestations, besides the rheumatologic findings (H&E, × 300).

agents (tuberculosis, syphilis, various fungi, bacteria, and viruses), tracheopathia osteoplastica, lymphoma, Wegener's granulomatosis, chondroma, and cricoarytenoid arthritis, with relapsing polychondritis included in this same differential diagnosis.[90,214,215] Histologic findings in the larynx are occasionally nonspecific for relapsing polychondritis. When combined with the appropriate clinical setting, however, the diagnosis can be made with confidence—especially if one or more of the six criteria of McAdam are present: (1) recurrent bilateral auricular chondritis, (2) inflammatory polyarthritis, (3) nasal chondritis, (4) ocular inflammation, (5) tracheal or laryngeal chondritis, and (6) cochlear and/or vestibular damage.[208] Systemic vasculitides (e.g., Wegener's granulomatosis), rheumatoid arthritis, and infectious perichondritis need to be excluded. The infectious agents include diphtheria, blastomycosis, actinomycosis, herpes, tuberculosis, syphilis, histoplasmosis, and other gram-negative bacilli.[206] There is no true perivascular predilection for the inflammatory response, which helps to exclude the systemic vasculitides, although both diseases have been described in the same patient.[217] Obtaining material for cultures or performing the necessary histochemical stains helps rule out infectious organisms, and performing clinical tests for cartilage matrix proteins or antibodies to type II collagen (found uniquely in cartilage) may help in defining relapsing polychondritis.[218-220] There is an association with HLA-DR4.[221] Cartilaginous tumors usually do not have the inflammatory component, nor is there a loss of basophilia.

Clinicopathologic Correlation

Other diseases may also be present in association with relapsing polychondritis (systemic chondromalacia), such as necrotizing sialometaplasia, Reiter's syndrome, Behçet's syndrome, systemic lupus erythematosus, rheumatoid arthritis, diabetes mellitus, ulcerative colitis, Sjögren's syndrome, lymphocytic thyroiditis, ulcerative colitis, glomerulonephritis, chondrosarcoma, and an increased frequency of myelodysplastic syndromes.[35,54,208,209,212,216,222-229] These entities usually have specific findings and are not a differential diagnostic difficulty. However, the finding of myelodysplastic syndromes may be associated with a specific immunologic imbalance and immunogenetic background, which plays a role in the pathogenesis of relapsing polychondritis.

Wegener's Granulomatosis

Gross Pathology

A reddish, friable to ulcerated, circumferential subglottic narrowing or stenosis is the typical gross finding, with pseudotumor formation and ulcerating tracheal lesions identified in a number of patients. Any portion of the larynx may be affected, but it is usually a subglottic disease with extension into the

trachea (the latter is especially more frequent in females). This nonspecific finding must be coupled with a histologic examination and additional studies as clinically warranted. Primary laryngeal presentation is uncommon, as the disease is generally systemic by the time laryngeal involvement is biopsied or suspected.[159,230-236]

Microscopic Pathology

The classic triad of granulomatous inflammation, necrosis, and vasculitis is ideal, but seldom identified on biopsy. The low-power depiction of widespread ischemic or geographic type necrosis is identified only in specimens of an adequate size. On small fragments of tissue, the necrosis may just be an overall basophilia to the biopsy section. A serpiginous border to the necrosis is often surrounded by granulomatous inflammation. True vasculitis—with inflammatory cells present within the small to medium-sized vessel walls, often with foci of fibrinoid necrosis (Fig. 8–53)—is requisite for definitive diagnosis of Wegener's granulomatosis (WG), but its absence does not exclude the diagnosis. Granulomatous vasculitis or infiltration by acute and/or chronic inflammatory elements without fibrinoid necrosis may also be seen in WG. The inflammatory cells include lymphocytes, histiocytes, eosinophils, and neutrophils. Microabscess formation may be present. Occasional multinucleated giant cells and exceptionally noncaseating granulomas may be identified. When a leukocytoclastic vasculitis or fibrosing vasculitis can be demonstrated, these findings may be associated with a more advanced form or late stage of the disease. Fibrosis, sometimes concentrically arranged around vessels, and chronic inflammation may be all that remains in the end-stages of the disease. Laryngeal WG seems to demonstrate a predominance of parenchymal changes (necrosis,

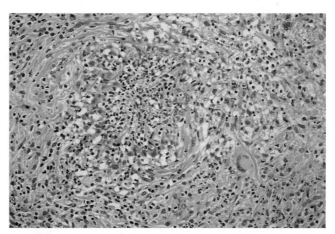

FIGURE 8–53. Perivascular inflammation with ultimate destruction of the vessel is characteristic for Wegener's granulomatosis, especially when combined with foreign-body giant cells, geographic type necrosis (seldom seen on laryngeal biopsies), and the clinical findings (including ANCA titers) (H&E, × 150).

granulomas, giant cells, and microabscesses), with infrequent vascular changes.[159,231,232,234,235,237,238]

Special Techniques

An elastic stain may aid in identifying the vessel wall in order to document a vasculitis. Cultures must be obtained during surgery, in addition to performing a variety of histochemical stains, to exclude an infectious etiology. These stains include GMS (fungal–*Sporothrix schenckii*, *Histoplasmosis*, and *Coccidioides immitis*); acid-fast stain (mycobacterial–tuberculosis and leprosy); PAS and mucicarmine (parasitic); and tissue gram stain (bacterial), combined with negative cultures obtained during the surgery. Immunohistochemical reactions for CD34, CD31, or Factor VIII may help but are generally unnecessary.

Electron microscopy will underscore the inflammatory and granulomatous nature of the disease but is impractical and unnecessary.[237,239]

Differential Diagnosis

The diagnosis of WG is usually a diagnosis of exclusion after ruling out other infectious diseases; foreign material; relapsing polychondritis; collagen-vascular disease (sarcoidosis); Churg-Strauss vasculitis (asthma, allergic nasal polyps, pulmonary infiltrates, peripheral eosinophilia, and systemic vasculitis); uremia; lymphoid diseases; and malignant diseases (usually lymphomas). Bacterial superinfection of the mucosal ulcerations must not be considered the singular cause of the symptoms. It is also quite possible that the characteristic histopathologic findings of WG may not be documented in the laryngeal or tracheal biopsies, even if multiple or repeated. Confirmation of the diagnosis with biopsies of other upper-aerodigestive-tract sites of involvement; clinical evidence of systemic disease (lung or kidney involvement, fever, malaise, arthralgias); or a positive antineutrophil cytoplasmic antibody titer may be necessary to document the diagnosis.[159,193,217,231,233–236,240–244] Although myospherulosis (granulomatous response to foreign material) is uncommon in the larynx, examination of the tissue for polarizable foreign material should be performed.[232,235]

Inflammatory cells, more specifically lymphocytes, are usually not atypical in WG, but the demonstration of a polymorphous cellular population with immunoreactivity for both B-cell and T-cell markers helps to exclude the possibility of a non-Hodgkin's malignant lymphoma (that would be monotypic/monoclonal). If necessary, additional molecular studies can be performed to exclude gene rearrangements in equivocal immunophenotypic findings. The terms polymorphic reticulosis and lymphomatoid granulomatosis have been included in the differential of WG. Although this disorder is thought to be a perivascular accumulation of polymorphous atypical lymphocytes, with angiodestruction, recent studies seem to indicate that this disorder is better considered under the rubric of a malignant lymphoma.[234,235,240,241]

Clinicopathologic Correlation

The larynx is more often involved in the setting of pre-existing disease elsewhere, and primary presentation with laryngeal WG is a rare event. An estimated 8% to 25% of patients with WG will develop disease referable to the larynx. Laryngeal involvement most often involves the subglottic region, primarily in women.

Laryngeal Manifestations of Cutaneous Diseases

A variety of cutaneous-based lesions may occur in the larynx concurrent with or independent of cutaneous disease. Both gross and microscopic findings of the laryngeal involvement are similar to their cutaneous counterpart.

EPIDERMOLYSIS BULLOSA

The gross findings in epidermolysis bullosa (EB) are bullae with ulceration extending to excoriation, depending upon the stage of the disease. Diffuse thickening of any part of the larynx with detachment of the epithelium, edema, and erythema with a fibropurulent exudate can be identified on laryngoscopy. The glottic disease is the most serious, as stenosis will have a more serious consequence. Stenosis may develop with scarring, especially in prolonged disease activity.[245–250] Tracheal disease has also been recognized, although it is rare.[247] Performing the laryngoscopy may be difficult, as the scope may produce vesicles or bullae.

DARIER'S DISEASE

Darier's disease, or keratosis follicularis, involves a gross thickening of the vocal cords with small hyperkeratotic nodules on the surface.[251] These nodules can also be identified elsewhere in the larynx. The changes identified histologically are similar to those seen in familial benign chronic pemphigus (Hailey Hailey disease). The distinction may be impossible based on specimens from the larynx. Lacunae and bullae in the laryngeal lesions of Darier's disease illustrate this point. Indeed, there are no recent reports of this disease occurring in the larynx.

PEMPHIGUS

Pemphigus can occur in the larynx, although it is rare. The larynx has an overall thickened or edematous appearance, with loss of the valleculae and aryepiglottic folds by a thickening of the mucosal surfaces. The overall luminal diameter is greatly diminished, resulting in laryngeal stenosis, with bands of adhesions seen in cases of long standing. Frequently, there are serous-filled bullae alternating with denuded areas. The ulcerated or eroded areas may be covered by a fibrinous exudate.[159,252–256] Pemphigus is histologically defined by the acantholysis, which is a disappearance of the intercellular bridges, most often in the suprabasal region. Acute inflammation is associated with the acantholysis. Pemphigus is generally distinguished from other bullous disease by the lack of dyskeratosis and the rich inflammatory infiltrate, usually containing eosinophils. There are a number of different types of pemphigus, and this distinction is difficult on laryngeal specimens. The clinical course of the disease helps to make these distinctions. Immunofluorescent studies for immunoglobulins and complement can also be performed but may be somewhat difficult to interpret in the mucosal specimens. Drugs that have been found to cause pemphigus should be discontinued as part of the treatment.[159,252–256]

STEVENS-JOHNSON SYNDROME

This syndrome may include pharyngeal and laryngeal lesions, but these may not occur at the same time as the other clinical manifestations. Stevens-Johnson is frequently confused with erythema multiforme (EM), Behçet's syndrome, and Reiter's syndrome and, in many instances, cannot be distinguished by the laryngeal biopsy specimen. Clinical correlation is always suggested in these diseases; the pattern of disease and type of cutaneous lesions assist with the diagnostic distinction.[257–260] The most frequent differential diagnosis problem is with herpes simplex infection. There is generally less inflammatory reaction, and the characteristic inclusion bodies can be identified or accentuated with immunohistochemical reactions. Stevens-Johnson is usually associated with drugs and almost never with a herpes infection, while EM is most commonly related to herpes infections. Balloon degeneration of the epithelium is usually an early finding in EM but can progress to total epithelial necrosis. This latter feature is seen more frequently in Stevens-Johnson syndrome, making separation of these diseases very difficult by histology alone. The acantholysis in pemphigus helps to exclude Stevens-Johnson. Reiter's syndrome will have urethritis and arthritis, which is generally not identified in Stevens-Johnson syndrome. Recurrent conjunctivitis and aphthous ulcers of the genitals, oral cavity, pharynx, and larynx, along with a pyodermia, help to document Behçet's syndrome.[257,258,260] Laryngeal and tracheal manifestations of uremia may show fibrinous exudate covering the surface of the mucosa, revealing a beefy red appearance beneath the crust. Clinical correlation with the history of renal failure is necessary to make the correct diagnosis.[134] Infectious agents can also be ruled out through culture, in situ hybridization, polymerase chain reaction, or clinical serum studies.[257,259]

MUCOUS MEMBRANE PEMPHIGOID

This condition does occur in the trachea and larynx, where it will produce cicatricial narrowing. The histologic findings in the larynx are nonspecific chronic inflammation with fibrosis, rarely demonstrating a subepithelial bullae. Immunofluorescence studies are more specific in developing the correct diagnosis, demonstrating linear immunofluorescence along the basement membrane zone, with C3 or IgG immunoglobulins, if they are present. There is no acantholysis within the epithelium in pemphigoid, helping to distinguish this entity from pemphigus vulgaris. Cicatricial pemphigoid is a progressive vesiculobullous disease with associated scar formation, usually without acantholysis or subepithelial bullae.[159,261]

SYSTEMIC LUPUS ERYTHEMATOSUS

Systemic lupus erythematosus (SLE) may manifest itself with laryngeal ulceration, erythema, and edema. Subglottic stenosis, rheumatoid nodules, and necrotizing vasculitis can be seen. As these findings are nonspecific in isolation, a biopsy differentiates other ulcerative or edema-producing lesions (hereditary angioneurotic edema, allergic angioedema, trauma, infections, radiation), coupled with appropriate laboratory tests to confirm the diagnosis. The vasculitis generally produces a thickened or hyalinized vessel wall without true destruction of the vessel wall, as would be seen in Wegener's granulomatosis. Rheumatoid type nodules have been seen in patients with SLE.[262]

LIGNEOUS CONJUNCTIVITIS

This disease primarily affects the conjunctivae and causes obstructive airway lesions. The hyaline material deposited in the larynx contains fibrin and mucopolysaccharides. These changes can be distinguished from those of amyloid by appropriate stains.[71]

PACHYONYCHIA CONGENITA

Pachyonychia congenita (or Jadassohn-Lewandowsky syndrome) generally involves abnormalities of the nails along with epithelial abnormalities. These epithelial abnormalities include exophytic, white lesions of the ventricles, true cords, and subglottic region. The epithelium is acanthotic with parakeratosis with characteristic intracellular vacuolization throughout the epithelium. The inflammatory infiltrate is generally mild.[263]

BLUE RUBBER BLEB NEVUS SYNDROME

Also called Bean syndrome, this presents with bleb-like cavernous hemangiomas, rarely presenting in the larynx as a supraglottic mass. The mass can be a bluish, dumbbell-shaped mass along the aryepiglottic fold or true vocal cord. The histologic appearance is a benign cavernous hemangioma with blood-filled lakes lined by flattened to cuboidal endothelial cells. Rendu-Osler-Weber syndrome can also have hemangiomas, but telangiectasias and subungual lesions will help distinguish between the two disorders.[264]

NECROBIOTIC XANTHOGRANULOMA

Necrobiotic xanthogranuloma with IgA paraproteinemia has been reported to involve the larynx, in which lipid-laden histiocytes are present in a necrotic background with polymorphonuclear neutrophils, nuclear dust, and occasional giant cells. There is no vasculitis. Immunofluorescence will demonstrate vascular immune reactants at the basement membrane (although this has not been demonstrated on laryngeal specimens). Clinical correlation with the dermatologic findings and the paraproteinemia for IgA will help elucidate the nature of the disease. Serum immunoglobulin levels and complement assays should also be evaluated.[265]

TUBEROUS SCLEROSIS

Although tuberous sclerosis is not a dermatologic disease alone, the dermatologic manifestations are often the initial presentation of the disease. Agenesis of the vocal cords and laryngeal polyposis have been described in tuberous sclerosis but there are generally no specific findings within the larynx.[266,267]

CROHN'S DISEASE

Laryngeal involvement by Crohn's disease is rarely encountered. On laryngoscopy the vocal cords demonstrate edema, erythema, and ulcerations with granulation tissue, although involvement of the epiglottis and other parts of the larynx are noted. Laryngeal obstruction can result. Microscopic examination reveals nonspecific inflammation with fibrosis. The diagnosis can be made with certainty only when combined with other features in the clinical presentation and confirmatory biopsy of a gastrointestinal site.[268]

DEVELOPMENTAL AND CONGENITAL LESIONS

Oncocytic Lesions

Gross Pathology

Oncocytic papillary proliferations generally present as a smooth submucosal polypoid mass in the supraglottic larynx, specifically the ventricle and false vocal cord (perhaps related to mucus gland distribution). The lesions reach up to 4 cm in greatest dimension and are frequently multifocal, although the multifocality may not be obvious on gross examination. These lesions are rarely found in the subglottis or vocal cord. The mass can be pink-red or blue, although a white keratotic surface reaction can be identified. The cut surface may reveal a fleshy to firm, brown to yellow solid nodule or a cyst filled with clear to brown fluid, occasionally tinged with blood.[132,269–282]

Microscopic Pathology

These lesions range from a solid proliferation to a thin-walled cyst, lined by multiple layers of cuboidal epithelium (occasionally respiratory type containing mucus) or thrown into papillary projections (Fig. 8–54). There may be true papillae with a delicate fibrovascular core, or the papillae may form due to degeneration of the surrounding cells. The cells are polyhedral to round with distinct cell borders, with cilia present on a few cells. The cytoplasm surrounds small, round, centrally situated, pyknotic to vesicular nuclei with small to moderately large, eosinophilic, round nucleoli. Abundant cytoplasm contains a varying number of fine to coarse eosinophilic granules (see Fig. 8–54). Focal nuclear and cytoplasmic variability can be observed, but mitotic activity, tumor necrosis, and invasive growth are not evident. In the more solid areas, the tumor cells are arranged in solid sheets, alveoli, or nests, separated by a delicate fibrovascular network. In some areas, there are pseudo-acinar arrangements with a small amount of debris in the "lumen." The cystic structures range from microscopic cysts to grossly visible cysts, either uni- or multilocular, occasionally filled with mucinous cellular debris. There may be separate cysts, distinct from a "main" mass grossly. A

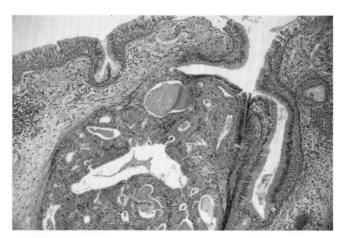

FIGURE 8–54. A papillary oncocytic proliferation within the larynx, composed of enlarged cells with abundant eosinophilic cytoplasm (H&E, × 150).

host response including lymphocytes and plasma cells can be seen adjacent to the cyst wall lining, but the lymphocytes are not arranged in follicular structures. Normal salivary gland tissue may be found in the region, occasionally demonstrating oncocytic metaplasia. There is generally no involvement of the cartilage, but there may be extension along the duct structures to include the surface epithelium.[132,269-273,276,277,279,280,282,283]

Special Techniques

A phosphotungstic acid hematoxylin (PTAH) stain illustrates distinctly positive, small, dark blue to black cytoplasmic granules, which represent mitochondria. A PAS-positive, diastase-sensitive reaction confirms the presence of glycogen. These lesions are immunoreactive for cytokeratin and epithelial membrane antigen. Electron microscopy reveals numerous mitochondria closely packed within the cytoplasm; these mitochondria are often enlarged and variably shaped, with many parallel, fine, tubular, lamellar cristae.[271,275,279,280]

Differential Diagnosis

Warthin's tumor (papillary cystadenoma lymphomatosum) generally has a more intimate association with lymphoid tissue, which will be arranged in follicles. Malignant change has not been described in laryngeal tumors, although radical treatment has been performed to obtain complete surgical resection. Squamous cell carcinoma has been described with oncocytic lesions, but there is no direct association or etiologic relationship.[270,271,273,276,277,281-283]

Clinicopathologic Correlation

Oncocytes can be present within a wide variety of lesions in the larynx, and a variety of names have been applied to oncocytic or oxyphilic lesions including, but not limited to, oncocytic papillary cystadenoma (OPC), oncocytic cyst, oncocytoma, oxyphilic adenoma, eosinophilic papillary cystadenoma, and oncocytic hyperplasia. Oncocytic lesions of the larynx manifest as a morphologic spectrum of changes, including surface oncocytic metaplasia of the respiratory or squamous epithelium, solitary solid oncocytic "adenoma" (neoplasm), multifocal "hyperplastic" masses, and cysts lined by oncocytes. Each of these entities is within the benign spectrum of oncocytic lesions, without any treatment implications. However, oncocytic change/metaplasia can be diagnosed if present diffusely or multifocally throughout the larynx. If there is a solid proliferation of oncocytes, the designation of adenoma can be used. Many cysts of the larynx may be lined by oncocytes, and a clear distinction between a saccular or ductal cyst and OPC may not always be possible.

Laryngeal Cysts

Gross Pathology

The gross appearance of cysts in the larynx is often determined by the point of origin in the larynx and the type of cyst (saccular, retention/inclusion, ductal, vascular, or traumatic). The cyst can be considered external or internal to the larynx based upon the degree of compression of the larynx by the cyst and the extent of disease within the larynx. Cysts generally do not communicate with the interior of the larynx. A laryngocele (an air-filled herniation or dilatation of the saccule) can be either internal or external to the larynx, communicating with the lumen. Saccular cysts (anterior or lateral) are submucosal and do not communicate with the lumen, but instead are filled with mucus or acute inflammatory elements. As air and fluid are forced into a laryngocele, the distinction between a laryngocele and other laryngeal cysts may be impossible. Since the saccule has great variability in size and contains a number of out-pouchings, the true nature of a laryngocele may be part of the normal variability of the larynx. That being said, cysts occur in all regions of the larynx, with retention types more frequent in the epiglottis, saccular cysts in the false cord, and traumatic type in the arytenoid region. The size of the cyst also depends on the location; small cysts are usually found on the vocal cords, while larger cysts are found attached to the epiglottis, pushing the larynx to one side, or projecting into the hypopharynx.[283-290] Eversion and prolapse of the ventricle and saccule have also been described, further complicating the classification of cysts of the larynx. The walls of the various cysts and/or laryngoceles may appear shiny and often thinned, containing fluctuant to firm contents, often streaked with blood vessels ranging in size from 0.5 cm to 8 cm. They are variably filled with thin serous fluid to tenacious thick, mucinous, gelatinous, or bloody fluid. They range from colorless to yellow, grey or red, and frequently are translucent.[283,285,286,289,290]

Microscopic Pathology

Cyst walls of fibrous connective tissue may vary in thickness. The lining helps to differentiate the cysts into a variety of subtypes. Most cysts are lined by squamous or respiratory epithelium (retention and saccular) (Fig. 8-55), while a few cysts are lined by fibrous connective tissue.[283,286,289] Those with an admixture of both mesodermal and endodermal layers qualify as congenital or embryonal cysts. This type of cyst contains squamous or respiratory epithelium along with some other mesodermal element, intimately associated with the epithelial component.[283,285,288,290,291] The microscopic appearance of rare vascular cysts formed by a localized collection of lymph or blood vessels in a subepithelial tissue

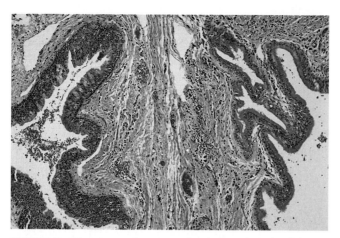

FIGURE 8–55. A saccular cyst is identified on the right of this photomicrograph with the normal respiratory epithelium identified on the left. Without the clinical information or any contents within the lumen a distinction cannot be made between a laryngocele and a laryngeal cyst on histology alone (H&E, × 75).

may be impossible to separate from a hemangioma, lymphangioma, or cystic hygroma.[291] The reimplantation or traumatic cyst is not common, but is described more frequently with increased surgical intervention in the larynx. Small islands of tissue are implanted deep in the stroma and undergo cystic degeneration. Any of the aforementioned cysts, when infected, are referred to as pyoceles, although still classified by the original cyst type. The larger the ventricular appendix, the more predisposed the individual is to infection or inflammation, which may be the presenting symptom.

Differential Diagnosis

The diagnosis of a laryngeal cyst is often straightforward by light microscopic evaluation. From a clinical standpoint, the differential diagnosis of laryngeal cysts may be rather involved. Histologic confirmation of the lesion is therefore mandatory to help define the type of cyst. A pharyngocele usually develops from the pyriform fossa, which should be suggested from the clinical examination, although it is frequently mistaken clinically for a laryngocele.[292,293] Prolapse of the ventricle can sometimes resemble a cyst on gross examination. However, prolapse can be replaced, while cysts cannot.[284] Large branchial cleft cysts and thyroglossal duct cysts may push into the laryngeal spaces, creating the illusion of a primary cyst of the larynx. Histologic examination, combined with the clinical site of origin, should help in distinguishing these other cysts of the region.[291,294] A dermoid cyst is generally thought to be a remnant of epithelial cells at the points of embryonic fusion or of displaced epithelium. A dermoid will generally contain two cell layers with mesenchymal and ectodermal structures.

This lesion is not a true teratoma, as it lacks all three layers and is different from the development cysts of the larynx.[291] An oncocytic cyst is merely a cyst of any type lined by cells with abundant eosinophilic cytoplasm.[283,285] External jugular phlebectasia (a congenital dilatation of the jugular vein) frequently presents as a neck mass, particularly during straining or crying (Valsalva's maneuver), similar to a laryngocele. Although often performed for cosmetic purposes, surgery is not required. The histologic appearance is of a dilated vascular space different from laryngocele or other laryngeal cysts.[295,296] Other clinical entities include laryngeal webs, vascular rings, hemangiomas, and foreign bodies. These entities can usually be excluded clinically or by biopsy.[81,290]

Clinicopathologic Correlation

Squamous cell carcinoma, usually supraglottic, can be associated with laryngoceles and may be induced by the carcinoma. Therefore, after surgical excision, it is important to exclude the possibility of a carcinoma, although laryngoceles are generally discovered during staging of a known cancer and are rarely the presenting symptom of a carcinoma.[287,297,298]

Hamartomas, Choristomas, and Ectopias

Gross Pathology

Hamartomas, choristomas, ectopias, and mesenchymomas are identified in the supraglottic and posterior commissure regions, although no region of the larynx or trachea is excluded. The lesions may have variable manifestations, encompassing a spherical, nodular, or polypoid mass; firm to soft; mobile or fixed; yellow, white, or red; measuring up to 5 cm in greatest dimension; often in a submucosal location. Without a characteristic gross appearance, histologic examination of the excised specimen is mandatory to confirm the diagnosis. Hamartomas have also been described in association with other congenital anomalies, including cleft larynx.[299–310]

Microscopic Pathology

Since a hamartoma is an excessive and abnormally arranged overgrowth of mature normal cells and tissues in an organ composed of the same cellular elements, it will have epithelial and mesenchymal components arranged in a haphazard fashion throughout the lesion. Squamous or respiratory-type epithelium, glandular elements (Fig. 8–56), adipose connective tissue, skeletal or smooth muscle, cartilage, fibrous connective tissue or collagen, nerves, lymphoid elements, and blood vessels can all be

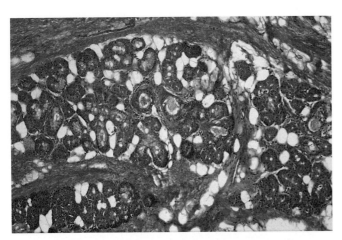

FIGURE 8–56. A collection of mucoserous glands out of proportion in number to that normally expected in the larynx comprises this hamartoma. No other elements are identified (H&E, × 75).

seen in variable combinations and degrees of disorganization. The lesions may not be encapsulated and will lack a demarcation from the rest of the tissue. Cartilaginous islands are frequently present, but in close approximation with other epithelial or mesenchymal elements.[302,306–311]

Choristoma and ectopic tissue represent tissues foreign to the location but normal in appearance. Any type of tissue may be present within these lesions, which usually can be separated from hamartomas, teratomas, and dermoid cysts by the type of tissue involved and the organization of the component parts. Thyroid may be present within the larynx or trachea if defects exist in these structures that allow the thyroid gland to protrude through.

A mesenchymoma is slightly different, having no epithelial component but at least two mesenchymal components not ordinarily found together, along with dense fibrous tissue. The most frequent mesenchymal elements are (in order of frequency) adipose tissue, smooth muscle, blood vessels, skeletal muscle, lymphoid and hematopoietic tissue, myxomatous tissue, and cartilage. These lesions may infiltrate into the surrounding tissues, but no malignant mesenchymoma has been described. In light of the insinuation, clear surgical margins must be obtained by wide excision.[300–302,304,312]

Differential Diagnosis

The differential diagnosis must include teratomas, dermoid cysts, chondroma, fibroma, and hemangiomas. An immature teratoma can be included in the differential diagnosis of hamartomas and ectopias. However, there are characteristically three germ layers represented—from ectoderm, mesoderm, and endoderm. All three germ layers should be identified before invoking the diagnosis of a teratoma, whether mature or immature. The tissues identified are usually foreign to the location, helping to exclude a hamartoma.[313–315] Rare examples of laryngeal blastoma occur, but this neoplasm has immature blastema-type tissue predominating, with transitions between blastemal, mesenchymal, and epithelial elements (similar to pulmonary blastoma).[316] A dermoid cyst has only two germ layers represented, including ectodermally derived squamous epithelium and keratin—usually the dominant finding—while cutaneous adnexa are found along the periphery. Since a choristoma represents tissues that are foreign to the location but normal in appearance, it usually can be readily separated from teratomas and dermoid cysts. A chondroma is a benign neoplastic proliferation of cartilage, demonstrating a well-circumscribed mass, often arising from cartilage (although soft-tissue forms have been noted) in the posterior subglottic region, without nuclear pleomorphism or other epithelial or mesenchymal elements.[317] Hemangiomas may be included in the differential diagnosis, but in contrast to hemangiomas, the vascular component in mesenchymomas is usually minor. If a single component of a hamartoma is dominant, such as the muscle component, other lesions such as rhabdoid tumor, granular cell tumor, or leiomyoma must be excluded. These lesions generally are made up of tumor cells only, while a hamartoma has a spectrum of various components.[299,318]

Tracheopathia Osteoplastica (Tracheobronchopathia Osteochondroplastica)

Gross Pathology

The mucosa is generally intact, stretched over a number of cartilaginous or bony nodules projecting into the lumen, usually sparing the posterior membranous portion of the tracheobronchial tree and frequently involving the bronchi. The bronchoscopic appearance is quite diagnostic. There is an overall rigidity to the trachea. Sometimes the radiographic appearance will demonstrate calcifications if ossification has occurred within the nodules.[128]

Microscopic Pathology

Heterotopic bone formation is seen in the soft tissue or stroma of the biopsy material (Fig. 8–57). These bony or cartilaginous protrusions often can be identified in continuity with the inner surface of the tracheal cartilage. The bony lamellae may protrude into the mucosa, thereby giving the characteristic appearance on bronchoscopy. The irregular bony spicules have thin walls surrounding fatty marrow. There is infrequent calcification and ossification of the trachea and larynx, most frequently seen in children.[319]

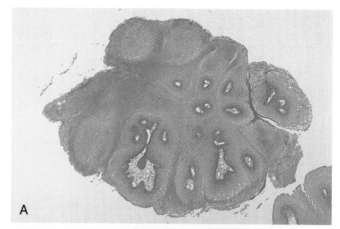

FIGURE 8–57. Submucosal bone deposition or metaplasia is found separated from the cartilage. This finding, combined with the clinical presentation, is distinctive for tracheopathia osteoplastica (H&E, × 15).

Differential Diagnosis

Although equally infrequent, laryngeal myositis ossificans can also be included in the differential diagnosis. The zonal phenomenon of a highly cellular inner zone with well-formed bone in the outer zone helps distinguish this lesion from tracheopathia osteoplastica. Difficulties may arise when the biopsy includes only material from the periphery or from the center of the lesion.[35,320] Bony stenosis as an isolated occurrence may also be seen, but it is generally associated with polyps or papillomas with associated chronic inflammation.[321]

In contrast to the rigidity of tracheopathia osteoplastica, tracheobronchiomegaly and tracheomalacia present with softening, flexibility, or dilatation of the trachea, resulting in obstructive symptoms. Tracheobronchiomegaly demonstrates absolute enlargement of the trachea and bronchi, with a histologic decrease in elastic longitudinal fibers and a thinning of the musculature of the tracheal wall.[73,322–324] Tracheomalacia is similar to laryngomalacia, where there is a softening of the cartilage or an abnormal pliability to the structure of the trachea. It may result from polychondritis or another disease entity.[73]

BENIGN NEOPLASMS

Papillomas

Gross Pathology

While papillomatosis can involve any part of the larynx, it most commonly begins in the glottis. The neoplasm forms glistening mulberry-like multinodular elevations that are grey to reddish-pink. The stalks may be narrowed or broad-based (Fig. 8–58A).

Microscopic Pathology

The histologic picture is that of rounded exophytic projections of nonkeratinizing squamous epithelium containing small fibrovascular stromal "cores" (Fig. 8–58B). The epithelium is moderately cellular and

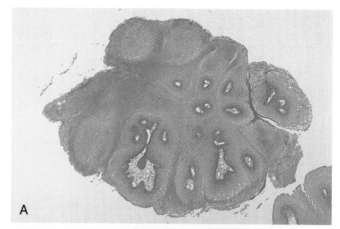

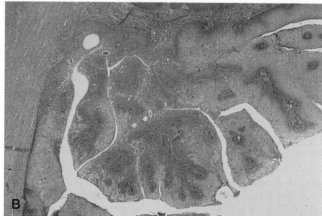

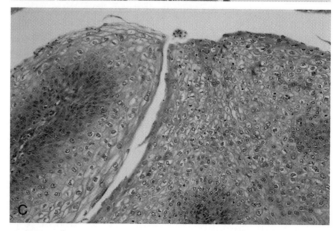

FIGURE 8–58. *A*, A low-power view of the fungiform growth pattern of a papilloma (H&E, × 30); *B*, The papillary fronds of this papilloma can be seen rising from a narrow stalk. There is an increase in the number of cell layers lining the filiform stalks (H&E, × 30); *C*, Koilocytic change (hyperchromatic nucleus with a perinuclear halo and prominent intracellular borders) can be quite prominent in many squamous papillomas of the larynx associated with human papilloma virus (H&E, × 150).

does not mature significantly from base to surface. Keratinization is typically absent, although there are occasional examples with minor amounts of keratin formation. Some degree of cytologic atypia is the rule rather than the exception.[327,328] In juveniles, even prominent atypia may occur and persist in recurrences without an apparent significantly increased risk of carcinomatous change (in the absence of prior irradiation). Although mitoses are infrequent, occasionally they may be easily found; their frequency may relate to degree of disease activity (i.e., frequency of recurrence of lesions and anatomic extent of involvement). In adults, especially older adults, prominent cytologic atypia should be interpreted circumspectly and cautiously with regard to possible premalignant or even malignant change. However, some adults have appreciable cytologic atypia in papillomas that does not necessarily imply malignancy.

Special Techniques

Many recent studies have concentrated on typing the human papilloma virus (HPV) genomes causing laryngeal papillomatosis. HPV generally causes a crenation of the nucleus with a perinuclear halo (cleared cytoplasm) with an accentuation of the cellular borders (Fig. 8–58C). The papillomavirus, part of the papovavirus family, is divided into a number of subtypes. The HPV virus can be detected by electron microscopy, immunohistochemical studies, polymerase chain reaction, in situ hybridization and dot blot analysis.[329,330,335–338] Type 6/11 is most common. Types 16 and 18 are possibly associated with more aggressive disease.[326,329,330,334,337,339] There are suggestions that viral typing may help delineate the risk of carcinomatous change subsequently occurring in the papillomatosis (primarily in adults), although viral typing and subtyping probably will continue to have only a limited role in the primary pathologic diagnosis of papillary or verruciform laryngeal lesions.[326,329,337,340] Since some laryngeal carcinomas contain an HPV genome, demonstrating the presence of such a genome is not significantly helpful (at this stage in the evolution of our knowledge) in determining whether or not an atypical papillary lesion is carcinomatous.[341]

Differential Diagnosis

The most important histologic differential diagnosis consists of distinguishing papillomatosis from benign hyperplasias (that may develop an irregular, slightly papillary architecture) and from verrucous carcinoma or papillary squamous cell carcinoma. The distinction of papilloma from hyperplasia rests on the lack of fibrovascular cores and the presentation of significant keratinization in hyperplasia. Papillomas usually have multiple small stromal fibrovascular cores and limited to absent keratinization.[342]

The distinction from a verrucous carcinoma can be made on the basis of three points. Verrucous carcinoma: (1) lacks the small fibrovascular stromal cores, (2) lacks the rounded surface projections of a papilloma and instead tends to have a filiform surface with sharply pointed projections, and (3) usually has very significant surface keratinization. Aside from rare instances of invasive papillomatosis, verrucous carcinoma differs from papillomatosis in the important point of having an invasive growth component.[331,333,343] However, this cannot reliably be judged from usually rather superficial laryngeal biopsies.

The diagnosis of atypical papilloma in older adults is a problematic type of lesion. Many of these subsequently prove to be, or perhaps develop into, carcinoma. It is likely that such lesions are very well-differentiated low-grade carcinomas from the outset and not papillomas.[344] This problem influences the statistics of how often papillomas might become carcinomatous in older adults, with the actual incidence probably much lower than is thought. The distinction of a well-differentiated papillary-verruciform squamous cell carcinoma from an atypical papilloma involves features similar to those already discussed—that is, the stromal cores of a papilloma and the dearth of keratinization in a papilloma. Papillary-verruciform carcinomas will frequently contain keratinization. Although a benign papilloma can have appreciable cytologic atypia, papillary-verruciform carcinomas sometimes have foci where the character of the dysplasia is much more than one would expect in a benign atypia.

Some papillary squamous cell carcinomas of the larynx have no keratinization, rounded surface projections, and a very papillary architecture. Such lesions can be especially difficult to distinguish from an atypical papilloma. Once again, the presence of the multiple small stroma cores of the papilloma can be helpful. However, confident distinction may rest on evaluating the subtle cytologic differences between the two types of lesions. Although benign papillomas can be moderately cellular, with the cells having a moderately increased N:C ratio, this ratio is usually higher for carcinomas. In the carcinoma, nuclei are more hyperchromatic and atypical. The mitotic rate for carcinomas may be higher than for papillomas, but not necessarily. Perhaps the most helpful feature in recognizing this type of carcinoma is the absence of normal maturation toward the surface, with a disordered growth pattern and a loss of nuclear "polarity," indicating a lack of "harmony" among the nuclei. Awareness of this potential pitfall in diagnosis dictates a cautious approach to each papillary laryngeal lesion with careful scrutiny to avoid misdiagnosis.

Clinicopathologic Correlation

Juvenile laryngeal papillomatosis is an important pediatric disease and represents the most common laryngeal neoplasm of children. The majority of the cases initially present in patients younger than 16 years, and more specifically in infants or children younger than 5 years. However, histologically identical tumors can develop at any age.[345] Laryngeal papillomata tend to recur numerous times and to become widespread and florid, extending into the tracheobronchial tree. This tendency for spread in adults, while significantly variable from patient to patient, is much less than it is in juveniles. An initial presentation in adulthood almost never becomes as florid as cases presenting in childhood.

Pleomorphic Adenoma (Benign Mixed Tumor)

Gross Pathology

The tumor usually presents as a subglottic or glottic mass, submucosal in location, focally cystic, measuring up to 4 cm in greatest dimension, although surface ulceration and resultant squamous metaplasia can be seen. The tumors are usually well-circumscribed, although often not encapsulated, with a rubbery consistency.[132,346-348]

Microscopic Pathology

The microscopic features of a pleomorphic adenoma are the same as would be expected in other locations. Tumors of the laryngeal minor salivary glands in general tend to be more cellular and contain less myxoid-chondroid material than their major gland counterparts. There may be a thin, delicate, fibrous capsule separating the tumor from the overlying epithelium and the rest of the submucosal tissues, although the capsule may be inconspicuous. Varying amounts of glandular, ductal, and squamous epithelial elements are intimately mixed with spindle, myxoid, and chondroid mesenchymal constituents. Morphologic diversity is the hallmark of pleomorphic adenoma, and few other neoplasms manifest a wider morphologic spectrum. Interlacing trabeculae or masses of loosely cohesive cells form numerous tubular or ductular structures (Fig. 8–59). Plump spindle-shaped cells or round cells with eosinophilic cytoplasm and eccentric nuclei (resembling plasma cells) may be the predominant feature. Atypical features are seen more frequently in the larynx due to the size of the biopsy taken (inadequate sampling of the tumor), nonencapsulation, and recurrence, which may be associated with incomplete excision.[346-351] Within the spectrum of pleomorphic adenoma is a myoepithelioma (myoepithelial proliferation without a biphasic appearance), which has been reported in the larynx but is exceptionally rare.[349]

Special Techniques

On the basis of H&E staining alone it may occasionally be difficult to distinguish these tumors from

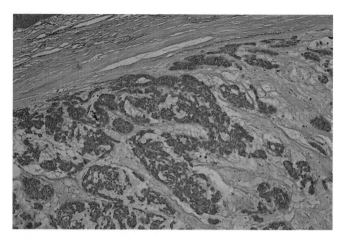

FIGURE 8–59. This pleomorphic adenoma (benign mixed tumor) is well circumscribed and contains an intimate admixture of epithelial cells floating in a chondroid-myxoid background matrix. A variety of architectural patterns is seen (H&E, × 75).

fibrous histiocytomas, neurilemmomas, or leiomyomas. Immunohistochemistry can be helpful, as myoepithelial cells are immunoreactive for keratin, S-100 protein, and smooth muscle actin and are sometimes reactive for glial fibrillary acidic protein and/or vimentin, while the epithelial cells are reactive with keratin.

Differential Diagnosis

Due to the extreme rarity of pleomorphic adenoma in the larynx, other lesions should be aggressively excluded. Direct extension of parotid gland tumors into the pharyngeal and hypopharyngeal space should be excluded. The differential diagnosis includes benign mesenchymal tumors (fibrous histiocytomas, neurilemmomas, or leiomyomas); malignant epithelial tumors (squamous cell carcinoma, mucoepidermoid carcinoma, mucinous adenocarcinoma, and adenoid cystic carcinoma); and mesenchymal tumors (chondrosarcoma). Fibrous histiocytomas, neurilemmomas, and leiomyomas do not usually demonstrate epithelial differentiation, nor will they be immunoreactive with keratin. Giant cells and xanthoma cells, peripheral palisading, and Verocay body formation and interlacing fascicles are not usually seen in a pleomorphic adenoma, while they are seen in the abovementioned benign mesenchymal tumors, respectively. Chondrosarcoma will likewise lack epithelial and myoepithelial differentiation both on histology and immunohistochemistries. Squamous metaplasia can be seen in pleomorphic adenomas as well as on the surface epithelium (depending on the location within the larynx), but is cytologically bland, a distinguishing feature from squamous cell carcinoma. Mucoepidermoid carcinoma and mucin-producing adenocarcinoma have no pseudocartilaginous matrix material. Adenoid cystic carcinoma tends to have an abrupt distinction between the stroma and the epithelial component, besides infiltrating into the surrounding tissues and presenting perineural invasion.[346,347,349–352] Although malignant mixed tumor of the vocal cord has been reported, the tumor may be an aggressive variant of squamous cell carcinoma, such as basaloid or adenosquamous, based on a review of the photographs and histologic description.[353]

Clinicopathologic Correlation

Pleomorphic adenomas of the larynx are nonencapsulated, may extend into surrounding tissues, and may recur after removal. Therefore, they have been confused with malignant tumors. Recurrences are generally associated with incomplete removal, often necessitating laryngectomy for adequate control of the benign tumor.

Granular Cell Tumor (Myoblastoma)

Gross Pathology

The tumor presents as a solitary polypoid or papillary to cystic, sessile lesion measuring up to 3 cm in maximum dimension (although most are less than 1 cm), with sporadic mucosal ulceration. The tumor is most frequently along the posterior true vocal cord, although any part of the larynx and trachea can be affected. The tumors are firm, pale white or grey-yellow, and homogenous on cut section.[132,354–359]

Microscopic Pathology

The tumors are usually unencapsulated and subepithelial in location, occasionally insinuating between the adjacent muscle fibers. A prominent pseudoepitheliomatous hyperplasia (PEH) is frequently seen in association with granular cell tumor, generally not extending beyond the limit of the lesion (Fig. 8–60A). The cells may be in close approximation with nerves, but this finding is not associated with malignancy. The cells are round to polygonal with hyperchromatic to vesicular nuclei enclosed by coarsely granular, faintly acidophilic, copious cytoplasm with indistinct cellular borders (Fig. 8–60B). The granules may aggregate to form large fragments within the cytoplasm (7μ). The cells are arranged in syncytial, trabecular, or nested growth patterns (see Fig. 8–60B). All of these patterns can be seen within a single tumor. Cellular pleomorphism may be marked, although uncommon, while necrosis and mitoses are ordinarily not seen. Angulate bodies (Bangle bodies, fibrillar bodies) can be seen in propinquity to vessels as PAS-positive needle-shaped bodies usually in spindle-shaped interstitial cells.[132,354–358,360]

Special Techniques

The granules within the cytoplasm are PAS-positive, diastase-resistant, and stain red with trichrome and

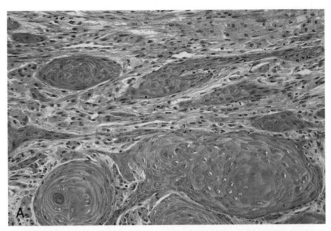
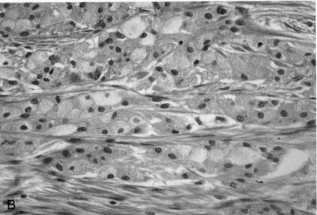
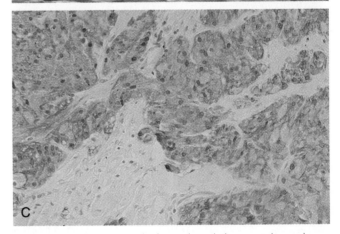

FIGURE 8–60. *A*, A marked pseudoepitheliomatous hyperplasia can obscure the underlying granular cell tumor, seen best at the top of this photomicrograph (H&E, × 150); *B*, The cells of a granular tumor are polygonal to spindled, with abundant, granular eosinophilic cytoplasm surrounding small to oval vesicular nuclei (H&E, × 300); *C*, Granular cell tumor cells will react strongly with S-100 protein immunohistochemical reaction (S-100 protein IHC, × 250).

blue with alcian blue at pH 2.5. Immunohistochemical stains show the granular cells to be immunopositive with S-100 protein (Fig. 8–60C), neuron-specific enolase, CD68, alpha-1-antitrypsin (A1AT), HLA-DR, and vimentin.[357,361–364] The reactivity with A1AT and CD68 may result from the intracytoplasmic accumulation of phagolysosomes and does not suggest a histiocytic origin, while HLA-DR expression may be associated with immunologic function.

If needed, ultrastructural studies will evince membrane-bound autophagic vacuoles with mitochondria, myelin figures, and myelinated and nonmyelinated lamellar mesoaxon-type structures. Angulate bodies, found in spindled cells, are elongated inclusions surrounded by a membrane, composed of a meshwork of fibrils and microtubules with a slightly beaded appearance.[355,357,360,361]

Differential Diagnosis

A malignant granular cell tumor is usually larger than 4 cm with histologic features of increased cellularity, prominent nucleoli, spindled cells, pleomorphism, necrosis, and increased mitotic figures, with obvious infiltration into skeletal muscle. Adequate biopsy size and sufficient sections of the tumor may be required to separate benign from malignant gran-

ular cell tumors, especially in clinically worrisome cases.[361,365] Although a granular cell tumor itself does not evoke the differential diagnosis of squamous cell carcinoma, the associated PEH can cause a mistaken diagnosis. PEH has fingers of epithelium that invade deep into the underlying stroma, but has no cytologic evidence of carcinoma. The lack of atypical cytologic features, a desmoplastic stromal response and inflammatory response, and rare mitotic figures should exclude a squamous cell carcinoma.[354,357] A rhabdomyoma, adult type, has polygonal cells with granular cytoplasm but has cytoplasmic vacuolization; a phosphotungstic acid–hematoxylin stain will readily demonstrate cross-striations. Desmin and myoglobin immunoreactivity will confirm the diagnosis. The fetal type of rhabdomyoma generally has immature spindle cells with a myxoid stroma and is rarely mistaken for a granular cell tumor. An alveolar soft-part sarcoma is arranged in a nested, alveolar, or organoid pattern with vascular channels and septa (Fig. 8–61A). Its cells have distinct borders containing eccentrically placed nuclei with prominent nucleoli surrounded by finely granular eosinophilic cytoplasm with frequent mitotic figures (Fig. 8–61B). The characteristic association with skeletal muscle, combined with immunoreactivity with desmin and muscle-specific actin, should help exclude this possibility.[366,367]

Paraganglioma

Gross Pathology

The gross appearance is generally a submucosal supraglottic smooth elevation, with an intact mucosa, often bluish or reddish in appearance, more frequently on the right side, ranging in size up to 6 cm. The tumor is usually encapsulated, separated from the tissues by a dense fibrous connective tissue, although this can be variable and not duplicated on microscopic sections. The tumors can be firm and rubbery or spongy with a nodular cut surface, periodically intersected with fibrous connective tissue and hemorrhage. The tumors are rarely functional or multiple.[368–373]

Microscopic Pathology

The cells of a paraganglioma are believed to be derived from the laryngeal nonchromaffin paraganglia (neural tissue), of which there are two pairs—a superior and an inferior set.[368] The tumor cells are arranged in characteristic cell nests (zellballen) or alveolar clusters, separated by a fibrovascular stroma (Fig. 8–62A). Capillaries are usually found within the fibrovascular septa, while thick-walled vessels are present in the fibrous connective tissue trabeculae, occasionally exposing hemosiderin pigment. There are generally two constituent cells in this neoplasm: polygonal to spindle-shaped chief

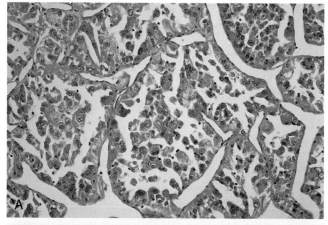

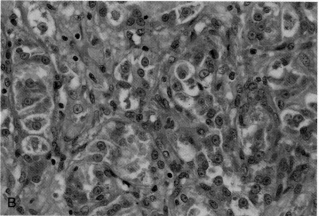

FIGURE 8–61. *A,* An alveolar soft part sarcoma is arranged in an alveolar pattern of growth, lined by eosinophilic cells with hyperchromatic to vesicular irregular nuclei (H&E, × 150); *B,* On higher power, the cells of an alveolar soft part sarcoma are arranged in small packages and have prominent nucleoli within the vesicular nuclei, while the cytoplasm has crystalline structures (H&E, × 300).

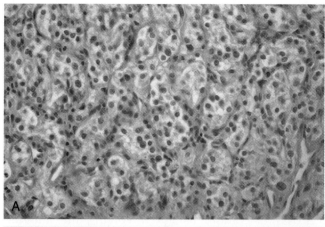

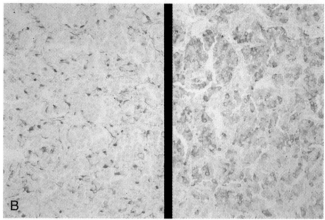

FIGURE 8–62. *A,* The characteristic "zellballen" growth pattern of a paraganglioma. The cells have slightly basophilic cytoplasm surrounding variably sized basophilic nuclei. The supporting sustentacular cells are not easily identified (H&E, × 300); *B,* The supporting sustentacular cells react with S-100 protein (*left,* S-100 protein [IHC] × 150), while the chief cells will react with chromogranin (*right,* chromogranin [IHC] × 150) in this laryngeal paraganglioma.

cells (with abundant pale eosinophilic to granular or cleared cytoplasm surrounding central, round to oval, vesicular to hyperchromatic nuclei), and spindled sustentacular cells (found at the periphery of the nests and composing the supporting framework of the tumor) (see Fig. 8–62*A*). The sustentacular cells are generally inconspicuous to absent and difficult to identify on standard H&E preparations. Mitotic activity can be seen but is rarely increased beyond two mitoses per 10 high-power fields. Necrosis is almost entirely absent and only rarely identified. Vascular or perineural invasion does not correlate with malignant behavior or a more biologically aggressive tumor.[368–375]

Special Techniques

The nested pattern of growth can be identified in other neoplasms, so the diagnosis of laryngeal paraganglioma is best supported by additional studies.

The chief cells are argyrophilic (brown to black intracytoplasmic granules within the cytoplasm with Grimelius stain) but not argentaffinic (negative Fontana-Masson stain). A reticulin stain demonstrates the nested growth pattern by outlining the fibrovascular stroma surrounding the nests of cells, rather than individual cell investment. There is a lack of epithelial mucin as demonstrated by either a mucicarmine or a periodic acid-Schiff stain.[369–373]

The chief cells will display immunoreactivity for chromogranin (Fig. 8–62*B*), synaptophysin, serotonin, and neuron-specific enolase, generally without reactivity for cytokeratin, calcitonin, carcinoembryonic antigen, GFAP, and desmin. The supporting sustentacular cells (nuclear and cytoplasmic) are accentuated by S-100 protein reactivity (see Fig. 8–62*B*). There have been numerous reports documenting a variety of other chief cell immunohistochemical reactions, but many of these reactions are nonspecific and will not be presented here. While cytokeratin has been reported rarely to occur in paragangliomas, this finding is most unusual and should instigate an investigation of a different type of neuroendocrine tumor (i.e., neuroendocrine carcinoma or carcinoid).[373,375–377] Initial studies seem to indicate that paragangliomas with sparse to absent sustentacular cells and scant immunoreactivity tend to behave more aggressively.[377,378]

Because the immunohistochemical profile can separate out the other neuroendocrine tumors from paraganglioma, electron microscopy is seldom needed. Ultrastructural analysis will illustrate membrane-bound dense-core neurosecretory granules and rare junctional desmosome-like complexes within the chief cells. However, these features do not discriminate between neuroendocrine carcinoma, carcinoid tumors, or paraganglioma. The sustentacular cells may or may not be identified.[371,377]

Differential Diagnosis

The differential diagnosis includes other neuroendocrine lesions, including carcinoid, atypical carcinoid, neuroendocrine carcinoma, medullary thyroid carcinoma, malignant melanoma (mucosal and secondary), extramedullary plasmacytoma, alveolar soft-part sarcoma, metastatic carcinoma, and hemangiopericytoma. These will be discussed in more detail in the section on neuroendocrine carcinoma, but a brief mention of the major differences in paraganglioma will be presented here.

Atypical carcinoid usually grows in a trabecular, cribriform, or solid pattern; an organoid or insular growth pattern is seen only infrequently, with the cells expressing pleomorphism from a mild to marked degree. Glandular differentiation is often seen (with positive mucicarmine reaction). Atypical carcinoid will manifest metastases, while in paraganglioma only rarely has metastatic disease been documented. Atypical carcinoid will usually present immunoreactivity with cytokeratin, CEA, and calcitonin, and rarely with S-100 protein (although not in a sustentacular cell pattern). These difference should help to distinguish atypical carcinoid from paraganglioma.

A small cell neuroendocrine carcinoma is an aggressive neoplasm, frequently demonstrating marked nuclear pleomorphism, necrosis, mitoses, and a different immunohistochemical reactivity than paraganglioma. Although it is academically sound to distinguish categories in the neuroendocrine tumors, it is much more realistic to view these tumors of the larynx in a spectrum, with the benign paraganglioma falling outside the spectrum of carcinoid, atypical carcinoid, and neuroendocrine carcinoma. The distinction between paraganglioma and neuroendocrine carcinoma should be easily established. When a diagnostic dilemma arises, cytokeratin is the most useful ancillary test to help distinguish between these two lesions.[368,370,373–375]

Medullary carcinoma of the thyroid gland may extend into the larynx or have laryngeal metastases. These tumors will generally be in a subglottic location and demonstrate amyloid material coupled with CEA, calcitonin, and cytokeratin immunoreactivity. An elevated serum level of calcitonin can be seen in thyroid medullary carcinoma and in primary neuroendocrine carcinomas of the larynx. Documentation of a negative thyroid scan or radiograph and discovery of a laryngeal lesion will help with this differential diagnostic dilemma.[379,380]

Malignant melanoma, both primary and secondary, can be distinguished by the prominent nucleolus, intranuclear cytoplasmic inclusions, and immunoreactivity with S-100 protein and HMB-45 in the tumor cells. Paragangliomas are not melanocytic in nature and will therefore not mark with HMB-45. A plasmacytoma is generally in a sheet-like or solid growth pattern, with a slightly different nuclear chromatin distribution. Plasmacytoma will frequently demonstrate light chain restriction or present with clinical manifestations and can be confirmed with serum or urine electrophoresis. Hemangiopericytoma is exceptionally rare and is a pattern diagnosis. The cells of a hemangiopericytoma will be encircled by reticulin, in addition to being negative for most immunomarkers except CD34 or CD31, which can be helpful in defining this entity.

Although the literature is replete with reports of malignant laryngeal paragangliomas, we believe that they are inaccurately classified neuroendocrine carcinomas or atypical carcinoids. If the lesions are correctly classified, there is a less than 2% metastatic potential in paragangliomas of the larynx.[368–370,373,381]

Clinicopathologic Correlation

Paragangliomas generally have a more benign clinical course and are the only tumor of the neuroendocrine system that is more frequent in females. An accurate diagnosis and distinction from other neuroendocrine tumors is essential in order to provide

appropriate treatment and suggest the more benign biologic behavior.

Chondroma

Gross Pathology

A chondroma is generally a lobulated, firm to hard, smooth and sessile, blue-grey, solitary submucosal mass usually less than 2 cm in size involving any of the laryngeal cartilages—most frequently the cricoid and thyroid cartilages and less frequently the tracheal rings (Fig. 8–63A). The tumors are usually on the endolaryngeal surface of these cartilages without mucosal ulceration, usually involving the anterior surface of the posterior lamina of the cricoid. The mucosal vessels may be engorged or prominent. Rarely a patient may present with a hard, nontender mass in the neck that is fixed to the larynx. Equally unusual is a chondroma attached to the vocal cord.[22,317,382–393]

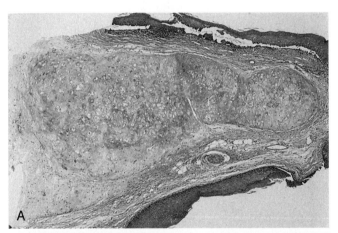

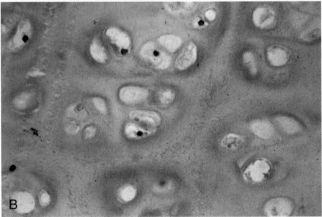

FIGURE 8–63. A, An abnormal proliferation of cartilage cells is seen in this low-power micrograph, but the mass is well delineated and hypocellular, similar to normal cartilage (H&E, × 30); B, High-power view of a chondroma reveals the small nuclei with the lacuna spaces without an increased nuclear : cytoplasmic ratio and no nuclear atypia (H&E, × 400).

Microscopic Pathology

Chondromas display cytologically bland chondrocytes growing in a fashion reminiscent of normal cartilage, either hyaline or elastic. The growth is confined to the perichondrium, which is still intact. The cells are found within lacunae that are widely separated by cartilaginous hyaline or fibroelastic substance. The cells are small, with hyperchromatic nuclei surrounded by clear cytoplasm (Fig. 8–63B). Only rarely are double-nucleated cells seen; in these cases the nuclei are still small and hyperchromatic. No giant cells are identified. There may be areas of calcification or ossification in addition to some areas of myxomatous degeneration.[22,317,382,384–389,391–393]

Differential Diagnosis

The principle differential diagnosis rests with chondrosarcoma, although cartilaginous hamartoma, teratoma, pleomorphic adenoma, amyloid tumor, chordoma, peripheral nerve sheath tumor, and tracheopathia osteoplastica are also included in the broader differential for this tumor.

Chondrosarcomas usually have increased cellularity, atypical cells, binucleated forms, and mitotic figures. The very low-grade chondrosarcoma may be extraordinarily difficult to distinguish from chondroma, but complete surgical excision is generally adequate treatment for both these lesions, with clinical follow-up suggested to identify local recurrence, as low-grade chondrosarcomas rarely, if ever, metastasize. Even though the distinction may be impossible in some cases, adequate surgical treatment is necessary as the airway compromise of either tumor can cause the patient's death.

Hamartomas are much more common in the location of Reinke's space, although a chondroma may arise in this soft-tissue location. It is prudent to consider the lesions of this soft-tissue location as hamartoma rather than chondroma; the latter is usually attached to a cartilage of the larynx, with vocal cord lesions an exception. Teratoma will contain all three germ layers, including immature blastema-type tissues, usually not identified in chondroma. Pleomorphic adenoma will have both epithelial and myoepithelial cells present in the myxoid-chondroid matrix material; this will exclude chondroma. The acellular, eosinophilic matrix material of an amyloid tumor, often rich in inflammatory cells, combined with a positive reaction with a Congo red stain, will eliminate chondroma. Chordoma will demonstrate nests of tumor cells arranged in trabeculae, myxoid or cartilaginous matrix material, and the characteristic physaliferous cells (bubbly cytoplasm surrounding indented nuclei). The keratin, along with the S-100 protein reactivity of these cells, will help to exclude a chondroma. A peripheral nerve sheath tumor (neurilemmoma) may have myxoid degeneration, but the nuclei are palisaded, there is a lack of lacunae, and the cells are generally spindled. Laryngeal

cysts (of all types) will generally have an epithelial lining, although laryngoceles may be air-filled and not specifically lined. This should rule out a chondroma, which generally does not have an epithelial lining of a cystic space. Tracheopathia osteoplastica has a characteristic clinical presentation with multiple submucosal nodules and, generally, attachment to the cartilages.[317,382,384,386,391–393]

Rhabdomyoma

Gross Pathology

The tumor is generally divided into two subtypes based on histologic features, not upon the patient's age at presentation. The adult-type rhabdomyoma is usually a well-delineated (nonencapsulated), solitary, smooth, submucosal mass. It may be lobulated, polypoid, or pedunculated and is tan-yellow to deep grey-red-brown. They may measure up to 7.5 cm in greatest dimension, although usually in the 1 to 3 cm range. The lesion is most frequent in the hypopharynx or supraglottis and vocal cord. The cut surface is circumscribed, rubbery, and pink-brown. The fetal-type rhabdomyoma is a solitary circumscribed polypoid nodule, measuring up to 8 cm in greatest dimension, (with an average of 3 cm), pink-tan to grey-white, with an overall mucoid-myxoid or cystic appearance. The tumor is usually submucosal, involving the true or false vocal cord, although the surface epithelium may be ulcerated, depending on the extent of tumor growth.[394–405]

Microscopic Pathology

The adult-type rhabdomyoma may be covered by granulation tissue, depending upon the degree of surface ulceration. Adult rhabdomyomas show numerous nests or lobules of large polygonal, globular, round, or spindled rhabdomyoblasts with abundant pale, eosinophilic, granular cytoplasm. The cells contain one or more peripherally encountered vesicular nuclei (Fig. 8–64A). The nuclei may contain conspicuous nucleoli, often peripherally located within the nuclei. One or more cytoplasmic vacuoles, typical for the neoplasm, may be identified in many cells, related to the removal of glycogen during processing. A "spider-web" appearance may be imparted to the cells if the strands of cytoplasm are accentuated between vacuoles. Mitoses are usually absent or scarce. The neoplastic cells are usually seen in a fibrous stroma, occasionally showing myxoid changes.

The fetal-type rhabdomyoma (either myxoid or cellular) is usually circumscribed, occasionally seeming to infiltrate into the surrounding tissue. It is composed of undifferentiated or primitive mesenchymal spindle cells and immature muscle fibers (myoblasts) within a rich myxoid stroma (Fig. 8–64B). A maturation phenomenon may occur within

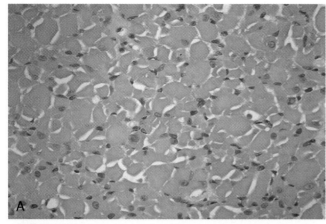

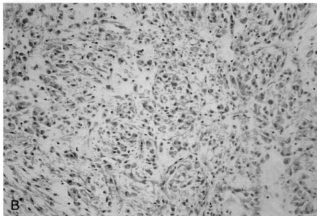

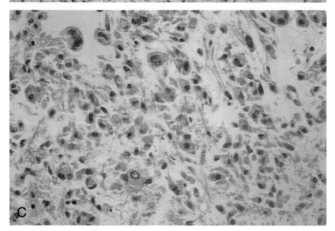

FIGURE 8–64. *A*, Adult-type rhabdomyoma is composed of sheets of mature-appearing muscle cells with peripherally placed nuclei and abundant eosinophilic cytoplasm (not granular) (H&E, × 300); *B*, Juvenile rhabdomyomas are quite cellular, recapitulating early embryonic development of skeletal muscle. The cells are arranged haphazardly, demonstrating wispy or tapered eosinophilic cytoplasm (H&E, × 150); *C*, Although there is nuclear pleomorphism and variability to some of the cells, there is no mitotic activity, no true necrosis, and no infiltrative growth pattern. The cells have tapered or eccentric eosinophilic cytoplasm (H&E, × 300).

this tumor, with the periphery demonstrating mature muscle fiber differentiation and the center being packed with immature mesenchymal cells. The ground substance, rich in acid mucopolysaccharides,

is more conspicuous in the center of the tumor. The cells are arranged in haphazard irregular bundles, with the cells demonstrating focally enlarged nuclei, irregular nuclear contours, and a variable amount of eosinophilic cytoplasm (Fig. 8–64C). Similar to the adult-type rhabdomyoma, mitoses, necrosis, and cellular pleomorphism are absent. This tumor is usually not a diagnostic dilemma in the larynx, as a fetal-type rhabdomyoma in that location is unique in histology and rare in occurrence.[394,395,397,398,400,406,407]

Special Techniques

A phosphotungstic acid–hematoxylin stain will reveal the cross-striations that are characteristic of adult-type rhabdomyoma. PAS-positive, diastase-sensitive cytoplasmic granules of glycogen can also be demonstrated, while crystal-like, rod-shaped particles can be seen in the cytoplasm of some cells.[394–396,398–403,405,407,408]

Cross-striations are usually difficult to define in fetal-type rhabdomyoma, although ganglion-like strap cells or rhabdomyoblasts can be seen, especially with a Masson's trichrome or PTAH stain.

Desmin, myoglobin, smooth muscle actin (SMA), and muscle-specific actin immunoreactivity can be demonstrated in adult-type rhabdomyoma cells, although the SMA may be rare. S-100 and Leu-7 can also be found, but reactivity is usually weak and focal. In addition to these antibodies, vimentin and fetal myosin are reactive in immature or fetal-type rhabdomyomas. Vimentin reactivity is variable, focal, and/or weak.

If ultrastructural investigation is needed, hypertrophied Z-bands with myofilament attachment and actin filaments will be identified. Myofilaments arranged in a haphazard fashion with abnormally hypertrophied Z-bands, represent the crystal-like structures seen on light microscopy. Occasional cells will illustrate more fully organized parallel arrays of cross-striations. Glycogen granules can also be detected, along with free ribosomes.[396–400,406,407,409]

Differential Diagnosis

Granular cell tumor, oncocytoma, paraganglioma, hibernoma, and alveolar soft-part sarcoma are the usual differential diagnoses for adult-type rhabdomyoma, while myxoid polyp, hamartoma, and rhabdomyosarcoma are included in the differential for fetal-type rhabdomyoma. Granular cell tumor demonstrates a similar histologic appearance to adult-type rhabdomyoma in the cytoplasm of the cells, although the cells are arranged in a syncytium, lack transverse cross-striations, and have no cytoplasmic glycogen or rod-shaped crystals. S-100 protein reactivity and a lack of desmin or myoglobin reactivity, combined with a lack of contractile elements on ultrastructural study, should help to separate these neoplasms. Overlying surface pseudoepitheliomatous hyperplasia is not seen in rhabdomyoma. The cells of an oncocytoma are filled with mitochondria that can be disclosed with histochemical (PAS-positive, diastase-resistant and PTAH or Luxol Fast Blue reactive), immunohistochemical (cytokeratin reactivity and S-100 protein negativity) or electronmicroscopy studies (cytoplasm stuffed with abnormal mitochondria). A paraganglioma has a slightly different architectural arrangement, with an organoid growth pattern, lined by cells with a more basophilic granular cytoplasm. Immunoreactivity with chromogranin in the tumor cells and S-100 protein in the sustentacular cells will discriminate between these tumors. Hibernoma contains distinct cell borders, and although the cytoplasm may be granular, it contains small uniform lipid vacuoles. An alveolar soft-part sarcoma has an alveolar growth pattern, generally displaying slightly greater nuclear pleomorphism and prominent nucleoli. The immunoreactivity is similar, but the crystals of rhabdomyoma are not identified in an alveolar soft-part sarcoma.[395,397,401,405,409,410]

A myxoid polyp will usually have scant cellularity and will certainly not demonstrate desmin reactivity, as is expected with myxoid fetal-type rhabdomyoma. The muscle components of a hamartoma are usually more mature than those of a fetal rhabdomyoma, which will help differentiate between these tumors. Embryonal rhabdomyosarcoma is the most frequent tumor to be distinguished from fetal-type rhabdomyoma. Nuclear and cellular pleomorphism, mitotic activity, and necrosis in a rhabdomyosarcoma will allow separation of these tumors, as will the invasive growth and destruction of the adjacent tissues. Strap cells, or cells with cross-striations, are extremely rare in rhabdomyosarcoma.[395,397,405,406,407.]

Clinicopathologic Correlation

Rhabdomyomas of the heart are usually associated with tuberous sclerosis, but this has not been documented with laryngeal lesions of the adult type.[395,405,408] Multifocal disease may also be seen with laryngeal lesions and should be ruled out in other locations.[400,404,411,412] These lesions are thought to be neoplasms based conclusively on recent documentation of a chromosomal translocation, t(15;17), rather than the cardiac hamartoma associated with tuberous sclerosis.[396]

Lipoma

Gross Pathology

Lipomas can arise in the supraglottis, hypopharynx, retropharynx or postcricoid region, and anywhere along the tracheobronchial tree, although the supraglottic larynx seems to be slightly more common. A lipoma is usually a solitary, smooth, submucosal pink-to-yellow, soft, rubbery mass, measuring up to 20 cm in maximum dimension, often pedunculated and mobile, causing occlusion of the larynx. The cut surface is yellow, fatty, greasy, and often surrounded by a capsule. The tumor is generally covered by an intact squamous epithelium.[132,413-420]

Microscopic Pathology

There is generally a circumscription or encapsulation to this benign tumor, but it may not be obvious, depending upon the type of resection. The microscopic appearance is of mature adipose cells arranged in a fine, often compressed, vascular network intersected by a reticular, collagenous, fibrous connective tissue, creating lobules of adipocytes. The lipocytes are uniform in appearance without evidence of atypia (Fig. 8-65). Minimal inflammation may be present, consisting of lymphocytes and plasma cells. Foci of myxoid stroma and areas of spindle-cell change can be seen. Secondary changes of hemorrhage, calcification, osseous or chondroid metaplasia, cyst formation, and infarction may be seen. The tumors do not contain lipoblasts, nor is there evidence of infiltration into the surrounding stroma. In the truest sense of the word, laryngeal lesions are really fibrolipomas, as there is a rich investment by fibrous connective tissue. (This is an academic distinction with no clinical implications.) A clinical correlation is needed, especially when adipose tissue is the only constituent, as it is a normal element of this region. To that end, radiographic imaging, especially. with MR or CT will document the lipomatous nature and extent of the mass.[413-415,417,419-422]

Special Techniques

While adipocytes have characteristic findings on histochemical (oil red-O, Sudan black), immunohistochemical (vimentin and S-100 protein), and electron

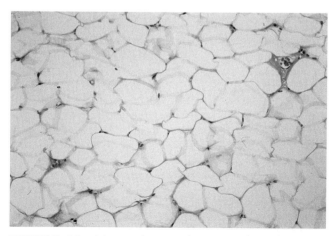

FIGURE 8-65. Mature adipose and compressed vessels are all that can be seen in a lipoma (H&E, × 150).

microscopy (central lipid vacuole with compressed peripheral nucleus), these adjuvant diagnostic aids are unnecessary for the diagnosis of a lipoma.

Differential Diagnosis

The major differential diagnostic dilemma arises with liposarcoma, especially well-differentiated liposarcoma. Myxoma, hamartoma, hibernoma, and chordoma are also included in the diagnostic differential. Liposarcoma will be discussed in depth in a later section, but generally it can be distinguished from lipoma by the identification of lipoblasts, an increased cellularity, nuclear pleomorphism, mitotic figures, and an infiltrative pattern with necrosis. While lipomas may have areas of myxoid change, a myxoma does not have fibrovascular septa, frequently contains mast cells mixed in with the stellate cells, and will usually have an unencapsulated "infiltrative" periphery. Hamartomas will usually have a haphazard arrangement of elements from all three germ layers, not just mature adipose tissue. A myxoid vocal cord polyp does not usually contain mature adipose tissue, but instead has a loose stroma. A hibernoma is composed of "brown fat," usually in the lateral neck, composed of cells with a finely reticulated cytoplasm filled with tiny lipid droplets. Chordoma (thought to be associated with notochord remnants) will demonstrate nests of tumor cells, vacuolization of the nuclei and cytoplasm, myxoid or cartilaginous matrix material, and characteristic physaliferous cells (bubbly cytoplasm surrounding indented nuclei). The keratin, along with the S-100 protein reactivity of these cells, help to exclude a lipoma.[22,34,410]

Clinicopathologic Correlation

Lipomas of the larynx have been found in association with symmetric lipomatosis.[423,424] Myxolipoma, fibrolipoma, infiltrating lipoma, and spindle cell lipoma in the larynx have been described but are rare. The interested reader is referred to a number of excellent reviews on the subject.[217,415,421,425–430]

Hemangioma

Gross Pathology

Hemangiomas in the pediatric population are more common in the posterior lateral subglottic area (Fig. 8–66A) while the vocal cords and supraglottic region predominate in adults. The gross appearance ranges from a diffuse flat mass to a bulging polypoid nodule, soft and compressible, usually submucosal with rare surface epithelial ulceration. The mass is pink-red to blue or grey-purple, often depending upon the degree of vascular congestion. The gross appearance of an adult hemangioma may mimic a hemorrhagic polyp; sessile lesions are more common in children. If the lesion is biopsied rather than excised, unusually excessive bleeding may suggest the type of lesion encountered.[19,22,84,132,431–435]

Microscopic Pathology

Hemangiomas can be divided into capillary (see Fig. 8–66A) and cavernous types (Fig. 8–66B) based on their histologic features; hemangiomatosis is a more widespread lesion involving contiguous structures around the larynx or the same tissue in multiple sites.[436,437] Hemangiomas demonstrate submucosal vascular spaces of variable sizes arranged in a circumscribed, although not encapsulated, architectural arrangement. Capillaries, veins, and arteries can be found in hemangiomas (an elastic stain will highlight the elastic lamina in the arteries). The vascular spaces are lined by benign-appearing endothelial cells, intersected by fibrous connective tissue, with

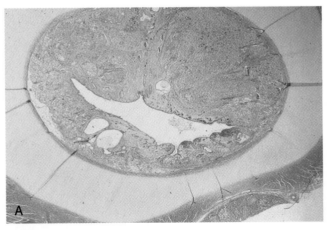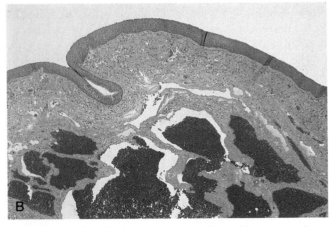

FIGURE 8–66.   *A*, Juvenile-type hemangiomas are usually found, as shown, in a subglottic location. A rich vascular proliferation can be seen growing into the laryngeal lumen (H&E, × 15); *B*, A cavernous hemangioma will reveal large dilated vascular spaces with intact surface epithelium. This type is more frequent in adults (H&E, × 30).

erythrocytes within the luminal spaces (see Fig. 8–66B). Mucous gland hyperplasia can also be identified in the background. Hemorrhage into the stroma is frequently seen, as is a variably intense chronic inflammatory infiltrate. Juvenile types of hemangioma are generally more cellular than adult types, the latter more often classified as cavernous hemangiomas.[19,22,132,431,434] Hemangiomatosis may frequently contain adipose tissue, suggesting a hamartomatous lesion rather than an exclusively vascular proliferation.[436]

Differential Diagnosis

Hemangiomas should be distinguished on histologic examination from telangiectasia, angiomatosis, vascular polyps (hemorrhagic type), granulation tissue, papillary endothelial hyperplasia, and other vascular neoplasms (lymphangioma, angiosarcoma).[30,438] The increased cellularity of pediatric hemangioma can often mimic angiosarcoma. However, angiosarcomas are very rare in children, usually have an anastamosing pattern of vascular channels with intraluminal tufting containing marked nuclear pleomorphism and frequent mitotic figures.[431,438] A laryngeal polyp generally has considerably less vascularity than a hemangioma, without the true neoplastic growth of vessels, but with more of a dilatation of the vessels that are present. Intravascular angiomatosis or organization within a thrombus can present with freely anastamosing vascular channels lined by endothelial cells with papillary projections. This lesion is more frequently misdiagnosed as angiosarcoma than hemangioma, but the thrombus and papillary growth pattern will help distinguish between these lesions.[132,439] The distinction between a hemangioma and telangiectasia may be difficult. However, in the correct clinical setting of a family history of hereditary hemorrhagic telangiectasia (Rendu-Osler-Weber [ROW] syndrome), typical lesions (in any location) and episodic bleeding can help to define ROW syndrome. Lesions are more often found in the pharynx than in the larynx.[440] If a hemangioma is identified in the larynx, the patient may have cutaneous hemangioma or other systemic diseases (e.g., Sturge-Weber disease and von Hippel-Lindau disease).[84]

Lymphangiomas (filled with thin, clear lymph fluid, nonerythrocyte-containing, with benign endothelial cell-lined spaces) can occur in the larynx but are extraordinary lesions. The distinction between a cystic hygroma with involvement of the larynx versus a primary lymphangioma underscores a semantic and clinical dilemma in this entity. The exact anatomic location and adequate neck examination are needed to exclude a primary lymphangioma.[19,132,418,441,442] Epithelioid hemangioma, bacillary angiomatosis, and other vascular lesions are included in the histologic differential diagnosis but have not been described in the larynx, warranting a mention only. Additional information is available in a review of the topic.[44,45,443]

Hemangiopericytoma

Gross Pathology

A supraglottic cyst-like mass is usually identified with a vascular-type appearance, although subglottic and tracheal lesions have been described. The mass is firm, solid, pedunculated or nodular, usually well-circumscribed, in a submucosal location, measuring up to 4 cm in greatest dimension. The surface is covered by an intact epithelium with dilated vessels, while the cut surface has a pale yellow-tan appearance.[444–448]

Microscopic Pathology

The tumors are generally quite well-circumscribed but not truly encapsulated. The pericytic cells are arranged in a streaming or whorling fashion, with thin-walled or endothelial-lined vascular spaces separating the tumor cells. These vessels have been described as having a "staghorn," antler, or branching configuration. The lesional cells are generally small, round to spindled, with oval to round vesicular nuclei surrounded by indistinct eosinophilic cytoplasm. A reticulin stain accentuates each individual cell or a very small group of cells, with the lesional cells located outside the basement membrane of the capillary. Mast cells can be seen sprinkled throughout the tumor. Mitotic activity is infrequent.[444–449] An increased cellularity with mitotic activity (>4 per 10 high-power fields), cellular pleomorphism, associated intratumoral hemorrhage, and necrosis (perhaps related to thrombosis) are features that have been associated with recurrences or metastases in other anatomic locations and may also apply in the larynx, although the criteria are not clear-cut.[449] Many of the tumors have recurred, with occasional metastases. However, there are so few reports in the literature that it may not be prudent to suggest a clinical outcome based on the histologic features alone.[450]

Special Studies

Immunohistochemical reactions for vimentin, factor XIIIa, CD31, CD34, CD57 (Leu-7), and class II major histocompatibility complex antigens have demonstrated tumor cell positivity, but there is no specific immunohistochemistry panel that is specific for this lesion. These reactions are usually different from true pericytic cells, raising the question of the origin of this tumor type. In any event, the tumor cells lack immunodeterminants of epithelial, neural, or myogenous differentiation.[449,451]

Although ultrastructural analysis is not specific for HPC, it will demonstrate tumor cells immediately surrounding the vascular spaces, containing rough endoplasmic reticulum, ribosomes, and mitochondria with a surrounding basal lamina, while lacking neurosecretory granules. There may also be areas of transition between pericytes, endothelial cells, smooth muscle cells, and fibroblasts, suggesting a relationship between these neoplasms or patterns within tumors.[447,452]

Differential Diagnosis

Controversy abounds in the literature relating to HPC-like growth and a true HPC. Hemangiopericytoma-like growth patterns can be seen in a number of different tumors and occasionally represent the dominant growth pattern. Therefore, it may be prudent to exclude the tumors in the differential diagnosis, using HPC as a diagnosis of exclusion. The differential diagnosis includes hemangioma, angiosarcoma, glomus tumor, fibrous histiocytoma, leiomyoma, synovial sarcoma, malignant melanoma, leiomyosarcoma, spindle squamous cell carcinoma, and mesenchymal chondrosarcoma.[447,449,451]

Angiosarcoma generally demonstrates a much more marked degree of cellular pleomorphism, with endothelial tufting and mitotic figures. The infiltrative nature of the tumor should be helpful in distinguishing between these lesions. A glomus tumor can be recognized by the perivascular distribution of the cells arranged in a organoid pattern, a regular appearance of their nuclei, and occasional smooth muscle elements. A glomous tumor frequently presents with exquisite pain, while HPC does not. The cells of a fibrous histiocytoma are usually arranged in a storiform or cartwheel pattern without a pronounced vascular network. The collagen deposition in HPC is generally immediately around the vessels—not a specific finding in fibrous histiocytoma. Synovial sarcoma is much more likely to be included in the differential diagnosis of malignant HPC than in the benign tumor. A monophasic synovial sarcoma can demonstrate an HPC-like pattern. However, there are often alternating patterns, with the more characteristic fibrosarcomatous pattern present in some areas. Focal calcifications can also be seen. Immunoreactivity with keratin or EMA will help to define a synovial sarcoma. Mesenchymal chondrosarcoma is associated with islands of cartilage or bone—not usually seen in HPC, although the vascular pattern may be identical. The cells of this extraskeletal chondrosarcoma are smaller and less well differentiated. A spindle squamous cell carcinoma is usually positive for keratin, occasionally demonstrating an overlying surface dysplasia or carcinoma in situ. Malignant melanoma may have a growth pattern like HPC, but the immunoreactivity with vimentin, S-100 protein, and occasionally HMB-45 will confirm the diagnosis, especially if melanosomes are found on ultrastructural study.

Leiomyoma

Gross Pathology

This extremely rare neoplasm usually occurs in the supraglottic larynx, with the ventricle and false vocal cord most often involved, although leiomyomas of the subglottis and trachea have been described. The tumors are usually sessile, bulging or polypoid red-brown masses, measuring up to 5 cm in maximum dimensions, with an average of about 1 to 2 cm. These masses are usually covered by an intact smooth surface epithelium, with a conspicuous vascular arborizing pattern, although ulceration is noted in larger lesions. The cut surface reveals an encapsulated soft to firm, grey-white, and fleshy or parenchymal tumor.[132,318,453–462]

Microscopic Pathology

Leiomyomas are distinctly encapsulated masses located in the submucosa, composed of spindled cells arranged in fascicles, whorls, and intersecting bundles. The smooth muscle cells have elongated, vesicular to stippled nuclei with blunt ends, surrounded by spindled, bipolar, fibrillar pink cytoplasm. Occasional cells may exhibit nuclear pleomorphism. Mitotic activity is scarce, while necrosis, hemorrhage, and invasion are completely absent. Mucinous degeneration can be seen but is usually focal. Vascular leiomyoma (angiomyoma) has also been described, containing capillary, cavernous, or venous vascular spaces in addition to the leiomyoma components. This tumor subtype is well circumscribed, but may have an inconspicuous capsule. There is usually an accentuation of the intertwining smooth muscle proliferation around the vascular channels. The vascular spaces may form a prominent component of these tumors, and their distinction from a hemangioma may be difficult. In other areas the vessels are compressed by the tumorigenesis.[132,453–464]

Special Techniques

Immunoreactivity for vimentin, desmin, and smooth muscle actin can be identified in the cytoplasm of the tumor cells. There is generally no reactivity with keratin, S-100 protein, or KP-1 (a histiocytic marker).

Electron microscopy identifies smooth muscle cells set in a background of amorphous material, endothelial cells, and fibrocytes or fibroblasts. In addition to pinocytotic vesicles, actin fibers, in parallel arrays, are also noted.[461]

Differential Diagnosis

Since the vascular leiomyomas or angioleiomyomas are composed of two mesenchymal tissues, they could be classified as hamartomas or mesenchymomas, but this distinction is often academic and artificial, and it has no clinical significance. As smooth muscle and blood vessels are constituent parts of the larynx, an abnormal collection of these components may be called a hamartoma. However, since there is a dominant smooth muscle component, which is encapsulated, seemingly fed by the predominant vascular component, calling these lesions benign leiomyomas seems more prudent.[312,318,459,462] The principal diagnostic differential rests with benign peripheral nerve sheath tumors (BPNST: neurilemmoma and neurofibroma), nodular fasciitis, fibroma, and leiomyosarcoma, although any of the spindle cell tumors (inflammatory myofibroblastic tumor, contact ulcer, fibrosarcoma, spindle squamous cell carcinoma, synovial sarcoma) can be included in the differential diagnosis. Although the distinction between PNST and leiomyoma may be impossible on light microscopic features in a small biopsy, the aid of immunohistochemical reactions will be invaluable in separating these lesions. Nodular fasciitis tends to have a more reactive or granulation-like tissue appearance, with inflammation and extravasated erythrocytes, often presenting a corroborating clinical history of an antecedent event. A leiomyosarcoma will have a similar growth pattern to a leiomyoma, but generally has greater cellularity, nuclear and cellular pleomorphism, necrosis, hemorrhage, and mitotic activity in addition to the invasive growth. A leiomyosarcoma of the larynx is truly extraordinary, and a spindle cell carcinoma must be excluded by examining the surface epithelium and performing immunohistochemical reactions, and perhaps even ultrastructural evaluation, to determine the type of tumor. Laryngeal leiomyoblastoma has been described but is exceedingly rare, composed of short, spindled, fusiform, epithelioid cells with clear cytoplasm, arranged in solid nests and sheets, demonstrating smooth muscle differentiation on immunohistochemical reactions (actin) and electron microscopy.[464]

Fibrous Histiocytoma

Gross Pathology

A fibrous histiocytoma (FH) is usually a solitary exophytic or nodular, white-grey to yellow-orange, firm, solid tumor mass, more often involving the supraglottic larynx, although the subglottic larynx and trachea are also affected. Focal hemorrhage and degenerative changes can be seen on cut surface. Lesions measure up to 3.5 cm in greatest dimension. The overlying epithelium is generally intact, although occasionally keratotic.[132,465–469]

Microscopic Pathology

A storiform (pinwheel, spiral nebular) submucosal proliferation of oval to spindle-shaped fibroblasts is identified in combination with histiocytes, collagenous stroma, and a variety of inflammatory elements, usually lymphocytes (Fig. 8–67). The right-angle abutment of one fascicle against another is the mark of true storiform arrangement. Multinucleated giant cells and foamy histiocytes can be seen, accompanied by hemosiderin (either intracellular or free in the stroma). The background stroma is frequently vascular, with some areas showing hyalinization or myxoid degeneration. There is a marked

variability of the proportions of histiocytic to fibroblastic cells. Cellular pleomorphism is minimal, there are few mitotic figures, no necrosis, no hemorrhage, and no invasion (see Fig. 8–67). There are no atypical mitotic figures in FH.[132,465,468,469]

Special Techniques

The lesional cells are usually reactive with vimentin, actin, alpha-1-antichymotrypsin, and KP-1 (the latter two are histiocytic markers), but these findings are not sensitive or specific. A panel of immunoreactions is necessary in order to rule out other spindle cell lesions, and a fibrous histiocytoma is usually diagnosed on the hematoxylin-and-eosin findings and negative findings on immunohistochemistries. Ultrastructural studies will demonstrate both the fibroblastic nature of the cells, as well as document the histiocytic and inflammatory elements present.[468,469]

Differential Diagnosis

The differential diagnosis obviously begins with the origin of this tumor. In short, the origin is still uncertain, but a fibroblastic cell with histiocytic differentiation seems to be the cell most frequently cited.[470] Benign FH is considerably less frequent than malignant fibrous histiocytoma (MFH), with the odds in favor of a malignant lesion if it is recognized. The distinction between FH, inflammatory myofibroblastic tumor, nodular fasciitis, contact ulcer, benign peripheral nerve sheath tumors (BPNST), smooth muscle tumors, MFH, metastatic sarcomatoid carcinoma, and spindle cell carcinoma is very difficult. No clear-cut criteria exist to separate each of these entities with 100% certainty. However, some guidelines can be used to separate them into more accurate groups. FH has limited nuclear and cellular variability, no tumor necrosis, no tumor hemor-

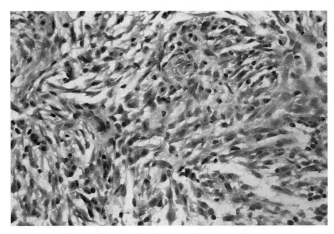

FIGURE 8–67. The pinwheel or storiform growth pattern is attributed to fibrous histiocytoma, although a number of other tumors can demonstrate this growth pattern focally. The spindle cells are not atypical in this example, nor is there much in the way of histiocytic or inflammatory infiltrate (H&E, × 300).

rhage, and no atypical mitotic figures. FH is usually circumscribed and does not demonstrate destructive invasive growth. The inflammatory myofibroblastic tumor does not usually have a storiform growth pattern and frequently has surface ulceration. There are usually more inflammatory elements, with less histiocytic cells, but this may be a subjective difference. The myofibroblastic nature of the cells may also help in separating these benign lesions. Fibromatosis usually has tight fascicles of monotonously bland-appearing cells set in a densely collagenized stroma. Mitotic activity is scarce. Nodular fasciitis is a proliferation of fibroblasts, often exhibiting a plump reactive appearance, arranged haphazardly or in loose fascicles in a collagenized stroma. A zonation or maturation is often noted toward the periphery. The nuclear chromatin is finely stippled with nucleoli. Multinucleated cells can be seen, containing the same type of nuclei as the surrounding fibroblasts. There is a rich vascularity, often with extravasated erythrocytes in a background of inflammatory elements. Hemosiderin may also be seen. While there may be many mitotic figures, they are not atypical. The distinction between nodular fasciitis and FH is often difficult, and all the features—including the point of origin, combined with the clinical presentation—need to be evaluated. BPNST tend to have an encapsulated growth pattern, more palisaded growth, an obvious association with a nerve, and no inflammatory component; they are usually reactive with S-100 protein. A leiomyoma has longer interlacing fascicles, is usually encapsulated with a limited amount of inflammatory response, and demonstrates desmin and smooth muscle actin reactivity. A benign juvenile xanthogranuloma contains Touton giant cells (wreath of nuclei around glassy cytoplasm) but is still within the spectrum of fibrohistiocytic lesions. An MFH should be excluded on the basis of the cytomorphologic features alone, with nuclear pleomorphism, mitotic activity, necrosis, hemorrhage, and destructive, infiltrative growth. On a similar note, the pleomorphism identified in spindle cell carcinomas and metastatic tumors should likewise distinguish between these tumors and FH. If needed, immunoreactivity with keratin or the demonstration of epithelial origin on electron microscopy can separate these tumors correctly.[131,465–469,471]

The most clinically relevant distinction between the various tumors in the differential diagnosis is between benign and malignant. Benign tumors may also recur if incompletely excised and therefore usually require a wide margin for complete removal.

Peripheral Nerve Sheath Tumor

Gross Pathology

Grossly, benign peripheral nerve sheath tumor (BPNST) can be a nodule affecting any location in the larynx, although a supraglottic location (related to the superior laryngeal nerve) is common, frequently involving the false cords and aryepiglottic fold. The tumors are smooth; round or lobulated to fusiform submucosal masses; pink, grey, or brown; firm or soft, depending upon the degree of cystic or mucinous degeneration; and measure up to 5 cm in greatest dimension. There is generally an intact epithelium, although larger tumors may cause ulceration. Neurilemmoma is usually encapsulated, round, solitary, and adherent or partially surrounded by a peripheral nerve; neurofibroma is nonencapsulated, fusiform, often multiple (especially when associated with neurofibromatosis), and intermixed with the nerve sheath rather than pushing the nerve aside.[22,132,418,435,472–482]

Microscopic Pathology

A neurilemmoma, much more common than other BPNSTs in the larynx, is well circumscribed, although not necessarily encapsulated, variably cellular, with densely cellular areas (Antoni A) alternating with hypocellular areas (Antoni B), situated within a variably hyalinized matrix (Fig. 8–68A). Cystic degeneration and hyalinization can be seen. There can be a number of small to medium-sized blood vessels with hyalinized walls (Fig. 8–68B). Occasional Verocay body formation can be seen with peripheral palisading of fusiform cells with elongated cytoplasmic extensions, presenting a wavy to spindled appearance (see Fig. 8–68A). The elongated nuclei have little pleomorphism, coarse nuclear chromatin distribution, and inconspicuous nucleoli. Nerve axons are not seen within the tumor; however, they may be identified at the periphery.[132,418,435,474,476,477,480]

A neurofibroma is nonencapsulated with vague borders and it is intimately intertwined with nerve axons (Fig. 8–69A). The Schwann cell proliferation is set in a densely collagenized stroma composed of haphazardly arranged elongated and spindled cells with cytologically bland nuclei (Fig. 8–69B). Twigs of axons or nerve fascicles are seen throughout the lesion, not just at the periphery as seen in a neurilemmoma (see Fig. 8–69A). Edema of the endoneurium may also be noted, but degenerative changes are unusual. Mitotic activity, pleomorphism, and necrosis are lacking, as is a destructive infiltrative growth or vascular invasion.[22,132,418,435,472,475,479,480]

Special Techiques

The tumor cells of all BPNST show immunoreactivity with S-100 protein (see Fig. 8–69B), vimentin, epithelial membrane antigen (EMA), and Leu-7 (Schwann cell marker). Neuron-specific enolase and actin are variably present and noncontributory. BPNSTs do not express reactivity with actin and desmin.[474,480,483]

By electron microscopy, features of Schwann cell

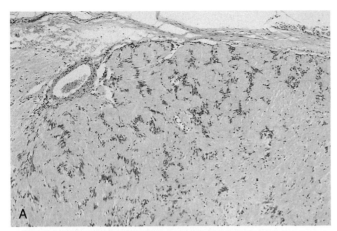

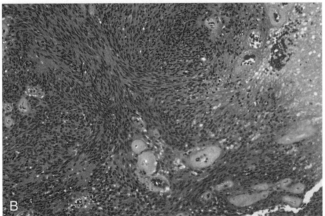

FIGURE 8-68. *A,* This schwannoma (neurilemmoma) of the epiglottis is submucosal, well circumscribed, and encapsulated, composed of hypercellular (Antoni A) and hypocellular or hyalinized (Antoni B) areas. Verocay body formation can be seen (H&E, × 75); *B,* The spindle cells of a neurilemmoma are arranged in a swirled pattern, with hyalinized vessels near an area of hypocellularity (H&E, × 150).

neurofibroma), but these are very rare.[473,478,484] It is imperative that a thorough clinical evaluation for the features of von Recklinghausen's disease (neurofibromatosis) be conducted, including the search for café au lait spots, in patients who have laryngeal neurofibroma. Although isolated neurofibromas of the larynx have been described, association with neurofibromatosis is much more likely.[435,475,476,481] Other lesions in the differential diagnosis for BPNST include inflammatory myofibroblastic tumor and pleomorphic adenoma.

Inflammatory myofibroblastic tumor will demonstrate a spindle cell proliferation with a variable inflammatory infiltrate but no peripheral palisading, Verocay bodies, or association with peripheral nerves. Schwann cell differentiation is absent. A pleomorphic adenoma may have spindle cells, but the dual cell population and the chondroid matrix material are different from benign PNST.

Malignant peripheral nerve sheath tumor (MPNST) presents as a single dominant mass, often quite large, with surface ulceration and infiltration

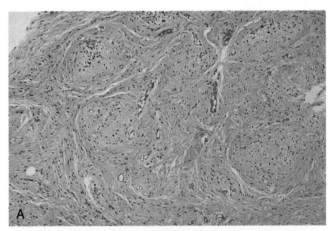

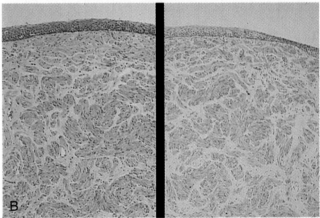

FIGURE 8-69. *A,* This neurofibroma demonstrates a number of nerve twigs intimately admixed with the proliferation of Schwann cells. There is a nodular or lobular growth pattern (H&E, × 75); *B,* The swirled growth pattern of a neurofibroma (*left,* H&E, × 75) characteristically reacts with S-100 protein (*right,* S-100 protein, IHC, × 75).

or perineurial cell derivation are identified with cells possessing narrow to broad entangled or interdigitating cell processes covered by a discrete reduplicated or redundant basement membrane substance. Collagen fibers are banded together and inserted into the basal lamina. Intermediate filaments are contained within the cytoplasm. Primitive junctions are identified between tumor cells. The so-called "fibrous long-spacing collagen," with its distinct periodicity, can be seen. Differentiation is not uniform between tumors or within a tumor.[483]

Differential Diagnosis

It is often impossible to tell the difference between neurilemmoma and neurofibroma, especially when presented with a small biopsy. In that setting, calling the lesion a BPNST is satisfactory, awaiting the definitive surgical specimen for accurate classification. Other variants of neurofibroma have also been identified (plexiform neurofibroma, ganglio-

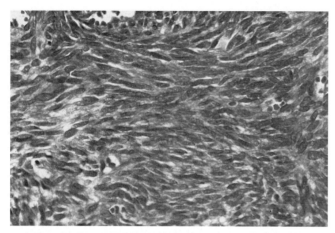

FIGURE 8-70. A malignant peripheral nerve sheath tumor is very hypercellular, with atypical spindle shaped cells arranged in fascicles. There is a hint of nuclear and cellular "waviness" or undulation. Additional studies would be required to confirm this diagnosis (immunohistochemical or electron microscopy) (H&E, × 300).

into the surrounding soft tissue. An attachment to a nerve should be sought, although it may not be obvious by the time the tumor is resected. The tumor cells are fusiform and plump, arranged in tightly packed fascicles woven into a vague herringbone-type pattern, while in other areas the cells are wavy, with fibrillar cytoplasmic extensions arranged in a loose myxoid background matrix. Focal palisading of the nuclei may be seen. In comparison to benign peripheral nerve sheath tumor, MPNST is highly cellular, composed of variably pleomorphic cells with a high nuclear:cytoplasmic ratio (Fig. 8–70). Numerous mitotic figures include atypical forms. Areas of necrosis and hemorrhage with a slight increase in cellularity immediately surround the vessels. Vascular invasion can be readily identified. There is generally no remaining benign PNST to demonstrate a point of origin or to help with the classification of the tumor. S-100 protein and EMA reactivity are usually less intense and less diffuse in distribution in malignant PNST, frequently altogether absent. Occasionally, poorly differentiated sarcomas will be S-100 protein negative but will show ultrastructural evidence of nerve sheath differentiation.[480,485,486]

PREMALIGNANT LESIONS AND MALIGNANT NEOPLASMS

Epithelial Dysplasia and Carcinoma In Situ

Gross Pathology

Grossly, the presentation of dysplasia or CIS is variable, without a distinctive or characteristic appearance. These lesions can be circumscribed or diffuse; appearing white, red, or grey, smooth to slightly raised, irregular, granular, or thickened. Any portion of the larynx may be involved, although the anterior cords are involved slightly more frequently and appear dry and roughened.[18,487–493]

Microscopic Pathology

The term dysplasia refers to all disturbances of differentiation of the surface epithelium, except for full thickness, which is usually referred to as carcinoma in situ. In keeping with other areas of pathology, the term laryngeal intraepithelial neoplasia (LIN) has been proposed and seems to have clinical and histologic utility.[494,495] These should perhaps be used instead of the more vague terms of keratosis, leukoplakia, hyperkeratosis, parakeratosis, pachydermia, dyskeratosis, and dysplasia.

The abnormalities of LIN, mild to moderate dysplasia, are confined to the lower half of the epithelium, with loss of polarity in the axis of the cells and a disturbance in maturation toward the surface (Fig. 8–71A). The variability in cell size and shape, nuclear features and mitotic activity will increase quantitatively in a continuous spectrum, until the entire thickness of the epithelium is involved (carcinoma in situ).

LIN, severe dysplasia, or carcinoma in situ is composed of the same histologic features identified in ordinary squamous cell cancers, with one exception: there is no evidence of penetration of the basement membrane. Instead, these neoplastic cells are increased in number (hypercellular) and spread into the surrounding epithelium, even though the epithelium may not necessarily be thickened. The lesions are frequently divided into basaloid, squamous, and bowenoid by the dominant cellular features. The bowenoid type of CIS shows an expanded or exaggerated rete peg (Fig. 8–71B). Although there are some clinically associated findings with each type, there is no clear-cut point to making these distinctions for prognostic purposes.[18,491,493,496]

The high-grade (LIN III, severe dysplasia, and carcinoma in situ) lesions demonstrate complete structural and cytologic abnormalities, occasionally showing surface keratinization, often with parakeratosis and dyskeratosis (Fig. 8–71B–D). The cells are disordered in their arrangement. Basal-type cells appear at different levels within the epithelium, showing no normal stratification or maturation toward the luminal surface and with an abrupt border between the adjacent normal epithelium. All the various layers begin to resemble the basal layer cells in size and shape as the lesion progresses from low-grade dysplasia toward carcinoma in situ. The cells may even take on a monotonous appearance, even though they are all atypical. Intercellular bridges become more difficult to detect, while mitotic figures become more frequent and are often atypical (see Fig. 8–71D). There is a poikilocytosis and anisonu-

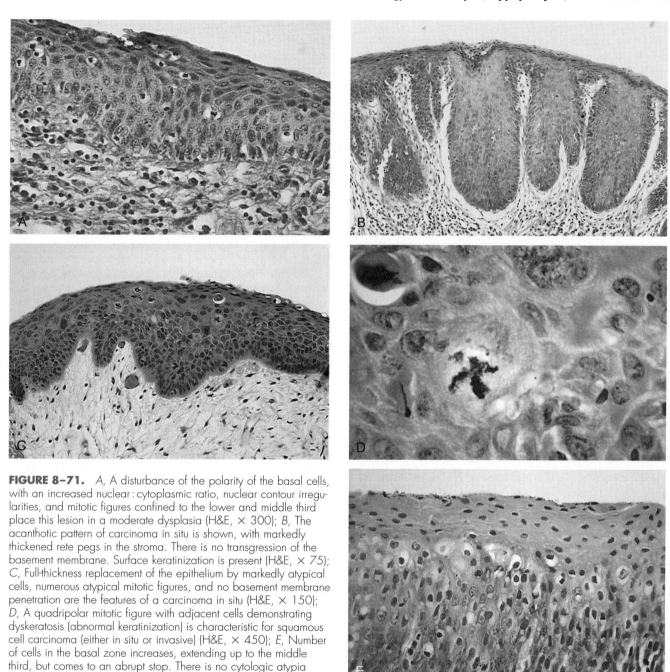

FIGURE 8–71. *A,* A disturbance of the polarity of the basal cells, with an increased nuclear : cytoplasmic ratio, nuclear contour irregularities, and mitotic figures confined to the lower and middle third place this lesion in a moderate dysplasia (H&E, × 300); *B,* The acanthotic pattern of carcinoma in situ is shown, with markedly thickened rete pegs in the stroma. There is no transgression of the basement membrane. Surface keratinization is present (H&E, × 75); *C,* Full-thickness replacement of the epithelium by markedly atypical cells, numerous atypical mitotic figures, and no basement membrane penetration are the features of a carcinoma in situ (H&E, × 150); *D,* A quadripolar mitotic figure with adjacent cells demonstrating dyskeratosis (abnormal keratinization) is characteristic for squamous cell carcinoma (either in situ or invasive) (H&E, × 450); *E,* Number of cells in the basal zone increases, extending up to the middle third, but comes to an abrupt stop. There is no cytologic atypia (H&E, × 300).

cleosis, with spindling of the nuclei. Nucleoli may become prominent. Disruption of the nuclear chromatin distribution with clumping and irregularities of the nuclear contours is evident (see Fig. 8–71C). Koilocytes can be present, with dense nuclear chromatin surrounded by a cleared zone with nuclear membrane accentuation. Tumor giant cells can also be seen. If the rete pegs are still present, they may be slightly wider, often surrounded by an inflammatory infiltrate (see Fig. 8–71B). Various substratifications within high-grade LIN have been suggested but are cumbersome, tedious to apply, and are of no significant benefit to patient outcome. Lesions that contain mitoses (usually in the upper one half to one third of the epithelium) and abnormal mitotic figures (misalignment of chromosomes, unbalanced distribution of chromosomes and multipolar figures) (see Fig. 8–71D), intense stromal inflammation, nuclear pleomorphism, and increased dyskeratosis (deep keratinization) (see Fig. 8–71D) seem to correlate more closely with disease progression than other histomorphologic criteria.[16–18,487–493,496–498]

Careful sectioning of the specimen is vital to avoid tangential sections. Additional deeper sections may be needed to demonstrate diagnostic features deeper in the block.[499] Biopsy of the transitional epithelium of the vocal cord can give a false appearance of LIN.

Special Techniques

DNA analysis has demonstrated aneuploid DNA histograms and has prognostic implications, but is not routinely performed.[489,494,500] An increased PCNA index has been linked to a high probability of further malignant progression, but this finding needs to be corroborated in larger groups before the index is incorporated into the diagnostic armamentarium.[501] Human papillomavirus capsid antigen has been identified in CIS but does not seem to affect clinical outcome.[502]

Differential Diagnosis

Basal and paranasal zone hyperplasia can be confused with LIN. The hyperplastic epithelium has a columnar arrangement to the basal cells that maintains a vertical polarity and hyperchromatic nuclei. The process terminates abruptly at the upper edge of the prickle-layer, with a horizontally oriented, very sharp zone of transition. There is no disruption of the arrangement and no nuclear features of malignancy (Fig. 8–71E).

Inflammatory conditions and granular cell tumor can cause atypical epithelial changes, and the characteristic histologic features of these lesions should be sought. Tuberculosis and other mycobacterial infections and fungal organisms should be ruled out by the application of special stains or by performing cultures. The inflammatory changes associated with previous irradiation or a previous biopsy site can falsely suggest the possibility of a malignant epithelial tumor. Granular cell tumor can be excluded through careful searching for the characteristic cells or the application of immunohistochemistry (S-100 protein).

Clinicopathologic Correlation

A number of studies document the association of human papillomavirus capsid antigen in carcinoma in situ of the larynx. However, there seems to be no independent prognostic implication between clinical course (histologic severity of the vocal cord lesion) and the presence of HPV. It does seem that the location within the glottis has prognostic significance, with 92% of the anterior commisure lesions converting to invasive squamous cell carcinoma, while other locations within the larynx tend to convert less frequently (17%).[503]

The microscopic changes found are often more extensive than clinically obvious. It is therefore imperative to biopsy lesions, especially in patients with chronic laryngitis changes or in patients with etiologically associated factors. The size of the biopsy can also make interpretation difficult. One part of the specimen may have normal or only an intraepithelial component, while another part may reveal the invasive disease. Similarly, involvement of the glandular ducts can be misinterpreted as infiltrating carcinoma. It is in this setting that multiple biopsies within the diseased areas and in the immediately surrounding regions are imperative for correct diagnosis. A negative biopsy does not preclude the presence of an invasive carcinoma elsewhere in the larynx! In fact, invasive carcinoma is a frequent synchronous occurrence with CIS, and should therefore be aggressively sought. Likewise, dysplasia or a carcinoma in situ does not have to be documented prior to the development of an invasive squamous cell carcinoma. In many instances, the overlying epithelium is unremarkable or demonstrates hyperplasia, but there will be no dysplasia. Since many of these changes seem to occur in a continuous spectrum of dysplasia, carcinoma in situ, and invasive carcinoma, close monitoring of a patient with any of these changes is recommended.[16,18,487,493,498,499,504]

Squamous Cell Carcinoma

Gross Pathology

Squamous cell carcinoma (SCC) can occur in any portion of the larynx or trachea and is the most common malignant tumor of these regions. The tumors can be ulcerative, flat, papillary, or exophytic in growth and can range from minute mucosal thickened areas to masses filling the laryngeal spaces. Most tumors arise in the glottis (vocal cord region). Tumors are generally divided into supraglottic, glottic, subglottic, and transglottic based on the exact anatomic location. Each of these locations has a different clinical outcome and therefore different treatment. The tumors are erythematous to white to tan, frequently feeling firm on palpation. Staging and prognostications about laryngeal and tracheal SCC are based upon the exact anatomic location, extension of the tumor into surrounding tissues, impairment of the cords (in supraglottic and glottic tumors), and the overall size of the tumor. Careful documentation, therefore, as described in the gross and frozen section procedures at the beginning of this chapter (including margin assessment), is imperative for accurate diagnosis and clinical staging, with obvious treatment implications.[3,490,505–508]

Microscopic Pathology

"Conventional" SCC (excluding verrucous or spindle squamous cell carcinomas) comprises about 99% of laryngeal carcinomas and is obviously the most important laryngeal cancer examined and treated by otolaryngologists.[13,506] Since it is also a very common cancer seen in other anatomic sites, all pathologists are familiar with the histologic diagnosis of this malignancy. This familiarity limits the need for comments here despite the great importance of this tumor type. SCC is composed of variable degrees of squamous differentiation, with well-differentiated cells almost perfectly recapitulating normal squamous epithelium, but demonstrating basement membrane violation by nests of tumor cells, a disorganized growth pattern, keratin pearls, intercellular bridges, a loss of polarity, dyskeratosis, an increased nuclear:cytoplasmic ratio, nuclear chromatin irregularities, prominent eosinophilic nucleoli, and mitotic figures (including atypical forms) (Fig. 8–72). Keratinizing SCC is seen less frequently than the nonkeratinizing or poorly differentiated types. Mitotic figures and necrosis tend to increase as the grade of the tumor becomes more poorly differentiated. A rich inflammatory infiltrate (usually of lymphocytes and plasma cells) is seen at the tumor-to-stroma

junction, along with a dense desmoplastic fibrous connective tissue (see Fig. 8–72B). The more poorly differentiated tumors may not have as brisk an inflammatory response. The histologic appearance can be associated with a carcinoma in situ (CIS) or may invade from an epithelium without evidence of CIS. The poorly differentiated lesions have only a vague resemblance to squamous epithelium, with only rare foci of squamous differentiation (see Fig. 8–72B). The malignant cells are arranged in cohesive clusters or sheets, with cells demonstrating dyskeratosis, intercellular bridges, and a dense opaque cytoplasm.[509–511] Perineural invasion can be noted, with a positive correlation to metastatic potential.[512] All the basic features of SCC are well inculcated into the armamentarium of a budding pathologist and need not be described further in this text. However, several facets of SCC deserve comment.

Special Techniques

Occasionally, additional special studies (specifically, immunohistochemical reactions) are needed to document the epithelial nature of the tumor. A number of studies have been performed, including DNA content (ploidy may be an independent prognostic indicator), E-Cadherin presence (dedifferentiation association), human papillomavirus association, epidermal growth factor or surface receptor (role in tumor progression with overexpression), proliferating cell nuclear antigen, and p53 gene mutations. However, these special technique results are generally not used in the diagnosis or staging of the tumors at this time.[328,513–516]

Differential Diagnosis

Depending on degree of tumor differentiation, the differential diagnosis is usually limited to papilloma and hyperplasias. The histologic distinction of atypical papilloma in adults from well-differentiated papillary or exophytic SCC has been discussed previously. This type of carcinoma is not rare, but it is insufficiently discussed in the literature; pathologists should keep this type of lesion in mind when examining laryngeal biopsies.

Although laryngeal granular cell tumors are rare, they are frequently misdiagnosed due to the associated marked pseudoepitheliomatous hyperplasia (PEH), which is mistakenly diagnosed as SCC. Granular cell tumors are rare enough that most pathologists do not routinely and consciously examine every laryngeal biopsy for granular cells before making a diagnosis of well-differentiated SCC. Since granular cell tumors are often yellowish-pink tumors in the posterior glottic region and clinically don't resemble typical laryngeal carcinomas, this clinical information should be communicated to the pathologist. This will help distinguish the lesion from carcinoma, thereby avoiding a total laryngectomy for a benign tumor.[356]

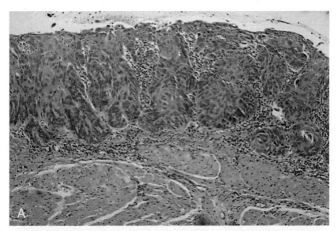

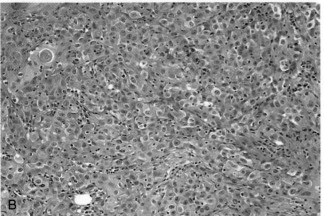

FIGURE 8–72. *A,* Intermediate-power view shows the uneven finger-like infiltration of the squamous cell carcinoma cells into the underlying stroma. Marked nuclear pleomorphism and cellular disarray are evident (H&E, × 100); *B,* Moderate to poorly differentiated squamous cell carcinoma featuring a single keratin pearl in a pavemented sheet of cells with prominent cell borders mixed with an inflammatory response (H&E, × 150).

Clinicopathologic Correlation

A clinically important distinction must be made between invasive carcinoma and carcinoma in situ. Squamous cell carcinomas showing only superficial or microinvasion from the same anatomic location and with the same degree of differentiation (well differentiated) will probably behave in a fashion quite similar to a carcinoma in situ, requiring similar clinical treatment. Some supraglottic carcinomas, especially if they are of wide field origin and not well differentiated, can metastasize while still in a superficially invasive stage. The degree of invasion seems to have clinical implications, with a deeply invading SCC having a much greater metastatic potential than a superficially invading SCC of the same anatomic site and degree of histologic differentiation. This is taken into consideration and partly compensated for by clinical staging, but such compensation is not perfect. Diagnostic qualifiers (minimal, superficial, incipient) should be used, when appropriate, in making a diagnosis or in communicating to the clinician exactly what is being seen on the slide. Circumspection and conservatism in labeling a carcinoma as invasive should be the approach.[517] Likewise, the clinician should clearly understand that there is hardly any detectable difference between what may be called severe dysplasia and carcinoma in situ, even though the formidable word "carcinoma" is being used in the latter instance. Overall, tumor location (transglottic), tumor size (large), histology (poorly differentiated), lymph node metastases (especially when there is extranodal spread), and multifocal disease all correlate with a poorer prognosis.[517–518]

The decision to ask for a frozen section examination of a laryngeal biopsy and judging the time interval between successive biopsies are two clinical decisions that influence histologic interpretation. Although there are rare instances (a large "obvious" carcinoma that warrants urgent surgery because of airway obstruction) where frozen section diagnosis is justified, these instances should be scarce. As already mentioned, laryngeal biopsies often contain artifacts because of unavoidable tangential sectioning and malorientation. When these are combined with cytologic and architectural distortions and the tissue consumption or "wastage" effect of frozen section examination, the biopsy that may have been diagnostic of carcinoma is rendered useless. Even with the best biopsy and tissue preservation, the separation of carcinoma from pseudoepitheliomatous hyperplasia can be a most difficult and challenging problem. Although rebiopsy may solve the problem, depending upon the time frame, the problem may escalate. If the rebiopsy is required from the same area as the previous biopsy, partial healing and epithelial regeneration effects, especially of an already abnormal epithelium, can produce a markedly atypical PEH that can be very difficult, if not impossible, to distinguish from carcinoma. For these reasons, it is important either to biopsy a different area (undisturbed by the previous biopsy) or wait, clinical conditions permitting, at least 10 to 12 weeks before rebiopsy of the same area. This will allow for adequate healing and a more accurate interpretation of the nature of the lesion.

Verrucous Carcinoma

Gross Pathology

The gross presentation in the larynx is usually of a large, broad-based, exophytic, wart-like, or fungating lesion that is firm to hard. The tumor may be tan to white, measuring up to 10 cm in greatest dimension. The papillary structures may show surface ulceration. The tumors are usually found in the glottic portion of the larynx, although no region of the larynx is exempt.[520–527]

Microscopic Pathology

On histologic examination, verrucous carcinoma (VC) is composed of an exophytic, warty tumor with multiple thickened club-shaped filiform projections lined by well-differentiated squamous epithelium (Fig. 8–73 A and B). The advancing margins of the tumor are usually of a pushing rather than an infiltrative pattern, with a dense inflammatory response in the subjacent tissues (see Fig. 8–73 A and B). The epithelium is extraordinarily well-differentiated with none of the normally associated malignant criteria identified in a squamous cell carcinoma (Fig. 8–73C). The cells are arranged in an orderly maturation toward the surface, lined by a "church-spire" keratosis (see Fig. 8–73A). These tumors are almost amitotic and are certainly without atypical forms.[520–528] There has been an association with human papillomavirus.[520] Since both a benign keratinizing hyperplasia (or verruca vulgaris) and a very well-differentiated, nonverrucous SCC can share all the previously described features throughout most of their structure (and certainly throughout all biopsy fragments), it is easy to understand how the determination of which biopsies to include within the spectrum of VC and which to exclude is a most vexing problem for the surgical pathologist.[529]

Special Techniques

The diagnosis of VC of the larynx is probably one of the most difficult and problematic in almost every instance. The challenge in diagnosis derives from the fact that the lesion is not cytologically malignant, and thus evidence of invasion is required for definitive diagnosis. However, definite histologic evidence of invasion for this type of lesion in the limited and small biopsies of the larynx is usually difficult or impossible to ascertain. With a large and mostly exophytic lesion in the larynx, the biopsies, even when

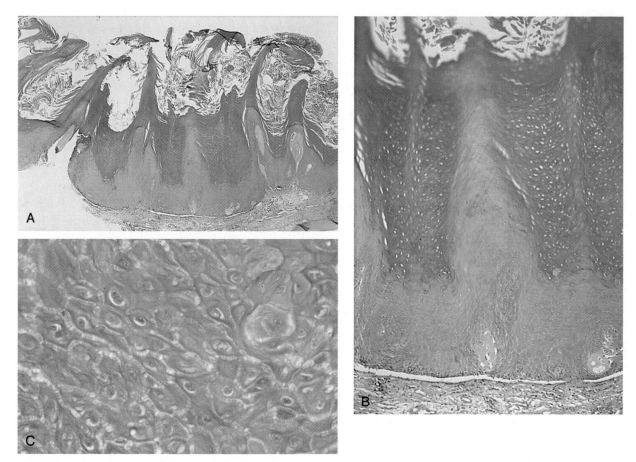

FIGURE 8–73.   *A,* Broad pushing infiltration at the base of a verrucous carcinoma, demonstrating "church spire" type hyperkeratosis with a bland epithelium (H&E, × 30); *B,* Even, broad border of infiltration with marked keratosis in a cytologically bland epithelium (H&E, × 75); *C,* No nuclear criteria of malignancy are identified in this squamous epithelium (H&E, × 300).

generous in volume of tissue, will usually not include much if any of the stromal interface at the lower portion of the lesion. Compounding this difficulty is the almost unavoidable tangential sectioning artifact of the curled, piecemeal, or fragmented biopsy. Attempts to judge whether or not there is invasion of broad sheets of squamous epithelium are almost routinely frustrating. This problem is not so bad in the oral cavity or skin, where it is more feasible to have a large intact well-oriented biopsy that demonstrates the architecture of the lower portion of the lesion.[530] Therefore, an adequate biopsy sample to include a stromal to epithelial junction is required for diagnostic purposes.

Differential Diagnosis

The differential diagnosis rests between verrucous hyperplasia and conventional SCC. It has been argued that the difference between verrucous hyperplasia and VC is only in stage and size, and that the lesions represent a developmental spectrum. Lesions that have not invaded may just be early-stage VC.[531]

The distinction on histologic features alone, even when specialized studies have been performed (including DNA analysis), is not possible. However, we believe that isolated true verrucous hyperplasia does exist.[532,533] If a superficial verrucoid lesion of the glottic larynx, has been adequately sampled and almost completely removed by the biopsy, and if there is no evidence of significant cytologic dysplasia, nor clinical or histologic evidence of invasion, such a lesion can be considered as verrucous hyperplasia (see Fig. 8–38A). Conservative management with close patient follow-up is warranted, however, as the lesion may recur or progress to VC, the untoward consequences of a hemi- or total laryngectomy have been temporarily avoided. In addition, a large majority of a conventional SCC may simulate VC, both clinically and histologically. However, focal to extensive areas of the invasive component may be ordinary SCC, highlighting the need for adequate sampling of all verrucoid lesions. This is an area where the judgments of both pathologist and clinician are tested, and communication between the two is of paramount importance.[506,521–523,525] The pathologist must be as thorough as possible to ensure that the clinician understands exactly what is present on the biopsy slides.

VC is often referred to as a "distinct entity," separable from conventional SCC, with a biologic behavior between non-neoplastic hyperplasias and conventional SCC.[521,533] However, occasional lesions of verrucous hyperplasia, VC, and very well-differentiated "ordinary" SCC form a continuum that is not completely amenable to our attempts at neat categorization. Therefore, it may be helpful to think of VC as "extremely well-differentiated squamous cell carcinoma" rather than a separate entity, as used in the title of this section to emphasize the relationship of this tumor to conventional SCC.

Clinicopathologic Correlation

From a clinical standpoint, there are a couple of incorrect beliefs regarding VC. One is that VC does not metastasize, the other that radiotherapy is contraindicated. Since many well-differentiated SCC of the glottis—even those with considerable cytologic atypia—have not metastasized at the time of initial treatment, it is not difficult to extrapolate that verrucous carcinoma (extremely well-differentiated SCC) at the same anatomic location would have a low metastatic rate.[534] Considering the superficial nondestructive invasion and the probability that many lesions reported in the literature as verrucous carcinomas may be verrucous hyperplasias, there is a very slight metastatic capacity in the group as a whole. This does not exclude the possibility of metastasis, especially if the lesion has been present for a long time and contains foci of conventional SCC.

Likewise, since conventional SCC can recur with a more poorly differentiated transformation after radiation therapy, the risk of transformation in a VC to a more poorly differentiated tumor has probably been overemphasized (see Fig. 8–38B). Well-differentiated SCC (including VC) does not generally respond significantly to radiation therapy and it should, therefore, probably not be used as a treatment modality. However, for patients who are not good surgical candidates, radiation therapy of a lesion diagnosed as VC is not absolutely contraindicated.[525–528]

Spindle Cell (Sarcomatoid)– Squamous Cell Carcinoma

Gross Pathology

Although spindle cell–squamous cell carcinoma can arise in the hypopharyngeal and supraglottic areas, laryngeal SCSCC are usually glottic lesions. The tumor presents as a polypoid or exophytic lesion, sometimes with a small stalk, often expanding to fill the larynx. Occasional infiltrative tumors will present as sessile or ulcerative. The cut surface is firm to friable, tan-white or grey to red, measuring up to 8 cm in maximum dimension.[535–544]

Microscopic Pathology

The exophytic or polypoid pattern of growth in an SCSCC will often show little invasion, although an invasive SCC component can usually be demonstrated. Requisite for the diagnosis in ideal cases, is the identification of a squamous cell carcinoma, either in situ or invasive in association with a malignant spindle cell pattern, often demonstrating an area of transition, transformation, or fusion (Fig. 8–74A). In some cases, diagnosis can be identified by a history of a conventional squamous cell carcinoma previously diagnosed at the same anatomic location and, if irradiated, the prior treatment interval being much too short (e.g., less than a year) for a post-irradiation-induced sarcoma. The squamous cell carcinoma may be well differentiated or poorly differentiated, frequently showing both patterns in the same tumor. In lesions that have eroded or ulcerated, the carcinomatous portion on the surface epithelium is absent (Fig. 8–74B). In the ulcerated tumors, an inflammatory infiltrate will frequently separate the tumor cells, yielding a more hypocellular appearance. Often the only portion that reveals the squamous component is in the stalk of the polypoid or pedunculated tumors. If surface epithelium is present, it may not manifest the carcinomatous area from which the tumor developed. It is also possible, and strongly suggested histologically, that the sarcomatoid tumor develops directly from the basal area of a benign-appearing surface epithelium with no significant dysplasia (with disruption of the basal lamina) in any portion of the epithelium (Fig. 8–74C). This notion is similar to that of "ordinary" squamous cell carcinoma, in which a cytologically malignant and invasive carcinoma grows off the basal layer of a surface epithelium that is otherwise not atypical or dysplastic. Spindle cell carcinomas often have become so remarkably transformed, with such a sarcomatoid appearance, as to make them virtually identical to a malignant fibrous histiocytoma (MFH) or fibrosarcoma. The spindle cell or sarcomatous portion is often extremely cellular, with a variable cytologic picture of very bland cells in dense fibrosis to marked pleomorphism. The spindle cell component can be arranged in a fascicular, storiform (see Fig. 8–74A), cartwheel, or pinwheel configuration with areas of degeneration or necrosis. The spindle cells can suggest a subtly rounded, more epithelioid quality, while other areas will have hyperchromatic nuclei, prominent nucleoli, and irregular cellular outlines (Fig. 8–74 A and D). Both bland-appearing osteoclast-like (or foreign-body type) and tumor giant cells can be seen within the tumor. Occasionally osteoid material is formed, suggesting osteosarcoma (although bone or cartilage has not been identified in metastatic foci, suggesting a metaplastic phenomenon) (Fig. 8–74E).[535–541,543–547]

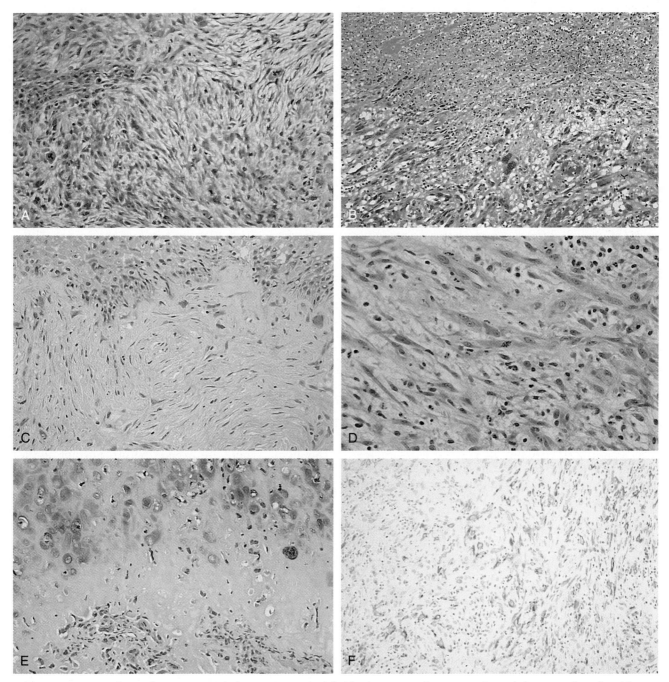

FIGURE 8–74. *A,* A focus of squamous epithelium is seen at the left, blending or transforming into the underlying spindle cell proliferation. Tripolar mitotic figures are identified within the haphazardly arranged, markedly atypical spindle cells (H&E, × 150); *B,* Complete loss of the surface epithelium is characteristic for this tumor, with markedly atypical, hyperchromatic nuclei identified within the spindle cells (H&E, × 300); *C,* Within the desmoplastic stromal response a number of markedly atypical spindle cells can be identified, a few dropping off from the overlying squamous epithelium (H&E, × 150); *D,* Mitotic figures can be found within the spindle cell component. These nuclei are not particularly atypical, which can mask the true nature of this malignant tumor (H&E, × 300); *E,* Metaplastic cartilage tissue has undergone malignant transformation into a chondrosarcoma within this spindle cell squamous cell carcinoma (H&E, × 150); *F,* Although it is unusual to find such a prominently positive stain in a spindle cell squamous cell carcinoma, the tumor cells in this case are richly decorated with keratin (Keratin, IHC, × 150).

Many of these carcinoma-associated factors are frequently absent in an individual case but can be confirmed with definite or compelling keratin reactivity in the sarcomatoid cells (Fig. 8–74F).

Special Techniques

The dual expression within single cells of epithelial and mesenchymal differentiation supports the notion of aberrance of epithelial differentiation and sarcomatoid transformation[542,543,545,546,548,549] Immunoreactivity of the spindle cells for keratin (or epithelial membrane antigen) and vimentin can confirm the diagnosis of SCSCC (see Fig. 8–74F). These tumor cells are negative for S-100 protein, HMB-45, and myoglobin, and are almost always negative for actin, desmin, KP-1, and alpha-1-antitrypsin. The latter two stains may be picked up passively by the tumor cells but are not truly expressed. It is the aggregate of findings that is useful, as the keratin is frequently negative in these tumors. Many of these tumors have become so completely transformed that they have entirely lost their keratin antigens.[543,545,547,549,550]

Ultrastructurally, the tumor cells demonstrate areas of epithelial differentiation, with desmosomes and tonofilaments, often demonstrating collagen production, while also occasionally demonstrating filaments with dense bodies and rough endoplasmic reticulum.

Differential Diagnosis

If there is no evidence of conventional carcinoma extant or by history, how is the diagnosis of carcinoma versus sarcoma made? In an individual case it may be impossible to scientifically "prove" that it is a sarcomatoid carcinoma. However, when considered as a group of tumors, particularly those of the glottis, the clinicopathologic entity seems to support a conclusion that virtually all spindle-cell sarcomatoid malignant tumors of the glottis in adults are sarcomatoid carcinomas rather than sarcomas. When similar spindle cell tumors of the glottic larynx are compared, the tumors are identical except for keratin reactivity, validating the conclusion. In particular, most tumors in both groups will present clinically as exophytic polypoid masses without any clinical evidence of invasion of the vocal ligament or vocalis muscle. If fibrosarcomas or MFH occurred with any frequency in the glottis, why would they almost always occur in an area in which there is very little soft tissue (Reinke's space) or superficial to the vocal ligament? One would expect such sarcomas to arise in the deeply seated paraglottic soft tissues. Contrary to this, virtually all of these glottic-area sarcomatoid tumors apparently arise from the vocal cord mucosa that is composed primarily of squamous epithelium—also the most common site of origin for laryngeal squamous cell carcinoma. When the tumors metastasize, they may present with either carcinomatous growth, sarcomatous growth, or a mixture of the two, but with no metaplastic elements (bone or cartilage).[535,538,541–544,549] While the conclusion may not be scientific proof for the origin of the sarcomatoid tumors from said epithelium, it is certainly based on a preponderance of evidence that adult spindle cell tumors of the glottis are most likely spindle cell carcinomas.

The distinction between a fibrosarcoma or MFH and SCSCC is not entirely academic from a clinical standpoint. Although a spindle cell carcinoma probably has a poor response to radiation therapy, similar to fibrosarcoma or MFH, any significant invasive component is more likely to metastasize to lymph nodes (similar to a carcinoma). This may influence the choice of elective neck dissection. However, polypoid glottic lesions do not metastasize so frequently as other sites of the larynx or nonpolypoid growth pattern.[539] Mucosal malignant melanoma can be spindled, frequently demonstrating a surface component. However, the S-100 protein and HMB-45 immunoreactivity, combined with ultrastructural melanosomes, will confirm the diagnosis of a melanoma.

Also included in the differential diagnosis is the mere recognition that the tumor is malignant. This is not often difficult, as most spindle cell carcinomas are moderately densely cellular tumors with many cells having significant malignant characteristics. However, some tumors develop a dense stromal connective tissue and are hypocellular. The cells in these tumors may be difficult or impossible to recognize as cytologically malignant. In this event, the distinction from a benign inflammatory myofibroblastic tumor can become very problematic. An inflammatory myofibroblastic tumor tends to be circumscribed without infiltration. Its cells have a slightly more prominent "myoid" and "feathery" cytoplasmic appearance (similar to that of the cells of nodular fasciitis) than do the cells of a sarcomatoid carcinoma. There are mitotic figures but not atypical forms (in both inflammatory myofibroblastic tumor and nodular fasciitis) (see Fig. 8–35 B and C). Actin immunostaining of the inflammatory myofibroblastic tumor can be of some help, although it must be remembered that some weak to moderate actin reactivity can often occur in the malignant cells of sarcomatoid carcinomas. However, keratin is not found in inflammatory myofibroblastic tumor.[113,543,547] An aneuploid stem line on ploidy analysis may help in distinguishing between benign and malignant tumors.[551]

Basaloid Squamous Cell Carcinoma

Gross Pathology

The tumor has a predilection for the hypopharynx and supraglottic larynx. It may be poorly defined to exophytic, nodular or polypoid, and is generally firm to hard, yellow to grey-white, frequently exhibiting central necrosis or surface ulceration, measuring up to 6 cm in greatest dimension.[552–559]

Microscopic Pathology

The infiltrating tumor offers a variety of growth patterns, including solid, lobular, cribriform, cords, trabeculae, nests and glands, or cysts (Fig. 8–75A). The depth of invasion may not be obvious on a shallow

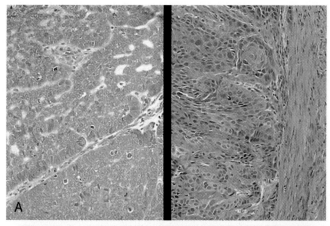

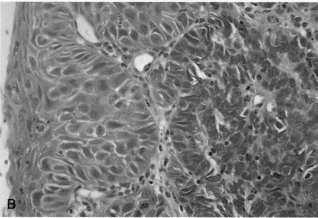

FIGURE 8–75. *A*, A conventional squamous cell carcinoma is seen (*right*) with the characteristic basaloid, small, peripherally palisaded nuclear architecture of a basaloid squamous cell carcinoma (*left*) (H&E, × 150); *B*, The squamous cell carcinoma on the left is seen blending imperceptibly with the basaloid cells, which are more hyperchromatic, smaller in size, with less cytoplasm (H&E, × 300).

biopsy; a generous biopsy is imperative for accurate interpretation of the neoplasm. Vascular or lymphatic perforation is common, while perineural invasion is less frequent. The basaloid component is the most diagnostic feature, incorporating small, closely opposed, moderately pleomorphic cells with hyperchromatic nuclei and scant cytoplasm. A lobular configuration with peripheral palisading, closely opposed to or involving the surface mucosa may be noted (Fig. 8–75B). These basaloid regions are in intimate association with areas of squamous differentiation, manifested as squamous cell carcinoma (invasive or in situ), dysplasia, or just squamous differentiation, frequently in abrupt apposition to the basaloid constituent (see Fig. 8–75 *A* and *B*). A spindled squamous cell carcinoma may also be seen in rare cases.[560] The basaloid component frequently demonstrates marked mitotic activity as well as comedonecrosis in the center of the neoplastic islands. The tumor cells are separated by a prominent dense pink hyaline material and small cystic spaces containing mucoid-type material. The hyaline material may be arranged in a cylinder, rimmed by cells. In metastatic disease, both basaloid- and squamous cell components can be seen, although the basaloid features predominate.[552–559,561]

Special Techniques

The mucinous-type material within the glandular spaces or cystic spaces will react with periodic acid-Schiff and variably with alcian blue preparations but not with mucicarmine. The immunohistochemical profile is that of a carcinoma, with immunoreactivity for cytokeratin, CAM 5.2, EMA, and CEA, with rare cases of reactivity with S-100 protein (perhaps isolated to the dendritic Langerhans' cells) and muscle-specific actin. There is generally no reactivity with vimentin, chromogranin, GFAP, or synaptophysin.[552,557,558,561]

Electron microscopy is not particularly specific, with epithelial features including desmosomes and isolated tonofilaments. There are no neurosecretory granules or myofilaments. The cystic spaces may contain a few loose stellate granules or reduplicated basal lamina.[559] Nuclear ploidy does not seem to provide any useful diagnostic or prognostic information; although a slightly better prognosis in a few of the aneuploid tumors has been reported.[554]

Differential Diagnosis

While the differential diagnosis includes neuroendocrine carcinoma, squamous cell carcinoma, adenoid cystic carcinoma, adenosquamous carcinoma, mucoepidermoid carcinoma, and spindle cell carcinoma, correct diagnosis is predicated on an adequate tissue sample of sufficient depth to demonstrate the heterogeneous nature of the tumor. Adenoid cystic carcinoma does not have any squamous differentiation (squamous carcinoma whether invasive or in situ, dysplasia, or squamous differentiation alone) and usually metastasizes to distant sites rather than cervical lymph nodes. Adenoid cystic carcinoma usually has no prominent pleomorphism, mitoses, or necrosis. A neuroendocrine carcinoma shows nuclear molding, finely granular nuclear chromatin, inconspicuous nucleoli, has immunoreactivity for neuroendocrine markers, and shows neurosecretory granules by ultrastructural studies. An adenosquamous carcinoma may involve acini and ducts, while basaloid squamous cell carcinoma does not. Actually, many carcinomas that have been labeled basaloid squamous cell carcinoma (BSCC) have a majority of cells that are moderately large and not all that "basaloid." Since many BSCC have an adenoid pattern (even having been misdiagnosed as adenoid cystic carcinoma), the distinction from adenosquamous carcinoma can be rather arbitrary. The basaloid component is generally not a feature in spindle cell carcinoma, mucoepidermoid carcinoma or adenoid squamous cell carcinoma.[552–557,559,561–563]

Clinicopathologic Correlation

When the diagnosis of a basaloid squamous carcinoma is made, there is an increased possibility (up to 25%) that there may be a second contemporaneous primary in the upper gastrointestinal or respiratory tract.[558] Nasopharyngeal BSCC has been shown to be associated with EBV, but this has not been revealed in BSCC of the hypopharynx and larynx.[564]

Adenosquamous Carcinoma

Gross Pathology

The tumor may offer an indurated submucosal nodule to an exophytic or polypoid mass, frequently friable and granular with surface ulceration, most frequently in the supraglottic or transglottic, measuring up to 5 cm in maximum dimension, though many are less than 1 cm.[562,565–569]

Microscopic Pathology

By definition, the tumor demonstrates biphasic components of adenocarcinoma and squamous cell carcinoma, with an undifferentiated cellular component in several tumors. The squamous cell carcinoma can be in situ or invasive ranging from well to poorly differentiated. Squamous differentiation is confirmed by pavemented growth with intercellular bridges, keratin pearl formation, dyskeratosis, or individual cell keratinization. The adenocarcinoma component can be tubular, alveolar, and glandular, although mucous cell differentiation is not essential for the diagnosis. The cells in the adenocarcinoma can be basaloid, and separation from basaloid squamous cell carcinoma can be arbitrary (Fig. 8–76). There may also be an in situ component to the adenocarcinoma, with these changes present in the neighboring ductal epithelium. The two carcinomas may be separate or intermixed, with areas of commingling and/or transition of the squamous cell carcinoma to adenocarcinoma. The undifferentiated area between the two distinct carcinomas is often composed of clear cells. Both carcinomas may demonstrate frequent mitoses, necrosis, and infiltration into the surrounding tissue with affiliated perineural invasion. There might be a sparse inflammatory cell infiltrate at the tumor-stromal interface.[562,565–568,570,571]

Special Techniques

The glandular component can be confirmed by illustrating Mayer mucicarmine or diastase-resistant, PAS-positive material in the cells or in the gland lumens.[562,565,566,568,570] Both tumor cell types are diffusely immunoreactive with cytokeratin, while low-molecular-weight cytokeratins and carcinoembryonic antigen are positive only in the glandular component.[571]

Differential Diagnosis

The differential diagnosis includes mucoepidermoid carcinoma, adenocarcinoma with squamous metaplasia, adenoid cystic carcinoma, basaloid squamous cell carcinoma, and adenoid squamous cell carcinoma. Although separation of adenosquamous from mucoepidermoid carcinoma may be impossible in some cases (and it has been stated that adenosquamous carcinoma is a high-grade mucoepidermoid carcinoma), a mucoepidermoid carcinoma demonstrates intermediate-type cells and generally has no true squamous cell differentiation.[566] There is no true adenocarcinoma and distinctly separate squamous cell carcinoma in a mucoepidermoid carcinoma. The demonstration of true mucous cells, with squashed, eccentrically placed nuclei, also helps segregate these neoplasms. An adenocarcinoma with squamous metaplasia generally does not demonstrate the nuclear criteria of a malignant squamous cell component. Adenoid cystic carcinoma is usually composed of smaller cells with hyperchromatic nuclei, arranged in the characteristic cribriform pattern, although the solid variant may be difficult to distinguish. The reduplicated basement membrane material can be accentuated with diastase-resistant PAS positivity. An adenoid squamous cell carcinoma (acantholytic squamous cell carcinoma) is a variant of squamous cell carcinoma, in which there is acantholysis of the squamous cells, a few of which can be clear, mimicking glandular differentiation. A mucicarmine stain will not react, discriminating between these two tumors.[562,563,566–568,570–572] A contemporaneous squamous cell carcinoma and adenocarcinoma may affect the larynx, but these lesions are usually temporally separated.[573,574]

Clinicopathologic Correlation

Adenosquamous carcinoma behaves aggressively, irrespective of the size of the lesion and the type of

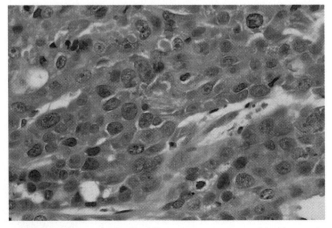

FIGURE 8–76. Small gland-like structures are seen blending with sheets of squamous epithelium (H&E, × 300).

therapy used, necessitating correct diagnosis at the time of surgery on an adequate tissue sample. Nearly 80% of cases demonstrate metastases, while adenoid squamous cell carcinoma and muco-epidermoid carcinomas rarely metastasize. The metastatic disease generally displays both components of the neoplasm, although one may predominate.[562,565–568]

Adenoid Cystic Carcinoma

Gross Pathology

Location within the larynx varies, with a slight majority of the tumors found in the subglottis and the remainder in the supraglottis, depending on which studies are reported. It also occurs in the trachea as the second most common malignant tumor (after squamous cell carcinoma). The tumor mass frequently presents as a diffuse thickening of the mucosa, although it may be a solid, rubbery to firm pink-grey mass still covered by an intact mucosa, measuring up to 5 cm in greatest dimension.[350,575–583]

Microscopic Pathology

The tumor is unencapsulated and infiltrative, with a proclivity to perineural invasion. The cribriform pattern is the most characteristic for this tumor, with uniform sheets of cells strikingly punctured with large pseudocystic spaces, resembling Swiss cheese; the pseudocystic spaces are filled with hyaline material (Fig. 8–77A). There is a vague degree of palisading around these spaces. The tubular pattern has well-formed ducts with a central lumen, which if cut longitudinally will give the trabecular pattern. If tumor cells are seen surrounding the matrix material, it is generally considered to be a cylindromatous pattern. The solid pattern has only rare lumen formation, sometimes demonstrating necrosis and small

nests within larger nests. Multiple growth patterns may be seen in the same tumor. Small round cells with large hyperchromatic nuclei with scant cytoplasm, in a syncytial type arrangement, are characteristically found in close approximation with the hyaline matrix material. The cells are generally bland cytologically (Fig. 8–77B). The stroma may be hyalinized into the cylindrical structures characteristic for the tumor, or it may be mucinous or myxoid, abruptly juxtaposed to the epithelial component (unlike pleomorphic adenoma in which there is a blending of the epithelium and stroma). The stroma is diastase-resistant PAS-positive.[350,576,577,579,581,582,584,585] A solid histology with necrosis has been associated with a more aggressive clinical course, as does infiltration into the surrounding region and the grade of the tumor.[577,583]

Special Techniques

The dual cell types (epithelial and myoepithelial) are confirmed with immunohistochemical analysis, although the undifferentiated cells observed by electron microscopy do not react with any specific antibodies. The cells found lining the true lumens express keratin, carcinoembryonic antigen, epithelial membrane antigen, vimentin, and S-100 protein, while the myoepithelial cells found at the stromal-tumor interface react with actin and, to a lesser and variable extent, with the previously mentioned antisera. There is some variability of staining based on the architectural pattern of growth. The replicated basal lamina react with antisera to type IV collagen and laminin.[561,584,586]

Undifferentiated, ductal, secretory, and myoepithelial cells can be found on ultrastructural study. The epithelial nature of the ductal and secretory cells is confirmed with small true lumens lined with microvilli and junctional complexes and secretory products in association with rough endoplasmic re-

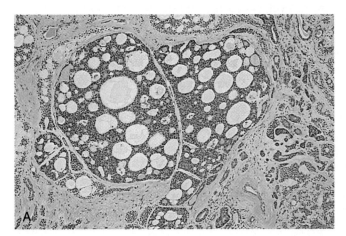
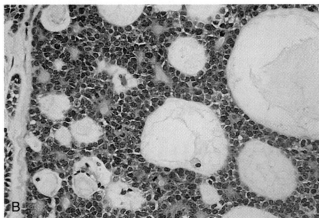

FIGURE 8–77. *A*, The characteristic "Swiss cheese" or cribriform pattern of an adenoid cystic carcinoma is seen in the center, with glandular and tubular profiles at the periphery (H&E, × 75); *B*, Small, hyperchromatic to vesicular nuclei are arranged around small rims of reduplicated basement membrane around the central cystic spaces. Mitotic figures are seen (H&E, × 300).

ticulum and Golgi complexes. Myoepithelial cells have myofilaments with focal densities and pinocytotic vesicles. The pleuripotent cell does not demonstrate any specific or characteristic findings. The cyst-like material is multilayered basal lamina or lamina lucida and lamina densa substance.[587]

Differential Diagnosis

The differential diagnosis is complicated by the variable histology of adenoid cystic carcinoma (formerly called cylindroma). The cells of pleomorphic adenoma are usually more variable and not quite so hyperchromatic. The background stroma of a pleomorphic adenoma is intimately admixed with the epithelial/myoepithelial component, in contrast to the abrupt interface in an adenoid cystic carcinoma. A lack of perineural invasion or invasive growth supports diagnosis of pleomorphic adenoma. A mucoepidermoid carcinoma has intermediate cells and mucous cells, which are not found in adenoid cystic carcinoma. A basaloid squamous cell carcinoma has not only the squamous differentiation, but it generally also has a greater degree of nuclear pleomorphism and is not arranged in a cribriform pattern. An adenoid squamous cell carcinoma has a characteristic acantholysis of the tumor cells, which demonstrate obvious squamous differentiation. Although neuroendocrine tumors are composed of small cells, they are usually not arranged in a cribriform architecture (although they may be), and immunoreactivity with neuroendocrine markers will help to separate these neoplasms.[350,552,572,582]

Clinicopathologic Correlation

Positive margins of resection are frequent in this type of tumor, especially when located in the trachea. The lesional cells may track along the nerves of the region, often for quite a distance from the gross tumor, thereby resulting in positive surgical margins. The tumor does not seem to metastasize frequently but will affect the adjacent lymph nodes and larynx or trachea through recurrence or direct extension. The type of treatment rendered postoperatively should be tailored due to the infrequent lymph node metastases but occasional systemic metastases. Adenoid cystic carcinomas tend to have a better prognosis than squamous cell carcinomas of the trachea.[578–580,582]

Mucoepidermoid Carcinoma

Gross Pathology

A mass lesion, often exophytic or fungating, is usually identified within the supraglottic (epiglottis) or less frequently in the glottic larynx. There are rare reports of tracheal involvement. The tumors are usually submucosal, with infrequent surface ulceration.

While there are no specific gross characteristics of the tumor, the cut surface is usually solid, firm, tan-white to pink with a mucoid material, measuring up to 5 cm in maximum dimension. Cystic spaces are present in the low-grade lesions, often filled with mucoid or blood-tinged fluid.[350,564,588–596]

Microscopic Pathology

The tumors are infiltrative, unencapsulated or poorly encapsulated masses, infrequently involving the nerves of the region. The triad of squamous cells, intermediate cells and mucin-producing cells sets the defining characteristics of this tumor, with the varying proportions of each of these cell types determining the grade of the tumor (Fig. 8–78A). In the low-grade tumors, which may arise from the surface epithelium, there is an admixture of mucus-producing cells with intermediate cells and squamous cells arranged around variable-sized cystic cavities.[350,595] Mucin-producing cells are not difficult to identify with their pale or foamy cytoplasm with a peripherally placed, small, dark nucleus (Fig. 8–78B). The intermediate or transitional cells are pavemented with distinct cellular borders separating the sheets of cells. The intermediate cells contain small round nuclei with limited eosinophilic cytoplasm, while the epidermoid cells have vesicular nuclei surrounded by ample amounts of eosinophilic cytoplasm. True keratinization of the cells and intercellular bridges is quite unusual in the epidermoid component, although these features can be seen. Mitoses and pleomorphism are unusual. The mucous cells may rupture, producing an inflammatory and desmoplastic stromal response, in addition to extracellular mucin pools.[350,569,588,591,593–596] Mucous cells are often difficult to find in the high-grade mucoepidermoid carcinoma, which is composed primarily of squamous and intermediate cells. Nuclear atypia and mitoses are much more frequent in this grade of tumor. Vascular invasion is usually easy to identify. The intermediate grade is identified by features intermediate between low-grade and high-grade mucoepidermoid carcinoma (MEC). The cysts are usually less numerous and smaller in size, having an increased cellularity, although not as cellular as the high-grade tumors. Clear cell changes can be seen in all grades of MEC and are thought to represent hydropic change within epidermoid cells (no PAS or mucicarmine reactivity).[569,588,589,592,595]

Special Techniques

The mucin-producing cells will reveal intracytoplasmic mucicarmine positivity (Fig. 8–78C) and PAS-positive, diastase-resistant material. The intermediate and epidermoid cells do not contain mucicarminophilic material. The cells are generally cytokeratin reactive, but will be negative with stains for S-100 protein, glial fibrillary acidic protein, and actin.

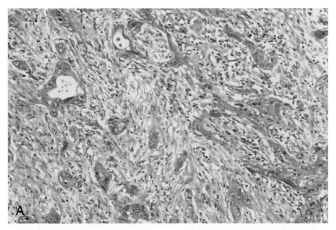

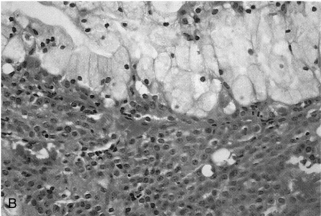

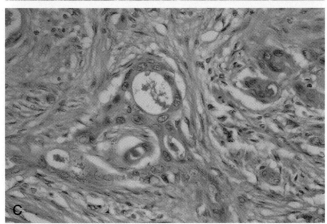

FIGURE 8-78. *A,* A moderately differentiated mucoepidermoid carcinoma with rare cysts lined by epidermoid cells. The epidermoid cells are seen infiltrating into the stroma (H&E, × 150); *B,* Mucous cells with peripherally compressed nuclei (*top*) lying above intermediate-type cells in the lower portion (H&E, × 300); *C,* Both intracytoplasmic and extracellular mucin material are present in this infiltrating, intermediate-grade mucoepidermoid carcinoma (Mucicarmine, × 300).

The ultrastructural findings are those of squamous and mucus-secreting cells, with abundant cytoplasmic tonofilaments and desmosomes in the squamous cells and membrane-bound, electron-lucent mucin granules in the mucous cells. Short microvilli are present in addition to tight junctions and desmosomes. Myoepithelial cells are not seen.[592,596,597]

Differential Diagnosis

Perhaps the differential diagnosis needs to be prefaced by a statement by Damiani and colleagues[566] in which they suggest the term "mucoepidermoid-adenosquamous carcinoma" to include the spectrum of changes identified in a pure squamous cell carcinoma on one aspect and a pure adenocarcinoma on the other. The differential therefore includes squamous cell carcinoma, adenosquamous carcinoma, adenoid cystic carcinoma, epithelial-myoepithelial carcinoma, and adenocarcinoma, not otherwise specified. A squamous cell carcinoma may be poorly differentiated and vaguely resemble mucoepidermoid carcinoma. However, intermediate cells and mucous cells are not present in a squamous cell carcinoma, the latter accentuated with a mucicarmine stain. Squamous cell carcinoma generally responds well to irradiation, while MEC does not, hence the importance of distinguishing between these two tumors.[589,590,595] Adenosquamous cell carcinomas demonstrate distinct foci of adenocarcinoma (glandular differentiation), and squamous cell carcinoma generally does not exhibit intermediate cells nor true mucus (goblet) cells. This is generally considered a highly aggressive malignancy.[350,562,588,591] Adenoid cystic carcinoma may have a myxoid stroma but does not usually exhibit true mucous cells, nor are there intermediate cells or epidermoid cells. Electron microscopy will reveal myoepithelial cells, which are absent in MEC. An epithelial-myoepithelial carcinoma has a distinctive dual cell population, with a mantle of clear cells surrounding the central cuboidal, dark staining cells.[350,588,598] An adenocarcinoma will generally contain mucin within the clear cells, while the clear cell variant of MEC in the larynx is usually negative. A metastatic renal cell carcinoma (RCC) also needs to be excluded. Metastatic RCC is not usually arranged in a cystic configuration, does not demonstrate intermediate cells, will have a distinctive rich vascular network, and will be diastase-sensitive, PAS-positive for glycogen. A clinical history or examination will demonstrate the renal primary.

Benign mucous gland hamartomas or proliferations can also be seen in the larynx, but usually they have no squamous or intermediate cell differentiation and do have much better gland formation.[350] Necrotizing sialometaplasia has been described in the larynx, but the lobular nature of the growth and the lack of nuclear atypia will exclude a mucoepidermoid carcinoma.[54]

Neuroendocrine Carcinoma

There is a great deal of confusion in the literature as to the correct terminology for neuroendocrine tumors of the larynx. In a recent description of the terminology used for the tumors, fully 43 different names were catalogued, followed by "etc.", which suggests only part of the terminology problem.[599] We will try to be uniform in our use of the terminology by supporting the terms suggested by the World Health Organization and by limiting the terms to carcinoid tumor, atypical carcinoid tumor, and small-cell carcinoma (oat cell and intermediate and combined cell types) for the malignant lesions (see previous discussion of paraganglioma). There are many articles relating to this topic, but we will include only the more recent reviews.[373,374,379,600–607] Although the tumors express neuroendocrine differentiation, rarely do any of the carcinoids or atypical carcinoids exhibit ectopic hormone production and are generally considered to be nonfunctional tumors.[373,601,605,608] However, small-cell carcinomas may be associated with paraneoplastic syndromes.[374,609]

Gross Pathology

Neuroendocrine tumors of the aforementioned three categories generally occur most frequently in the supraglottic region, presenting as a submucosal mass in the aryepiglottic fold, arytenoid, or laryngeal side of the epiglottis. It is proposed that carcinoids and atypical carcinoids arise in the seromucous gland-duct apparatus, since most of the tumors are supraglottic in location and that is where the most seromucus glands are found. The histogenesis is unsettled, with either a pluripotential stem cell or the Kulchitsky-like cell being the cell of origin.[373,602,605–607,609–611] Paraganglioma is thought to be of neural origin, while neuroendocrine carcinomas are thought to be of epithelial origin.[373,374,599,605,606] The gross appearance ranges from polypoid, pedunculated to ulcerated, often appearing blue or red, ranging in size up to 4 cm, but on average are 1.8 cm for carcinoids, 1.6 cm for atypical carcinoids, and 1.8 cm for small-cell carcinoma.[372,373,379,602,603,605–607,609,612–614]

Microscopic Pathology

Neuroendocrine tumors are usually unencapsulated, although carcinoids and atypical carcinoids are circumscribed, covered by an uninvolved surface mucosa. The atypical carcinoid and small-cell carcinoma may demonstrate surface ulceration. The tumors present with a variety of histologic patterns, including an organoid or trabecular growth in the carcinoid tumors (Fig. 8–79A); the addition of cords, and solid, single-file, and cribriform patterns in the atypical carinoids (Fig. 8–79B; 8–80 A and B). All the aforementioned patterns, along with sheets, ribbons, pseudoglands, and rosette formations, occur in small-cell carcinoma. A cell nest pattern may also occur, mimicking a paraganglioma. A fibrovascular stroma is generally absent in small-cell carcinoma,

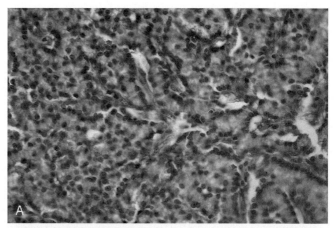

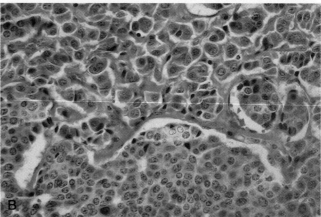

FIGURE 8–79. *A,* Well-differentiated cells with pale cytoplasm surrounding round nuclei with granular, coarse nuclear chromatin are seen in this carcinoid (H&E, × 300); *B,* The upper portion of the field demonstrates moderately pleomorphic cells with coarse, hyperchromatic nuclei, while the lower portion shows better differentiated tumor cells, with a glandular-type arrangement of small cells with stippled chromatin and ample, eosinophilic cytoplasm (H&E, × 300).

although it is seen in carcinoids and atypical carcinoids. Vascular or lymphatic invasion, perineural invasion, and soft-tissue infiltration is seen in the atypical carcinoids or small-cell carcinomas.[374,373,379,602,603,605–607,611–614]

The cytologic appearance of the cells is determined by the subtype of neuroendocrine carcinoma. Epithelial differentiation as evidenced by glandular (with mucin production) or squamous nests has been seen in carcinoid (see Fig. 8–79A), is often present in atypical carcinoid, and is occasionally identified in small-cell carcinoma. Within the spectrum of neuroendocrine tumors, the degree of cellular pleomorphism and mitotic activity and necrosis increases as the tumor becomes more poorly differentiated (small-cell carcinoma). There is virtual absence of pleomorphism, necrosis, and mitoses in a carcinoid; all these are prominent in a small-cell carcinoma; and atypical carcinoid exhibits intermediate features (see Figs. 8–79B; 8–80 A and B). Due to the

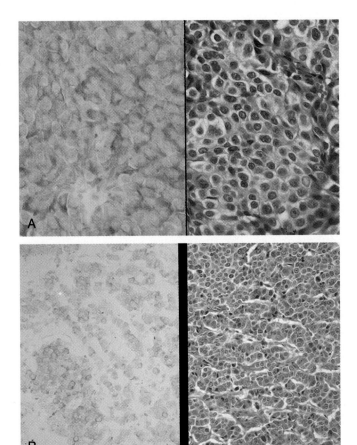

FIGURE 8–80. A, The cytoplasm of the tumor cells mark with chromogranin (left, × 300). The cells are small, with round nuclei with prominent nucleoli (right, H&E, × 300); B, Many of the cells are arranged in trabeculae or cords with cellular engulfment by other cells seen in a number of foci (right, H&E, × 150). There is strong reactivity with calcitonin, a frequent finding in neuroendocrine carcinomas (left, calcitonin, × 150).

fragility of the cells, crush artifact is frequently prominent in small-cell carcinoma.

Carcinoid tumors have small, monotonous cells with a low nuclear:cytoplasmic ratio, round to oval vesicular and centrally placed nuclei surrounded by eosinophilic to clear cytoplasm. The nuclei may demonstrate finely stippled chromatin. There are usually no nucleoli (see Fig. 8–79A). Atypical carcinoid tumors usually have a more pleomorphic cell population than is seen in carcinoid tumors, with vesicular to hyperchromatic nuclei within polygonal cells that have an increased nuclear:cytoplasmic ratio. The location of the nucleus is variable, surrounded by amphophilic to eosinophilic cytoplasm. Nucleoli are variable, from absent to prominent[373,602,605] (see Figs. 8–79B; 8–80 A and B). Increased mitotic activity is seen.

The small-cell carcinoma has cells that demonstrate a high nuclear:cytoplasmic ratio with minimal cytoplasm, generally no nucleoli within the intensely

hyperchromatic oval to spindled nuclei. Necrotic nuclear debris may be found, as well as occasional neoplastic multinucleated giant cells. The intermediate cell type of small-cell carcinoma has slightly larger nuclei with obvious, more abundant, cytoplasm. There is usually limited stroma, which may be mucoid. A combined small-cell carcinoma has an associated squamous cell carcinoma, adenocarcinoma, or other tumor type.[609,611,613] It is apparent from this description that there is a definite spectrum from the more indolent carcinoid to the high-grade small-cell carcinoma. Although each feature by itself is not diagnostic, in aggregate the distinction between each of these tumors becomes manifest.[373,374,379,603,605–607,609,612–614]

Special Techniques

Carcinoids and atypical carcinoids will demonstrate argyrophilia (Grimelius method), but are only rarely agentaffinic, while small-cell carcinomas almost never demonstrate either.[373,374,379,605–607,609,611–614]

Carcinoids react with neuron-specific enolase, chromogranin, keratin (low-molecular-weight), EMA, CEA, somatostatin, serotonin, and calcitonin. However, immunohistochemistries have only been performed in a few cases.[372,374,379,602,606,612,615,616] Atypical carcinoids mark most frequently with the following immunohistochemical reactions: chromogranin (94%) (see Fig. 8–80A), synaptophysin (100%), keratin (low-molecular-weight) (96%), calcitonin (80%) (see Fig. 8–80B), CEA (75%), and somatostatin (50%).[372–374,603,605,606,614,615] Small-cell neuroendocrine carcinomas express keratin, CAM 5.2, CEA, chromogranin, calcitonin, NSE, and synaptophysin.[372–374,379,603,605–607,609,615] A complete spectrum of immunoreactivities for a variety of markers has been found in individual case reports, but are not specific or sensitive for the tumors. Almost all the neuroendocrine carcinomas (all three types) were negative for S-100 protein, GFAP, and met-enkephalins, although there have been reports of S-100 protein reactivity in isolated cases.[372,617] Perhaps this finding serves to underscore the heavy reliance on immunohistochemistries for this category of tumors. However, suffice it to say there needs to be a correlation between the histologic features and the immunoreactivity in order to achieve useful clinical treatment and prognosis.

Electron microscopy of carcinoid and atypical carcinoid tumors will demonstrate abundant membrane-bound electron-dense neurosecretory granules, ranging from 100 μm to 250 μm. Complex intercellular digitation and occasional intercellular junctions are present.[373,379,603,605–607,612,616] Small-cell carcinoma usually has fewer neurosecretory granules, ranging in size from 50 μm 200 μm, desmosomes, and tonofilament bundles.[373,379,605–607,609,611,618] Nuclear ploidy analysis does not provide any useful diagnostic or prognostic information.[619]

Differential Diagnosis

The differential diagnosis includes undifferentiated carcinoma, squamous cell carcinoma, malignant melanoma, poorly differentiated adenoid cystic carcinoma, lymphoma, mycosis fungoides, metastatic carcinoma, medullary carcinoma, and paraganglioma.

Part of the reason for making a definitive diagnosis regarding neuroendocrine tumors is the difference in treatment protocols and patient outcome. A poorly differentiated squamous cell carcinoma (which will be negative for neuroendocrine immunohistochemistries and will not be argyrophilic) will respond to radiation therapy, while atypical carcinoid is generally insensitive to this modality. Paraganglioma is a benign tumor with an excellent prognosis, responding to surgical excision alone. The rich vascularity, cell nest growth, S-100 protein reactivity of the sustentacular cells, and negative calcitonin reaction will define a paraganglioma. A typical carcinoid is quite rare, demonstrating a lack of pleomorphism, necrosis, and mitosis, with uniform bland features in an organoid arrangement. A mucosal melanoma may have melanin pigment, more frequently involves the surface epithelium, will demonstrate more atypia in the nuclear and cellular features, and will have S-100 protein and HMB-45 reactivity in the tumor cells (rather than the sustentacular cells of a paraganglioma).[373,605-607,611,612,614,620] It is imperative to exclude a metastatic tumor to the larynx, especially in small-cell carcinoma, where a lung primary may have metastasized. Medullary carcinoma of the thyroid may metastasize to the larynx; however, the distinction between medullary carcinoma of the thyroid and neuroendocrine carcinoma of the larynx is nearly impossible, with the exception of an increased serum calcitonin level being much more likely in a thyroid medullary carcinoma and usually a lack of amyloid in the laryngeal lesions.[380,606,607,621,622] Lymphomas, with crush artifact and a submucosal location, can be separated by lacking neuroendocrine differentiation (either immunohistochemically or ultrastructurally). Mycosis fungoides specifically demonstrates cerebriform nuclei and Pautrier's mucosal microabscesses and a polymorphic lymphocytic infiltrate.

Clinicopathologic Correlation

The reason for the distinction between of these tumor types relates to the differences in treatment and prognosis. Large-cell neuroendocrine carcinomas are usually treated with surgery alone, as they are rather insensitive to radiation or chemotherapy.

Mucosal Malignant Melanoma

Gross Pathology

Most laryngeal mucosal malignant melanomas (MMM) arise within the supraglottic region, presenting as a nodular, sessile, pedunculated, polypoid or exophytic growth. Ulceration of the surface epithelium can be present. A variety of colors can be seen from black to red, tan, or white. The tumors measure up to 6 cm in greatest dimensions.[620,623-630]

Microscopic Pathology

Although malignant melanomas of the mucosa are not categorized as their cutaneous counterparts, a specific cell type—spindle-shaped, epithelioid, plasmacytoid—can be utilized in the description of the tumor (Fig. 8–81 A and B). A solid, infiltrative growth pattern is identified in these hypercellular tumors, with occasional pseudoglands and rare squamous foci. The tumor may invade into the surrounding adipose connective tissue, muscle, cartilage, and/or nerves. The cells are customarily large epithelioid cells containing large round to oval nuclei surrounded by variable amounts of eosinophilic cytoplasm. The nuclei are vesicular to hyperchromatic with prominent eosinophilic nucleoli (see Figs. 8–81 A and B). When spindle cells are present, they are arranged in a fascicular or storiform growth pattern. The cells are elongated, with similar nuclear and cytoplasmic features. The plasmacytoid pattern exhibits an eccentrically located vesicular to basophilic nucleus without any clearing in the paranuclear zone (hof region). Cellular pleomorphism is common, accompanied by necrosis and mitoses, many of which can be atypical (see Fig. 8–81 A and B).[620,625,626,628-630]

Special Techniques

If melanin pigment is observed, it is granular and black to brown (see Fig. 8–81A). An argentaffin stain (Fontana-Masson) will expose the melanin as fine, black intracytoplasmic granules (Fig. 8–81C), with a more granular black to brown inclusion revealed by an argyrophil stain (Grimelius or Churukian-Schenk). Hemosiderin can look similar to melanin on H&E, but Prussian blue will react with the iron in hemosiderin pigment, yielding a blue reaction.[624,626,629,630]

While a number of immunoreactions have been demonstrated in melanoma, S-100 protein (cytoplasmic or nuclear) and melanoma antigen using antibody HMB-45 (cytoplasmic) are the most helpful in the differential diagnosis with other tumors. Melanoma antigen has been demonstrated in other neoplasms but, in combination with the S-100 protein, usually excludes most of the possibilities in the larynx.[631] The spindle cell variant of melanoma tends to be nonreactive with HMB-45.[632] Inasmuch as MMM is a great mimic of other neoplasms, a panel of antibodies should be utilized, including cytokeratin, chromogranin, synaptophysin, leukocyte common antigen, B- and T-cell markers, vimentin, actin, and desmin, with κ and λ in the plasmacytoid tumor types.[625,629,630]

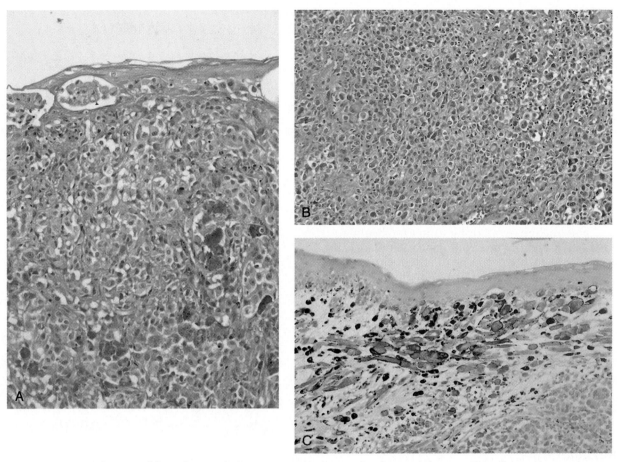

FIGURE 8–81. *A,* Involvement of the surface epithelium is seen in this mucosal malignant melanoma. The cells are pleomorphic, arranged in epithelioid packages with abundant melanin pigment present (H&E, × 150); *B,* Enlarged cells with hyperchromatic nuclei, opaque cytoplasm, and an overall epithelioid pattern. Mitotic figures and apoptosis are seen (H&E, × 200); *C,* Melanoma cells react with Fontana Masson stain to demonstrate a positive argentaffin reaction (Fontana Masson, × 250).

Equivocal immunohistochemistries may necessitate the adoption of electron microscopy, which will demonstrate unique membrane-bound vesicles containing helical structures with a characteristic transverse and zigzag 8 to 10 nm periodicity, referred to as premelanosomes or melanosomes. There are generally no desmosomes or cell junctions.[625,630,633]

Differential Diagnosis

Melanocytes within the epithelium give rise to MMM in the larynx, and a junctional or in situ component may be identified in the surface epithelium so long as there is no ulceration of the surface (see Fig. 8–81*A*).[620,630,634–636] However, in the absence of a documented origin in the mucosa, a metastatic tumor to the larynx must be excluded.[620,624,629,630,637,638] The protean manifestations of MMM evoke a wide differential diagnosis of pleomorphic and spindle cell tumors, including SCC, SCSCC, neuroendocrine carcinoma (NEC), extramedullary plasmacytoma, malignant lymphoma, and a variety of sarcomas. SCC may demonstrate a surface or in situ component or rare foci of keratinization,

which should be carefully sought. Poorly differentiated squamous carcinoma may not show cytokeratin immunoreactivity, but it is negative for S-100 protein or melanoma antigen. SCSCC is usually associated with squamous cell carcinoma (in situ or invasive), often requiring multiple sections to document the conventional SCC. These efforts may be confounded by ulceration and loss of the surface epithelium. The spindle cell component may vary from bland to markedly pleomorphic. Immunoreactivity with cytokeratin may be absent in up to 40% of cases, but a full panel, including S-100 protein and antibody HMB-45, will help to segregate these neoplasms.[550]

A malignant lymphoma can usually be differentiated by light microscopy coupled with the clinical history, expressing immunoreactivity with LCA and either B- or T-cell lineage markers. An extramedullary plasmacytoma may have a similar histology to the plasmacytoid variant of MMM. The nuclear chromatin in a plasmacytoma tends to be more stippled and "clock-face" than in MMM and will present a classic paranuclear clear zone (hof). Plasmacytomas tend to be less pleomorphic, with fewer mitotic figures. Histochemical (intracytoplasmic red staining with methyl green pyronine) and immuno-histochemical reactions (κ, λ) can be used to confirm the nature of the tumor.

NEC, specifically the atypical carcinoid type, share histologic similarities with MMM. NEC will often have a glandular growth pattern and demonstrate epithelial mucin (mucicarmine or diastase-resistant PAS-positive) but no argentaffinity (Fontana-Masson). NEC will also react with antibodies for keratin, chromogranin, and calcitonin; is infrequently S-100 protein positive but is negative with HMB-45. While laryngeal sarcomas are extraordinary (chondrosarcoma is not included in this differential), malignant fibrous histiocytoma (MFH), leiomyosarcoma, fibro-sarcoma, and malignant peripheral nerve sheath tumors (MPNST) yield a morphologic resemblance to spindled MMM, which can be distinguished with the aid of immunophenotyping. Vimentin will be reactive in fibrosarcoma and MFH, while KP-1 (his-tiocytic marker) will be reactive in MFH. Leiomyo-sarcoma will react with vimentin, desmin, and actin, but not with HMB-45. MPNST will, by definition, react with S-100 protein, although not as intensely or diffusely as MMM, but does not reveal HMB-45 immunoreactivity. The histologic appearance, united with the immunophenotype, will help to establish a correct diagnosis.[620,629,630]

Chondrosarcoma

Gross Pathology

The tumor most commonly occurs on the anterior surface of the posterior lamina of the cricoid carti-lage (usually subglottic in location), with the thyroid cartilage and arytenoid affected slightly less com-monly, and the trachea only rarely. Patients might present with a neck mass. The tumor is usually a smooth, lobulated or rounded, hard (may have de-generative softening) submucosal mass, expanding into the larynx, hypopharyx, or trachea, measuring greater than 2 cm in greatest dimension. The mucosa is ordinarily intact, although it may be erythematous and ulcerated in advanced tumors (Fig. 8–82A). Many patients demonstrate impairment of the vocal cords.[22,317,384,386,393,639–646]

Microscopic Pathology

The tumor is composed of lobules of hypercellular hyaline (not elastic) basophilic cartilage, the chon-droid lacunae filled with pleomorphic nuclei and binucleated and multinucleated forms. There is an increased nuclear:cytoplasmic ratio, with delicate to hyperchromatic and enlarged nuclei, many of them featuring prominent nucleoli. Although the tumor may appear quite pleomorphic, there are usually few mitotic figures (Fig. 8–82B). The increase in cel-lularity results in a relative decrease in the amount

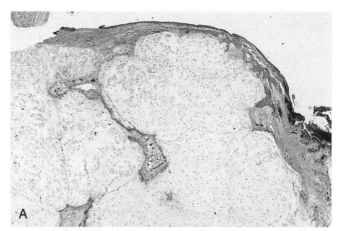

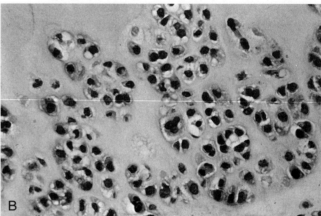

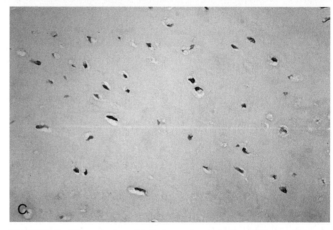

FIGURE 8–82. *A*, A multilobular, submucosal cartilaginous neo-plasm can be seen in this specimen, with focal surface ulceration (H&E, × 15); *B*, Marked nuclear pleomorphism, multinucleation, and hyperchromatic nuclei in high-grade chondrosarcoma. Mitotic figures can be seen (H&E, × 450); *C*, Increased cellularity, only mild nuclear pleomorphism, and increased nuclear:cytoplasmic ra-tio are changes characteristic of a low-grade chondrosarcoma (H&E, × 300).

of stroma between the lacunae. Areas of necrosis, calcification, and osteoid matrix can be found in these tumors, but these findings do not change the diagnosis or the prognosis. There is not true bone formation by the tumor cells, but non-neoplastic bone can be identified. Spindled cell regions may be seen in higher-grade tumors, resembling fibrosarcoma. Chondrosarcomas are usually divided into low-, medium-, and high-grade tumors, although a two-tiered classification is also used (Fig. 8–82 *B* and *C*) These grades are based on an increasing cellularity; greater variability in the size, shape, and nuclear hyperchromasia; as well as necrosis and a greater number of bi- and multinucleated cells. The extent of atypical nuclei does not have to be great in order to qualify the whole lesion as a low-grade chondrosarcoma (see Fig. 8–82C). The intermediate- and high-grade tumors tend to recur and metastasize more frequently than the low-grade tumors, as do tumors of the thyroid cartilage. However, the rate of metastasis is usually below 10%. Overall prognosis is determined by the site, grade, and tumor resectability, especially in the head and neck, and specifically in the larynx. Myxoid and dedifferentiated chondrosarcomas may portend a more aggressive clinical course.[22,317,384,386,640,641,643–648]

Special Techniques

Although usually not needed, immunoreactivity for S-100 protein and vimentin can be documented.[646] Ultrastructurally, round to spindle-shaped chondrocytes with short processes and scalloped membranes are found on ultrastructural analysis of chondrosarcomas, similar to other body sites. The nuclei are indented with dispersed chromatin and nucleoli. Flocculent material can be found within distended short segments of rough endoplasmic reticulum. Glycogen, often in rosette formation, can be seen in the cytoplasm. Extralacunar matrix vesicles and proteoglycan granules are found enmeshed in fine fibrils of matrix material.[640,649,650]

DNA ploidy has been equivocal in distinguishing between chondromas and low-grade chondrosarcomas, although most high-grade chondrosarcomas are aneuploid.[644]

Differential Diagnosis

A variety of chondroid or myxoid tumors are included in the differential diagnosis (although sarcomas as a whole are rare in the larynx), with chondroma, chondromatous hamartoma/metaplasia, pleomorphic adenoma, and myxoma constituting the benign lesions and fibrosarcoma, liposarcoma, osteosarcoma, and spindle squamous cell carcinoma with cartilaginous metaplasia completing the malignant differential diagnoses. Chondroma has been previously discussed. Cartilaginous tissues can be present in hamartomas or pleomorphic adenoma, but there is usually no atypia to the cells or increased cellularity, and epithelial or myoepithelial components are present. Myxoma is extraordinarily rare in the larynx and generally has stellate cells with bland nuclei, a reticular fiber network, and mast cells within the myxoid background material.[22,34] Liposarcomas

demonstrate lipoblasts and often have a characteristic vascular pattern not seen in chondrosarcomas. Osteosarcomas are rare as primary tumors of the larynx, demonstrating osteoid matrix deposition by the malignant osteoblasts. Histochemical studies of alkaline phophatase (positive in osteosarcoma) may be necessary to separate these tumors. A spindle squamous cell carcinoma often demonstrates a surface carcinoma in situ or an invasive squamous cell carcinoma intimately associated with the spindled component. The areas of chondroid metaplasia may undergo malignant transformation and become a chondrosarcoma. In this setting, the features of chondrosarcoma are present within the cartilaginous foci.[317,393,641]

Fibrosarcoma and Malignant Fibrous Histiocytoma

Review of the literature about fibrosarcoma and malignant fibrous histiocytoma (MFH) is fraught with inconsistencies. Many cases of MFH and fibrosarcoma do not include the gross description, often have surface epithelium ulceration, and were reported prior to the widespread use of immunohistochemistries. It is, therefore, this author's contention that most if not all of these reports are in fact examples of spindle squamous cell carcinoma. As there is no way to prove this assertion, these tumors will be discussed, for illustrative and differential purposes only, realizing that these tumors are exceedingly rare in the larynx and trachea.

Gross Pathology

Most of these tumors are found along the anterior vocal cords or the anterior commissure, although any portion of the larynx and trachea can be involved. The tumors generally present as smooth, nodular, or pedunculated masses, with a number presenting as fungating or ulcerating masses. The lesions are often mucosal or submucosal in location, the cut surface revealing a fleshy, homogeneous white-tan to yellow-pink mass, measuring up to 5 cm in maximum dimension.[467,651–663]

Microscopic Pathology

Malignant fibrous histiocytoma is divided into a number of different subtypes based on the predominant feature (myxoid, inflammatory, giant cell, pleomorphic, angiomatoid), but subtyping in the larynx is not related to outcome. The cellular tumors are unencapsulated, sometimes sharply circumscribed, although often infiltrating out into the submucosa and occasionally ulcerating through the surface epithelium. Spindle cells are arranged in compact fascicles, intersected by various amounts of collagen. The cell bundles may be arranged at abrupt angles to one another, giving a herringbone or a storiform appearance, while in other areas there is a gentle undulation of the cells. The areas of cartwheel, pinwheel, or haphazard matted appearance often blend with cellular and myxoid areas. There is a marked variability in the cellularity within and between tumors (Fig. 8–83). The cells are fusiform and elongated with a centrally placed vesicular, needle-like nucleus surrounded by tapering cytoplasm that is often indistinct, giving a syncytial appearance to the fascicles. Giant cells can be found, including tumor giant cells, containing multiple nuclei, different from those contained within the spindled tumor cells. There can be marked nuclear pleomorphism, with high nuclear:cytoplasmic ratios. The nuclei in these areas are often hyperchromatic and irregular in contour. Histiocytes with large, vacuolated cells with round nuclei can be identified, but the number and location vary from tumor to tumor. In either tumor type, the cells are not usually wavy and there are no cross-striations. Mitotic figures can be found in varying numbers, with the more poorly differentiated tumors containing atypical forms. Hemorrhage and necrosis can be found in the poorly differentiated forms, with areas of myxoid degeneration (see Fig. 8–83).[467,536,651–653,655,659–661,663]

Special Techniques

A true malignant fibrous histiocytoma of the larynx would demonstrate polygonal and spindle cells and bizarre giant cells. The cells react with vimentin, lysosomal enzymes, Fc receptors, and mesenchymal antigens, but do not usually demonstrate true histiocytic lineage. Instead, there seems to be a modification to the histiocytes that demonstrate mesenchymal differentiation as well, either representing facultative histiocytes or facultative fibroblasts. There is usually no reactivity with myoglobin, actin, S-100 protein, or keratin.[470,652,658]

Electron microscopy (EM) is difficult to interpret, as the lesional cells are ill-defined and poorly understood. Fibroblastic cells, histiocytic cells, and undifferentiated cells are all identified. Depending upon the differentiation of the tumor, intercellular bridges and tonofilaments are not identified. Fibrosarcomas demonstrate similar findings, although they do not have histiocytic cells by EM or immunohistochemistry. The fusiform cells recapitulate normal fibroblasts without epithelial differentiation.[664] Karyotypic abnormalities are also noted, but are not specific for MFH.[470]

Differential Diagnosis

As previously stated, the differential diagnosis between MFH and fibrosarcoma rests most importantly with SCSCC, while other spindle cell tumors (liposarcoma, rhabdomyosarcoma, hemangiopericytoma, and malignant peripheral nerve sheath tumor) are included in the differential diagnosis for the sake of completeness. The clinical manifestations of the tumor may also contribute to the correct diagnosis, including the exact location, surface appearance, lymph node involvement, and evidence of systemic disease. The performance of an immunohistochemical panel of antibodies helps to distinguish the undifferentiated appearance of these tumors on histomorphologic appearance. A SCSCC will frequently demonstrate an in situ or invasive squamous cell component. Surface ulceration may obscure the true nature of the tumor. Obtaining deeper sections or serial sections on the block may help to illustrate the surface involvement. Focal dyskeratosis or intercellular bridges may be identified within the tumor. Immunoreactivity for keratin will certainly help to define the nature of the tumor, but immunoreactivity is identified in less than 50% of cases. The overall histomorphologic appearance, combined with the polypoid, mucosa-associated location of the tumor, often allows for a distinction between these tumors. The only instance of a true fibrosarcoma developing may be in the setting of previous irradiation, but since the radiation is usually performed for a squamous cell carcinoma, it may represent a recurrence.[665] Fibrosarcomatous growth can also be identified in a synovial sarcoma, and an epithelial or glandular component should be sought. Epithelial membrane antigen may be reactive in monophasic synovial sarcoma, but usually not keratin. Rhabdomyosarcoma will have cross-striations and reactivity with desmin, actin, and myoglobin. Liposarcoma will have lipoblasts and demonstrate an S-100 protein reactivity. Malignant peripheral nerve sheath tumors are usually highly cellular, compact, and demonstrate focal S-100 protein immunoreactivity. A benign fibrous histiocytoma should also be considered, but the subtle changes seen in a malignant

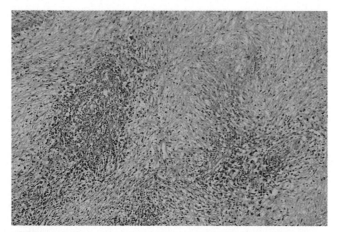

FIGURE 8–83. This poorly differentiated spindle cell malignant tumor was not associated with the surface (there was ulceration), had extensive necrosis and numerous mitotic figures, and did not react with any immunohistochemical reactions except vimentin. Possibly MFH, spindle cell squamous cell carcinoma cannot be excluded (H&E, × 75).

tumor may be overlooked, allowing the inappropriate therapeutic intervention.

Synovial Sarcoma

Gross Pathology

The tumor mass is usually poorly circumscribed or partially encapsulated, with surface lobulation or bosselation in a submucosal location, most frequently in the retropharynx or hypopharynx and arytenoid, measuring up to 10 cm in size. The tumor may be exophytic or pedunculated, occasionally with surface ulceration. The cut surface is yellow or grey-white with a consistency that is firm, gritty, and friable to soft, boggy, and rubbery. The cut surface reveals a whorled fibrous appearance with areas of cystic, mucoid, or hemorrhagic degeneration.[349,666-672]

Microscopic Pathology

Synovial sarcoma (SS) generally has two components in the classic form—a mesenchymal spindle component and a glandular epithelioid constituent, in variable proportions (Fig. 8–84A). However, a monophasic variant will only unveil the spindle or the epithelioid component. The spindle cells are arranged in orderly, densely packed, short, interlacing fascicles of plump cells with oval to spindle, vesicular to hyperchromatic nuclei, and scant cytoplasm with indistinct cellular boundaries (Fig. 8–84). The epithelioid cells are cuboidal to columnar, with round to oval vesicular nuclei encompassed by abundant pale or clear cytoplasm arranged in gland-like spaces, cords, nests, whorls, or papillary structures, with distinct cell membranes (see Fig. 8–84). The fibrovascular cores are occupied by the malignant spindled cells, expanding the core beyond the usual delicate fibrovascular cores identified in other papillary tumors. Mitotic activity is easily identified although not excessive (see Fig. 8–84C). Mast cells and exceptional calcifications can be seen in the spindle cell regions, more easily recognized in hypocellular foci or in areas of myxoid change or necrosis. A rich vascularity is often present. There is usually little collagen deposition.[349,666,667,669-676]

Special Techniques

Mucicarmine-positive and diastase-resistant PAS-positive epithelial mucin can be seen within the cytoplasm of the epithelial cells, within the glandular lumens, and in intracellular areas, while hyaluronidase-sensitive alcian blue and colloidal iron mesenchymal mucin can be identified in the spindle cell and myxoid areas.[349,668,672,675]

The immunoreactivity is compartmented by the type of cells seen: both the epithelial and spindle cells will be reactive with cytokeratin and epithelial

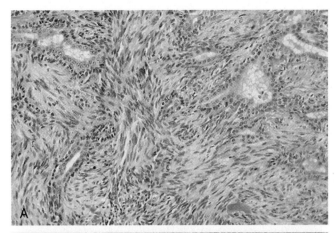

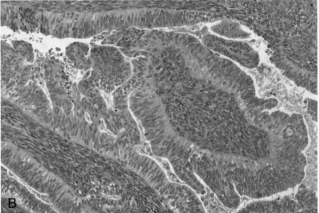

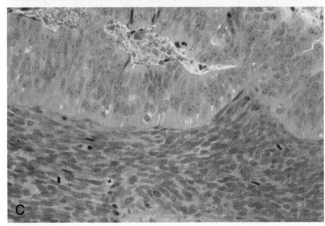

FIGURE 8–84. *A,* Glandular-type epithelium intermingled with the spindle cell component is classic for a biphasic synovial sarcoma (H&E, × 150); *B,* Marked nuclear stratification of epithelial cells is seen as it surrounds the atypical, dense spindle cell portion of the tumor (H&E, × 150); *C,* the epithelial component is well differentiated, arranged in a pseudostratified configuration. The spindle cell component is hypercellular with numerous mitotic figures and mild nuclear pleomorphism (H&E, × 300).

membrane antigen (EMA), while only the spindle cells will be vimentin positive. The spindle cell staining with epithelial markers may be focal, weak, or absent, depending upon the individual case. Due to vagaries of reactivity, both epithelial markers should be performed.[667,670,674,676,677] S-100 protein has been demonstrated in a few synovial sarcomas, but not of the larynx.[674,678]

Electron microscopy demonstrates glandular differentiation with microvilli, intercellular junctions, tonofilaments, and an intact basal lamina in the glandular portions, while the spindle cells demonstrate poorly formed rudimentary cellular junctions, nonbranching cytoplasm, intermediate filaments, and perhaps focal short cell processes surrounded by an external lamina.[349,670,673,674,677,679]

In addition to ultrastructural study and immunohistochemistry, molecular studies can be performed to document a translocation [usually t(X;18)] through reverse transcriptase polymerase chain reaction or fluorescence in situ hybridization.[680,681]

Differential Diagnosis

The biphasic tumor presents a unique differential diagnosis related to each of the components, although the monophasic SS presents more of a challenge. The tumors included in the differential are hemangiopericytoma, fibrous histiocytoma, spindle cell carcinoma, malignant peripheral nerve sheath tumors, fibrosarcoma, leiomyosarcoma, malignant melanoma, epithelioid sarcoma, angiosarcoma, and papillary thyroid carcinoma or other metastatic adenocarcinomas. SS can have a hemangiopericytomatous growth pattern, especially in the monophasic variant, but it is usually focal. The cells of a hemangiopericytoma tend to be smaller and not as fascicular in arrangement; they will not demonstrate immunopositivity with epithelial markers but may react with CD34 or CD31. A fibrous histiocytoma has histiocytic cells sprinkled between a storiform and whorled fibrohistiocytic proliferation, frequently with giant cells. The benign nature of this tumor usually removes it from diagnostic consideration. A spindle cell carcinoma frequently demonstrates an in situ or invasive squamous cell carcinoma in addition to the spindled component and will not have a glandular configuration. The immunohistochemical reactivity may be the same in both lesions, but the focal nature of the reactivity in synovial sarcoma may help to distinguish between the tumors. The distinction may be quite difficult. MPNST may have a similar growth pattern, but has nuclei that are more wrinkled and hyperchromatic and, perhaps, nuclear palisading. MPNST is usually S-100 positive and negative with epithelial markers, although crossreactivity with both tumors has been described. EM will demonstrate the interdigitating processes indicating Schwann cell derivation. Both tumor types (SS and MPNST) are extraordinarily rare in this location. Fibrosarcoma is usually a term reserved for tumors with a chevron-like pattern with long, tapered nuclei and tapering cytoplasm. Ultrastructural examination will reveal abundant rough endoplasmic reticulum and no intercellular junctions. A

leiomyosarcoma usually has fascicles at right angles, composed of cells with abundant cytoplasm, cytoplasmic vacuolization, and actin or desmin immunoreactivity. EM demonstrates pinocytosis and dense bodies within the myofilaments. Malignant melanoma usually has a more epithelioid appearance with prominent eosinophilic nucleoli, may have overlying surface mucosal (junctional) involvement, and will be reactive with S-100 protein and/or antibody HMB-45. Of course, if the melanoma is spindled, the HMB-45 may be unhelpful. Ultrastructural identification of melanosomes or premelanosomes will confirm the diagnosis. A papillary thyroid carcinoma does not have malignant spindle cells within the fibrovascular cores of the papillae, and a thyroglobulin reaction will confirm the nature of the metastatic tumor. A history of adenocarcinoma elsewhere or a lack of the biphasic pattern should assist in defining a metastatic adenocarcinoma.[349,667,670,674,676]

When the tumor is identified in recurrent or metastatic foci, the histologic appearance may be quite different, yielding only a single component, most usually the fibrous mesenchymal part. The same immunohistochemical results can be expected in the metastatic foci. There has been a reportedly better prognosis with the calcifying synovial sarcoma, but this variant is not seen in the larynx or hypopharynx.[682]

Rhabdomyosarcoma

Gross Pathology

The tumors are usually polypoid or sessile, firm, pale to grey masses of the glottis, frequently filling the laryngeal space, usually measuring greater than 2 cm, reaching 6 cm in maximum dimension. The cut surface may have a glistening, mucinous appearance. The tumors are usually submucosal swellings, with surface epithelial keratosis or hyperplasia, while surface ulceration has been described in larger tumors. The botryoid type (usually in adults) may have the classic grape-like tumor growth. No site in the larynx or trachea is exempt from rhabdomyosarcoma (RMS).[459,683–692]

Microscopic Pathology

RMS of the larynx can be separated into embryonal, botryoid, alveolar, and pleomorphic subtypes depending upon the pattern of growth, cellularity, and degree of differentiation. Although all types can occur in the larynx, embryonal RMS is the most frequent, the pleomorphic type the second most common. Rhabdomyoblasts, recapitulating embryonic muscle development, are generally the defining characteristic of the tumor, but are less frequently identified or difficult to find in the poorly differentiated tumors. The cross-striations within the cytoplasm are usually identified in the elongated cells and those with abundant cytoplasm. The tumors are variably cellular, with myxoid stroma identified in the less cellular areas. A variable amount of dense, eosinophilic, opaque cytoplasm is found around a central or eccentrically placed hyperchromatic nucleus, which is frequently oval to elongated. Small "blue" round cells can be seen, often with an increased mitotic count (Fig. 8–85). The botryoid type has a characteristic alternating pattern of hyper- and hypocellular regions, with a condensation of cells immediately below the epithelial layer (cambium layer), while the alveolar type has noncohesive round to oval cells (similar to embryonal type) attached to fibrous septa in a characteristic alveolar growth pattern (see Fig. 8–85). Pleomorphic type, as the name implies, can have all shapes and sizes of cells identified within the tumor, many of which will have the cross-striations of mature adult muscle. There is generally abundant eosinophilic cytoplasm, surrounding markedly atypical nuclei, often with prominent nucleoli. A lymphohistiocytic infiltrate can be seen within the tumor.[459,683,685–689,692]

Special Techniques

Rhabdomyoblasts can be accentuated with a phosphotungstic acid–hematoxylin or a trichrome stain to bring out the cross-striations in the immature muscle cells. A periodic acid–Schiff (PAS) recognizes the glycogen present within the cytoplasm of the tumor cells. Desmin, myoglobin, muscle-specific actin (MSA), myo-D1, and myogenin are expressed in the tumor cells, especially those with abundant cytoplasm, in varying degrees, with desmin usually reactive in more cells and more strongly than the other markers. Myosin (fast) can be identified, but is

not more sensitive or specific than the previously described panel. Vimentin is variably present and a nonspecific marker for mesenchymal differentiation. A combination of desmin and MSA yields the most helpful results.

The cytoplasm of the tumor cells contains mitochondria, glycogen granules, and lipoid granules, in addition to the haphazardly arranged filaments. Whether the tumor cells are round with irregular nuclei, rhabdomyoblasts with regular thin and thick filament arrangement, or spindled bipolar cells, they all contain actin (thin) and myosin (thick) filaments with associated regular, distorted, or haphazard Z-bands. The cells are surrounded by a basement membrane. Background fibroblasts, collagen fibers, and endothelial cells can be identified in the myxoid or less cellular areas.[683,685,686,688,693–696] The t(2;13) (q35;q14) chromosomal rearrangement can be identified in a number of alveolar type RMS.[697]

Differential Diagnosis

The tumor should be differentiated from a variety of small round cell tumors, such as lymphoma, leukemia, melanoma, carcinoma, leiomyosarcoma, malignant fibrous histiocytoma (MFH), Ewing's sarcoma, retinoblastoma, and olfactory neuroblastoma (although the latter two are most unlikely in the larynx), and from benign conditions, such as fetal rhabdomyoma, granular cell tumor, myxoma, myxoid polyp, polyp with stromal atypia, contact ulcer, and granulation tissue. The rhabdomyoblastic differentiation of RMS is defined by the "strap" cell, with accentuation of the cross-striations achieved by performing a PTAH or trichrome stain. If there are limited cross-striations, the differential diagnosis is much broader and will include the entities described above. Hematologic malignancies may be incorrectly diagnosed in small round cell tumors, especially with marrow or systemic involvement by a rhabdomyosarcoma. The undifferentiated appearance of embyronal RMS is particularly difficult to distinguish from leukemia or lymphoma on small biopsies. After careful search, identification of spindled cells, combined with an immunohistochemical panel of markers (including LCA), will elucidate the nature of a round cell tumor. LCA is nonreactive in rhabdomyosarcomas. A panel of markers is indispensable and cardinal in undifferentiated neoplasms in order to avoid anomalous reactivity with a specific marker in other neoplasms. Melanoma may have an identical histologic appearance but often has prominent nucleoli, cytoplasmic pigment, and an HMB-45 and S-100 protein immunoreactivity. A leiomyosarcoma is usually composed of spindled cells, arranged in interlacing fascicles, usually with cigar-shaped, blunt, vesicular nuclei. MSA, smooth muscle actin, and desmin immunoreactivity and differences on ultrastructural study (parallel actin filaments, dense bodies, and pinocytotic vesicles)

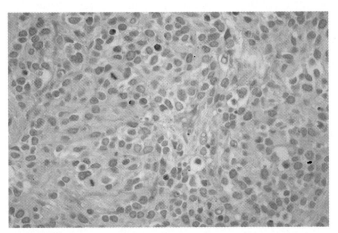

FIGURE 8–85. Intermediate-sized cells have moderate nuclear pleomorphism with variable amounts of eosinophilic cytoplasm and mitotic figures. Additional special studies would be required to prove this is a rhabdomyosarcoma (H&E, × 300).

should help exclude RMS. MFH usually has a variable histologic picture, with storiform architecture, marked variability to the cells, giant cell formation, histiocytic cells, and abundant mitotic figures. The immunoreactivity may overlap RMS, although alpha-1-antichymotrypsin and alpha-1-antitrypsin are reactive in MFH. The identification of thick and thin filaments and Z-bands on ultrastructural analysis should exclude MFH. The distinction between Ewing's sarcoma and RMS may be very difficult, especially on limited biopsy material. Extraskeletal Ewing's sarcoma will be nonreactive with myo-D1 and myogenin. On electron microscopy Ewing's sarcoma will demonstrate light and dark cells, finely dispersed nuclear chromatin, a lack of cytoplasmic organelles, only a few cytoplasmic glycogen granules, no myosin/ribosome complexes, no basement membrane investment, and no filaments (thick, intermediate, or thin). The distinction may be academic, as the treatment protocols are similar. A poorly differentiated carcinoma will usually involve the surface mucosa, and keratin reactivity may be helpful. A thyroid papillary carcinoma, although arranged in an "alveolar" pattern in some cases, generally has open nuclear chromatin, irregular nuclear outlines, intranuclear inclusions, nuclear grooves, and a positive reaction with keratin and thyroglobulin immunohistochemical antibodies. Discussed earlier, a rhabdomyoma is a benign condition and does not have nuclear pleomorphism. Granular cell tumor does not contain cross-striations, usually contains a granular cytoplasm, demonstrates surface pseudoepitheliomatous hyperplasia, and is S-100 protein immunoreactive. Close examination of a biopsy should exclude a polyp and a myxoma, as they do not have atypical cells, nor is the cellularity so dense. In polyps with stromal atypia, there is no associated increased mitotic activity or condensation of the atypical cells near the mucosal surface. Immunoreactivity of atypical stromal cells with keratin, actin, and histiocytic markers (CD68 or KP-1) will help to further define the nature of the cells (myofibroblastic). A contact ulcer and granulation tissue may have an exuberant proliferation of spindled cells, but the rich vascularity, the associated inflammatory elements, and the lack of nuclear atypicality should help to exclude an RMS.[35,123,124,684,686,692,693,698,699]

Clinicopathologic Correlation

The tumors are divided into clinically significant groups, with divisions based upon the completeness of resection, degree of residual disease, and the status of the lymph nodes or metastatic disease. Treatment is based upon the identification by pathology of residual disease and the extent of tumor. There is a survival or prognostic difference between the various types of RMS, but the primary site, tumor size, resectability, invasiveness, and vascular supply seem to be the dominant factors in long-term survival.[700,701]

Liposarcoma

Gross Pathology

The tumors usually present as a supraglottic or hypopharyngeal firm, polypoid, pedunculated or exophytic, yellow to pink-white, ill-defined mass, measuring up to 9 cm in greatest dimension, with 2 to 4 cm as the average. Smaller satellite masses can be found around the base of the pedunculated mass. These tumors are usually covered by an intact surface epithelium. Submucosal lesions are also identified. The cut surface will demonstrate grey-yellow firm tissue with a lobulated, glistening, translucent appearance, with bands of tissue seen intersecting the tumor mass. Tracheal tumors are exceptionally rare.[702-712]

Microscopic Pathology

The microscopic appearance of liposarcoma can be divided into a variety of subtypes, based on the degree of differentiation and the background material. These types include well differentiated, myxoid, round cell, pleomorphic, and dedifferentiated types. Although each of these has been found in the larynx, the most common is the well-differentiated sclerosing variant. Liposarcomas are usually submucosal with an intact overlying surface epithelium. The well-differentiated sclerosing variant is unencapsulated with infiltration into the surrounding soft tissues, intersected by dense bands of varying amounts of fibrous connective tissue, creating lobules. The lobules have a delicate plexiform capillary network, often compressed by the adipocytes (Fig. 8–86A). The mature-appearing lipocytes are variable in size and shape, containing hyperchromatic enlarged nuclei (Fig. 8–86B). The striking difference between a lipoma and a liposarcoma is the identification of a lipoblast, which is a lipocyte with multiple tiny lipid vacuoles or irregular droplets indenting or notching the nucleus, creating a multilobated appearance (Fig. 8–86C). Occasionally cells can contain multiple nuclei in a ring-like pattern around the periphery, typically called a "floret cell." Lipoblasts may be few and far between, necessitating the cutting of multiple sections and the careful examination of the tumor under high power. Mitotic figures can be seen, but are not usually numerous, while necrosis is absent. Bone and cartilage metaplasia can be seen.[702,705,706,708,709,711–714]

The other variants are rare. In addition to the histologic features described above, the myxoid variant has an abundant myxoid background matrix material (mucopolysaccharide) arranged around a capillary network. The pleomorphic type shows marked nuclear and cellular pleomorphism, often containing tumor giant cells (see Fig. 8–86B). These cells may also have opaque eosinophilic cytoplasm, making the determination of the lipid origin of the cells quite difficult. However, lipid or fat droplets

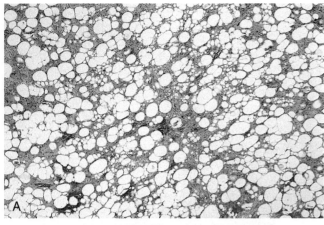

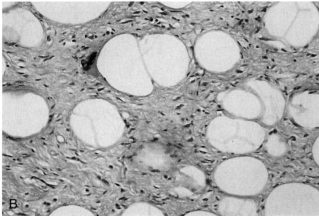

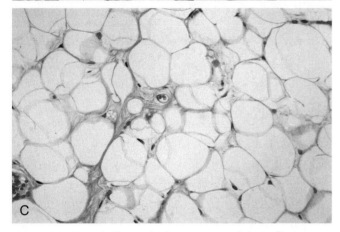

FIGURE 8–86. *A,* The marked increase in cellularity, fibrous bands, and vascularity, along with the increased nuclear : cytoplasmic ratio, even at this relatively low power is highly suggestive of liposarcoma (H&E, × 30); *B,* Markedly atypical cells can be seen in liposarcoma along with a fibrous connective tissue separating adipocytes (H&E, × 300); *C,* Lipoblasts *(left)* are diagnostic of a liposarcoma, but may be inconspicuous (H&E, × 300).

within the cytoplasm will clinch the diagnosis of pleomorphic liposarcoma. This tumor type demonstrates prominent mitotic activity, hemorrhage, and necrosis.[703,704,707,714]

Special Techniques

The need for special histochemical or immunohistochemical stains in liposarcoma is rare. Although the intracytoplasmic lipid may appear by light microscopy to be mucin, it is mucicarmine negative. Lipid stains can be used, but breakdown of any cell's membrane, taken up by a histiocyte, will give a false positive reaction. Alcian blue will accentuate the myxoid nature of the background material. Mast cells can be appreciated with a Giemsa stain. However, these stains are not really contributory to the diagnosis.

S-100 protein and vimentin can be demonstrated in the adipocytes (S-100 protein in the cytoplasm and nucleus), but their use is seldom warranted, except for the most poorly differentiated tumors. However, in the poorly differentiated cases, S-100 protein may not be reactive anyway.

The ultrastructure of lipoblasts shows nonmembrane-bound lipid droplets, often compressing or indenting the hyperchromatic nucleus, usually peripherally located. Fibroblasts and loose-ground substance containing collagen can also be seen.[705–708,710,712]

Differential Diagnosis

Laryngeal lipomas are the most frequent tumor included in the differential diagnosis. However, lipomas are encapsulated, noninfiltrative, lack nuclear pleomorphism, do not have lipoblasts, and do not manifest necrosis, hemorrhage, or mitoses. A myxoid polyp may be included in the differential diagnosis for a pedunculated or polypoid mass, but the histologic nuclear features and lipoblasts will exclude a polyp. A variety of other malignant tumors may contain cells with vacuolated cytoplasm, which may simulate a lipoblast. However, the overall architecture of malignant fibrous histiocytoma, poorly differentiated carcinoma, malignant melanoma, and chordoma should help in differentiation. A chordoma will have physaliferous cells, which are also multilocular or multivacuolated cells. However, the overall glandular and trabecular arrangement to these cells, combined with a reactivity with keratin immunohistochemistry, should aid in classifying this tumor correctly. A malignant melanoma is usually a tumor close to the mucosal surface, if not involving the surface, which may demonstrate pigment, usually has a more opaque dense cytoplasm, often has intranuclear cytoplasmic inclusions, and will be S-100 protein, HMB-45, and vimentin reactive.[712]

Clinicopathologic Correlation

In the tumors of the larynx that are difficult to separate into lipoma or well-differentiated lipoma-like liposarcoma, multiple recurrences or difficulty in obtaining complete resection should tend to favor a liposarcoma. However, the low-grade liposarcomas of the larynx tend not to metastasize, nor are they usually lethal. Although these tumors could be classified as atypical lipomatous tumors rather than liposarcomas, the difficulty in treating these patients relates to obtaining adequate surgical margins, and multiple surgeries may be necessary in order to obtain adequate resection of the tumor. Therefore, it seems more prudent to designate these lesions as liposarcomas to alert the surgeon and help to ensure adequate treatment for these patients. Radiographic imaging, especially with MR or CT, will document the lipomatous nature and extent of the mass. The tumor size, histologic type (synonymous with tumor grade), site, operability, and treatment employed all seem to influence the clinical outcome, with small well-differentiated laryngeal lesions completely excised having a better prognosis than liposarcomas elsewhere in the body.[712–717]

Lymphoproliferative Neoplasms

A variety of hematologic neoplasms can involve the larynx or trachea, generally as a part of disseminated disease (either lymphoma or leukemia), but isolated laryngeal or tracheal involvement can certainly occur.[718–729] Primary extramedullary plasmacytoma and primary extranodal non-Hodgkin's malignant lymphomas are the most frequent lymphoid tumors of the larynx. (Fig. 8–87). Given the disseminated clinical manifestations of hematologic neoplasms, one would think that the larynx would frequently be involved; however, the number of reports in the literature relating to lymphomas of the larynx suggest the opposite. Likewise, there are only exceptional reports of primary myelogenous tumors (granulocytic sarcoma and mast cell sarcoma) and no convincing report of primary Hodgkin's disease. The rarity of these lesions warrants only passing mention, but we refer the interested reader to the specific articles.[718–720] The stages of lymphoma are divided into categories based on isolated laryngeal involvement (IE), larynx and regional lymph node involvement (IIE), disseminated disease of the head and neck (IIIE), and secondary involvement of the larynx by disseminated disease (IV).[721–729]

A variety of other lymphoproliferative disorders can also be identified in the larynx, including angiofollicular hyperplasia (Castleman's disease), sinus histiocytosis with massive lymphadenopathy (Rosai-Dorfman) (Fig. 8–88), and Langerhans' cell histiocytosis.[730–739]

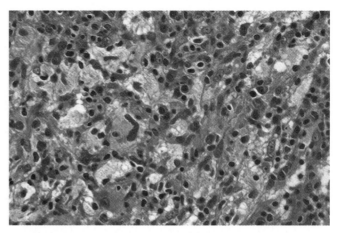

FIGURE 8–88.   Identifying mature lymphocytes within the cytoplasm of histiocytes (emperipolesis) is characteristic for Rosai-Dorfman disease (sinus histiocytosis with massive lymphadenopathy). The histiocytes are characteristically S-100 protein positive (H&E, × 300).

Secondary Tumors

Gross Pathology

Although any portion of the larynx and trachea can be involved by a metastatic tumor, a submucosal supraglottic mass is the most frequent presentation; isolated cartilaginous involvement has also been reported (Table 8–4).[637,638,740–747]

Microscopic Pathology

There is obviously no single histologic picture that will encompass all the various tumors that have been shown to metastasize to the larynx and trachea. Although many of the case reports do not have pathologic illustrations, good faith presumes that almost any tumor can metastasize to the larynx. While this dictum is true, clear cell renal cell adenocarcinoma and cutaneous malignant melanoma account for the majority of tumors that are secondary to the larynx and trachea.[637,638,740,743–745,747–752]

Other tumors known to metastasize to the larynx include (to name only a few): choriocarcinoma[691]

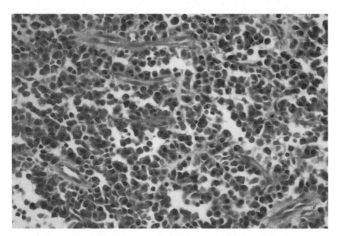

FIGURE 8–87.   The "alveolar" degenerative change associated with a plasmacytoma is quite characteristic. The cells have centrally placed nuclei, pale paranuclear regions, and clock-face type chromatin (H&E, × 300).

TABLE 8-4	MOST FREQUENT PRIMARY SITES WHICH METASTASIZE TO THE LARYNX AND THE ORDER OF FREQUENCY OF LOCATION WITHIN THE LARYNX TO WHICH METASTASES OCCUR

PRIMARY SITE	LOCATION WITHIN LARYNX
Melanoma of cutaneous origin	Supraglottis
Kidney	Subglottis
Genitourinary	Cartilage
Lung, breast, and gastrointestinal system	Glottis and transglottic

ovarian carcinoma,[740,741,743] uterine carcinoma,[753] prostate,[740,754–756] colon carcinoma,[740,747,757,758] pancreatic adenocarcinoma,[759] breast carcinoma,[740,742,746,757,760] nasopharynx,[743] lung,[740,761] stomach adenocarcinoma,[740] testes,[762] liver,[763] and osteosarcoma.[764] Sarcomas are obviously most scarce in their presentation in the larynx and trachea. Direct extension of a thyroid malignancy through the thyroid cartilage and thyroid carcinoma developing in an ectopic thyroid fragment within the larynx must be excluded, as does direct extension from the esophagus.[765] However, the clinical presentation should help to define these lesions, especially in light of preoperative radiographic imaging. Generally, involvement by lymphoma and leukemia is not considered metastatic disease, but rather part of the systemic manifestations of these tumors.

Differential Diagnosis

Metastatic disease to the larynx from other primaries is generally a late manifestation of the primary tumor, obviously bearing an ominous prognostic implication. Therefore, separating a metastatic lesion from a primary lesion is essential in order to avoid unnecessary surgery or other therapeutic intervention. Combining a careful histologic examination with an accurate clinical history and other immunohistochemical or ultrastructural studies should allow for a correct diagnosis.

REFERENCES

1. Michaels L. Examination of specimens of the larynx. *J Clin Pathol*. 1990; 43:792.
2. Fu Y-S. Larynx sectioning. Personal communication, 1997.
3. Ackerman LV, Ramirez GA. The indications for and limitations of frozen section diagnosis. A review of 1269 consecutive frozen section diagnoses. *Br J Surg*. 1957; 44:336.
4. Gnepp DR. Uses, abuses and pitfalls of frozen section diagnoses. In: Ferlito A, ed. *Surgical Pathology of Laryngeal Neoplasms*. London: Chapman Hall; 1996:9.
5. Barney PL. Histopathologic problems and frozen section diagnosis in diseases of the larynx. *Otolaryngol Clin North Am*. 1970; 3:493.
6. Saltzstein SL, Nahum AM. Frozen section diagnosis: Accuracy and errors; uses and abuses. *Laryngoscope*. 1973; 83:1128.
7. Holaday WJ, Assor D. Ten thousand consecutive frozen sections. A retrospective study focusing on accuracy and quality control. *Am J Clin Pathol*. 1974; 61:769.
8. Gandour-Edwards RF, Donald PJ, Lie JT. Clinical utility of intraoperative frozen section diagnosis in head and neck surgery: A quality assurance perspective. *Head Neck*. 1993; 15:373.
9. Lee JG. Detection of residual carcinoma of the oral cavity, oropharynx, hypopharynx, and larynx: A study of surgical margins. *Trans Am Acad Ophthalmol Otolaryngol*. 1974; 78:49.
10. Bauer WC, Lesinski SG, Ogura JH. The significance of positive margins in hemilaryngectomy specimens. *Laryngoscope*. 1975; 85:1.
11. Kirchner JA. Pathways and pitfalls in partial laryngectomy. *Ann Otol*. 1984; 93:301.
12. Kirchner JA. What have whole organ sections contributed to the treatment of laryngeal cancer? *Ann Otol*. 1989; 98:661.
13. Barnes L, Johnson JT. Pathologic and clinical considerations in the evaluation of major head and neck specimens resected for cancer. In: Sommers SC, Rosen PP, Fechner RE, eds. *Pathology Annual*. vol. 21, pt 1. Norwalk, CT: Appleton-Century-Crofts; 1986:217.
14. Browning GG, Busuttil A, McLay A. An improved method of report on laryngectomy specimens. *J Pathol*. 1976; 119:101.
15. Gregor RT, Lloyd GAS, Michaels L. Computed tomography of the larynx: A clinical and pathologic study. *Head Neck Surg*. 1981; 3:284.
16. Gillis TM, Incze J, Strong MS, Vaughan CW, Simpson GT. Natural history and management of keratosis, atypia, carcinoma in situ and microinvasive cancer of the larynx. *Am J Surg*. 1983; 146:512.
17. Goodman ML. Keratosis (leukoplakia) of the larynx. *Otolaryngol Clin North Am*. 1984; 17:179.
18. Hellquist H, Lundgren J, Olofsson J. Hyperplasia, dysplasia and carcinoma in situ of the vocal cords: A follow-up study. *Clin Otolaryngol*. 1982; 7:11.
19. Holinger PH, Johnston KC. Benign tumors of the larynx. *Ann Otol Rhinol Laryngol*. 1951; 60:496.
20. McGavran MH, Bauer WC, Ogura JH. Isolated laryngeal keratosis. Its relation to carcinoma of the larynx based on a clinicopathologic study of 87 consecutive cases with long-term follow-up. *Laryngoscope*. 1960; 70:932.
21. Michaels L. The metaplastic process in epithelial strata. *Cholest Mast Surg Proc*. 1982; 14:299.
22. New GB, Erich JB. Benign tumors of the larynx: A study of 722 cases. *Arch Otolaryngol*. 1938; 28:841.
23. Norris CM, Peale AR. Keratosis of the larynx. *J Laryngol Otol*. 1963; 77:635.
24. Sataloff RT, Spiegel JR, Hawkshaw MJ, Heuer RJ. Vocal fold masses associated with leukoplakia. *Ear Nose Throat J*. 1995; 74:316.
25. Sllamniku B, Bauer W, Painter C, Sessions D. The transformation of laryngeal keratosis into invasive cancer. *Am J Otolaryngol*. 1989; 10:42.
26. Barnes L, Yunis EJ, Krebs FJ III, Sonmez-Alpan E. Verruca vulgaris of the larynx. Demonstration of human papillomavirus types 6/11 by in-situ hybridization. *Arch Pathol Lab Med*. 1991; 115:895.
27. Kambic V, Radsel Z, Zargi M, Acko M. Vocal cord polyps: Incidence, histology and pathogenesis. *J Laryngol Otol*. 1981; 95:609.
28. Strong MS, Vaughan CW. Vocal cord nodules and polyps. The role of surgical treatment. *Laryngoscope*. 1971; 81:911.
29. Sataloff RT, Hawkshaw M, Rosen DC. Vocal cord polyp and varicosity. *Ear Nose Throat J*. 1993; 72:780.
30. Sataloff RT, Spiegel JR, Emerich KA, Rosen DC. Post-hemorrhagic vocal fold polyps. *Ear Nose Throat J*. 1994; 73:883.
31. Yanagisawa E, Hausfeld JN, Pensak ML. Sudden airway ob-

struction due to pedunculated laryngeal polyps. *Ann Otol.* 1983; 92:340.

32. Werner JA, Schünke M, Rudert H, Tillmann B. Description and clinical importance of the lymphatics of the vocal fold. *Otolaryngol Head Neck Surg.* 1990; 102:13.

33. Gray SD, Hammond E, Hanson DF. Benign pathologic responses of the larynx. *Ann Otol.* 1995; 104:13.

34. Sena T, Brady MS, Huvos AG, Spiro RH. Laryngeal myxoma. *Arch Otolaryngol Head Neck Surg.* 1991; 117:430.

35. Wenig BM, Devaney K, Wenig BL. Pseudoneoplastic lesions of the oropharynx and larynx simulating cancer. *Pathol Annu.* 1995; 30 (pt 1):143.

36. Keane WM, Denneny JC, Rowe LD, Atkins JP Jr. Complications of intubation. *Ann Otol.* 1982; 91:584.

37. McFerran DJ, Abdullah V, Gallimore AP, Pringle MB, Croft CB. Vocal process granulomata. *J Laryngol Otol.* 1994; 108: 216.

38. New GB, Devine KD. Contact ulcer granuloma. *Ann Otol.* 1949; 58:548.

39. Ward PH, Zwitman D, Hanson D, Berci G. Contact ulcers and granulomas of the larynx: New insights into their etiology as a basis for more rational treatment. *Otolaryngol Head Neck Surg.* 1980; 88:262.

40. Wenig BM, Heffner DK. Contact ulcers of the larynx: A reacquaintance with the pathology of an often underdiagnosed entity. *Arch Pathol Lab Med.* 1990; 114:825.

41. Hilding AC. Laryngotracheal damage during intratracheal anesthesia. Demonstration by staining the unfixed specimen with methylene blue. *Ann Otol.* 1971; 80:565.

42. Johansen H, Kiaer W. Contact ulcers and laryngeal tuberculosis. *Arch Otol Rhinol Laryngol.* 50:264, 1949

43. Fechner RE, Cooper PH, Mills SE. Pyogenic granuloma of the larynx and trachea. A causal and pathologic misnomer for granulation tissue. *Arch Otolaryngol.* 1981; 107:30.

44. LeBoit PE, Berger TG, Egbert BM, et al. Bacillary angiomatosis. The histopathology and differential diagnosis of a pseudoneoplastic infection in patients with human immunodeficiency virus disease. *Am J Surg Pathol.* 1989; 13:909.

45. Fetsch JF, Weiss SW. Observations concerning the pathogenesis of epithelioid hemangioma (angiolymphoid hyperplasia). *Mod Pathol.* 1991; 4:449.

46. Marcusen DC, Sooy CD. Otolaryngologic and head and neck manifestations of acquired immunodeficiency syndrome (AIDS). *Laryngoscope.* 1985; 95:401.

47. Peppard SB, Dickens JH. Laryngeal injury following short-term intubation. *Ann Otol.* 1983; 92:327.

48. Delahunty JE. Acid laryngitis. *J Laryngol Otol.* 1972; 86:355.

49. Koufman JA. The otolaryngologic manifestations of gastroesophageal reflux disease (GERD): A clinical investigation of 225 patients using ambulatory 24-hr pH monitoring and an experimental investigation of the role of acid and pepsin in the development of laryngeal injury. *Laryngoscope.* 1991; 101(suppl):1.

50. Wiener GJ, Koufman JA, Wu WC, et al. Chronic hoarseness secondary to gastroesophageal reflux disease: Documentation with 24-h ambulatory pH monitoring. *Am J Gastroenterol.* 1989; 84:1503.

51. Littman CD. Necrotizing sialometaplasia (adenometaplasia) of the trachea. *Histopathology.* 1993; 22:298.

52. Romagosa V, Bella MR, Truchero C, Moya J. Necrotizing sialometaplasia (adenometaplasia) of the trachea. *Histopathology* 1992; 21:280.

53. Walker GK, Fechner RE, Johns ME, Teja K. Necrotizing sialometaplasia of the larynx secondary to atheromatous embolization. *Am J Clin Pathol.* 1982; 77:221.

54. Wenig BM. Necrotizing sialometaplasia of the larynx. A report of two cases and a review of the literature. *Am J Clin Pathol.* 1995; 103:609.

55. Abrams AM, Melrose RJ, Howell FV. Necrotizing sialometaplasia. A disease simulating malignancy. *Cancer.* 1973; 32:13.

56. Brannon RB, Fowler CB, Hartman KS. Necrotizing sialometaplasia. A clinicopathologic study of sixty-nine cases and review of the literature. *Oral Surg Oral Med Oral Pathol.* 1991; 72:317.

57. Ben-Izhak O, Ben-Arieh Y. Necrotizing sialometaplasia of the larynx [letter]. *Am J Clin Pathol.* 1996; 105:251.

58. Ben-Izhak O, Ben-Arieh Y. Necrotizing squamous metaplasia in herpetic tracheitis following prolonged intubation: A lesion similar to necrotizing sialometaplasia. *Histopathology.* 1993; 22:265.

59. Pillsbury HC III, Sasaki CT. Granulomatous diseases of the larynx. *Otolaryngol Clin North Am.* 1982; 15:539.

60. Barnes EL Jr, Zafar T. Laryngeal amyloidosis. Clinicopathologic study of seven cases. *Ann Otol.* 1977; 86:856.

61. Berg AM, Troxler RF, Grillone G, et al. Localized amyloidosis of the larynx: Evidence for light chain composition. *Ann Otol.* 1993; 102:884.

62. Chow LT-C, Chow W-H, Shum BS-F. Fatal massive upper respiratory haemorrhage: An unusual complication of localized amyloidosis of the larynx. *J Laryngol Otol.* 1993; 107:51.

63. Ferrara G, Boscaino A. Nodular amyloidosis of the larynx. *Pathologica.* 1995; 87:94.

64. Heinritz H, Kraus TH, Iro H. Localized amyoidosis in the head and neck. A retrospective study. *HNO.* 1994; 42:744.

65. Lewis JE, Olsen KD, Kurtin PJ, Kyle RA. Laryngeal amyloidosis: A clinicopathologic and immunohistochemical review. *Otolaryngol Head Neck Surg.* 1992; 106:372.

66. Michaels L, Hyams VJ. Amyloid in localised deposits and plasmacytomas of the respiratory tract. *J Pathol.* 1979; 128:29.

67. O'Halloran LR, Lusk RP. Amyloidosis of the larynx in a child. *Ann Otol.* 1994; 103:590.

68. Stark DB, New GB. Amyloid tumors of the larynx, trachea or bronchi. A report of 15 cases. *Ann Otol.* 1949; 58:117.

69. Thompson LDR, Derringer GA, Wenig BM. Amyoidosis of the larynx: A clinicopathologic study of 11 cases. *Modern Pathol.* 2000; 13:528.

70. Creston JE. The otolaryngologic manifestations of multiple myeloma. *Laryngoscope.* 1978; 88:1320.

71. Cohen SR. Ligneous conjunctivitis: An ophthalmic disease with potentially fatal tracheobronchial obstruction. Laryngeal and tracheobronchial features. *Ann Otol.* 1990; 99:509.

72. Richards SH, Bull PD. Lipoid proteinosis of the larynx. *J Laryngol Otol.* 1973; 87:187.

73. Holinger PH, Johnston KC, Parchet VN, Zimmerman AA. Congenital malformations of the trachea, bronchi and lung. *Ann Otol.* 1952; 61:1159.

74. Blumberg JB, Stevenson JK, Lemire RJ, Boyden EA. Laryngotracheoesophageal cleft, the embryologic implications: Review of the literature. *Pediatr Surg.* 1965; 57:559.

75. Harpman JA. Cricoid cartilage abnormalities. *Arch Otolaryngol.* 1969; 90:118.

76. Imbrie JD, Doyle PJ. Laryngotracheoesophageal cleft. *Laryngoscope.* 1969; 79:1252.

77. Morimitsu T, Matsumoto I, Okada S, Takahashi M, Kosugi T. Congenital cricoid stenosis. *Laryngoscope.* 1981; 91:1356.

78. Strome M. Subglottic stenosis: Therapeutic considerations. *Otolaryngol Clin North Am.* 1984; 17:63.

79. Tucker GF, Ossoff RH, Newman AN, Holinger LD. Histopathology of congenital subglottic stenosis. *Laryngoscope.* 1979; 89:866.

80. Woo P, Karmody CS. Congenital laryngeal atresia. Histopathologic study of two cases. *Ann Otol.* 1983; 92:391.

81. Benjamin B. Congenital laryngeal webs. *Ann Otol.* 1983; 92: 317.

82. Belmont JR, Grundfast KM, Heffner DK, Hyams VJ. Laryngeal dysgenesis. *Ann Otol.* 1985; 94:602.

83. Brandenburg JH. Idiopathic subglottic stenosis. *Trans Am Acad Ophthalmol Otol.* 1972; 76:1402.

84. McGill T. Congenital diseases of the larynx. *Otolaryngol Clin North Am.* 1984; 17:57.

85. Shearer WT, Biller HF, Ogura JH, Goldring D. Congenital laryngeal web and interventricular septal defect. *Am J Dis Child.* 1972; 123:605.

86. Smith II, Bain AD. Congenital atresia of the larynx. A report of nine cases. *Ann Otol.* 1965; 74:338.

87. Belmont JR, Grundfast KM. Congenital laryngeal stridor (laryngomalacia): Etiologic factors and associated disorders. *Ann Otol.* 1984; 93:430.

88. Ferguson CP. Treatment of airway problems in the newborn. *Ann Otol.* 1967; 76:762.

89. Templer J, Hast M, Thomas JR, Davis WE. Congenital laryngeal stridor secondary to flaccid epiglottis, anomalous accessory cartilages and redundant aryepiglottic folds. *Laryngoscope.* 1981; 91:394.

90. Bhalla M, Grillo HC, McLoud TC, et al. Idiopathic laryngotracheal stenosis: Radiologic findings. *Am J Roentgenol.* 1993; 161:515.

91. Goff WF. Teflon injection for vocal cord paralysis. *Arch Otolaryngol.* 1969; 90:124.

92. Kasperbauer JL, Slavit DH, Maragos NE. Teflon granulomas and overinjection of Teflon: A therapeutic challenge for the otorhinolaryngologist. *Ann Otol.* 1993; 102:748.

93. Nakayama M, Ford CN, Bless DM. Teflon vocal cord augmentation: Failures and management in 28 cases. *Otolaryngol Head Neck Surg.* 1993; 109:493.

94. Stone JW, Arnold GE. Human larynx injected with Teflon paste. Histologic study of innervation and tissue reaction. *Arch Otolaryngol.* 1967; 86:98.

95. Tsuzuki T, Fukuda H, Fujioka T. Response of the human larynx to silicone. *Am J Otolaryngol.* 1991; 12:288.

96. Wenig BM, Heffner DK, Oertel YC, Johnson FB. Teflonomas of the larynx and neck. *Hum Pathol.* 1990; 21:617.

97. Reiman HM. Use of energy-dispersive X-ray analysis for detection of Teflon in tissue sections. *Hum Pathol.* 1990; 21: 1190.

98. Varvares MA, Montgomery WW, Hillman RE. Teflon granuloma of the larynx: Etiology, pathophysiology, and management. *Ann Otol.* 1995; 104:511.

99. Bauer CA, Valentino J, Hoffman HT. Long-term result of vocal cord augmentation with autogenous fat. *Ann Otol.* 1995; 104:871.

100. Lemberg PS, Darrow DH, Holinger, LD. Aerodigestive tract foreign bodies in the older child and adolescent. *Ann Otol.* 1996; 105:267.

101. Reilly JS, Walter MA, Beste D, et al. Size/shape analysis of aerodigestive foreign bodies in children: A multi-institutional study. *Am J Otolaryngol.* 1995; 16:190.

102. Rimell FL, Thome A Jr, Stool S, et al. Characteristics of objects that cause choking in children. *JAMA.* 1995; 274:1763.

103. Weston JT. Airway foreign body fatalities in children. *Ann Otol.* 1965; 74:1144.

104. Baker DC Jr, Karlan MS. Laryngolith. *Ann Otol.* 1972; 81:840.

105. Albizzati KC, Ramesar KCRB, Davis BC. Plasma cell granuloma of the larynx. Case report and review of the literature. *J Laryngol Otol.* 1988; 102:187.

106. Barker AP, Carter MJ, Matz LR. Armstrong JA. Plasma-cell granuloma of the trachea. *Med J Aust.* 1987; 146:443.

107. Coffin CM, Watterson J, Priest JR, Dehner LP. Extrapulmonary inflammatory myofibroblastic tumor (inflammatory pseudotumor). A clinicopathologic and immunohistochemical study of 84 cases. *Am J Surg Pathol.* 1995; 19:859.

108. Fonseca CA, Suarez RV. Plasma cell granuloma of the larynx as a cause of sudden asphyxial death. *Am J Forensic Med Pathol.* 1995; 16:243.

109. Ishii Y, Inoue F, Kamikawa Y, et al. A case report of tracheal inflammatory pseudotumor. *Nippon Kyobu Geka Gakkai Zasshi.* 1993; 41:672.

110. Keen M, Cho HT, Savetsky L. Pseudotumor of the larynx—An unusual cause of airway obstruction. *Otolaryngol Head Neck Surg.* 1986; 94:243.

111. Manni JJ, Mulder JJS, Schaafsma HE, van Hœlst UJGM. Inflammatory pseudotumor of the subglottis. *Eur Arch Otorhinolaryngol.* 1992; 249:16.

112. Satomi F, Mori H, Ogasawara H, Kumoi T, Uematsu K. Subglottic plasma cell granuloma: Report of a case. *Auris Nasus Larynx.* 1991; 18:391.

113. Wenig BM, Devaney K, Bisceglia M. Inflammatory myofibroblastic tumor of the larynx. A clinicopathologic study of eight cases simulating a malignant spindle neoplasm. *Cancer.* 1995; 76:2217.

114. Williams SB, Foss RD, Ellis GL. Inflammatory pseudotumors of the major salivary glands. Clinicopathologic and immu-

nohistochemical analysis of six cases. *Am J Surg Pathol.* 1992; 16:896.

115. Zapatero J, Lago J, Madrigal L, et al. Subglottic inflammatory pseudotumor in a 6-year-old child. *Pediatr Pulmonol.* 1989; 6:268.

116. Zbären P, Läng H, Beer K, Becker M. Plasma cell granuloma of the supraglottic larynx. *J Laryngol Otol.* 1995; 109:895.

117. Anthony PP. Inflammatory pseudotumour (plasma cell granuloma) of lung, liver and other organs. *Histopathology.* 1993; 23:501.

118. Hytiroglou P, Brandwein MS, Strauchen JA, et al. Inflammatory pseudotumor of the parapharyngeal space: Case report and review of the literature. *Head Neck.* 1992; 14:230.

119. Pettinato G, Manivel JC, DeRosa N, Dehner LP. Inflammatory myofibroblastic tumor (plasma cell granuloma). Clinicopathologic study of 20 cases with immunohistochemical and ultrastructural observations. *Am J Clin Pathol.* 1990; 94:538.

120. Nochomovitz LE, Orenstein JM. Inflammatory pseudotumor of the urinary bladder—possible relationship to nodular fasciitis. Two case reports, cytologic observations, and ultrastructural observations. *Am J Surg Pathol.* 1985; 9:366.

121. Spencer H. The pulmonary plasma cell/histiocytoma complex. *Histopathology.* 1984; 8:903.

122. Tang TT, Segura AD, Oechler HW, et al. Inflammatory myofibrohistiocytic proliferation simulating sarcoma in children. *Cancer.* 1990; 65:1626.

123. Ferlito A. Vocal cord polyp with stromal atypia: A pseudosarcomatous lesion. *Acta Otorhinolaryngol.* 1980; 39:955.

124. Nakayama M, Wenig BM, Heffner DK. Atypical stroma cells in inflammatory nasal polyps: Immunohistochemical and ultrastructural analysis in defining histogenesis. *Laryngoscope.* 1995; 105:127.

125. Arber DA, Kamel OW, van de Rijn M, et al. Frequent presence of the Epstein-Barr virus in inflammatory pseudotumor. *Hum Pathol.* 1995; 26:1093.

126. Coffin CM, Hussong J, Perkins S, Griffin CA, Perlman EJ. ALK and p80 expression in inflammatory myofibroblastic tumor (IMT). *Mod Pathol* 2000; 13:8A.

127. Rubin BP, Lawrence BD, Perez-Atayde A, et al. TPM-ALK fusion genes and ALK expression in inflammatory myofibroblastic tumor. *Mod Pathol.* 2000; 13:15A.

128. D'Aunoy R, Zoeller A. Primary tumors of the trachea. Report of a case and review of the literature. *Arch Pathol.* 1931; 11:589.

129. Myerson MC. Smoker's larynx. *Ann Otol Rhinol Laryngol.* 1950; 5:541.

130. Tsui HN, Loré JM Jr. Congenital subglottic fibroma in the newborn. *Laryngoscope.* 1976; 86:571.

131. Dahl I, Jarlstedt J. Nodular fasciitis in the head and neck. A clinicopathologic study of 18 cases. *Acta Otolaryngol.* 1980; 90:152.

132. Jones SR, Myers EN, Barnes L. Benign neoplasms of the larynx. *Otolaryngol Clin North Am.* 1984; 17:151.

133. Szpunar J, Glowacki J, Laskowski A, Miszke A. Fibrinous laryngotracheobronchitis in children. *Arch Otolaryngol.* 1971; 93:173.

134. Myerson MC. A manifestation of uremia in the pharynx, larynx, trachea and bronchi. *JAMA.* 1927; 89:685.

135. Nash G, Foley FD. Herpetic infection of the middle and lower respiratory tract. *Am J Clin Pathol.* 1970; 54:857.

136. Yeh V, Hopp ML, Goldstein NS, Meyer RD. Herpes simplex chronic laryngitis and vocal cord lesions in a patient with acquired immunodeficiency syndrome. *Ann Otol.* 1994; 103: 726.

137. Baxter JD. Acute epiglottitis. In: English GM, ed. *Otolaryngology.* Vol. 3. Philadelphia: Lippincott-Raven; 1996:Chapt. 39.

138. Davison FW. Inflammatory diseases of the larynx of infants and small children. *Ann Otol.* 1967; 76:753.

139. Hawkins DB, Miller AH, Sachs GB, Benz RT. Acute epiglottitis in adults. *Laryngoscope.* 1973; 83:1211.

140. Hazard GW, Porter P, Ingall D. Pneumococcal laryngitis in the newborn infant. Report of a case. *N Engl J Med.* 1964; 271:361.

141. Johnson GK, Sullivan JL, Bishop LA. Acute epiglottitis. Re-

view of 55 cases and suggested protocol. *Arch Otolaryngol.* 1974; 100:333.

142. Lederer FJ, Soboroff BJ. Medical problems related to diseases of the larynx. *Otolaryngol Clin North Am.* 1970; 3:599.

143. Liston SL, Gehrz RC, Jarvis CW. Bacterial tracheitis. *Arch Otolaryngol.* 1981; 107:561.

144. Schloss MD, Hannallah R, Baxter JD. Acute epiglottitis: 26 years' experience at the Montreal Children's Hospital. *J Otolaryngol.* 1979; 8:259.

145. Vrabec DP. Inflammatory diseases of the larynx. In: English GM, ed. *Otolaryngology.* Vol. 3. Philadelphia: Lippincott-Raven; 1996: Chapt. 37.

146. Wurtele P. Acute epiglottitis in children and adults: A large-scale incidence study. *Otolaryngol Head Neck Surg.* 1990; 103:902.

147. Lang WS. Diphtheria at the present time. *Laryngoscope.* 1965; 75:1092.

148. Heeneman H, Ward KM. Epiglottic abscess: Its occurrence and management. *J Otolaryngol.* 1977; 6:31.

149. Kernan JD, Schugt HP. Abscess of the larynx and its treatment. *Trans Am Laryngol Assoc.* 1934; 55:180.

150. Sopher IM, Fisher RS. Epiglottic abscess. Fatal acute airway obstruction in an adult. *Arch Otolaryngol.* 1971; 93:533.

151. Yeo TC. Acute stridor in childhood: Retropharyngeal abscess. *Med J Malaysia.* 1988; 43:65.

152. Auerbach O. Laryngeal tuberculosis. *Arch Otolaryngol.* 1946; 44:191.

153. Couldery AD. Tuberculosis of the upper respiratory tract misdiagnosed as Wegener's granulomatosis—an important distinction. *J Laryngol Otol.* 1990; 104:255.

154. Kahn I. Tuberculous granuloma of the epiglottis. *J Laryngol Otol.* 1983; 97:969.

155. Klimala KJ. Tuberculosis of the larynx in material from the ORL ward of the District General Hospital in Czestochowa in the years 1980–1992. *Pneumonol Alergol Pol.* 1996; 64:68.

156. Maloney WH. Laryngeal manifestations of systemic disease. *Ann Otol.* 1960; 69:421.

157. Muñoz-MacCormick CE. The larynx in leprosy. *Arch Otolaryngol.* 1957; 66:138.

158. O'Keefe JJ. Tuberculous laryngitis and tracheobronchitis. *Ann Otolaryngol.* 1949; 58:441.

159. Lerner DM, Deeb Z. Acute upper airway obstruction resulting from systemic diseases. *South Med J.* 1993; 86:623.

160. Amoils CP, Shindo ML. Laryngotracheal manifestations of rhinoscleroma. *Ann Otol.* 1996; 105:336.

161. Miller RH, Shulman JB, Canalis RF, Ward TH. Klebsiella rhinoscleromatis: A clinical and pathogenic enigma. *Otolaryngol Head Neck Surg.* 1979; 87:212.

162. Miller AH. Scleroma of the larynx, trachea and bronchi. *Laryngoscope.* 1949; 59:506.

163. Bartels LJ, Vrabec DP. Cervicofacial actinomycosis. A variable disorder. *Arch Otolaryngol.* 1978; 104:705.

164. Vrabec DP. Fungal infections of the larynx. *Otolaryngol Clin North Am.* 1993; 26:1091.

165. Benson-Mitchell R, Tolley N, Croft CB, Gallimore A. Aspergillosis of the larynx. *J Laryngol Otol.* 1994; 108:883.

166. Boyle JO, Coulthard SW, Mandel RM. Laryngeal involvement in disseminated coccidioidomycosis. *Arch Otolaryngol Head Neck Surg.* 1991; 117:433.

167. Cody CC. Moniliasis of the larynx: Report of two cases. *Ann Otolaryngol.* 1948; 57:371.

168. Donegan JO, Wood MD. Histoplasmosis of the larynx. *Laryngoscope.* 1984; 94:206.

169. Gori S, Scasso A. Cytologic and differential diagnosis of rhinosporidiosis. *Acta Cytol.* 1994; 38:361.

170. Isaacson JE, Frable MAS. Cryptococcosis of the larynx. *Otolaryngol Head Neck Surg.* 1996; 114:106.

171. King HC, Cline JFX. Histoplasmosis involving the larynx. *Arch Otolaryngol.* 1958; 67:649.

172. Richardson BE, Morrison VA, Gapany M. Invasive aspergillosis of the larynx: Case report and review of the literature. *Otolaryngol Head Neck Surg.* 1996; 114:471.

173. Stachowsky LN. Primary paracoccidioidomycosis of the larynx. Report of a case. *Arch Otolaryngol.* 1963; 78:205.

174. Thornell WC. Blastomycosis of the larynx. *Ann Otolaryngol.* 1955; 64:1155.

175. Ward PH, Berci G, Morledge D, Schwartz H. Coccidioidomycosis of the larynx in infants and adults. *Ann Otol.* 1977; 86;655.

176. Withers BT, Pappas JJ, Erickson EE. Histoplasmosis primary in the larynx. Report of a case. *Arch Otolaryngol.* 1963; 77:25.

177. Goldner AI. Tertiary syphilis of ear, nose and throat. *Arch Otolaryngol.* 1947; 45:463.

178. Lacy PD, Alderson DJ, Parker AJ. Late congenital syphilis of the larynx and pharynx presenting at endotracheal intubation. *J Laryngol Otol.* 1994; 108:688.

179. Mollo J-L, Groussard O, Baldeyrou P, et al. Tracheal malacoplakia. *Chest.* 1994; 105:608.

180. Gabriel CE, Jones DG. The importance of chronic laryngitis. *J Laryngol.* 1960; 74:349.

181. Brunner H. Superficial epidermoid carcinoma of the larynx. *Arch Otolaryngol.* 1949; 51:49.

182. Jaffé L. Otorhinolaryngology in the tropics. *Otolaryngology.* 1955; 5:1.

183. Lewy RB. Carcinoma of larynx and trichinosis. *Arch Otolaryngol.* 1964; 80:320.

184. Regezi JA, Taylor CG, Spinelli FR Jr, Lucas RN. Allergic gingivostomatitis with laryngeal manifestations: Report of case. *J Oral Surg.* 1972; 30:373.

185. Williams RI. Allergic laryngitis. *Ann Otol.* 1972; 81:558.

186. Bicknell PG. Mild hypothyroidism and its effects on the larynx. *J Laryngol Otol.* 1973; 87:123.

187. Hilger JA. Otolaryngologic aspects of hypometabolism. *Ann Otol.* 1956; 65:395.

188. Alexander FW. Micropathology of radiation reaction in the larynx. *Ann Otol.* 1963; 72:831.

189. Calcaterra TC, Stern F, Ward PH. Dilemma of delayed radiation injury of the larynx. *Ann Otol.* 1972; 81:501.

190. Kashima HK, Holliday MJ, Hyams VJ. Laryngeal chondronecrosis: Clinical variations and comments and recognition and management. *Trans Am Acad Ophthalmol Otolaryngol.* 1977; 84:878.

191. Stell PH, Morrison MD. Radiation necrosis of the larynx. Etiology and management. *Arch Otolaryngol.* 1973; 98:111.

192. Benjamin B, Dalton C, Croxson G. Laryngoscopic diagnosis of laryngeal sarcoid. *Ann Otol.* 1995; 104:529.

193. DeRemee RA. Sarcoidosis and Wegener's granulomatosis: A comparative analysis. *Sarcoidosis.* 1994; 11:7.

194. Devine KD. Sarcoidosis and sarcoidosis of the larynx. *Laryngoscope.* 1965; 75:533.

195. Gallivan GJ, Landis JN. Sarcoidosis of the larynx: Preserving and restoring airway and professional voice. *J Voice.* 1993; 7:81.

196. Lindsay JR, Perlman HB. Sarcoidosis of the upper respiratory tract. *Ann Otol.* 1951; 60:549.

197. McHugh K, de Silva M, Kilham HA. Epiglottic enlargement secondary to laryngeal sarcoidosis. *Pediatr Radiol.* 1993; 23:71.

198. Neel HB III, McDonald TJ. Laryngeal sarcoidosis. Report of 13 patients. *Ann Otol.* 1982; 91:359.

199. Webb J, Payne WH. Rheumatoid nodules of the vocal cords. *Ann Rheum Dis.* 1972; 31:122.

200. Woo P, Mendelsohn J, Humphrey D. Rhematoid nodules of the larynx. *Otolaryngol Head Neck Surg.* 1995; 113:147.

201. Montgomery WW, Lofgren RH. Usual and unusual causes of laryngeal arthritis. *Arch Otolaryngol.* 1963; 77:29.

202. Wolman L, Darke CS, Young A. The larynx in rheumatoid arthritis. *Laryngol Otol.* 1965; 79:403.

203. Goodman M, Montgomery W, Minnette L. Pathologic findings in gouty cricoarytenoid arthritis. *Arch Otolaryngol.* 1976; 102:27.

204. Okada T. Hoarseness due to gouty tophus in vocal cords. *Arch Otolaryngol.* 1964; 79:407.

205. Stark TW, Hirokawa RH. Gout and its manifestations in the head and neck. *Otolaryngol Clin North Am.* 1982; 15:659.

206. Damiani JM, Levine HL. Relapsing polychondritis—report of ten cases. *Laryngoscope.* 1979; 89:929.

207. Hussain SSM. Relapsing polychondritis presenting with stri-

dor from bilateral vocal cord palsy. *J Laryngol Otol.* 1991; 105:961.

208. McAdam LP, O'Hanlan MA, Bluestone R, Pearson CM. Relapsing polychondritis. Prospective study of 23 patients and a review of the literature. *Medicine.* 1976; 55:193.

209. McCaffrey TV, McDonald TJ, McCaffrey LA. Head and neck manifestations of relapsing polychondritis: Review of 29 cases. *Otolaryngology.* 1978; 86:473.

210. Purcelli FM, Nahum A, Monell C. Relapsing polychondritis with tracheal collapse. *Ann Otol.* 1962; 71:1120.

211. Mahindrakar NH, Libman LJ. Relapsing polychondritis. *J Laryngol Otol.* 1970; 84:337.

212. Dolan DL, Lemmon GB, Teitelbaum SL. Relapsing polychondritis. Analytical literature review and studies on pathogenesis. *Am J Med.* 1966; 41:285.

213. Eng J, Sabanathan S. Airway complications in relapsing polychondritis. *Ann Thorac Surg.* 1991; 51:686.

214. Moloney JR. Relapsing polychondritis—its otolaryngological manifestations. *J Laryngol Otol.* 1978; 92:9.

215. Swain RE, Stroud MH. Relapsing polychondritis. *Laryngoscope.* 1972; 82:891.

216. Kaye RL, Sones DA. Relapsing polychondritis. Clinical and pathologic features in 14 cases. *Ann Intern Med.* 1964; 60:653.

217. Cauhape P, Aumaitre O, Papo T, et al. A diagnostic dilemma: Wegener's granulomatosis, relapsing polychondritis or both? *Eur J Med.* 1993; 2:497.

218. Saxne T, Heinegard D. Serum concentrations of two cartilage matrix proteins reflecting different aspects of cartilage turnover in relapsing polychondritis. *Arthritis Rheum.* 1995; 38:294.

219. Anstey A, Mayou S, Morgan K, Clague RB, Munro DD. Relapsing polychondritis: Autoimmunity to type II collagen and treatment with cyclosporin A. *Br J Dermatol.* 1991; 125:588.

220. McCune WJ, Schiller AL, Dynesius-Trentham RA, Trentham DE. Type II collagen-induced auricular chondritis. *Arthritis Rheum.* 1982; 25:266.

221. Lang B, Rothenfusser A, Lanchbury JS, et al. Susceptibility to relapsing polychondritis is associated with HLA-DR4. *Arthritis Rheum.* 1993; 36:660.

222. Silva J, Branco JA, de Matos AA, et al. Relapsing polychondritis and Reiter's syndrome. *J Rheumatol.* 1991; 18:908.

223. Miller PK, Rogers RS III. Polychondritis and Behçet's disease. *Curr Opin Rheumatol.* 1990; 2:70.

224. Harisdangkul V, Johnson WW. Association between relapsing polychondritis and systemic lupus erythematosus. *South Med J.* 1994; 87:753.

225. Krasovskii II, Shkodkin IV, Vladimirova NN. The combined treatment of relapsing polychondritis (systemic chondromalacia) developing against a background of severe diabetes mellitus. *Ter Arkh.* 1994; 66:64.

226. Harada M, Yoshida H, Mimura Y, et al. Relapsing polychondritis associated with subclinical Sjögren's syndrome and phlegmon of the neck. *Intern Med (Jpn).* 1995; 34:768.

227. Fransen HR, Ramon FA, De Schepper AM, et al. Chondrosarcoma in a patient with relapsing polychondritis. *Skeletal Radiol.* 1995; 24:477.

228. Diebold L, Rauh G, Jager K, Lohrs U. Bone marrow pathology in relapsing polychondritis: High frequency of myelodysplastic syndromes. *Br J Haematol.* 1995; 89:820.

229. Enright H, Jacob HS, Vercellotti G, et al. Paraneoplastic autoimmune phenomena in patients with myelodysplastic syndromes: Response to immunosuppressive therapy. *Br J Haematol.* 1995; 91:403.

230. Arauz JC, Fonseca R. Wegener's granulomatosis appearing initially in the trachea. *Ann Otol.* 1982. 91:593.

231. Daum TE, Specks U, Colby TV, et al. Tracheobronchial involvement in Wegener's granulomatosis. *Am J Respir Crit Care Med.* 1995; 151:522.

232. Devaney KO, Travis WD, Hoffman G, et al. Interpretation of head and neck biopsies in Wegener's granulomatosis: A pathologic study of 126 biopsies in 70 patients. *Am J Surg Pathol.* 1990; 14:555.

233. Hoare TJ, Jayne D, Evans PR, Croft CB, Howard DJ. Wegener's granulomatosis, subglottic stenosis and antineutrophil cytoplasm antibodies. *J Laryngol Otol.* 1989; 103:1187.

234. McDonald TJ, Neel HB III, DeRemee RA. Wegener's granulomatosis of the subglottis and upper portion of the trachea. *Ann Otol.* 1982; 91:588.

235. McDonald TJ, DeRemee RA. Wegener's granulomatosis. *Laryngoscope.* 1983; 93:220.

236. Waxman J, Bose WJ. Laryngeal manifestations of Wegener's granulomatosis: Case reports and review of the literature. *J Rheumatol.* 1986; 13:408.

237. Gindre D, Peyrol S, Raccurt M. Fibrosing vasculitis in Wegener's ganulomatosis: Ultrastructural and immunohistochemical analysis of the vascular lesions. *Virch Arch [A].* 1995; 427:385.

238. Matsubara O, Yoshimura N, Doi Y, Tamura A, Mark EJ. Nasal biopsy in the early diagnosis of Wegener's granulomatosis. Significance of palisading granuloma and leukocytoclastic vasculitis. *Virch Arch [A].* 1996; 428:13.

239. Friedmann I. Midline granuloma. *Proc R Soc Med.* 1964; 57:289.

240. Lipford EH Jr, Margolick JB, Longo DL, Fauci AS, Jaffe ES. Angiocentric immunoproliferative lesions: A clinicopathologic spectrum of post-thymic T-cell proliferations. *Blood.* 1988; 72:1674.

241. Lippman SM, Grogan TM, Spier CM, et al. Lethal midline granuloma with a novel T-cell phenotype as found in peripheral T-cell lymphoma. *Cancer.* 1987; 59:936.

242. Olsen KD, Neel HB III, DeRemee RA, Weiland LH. Nasal manifestations of allergic granulomatosis and angiitis (Churg-Strauss syndrome). *Otolaryngol Head Neck Surg.* 1980; 88:85.

243. Rao JK, Weinberger M, Oddone EZ, et al. The role of antineutrophil cytoplasmic antibody (c-ANCA) testing in the diagnosis of Wegener granulomatosis. A literature review and meta-analysis. *Ann Intern Med.* 1995; 123:925.

244. Talerman A, Wright D. Laryngeal obstruction due to Wegener's granulomatosis. *Arch Otolaryngol.* 1972; 96:376.

245. Berson S, Lin AN, Ward RF, Carter DM. Junctional epidermolysis bullosa of the larynx. Report of a case and literature review. *Ann Otol.* 1992; 101:861.

246. Cohen SR, Landing BH, Isaacs H. Epidermolysis bullosa associated with laryngeal stenosis. *Ann Otol.* 1978; 87(suppl 52):25.

247. Gonzalez C, Roth R. Laryngotracheal involvement in epidermolysis bullosa. *Int J Pediatr Otorhinolaryngol.* 1989; 17:305.

248. Hester JE, Arnstein DP, Woodley D. Laryngeal manifestations of epidermolysis bullosa acquisita. *Arch Otolaryngol Head Neck Surg.* 1995; 121:1042.

249. Lyos AT, Levy ML, Malpica A, Sulek M. Laryngeal involvement in epidermolysis bullosa. *Ann Otol.* 1994; 103:542.

250. Schaffer SR. Head and neck manifestations of epidermolysis bullosa. *Clin Pediatr.* 1992; 31:81.

251. Fisher ER, Kyler SL. Darier's disease of the larynx. *Arch Otolaryngol.* 1955; 62:438.

252. Charow A, Pass F, Ruben R. Pemphigus of the upper respiratory tract. *Arch Otolaryngol.* 1971; 93:209.

253. Frangogiannis NG, Gangopadhyay S, Cate T. Pemphigus of the larynx and esophagus. *Ann Intern Med.* 1995; 122:803.

254. New GB, O'Leary P. Pemphigus from the laryngologist's standpoint. *Arch Otolaryngol.* 1925; 1:617.

255. Obregon G. Pemphigus of the larynx. *Ann Otol.* 1957; 66:649.

256. Weinstein S, Sachs AR. Pemphigus of the oropharynx and larynx. *Arch Otolaryngol.* 1955; 62:214.

257. Assier H, Bastuji-Garin S, Revuz J, Roujeau J-C. Erythema multiforme with mucous membrane involvement and Stevens-Johnson syndrome are clinically different disorders with distinct causes. *Arch Dermatol.* 1995; 131:539.

258. Bosma JF, Graykowski EA, Trygstad CW. Chronic ulcerative pharyngitis. Radiographic studies of progressive dysphagia in five patients. *Arch Otolaryngol.* 1968; 87:85.

259. Calcaterra TC, Strahan RW. Stevens-Johnson syndrome. Oropharyngeal manifestations. *Arch Otolaryngol.* 1971; 93:37.

260. Nonomura N, Nishiwaki C, Hasegawa S, Ikarashi F, Nakano Y: A case of pharyngolaryngeal stenosis in Behçet's disease. *Auris Nasus Larynx.* 1992; 19:55.

261. Hanson RD, Olsen KD, Rogers RS III. Upper aerodigestive tract manifestations of cicatricial pemphigoid. *Ann Otol.* 1988; 97:493.

262. Teitel AD, MacKenzie CR, Stern R, Paget SA. Laryngeal involvement in systemic lupus erythematosus. *Semin Arthritis Rheum.* 1992; 22:203.

263. Cohn AM, McFarlane JR, Knox J. Pachyonychia congenita with involvement of the larynx. *Arch Otolaryngol.* 1976; 102: 233.

264. Crepeau J, Poliquin J. The blue rubber bleb nevus syndrome. *J Otolaryngol.* 1981; 10:387.

265. Fortson JS, Schroeter AL: Necrotiotic xanthogranuloma with IgA paraproteinemia and extracutaneous involvement. *Am J Dermatopathol.* 1990; 12:579.

266. Jordan WM. Laryngeal polyposis in tuberous sclerosis. *Br Med J.* 1956; 2:132.

267. Lautch H, Trethowan WH. Agenesis of vocal cords in a case of tuberous sclerosis. *J Laryngol Otol.* 1971; 85:871.

268. Gianoli GJ, Miller RH. Crohn's disease of the larynx. *J Laryngol Otol.* 1994; 108:596.

269. Barton RT. Oxyphilic adenoma of the larynx. *Ann Otol.* 1972; 81:256.

270. Capo OA. Oxyphilic adenoma (oncocytoma) of the larynx. *Arch Otolaryngol.* 1965; 82:42.

271. Dhingra JK, Aqel NM, McEwen J, Bleach NR. Multiple oncocytic cysts of the larynx. *J Laryngol Otol.* 1995; 109:1226.

272. Ekedahl C, Schnürer L-B. Eosinophilic papillary cystadenoma of the larynx. *Acta Otolaryngol.* 1969; 67:467.

273. Gallagher JC, Puzon BQ. Oncocytic lesions of the larynx. *Ann Otol.* 1969; 78:307.

274. Kleidermacher P, Mastros NP, Miller FR, Jones EW, Wood BG. Oncocytic cyst of the larynx. *Arch Otolaryngol Head Neck Surg.* 1995; 121:1430.

275. Kroe DJ, Pitcock JA, Cocke EW. Oncocytic papillary cystadenoma of the larynx. Presentation of two cases. *Arch Pathol.* 1967; 84:429.

276. Lundgren J, Olofsson J, Hellquist H. Oncocytic lesions of the larynx. *Acta Otolaryngol.* 1982; 94:335.

277. Martin-Hirsch DP, Lannigan FJ, Irani B, Batman P. Oncocytic papillary cystadenomatosis of the larynx. *J Laryngol Otol.* 1992; 106:656.

278. Nassar VH, Bridger GP. Topography of the laryngeal mucous glands. *Arch Otolaryngol.* 1971; 94:490.

279. Oliveira CA, Roth JA, Adams GL. Oncocytic lesions of the larynx. *Laryngoscope.* 1977; 87:1718.

280. Robinson AC, Kaberos A, Cox PM, Stearns MP. Oncocytoma of the larynx. *J Laryngol Otol.* 1990; 104:346.

281. Thawley SE, Berlin BP, Berkowitz WP. Oncocytic hyperplasia of the larynx. *J Laryngol Otol.* 1977; 91:619.

282. Yamase HT, Putman HC III. Oncocytic papillary cystadenomatosis of the larynx: A clinicopathologic entity. *Cancer.* 1979; 44:2306.

283. DeSanto LW, Devine KD, Weiland LH. Cysts of the larynx. Classification. *Laryngoscope.* 1970; 80:145.

284. Civantos FJ, Holinger LD. Laryngoceles and saccular cysts in infants and children. *Arch Otolaryngol Head Neck Surg.* 1992; 118:296.

285. DeSanto LW. Laryngocele, laryngeal mucocele, large saccules and saccular cysts: A developmental spectrum. *Laryngoscope.* 1974; 84:1291.

286. Holinger PH, Johnson KC, Schiller F. Congenital anomalies of the larynx. *Ann Otol.* 1954; 63:581.

287. Matiño Soler E, Martinez Vecina V, Leon Vintro X, et al. Laringoceles: Estudio clinico y terapéutico de 60 casos. *Acta Otorrinolaringol Esp.* 1995; 46:279.

288. New GB, Erich JB. Congenital cysts of the larynx. *Arch Otolaryngol.* 1939; 30:943.

289. Richards L. Laryngocele. *Ann Otol.* 1951; 60:510.

290. Suehs OW, Powell DB Jr. Congenital cyst of the larynx in infants. *Laryngoscope.* 1967; 77:654.

291. New GB. Congential cysts of the tongue, the floor of the mouth, the pharynx and the larynx. *Arch Otolaryngol.* 1947; 45:145.

292. Norris CW. Pharyngoceles of the hypopharynx. *Laryngoscope.* 1979; 89:1788.

293. van der Ven PM, Schutte HK. The pharyngocele: infrequently encountered and easily misdiagnosed. *J Laryngol Otol.* 1995; 109:247.

294. Shaari CM, Ho BT, Som PM, Urken ML. Large thyroglossal duct cyst with laryngeal extension. *Head Neck.* 1994; 16:586.

295. Balik E, Erdener A, Taneli C, et al. Jugular phlebectasia in children. *Eur J Pediatr Surg.* 1993; 3:46.

296. Pul N, Pul M. External jugular phlebectasia in children. *Eur J Pediatr.* 1995; 154:275.

297. Celin SE, Johnson J, Curtin H, Barnes L. The association of laryngoceles with squamous cell carcinoma of the larynx. *Laryngoscope.* 1991; 101:529.

298. Micheau C, Luboinski B, Lanchi P, Cachin Y. Relationship between laryngoceles and laryngeal carcinomas. *Laryngoscope.* 1978; 88:680.

299. Archer SM, Crockett DM, McGill TJI. Hamartoma of the larynx: Report of two cases and review of the literature. *Int J Pediatr Otorhinolaryngol.* 1988; 16:237.

300. Bone RC, Biller HF, Irwin TM. Intralaryngotracheal thyroid. *Ann Otol.* 1972; 81:424.

301. Bures C, Barnes L. Benign mesenchymomas of the head and neck. *Arch Pathol Lab Med.* 1978; 102:237.

302. Cenik Z, Uyar Y, Özer B, Güngör S, Bulun E. An unusual laryngeal hamartoma: Lipofibroleiomyoma. *J Otolaryngol.* 1993; 22:136.

303. Cohen SR. Posterior cleft larynx associated with hamartoma. *Ann Otol.* 1984; 93:443.

304. Feenstra L, Houthoff HJ. An unusual hypopharyngeal tumour. *J Laryngol Otol.* 1972; 86:1177.

305. Holinger LD, Tansek KM, Tucker GF Jr. Cleft larynx with airway obstruction. *Ann Otol.* 1985; 94:622.

306. Patterson HC, Dickerson GR, Pilch BZ, Bentkover SH. Hamartoma of the hypopharynx. *Arch Otolaryngol.* 1981; 107: 767.

307. Weinberger J, Kassim O, Birt BD. Hamartoma of the larynx. *J Otolaryngol.* 1985; 14:305.

308. Wind J, Lecluse FLE. Een slokdarmpoliep of een hamartoom van de hypopharynx. *Ned Tijdschr Geneeskd.* 1980; 124:1467.

309. Wind J, Lecluse FLE. Hamartoma of the hypopharynx. *Arch Otolaryngol.* 1983; 109:495.

310. Zapf B, Lehmann WB, Snyder GG III. Hamartoma of the larynx: An unusual cause for stridor in an infant. *Otolaryngol Head Neck Surg.* 1981; 89:797.

311. Lyons TJ, Variend S. Posterior cleft larynx association with hamartoma: A case report and literature review. *J Laryngol Otol.* 1988; 102:471.

312. Le Ber MS, Stout AP. Benign mesenchymomas in children. *Cancer.* 1962; 15:598.

313. Abemayor E, Newman A, Bergstrom L, et al. Teratomas of the head and neck in childhood. *Laryngoscope.* 1984; 94:1489.

314. Cannon CR, Johns ME, Fechner RE. Immature teratoma of the larynx. *Otolaryngol Head Neck Surg.* 1987; 96:366.

315. Johnson LF, Strong MS. Teratoma of the larynx. *Arch Otolaryngol.* 1953; 58:435.

316. Eble JN, Hull MT, Bojrab D. Laryngeal blastoma. A light and electron microscopic study of a novel entity analogous to pulmonary blastoma. *Am J Clin Pathol.* 1985; 84:378.

317. Hyams VJ, Rabuzzi DD. Cartilagenous tumors of the larynx. *Laryngoscope.* 1970; 80:755.

318. Evans KL, Lowe DG, Keene MH. Vallecula angioleiomyoma: An unusual cause of adult airway obstruction. *J Laryngol Otol.* 1990; 104:341.

319. Marchal G, Baert AL, van der Hauwaert L. Calcification of larynx and trachea in infancy. *Br J Radiol.* 1974; 47:896.

320. Pappas DG, Johnson LA. Laryngeal myositis ossificans. A case report. *Arch Otolaryngol.* 1965; 81:227.

321. Canfield N. Bony stenosis of the larynx. *Ann Otol.* 1949; 58: 559.

322. Fisher F, Tomanek A, Rimonava Seelevy V. Tracheobronchomegaly. *Scand J Respir Dis.* 1969; 50:147.

323. Himalstein MR, Gallagher JC. Tracheobronchiomegaly. *Ann Otol.* 1973; 82:223.

324. Levin SJ, Adler P, Scherer RA. Collapsible trachea (tracheomalacia). A non-allergic cause of wheezing in infancy. *Ann Allerg.* 1964; 22:20.

325. Batsakis JG, Raymond AK, Rice DH. The pathology of head and neck tumors: Papillomas of the upper respiratory tracts, pt. 18. *Head Neck Surg.* 1983; 5:332.

326. Kashima H, Wu T-C, Mounts P, et al. Carcinoma ex-papilloma: Histologic and virologic studies in whole-organ sections of the larynx. *Laryngoscope.* 1988; 98:619.

327. Johnson JT, Barnes EL. Adult onset laryngeal papillomatosis. *Otolaryngol Head Neck Surg.* 1981; 89:867.

328. Runckel D, Kessler S. Bronchogenic squamous carcinoma in nonirradiated juvenile laryngotracheal papillomatosis. *Am J Surg Pathol.* 1980; 4:293.

329. Abramson AL, Steinberg BM, Winkler B. Laryngeal papillomatosis: Clinical, histopathologic and molecular studies. *Laryngoscope.* 1987; 97:678.

330. Arends MJ, Wyllie AH, Bird CC. Papillomaviruses and human cancer. *Hum Pathol.* 1990; 21:686.

331. Gaylis B, Hayden RE. Recurrent respiratory papillomatosis: Progression to invasion and malignancy. *Am J Otolaryngol.* 1991; 12:104.

332. Quick CA, Foucar E, Dehner LP. Frequency and significance of epithelial atypia in laryngeal papillomatosis. *Laryngoscope.* 1979; 89:550.

333. Schnadig VJ, Clark WD, Clegg TJ, Yao CS. Invasive papillomatosis and squamous carcinoma complicating juvenile laryngeal papillomatosis. *Arch Otolaryngol Head Neck Surg.* 1986; 112:966.

334. Steinberg BM. Human papillomaviruses and upper airway oncogenesis. *Am J Otolaryngol.* 1990; 11:370.

335. Boyle WF, Riggs JL, Oshiro LS, Lennette EH. Electron microscopic identification of papovavirus in laryngeal papilloma. *Laryngoscope.* 1973; 83:1102.

336. Braun L, Kashima H, Eggleston J, Shah K. Demonstration of papillomavirus antigen in paraffin sections of laryngeal papillomas. *Laryngoscope.* 1982; 92:640.

337. Johnson TL, Plieth DA, Crissman JD, Sarkar FH. HPV detection by polymerase chain reaction (PCR) in verrucous lesions of the upper aerodigestive tract. *Mod Pathol.* 1991; 4:461.

338. Lack EE, Jenson AB, Smith HG, et al. Immunoperoxidase localization of human papillomavirus in laryngeal papillomas. *Intervirology.* 1980; 14:148.

339. Pou AM, Rimell FL, Jordan JA, et al. Adult respiratory papillomatosis: Human papillomavirus type and viral coinfections as predictors of prognosis. *Ann Otol.* 1995; 104:758.

340. Mounts P, Kashima H. Association of human papilloma virus subtype and clinical course in respiratory papillomatosis. *Laryngoscope.* 1984; 94:28.

341. Clayman GL, Stewart MG, Weber RS, et al. Human papillomavirus in laryngeal and hypopharyngeal carcinomas. *Arch Otolaryngol Head Neck Surg.* 1994; 120:743.

342. Hollinger PH, Johnston KC, Conner GH, Conner BR, Holper J. Studies of papilloma of the larynx. *Ann Otol.* 1962; 71:443.

343. Fechner RE, Goepfert H, Alford BR. Invasive laryngeal papillomatosis. *Arch Otolaryngol.* 1974; 99:147.

344. Friedberg SA, Stagman R, Hass GM. Papillary lesions of the larynx in adults. *Ann Otol.* 1971; 80:683.

345. Hollinger PH, Schild JA, Maurizi DG. Laryngeal papilloma: Review of etiology and therapy. *Laryngoscope.* 1968; 78:1462.

346. Cotelingam JD, Barnes L, Nixon VB. Pleomorphic adenoma of the epiglottis. Report of a case. *Arch Otolaryngol.* 1977; 103:245.

347. MacMillan RH III, Fechner RE. Pleomorphic adenoma of the larynx. *Arch Pathol Lab Med.* 1986; 110:245.

348. Som PM, Nagel BD, Feuerstein SS, Strauss L. Benign pleomorphic adenoma of the larynx. A case report. *Ann Otol Rhinol Laryngol.* 1979; 88:112.

349. Batsakis JG, Hyams VJ, Morales AR. *Special Tumors of the Head and Neck.* Proceedings, 48th Annual Seminar. Chicago: ASCP Press; 1983:37.

350. Heffner DK. Sinonasal and laryngeal salivary gland lesions. In: Ellis GL, Auclair PL, Gnepp DR, eds. *Surgical Pathology of the Salivary Glands.* Philadelphia: WB Saunders; 1991:554.

351. Putney, FJ. Borderline malignant lesions of the larynx. *Arch Otolaryngol.* 1955; 61:381.

352. Work WP, Habel DW. Mixed tumors of the parotid gland with extension to the lateral pharyngeal space. *Ann Otol.* 1963; 72:842.

353. Sabri JA, Hajjar MA. Malignant mixed tumor of the vocal cord. Report of a case. *Arch Otolaryngol.* 1967; 85:118.

354. Agarwal RK, Blitzer A, Perzin KH. Granular cell tumors of the larynx. *Otolaryngol Head Neck Surg.* 1979; 87:807.

355. Booth JB, Osborn DA. Granular cell myoblastoma of the larynx. *Acta Otolaryngol.* 1970; 70:279.

356. Compango J, Hyams NJ, Ste-Marie P. Benign granular cell tumors of the larynx: A review of 36 cases with clinicopathologic data. *Ann Otol.* 1975; 84:308.

357. Cree IA, Bingham BJG, Ramesar KCRB. Granular cell tumour of the larynx. *J Laryngol Otol.* 1990; 104:159.

358. Pope TH. Laryngeal myoblastoma. *Arch Otolaryngol.* 1965; 81: 80.

359. Thawley SE, Ogura JH. Granular cell myoblastoma of the trachea. *Arch Otolaryngol.* 1974; 100:393.

360. Sobel HJ, Schwarz R, Marquet E. Light- and electron-microcope study of the origin of granular-cell myoblastoma. *J Pathol.* 1973; 109:101.

361. Al-Sarraf M, Loud AV, Vaitkevicius VK. Malignant granular cell tumor. *Arch Pathol.* 1971; 91:550.

362. Filie AC, Lage JM, Azumi N. Immunoreactivity of S100 protein, alpha-1-antitrypsin, and CD68 in adult and congenital granular cell tumors. *Mod Pathol.* 1996; 9:888.

363. Regezi JA, Zarbo RJ, Courtney RM, Crissman JD. Immunoreactivity of granular cell lesions of skin, mucosa and jaw. *Cancer.* 1989; 64:1455.

364. Stefansson K, Wollmann RL. S-100 protein in granular cell tumors (granular cell myoblastomas). *Cancer.* 1982; 49:1834.

365. Thunold S, von Eyben FE, Mæhle B. Malignant granular cell tumor of the neck: Immunohistochemical and ultrastructural studies. *Histopathology.* 1989; 14:655.

366. Christopherson WM, Foote FW Jr, Stewart FW. Alveolar soft-part sarcomas. Structurally characteristic tumors of uncertain histogenesis. *Cancer.* 1952; 5:100.

367. Miettinen M, Ekfors T. Alveolar soft part sarcoma. Immunohistochemical evidence for muscle cell differentiation. *Am J Clin Pathol.* 1990; 93:32.

368. Barnes L. Paraganglioma of the larynx. A critical review of the literature. *ORL J Otorhinolaryngol Relat Spec.* 1991; 53:220.

369. Batsakis JG. Diagnosis, classification, treatment, and prognosis of laryngeal paraganglioma. *Adv Anat Pathol.* 1995; 2:237.

370. Ferlito A, Barnes L, Wenig BM. Identification, classification, treatment, and prognosis of laryngeal paraganglioma: Review of the literature and eight new cases. *Ann Otol.* 1994; 103:525.

371. Lack EE, Cubilla AL, Woodruff JM. Paragangliomas of the head and neck region. A pathologic study of tumors from 71 patients. *Hum Pathol.* 1979; 10:191.

372. Milroy CM, Rode J, Moss E. Laryngeal paragangliomas and neuroendocrine carcinomas. *Histopathology.* 1991; 18:201.

373. Wenig BM, Gnepp DR. The spectrum of neuroendocrine carcinoma of the larynx. *Semin Diagn Pathol.* 1989; 6:329.

374. Batsakis JG, El-Naggar AK, Luna MA. Neuroendocrine tumors of the larynx. *Ann Otol.* 1992; 101:710.

375. Martinez-Madrigal F, Bosq J, Micheau CH, Nivet P, Luboinski B. Paragangliomas of the head and neck. Immunohistochemical analysis of 16 cases in comparison with neuroendocrine carcinomas. *Pathol Res Pract.* 1991; 187:814.

376. Johnson TL, Zarbo RJ, Lloyd RV, Crissman JD. Paragangliomas of the head and neck: Immunohistochemical neuroendocrine and intermediate filament typing. *Mod Pathol.* 1988; 1: 216.

377. Kliewer KE, Wen D-R, Cancilla PA, Cochran AJ. Paragangliomas: Assessment of prognosis by histologic, immunohistochemical, and ultrastructural techniques. *Hum Pathol.* 1989; 20:29.

378. Linnoila RI, Lack EE, Steinberg SM, Keiser HR. Decreased

expression of neuropeptides in malignant paragangliomas: An immunohistochemical study. *Hum Pathol.* 1988; 19:41.

379. Googe PB, Ferry JA, Bhan AK, et al. A comparison of paraganglioma, carcinoid tumor, and small-cell carcinoma of the larynx. *Arch Pathol Lab Med.* 1988; 112:809.

380. Sweeney EC, McDonnell L, O'Brien C. Medullary carcinoma of the thyroid presenting as tumours of the pharynx and larynx. *Histopathology.* 1981; 5:263.

381. Marks PV, Brookes GB. Malignant paraganglioma of the larynx. *J Laryngol Otol.* 1983; 97:1183.

382. Cocke EW Jr. Benign cartilaginous tumors of the larynx. *Laryngoscope.* 1962; 72:1678.

383. Damiani KK, Tucker HM. Chondroma of the larynx. Surgical technique. *Arch Otolaryngol.* 1981; 107:399.

384. Devaney KO, Ferlito A, Silver CE. Cartilaginous tumors of the larynx. *Ann Otol.* 1995; 104:251.

385. Moore I. Cartilaginous turnours of the larynx. A study of all the recorded cases. *J Laryngol Otol.* 1925; 40:145.

386. Neel HM III, Unni KK. Cartilaginous tumors of the larynx: A series of 33 cases. *Otolaryngol Head Neck Surg.* 1982; 90:201.

387. New GB. Cartilaginous tumors of the larynx. *Laryngoscope.* 1918; 28:367.

388. Rosedale RS. Laryngeal chondroma. *Arch Otolaryngol.* 1947; 45:543.

389. Schiff M, Bender MS. Chondroma of the larynx. *Arch Otolaryngol.* 1959; 69:459.

390. Schittek A, James AG. Chondroma of the larynx. *J Surg Oncol.* 1982; 21:176.

391. Singh J, Black MJ, Fried I. Cartilaginous tumors of the larynx: A review of the literature and two case experiences. *Laryngoscope.* 1980; 90:1872.

392. Swerdlow RS, Som ML, Biller HF. Cartilaginous tumors of the larynx. *Arch Otolaryngol.* 1974; 100:269.

393. Zizmor J, Noyek AM, Lewis JS. Radiologic diagnosis of chondroma and chondrosaroma of the larynx. *Arch Otolaryngol.* 1975; 101:232.

394. Di Sant'Agnese PA, Knowles DM II. Extracardiac rhabdomyoma: A clinicopathologic study and review of the literature. *Cancer.* 1980; 46:780.

395. Ferlito A, Frugoni P. Rhabdomyoma purum of the larynx. *J Laryngol Otol.* 1975; 89:1131.

396. Gibas Z, Miettinen M. Recurrent parapharyngeal rhabdomyoma. Evidence of neoplastic nature of the tumor from cytogenetic study. *Am J Surg Pathol.* 1992; 16:721.

397. Granich MS, Pilch BZ, Nadol JB, Dickersin GR. Fetal rhabdomyoma of the larynx. *Arch Otolaryngol.* 1983; 109:821.

398. Helliwell TR, Sissons MCJ, Stoney PJ, Ashworth MT. Immunochemistry and electron microscopy of head and neck rhabdomyoma. *J Clin Pathol.* 1988; 41:1058.

399. Johansen ECJ, Illum P. Rhabdomyoma of the larynx: A review of the literature with a summary of previously described cases of rhabdomyoma of the larynx and a report of a new case. *J Laryngol Otol.* 1995; 109:147.

400. Kapadia SB, Meis JM, Frisman DM, et al. Adult rhabdomyoma of the head and neck. A clinicopathologic and immunophentoypic study. *Hum Pathol.* 1993; 24:608.

401. Modlin B. Rhabdomyoma of the larynx. *Laryngoscope.* 1982; 92:580.

402. Roberts DN, Corbett MJ, Breen D, Jonathan DA, Smith CET. Rhabdomyoma of the larynx: A rare cause of stridor. *J Laryngol Otol.* 1994; 108:713.

403. Shapiro RS, Stool SE, Snow JB Jr, Chamorro H. Parapharyngeal rhabdomyoma. *Arch Otolaryngol.* 1975; 101:323.

404. Shemen L. Spiro R. Tuazon R, Multifocal adult rhabdomyomas of the head and neck. *Head Neck.* 1992; 14:395.

405. Winther LK. Rhabdomyoma of the hypopharynx and larynx. Report of two cases and a review of the literature. *J Laryngol Otol.* 1976; 90:1041.

406. Dehner LP, Enzinger FM, Font RL. Fetal rhabdomyoma. An analysis of nine cases. *Cancer.* 1972; 30:160.

407. Eusebi V, Ceccarelli C, Daniele E, et al. Extracardiac rhabdomyoma: An immunocytochemical study and review of the literature. *Appl Pathol.* 1988; 6:197.

408. Moran JJ, Enterline HT. Benign rhabdomyoma of the pharynx. A case report, review of the literature, and comparison with cardiac rhabdomyoma. *Am J Clin Pathol.* 1964; 42:174.

409. Battifora HA, Eisenstein R, Schild JA. Rhabdomyoma of the larynx. Ultrastructural study and comparison with granular cell tumours (myoblastomas). *Cancer.* 1969; 23:183.

410. Sellari Franceschini S, Segnini G, Berrettini S, et al. Hibernoma of the larynx. Review of the literature and a new case. *Acta Otorhinolaryngol Belg.* 1993; 47:51.

411. Assor D, Thomas JR. Multifocal rhabdomyoma. *Arch Otolaryngol.* 1969; 90:489.

412. Gardner DG, Corio RL. Multifocal adult rhabdomyoma. *Oral Surg Oral Med Oral Pathol.* 1983; 56:76.

413. Aland JW Jr. Retropharyngeal lipoma causing symptoms of obstructive sleep apnea. *Otolaryngol Head Neck Surg.* 1996; 114:628.

414. Beaton AH, Heatly CA. Fat in the tracheo-bronchial tree with report of a case of true lipoma of the bronchus. *Ann Otol.* 1952; 61:1206.

415. Davison FW. Fibrolipoma of the laryngopharynx. *Ann Otol.* 1942; 51:853.

416. Di Bartolomeo JR, Olsen AR. Pedunculated lipoma of the epiglottis. *Arch Otolaryngol.* 1973; 98:55.

417. Eagle WW. Lipoma of the epiglottis and lipoma of the hypopharynx in the same patient. *Ann Otol.* 1965; 74:851.

418. El-Serafy S. Rare benign tumours of the larynx. *J Laryngol Otol.* 1971; 85:837.

419. Wenig BM. Lipomas of the larynx and hypopharynx: A review of the literature with the addition of three new cases. *J Laryngol Otol.* 1995; 109:353.

420. Zakrzewski A. Subglottic lipoma of the larynx. *J Laryngol Otol.* 1965; 79:1039.

421. Jesberg N. Fibrolipoma of the pyriform sinus: Thirty-seven year follow-up. *Laryngoscope.* 1982; 92:1157.

422. Ortiz CL, Weber AL. Laryngeal lipoma. *Ann Otol Rhinol Laryngol.* 1991; 100:783.

423. Moretti JA, Miller D. Laryngeal involvement in benign symmetric lipomatosis. *Arch Otolaryngol* 1973; 97:495.

424. Pahor AL. Lipoma of the larynx. *Ear Nose Throat J.* 1976; 55:341.

425. Chen KTK, Weinberg RA. Intramusclar lipoma of the larynx. *Am J Otolaryngol.* 1984; 5:71.

426. Dinsdale RC, Manning SC, Brooks DJ, Vuitch F. Myxoid laryngeal lipoma in a juvenile. *Otolaryngol Head Neck Surg.* 1990; 103:653.

427. Dionne GP, Seemayer TA. Infiltrating lipomas and angiolipomas revisted. *Cancer.* 1974; 33:732.

428. Enzinger FM, Harvey DA. Spindle cell lipoma. *Cancer.* 1975; 36:1852.

429. Fletcher CDM, Martin-Bates E. Spindle cell lipoma: A clinicopathological study with some original observations. *Histopathology.* 1987; 11:803.

430. Nonako S, Enomoto K, Kawabori S, Unno T, Muraoko S. Spindle cell lipoma within the larynx: A case report with correlated light and electron microscopy. *ORL J Otol Rhinol Laryngol Rel Spec.* 1993; 55:147.

431. Brodsky L, Yoshpe N, Ruben RJ. Clinical-pathological correlates of congenital subglottic hemangiomas. *Ann Otol.* 1983; 92:4.

432. Kärjä J. Benign neoplastic tumours and space-occupying tumours lesions of the larynx in children. *Acta Otolaryngol.* 1982; 386:181.

433. Sataloff RT, Spiegel JR, Rosen DC, Hawkshaw MJ. Capillary hemangioma of the vocal cord. *Ear Nose Throat J.* 1995; 74:390.

434. Shikhani AJ, Jones MM, Marsh BR, Holliday MJ. Infantile sublottic hemangiomas. An update. *Ann Otol.* 1986; 95:336.

435. Thomas RL. Non-epithelial tumours of the larynx. *J Laryngol Otol.* 1979; 93:1131.

436. Rao VK, Weiss SW. Angiomatosis of soft tissue. An analysis of the histologic features and clinical outcome in 51 cases. *Am J Surg Pathol.* 1992; 16:764.

437. Wallis LA, Asch T, Maisel BW. Diffuse skeletal hemangioma-

tosis. Report of two cases and review of the literature. *Am J Med.* 1964; 37:545.

438. Pratt LW, Goodof II. Hemangioendotheliosarcoma of the larynx. *Arch Otolaryngol.* 1968; 87:484.

439. Salyer WR, Salyer DC. Intravascular angiomatosis: Development and distinction from angiosarcoma. *Cancer.* 1975; 36:995.

440. Stecker RH, Lake CF. Hereditary hemorrhagic telangiectasia. *Arch Otolaryngol.* 1965; 82:522.

441. Claros P, Viscasillas S, Claros A Sr, Claros A Jr. Lymphangioma of the larynx as a cause of progressive dyspnea. *Int J Pediatr Otorhinolaryngol.* 1985; 9:263.

442. Jaffe BF. Unusual laryngeal problems in children. *Ann Otol.* 1973; 82:637.

443. Tsang WYW, Chan JKC, Fletcher CDM. Recently characterized vascular tumors of skin and soft tissues. *Histopathology.* 1991; 19:489.

444. Ballard RW, Yarington CT Jr. Hemangiopericytoma of the tracheal wall. *Arch Otolaryngol.* 1981; 107:558.

445. Hertzanu Y, Mendelsohn DB, Kassner G, Hockman M. Haemangiopericytoma of the larynx. *Br J Radiol.* 1982; 55:870.

446. Pesavento G, Ferlito A. Haemangiopericytoma of the larynx: A clinicopathologic study with review of the literature. *J Laryngol Otol.* 1982; 96:1065.

447. Schwartz MR, Donovan DT. Hemangiopericytoma of the larynx: A case report and review of the literature. *Otolaryngol Head Neck Surg.* 1987; 96:369.

448. Taguchi K, Yoda M, Maruyama Y. Hemangiopericytoma of the larynx: A case report. *Otolaryngology.* 1974; 46:21.

449. Enzinger FM, Smith BH. Hemangiopericytoma. An analysis of 106 cases. *Hum Pathol.* 1976; 7:61.

450. Ferlito A. Primary malignant haemangiopericytoma of the larynx (a case report with autopsy). *J Laryngol Otol.* 1978; 92:511.

451. Nappi O, Ritter JH, Pettinato G, Wick MR. Hemangiopericytoma: Histopathological pattern or clinicopathologic entity? *Semin Diagn Pathol.* 1995; 12:221.

452. Battifora H. Hemangiopericytoma: Ultrastructural study of five cases. *Cancer.* 1973; 31:1418.

453. Chen KTK. Leiomyoma of the trachea. *Am J Otolaryngol.* 1983; 4:144.

454. Harris PF, Maness GM, Ward PH. Leiomyoma of the larynx and trachea: Case reports. *South Med J.* 1967; 60:1223.

455. Hirakawa K, Harada Y, Tatsukawa T, Nagasawa A, Fujii M. A case of vascular leiomyoma of the larynx. *J Laryngol Otol.* 1994; 108:593.

456. Iqbal SM, Bhogoliwal SK. Nandi NB. Laryngeal leiomyoma. *J Laryngol Otol.* 1986; 100:723.

457. Kamata T, Ogawa Y, Iguchi Y, Nakamura Y, Mochizuki T. A case of vascular leiomyoma in the larynx. *Nippon Jibiinkoka Gakkai Kaiho.* 1995; 98:1119.

458. Karma P, Hyrynkangas K, Räsänen O. Laryngeal leiomyoma. *J Laryngol Otol.* 1978; 92:411.

459. Kleinsasser O, Glanz H. Myogenic tumours of the larynx. *Arch Otorhinolaryngol.* 1979; 225:107.

460. Nuutinen J, Syrjänen K. Angioleiomyoma of the larynx. Report of a case and review of the literature. *Laryngoscope.* 1983; 93:941.

461. Shibata K, Komune S. Laryngeal angiomyoma (vascular leiomyoma): Clinicopathological findings. *Laryngoscope.* 1980; 90:1880.

462. Wolfowitz BL, Schmaman A. Smooth-muscle tumours of the upper respiratory tract. *S Afr Med J.* 1973; 47:1189.

463. Hellquist HB, Hellqvist H, Vejlens L, Lindholm CE. Epithelioid leiomyoma of the larynx. *Histopathology.* 1994; 24:155.

464. Mori H, Kumoi T, Hashimoto M, Uematsu K. Leiomyoblastoma of the larynx: Report of a case. *Head Neck.* 1992; 14:148.

465. Cohen SR, Landing BH, Isaacs H. Fibrous histiocytoma of the trachea. *Ann Otol.* 1978; 87(suppl 52):2.

466. Jordan MB, Soames JV. Fibrous histiocytoma of the larynx. *J Laryngol Otol.* 1989; 103:216.

467. Rolander T, Kim OJ, Shumrick DA. Fibrous histiocytoma of the larynx. *Arch Otolaryngol.* 1972; 96:168.

468. Sanstrom RE, Propper KH, Trelstad RL. Fibrohistiocytoma of the trachea. *Am J Clin Pathol.* 1978; 70:429.

469. Wetmore RF. Fibrous histiocytoma of the larynx in a child. *Clin Pediatr.* 1987; 26:200.

470. Iwasaki H, Isayama T, Ohjimi Y, et al. Malignant fibrous histiocytoma. A tumor of facultative histiocytes showing mesenchymal differentiation in cultured cell lines. *Cancer.* 1992; 69:437.

471. Benjamin B, Motbey J, Ivers C, Kan A. Benign juvenile xanthogranuloma of the larynx. *Int J Pediatr Otorhinolaryngol.* 1995; 32:77.

472. Cohen SR, Landing BH, Isaacs H. Neurofibroma of the larynx in a child. *Ann Otol.* 1978; 87(suppl 52):29.

473. Cummings CW, Montgomery WW, Balogh K Jr. Neurogenic tumors of the larynx. *Ann Otol.* 1969; 78:76.

474. Dekker PJ, Haidar A. Neurilemmoma of the larynx. *Br J Clin Pract.* 1994; 48:159.

475. Ejnell H, Järund M, Bailey M, Lindeman P. Airway obstruction in children due to plexiform neurofibroma of the larynx. *J Laryngol Otol.* 1996; 110:1065.

476. Gooder P, Farrington T. Extracranial neurilemmomata of the head and neck. *J Laryngol Otol.* 1980; 94:243.

477. Jamal MN. Schwannoma of the larynx: Case report, and review of the literature. *J Laryngol Otol.* 1994; 108:788.

478. Martin DS, Stith J, Awwad EE, Handler S. MR in neurofibromatosis of the larynx. *Am J Neuroradiol.* 1995; 16:503.

479. Supance JS, Quenelle DJ, Crissman J. Endolaryngeal neurofibromas. *Otolaryngol Head Neck Surg.* 1980; 88:74.

480. Swanson PE, Scheithauer BW, Wick MR. Peripheral nerve sheath neoplasms. Clinicopathologic and immunochemical observations. *Pathol Annu.* 1995; 30:1.

481. Thomas AB, Rees L. Neurilemmoma of the larynx. *J Laryngol Otol.* 1969; 83;189.

482. Whittam DE, Morris TMO. Neurilemmoma of the larynx. *J Laryngol Otol.* 1970; 84:747.

483. Fisher C, Carter RL, Ramachandra S, Thomas DM. Peripheral nerve sheath differentiation in malignant soft tissue tumours: An ultrastructural and immunohistochemical study. *Histopathology.* 1992; 20:115.

484. Chang-Lo M. Laryngeal involvement in von Recklinghausen's disease: A case report and review of the literature. *Laryngoscope.* 1977; 87:435.

485. DeLozier HL. Intrinsic malignant schwannoma of the larynx. A case report. *Ann Otol.* 1982; 91:336.

486. Giangaspero F, Fratamico FCM, Ceccarelli C, Brisigotti M. Malignant peripheral nerve sheath tumors and spindle cell sarcomas: An immunohistochemical analysis of multiple markers. *Appl Pathol.* 1989; 7:134.

487. Altmann F, Ginsberg I, Stout AP. Intraepithelial carcinoma (cancer in situ) of the larynx. *Arch Otolaryngol.* 1952; 56:121.

488. Crissman JD, Gnepp DR, Goodman ML, Hellquist H, Johns ME. Preinvasive lesions of the upper aerodigestive tract: Histologic and clinical implications. In: Rosen PP, Fechner RE, eds. *Pathology Annual.* vol 22. pt. 1. Norwalk, CT: Appleton-Century-Crofts; 1987:311.

489. Hellquist H, Olofsson J, Gröntoft O. Carcinoma in situ and severe dysplasia of the vocal cords: A clinicopathological and photometric investigation. *Acta Otolaryngol.* 1981; 92:543.

490. Hyams VJ, Batsakis JG, Michaels L. Tumors of the upper respiratory tract and ear. *Atlas of Pathology.* fascicle 25, 2nd series. Washington, DC: Armed Forces Institute of Pathology; 1988.

491. McNelis FL, Esparza AR. Carcinoma in situ of the larynx. *Laryngoscope.* 1971; 81:924.

492. Miller AH, Fisher HR. Carcinoma-in-situ of the larynx. *Arch Otorhinolaryngol.* 1956; 60:358.

493. Miller AH. Carcinoma in situ of the larynx. *Am J Surg.* 1970; 120:492.

494. Crissman JD, Zarbo RJ. Quantitation of DNA ploidy in squamous intraepithelial neoplasia of the laryngeal glottis. *Arch Otolaryngol Head Neck Surg.* 1991; 117:182.

495. Friedmann I, Ferlito A. Precursors of squamous cell carci-

noma. In: Ferlito A, ed. *Neoplasms of the Larynx*. Edinburgh: Churchill Livingstone; 1993.

496. Bauer WC, McGavran MH. Carcinoma in situ and evaluation of epithelial changes in laryngopharyngeal biopsies. *JAMA.* 1972; 221:72.

497. Blackwell KE, Fu Y-S, Calcaterra TC. Laryngeal dysplasia. A clinicopathologic study. *Cancer.* 1995; 75:457.

498. Elman AJ, Goodman M, Wang CC, Pilch B, Busse J. In situ carcinoma of the vocal cords. *Cancer.* 1979; 43:2422.

499. Michaels L. Pitfalls in the histological diagnosis of premalignant lesions and carcinoma in situ of the larynx. In: Surjan L, Bodo GY, eds. *Proceedings of the XIIth ORL World Congress.* Budapest; 1981:99.

500. Crissman JD, Fu Y-S. Intraepithelial neoplasia of the larynx: A clinicopathologic study of six cases with DNA analysis. *Arch Otolaryngol Head Neck Surg.* 1986; 112:522.

501. Pignataro LD, Broich G, Lavezzi A-M, Biondo B, Ottaviani F. PCNA—A cell proliferation marker in vocal chord cancer. Part I: Premalignant laryngeal lesions. *Anticancer Res.* 1995; 15:1517.

502. Kashima H, Mounts P, Kuhajda F, Loury M. Demonstration of human papillomavirus capsid antigen in carcinoma in situ of the larynx. *Ann Otol.* 1986; 95:603.

503. Myssiorek D, Vambutas A, Abramson AL. Carcinoma in situ of the glottic larynx. *Laryngoscope.* 1994; 104:463.

504. Bauer WC. Concomitant carcinoma in situ and invasion carcinoma of the larynx. In: Alberti PW, Bryce DP, eds. *Centennial Conference on Laryngeal Cancer.* New York: Crofts; 1976: 127.

505. Elias MM, Hilgers FJM, Keus RB, et al. Carcinoma of the pyriform sinus: A retrospective analysis of treatment results over a 20-year period. *Clin Otolaryngol.* 1995; 20:249.

506. Hyams VJ, Heffner DK. Laryngeal pathology. In: Tucker HM, ed. *The Larynx.* 2nd ed. New York:Thieme Medical Publishers; 1993:35.

507. Lam KY, Yuen APW. Cancer of the larynx in Hong Kong: A clinico-pathological study. *Eur J Surg Oncol.* 1996; 22:166.

508. Tucker GF Jr. The anatomy of laryngeal cancer. *Can J Otolaryngol.* 1974; 3:417.

509. Kleinsasser O, Glanz H. Microcarcinoma and microinvasive carcinoma of the vocal cords. *Clin Oncol.* 1982; 1:479.

510. Pesch H-J, Steiner W, Münch E. Microcarcinoma of the upper aerodigestive tract. *Clin Oncol.* 1982; 1:495.

511. Sala O, Ferlito A. Morphological observations of immunobiology of laryngeal cancer. Evaluation of the defensive activity of immunocompetent cells present in tumour stroma. *Acta Otolaryngol.* 1976; 81:353.

512. Goepfert H, Dichtel WJ, Medine JE, Lindberg RD, Luna MD. Perineural invasion in squamous cell carcinoma of the head and neck. *Am J Surg.* 1984; 148:542.

513. Ruá S, Comino A, Fruttero A, et al. Relationship between histologic features, DNA flow cytometry, and clinical behavior of squamous cell carcinomas of the larynx. *Cancer.* 1991; 67:141.

514. Sorscher SM, Russack V, Cagle M, Feramisco JR, Green MR. Immunolocalization of E-Cadherin in human head and neck cancer. *Arch Pathol Lab Med.* 1995; 119:82.

515. Wen QH, Nishimura T, Miwa T, Nagayama I, Furukawa M. Expression of EGF, EGFR and PCNA in laryngeal lesions. *J Laryngol Otol.* 1995; 109:630.

516. Zhang L-F, Hemminki K, Szyfter K, Szyfter W, Söderkvist P. p53 mutations in larynx cancer. *Carcinogenesis.* 1994; 15:2949.

517. Crissman JD, Zarbo RJ, Drozdowicz S, et al. Carcinoma insitu and microinvasive squamous carcinoma of the laryngeal glottis. *Arch Otolaryngol Head Neck Surg.* 1988; 114:299.

518. Putney FJ, Chapman CE. Carcinoma of the larynx: Analysis of 311 cases treated surgically. *Ann Otol.* 1972; 81:455.

519. Sessions DG. Surgical pathology of cancer of the larynx and hypopharynx. *Laryngoscope.* 1976; 86:814.

520. Abramson AL, Brandsma J, Steinberg B, Winkler B. Verrucous carcinoma of the larynx. *Arch Otolaryngol.* 1985; 111:709.

521. Batsakis JG, Hybels R, Crissman JD, Rice DH. The pathology of head and neck tumors: Verrucous carcinoma. pt 15. *Head Neck Surg.* 1982; 5:29.

522. Biller HF, Ogura JH, Bauer WC. Verrucous cancer of the larynx. *Ann Otol.* 1971; 80:1323.

523. Ferlito A, Recher G. Ackerman's tumor (verrucous carcinoma) of the larynx: A clinicopathologic study of 77 cases. *Cancer.* 1980; 46:1617.

524. Kraus FT, Perez-Mesa C. Verrucous carcinoma: Clinical and pathologic study of 105 cases involving oral cavity, larynx and genitalia. *Cancer.* 1966; 19:26.

525. Longarela Herrero Y, Morales Angulo C, Rubio Suarez A, Gonzalez-Rodilla I, Rama Quintela J. Laryngeal verrucous carcinoma. *Acta Otorrinolaringol Esp.* 1995; 46:49.

526. Ryan RE, DeSanto LW, Devine KD, Weiland LH. Verrucous carcinoma of the larynx. *Laryngoscope.* 1977; 87:1989.

527. van Nostrand AWP, Olofsson J. Verrucous carcinoma of the larynx: A clinical and pathologic study of 10 cases. *Cancer.* 1972; 30:691.

528. Ackerman LV. Verrucous carcinoma of the oral cavity. *Surgery.* 1948; 23:670.

529. Fechner RE, Mills SE. Verruca vulgaris of the larynx: A distinctive lesion of probable viral origin confused with verrucous carcinoma. *Am J Surg Pathol.* 1982; 6:357.

530. Goethals PL, Harrison EG, Devine KD. Verrucous carcinoma of the oral cavity. *Am J Surg.* 1963; 106:845.

531. Slootweg PJ, Müller H. Verrucous hyperplasia or verrucous carcinoma. An analysis of 27 patients. *J Maxillofac Surg.* 1983; 11:13.

532. Ferlito A, Antonutto G, Silvestri F. Histological appearances and nuclear DNA content with verrucous squamous cell carcinoma of the larynx. *ORL J Otorhinolaryngol Relat Spec.* 1976; 38:65.

533. Prioleau PG, Santa Cruz DJ, Meyer JS, Bauer WC. Verrucous carcinoma: A light and electron microscopic, autoradiographic, and immunofluorescence study. *Cancer.* 1980; 45: 2849.

534. Bauer WC. Varieties of squamous carcinoma—biologic behavior. Therapeutic implications and prognostic significance in the upper aerodigestive tract. *Front Radiat Ther Oncol.* 1974; 9:164.

535. Appelman HD, Oberman HA. Squamous cell carcinoma of the larynx with sarcoma-like stroma. A clinicopathologic assessment of spindle cell carcinoma and pseuosarcoma. *Am J Clin Pathol.* 1965; 44:135.

536. Batsakis JG, Rice DH, Howard DR. The pathology of head and neck tumors: Spindle cell lesions (sarcomatoid carcinomas, nodular fasciitis, and fibrosarcoma) of the aerodigestive tracts, pt 14. *Head Neck Surg.* 1982; 4:499.

537. Giordano AM, Ewing S, Adams G, Maisel R. Laryngeal pseudosarcoma. *Laryngoscope.* 1983; 93:735.

538. Hyams VJ. Spindle cell carcinoma of the larynx. *Can J Otolaryngol.* 1975; 4:307.

539. Lambert PR, Ward PH, Berci G. Pseudosarcoma of the larynx. *Arch Otolaryngol.* 1980; 106:700.

540. Lane N. Pseudosarcoma (polypoid sarcoma-like masses) associated with squamous-cell carcinoma of the mouth, fauces, and larynx. Report of ten cases. *Cancer.* 1957; 10:19.

541. Leventon GS, Evans HL. Sarcomatoid squamous cell carcinoma of the mucous membranes of the head and neck: A clinicopathologic study of 20 cases. *Cancer.* 1981; 48:994.

542. Minckler DS, Meligro CH, Norris HT. Carcinosarcoma of the larynx. Case report with metastases of epidermoid and sarcomatous elements. *Cancer.* 1970; 26:195.

543. Nappi O, Wick MR. Sarcomatoid neoplasms of the respiratory tract. *Semin Diagn Pathol.* 1993; 10:137.

544. Recher G. Spindle cell squamous carcinoma of the larynx: Clinico-pathologic study of seven cases. *J Laryngol Otol.* 1985; 99:871.

545. Balercia G, Bhan AK, Dickersin GR. Sarcomatoid carcinoma: An ultrastructural study with light microscopic and immunohistochemical correlation of 10 cases from various anatomic sites. *Ultrastruct Pathol.* 1995; 19:249.

546. Lichtiger B, Mackay B, Tessmer CF. Spindle-cell variant of squamous carcinoma. A light and electron microscopic study of 13 cases. *Cancer.* 1970; 26:1311.

547. Nakhleh RE, Zarbo RJ, Ewing S, Carey JL, Gown AM. Myo-

genic differentiation in spindle cell (sarcomatoid) carcinomas of the upper aerodigestive tract. *Appl Immunohistochem.* 1993; 1:58.

548. Battifora H. Spindle cell carcinoma. Ultrastructural evidence of squamous origin and collagen production by the tumor cells. *Cancer.* 1976; 37:2275.

549. Zarbo RJ, Crissman JD, Venkat H, Weiss MA. Spindle-cell carcinoma of the upper aerodigestive tract mucosa: An immunohistochemical and ultrastructural study of 18 biphasic tumors and comparison with seven monophasic spindle-cell tumors. *Am J Surg Pathol.* 1986; 10:741.

550. Ellis GL, Langloss JM, Heffner DK, Hyams VJ. Spindle cell carcinoma of the aerodigestive tract: An immunohistochemical analysis of 21 cases. *Am J Surg Pathol.* 1987; 11:335.

551. Cassidy M, Maher M, Keogh P, Leader M. Pseudosarcoma of the larynx: The value of ploidy analysis. *J Laryngol Otol.* 1994; 108:525.

552. Banks ER, Frierson HF Jr, Mills SE, et al. Basaloid squamous cell carcinoma of the head and neck. A clinicopathologic and immunohistochemical study of 40 cases. *Am J Surg Pathol.* 1992; 16:939.

553. Ereño C, Lopez JI, Sanchez JM, Toledo JD. Basaloid-squamous cell carcinoma of the larynx and hypopharynx. A clinicopathologic study of 7 cases. *Pathol Res Pract.* 1994; 190:186.

554. Luna MA, El Naggar A, Parichatikanond P, Weber RS, Batsakis JG. Basaloid squamous cell carcinoma of the upper aerodigestive tract. Clinicopathologic and DNA flow cytometric analysis. *Cancer.* 1990; 66:537.

555. McKay MJ, Bilous AM. Basaloid-squamous carcinomas of the hypopharynx. *Cancer.* 1989; 63:2528.

556. Raslan WF, Barnes L, Krause JR, et al. Basaloid squamous cell carcinoma of the head and neck: A clinicopathologic and flow cytometry study of 10 new cases with review of the English literature. *Am J Otolaryngol.* 1994; 15:204.

557. Saltarelli MG, Fleming MV, Wenig BM, et al. Primary basaloid squamous cell carcinoma of the trachea. *Am J Clin Pathol.* 1995; 104:594.

558. Seidman JD, Berman JJ, Yost BA, Iseri OA. Basaloid squamous carcinoma of the hypopharynx and larynx associated with second primary tumors. *Cancer.* 1991; 68:1545.

559. Wain SL, Kier R, Vollmer RT, Bossen EH. Basaloid-squamous carcinoma of the tongue, hypopharynx and larynx: Report of 10 cases. *Hum Pathol.* 1986; 17:1158.

560. Muller S, Barnes L. Basaloid squamous cell carcinoma of the head and neck with spindle cell component. *Arch Pathol Lab Med.* 1995; 119:181.

561. Klijanienko J, El-Naggar A, Ponzio-Prion A, et al. Basaloid squamous carcinoma of the head and neck. Immunohistochemical comparison with adenoid cystic carcinoma and squamous cell carcinoma. *Arch Otolaryngol Head Neck Surg.* 1993; 119:887.

562. Gerughty RM, Hennigar GR, Brown FM. Adenosquamous carcinoma of the nasal, oral and laryngeal cavities. A clinicopathologic survey of 10 cases. *Cancer.* 1968; 22:1140.

563. Ferlito A, Devaney KO, Rinaldo A, Milroy CM, Carbone A. Mucosal adenoid squamous cell carcinoma of the head and neck. *Ann Otol.* 1996; 105:409.

564. Wan S-K, Chan JKC, Lau W-H, Yip TTC. Basloid-squamous carcinoma of the nasopharynx. An Epstein-Barr virus-associated neoplasm compared with morphologically identical tumors occurring in other sites. *Cancer.* 1995; 76:1689.

565. Aden KK, Adams GL, Niehans G, Abdel-Fattah HMMI. Adenosquamous carcinoma of the larynx and hypopharynx with five new case presentations. *Trans Am Laryngol Assoc.* 1988; 190:216.

566. Damiani JM, Damiani KK, Hauck K, Hyams VJ. Mucoepidermoid-adenosquamous carcinoma of the larynx and hypopharynx: A report of 21 cases and a review of the literature. *Otolaryngol Head Neck Surg.* 1981; 89:235.

567. Ferlito A. A pathologic and clinical study of adenosquamous carcinoma of the larynx. Report of four cases and review of the literature. *Acta Otorhinolaryngol Belg* 1976; 30:379.

568. Fujino K, Ito J, Kanaji M, Shiomi Y, Saiga T. Adenosquamous carcinoma of the larynx. *Am J Otolaryngol.* 1995; 16:115.

569. Sanderson RJ, Rivron RP, Wallace WA. Adenosquamous carcinoma of the hypopharynx. *J Laryngol Otol.* 1991; 105:678.

570. Ferlito A. Histological classification of larynx and hypopharynx cancers and their clinical implications. Pathologic aspects of 2052 malignant neoplasms diagnosed at the ORL Department of Padua University from 1966 to 1976. *Acta Otolaryngol.* 1976; 342:1.

571. Martinez-Madrigal F, Baden E, Casiraghi O, Micheau C. Oral and pharyngeal adenosquamous carcinoma. Report of four cases with immunohistochemical studies. *Eur Arch Otorhinolaryngol.* 1991; 248:255.

572. Batsakis JG, Huser J. Squamous carcinomas with glandlike (adenoid) features. *Ann Otol.* 1990; 99:87.

573. Komorn RM, Fechner RE, Alford BR, Ramey JA, Stiernberg C. Simultaneous squamous carcinoma and adenocarcinoma of the larynx. *Arch Otolaryngol.* 1973; 97:420.

574. Obermyer NE, Ramadan HH. Adenocarcinoma with simultaneous squamous carcinomas of the larynx. *Head Neck.* 1994; 16:453.

575. Bignardi L, Aimoni C, Franceschetti E, Galceran M, Rabitti C. Carcinoma adenoide quístico de laringe: Revisión de la literatura y aportación casuística. *Acta Otorrinolaringol Esp.* 1993; 44:141.

576. Diaz Caparros F, Pastor Quirante FA, Perez Martinez F, Calero del Castillo JB. Carcinoma adenoide quistico. Revision de los ultimos cinco anos en nuestro servicio de ORL (1987–1991). *An Otorrinolaringol Ibero Am.* 1995; 22:557.

577. Dueñas Parrilla JM, Alvarez Bautista A, Sanchez Gomez S, Tirado Zamora I. Carcinoma adenoide quístico de laringe. Presentación de un caso y revisión de la literatura. *Acta Otorrinolaringol Esp.* 1991; 42:67.

578. Ferlito A, Caruso G. Biological behavior of laryngeal adenoid cystic carcinoma. Therapeutic considerations. *ORL J Otorhinolaryngol Relat Spec.* 1983; 45:245.

579. Olofsson J, van Nostrand AWP. Adenoid cystic carcinoma of the larynx. A report of four cases and a review of the literature. *Cancer.* 1977; 40:1307.

580. Regnard JF, Fourquier P, Levasseur P. Results and prognostic factors in resections of primary tracheal tumors: A multicenter retrospective study. *J Thorac Cardiovasc Surg.* 1996; 111:808.

581. Ross DE, Sukis AE. Salivary gland tumors in ectopic sites. *Laryngoscope.* 1971; 81:558.

582. Soboroff BJ. Clindroma of the upper digestive and respiratory passages. A correlative study of their histologic patterns, clinical findings and modes of therapy. *Laryngoscope.* 1959; 69:1381.

583. Wilson RW, Wenig BM. Adenoid cystic carcinoma (ACC) of the larynx (LACC). Abstract. *Mod Pathol.* 1997; 10:118.

584. Azumi N, Battifora H. The cellular composition of adenoid cystic carcinoma. An immunohistochemical study. *Cancer.* 1987; 60:1589.

585. Leafstedt SW, Gaeta JF, Sako K, Marchetta FC, Shedd DP. Adenoid cystic carcinoma of major and minor salivary glands. *Am J Surg.* 1971; 122:756.

586. Chen J-C, Gnepp DR, Bedrossian CWM. Adenoid cystic carcinoma of the salivary glands: An immunohistochemical analysis. *Oral Surg Oral Med Oral Pathol.* 1988; 65:316.

587. Chaudhry AP, Leifer C, Culter LS. Histogenesis of adenoid cystic carcinoma of the salivary glands. Light and electronmicroscopic study. *Cancer.* 1986; 58:72.

588. Ferlito A, Recher G, Bottin R. Mucoepidermoid carcinoma of the larynx. A clinicopathologic study of 11 cases with review of the literature. *ORL J Otorhinolaryngol Relat Spec.* 1981; 43:280.

589. Kaznelson DJ, Schindel J. Mucoepidermoid carcinoma of the air passages. Report of three cases. *Laryngoscope.* 1979; 89:115.

590. Lipper BM, Werner JA, Schlüter E, Rudert H. Mukoepidermoides karzinom des larynx. Fallbericht und literaturübersicht. *Laryngorhinootol.* 1992; 71:495.

591. Martínez-Barona T, Regadera J, Gavilán J, Vicandi B, Patrón M. Carcinoma mucoepidermoide de la laringe de alto grado de malignidad. Estudio clinico-patológico de un caso y revisión de la literatura. *Ann Otorrinolaryngol Ibero Am.* 1986; 13:455.

592. Seo IS, Tomich CE, Warfel KA, Hull MT. Clear cell carcinoma of the larynx. A variant of mucoepidermoid carcinoma. *Ann Otol.* 1980; 89:168.

593. Spiro RH, Lewis JS, Hajdu SI, Strong EW. Mucus gland tumors of the larynx and laryngopharynx. *Ann Otol.* 1976; 85:498.

594. Supiyaphun P, Vaewvichit K, Pongsupat T, Yenrudi S, Boonyapipat P. Mucoepidermoid carcinoma of the larynx: Report of two cases. *J Med Assoc Thai.* 1986; 69:500.

595. Thomas K. Mucoepidermoid carcinoma of the larynx. *J Laryngol Otol.* 1971; 85:261.

596. Tomita T, Lotuaco L, Talbott L Watanabe I. Mucoepidermoid carcinoma of the subglottis. An ultrastructural study. *Arch Pathol Lab Med.* 1977; 101:145.

597. Ho K-J, Jones JM, Herrera GA. Mucoepidermoid carcinoma of the larynx: A light and electron microscopic study with emphasis on histogenesis. *South Med J.* 1984; 77:190.

598. Mikaelian DO, Contrucci RB, Batsakis JG. Epithelial-myoepithelial carcinoma of the subglottic region: A case presentation and review of the literature. *Head Neck Surg.* 1986; 95:104.

599. Ferlito A, Rosai J. Terminology and classification of neuroendocrine neoplasms of the larynx. *ORL J Otorhinolaryngol Relat Spec.* 1991; 53:185.

600. Baugh RF, Wolf GT, Lloyd RV, McClatchey KD, Evans DA. Carcinoid (neuroendocrine carcinoma) of the larynx. *Ann Otol.* 1987; 96:315.

601. Ferlito A, Friedmann I. Review of neuroendocrine carcinomas of the larynx. *Ann Otol.* 1989; 98:780.

602. Ferlito A, Friedmann I, Goldman NC. Primary carcinoid tumors of the larynx. *ORL J Otorhinolaryngol Relat Spec.* 1988; 50:129.

603. Gripp FM, Risse EKJ, Leverstein H, Snow GB, Meijer CJLM. Neuroendocrine neoplasms of the larynx. Importance of the correct diagnosis and differences between atypical carcinoid tumors and small-cell neuroendocrine carcinoma. *Eur Arch Otorhinolaryngol.* 1995; 252:280.

604. Overholt SM, Donovan DT, Schwartz MR, et al. Neuroendocrine neoplasms of the larynx. *Laryngoscope.* 1995; 105:789.

605. Wenig BM, Hyams VJ, Heffner DK. Moderately differentiated neuroendocrine carcinoma of the larynx. A clinico-pathologic study of 54 cases. *Cancer.* 1988; 62:2658.

606. Wenig BM, Gnepp DR. The spectrum of neuroendocrine carcinomas of the larynx. *Semin Diagn Pathol.* 1989; 6:329.

607. Woodruff JM, Huvos AG, Erlandson RA, Shah JP, Gerold FP. Neuroendocrine carcinomas of the larynx. A study of two histologic types, one of which mimics thyroid medullary carcinoma. *Am J Sug Pathol.* 1985; 9:771.

608. Gould VE, Banner BF, Baerwaldt M. Neuroendocrine neoplasms in unusual primary sites. *Diagn Histopathol.* 1981; 4:263.

609. Gnepp DR. Small cell neuroendocrine carcinoma of the larynx. A critical review of the literature. *ORL J Otorhinolaryngol Relat Spec.* 1991; 53:210.

610. Doglioni C, Ferlito A, Chiamenti C, Viale G, Rosai J. Laryngeal carcinoma showing multidirectional epithelial, neuroendocrine and sarcomatous differentiation. *ORL J Otorhinolaryngol Relat Spec.* 1990; 52:316.

611. Ferlito A. Diagnosis and treatment of small cell carcinoma of the larynx: A critical review. *Ann Otol.* 1986; 95:590.

612. El-Naggar AK, Batsakis JG. Carcinoid tumor of the larynx. A critical review of the literature. *ORL J Otorhinolaryngol Relat Spec.* 1991; 53:188.

613. Gnepp DR, Ferlito A, Hyams V. Primary anaplastic small cell (oat cell) carcinoma of the larynx. *Cancer.* 1983; 51:1731.

614. Woodruff JM, Senie RT. Atypical carcinoid tumor of the larynx. A critical review of the literature. *ORL J Otorhinolaryngol Relat Spec.* 1991; 53:194.

615. Ferlito A, Friedmann I. Contribution of immunohistochemistry in the diagnosis of neuroendocrine neoplasms of the larynx. *ORL J Otorhinolaryngol Relat Spec.* 1991; 53:235.

616. Dieler R, Dämmrich J. Immunohistochemical and fine structural characterization of primary carcinoid tumors of the larynx. *Eur Arch Otorhinolaryngol.* 1995; 252:229.

617. Watters GWR, Molyneux AJ, Path MRC. Atypical carcinoid tumour of the larynx. *J Laryngol Otol.* 1995; 109:455.

618. Nirchio V, Bisceglia M, Bosman C, et al. Microcitoma primitivo della laringe. Segnalazione di un caso, studio ultrastrutturale e rassegna della letteratura. *Pathologica.* 1995; 87:171.

619. Milroy CM, Williams RA, Charlton IG, Moss E, Rode J. Nuclear ploidy in neuroendocrine neoplasms of the larynx. *ORL J Otorhinolaryngol Relat Spec.* 1991; 53:245.

620. Reuter VE, Woodruff JM. Melanoma of the larynx. *Laryngoscope.* 1986; 94:389.

621. Duvall E, Johnston A, McLay K, et al. Carcinoid tumor of the larynx: A report of two cases. *J Laryngol Otol.* 1983; 97:1073.

622. El-Naggar AK, Batsakis JG, Vassilopoulou-Sellin R, Ordóñez NG, Luna MA. Medullary (thyroid) carcinoma-like carcinoids of the larynx. *J Laryngol Otol.* 1991; 105:683.

623. Blatchford SJ, Koopmann CF Jr, Coulthard SW. Mucosal melanoma of the head and neck. *Laryngoscope.* 1986; 96:929.

624. El-Barbary AE-S, Fouad HA, El-Sayed AF-H. Malignant melanoma involving the larynx. Report of two cases. *Ann Otol.* 1968; 77:338.

625. Hussain SSM, Whitehead E. Malignant melanoma of the larynx. *J Laryngol Otol.* 1989; 103:533.

626. Kim H, Park CI. Primary malignant laryngeal melanoma. Report of a case with review of literature. *Yonsei Med J.* 1982; 23:118.

627. Moore ES, Martin H. Melanoma of the upper respiratory tract and oral cavity. *Cancer.* 1955; 8:1167.

628. Shah JP, Huvos AG, Strong EW. Mucosal melanomas of the head and neck. *Am J Surg.* 1977; 134:531.

629. Smith BC, Wenig BM. Neurogenic neoplasms including melanoma. In: Ferlito A, ed. *Surgical Pathology of Laryngeal Neoplasms.* London: Chapman & Hall; 1996:195.

630. Wenig BM. Laryngeal mucosal malignant melanoma. A clinicopathologic, immunohistochemical, and ultrastructural study of four patients and a review of the literature. *Cancer.* 1995; 75:1568.

631. Kornstein MJ, Franco AP. Specificity of HMB-45. *Arch Pathol Lab Med.* 1990; 114:450.

632. Wick MR, Swanson PE, Rocamora A. Recognition of malignant melanoma by monoclonal antibody HMB-45. An immunohistochemical study of 200 paraffin-embedded cutaneous tumors. *J Cutan Pathol.* 1988; 15:201.

633. Ghadially FN. Is it melanoma? In: *Diagnostic Electron Microscopy of Tumours.* 2nd ed. London: Butterworths; 1982:78.

634. Barton RT. Mucosal melanomas of the head and neck. *Laryngoscope.* 1974; 73:93.

635. Pesce C, Toncini C. Melanin pigmentation of the larynx. *Acta Otolaryngol.* 1983; 96:189.

636. Seals JL, Shenefelt RE, Babin RW. Intralaryngeal nevus in a child. A case report. *Int J Pediatr Otorhinolaryngol.* 1986; 12:55.

637. Ferlito A, Caruso G. Secondary malignant melanoma of the larynx. Report of 2 cases and review of 79 laryngeal secondary cancers. *ORL J Otorhinolaryngol Relat Spec.* 1984; 46:117.

638. Ferlito A, Caruso G, Recher G. Secondary laryngeal tumors. *Arch Otolaryngol Head Neck Surg.* 1988; 114:635.

639. Fallahnejad M, Harrell D, Tucker J, Forest J, Blakemore WS. Chondrosarcoma of the trachea. Report of a case and five-year follow-up. *J Thorac Cardiovasc Surg.* 1973; 65:210.

640. Ferlito A, Nicolai P, Montaguti A, Cecchetto A, Pennelli N. Chondrosarcoma of the larynx: Review of the literature and report of three cases. *Am J Otolaryngol.* 1984; 5:350.

641. Finn DG, Goepfert H, Batsakis JG. Chondrosarcoma of the head and neck. *Laryngoscope.* 1984; 94:1539.

642. Gasior RM, Remine WH. Cartilaginous tumors of the larynx. Chondrosarcoma of the larynx. *Minn Med.* 1967; 50:1197.

643. Goethals PL, Dahlin DC, Devine KD. Cartilaginous tumors of the larynx. *Surg Gynecol Obstet.* 1963; 117:77.

644. Hellquist H, Olofsson J, Gröntoft O. Chondrosarcoma of the larynx. *J Laryngol Otol.* 1979; 93:1037.

645. Huizenga C, Balogh K. Cartilaginous tumors of the larynx. A clinicopathologic study of 10 new cases and a review of the literature. *Cancer.* 1970; 26:201.

646. Nicolai P, Ferlito A, Sasaki CT, Kirchner JA. Laryngeal chondrosarcoma: Incidence, pathology, biological behavior, and treatment. *Ann Otol.* 1990; 99:515.

647. Lichtenstein L, Jaffe HL. Chondrosarcoma of bone. *Am J Pathol.* 1943; 19:553.

648. Burkey BB, Hoffman HT, Baker SR, Thornton AF, McClatchey KD. Chondrosarcoma of the head and neck. *Laryngoscope.* 1990; 100:1301.

649. Erlandson RA, Huvos AG. Chondrosarcoma: A light and electron microscopic study. *Cancer.* 1974; 34:1642.

650. Fu Y-S, Kay S. A comparative ultrastructural study of mesenchymal chondrosarcoma and myxoid chondrosarcoma. *Cancer.* 1974; 33:1531.

651. Batsakis JG, Fox JE. Supporting tissue neoplasms of the larynx. *Surg Gynecol Obstet.* 1970; 131:989.

652. Bernáldez R, Nistal M, Kaiser C, Gavilán J. Malignant fibrous histiocytoma of the larynx. *J Laryngol Otol.* 1991; 105: 130.

653. Ferlito A, Nicolai P, Recher G, Narne S. Primary laryngeal malignant fibrous histiocytoma: Review of the literature and report of seven cases. *Laryngoscope.* 1983; 93:1351.

654. Godoy J, Jacobs JR, Crissman J. Malignant fibrous histiocytoma of the larynx. *J Surg Oncol.* 1986; 31:62.

655. Gorenstein A, Neel HB III, Weiland LH, Devine KD. Sarcomas of the larynx. *Arch Otolaryngol.* 1980; 106:8.

656. Hacihanefioglu U, Öztürk AS. Sarcomas of the larynx. Report of ten cases. *Ann Otol.* 1983; 92:81.

657. Johnson JT, Poushter DL. Fibrous histiocytoma of the subglottic larynx. *Ann Otol.* 1977; 86:243.

658. Keenan JP, Synder GG III, Toomey JM. Malignant fibrous histiocytoma of the larynx. *Otolaryngol Head Neck Surg.* 1979; 87:599.

659. Majumder NK, Sharma HS, Srinivasan V. Malignant fibrous histiocytoma of larynx. *J Laryngol Otol.* 1989; 103:219.

660. Ogura JH, Toomey JM, Setzen M, Sobol S. Malignant fibrous histiocytoma of the head and neck. *Laryngoscope.* 1980; 90: 1429.

661. Ramadass T, Balasubramaniam VC, Annamalai L. Malignant pleomorphic fibrous histiocytoma of the larynx. A case report with review of literature. *J Laryngol Otol.* 1984; 98:93.

662. Saha AM, Mukherjee, Chatterjee DN, Mukherjee AL, Mondal A. Malignant fibrous histiocytoma of larynx. *J Indian Med Assoc.* 1989; 87:73.

663. Tan-Lui NS, Matsubara O, Grillo HC, Mark EJ. Invasive fibrous tumor of the tracheobronchial tree: Clinical and pathologic study of seven cases. *Hum Pathol.* 1989; 20:180.

664. Tobey DN, Wheelis RF, Yarington CT Jr. Electron microscopy in the diagnosis of liposarcoma and fibrosarcoma of the larynx. *Ann Otol.* 1979; 88:867.

665. Donaldson I. Fibrosarcoma in a previously irradiated larynx. *J Laryngol Otol.* 1978; 92:425.

666. Amble FR, Olsen KD, Nascimento AG, Foote RL. Head and neck synovial sarcoma. *Otolaryngol Head Neck Surg.* 1992; 107:631.

667. Ferlito A, Caruso G. Endolaryngeal synovial sarcoma. An update of diagnosis and treatment. *ORL J Otorhinolaryngol Relat Spec.* 1991; 53:116.

668. Gatti WM, Strom CG, Orfei E. Synovial sarcoma of the laryngopharynx. *Arch Otolaryngol.* 1975; 101:633.

669. Miller LH, Santaella-Latimer L, Miller T. Synovial sarcoma of the larynx. *Trans Am Acad Ophthalmol Otolaryngol.* 1975; 80: 448.

670. Pruszczynski M, Manni JJ, Smedts F. Endolaryngeal synovial sarcoma: Case report with immunohistochemical studies. *Head Neck.* 1989; 11:76.

671. Quinn HJ Jr. Synovial sarcoma of the larynx treated by partial laryngectomy. *Laryngoscope.* 1984; 94:1158.

672. Roth JA, Enzinger FM, Tannenbaum M. Synovial sarcoma of the neck: A follow-up study of 24 cases. *Cancer.* 1975; 35: 1243.

673. Krall RA, Kostianovsky M, Patchesfsky AS. Synovial sarcoma. A clinical, pathological and ultrastructural study of 26 cases supporting the recognition of a monophasic variant. *Am J Surg Pathol.* 1981; 5:137.

674. Ordóñez NG, Mahfouz SM, Mackay B. Synovial sarcoma: An immunohistochemical and ultrastructural study. *Hum Pathol.* 1990; 21:733.

675. Palmer BV, Levene A, Shaw HJ. Synovial sarcoma of the pharynx and oesophagus. *J Laryngol Otol.* 1983; 97:1173.

676. Ramamurthy L, Nassar WY, Hasleton PS, Gattamaneni HR, Orton CI. Synovial sarcoma of the pharynx. *J Laryngol Otol.* 1995; 109:1207.

677. Fisher C. Synovial sarcoma: Ultrastructural and immunohistochemical features of monophasic and biphasic tumours. *Hum Pathol.* 1986; 17:996.

678. Fisher C, Schofield J. S-100 protein positive synovial sarcoma. *Histopathology.* 1991; 19:375.

679. Mickelson MR, Brown GA, Maynard JA, Cooper RR, Bonfiglio M. Synovial sarcoma. An electron microscopic study of monophasic and biphasic forms. *Cancer.* 1980; 45:2109.

680. Fligman I, Lonardo F, Jhanwar SC, et al. Molecular diagnosis of synovial sarcoma and characterization of a variant SYT-SSX2 fusion transcript. *Am J Pathol.* 1995; 147:1592.

681. Shipley J, Crew J, Birdsall S, et al. Interphase fluorescence in situ hybridization and reserve transcription polymerase chain reaction as a diagnostic aid for synovial sarcoma. *Am J Pathol.* 1996; 148:559.

682. Varela-Duran J, Enzinger FM. Calcifying synovial sarcoma. *Cancer.* 1982; 50:345.

683. Balázs M, Egerszegi P. Laryngeal botryoid rhabdomyosarcoma in an adult. Report of a case with electron microscopic study. *Pathol Res Pract.* 1989; 184:643.

684. Batsakis JG, Fox JE. Rhabdomyosarcoma of the larynx. Report of a case. *Arch Otolaryngol.* 1970; 91:136.

685. Canalis RF, Platz CE, Cohn AM. Laryngeal rhabdomyosarcoma. *Arch Otolaryngol.* 1976; 102:104.

686. Da Mosto MC, Marchiori C, Rinaldo A, Ferlito A. Laryngeal pleomorphic rhabdomyosarcoma. A critical review of the literature. *Ann Otol.* 1996; 105:289.

687. Diehn KW, Hyams VJ, Harris AE. Rhabdomyosarcoma of the larynx: A case report and review of the literature. *Laryngoscope.* 1984; 94:201.

688. Dodd-O JM, Wieneke KF, Rosman PM. Laryngeal rhabdomyosarcoma. Case report and literature review. *Cancer.* 1987; 59: 1012.

689. Haerr RW, Turalba CIC, El-Mahdi AM, Brown KL. Alveolar rhabdomyosarcoma of the larynx: Case report and literature review. *Laryngoscope.* 1987; 97:339.

690. Kato MADP, Flamant F, Terrier-Lacombe MJ, et al. Rhabdomyosarcoma of the larynx in children: A series of five patients treated in the Institut Gustave Roussy (Villejuif, France). *Med Pediatr Oncol.* 1991; 19:110.

691. Ohlms LA, McGill T, Healy GB. Malignant laryngeal tumors in children: A 15-year experience with four patients. *Ann Otol.* 1994; 103:686.

692. Winther LK, Lorentzen M. Rhabdomyosarcoma of the larynx. Report of two cases and a review of the literature. *J Laryngol Otol.* 1978; 92:417.

693. Erlandson RA. The ultrastructural distinction between rhabdomyosarcoma and other undifferentiated "sarcomas." *Ultra Pathol.* 1987; 11:83.

694. Eusebi V, Caccarelli C, Gorza L, Schiaffino S, Bussolati G. Immunocytochemistry of rhabdomyosarcoma: The use of four different markers. *Am J Surg Pathol.* 1986; 10:293.

695. Parham DM, Webber B, Holt H, Williams WK, Maurer H. Immunohistochemical study of childhood rhabdomyosarcoma and related neoplasms. Results of an Intergroup Rhabdomyosarcoma Study Project. *Cancer.* 1991; 67:3072.

696. Skalli O, Gabbiani G, Babaï F, et al. Intermediate filament proteins and actin isoforms as markers for soft tissue tumor differentaition and origin. II. Rhabdomyosarcoma. *Am J Pathol.* 1988; 130:515.

697. Douglass ED, Shapiro DN, Valentine M, et al. Alveolar rhabdomyosarcoma with the t(2;13): cytogenetic findings and clinicopathologic correlations. *Med Pediatr Oncol.* 1993; 21:83.

698. Abramowsky CR, Witt WJ. Sarcoma of the larynx in a newborn. *Cancer.* 1983; 51:1726.

699. Rowe-Jones JM, Solomons NB, Ratcliffe NA. Leiomyosarcoma of the larynx. *J Laryngol Otol.* 1994; 108:359.

700. Maurer HM, Beltangady M, Gehan EA, et al. The Intergroup Rhabdomyosarcoma study—I: A final report. *Cancer.* 1988; 61:209.

701. Wharam MD, Beltangady MS, Heyn RM, et al. Pediatric orofacial and laryngopharyngeal rhabdomyosarcoma. An Intergroup Rhabdomyosarcoma Study report. *Arch Otolaryngol Head Neck Surg.* 1987; 113:1225.

702. Allsbrook WC Jr, Harmon JD, Chongchitnant N, Erwin S. Liposarcoma of the larynx. *Arch Pathol Lab Med.* 1985; 109: 294.

703. Ferlito A. Primarily pleomorphic liposarcoma of the larynx. *J Otolaryngol.* 1978; 7:161.

704. Gaynor EB, Raghausan UMA, Weisbrot IM. Primary myxoid liposarcoma of the larynx. *Otolaryngol Head Neck Surg.* 1984; 92:476.

705. Gertner R, Podoshin L, Fradis M, Misselevitch I, Boss J. Liposarcoma of the larynx. *J Laryngol Otol.* 1988; 102:838.

706. Hurtado JF, Lopes JJ, Aranda FI, Talavera J. Primary liposarcoma of the larynx. Case report and literature review. *Ann Otol.* 1994; 103:315.

707. Krausen AS, Gall AM, Garza RG, Spector GJ, Ansel DG. Liposarcoma of the larynx: A multicentric or a metastatic malignancy. *Laryngoscope.* 1977; 87:1116.

708. Meis JM, Mackay B, Goepfert H. Liposarcoma of the larynx: Case report and literature review. *Arch Otolaryngol Head Neck Surg.* 1986; 112:1289.

709. Miller D, Goodman M, Weber A, Goldstein A. Primary liposarcoma of the larynx. *Trans Am Acad Ophthalmol Otol.* 1975; 80:444.

710. Tobey DN, Wheelis RF, Yarington CT Jr. Electron microscopy in the diagnosis of liposarcoma and fibrosarcoma of the larynx. *Ann Otol.* 1979; 88:867.

711. Velek JP: Liposarcoma of the larynx. *Trans Am Acad Ophthalmol Otol.* 1976; 82:569.

712. Wenig BM, Weiss SW, Gnepp DR. Laryngeal and hypopharyngeal liposarcoma. A clinicopathologic study of 10 cases with a comparison to soft-tissue counterparts. *Am J Surg Pathol.* 1990; 14:134.

713. Esclamado RM, Disher MJ, Ditto JL, Rontal E, McClatchey KD. Laryngeal liposarcoma. *Arch Otolaryngol Head Neck Surg.* 1994; 120:422.

714. Evans HL. Liposarcomas and atypical lipomatous tumors: A study of 66 cases followed for a minimum of 10 years. *Surg Pathol.* 1988; 1:41.

715. Evans HL. Liposarcoma. A study of 55 cases with reassessment of its classification. *Am J Surg Pathol.* 1979; 3:507.

716. Golledge J, Fisher CY, Rhys-Evans PH. Head and neck liposarcoma. *Cancer.* 1995; 76:1051.

717. Reitan JB, Kaalhus O, Brennhovd IO, et al. Prognostic factors in liposarcoma. *Cancer.* 1985; 55:2482.

718. Horny H-P, Parwaresch MR, Kaiserling E, et al. Mast cell sarcoma of the larynx. *J Clin Pathol.* 1986; 39:596.

719. Shilling BB, Abell MR, Work WP. Leukemic involvement of larynx. *Arch Otolaryngol.* 1967; 85:102.

720. Vassallo J, Altemani A, Cardinalli IA, et al. Granulocytic sarcoma of the larynx preceding chronic myeloid leukemia. *Pathol Res Pract.* 1993; 198:1084.

721. Bickerton RC, Brockbank MJ. Lymphoplasmacytic lymphoma of the larynx, soft palate and nasal cavity. *J Laryngol Otol.* 1988; 102:468.

722. DeSanto LW, Weiland LH. Malignant lymphoma of the larynx. *Laryngoscope.* 1970; 80:966.

723. Fidias P, Wright C, Harris NL, Urba W, Grossbard ML. Primary tracheal non-Hodgkin's lymphoma. A case report and review of the literature. *Cancer.* 1996; 77:2332.

724. Gregor RT. Laryngeal malignant lymphoma—An entity? *J Laryngol Otol.* 1981; 95:81.

725. Hessan H, Houck J, Harvey H. Airway obstruction due to lymphoma of the larynx and trachea. *Laryngoscope* 1988; 98: 176.

726. Horny H-P, Kaiserling E. Involvement of the larynx by hemopoietic neoplasms. An investigation of autopsy cases and review of the literature. *Pathol Res Pract.* 1995; 191:130.

727. Horny H-P, Ferlito A, Carbone A. Laryngeal lymphoma derived from mucosa-associated lymphoid tissue. *Ann Otol.* 1996; 105:577.

728. Swerdlow JB, Merl SA, Davey FR, Gacek RR, Gottlieb AJ. Non-Hodgkin's lymphoma limited to the larynx. *Cancer.* 1984; 53:2546.

729. Wang CC. Malignant lymphoma of the larynx. *Laryngoscope.* 1972; 82:97.

730. Biller HF, Pilch BZ, Scully RE, Mark EJ, McNeely BU. A 51 year old male with upper airway obstruction and lymphadenopathy. *N Engl J Med* 1981; 305:1572.

731. Courtney-Harris RG, Goddard MJ. Extranodal sinus histiocytosis with massive lymphadenopathy (Rosai-Dorfman disease): A rare cause of subglottic narrowing. *J Laryngol Otol.* 1992; 106:61.

732. Foucar E, Rosai J, Dorfman RF. Sinus histiocytosis with massive lymphadenopathy: Ear, nose and throat manifestations. *Arch Otolaryngol.* 1978; 104:687.

733. Foucar E, Rosai J, Dorfman RF. Sinus histiocytosis with massive lymphadenopathy (Rosai-Dorfman disease): Review of the entity. *Semin Diagn Pathol.* 1990; 7:19.

734. Wenig BM, Abbondanzo SL, Childers EL, Kapadia SB, Heffner DK. Extranodal sinus histiocytosis with massive lymphadenopathy (Rosai-Dorfman disease) of the head and neck. *Hum Pathol.* 1993; 24:483.

735. Eisen RN, Buckley PJ, Rosai J. Immunophenotypic characterization of sinus histiocytosis with massive lymphadenopathy (Rosai-Dorfman disease). *Semin Diagn Pathol.* 1990; 7:74.

736. Booth JB, Thomas RSA. Histiocytosis X. *J Laryngol Otol.* 1970; 84:1123.

737. Friedmann I, Ferlito A. Primary eosinophilic granuloma of the larynx. *J Laryngol Otol.* 1981; 95:1249.

738. Lhoták J, Dvoracková I. Histiocytosis X of the larynx. *J Laryngol Otol.* 1975; 89:771.

739. Nolph MB, Luikin GA. Histiocytosis X. *Otolaryngol Clin North Am.* 1982; 15:635.

740. Batsakis JG, Luna MA, Byers RM. Metastases to the larynx. *Head Neck Surg.* 1985; 7:458.

741. Cullen JR. Ovarian carcinoma metastatic to the larynx. *J Laryngol Otol.* 1990; 104:48.

742. Ellis M, Winston P. Secondary carcinoma of the larynx. *J Laryngol Otol.* 1957; 71:16.

743. Freeland AP, van Nostrand AWP, Jahn AF. Metastases to the larynx. *J Otolaryngol.* 1979; 8:448.

744. Friedmann I, Osborn DA. Metastatic tumours in the ear, nose and throat region. *J Laryngol Otol.* 1965; 79:576.

745. Glanz H, Kleinsasser O. Metastasen in Kehrkopf. *HNO.* 1978; 26:163.

746. Mazzarella LA, Pina LH, Wolff D. Asymptomatic metastasis to the larynx. *Laryngoscope.* 1966; 76:1547.

747. Whicker JH, Carder GA, Devine KD. Metastasis to the larynx. Report of a case and review of the literature. *Arch Otolaryngol.* 1972; 96:182.

748. Chamberlain D. Malignant melanoma, metastatic to the larynx. *Arch Otolaryngol.* 1966; 83:63.

749. Loughead JR, Bushnell J. Metastasis of malignant tumors to the larynx. *Laryngoscope.* 1954; 64:50.

750. Loughead JR. Malignant melanoma of the larynx. *Ann Otol.* 1952; 61;154.

751. Miyamoto R, Helmus C. Hypernephroma metastatic to the head and neck. *Laryngoscope.* 1973; 83:898.

752. Mochimatsu I, Tsukuda M, Furukawa S, Sawaki S. Tumours metastasizing to the head and neck—a report of seven cases. *J Laryngol Otol.* 1993; 107:1171.

753. Ritchie WW, Messmer JM, Whitley DP, Gopelrud DR. Uterine carcinoma metastatic to the larynx. *Laryngoscope.* 1985; 95:97.

754. Grignon DJ, Ro JY, Ayala AG, et al. Carcinoma of the prostate metastasizing to vocal cord. *Urology.* 1990; 36:85.

755. Quinn FB Jr, McCabe BF. Laryngeal metastases from malignant tumors in distant organs. *Ann Otol.* 1957; 66:139.

756. Park YW, Park MH. Vocal cord paralysis from prostatic carcinoma metastasizing to the larynx. *Head Neck.* 1993; 15:455.

757. Abemayor E, Cockran AJ, Calcaterra TC. Metastatic cancer to the larynx. Diagnosis and management. *Cancer.* 1983; 52: 1944.

758. Cavicchi O, Farneti G, Occhiuzzi L, Sorrenti G. Laryngeal metastasis from colonic adenocarcioma. *J Laryngol Otol.* 1990; 104:730.

759. Oku T, Hasegawa M, Watanabe I, Nasu M, Aoki N. Pancreatic cancer with metastasis to the larynx. *J Laryngol Otol.* 1980; 94:1205.

760. Wanamaker JR, Kraus DH, Eliachar I, Lavertu P. Manifestations of metastatic breast carcinoma to the head and neck. *Head Neck.* 1993; 15:257.

761. Ogata H, Ebihara S, Mukai K, et al. Laryngeal metastasis from a pulmonary papillary adenocarcinoma: A case report. *Jpn J Clin Oncol.* 1993; 23:199.

762. Bolognesi C, Caliceti G. Seminoma metastatico della laringe. *Otorinolaringol Ital.* 1960; 29:15.

763. Nambu T, Shinohara M, Takada A, et al. A case of icteric hepatoma with laryngeal metastasis and coexisting pancreatic cancer. *Gan No Rinsho.* 1990; 36:515.

764. Shimizu KT, Selch MY, Fu Y-S, Anzai Y, Lufkin RB. Osteosarcoma metastatic to the larynx. *Ann Otol.* 1994; 103:160.

765. Rotenberg D, Lawson VG, van Nostrand AWP. Thyroid carcinoma presenting as a tracheal tumor. Case report and literature review with reflections on pathogenesis. *J Otolaryngol.* 1979; 8:401.

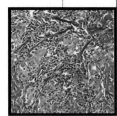

CHAPTER 9

Oral Cavity

I. CLINICAL CONSIDERATIONS FOR NON-NEOPLASTIC LESIONS OF THE ORAL CAVITY

■ LOUIS G. PORTUGAL

■ JOHN GOLDENBERG

The differential diagnosis for lesions presenting within the oral cavity includes a number of non-neoplastic conditions. Understanding the clinical manifestations of each of these lesions is essential for differentiating primary lesions from lesions related to systemic disease. The latter group of diseases is particularly significant given the potential for diseases, such as sarcoidosis or human immunodeficiency virus (HIV) infections, to manifest initially within the oral cavity. This chapter reviews the clinical manifestations of non-neoplastic lesions presenting within the oral cavity.

DEVELOPMENTAL LESIONS

Hamartomas, Choristomas, and Ectopias

Hamartomas are benign overgrowths of tissue normally present at a given anatomic location. These lesions have been described throughout the oral cavity and oropharynx, but are commonly reported to involve the tongue base in particular. The clinical presentation of affected patients is related to the size and location of the lesion; the condition is often associated with feeding difficulties in a neonate or infant. Hamartomas have also been reported to be the etiologic agent for globus pharyngeus and dysphagia in adults with oropharyngeal involvement.

Choristoma is a pathologic term for a mass of normal-appearing tissue in an aberrant location. These are not neoplasms, but rather embryologic rests of tissue secondary to dysgenesis. Examples of these lesions within the oral cavity are glial, cartilaginous, or osseous masses arising from the tongue or buccal mucosa. Treatment is complete excision of the mass. Recurrence is extremely rare.

Congenital heterotopic gastrointestinal cysts have been reported in the oral cavity of neonates and children. These are almost exclusively found in the floor of the mouth or tongue and may result in respiratory compromise or feeding difficulties. The etiology of these lesions is an entrapment of endoderm within the oral cavity during the third to fourth week of embryogenesis.

Lingual Thyroid

The thyroid anlage arises at the foramen caecum of the tongue and descends into the neck during embryologic development. Arrest of this migration, with a resulting mass of thyroid tissue overlying the base of tongue, is termed a lingual thyroid. The lingual thyroid may be the only functioning thyroid tissue, although commonly, thyroid gland is present in the normal cervical location as well.

Women appear to manifest symptoms of a lingual thyroid more often than do men. Related symptoms include dysphagia, odynophagia, and dysarthria. Rarely, airway obstruction may result from a lingual thyroid in a neonate. Patients are typically euthyroid or hypothyroid, and on pathologic examination, the tissue mimics that of thyroid in the normal cervical location.

Work-up of this lesion often includes a biopsy to confirm the diagnosis and radioactive iodine scanning to confirm the presence of functioning thyroid tissue in the neck. Treatment includes suppression with exogenous thyroid hormone or total excision via a transoral approach. If the lingual thyroid is the only functioning tissue, surgical treatment should include autotransplantation of a portion of the removed gland within the strap musculature.

Epidermoid and Dermoid Cysts

The oral cavity and oropharynx are host to a number of cystic growths that may be either congenital or acquired. Epidermoid cysts are considered to be true cysts in that they have a complete epidermal lining, which may occur in the oral cavity. These cysts, when present, tend to be superficially located in the buccal mucosa or floor of the mouth. They sometimes occur in very young patients without a history of trauma, but are most commonly seen in older patients, often in association with a history of previous trauma. These cysts are easily enucleated, and their recurrence rate is negligible.

Dermoid cysts have a similar clinical appearance but histopathologic examination reveals that they are composed of stratified squamous epithelium and adnexal structures. These cysts are removed in a similar fashion to epidermoid cysts. As mucoceles are the more commonly acquired oral cavity cysts, they are discussed later in this chapter in greater detail.

INFECTIOUS LESIONS

Bacterial Infection

Bacterial pharyngitis and tonsillitis are the primary bacterial infections affecting the oral cavity and pharynx. Common presenting symptoms include dysphagia, odynophagia, fever, and malaise. Incubation periods tend to be short (on the order of a few days), and associated lymphadenopathy is common. Group A β-hemolytic streptococcus is the most common pathogen and is readily identified on culture. Common pathogens also include *Streptococcus pneumoniae*, *Staphylococcus aureus*, and *Haemophilus influenzae*. Less common etiologic agents include *Corynebacterium diphtheriae* (diphtheria), *Bordetella pertussis* (whooping cough), *Treponema pallidum* (syphilis), *Neisseria gonorrhoea*, and *Klebsiella pneumoniae rhinoscleromatis*. Oral anaerobic flora may also be involved in pathologic infections, such as those caused by *Bacteroides fragilis* and Peptostreptococcus. Treatment of bacterial pharyngitis involves administration of penicillin, erythromycin, and/or first-generation cephalosporins.

Viral Infection

Viral pathogens may involve multiple sites within the oral cavity and oropharynx. They most commonly include herpesvirus, Epstein-Barr virus, human papillomavirus, and cytomegalovirus.

HERPES SIMPLEX VIRUS

Herpes simplex virus (HSV) produces an inflammatory lesion of the oral cavity and pharynx. HSV type I, the type most commonly responsible for stomatitis, is often primarily acquired before the age of 5 years. During the initial infection (primary herpetic gingivostomatitis), patients often present with fever, malaise, sore throat, and cervical lymphadenopathy.

The lesions of the oral mucosa are typically well-circumscribed ulcers, 3 mm in diameter, with a surrounding erythematous halo. The hard palate and gingival surfaces are most frequently involved, which distinguishes them from recurrent aphthous ulcers which do not typically involve these areas (see later section).

HSV remains latent in the trigeminal nerve ganglia and may reactivate throughout life. This recurrent herpetic infection results in self-limited oral ulcers without the associated systemic symptoms. Reactivation in immunocompromised patients may result in an aggressive course with a high mortality rate. Treatment is largely symptomatic. Topical or oral antiviral agents, such as acyclovir, have been used with success to shorten the clinical course and to treat immunosuppressed patients.

CYTOMEGALOVIRUS

Cytomegalovirus (CMV) is a well-known cause of congenital deafness, blindness, and mental retardation. However, in adults, the acquired form of CMV results in less dramatic sequelae, and the disease is usually asymptomatic in immunocompetent hosts. Cytomegalovirus can result in a mononucleosis-like pharyngitis with associated malaise, lymphadenopathy, and lymphocytosis. Alternatively, a single ulcerative lesion of the tongue or oropharynx in a diabetic or a patient with acquired immunodeficiency syndrome (AIDS) may be secondary to CMV.[1]

EPSTEIN-BARR VIRUS

Epstein-Barr virus (EBV) rarely involves the oral cavity, but is a common cause of pharyngitis in young adults, mimicking the clinical picture of infectious mononucleosis. The clinical presentation is similar to that of acute bacterial tonsillitis and includes fever, malaise, and sore throat. Additionally, prominent cervical lymphadenopathy, hepatosplenomegaly, elevated liver enzymes, and lymphocytosis may be present. EBV is responsible for 90% of cases of infectious mononucleosis, although other viral agents have been implicated.

HUMAN PAPILLOMAVIRUS

Human papillomavirus (HPV) comprises more than 55 identifiable types and is found in locations with predominantly squamous epithelium. HPV types 16, 18, 31, and 33 encode viral oncogenes and have been implicated in oral cavity and oropharyngeal malignant disease.[2] The more common benign types (6 and 11) are found within verrucous lesions of the tonsillar pillars. These lesions are typically asymptomatic and are treated with simple excision. No serologic tests are available to identify HPV, and no effective medical therapy exists to treat these lesions.

Fungal Infection

Candida albicans is frequently present in the oral cavity as normal flora but is also the most common fungal pathogen involving the oral cavity and oropharynx. This infection, referred to as candidiasis, typically affects diabetics, patients receiving broad-spectrum antibiotics, and immunocompromised individuals. Pseudomembranous candidiasis is the most common form of oral candidiasis, presenting as a white, thick plaque overlying an erythematous base. Oral candidiasis may also present in other forms. The atrophic or erythematous form of this infection presents as a tender, erythematous, or hyperemic lesion of the mucosa without the presence of white plaques. The hyperplastic form of oral candidiasis is associated with thick, white plaque similar to that characterizing hairy leukoplakia. Biopsy studies may be necessary to establish the diagnosis. The buccal mucosa is the most common site for hyperplastic candidiasis. Finally, oral candidiasis may present as angular cheilitis. This lesion appears as an erythematous erosion at the oral commissure, associated with adjacent erythema. Confirmation of the diagnosis is based on the presence of hyphae on KOH stain.

Treatment, which is generally initiated at the time of suspected diagnosis, usually involves use of a topical nystatin solution or clotrimazole. If this approach is ineffective, if there is multisystem involvement, or if the patient is immunosuppressed, then systemic treatment is initiated with ketoconazole, fluconazole, or amphotericin. Amphotericin is the most potent of the systemic antifungal agents, but it also has the greatest side effect profile, including nephrotoxicity, bone marrow suppression, nausea, vomiting, anorexia, and cardiac toxicity.

IMMUNOLOGIC AND SYSTEMIC DISEASES

Recurrent Aphthous Ulcers

Recurrent aphthous ulcers (RAUs) are very common lesions affecting up to 20% of the general population.[3] The RAU appears as a discrete, painful, shallow, recurrent ulcer covered by fibrinous exudate surrounded by an erythematous halo (Fig. 9–1). The ulcers are typically less than 1 cm in diameter, but in certain instances, they may present as more severe, symptomatic, large, coalescent ulcers lasting for months. These ulcers are confined to the nonkeratinized mucosa of the mouth, including the labial and buccal mucosa, maxillary and mandibular sulci, nonattached gingiva, floor of the mouth, ventral surface of the tongue, soft palate, and tonsillar fossae. RAUs typically spare the dorsum of the tongue, the attached gingiva, and the hard palate, which are

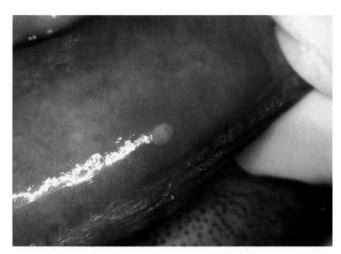

FIGURE 9–1 Recurrent aphthous ulcer involving the lower lip. Courtesy of Dr. Robert Kelsch, University of Illinois at Chicago College of Dentistry.

keratinized. Aggressive lesions may heal with scarring.

Numerous conditions are associated with aphthous ulcers. The classic triad of RAUs, genital ulcers, and ocular lesions is seen in individuals with Behçet's syndrome (see later section). Crohn's disease, which is an inflammatory disease of the gastrointestinal tract, is sometimes characterized by multiple, aphthous-like oral ulcers. However, unlike the ulcers in RAUs or Behçet's syndrome, which are histologically nonspecific, those in Crohn's disease may show noncaseating granulomas on histologic examination. Recently, an association between aphthous ulcers and HIV infection has been described.[4] Unlike the more common forms of RAU, HIV-associated aphthous ulcers are often larger than 1 cm in diameter and may persist for several months. Cultures or biopsy studies may be necessary to rule out HSV or CMV infections, or even a malignant lesion in HIV-infected patients with mucosal ulcerations. In general, recurrent oral HSV infections occur most commonly at the junction of the vermilion border of the lip and the skin and intraorally on the keratinized mucosa of the attached gingiva and hard palate mucosa; this distribution differentiates their clinical presentation from RAU.

The first step in managing RAU is to rule out an oral manifestation of systemic disease. Important information derived from the clinical history includes evidence of ocular, genital, or gastrointestinal symptoms; if necessary, culture or biopsy studies of the ulcer itself help to rule out less common causes of RAU. In general, management is directed toward reducing local pain and reducing the frequency of recurrences. The mainstay of treatment for RAU includes topical steroids, applied directly to the ulcer in small amounts once the ulcer has dried. Although topical steroids have been shown to reduce the period of ulceration and pain, they have not consist-

ently reduced the frequency of recurrences. Patients with more severe disease may require systemic steroids.

Behçet's Syndrome

Behçet's syndrome is a multisystem disorder with a primary presentation of recurrent oral ulcerations. Establishment of the diagnosis of Behçet's syndrome is based on the clinical manifestation of recurrent oral ulcerations plus both of the following diagnostic criteria: (1) recurrent genital ulcers, eye lesions, or skin lesions, and (2) a positive pathergy test.[5] This disease affects all races, mainly affecting young adults in the third decade of life. Men tend to have more severe disease than women. Although this disease is considered to be an autoimmune process because of the presence of autoantibodies to oral mucosa, the exact pathogenesis still remains unclear. The oral ulcers associated with Behçet's syndrome are usually painful, 2 to 10 mm in diameter, shallow, and covered with fibrinous exudate. However, unlike recurrent aphthous stomatitis, the oral lesions of Behçet's syndrome may be large and deep and may involve any portion of the oral cavity, including the keratinized mucosa.

The genital ulcers resemble the oral ulcers in appearance and, like the oral ulcers, they heal after 1 to 2 weeks with the potential for scarring. Genital ulcers most commonly affect the scrotum, but may affect any portion of the genitalia. External genital ulcers may be painful, whereas ulcers of the vagina are usually painless. Ocular involvement is usually present at the onset of disease and ranges in presentation from mild iritis and uveitis to optic neuritis and visual deterioration. Although hypopyon uveitis is often considered to be a hallmark of this disease, it is, in fact, a rare manifestation. Skin lesions include folliculitis and erythema nodosum. Nonspecific inflammatory reactions to scratches or intradermal saline injection (pathergy test) are common manifestations of this disease.

The severity of the syndrome usually lessens with time. Although serious complications may include blindness, or even death from neurologic complications, the life expectancy of an affected individual appears to be normal. Treatment of Behçet's syndrome is based upon symptoms. Mucous membrane involvement may respond to topical steroids. In general, the treatment of Behçet's syndrome is associated with a varied and unpredictable response.[5,6]

Oral Manifestations of Human Immunodeficiency Virus Infection

Oral manifestations are common among patients infected with the HIV virus. Because the oral manifestations of HIV infection often precede the development of AIDS, the clinician should be familiar with the oral findings in these patients.

ORAL CANDIDIASIS

Oral candidiasis is the most common abnormal finding in patients infected with HIV.[7-9] Although oral candidiasis occurs in patients with diabetes or patients taking broad-spectrum antibiotics, its appearance in otherwise unexplained circumstances should prompt a thorough work-up to determine the possibility of infection with HIV. The different manifestations of oral candidiasis have been described previously in this chapter. In general, pseudomembranous candidiasis is the most common form of oral Candida occurring in HIV-infected individuals. Typically, the lesions appear as white plaques that may easily be removed with scraping, leaving an erythematous or bleeding base. HIV-infected patients with oral candidiasis have significant potential for pharyngeal or esophageal involvement as well.

Treatment of oral candidiasis in HIV-infected patients frequently involves courses of topical antifungal medications. Oral candidiasis in more severely immunocompromised patients may require systemic antifungal agents. Prophylactic use of antifungals may be indicated, particularly in the later stages of HIV infection.

HAIRY LEUKOPLAKIA

Hairy leukoplakia is a common manifestation of patients with HIV infection, occurring in as many as 25% of cases.[10] Hairy leukoplakia is a lesion clearly unique to the HIV-infected individual. Nearly all patients with hairy leukoplakia are confirmed HIV positive. Hairy leukoplakia most commonly involves the lateral surface of the tongue. However, it may also appear elsewhere in the oral cavity, including the floor of the mouth and the buccal and labial mucosa. The lesion is typically white and is slightly raised, with a filiform or corrugated appearance (Fig. 9–2). It is often mistaken for the hyperplastic form of oral candidiasis; the correct diagnosis can be confirmed by biopsy. It appears that Epstein-Barr virus may be the causative agent for hairy leukoplakia. This lesion has been found to disappear upon treatment with high doses of antiviral agents, including acyclovir.

Hairy leukoplakia is generally asymptomatic. Its significance centers on its diagnostic and prognostic value in HIV-infected individuals. Any patient with this lesion should be tested for HIV, as more than 80% of HIV-infected patients identified with hairy leukoplakia develop full manifestations of AIDS within 3 years of diagnosis. Patients with hairy leukoplakia who develop AIDS appear to have a more rapidly progressive course than those without hairy leukoplakia.[11]

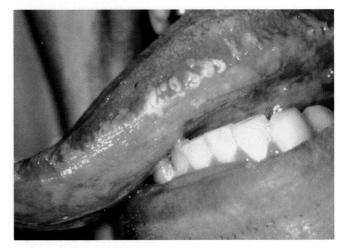

FIGURE 9–2　Hairy leukoplakia involving the lateral tongue in a patient with HIV infection. Courtesy of Dr. Robert Kelsch, University of Illinois at Chicago College of Dentistry.

HERPES SIMPLEX VIRUS INFECTIONS

HSV infections have been described previously in this chapter. In general, the lesions of herpes stomatitis in HIV-infected patients are more severe, recur more frequently, and persist longer than in the HIV-negative population.[9] Lesions may become extensive and may involve the adjacent skin of the face, resulting in giant herpetic lesions.

In general, herpetic lesions will respond to treatment with antiviral agents, such as acyclovir, if the treatment is initiated within the initial few days of the infection. High-dose treatment may be required for significant lesions. Antiviral agents may be used as a prophylactic agent in severe recurrent cases.

GINGIVITIS AND PERIODONTAL DISEASE

Gingivitis and periodontitis are much more severe, both in terms of symptoms and tissue loss, in HIV-infected individuals than in individuals not infected with HIV. There can be a rapid progression from mild gingivitis to a necrotizing process with soft tissue loss, bone exposure, and sequestration within the alveolar bone. The most severe form of this disease is acute necrotizing ulcerative gingivitis (ANUG), which is associated with significant destruction of the periodontal soft tissues and can lead to more severe and potentially life-threatening necrotizing stomatitis.[9] The etiologic agents for this spectrum of periodontal diseases are not always clear, but may be associated with a multiorganism infection of gram-negative anaerobic bacteria and Candida species. Proper dental care, including oral rinses with povidone-iodine or chlorhexidine, is important in preventing progression of this disease. Antibiotic therapy is directed against anaerobic organisms in patients with ANUG or necrotizing stomatitis.

Sarcoidosis

Sarcoidosis is a chronic, multisystemic disorder of unknown etiology. Although it can affect individuals of both sexes and all ages and races, most affected individuals in the United States are African-Americans and 20 to 40 years of age; there is a slight female preponderance. The lesion of sarcoidosis is the result of an exaggerated helper T-cell phenomenon of unknown etiology. This inflammatory process leads to the formation of noncaseating granulomas. Organ dysfunction occurs because of architectural distortion of involved tissue. The organ most frequently affected by this disease is the lung; signs and symptoms may include dyspnea, dry cough, and hilar adenopathy noted on chest x-ray studies.

Otolaryngologic manifestations are seen in 10% to 15% of cases of sarcoidosis and may, at times, be the initial manifestations of this disease.[12,13] Cervical adenopathy is the most common presentation in the head and neck.[14] Other manifestations include uveitis, intranasal involvement resulting in chronic rhinitis, salivary gland enlargement, laryngeal involvement resulting in hoarseness, and facial nerve paralysis secondary to temporal bone involvement. Oral manifestations include granulomatous involvement, resulting in nodular lesions of the tonsillar fossa and palate.

The diagnosis of sarcoidosis is made on the basis of a combination of clinical, radiographic, and histologic findings. Common laboratory abnormalities include increased erythrocyte sedimentation rate and an elevated level of angiotensin-converting enzyme. Ultimately, the definitive diagnosis of sarcoidosis is based on biopsy studies. The most common site for a biopsy to be performed is the lung, usually through a fiberoptic bronchoscope. If there are head and neck manifestations, fine-needle aspiration biopsy or open biopsy of neck nodes, enlarged salivary glands, or mucosal nodules may reveal the typical noncaseating granuloma. If no specific lesions are readily accessible, random lip biopsy of minor salivary glands may reveal the granulomatous lesions in up to 50% of patients who have associated hilar adenopathy.

Overall, the prognosis of patients with sarcoidosis is good. Most patients who present with the acute form of the disease do not manifest other sequelae, and many affected patients experience spontaneous remission. Topical internasal steroid treatment is useful in patients with chronic nasal involvement. Systemic steroids are indicated in patients with more advanced stages of this disease.[15]

Sjögren's Syndrome

Sjögren's syndrome is a chronic, progressive, autoimmune disease characterized by lymphocytic infiltration of the salivary and lacrimal glands. The disease predominantly affects middle-aged women. The disease may present as primary Sjögren's syndrome or as secondary Sjögren's syndrome in association with other autoimmune disorders, most commonly, rheumatoid arthritis.[16]

The main oral symptom of Sjögren's syndrome is xerostomia.[16,17] This symptom is associated with difficulty swallowing dry food, inability to speak continuously, and an increase in dental caries. Physical examination reveals atrophy of the filiform papillae on the dorsum of the tongue and decreased or absent expression of saliva from the glands. Enlargement of the major salivary glands is seen in most patients with primary Sjögren's syndrome, but is uncommon in those with the secondary syndrome. Ocular manifestations include dry eyes with a feeling of sand beneath the eyelids. There is decreased tearing, and slit-lamp examination of the cornea commonly reveals filamentary keratitis, which is specific for Sjögren's syndrome.

Other diagnoses may mimic the presentation of Sjögren's, including HIV infection or sarcoidosis. Sjögren's syndrome can be distinguished from other causes of sicca-like syndrome by a mucosal biopsy study of the lower lip. A so-called focus score is determined from the biopsy. A focus equals 50 or more inflammatory cells, and the focus score is determined by the number of foci in a 4-mm area. A score of greater than 1 is characteristic of Sjögren's syndrome but not of other sicca-like syndromes.

In addition to establishing the presence of autoimmune diseases, diagnostic tests may help to distinguish between primary and secondary Sjögren's syndrome. Circulating ss-A and ss-B autoimmune antibodies are found in 60% and 50% of primary Sjögren's cases, respectively, but are not found in secondary Sjögren's syndrome. Antibodies to human leukocyte antigens (HLAs) can also be helpful in differentiation, as HLA-B8 and HLA-DW3 are associated with primary Sjögren's syndrome, whereas HLA-DW4 is associated with secondary Sjögren's syndrome.

Treatment of Sjögren's syndrome is largely symptomatic and involves replacement of saliva and tears to limit the damaging local effects produced by missing these secretions. Severe cases may require treatment with steroids or an immunosuppressive agent.[18]

Wegener's Granulomatosis

Wegener's granulomatosis is an idiopathic inflammatory disorder characterized by granulomatous vasculitis of the upper and lower airways, together with glomerulonephritis of the kidneys. This is an uncommon disease affecting Caucasians more often than African-Americans and presenting at any age, with the mean age at onset being approximately 40 years. Pulmonary lesions range from asymptomatic infiltrates to multiple cavitary lesions associated with dyspnea and hemoptysis. Renal involvement generally dominates the clinical picture. Glomerulonephritis may manifest as proteinuria or hematuria and, if left untreated, will lead to rapidly progressive renal failure.

Up to 90% of affected patients have otolaryngologic symptoms at the time of presentation.[19] The most common site of involvement in the head and neck is the nose and sinuses, resulting in epistaxis, pain, obstruction, and chronic sinusitis. Progressive nasal involvement leads to septal destruction and saddle nose deformity. Oral cavity manifestations include hyperplastic gingivitis originating in the interdental papillary areas.[20] Conductive hearing loss secondary to serous otitis media can precede upper airway involvement by many months. Vasculitis within the inner ear vessels can result in a profound, but potentially reversible, sensorineural hearing loss. Subglottic stenosis can result from granulomatous inflammation of the larynx and trachea.

Characteristic laboratory findings include a markedly elevated sedimentation rate, mild anemia, and leukocytosis. In a high percentage of patients with Wegener's granulomatosis, antineutrophil cytoplasmic antibodies (ANCAs) are noted.[21] Although perinuclear ANCAs have been described in other vasculitis-associated disorders, cytoplasmic ANCAs are both specific and sensitive for Wegener's. Histopathologic findings of necrotizing granulomatous vasculitis affecting small vessels are characteristic for Wegener's granulomatosis, with open lung biopsy providing the highest diagnostic yield. Biopsy study of nasal lesions usually demonstrates inflammatory granulomatosis with necrosis, but may not show vasculitis.

The well-established treatment of choice is cyclophosphamide. Complete remission is achieved in up to 75% of patients with this disease. For additional symptomatic improvement, steroids may be added during initiation of the cyclophosphamide treatment.[22]

Amyloidosis

Amyloidosis is a rare disease characterized by the deposition of fibrous protein, amyloid, in different sites of the body, resulting in a wide variety of clinical manifestations. A classification scheme is used to distinguish the different clinical presentations. Primary amyloidosis is associated with systemic involvement with no identifiable etiology. Secondary amyloidosis refers to systemic amyloidosis that is associated with chronic disease, such as tuberculosis, osteomyelitis, or rheumatoid arthritis. A third category includes amyloid deposition in association with multiple myeloma. In systemic forms of amyloidosis, the morbidity and potential mortality relates primarily to the amyloid involvement of the renal and cardiac systems.

Up to 90% of patients with amyloidosis present with head and neck manifestations.[23] The most common site of involvement is the tongue, resulting in macroglossia (Fig. 9–3). Twenty-six percent of patients with multiple myeloma develop secondary amyloid deposition within the tongue. Surgical reduction of amyloid macroglossia can alleviate debilitating deglutition and dysarthria. In the respiratory tract, amyloidosis may be confined to the larynx, or it may infiltrate the tracheobronchial tree. Laryngeal manifestations range from tumor-like nodules to diffuse submucosal involvement. Localized amyloid deposition also may affect the tonsils, hard palate, and salivary glands. Localized forms of amyloidosis in the head and neck may be treated successfully without development of major sequelae. However, generalized amyloidosis is usually slowly progressive, leading to death within several years.

Positive results on tissue biopsy studies confirm the diagnosis of amyloidosis. In 75% to 90% of patients with systemic amyloidosis, abdominal fat aspirate or rectal biopsy specimens test positive. Amyloid deposits display a characteristic eosinophilic appearance on hematoxylin-eosin staining and demonstrate a unique green birefringence when viewed under polarized light microscopy after staining with Congo red.

Medical therapy for patients with systemic amyloidosis generally yields unsatisfactory results. Colchicine and melphalan have been used in an attempt to inhibit amyloid deposition. However, medical

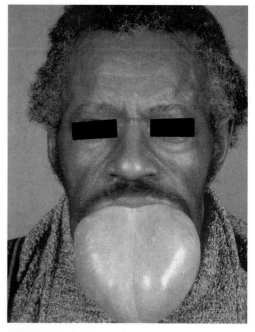

FIGURE 9–3 Severe macroglossia secondary to amyloidosis.

therapy generally has not been found to make a difference in the overall survival of patients with systemic amyloidosis. Treatment for localized head and neck disease is largely directed toward relieving the symptoms of macroglossia which, as stated, may be treated with surgical reduction of the involved tongue.

OTHER LESIONS

Mucocele

Mucoceles (mucus-retention cysts) may occur anywhere in the oral cavity or pharynx, but are most commonly found on the mucosa of the lower lip and floor of the mouth. These lesions are thought to occur secondary to the escape of saliva and mucus from a minor salivary gland duct into the surrounding connective tissue. These are not true cysts, as there is no complete epithelial lining. Trauma is the likely predisposing factor for cyst development, although such a history cannot be elicited in all patients. Lesions arise rather quickly as small, bluish cysts and are generally asymptomatic. They may spontaneously rupture and recur. Definitive management is best accomplished with complete surgical excision.

Ranula

Ranula is a term used for a mucocele involving the floor of the mouth. This asymptomatic lesion is typically a few centimeters in diameter. Marsupialization has been used to treat these lesions, but often results in an unacceptably high rate of recurrence. Therefore, complete excision, along with removal of the associated salivary gland, is the treatment of choice. When a ranula enlarges, it may extend deep to the mylohyoid, in which case it is referred to as a "plunging" ranula. This lesion may present as a unilateral neck mass in the submandibular triangle. Examination of the floor of the mouth may rarely yield normal findings; more commonly, a bulge is noted. Surgical treatment of these lesions involves both an external, as well as an intraoral, approach.

Condyloma Acuminatum

Condyloma acuminatum is an HPV lesion with a raised, warty appearance. It is most commonly found in the anogenital region but may also appear on the oral mucosa. These lesions are spread via direct contact, most frequently during sexual encounters (venereal spread). Condyloma acuminatum appears as multiple, small, papillomatous lesions that range in color from pink to white. Excision, cryosurgery, and electrodesiccation are all effective means of eradication. Recurrences are common.

Verruca Vulgaris

Oral verruca vulgaris (wart) is a lesion that is also caused by HPV infection. Clinically, these lesions appear identical to warts on other cutaneous surfaces. These raised, white lesions may be single or multiple and may regress spontaneously. However, definitive management consists of simple excision, curettage, or cryosurgery.

Verruciform Xanthoma

Verruciform xanthoma may mimic the appearance of a papillomatous oral lesion or an epithelial malignant lesion. Clinically, the most characteristic appearance is an asymptomatic, warty, or granular lesion on the alveolar ridge or gingival mucosa that measures 0.25 to 2 cm in diameter. Male individuals are affected more frequently than female patients, and the average age at presentation is the third to fourth decade. The etiology is unknown, although recent immunohistochemical evidence suggests that an underlying immune response is a factor in the pathogenesis of these lesions. The lesions are uniformly benign and are histologically characterized by foam cells in the papillae. Treatment is simple surgical excision.

Verrucous Hyperplasia

The clinical appearance of verrucous hyperplasia is that of red papules distributed over the surface of the hard palate. The lesions are often associated with maxillary denture use and are presumably due to repeated trauma. The characteristic gross and histologic findings may suggest a cancerous lesion, but no malignant potential has been found to be associated with verrucous hyperplasia. Treatment consists of remaking poorly fit dentures or wearing properly fit dentures only a portion of the day. Surgical treatment is rarely indicated.

A variant of oral verrucous hyperplasia characterized by marked hyperkeratosis and endophytic growth pattern was recognized by Shear and Pindborg[24] as potential precursor of verrucous carcinoma. Later Hansen et al[25] applied the term proliferative verrucous leukoplakia for similar lesions and observed a series of progression to dysplasia, verrucous carcinoma, and other invasive squamous cell carcinomas. These lesions tend to persist or recur following a variety of treatment modalities. Development of new lesions is common. This lesion is discussed further in the pathology section under Leukoplakia (see pages 530–531).

Necrotizing Sialometaplasia

Necrotizing sialometaplasia is an inflammatory process of ischemic etiology involving the salivary glands. Most commonly, this disease presents with a painful ulcerative lesion covering a few centimeters of the hard palate. As the gross appearance may mimic that of an epithelial malignant lesion, microscopic evaluation may be required to establish the diagnosis. Other sites within the oral cavity and oropharynx may be involved and are more likely to be associated with a predisposing traumatic event. The histologic appearance of necrotizing sialometaplasia suggests an ischemic vascular event as the underlying cause of these lesions. Treatment is supportive, as these lesions are self-limiting and heal by secondary intention over a period of 1 to 3 months.

REFERENCES

1. Kanas RJ, Jensen JL, Abrams AM, Wuerker RB. Oral mucosal cytomegalovirus as a manifestation of the acquired immune deficiency syndrome. *Oral Surg Oral Med Oral Pathol.* 1987; 64: 183–189.
2. Portugal LG, Goldenberg JD, Wenig BL, et al. Human papillomavirus expression and p53 gene mutations in squamous cell carcinoma. *Arch Otolaryngol Head Neck Surg.* 1997; 123:1230–1234.
3. Woo SB, Sonis ST. Recurrent aphthous ulcers: A review of diagnosis and treatment. *J Am Dent Assoc.* 1996; 127:1202–1213.
4. Phelan JA, Eisig S, Freedman PD, Newsome N, Klein RS. Major aphthous-like ulcers in patients with AIDS. *Oral Surg Oral Med Oral Pathol.* 1991; 71:68–72.
5. International Study Group for Behçet's Disease. Criteria for diagnosis of Behçet's disease. *Lancet.* 1990; 335:1078–1080.
6. Arbesfeld SJ, Kurban AK. Behçet's disease: New perspectives on an enigmatic syndrome. *J Am Acad Dermatol.* 1988; 19:767–779.
7. Phelan JA, Saltzman BR, Friedland GH, Klein RS. Oral findings in patients with acquired immunodeficiency syndrome. *Oral Surg Oral Med Oral Pathol.* 1987; 64:50–56.
8. Greenspan JS, Greenspan D, Winkler JR. Diagnosis and management of the oral manifestations of HIV infection and AIDS. *Infect Dis Clin North Am.* 1988; 2:373–385.
9. Dichtel WJ. Oral manifestations of immunodeficiency virus infection. *Otolaryngol Clin North Am.* 1992; 25:1211–1227.
10. Greenspan D, Greenspan JS, Hearst NG, et al. Relation of oral hairy leukoplakia to infection with the human immunodeficiency virus and the risk of developing AIDS. *J Infect Dis.* 1987; 155:475–481.
11. Centers for Disease Control and Prevention. Oral viral lesion (hairy leukoplakia) associated with acquired immunodeficiency syndrome. *MMWR Morb Mortal Wkly Rep.* 1985; 34: 549–550.
12. McCaffrey TV, McDonald TJ. Sarcoidosis of the nose and paranasal sinuses. *Laryngoscope.* 1983; 93:1281–1284.
13. Shah UK, White JA, Gooey JE, Hybels RL. Otolaryngologic manifestations of sarcoidosis: Presentation and diagnosis. *Laryngoscope.* 1997; 107:67–75.
14. Dash GI, Kimmelman CP. Head and neck manifestations of sarcoidosis. *Laryngoscope.* 1988; 98:50–53.
15. Crystal RG. Sarcoidosis. In: Braunwald E, et al. eds: *Harrison's Principles of Internal Medicine.* 14th ed. New York:McGraw-Hill; 1999:320.
16. Campbell SM, Montanaro A, Bardana EJ. Head and neck manifestations of autoimmune disease. *Am J Otolaryngol.* 1983; 4:187–216.
17. Doig JA, Whaley K, Dick WC, Nuki G, Williamson J, Buchanan WW. Otolaryngological aspects of Sjögren's syndrome. *Br Med J.* 1971; 4:460–463.
18. Moutsopoulos HM. Sjögren's syndrome. In: Braunwald E, et al. eds: *Harrison's Principles of Internal Medicine.* 14th ed. New York:McGraw-Hill; 1999:316.
19. Burlacoff SG, Wong FSH. Wegener's granulomatosis. The great masquerade: A clinical presentation and literature review. *J Otolaryngol.* 1993; 22:94–105.
20. Handlers JP, Waterman J, Abrams AM, Melrose RJ. Oral features of Wegener's granulomatosis. *Arch Otolaryngol.* 1985; 111:267–270.
21. Fukase S, Ohta N, Inamura K, Kimura Y, Aoyagi M, Koike Y. Diagnostic specificity of antineutrophil cytoplasmic antibodies (ANCA) in otorhinolaryngological diseases. *Acta Otolaryngol.* 1994; 511(suppl):204–207.
22. Fauci AS. The vasculitis syndromes: Wegener's granulomatosis. In: Braunwald E, et al. eds: *Harrison's Principles of Internal Medicine.* 14th ed. New York:McGraw-Hill; 1999:319.
23. Kerner MM, Wang MB, Angier G, Calcaterra TC, Ward PH. Amyloidosis of the head and neck: A clinicopathologic study of the UCLA experience, 1955–1991. *Arch Otolaryngol Head Neck Surg.* 1995; 121:778–782.
24. Shear M, Pindborg JJ. Verrucous hyperplasia of the oral mucosa. *Cancer.* 1980; 46:1855–1862.
25. Hansen LS, Olson JA, Silverman S. Proliferative verrucous leukoplakia. *Oral Surg Oral Med Oral Pathol.* 1985; 60:285–298.

II. CLINICAL CONSIDERATIONS FOR NEOPLASMS OF THE ORAL CAVITY AND OROPHARYNX

- SCOTT E. PHILLIPS
- PETER D. COSTANTINO
- GLEN D. HOUSTON

Most head and neck neoplasms develop within the oral cavity and oropharynx. Both benign and malignant tumors arising from all stem cell lines are represented. This wide variety of tumor types, coupled with the complex anatomy and multiple structures within these regions, makes the diagnosis and treatment of these lesions particularly challenging. As a result, a functional understanding of tumors that develop in the oral cavity and oropharynx is critical in achieving a timely diagnosis, usually by means of a biopsy study. The purposes of this chapter are to provide that knowledge base and to highlight the clinically relevant features of these tumors. The presentation of this information will be organized based on the stem cell line from which the tumors arise, as well as their potential for benign versus malignant behavior. In this manner, a more generalized understanding of oral cavity and oropharyngeal tumors can be gained.

ANATOMY

The oral cavity is bounded anteriorly by the vermilion border of the lips, posteriorly by a plane visualized between the line of circumvallate papillae on the tongue inferiorly, and the junction between the hard and soft palates superiorly. Laterally, the oral cavity is bounded on either side by the buccal mucosa, which is the epithelial lining of the inner surface of the cheeks and lips. Structures of note within these boundaries include the lips, the upper and lower alveolar ridges, the retromolar trigone, the floor of the mouth, the anterior two thirds of the tongue, the hard palate, the gingivae, the teeth, and the buccal mucosa.[1,2]

The oropharynx begins at the posterior border of the oral cavity and continues superiorly to a plane extending posteriorly from the hard palate and inferiorly to the pharyngoepiglottic folds and the upper border of the epiglottis. The palatopharyngeal arches make up the lateral borders. Structures included within these boundaries include the soft palate and uvula; base of the tongue, including the lingual tonsils, tonsillar fossae, and pillars (including the palatine tonsils); and the posterior pharyngeal wall between the planes described (Fig. 9–4).

Neoplasms of the oral cavity and oropharynx, both benign and malignant, can originate from the mucosal lining or any of the underlying supporting tissues. Thus, when considering the differential diagnosis for this area, one must consider lesions of squamous epithelium; blood vessels; mucous, serous,

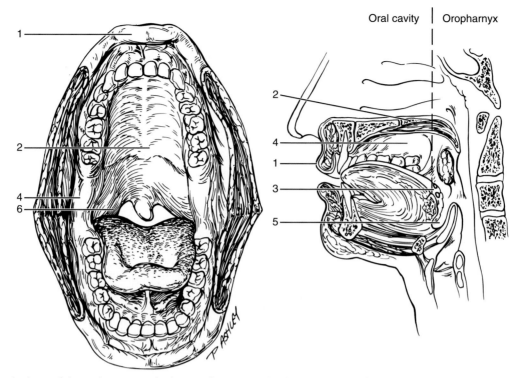

Oral cavity | Oropharynx

FIGURE 9–4 The limits of the oral cavity are the lip vermilion (anteriorly), the posterior hard palate and circumvallate papillae (posteriorly), and the buccal mucosa (laterally). The oropharynx then extends posteriorly from the oral cavity, bounded superiorly by a plane extending back from the hard palate, inferiorly by the pharyngoepiglottic folds, and laterally by the palatopharyngeal arches.

and sebaceous glands; nerve; bone; cartilage; and skeletal muscle.

Of clinical concern when evaluating many neoplasms of the oral cavity and oropharynx is the lymphatic drainage from the site of the neoplasm. The patterns of lymphatic drainage are of predictive value in the evaluation of a patient for metastases. Each of the structures listed previously has characteristic drainage patterns that must be considered individually. These patterns are outlined in Table 9–1 and Figure 9–5. It is important to note that, when nearing the midline of the oral cavity and oropharynx, the lymphatics decussate; thus, the propensity for bilateral metastasis increases. These decussations are very prominent in the tongue (both anterior and posterior), the posterior pharynx, the soft palate, and the lower lip. They are somewhat less prominent in the upper lip and hard palate.[1–5]

BENIGN NEOPLASMS

Epithelial Lesions

SQUAMOUS PAPILLOMA

Squamous papillomas are considered by many to be the most common benign neoplasm of the oral cav-

ity. They usually present as asymptomatic, well-circumscribed growths that exhibit a pedunculated, cauliflower-like appearance, often displaying many finger-like projections. Usually, squamous papillomas present as solitary, relatively small lesions, rarely growing to more than 1 cm in size. There is a slight predilection for their development in male individuals in their third to fifth decade. The most common location for these lesions is the palate or tongue, although they can present on any area of the intraoral mucosa, including the vermilion.

Some researchers believe that there is a viral etiology to these lesions in humans but this has never been proven, despite the fact that a viral origin has been identified for oral papillomas in other species. The clinical course is usually characterized by slow growth, and there is no proclivity for malignant transformation. Treatment is aimed at complete surgical excision; the base of the stalk, when present, must always be included with the excised specimen to prevent recurrence.

Rare syndromes associated with oral squamous cell papillomas include oral papillomatosis (also known as Gottron's papillomatosis cutis carcinoides) and Cowden's disease. The former is idiopathic, being characterized by a confluence of oral squamous papillomas, and is associated with multiple gastroduodenal polyps. The latter is an autosomal dominant condition with incomplete penetrance that, in

TABLE 9 – 1   PATTERNS OF LYMPHATIC METASTASIS OF ORAL CAVITY AND OROPHARYNX LESIONS BY SITE OF TUMOR ORIGIN

	PREAURICULAR	PAROTID	SUBMENTAL	SUBMANDIBULAR	UPPER DEEP JUGULAR	JUGULO-DIGASTRIC	JUGULO-OMOHYOID	POSTERIOR CERVICAL	RETROPHARYNGEAL
Upper lip	X	X		X					
Medial lower lip			X						
Lateral lower lip		X		X					
Buccal mucosa		X	X	X					
Buccal alveolar ridges			X	X					
Lingual alveolar ridges					X				X
Anterior oral tongue			X				X		
Lateral oral tongue				X	X				
Superficial floor of the mouth				X					
Deep floor of the mouth				X	X				
Posterior floor of the mouth						X			
Retromolar trigone				X	X				
Hard palate					X				X
Soft palate						X			
Tonsil						X		X	
Oropharynx wall						X			
Base of tongue						X			

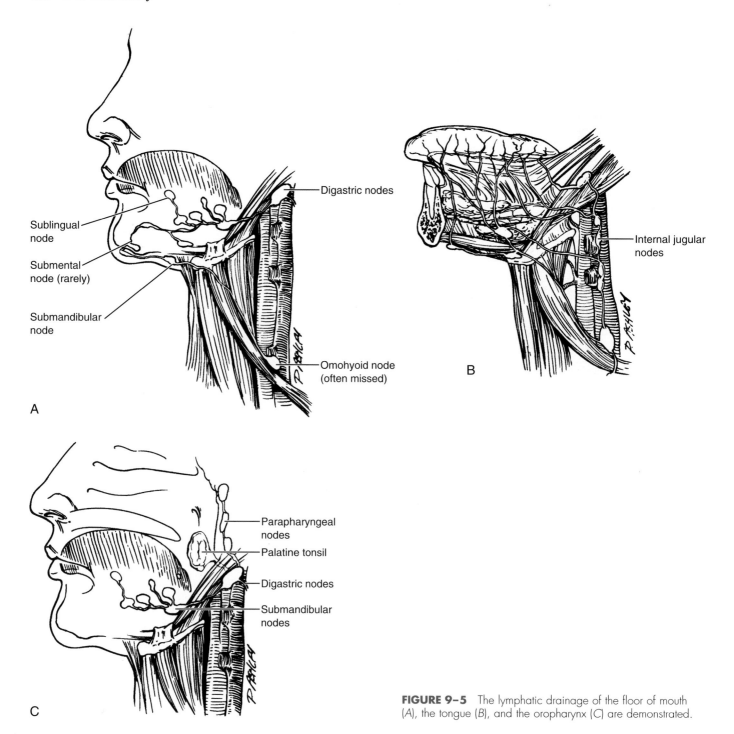

FIGURE 9–5 The lymphatic drainage of the floor of mouth (*A*), the tongue (*B*), and the oropharynx (*C*) are demonstrated.

addition to oral papillomas, is associated with hamartomas of the gastrointestinal tract, ovarian cysts, thyroid adenomas, and fibrocystic breast lesions. The thyroid and breast lesions of this disease have been considered to be premalignant, and the incidence of breast cancer in these patients is as high as 25%.[6–13]

BENIGN MIXED TUMOR

Benign mixed tumor (Fig. 9–6), or pleomorphic adenoma, is the most common benign salivary gland neoplasm. Approximately 5.5% of pleomorphic adenomas arise from an intraoral minor salivary gland, most commonly of the hard palate, the soft palate,

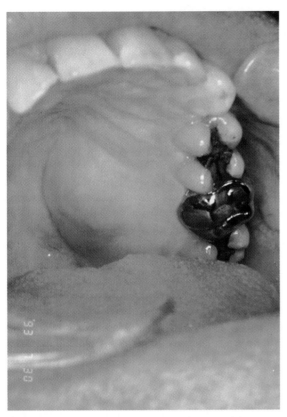

FIGURE 9–6 Slow-growing benign mixed tumor of the minor salivary glands of the palate.

or the upper lip. The typical history upon presentation is that of a smooth-surfaced, painless, slowly growing mass, although bursts of rapid growth are not uncommon. The age at presentation can range from 6 to 85 years, but the tumor is most commonly seen in individuals in their fifth decade. The lesions tend to be relatively small, rarely exceeding 1 to 2 cm at the time of presentation.

Complete surgical excision is the treatment of choice, and recurrence is rare. Owing to extension of the tumor through its incomplete fibrous capsule, enucleation or "shelling out" is ill-advised. Malignant transformation of mixed tumors, although uncommon, has been reported.[7,14–16]

Mesenchymal Lesions

PYOGENIC GRANULOMA

Pyogenic granuloma (Fig. 9–7) is the most common benign gingival growth encountered. It is a lesion that is thought to arise secondary to local trauma and irritation of the mucosa, followed by bacterial invasion and subsequent formation of exuberant granulation tissue. Known irritants believed to be causative include calculus, defective dental restorations, food debris, and endotracheal intubation. At one time, these lesions were thought to be transmitted from horses to humans as a botryomycotic disease, but this has since been disproven.

Although pyogenic granuloma may occur anywhere on the body, the oral cavity, with its rich microflora, is an excellent environment for its development. As it is associated with neither purulence nor granulomatous disease, the name pyogenic granuloma is somewhat misleading. It usually presents as an elevated, soft, painless, sessile, or pedunculated growth with a smooth red surface. Often, there is surface ulceration.

On radiographic examination, bone resorption is not seen; this can be useful in differentiating the lesion from a periodontal abscess. These lesions may also mimic early Kaposi's sarcoma, which must be considered in the differential diagnosis, particularly in HIV-positive individuals or patients with AIDS. These patients have an increased propensity for the development of both pyogenic granulomas and Kaposi's sarcoma. Treatment by conservative excision is usually curative, although recurrences can occur (particularly if the causative irritant is not removed).

Pyogenic granulomas have been associated with bone marrow transplants and pregnancy. The latter is termed a "pregnancy tumor" or "granuloma gravidarum." In this case, the lesions usually occur in the first trimester of pregnancy, often regressing after termination of gestation. If postpartum regression does not occur, the treatment is conservative excision. Tumors may recur at the same site with subsequent pregnancies.[7,10,16–19]

PERIPHERAL GIANT CELL GRANULOMA

The second most common benign gingival growth is referred to by many names, including peripheral giant cell granuloma, peripheral giant cell tumor, gingival giant cell granuloma, giant cell epulis, myeloid epulis, and osteoclastoma (Fig. 9–8). Like pyogenic

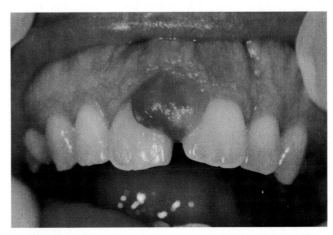

FIGURE 9–7 Pyogenic granuloma. Nodular mass of the maxillary gingiva.

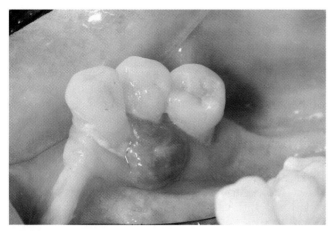

FIGURE 9–8 *Peripheral giant cell granuloma. Ulcerated mass of the mandibular gingiva.*

granuloma, it is thought to be due to tissue trauma; unlike pyogenic granuloma, it occurs only in tooth-bearing areas (or on the soft tissue over the alveolar ridge in edentulous areas) and may originate from osteoclasts at either the periodontal ligament or mucoperiosteum. It presents as a sessile, red-purple, vascular, hemorrhagic or easily bleeding mass that is usually singular but sometimes multilobulated, and that often arises anterior to the first molars. The size of these lesions varies, but usually ranges from 0.5 to 1.5 cm, and surface ulceration is often seen.

On radiographic examination, this lesion is seen to erode the underlying bone, which helps to differentiate it from a pyogenic granuloma. Treatment for this lesion is excision; owing to its bone-eroding properties, resection should be performed as quickly as possible. Recurrences, although reported, are rare.[10,16,17]

PALISADED ENCAPSULATED NEUROMA

Palisaded encapsulated neuroma is a small, solitary, peripheral nerve lesion that was first described in 1972.[18,19] Most reported examples of this rare lesion have involved the skin of the face, but the lesion has also been reported to occur on the oral mucosa, predominantly that of the hard palate. Currently, the cause of palisaded encapsulated neuroma is unknown, but local tissue injury may be contributory. This entity presents in the oral cavity as a small, firm, solitary, sessile nodule that may be partially or completely encapsulated. Usually, persons in their fifth or sixth decade of life are affected. In one study, excluding traumatic neuromas, this lesion represented 22% of the intraoral tumors of peripheral nerve origin.[20] These neuromas have been confused with the mucosal neuromas of multiple endocrine neoplasia (MEN) type 3 and with neurofibromas. Although the treatment of choice for neuromas in general is surgical excision, no long-term follow-up studies have been reported to document the effective control of this lesion.

BENIGN SCHWANNOMA

Benign schwannoma, also called Schwann cell tumor or neurilemmoma, is a benign, encapsulated, perineural tumor that arises from Schwann cells. It can occur in any nerve tissues that possess Schwann cells, including the cranial nerves (except cranial nerves I and II), peripheral nerves, spinal nerves, and the nervous tissue of the autonomic nervous system. Although relatively uncommon, it is the most common peripheral nerve sheath tumor in the oral cavity.

Benign schwannomas may involve either the soft tissues or bone, but most commonly originate in the tongue. Usually, these lesions appear as sessile, smooth-surfaced, well-circumscribed, firm lesions. They are slow-growing and painless. If, however, the tumor pushes on adjacent nerves, pain or paresthesias may be present. Symptoms are usually attributable to mechanical effects of the expanding tumor, and include speech and swallowing difficulties, tooth migration, or denture instability. Epidemiologic studies have shown that schwannomas can occur at any age, although oral schwannomas tend to occur in the second and third decades. Some studies demonstrate a female preponderance, whereas others report equal incidence among the sexes.

When present in bone, schwannomas create a sharply defined, unilocular or multilocular radiolucency, often with bone resorption around tooth roots. Magnetic resonance imaging (MRI) may be helpful in further narrowing the diagnosis. Treatment is surgical excision. Because schwannomas are encapsulated, they can usually be separated away from the nerve. However, great care must be exercised in removing the tumor to avoid permanent neurologic sequelae. Recurrence has been reported following incomplete excision; malignant transformation is extremely rare, and some authors have questioned that it occurs at all.[20–28]

NEUROFIBROMA AND MULTIPLE MUCOSAL NEUROMA SYNDROME

The neurofibroma can present as a solitary nodule or as a feature of the many neurofibromatosis syndromes. Additionally, there has been an association reported between neurofibromas and MEN type 3 (also called multiple mucosal neuroma syndrome). Neurofibromas are far more common than neuromas (by a ratio of 8:1) and, like neuromas, are of nerve sheath or Schwann cell origin. In contrast to schwannomas, which are typically well-encapsulated, neurofibromas do not possess a capsule, although they may be well circumscribed. This factor has implications when considering surgical treatment, as these lesions usually cannot be separated from the nerve during resection.

Solitary neurofibromas of the oral cavity occur more frequently in whites and, although they can occur at any age, are more commonly seen in the third or fourth decades of life. They usually present as asymptomatic, small, smooth-surfaced, sessile nodules. In order of frequency, these lesions may be found in the cheek, palate, tongue, lips, and alveolar ridge. These tumors characteristically grow very slowly, and treatment alternatives include clinical observation and surgical excision.

As many as seven different subtypes of neurofibromatosis have been described; however, only the most common—neurofibromatosis type 1—will be discussed here. Neurofibromatosis type 1, or von Recklinghausen's disease, is an autosomal dominant disease characterized by the presence of multiple neurofibromas in the skin, oral cavity, gastrointestinal tract, bones, and central nervous system. Although this disorder is autosomal dominant, only half of those afflicted will have a positive family history; the remainder of cases are attributable to spontaneous mutation. There is a slight male predominance, and the condition usually presents before the age of 1 year, almost always by early adulthood. Pigmented skin patches, known as café au lait spots, axillary or inguinal freckling, and multiple neurofibromas are the hallmarks of neurofibromatosis type 1. Although oral lesions associated with this disease were once considered rare,[27] incidence rates as high as 95% have recently been reported.[28] The tongue is the most common location for multiple oral neurofibromas.

Malignant degeneration has been reported in as many as 15% of cases. Although there are no curative treatments for this disease, conservative excision may be performed when practical. Individuals with oral involvement should be watched closely for early signs of disease progression that might lead to facial disfigurement and oral dysfunction. If such lesions are detected, surgical excision should be considered. As previously mentioned, separation of these lesions from the adjacent nerve is usually not possible, and permanent deficit of the adjacent nerve is to be expected.[28,29]

Multiple mucosal neuroma syndrome, also known as MEN type 2b or 3 is inherited in an autosomal dominant pattern. Like neurofibromatosis type 1, about 50% of cases are the result of sporadic mutation. This syndrome's most significant feature is medullary thyroid carcinoma, which is present in more than 90% of cases. Other associated disease processes include marfanoid habitus (but not Marfan syndrome), pheochromocytoma, medullated corneal nerves, and gastrointestinal ganglioneuromatosis. Unlike MEN 1 (Werner's syndrome), it is not associated with pituitary, parathyroid, or pancreatic island lesions; unlike MEN 2a (Sipple's syndrome) hyperparathyroidism is not seen. Multiple mucosal neuroma syndrome and MEN 2a do have medullary thyroid carcinoma and pheochromocytoma in common, however.

Multiple mucosal neuromas, which are often noted at birth and almost always by the age of 10 years, are likely to be present on the anterior tongue or the lips, but can present anywhere in the mucosa of the upper aerodigestive tract. These lesions are also seen on the eyelids, the corneas, and the skin. The medullary thyroid carcinoma associated with this syndrome occurs most commonly during the adolescent years and may be more aggressive than in sporadically appearing cases. More than 90% of patients with a palpable thyroid nodule have metastatic disease as well. One test used for screening is the measurement of serum calcitonin levels after either calcium or pentagastrin challenge. Metastases can be detected with computed tomography (CT) scans, ultrasonography, and radionuclide scanning. Total thyroidectomy for medullary thyroid carcinoma is the treatment of choice. Because of the association between multiple mucosal neuroma syndrome and this aggressive carcinoma, anyone suspected of having this syndrome, as well as all first-degree relatives, should undergo careful screening.[30]

MELANOTIC NEUROECTODERMAL TUMOR OF INFANCY

The melanotic neuroectodermal tumor of infancy (MNTI) is a rare tumor that has been called by as many as 23 different names in the past. This plethora of titles is due, in part, to the confusion of the tumor's origin. In the past, these tumors were thought to have been derived from ectopic retinal cells or from odontogenic structures. Modern staining techniques, however, indicate that MNTI is a neural crest cell tumor. This theory has been substantiated by the tumor's clinical characteristics, as well as immunohistochemical studies.

MNTI presents almost exclusively in the head and neck and shows no predilection for either sex. The most frequent site of origin is the maxilla (accounting for almost 70% of cases), followed by the skull, mandible, and brain. The tumor usually appears as a pigmented, fast-growing, nonulcerating soft-tissue lesion that displaces the upper lip.

Most cases of MNTI present by the age of 3 months, and nearly all are manifest by the age of 1 year. CT scans show an expansile or erosive hyperdense mass, often with a sharply demarcated bony rim. Although these lesions usually follow a benign course, malignant change occurs in up to 4% of cases. Complete, conservative resection is the standard treatment, although it has been reported that local excision with curettage of the underlying bone is sufficient in cases in which a more extensive resection would be mutilating. Local recurrence, expected in 10% to 15% of cases, is treated by repeated conservative excision.[8,31–34]

CONGENITAL EPULIS AND GRANULAR CELL TUMOR

Granular cell tumors (Fig. 9–9) are benign lesions of enigmatic origin, but the most favored candidate for

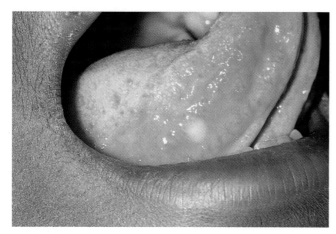

FIGURE 9–9 Granular cell tumor. Submucosal nodule on the ventral tongue.

the parent cell line is the Schwann cell or its undifferentiated mesenchymal precursor. Some researchers theorize that multiple cell lines can give rise to granular cell tumors. It is classically taught that the "mucosal" or "noninfantile" granular cell tumor and congenital epulis are both subtypes of granular cell tumors; some, however, emphasize that congenital epulis is not a variation of the granular cell tumor, but rather a distinct clinical and histopathologic entity.[2,35–37]

Congenital epulis (Fig. 9–10) presents in females eight times more frequently than in males and is found in the maxilla three times as often as in the mandible, usually at the site of eventual canine or lateral incisor tooth eruption. The underlying bone and unerupted teeth are usually not involved. The congenital epulis often appears as a firm, pink, or fleshy, broad-based, polypoid, mucosa-covered lesion varying in diameter from several millimeters to 9 cm. The smaller tumors are asymptomatic, but the

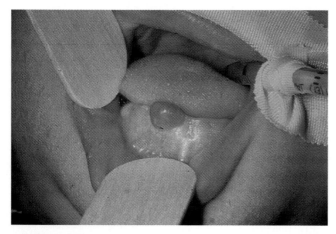

FIGURE 9–10 Congenital epulis. Polypoid mass on the anterior mandibular alveolar ridge in a newborn.

larger ones may cause airway or feeding difficulties. Occasionally, the lesions can be multicentric, and they have been reported to occur simultaneously in both the mandible and maxilla. They are not known to grow after birth, implicating possible in utero maternal hormonal stimulation as a factor, and occasionally, they have been reported to undergo spontaneous regression. Treatment is complete surgical excision.[36–39]

The mucosal or noninfantile granular cell tumor most commonly presents in adults in the second to sixth decades of life and shows a 2:1 female predominance over males. The lateral border of the tongue is the most common site in the oral cavity, followed by the hard palate, floor of the mouth, gingiva, and lip. It is usually a painless, solitary, mucosa-covered nodule measuring less than 2 cm in diameter, but it may be multifocal in up to 16% of cases. As in congenital epulis, treatment is complete excision. Although recurrence of these tumors occurs in approximately 8% of cases, not all those with positive margins will lead to recurrence. Further excision is generally curative.[40]

Malignant variants of granular cell tumor exist, but are quite rare. Clinically, metastasis is the primary indicator of malignancy, as benign and malignant varieties appear the same on histologic examination. Metastasis involves the regional lymph nodes, lungs, viscera, and bones. The mean age at presentation is 48 years of age, which is 16 years older than patients with benign granular cell tumors. Treatment is surgical excision, but the prognosis is poor, with death usually ensuing within 2 years.[35,37]

HEMANGIOMA

Although many classification systems for vascular lesions have been proposed, one well-accepted system that is based on biological behavior, as well as histologic appearance, divides them into hemangiomas and vascular malformations. Vascular malformations may be further subclassified by their vessel of origin; that is, arterial, venous, capillary, lymphatic, or combined.[41–43]

Hemangiomas (Fig. 9–11) are the most common tumors of childhood[44] and represent benign vascular neoplasms that enlarge by rapid cellular proliferation. These lesions are frequently seen in the oral cavity, and, although present at birth, may not appear clinically until 4 weeks of age. Female individuals are affected more commonly than male subjects by a ratio of 3:1. Initially, hemangiomas may present as erythematous macular patches or as localized telangiectasias. The consistency of hemangiomas is firm or rubbery, and they are not readily compressed or drained of blood. They usually grow rapidly until the age of 6 to 8 months (the proliferation phase), and then slowly and spontaneously resolve over the next several years (the involution phase). In general,

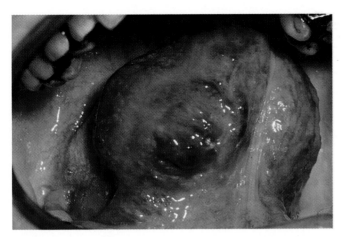

FIGURE 9–11 Hemangioma. Exophytic bluish-purple mass on the ventral surface of the tongue.

50% of hemangiomas will involute completely by the age of 5 years, 70% by the age of 7 years, and nearly all will spontaneously involute by the age of 12 years, although no known factor can predict the time course of involution.

Complications include ulceration, local obstruction, recurrent hemorrhage, and profound thrombocytopenia secondary to platelet trapping within the lesion (Kasabach-Merritt syndrome). As hemangiomas spontaneously involute, the treatment of such lesions is observation, unless the size, location, or complications associated with the lesion cause significant morbidity. Systemic steroids have been reported to accelerate the involutional process.[42] On a case-by-case basis, excision, embolization, laser photocoagulation, and sclerotherapy may also be considered, either alone or in combination.

By contrast, vascular malformations do not represent true neoplasms, but instead are hamartomas that occur secondary to an aberration in the development of the primitive vascular system (retiform plexus). These lesions, like hemangiomas, are physically present at birth but are usually subclinical; they may become clinically apparent at any age. They may be either low- or high-flow lesions. *Capillary* malformations are usually noted at birth, as are *lymphatic* vascular malformations. The appearance of *venous* malformations may be linked to times of hormonal flux, including puberty, pregnancy, and the initial use of birth control pills. *Arterial* and *arteriovenous* malformations usually present later in life. Malformations generally are soft, compressible, and can be emptied of their blood supply with gentle pressure. Growth of these malformations is commensurate with the patient's growth, and these lesions typically will not involute spontaneously. Treatment must be individualized and may include embolization, sclerotherapy, cryotherapy, laser photocoagulation, or surgical excision either alone or in combination.[41–49]

OSTEOMA

Although osteomas are more commonly seen in the paranasal sinuses, in rare cases they may present as tumors of the maxilla and mandible, the latter being the more frequent oral site. They can appear at any age, but are most commonly found in the young adult. As the tumor is slow-growing, it usually presents as a painless, hard, expansile mass. The endosteum or periosteum can be the source of the lesion; periosteal lesions grow more rapidly than the former and may be clinically apparent earlier. On radiographic studies, a well-circumscribed, expansile, sclerotic, radio-opaque mass of mature bone is usually seen.

Multiple lesions, especially in the mandibular ramus, may be seen in association with Gardner's syndrome. This condition is characterized also by autosomal dominant heredity, colonic polyps that are prone to adenocarcinomatous transformation, odontomas, subcutaneous fibrous tumors, and skin epidermal inclusion cysts. An even more rare subtype—the "soft-tissue osteoma" of the oral cavity—has appeared as an osteoma within the tongue or buccal mucosa. Of the two, the tongue is the more common site. These lesions may present with a sensation of gagging or throat irritation.

The growth of osteomas will often arrest; therefore, observation is often adequate treatment. If, however, the lesion continues to grow or is symptomatic, conservative excision is the treatment of choice.[2,10,16,50–52]

CHONDROMA

Although rare, oral cavity chondromas have been reported to occur in extraosseous and intraosseous locations. They are thought to arise from a residuum of Meckel's cartilage or vestigial cartilaginous rests, but they have also been postulated to occur as a result of trauma secondary to ill-fitting dentures. Extraosseous lesions are found most commonly on the lateral tongue, but have also been reported to occur, albeit rarely, in the soft tissue of the cheek. They tend to present in the third and fourth decades of life as firm, painless, mucosa-covered nodules. Extraosseous chondromas are seen in equal distribution between the sexes. Intraosseous chondromas have been reported to be seen more commonly both in the maxilla and the mandible by different authors; when presenting in the mandible, the coronoid and condylar processes, as well as the area behind the cuspids, are favored sites of presentation. Like their extraosseous counterparts, these lesions have no sex predilection, but they tend to occur most frequently in the sixth decade of life. These tumors grow slowly and are characterized by painless, localized swelling, malocclusion, loosened teeth, or decreased mandibular range of motion.

Irregular areas of radiolucency, mottled areas, and

TABLE 9-2	APPROXIMATE 5-YEAR SURVIVAL OF SQUAMOUS CELL CARCINOMA, BY SITE OF PRIMARY LESION

SITE	5-YEAR SURVIVAL(%)
Lip	75
Tongue	>30
Floor of mouth	21–66
Gingiva	26
Palate	35
Tonsil	12–48
Buccal mucosa	16–89

local destruction with adjacent tooth root resorption may all be seen on plain radiographs. Chondromas can become malignant, locally infiltrative, and difficult to eradicate. At times, they may behave as low-grade chondrosarcomas. Treatment should consist of radical local excision with a wide cuff of normal tissue and histologically cleared margins.[10,16,52–54]

MALIGNANT NEOPLASMS

Epithelial Lesions

SQUAMOUS CELL CARCINOMA

Squamous cell carcinomas (SCC) of the oral cavity and oropharynx constitute approximately 5% of all newly diagnosed cancers and are responsible for up to 15,000 deaths annually. Approximately 90% of the malignant lesions in the oral cavity and oropharynx are of this histologic type. In general, SCC is more common in men than in women, and is most commonly seen in individuals older than 50 to 60 years of age. Clearly, the most commonly cited risk factors for this lesion are the use of alcohol and tobacco products. Other, less clear associations have also been identified and include syphilis, herpesvirus, cytomegalovirus, HIV, chronic trauma and irritation (including that caused by ill-fitting dental appliances), malnutrition, and poor oral hygiene. The risk of developing an additional oral cavity or pharyngeal cancer has been found to increase 74-fold in male patients with SCC of the oral cavity, whereas the increase in risk for women is 190-fold. Lesions are usually firm and can ulcerate. Fungating, exophytic masses are also seen. Pain is rarely a symptom, unless ulceration and bacterial inflammation occur.

The site of presentation in order of frequency is as follows: lip (30% to 40%), tongue (15% to 25%), floor of the mouth (20%), gingiva (6%), palate (5% to 6%), tonsil (5%), and buccal mucosa (2%). Treatment involves both surgical excision and radiotherapy in various combinations. Treatment protocols must be tailored to the individual patient based on the exact anatomic site of involvement. Prognosis varies by tumor location (Table 9–2), tumor thickness, presence and extent of vascular and perineural invasion, age, sex, histologic grade, and TNM classification, with the latter being the most important (Tables 9–3 and 9–4; Fig. 9–12). The presence of metastasis, which varies by site (see Table 9–1) cuts the survival rate by half.

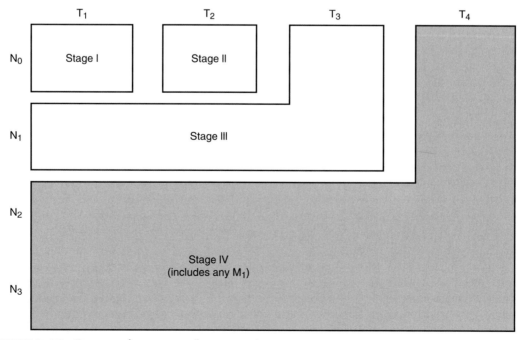

FIGURE 9-12 Grouping of squamous cell carcinoma by stage. Data from the American Joint Committee on Cancer, 1995.

T A B L E 9 – 3	**TNM CLASSIFICATION, LIP AND ORAL CAVITY**

PRIMARY TUMOR (T)

TX	Primary tumor cannot be assessed
T0	No evidence of primary tumor
Tis	Carcinoma in situ
T1	Tumor ≤2 cm in greatest dimension
T2	Tumor >2 cm but ≤4 cm in greatest dimension
T3	Tumor >4 cm in greatest dimension
T4	Lip tumor invades adjacent structures (e.g., through cortical bone, tongue, skin of neck)
T4	Oral cavity tumor invades adjacent structures (e.g., through cortical bone, into deep [extrinsic] muscle of tongue, maxillary sinus, skin)

REGIONAL LYMPH NODES (N)

NX	Regional lymph nodes cannot be assessed
N0	No regional lymph node metastasis
N1	Metastasis in a single ipsilateral lymph node, ≤3 cm in greatest dimension
N2	Metastasis in a single ipsilateral lymph node, >3 cm but ≤6 cm in greatest dimension; or in multiple ipsilateral lymph nodes, none >6 cm in greatest dimension; or
	N2a Metastasis in a single ipsilateral lymph node, >3 cm but ≤6 cm in greatest dimension
	N2b Metastasis in multiple ipsilateral lymph nodes, none >6 cm in greatest dimension
	N2c Metastasis in bilateral or contralateral lymph nodes, none >6 cm in greatest dimension
N3	Metastasis in a lymph node >6 cm in greatest dimension

DISTANT METASTASIS (M)

MX	Presence of distant metastasis cannot be assessed
M0	No distant metastasis
M1	Distant metastasis

Data from *Manual for Staging of Cancer*. 5th ed. American Joint Committee on Cancer. 1995.

T A B L E 9 – 4	**TNM CLASSIFICATION, OROPHARYNX**

PRIMARY TUMOR (T)

TX	Primary tumor cannot be assessed
T0	No evidence of primary tumor
Tis	Carcinoma in situ
T1	Tumor ≤2 cm in greatest dimension
T2	Tumor >2 cm but ≤4 cm in greatest dimension
T3	Tumor >4 cm in greatest dimension
T4	Tumor invades adjacent structures (e.g., through cortical bone, soft tissues of neck, deep [extrinsic] muscle of tongue

REGIONAL LYMPH NODES (N)

NX	Regional lymph nodes cannot be assessed
N0	No regional lymph node metastasis
N1	Metastasis in a single ipsilateral lymph node, ≤3 cm in greatest dimension
N2	Metastasis in a single ipsilateral lymph node, >3 cm but ≤6 cm in greatest dimension; or in multiple ipsilateral lymph nodes, none >6 cm in greatest dimension; or
	N2a Metastasis in a single ipsilateral lymph node, >3 cm but ≤6 cm in greatest dimension
	N2b Metastasis in multiple ipsilateral lymph nodes, none >6 cm in greatest dimension
	N2c Metastasis in bilateral or contralateral lymph nodes, none >6 cm in greatest dimension
N3	Metastasis in a lymph node >6 cm in greatest dimension

DISTANT METASTASIS (M)

MX	Presence of distant metastasis cannot be assessed
M0	No distant metastasis
M1	Distant metastasis

Data from *Manual for Staging of Cancer*. 5th ed. American Joint Committee on Cancer. 1995.

Several site-specific variations in tumor behavior have been elaborated. The lip is the most common site for oral carcinomas, and greater than 90% of these occur on the lower lip. In addition to the use of tobacco (especially pipe smoking) and alcohol, chronic exposure to sunlight is also considered to be a risk factor. The most common area of lip involvement is the paramedian vermilion border. Clinically, these lesions are slow-growing, but if left untreated, they eventually invade adjacent structures and metastasize.

The tongue is the next most common site for SCC; and, excluding the lip, it is the site of involvement for half of all intraoral carcinomatous lesions. The anterior two thirds of the lateral/ventral tongue is most commonly affected; lesions of the posterior third tend to present in a more advanced stage. Patients with lesions of the tongue base often present initially with an enlarging neck mass. Of special note is that metastasis from anterior tongue lesions is known to skip directly to the jugulodigastric nodes; thus, this area of the neck must always be addressed when treating metastatic disease.

SCCs involving the floor of the mouth (Fig. 9–13) are most likely to appear in men older than 60 years of age, and in this group, the anterior floor of mouth is most commonly affected. These carcinomas tend to exhibit extension to adjacent tissues at the time of diagnosis; if so, the individual's prognosis is much poorer.

SCC is more likely to involve the gingiva of the mandible than the gingiva of the maxilla, and usually, lesions are found posterior to the canine teeth. Edentulous areas are at increased risk. As with floor of the mouth lesions, gingival SCC tends to present in men older than 60 years of age and is likely to involve adjacent structures, such as the periosteum and underlying bone, at the time of diagnosis. Often, the diagnosis is delayed, as early lesions may mimic or be masked by dental infection.

The palate (including the hard palate, soft palate, and uvula) is a less common site of these cancers. Of all palatal lesions, however, SCC is still the most common type. The uvula is a rather rare site of SCC, comprising less than 1% of cases. Invasion of the underlying bone in hard palate lesions is relatively common.

Tonsillar lesions usually appear in the sixth decade, but in rare instances, they may occur in younger individuals. In this younger subset, the prognosis is poorer, as the disease process is noted to be more rapidly and relentlessly progressive. As with tongue base lesions, presentation with an enlarging neck mass is not uncommon.

The least common site for SCC is the buccal mucosa. Most buccal lesions involve the area below the occlusal plane and may readily invade the adjacent soft tissues. Unlike most SCCs, these lesions are often painful. Metastasis at the time of presentation is common and, when present, portends a poorer prognosis.

As previously mentioned, the primary treatment modalities for SCC are radiation therapy and surgery, with chemotherapy usually being reserved for palliation or research protocols. Literally volumes have been written regarding the management of these lesions. In addition to stage and location, factors to be considered when selecting a specific therapy also include the physical, social, and emotional status of the patient. For smaller lesions, irradiation and surgery may yield equal rates of cure. The disadvantages of irradiation include post-treatment mucositis, xerostomia, and osteoradionecrosis, but the risk of long-term disability may be less. Radiation therapy typically does not yield as great a cure rate as surgery or combined therapy for larger lesions or for metastatic disease. Brachytherapy has been especially successful as a treatment for tongue base lesions in individuals in whom operative morbidity would likely be very high. Surgical treatment is usually preferred for large yet curable lesions, especially those with bony involvement. The disadvantages of surgery include anesthetic risks and postoperative functional disability. Combined therapy may offer the best chance of cure in advanced lesions; no studies have shown a difference in survival between the use of preoperative versus postoperative irradiation. In any case, a team approach, involving the otolaryngologist, radiation oncologist, medical oncologist, dentist, prosthodontist, and speech pathologist, is advised.[1,2,7,16,55–63]

VERRUCOUS CARCINOMA

Verrucous carcinoma presents as a relatively uncommon variant of well-differentiated SCC (Fig. 9–14). This lesion is seen primarily in the oral cavity, although extraoral sites of presentation, including the larynx, trachea, major bronchi, nasal mucosa, bladder, esophagus, skin, and anogenital regions, have

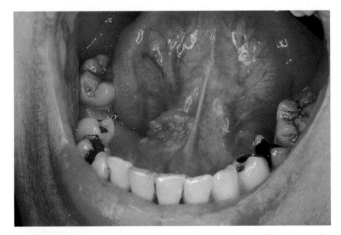

FIGURE 9–13 Squamous cell carcinoma. Ulcerated lesion involving the right floor of the mouth.

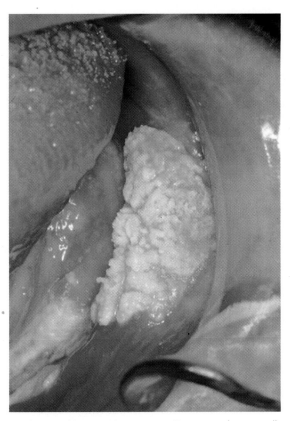

FIGURE 9–14 Verrucous carcinoma. Extensive white, papillary lesion of the mandibular gingiva.

been reported. Most commonly found on the buccal mucosa (>40%), followed, in order of frequency, by the alveolar mucosa, palate, and floor of the mouth, verrucous carcinoma accounts for 2% to 9% of all oral SCCs. Male patients older than 50 years of age are most frequently affected and, although the etiology is unclear, there have been reports of an association with ill-fitting dentures, poor oral hygiene, and the use of snuff, chewing tobacco, betel nut mixtures, and cigars. There is a variable relationship with HPV, which in some series has been noted to be present in up to 41% of cases. There may be a causal relationship, but in many cases the sensitivity of assays to detect the virus may be inadequate. A related lesion—verrucous hyperplasia—can only be differentiated by histologic examination and is thought by some to be an antecedent lesion to verrucous carcinoma.

Lesions of verrucous carcinoma may have a variable appearance, but usually are found to be nonulcerated, white growths with papillary, pebbly, or warty surfaces. They may vary in size from a few millimeters to several centimeters and are usually painless. Central ulcerations can occasionally occur. Verrucous carcinoma is characterized by slow and persistent local growth, with spread occurring by local invasion and tissue destruction; fortunately, metastasis is exceedingly rare. Diagnosis often may require multiple biopsy studies, and the biopsy must be sufficiently deep and peripheral to allow the relationship of the tumor to the normal surrounding tissue to be studied.

Although many lesions may be radiosensitive, surgical excision is the treatment of choice. In the past, there has been great controversy regarding the use of radiotherapy to treat this entity because of reports of anaplastic transformation after treatment with this modality. The average incidence of such transformation is reported to be only 7%, and it usually occurs within the first 6 months after therapy. Many now believe that the importance of radiotherapeutic malignant transformation has been overstated and that radiotherapy has a place in the treatment of selected cases. Primary lesion control rates for irradiation alone are reported to be slightly less than 50%. By comparison, surgery alone yields much better local control, with recurrence rates reported to be between 0% and 18%.[64–71]

ADENOID CYSTIC CARCINOMA

In the oral cavity, it is estimated that there are 500 to 700 minor salivary glands. Many sources list mucoepidermoid carcinoma as the most frequent malignant lesion involving these glands; however, conflicting reports indicate that adenoid cystic carcinoma is actually the most common. Adenoid cystic carcinoma accounts for approximately 30% of all minor salivary gland tumors and 16% of all intraoral tumors. Most commonly, these lesions present as smooth, painless masses, usually of the palate, and almost never in the midline. Other, less frequent sites of occurrence include the tongue, cheek, and alveolar ridges. A feeling of pressure or swelling is also common, and pain may rarely be present as well. These carcinomas are biologically aggressive, following a clinical course of indolent but relentless progression. Perineural invasion is a prevalent feature, often making curative resection difficult. It is not uncommon for metastases, usually involving the lungs or bone, to present many years after treatment of the primary lesion. Regional lymphatic spread is rarely seen. Radiographs may be helpful in assessing the degree of spread, as invasion beyond the skull base may be inferred by enlargement of the foramen ovale or foramen rotundum. The primary treatment for adenoid cystic carcinoma is wide local excision, often followed by radiation therapy, especially if tissue margins are positive. As regional lymphatics are not commonly involved, elective neck dissection is not indicated. Excision of local recurrences or isolated distant metastases, however, may prolong survival. Reported 5-year survival rates are as high as 58%; nevertheless, 20-year survival rates are less than 10%, so lifelong clinical follow-up is essential.[72–78]

POLYMORPHOUS LOW-GRADE ADENOCARCINOMA

First described by the term polymorphous low-grade adenocarcinoma in 1983, this salivary gland neoplasm was previously known as terminal duct adenocarcinoma and lobular carcinoma. It is a rare tumor, affecting patients between the ages of 30 and 70 years, with a mean age at presentation of 60 years. There is a female preponderance by a ratio ranging from 2:1 to 4:1. In the past, these tumors were confused with other neoplasms, such as carcinoma ex pleomorphic adenoma, adenocarcinoma not otherwise specified, pleomorphic adenoma, or adenoid cystic carcinoma.

A painless, firm, nonulcerated, raised, 1- to 4-cm mass that has been present for weeks to years is the usual presentation. The most common site for polymorphous low-grade adenocarcinoma, as with many other minor salivary gland neoplasms, is the palate, followed by the upper lip and buccal mucosa. The treatment of choice is complete surgical excision. The recurrence rate is 17% to 24%. Metastasis to the regional lymph nodes occurs in less than 10% of cases, so elective lymph node dissection is not warranted. The prognosis, in general, is favorable.[74,79-84]

MUCOEPIDERMOID CARCINOMA

As noted in the discussion of adenoid cystic carcinoma, mucoepidermoid carcinoma (Fig. 9–15) is thought by many to be the most common malignant lesion involving the minor salivary glands. Although there may be controversy regarding its incidence in adults, this lesion is definitely the most common malignant lesion in the pediatric population. An association with previous radiotherapy to the head and neck has been reported, sometimes antedating the tumor by more than 30 years. Male and female patients are equally affected, and although the tumor can occur at any age, it is most commonly seen in adults in the third to sixth decade. There are two main subsets of mucoepidermoid carcinoma, low- and high-grade, which are considered separately. There is also an intermediate grade, which shares characteristics with both groups.

Low-grade mucoepidermoid carcinomas usually appear as slow-growing, smooth, painless masses, usually measuring less than 5 cm in diameter and sometimes resembling a mucocele. The most common site of involvement for these lesions is the palate, but they can occur at any intraoral location. Most children with mucoepidermoid carcinoma have the low-grade variety. These tumors usually follow a benign pattern of behavior and rarely metastasize. Treatment for these lesions is complete, wide, local excision. Although these tumors are prone to local recurrence, especially if incompletely excised, metastasis is very rare. The prognosis for cure is excellent.

By contrast, high-grade mucoepidermoid carcinoma presents as a rapidly growing, painful mass whose behavior may mimic that of SCC. It can readily infiltrate surrounding structures and frequently metastasizes to regional lymph nodes, lung, bone, skin, and brain. Radical, wide, local excision is the treatment of choice for these lesions, followed by postoperative radiation therapy. Prophylactic lymph node dissection may be indicated, but is definitely warranted for clinically palpable disease. Prognosis is relatively poor, with a maximum 5-year survival rate of approximately 40%.[2,7,10,16,85,86]

MALIGNANT MELANOMA

The oral cavity is a rare site for the occurrence of malignant melanoma. The incidence has been variously reported to be 0.1% to 8% of all melanomas, with most studies favoring the lower figure. The percentages are somewhat higher in certain populations, notably the Japanese, in whom the incidence approaches 7%, and Ugandans, in whom oral mucosal melanoma accounts for 8% of all melanomas. Other groups that exhibit an increased incidence of oral mucosal melanomas include southwestern Native Americans and Hispanics. Some researchers have reported a higher rate in whites as compared to blacks, but others dispute this. Men are more commonly affected than women by a ratio of 2:1. Many authors have tried to correlate risk factors to the appearance of these tumors, but with the small number of cases, meaningful data are sparse. There does, however, appear to be a correlation with pre-existing pigmented lesions of the palate, for which numerous etiologies have been identified (Table 9–5).

Oral cavity melanomas tend to present during the fourth to seventh decade, with an average age at presentation of 50 years. The most common site of presentation in the oral cavity is the palate, followed by the maxillary gingiva. Together, these sites account for nearly 80% of primary lesions. The remaining 20% involve the gingiva of the mandible, buccal mucosa, floor of the mouth, tongue, and lips.

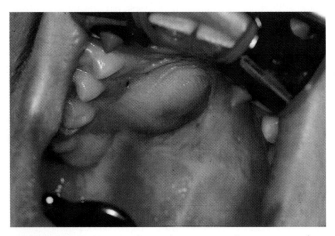

FIGURE 9–15   Mucoepidermoid carcinoma. Fluctuant mass of the soft palate.

TABLE 9 – 5	ETIOLOGIES OF FOCAL PIGMENTATION IN THE ORAL CAVITY			
FOREIGN BODIES	**DRUGS**	**ECCHYMOSES**	**NEOPLASMS**	**SYSTEMIC DISORDERS**
amalgam tattoos	antimalarials	trauma	nevi	Addison's disease
lead pencils	minocycline	bleeding diathesis	oral melanotic macule	Albright's syndrome
carbon	chlorpromazine		Kaposi's sarcoma	Peutz-Jegher's syndrome
dyes	amiodarone		malignant melanoma	neurofibromatosis
ink	phenolphthalein			hemochromatosis
	oral contraceptives			β-thalassemia
				Wilson's disease
				acromegaly
				porphyria

Modified from Eisen D, Voorhees JJ. Oral melanoma and other pigmented lesions of the oral cavity. *J Am Acad Dermatol.* 1991; 24:527.

Presentation is variable, but usually the lesions are pigmented, soft, painless, irregular, and ulcerated. Often, the painless nature of these lesions will cause a patient to delay seeking evaluation. Loosening of teeth and bony destruction does occur. Occasionally, there is a rapid growth phase during which the lesion becomes painful and circumscribed by erythema, and then begins to bleed. Amelanotic melanomas, which account for 5% to 15% of oral cavity melanomas, have a similar presentation except that they are usually pink. The possibility of metastatic lesions to the oral cavity must also be considered when establishing the diagnosis. Metastasis of oral melanomas may involve the regional lymphatics or may occur via hematogenous routes to the liver and bone. Demonstrable lymph node metastasis is present in approximately 50% of all cases at the time of diagnosis.

The treatment for melanomas of the oral cavity is radical surgical excision, usually accompanied by lymph node dissection. Prophylactic lymph node dissection in the absence of clinically apparent regional metastasis is a controversial procedure, but should be performed if the tumor thickness exceeds 3 mm (in the absence of distant metastasis). Radiotherapy and chemotherapy may play a minor adjuvant or palliative role in treatment. The prognosis is uniformly poor and does not correlate to cutaneous melanomas with regard to thickness (i.e., Clark's levels). Most affected patients succumb to their disease within 2 years; 5-year survival rates are as low as 2.9% to 5.9%. With the knowledge that approximately two thirds of these lesions will present in a pre-existing, focally pigmented area, a low threshold for excisional biopsy of pigmented oral lesions is appropriate.[87–92]

Mesenchymal Lesions

KAPOSI'S SARCOMA

This sarcoma, rare prior to the advent of AIDS, is now found most commonly in homosexual and bisexual men infected with HIV. In fact, it is the most frequent oral cavity malignancy in this population. The incidence has been steadily decreasing since 1983, when it involved 33% of these patients. At present it affects less than 15% of HIV-infected individuals; in the United States the male:female ratio is approximately 20:1. Four variants of Kaposi's sarcoma are known to occur in the oral cavity (Table 9–6). Only AIDS-associated Kaposi's sarcoma (Fig. 9–16) is commonly seen, however. The primary mechanism postulated in the etiology of this malignant tumor, as in many others, is the failure of immune surveillance. Because 2% of homosexual men with this tumor do not have HIV, and because they are 10 times more likely to develop the tumor than patients who contracted HIV through heterosexual contact or blood-product exposure, Kaposi's sarcoma may be, in part, due to another transmissible agent.

Kaposi's sarcoma can appear at any stage of the HIV infection; the oral cavity, which may be the initial and sole site in 22% of patients with AIDS, eventually becomes involved in nearly half of patients with these tumors. They may appear as isolated or multiple; as blue, red, or purple; as nodules, macules, or plaques, most often with exophytic surfaces that are occasionally ulcerated. The size of these lesions varies from a few millimeters to several centimeters. They tend not to blanch, which may be helpful in differentiating them from vascular neoplasms. Nonpigmented lesions have rarely been reported. Initially these lesions are asymptomatic, but in as many as 33% of patients, they may become painful or obstructive as they grow. While any area of the oral cavity and oropharynx may be involved, there is a predilection for the attached mucosa of the palate and gingiva. Although growth of these lesions is inevitable, the rate of progression is highly variable. Treatment is aimed at palliation and may include cryotherapy, laser ablation, surgical excision, radiation therapy, and chemotherapy. Chemotherapeutic methods include the use of single or multiple parenteral agents as well as intralesional agent injec-

TABLE 9 – 6	CLASSIC	AFRICAN	IATROGENIC	AIDS-ASSOCIATED
COMPARISON OF CLINICAL VARIANTS OF KAPOSI'S SARCOMA				
Population at Risk	Mediterranean basin	Africa	immunosuppressed and renal transplantees	homosexual and bi-sexual males, others with AIDS
Prevalence	rare	endemic	rare	10% of all patients with AIDS
Age at Onset	50–80	children 2–15 adults 25–50	any age	any age
M:F Ratio	10–15:1	children 3:1 adults 17:1	2.3:1	20:1[a]
Skin Lesions	lower extremities	all extremities, internal viscera, lymph nodes	any area	any area
Oral Lesions	rare	rare	rare	common, especially attached mucosa
Prognosis	good	fair to poor	good	poor

[a] An epidemiologic average. Reports vary from as low as 2.3:1 to as high as 106:1.
  Data from Epstein JB, Siverman S Jr. Head and neck malignancies associated with HIV infection. *Oral Surg Oral Med Oral Pathol.* 1992; 73:193 and Regezi JA, MacPhail LA, Daniels TE, et al. Oral Kaposi's sarcoma: A 10-year retrospective histopathologic study. *J Oral Pathol Med.* 1993; 22:292.

tion. Sclerosing agents may also be injected around the lesion.

The prognosis of patients with AIDS-associated Kaposi's sarcoma is poor, ranging from 3 months to 5 years, with an average survival rate of 21 months. Negative prognostic variables include the presence of opportunistic infections, other constitutional symptoms of HIV, CD4+ counts of less than $300/mm^3$, and female sex. Treatment of these lesions has not been shown to affect survival, and the effects of chemotherapy may further suppress the patient's immune system. The risks and benefits of all treatment options, therefore, must be carefully weighed.[92–99]

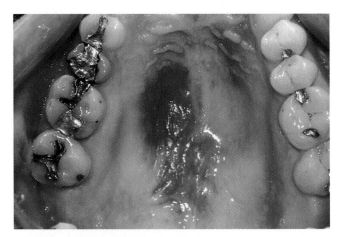

FIGURE 9–16 Large areas of Kaposi's sarcoma presenting a flat, brownish discoloration of the hard palate.

OSTEOSARCOMA

With the exception of multiple myeloma, osteosarcoma (osteogenic sarcoma) is the most common malignancy of bone. These tumors generally arise in the long bones of young adults and adolescents. Only about 4% to 6% arise within the bony structures of the oral cavity, with the most common site being the mandible. Within the mandible, osteosarcomas may occur (in decreasing order of frequency) in the body, symphysis, angle, or ramus. Unlike patients with long-bone tumors, those with oral cavity lesions present at a mean age of 30 years. Males are slightly more often afflicted than females, and—while most occur spontaneously—reported associations link osteosarcoma to a history of trauma, Paget's disease of bone, fibrous dysplasia, prior radiotherapy, and injection of Thorotrast (an intravenous radioactive contrast material). Two subtypes occur outside the medullary space of bones. The first is juxtacortical (paraosteal or periosteal) osteosarcoma. It accounts for approximately 5% of all skeletal osteosarcomas and is exceedingly rare in the oral cavity. Second, and rarer still, are the soft-tissue osteosarcomas, which can occur in extraskeletal sites including the heart, bladder, and tongue.

These aggressive tumors often present with either asymptomatic or painful swelling around the mandible or maxilla, sometimes with accompanying paresthesias. Often there is an antecedent history of tooth extraction, as it is common for teeth to loosen near the tumor. Invasion of the overlying gingiva is unusual. Two characteristic radiographic findings are of note. One of the earliest and most specific findings for this malignancy is symmetric widening of the periodontal ligament space on a periapical dental film. The osteoblastic (or sclerosing) form of osteosarcoma will yield a "sunburst" appearance on plain radiographs, due to the trabeculae and spicules of new bone being produced by the tumor. This is seen in about 25% of osteosarcomas. The osteolytic form may show a nondescript radiolucency with expansion or destruction of the cortical plates. Regarding laboratory studies, an elevation of serum alkaline phosphatase is often found.

Treatment for these lesions is radical surgical excision; some studies report a benefit from the use of combined modalities, adding radiation and/or chemotherapy, but these series are small. Metastasis, which occurs in about half of these cases, is most often by the hematogenous route to the lungs and brain. As it is less commonly seen in regional lymphatics, *prophylactic* neck dissection is not recommended. *Therapeutic* neck dissections, however, have been shown to be of benefit. Mandibular osteosarcomas appear to have a slightly better prognosis than those from the maxilla, with 5-year survival rates of 41% and 25%, respectively.[2,7,10,16,52,100-106]

CHONDROSARCOMA

Chondrosarcoma is a rare tumor of the mandible and maxilla; compared to its benign counterpart, the chondroma, it is much more common. The sexes are equally affected. This tumor is more likely to occur in the maxilla, especially the anterior alveolar ridge. When occurring in the mandible, the premolar and molar regions are most often involved. The mean age for individuals to present with these tumors is 55 years with a range of 10 to 80 years; they usually present as painless masses. Other less common symptoms include loosening or eruption of teeth and local paresthesias. Growth is usually relatively slow but can be unpredictable. Tumors that occur in those younger than 21 years of age tend to grow more rapidly and be more destructive. Radiographs show localized bone destruction without erosion of the cortex. Except for the lack of the sun-ray effect, these lesions appear similar to osteosarcomas.

A distinct subclass of this lesion, the mesenchymal chondrosarcoma, deserves special note. It is extraordinarily rare and appears in persons aged 10 to 30 years. It has a predilection for the ribs and the jaws and presents as a painless swelling of the bone. Radiographs show an osteolytic lesion that may be stippled by calcifications. Its course is highly variable but often prolonged, and metastases may appear many years after the primary tumor.

The treatment of chondrosarcomas is wide local excision. In one third to one half of cases, hematogenous metastasis or local recurrence occurs. Metastatic spread is most frequent to the lungs or bone. Local extension by mandibular lesions into the mediastinum and by maxillary lesions to the skull base will lead to the patient's death in many cases.

Five-year survival and long-term survival may be as low as 17%—much lower than that of osteosarcoma.[2,7,10,16,52,107-110]

CONCLUSION

A wide variety of benign and malignant tumors are known to present in the oral cavity and oropharynx, arising from most embryonic cell lines. The list presented in this chapter is far from complete. Regardless of the type of lesion, though, early detection and diagnosis are paramount. Careful examination of the region is the key to early detection of such lesions and, in the case of malignancy, almost certainly yields a more favorable prognosis for the patient. As the clinical presentation of these lesions is often similar, the need for early biopsy in order to achieve a definitive diagnosis cannot be overemphasized. For the majority of lesions, surgery is the mainstay of therapy, often augmented by adjunct therapeutic methods.

REFERENCES

1. Alvi A, Meyers E, Johnson J. Cancer of the oral cavity. In: Meyers E, Suen J, eds. *Cancer of the Head and Neck.* 3rd ed. Philadelphia: WB Saunders; 1996:321.
2. Wenig BM. *Atlas of Head and Neck Pathology.* Philadelphia: WB Saunders; 1993.
3. Civantos FJ, Goodwin WJ Jr. Cancer of the oral cavity. In: Meyers E, Suen J, eds. *Cancer of the Head and Neck.* 3rd ed. Philadelphia: WB Saunders; 1996:361.
4. Ossof RH, Bytell DE, Hast MH, Sisson GA. Lymphatics of the floor of the mouth and periosteum: Anatomic studies with possible clinical correlations. *Otolaryngol Head Neck Surg.* 1980; 88:652.
5. Lindberg R. Distribution of cervical lymph node metastasis from squamous cell carcinoma of the upper respiratory and digestive tracts. *Cancer.* 1972; 29:1146.
6. Yeatts D, Burns J. Common oral mucosal lesions in adults. *Am Fam Physician.* 1991; 44:2043.
7. Batsakis JG. *Tumors of the Head and Neck, Clinical and Pathological Considerations.* 2nd ed. Baltimore: Williams & Wilkins; 1979.
8. Wood NK, Goaz PW. *Differential Diagnosis of Oral Lesions.* 2nd ed. St Louis: Mosby; 1980.
9. Welch TB, Baker BF, Williams C. Perioxidase-antiperoxidase evaluation of human oral squamous cell papillomas. *Oral Surg.* 1986; 61:603.
10. Shafer WG, Hine MK, Levy BM. *A Textbook of Oral Pathology.* 4th ed. Philadelphia: WB Saunders; 1983.
11. Rock JA, Fisher ER. Florid papillomatosis of the oral cavity and larynx. *Arch Otolaryngol.* 1960; 72:593.
12. Mosovich B, Gatot A, Zirkin H. Widespread oral papillomatosis due to chronic buccal trauma. *Cutis.* 1989; 43:254.
13. Devlin MF, Barrie R, Ward-Booth RP. Cowden's disease: A rare but important manifestation of oral papillomatosis. *Br J Oral Maxillofac Surg.* 1992; 30:335.
14. Miles DA, Lovas JG, Daley TD. Intraoral pleomorphic adenoma, report of a case presenting in an unusual location. *J Can Dent Assoc.* 1986; 1:75.
15. Eneroth CM, Blanck C, Jacobson RA. Carcinoma in pleomorphic adenomas of the parotid gland. *Acta Otolaryngol.* 1968; 66:477.
16. Bhaskar SN. *Synopsis of Oral Pathology.* St. Louis: Mosby; 1986.
17. Brown FH, Houston GD. Differential diagnosis of localized

tumors of the gingiva. *Compend Cont Ed Gen Dent.* 1990; 11: 700.

18. Regezi JA, MacPhail LA, Daniels TE, et al. Oral Kaposi's sarcoma: A 10-year retrospective histopathologic study. *J Oral Pathol Med.* 1993; 22:292.

19. Lee L, Miller PA, Maxymiw WG, et al. Intraoral pyogenic granuloma after allogeneic bone marrow transplant. *Oral Surg Oral Med Oral Pathol.* 1994; 78:607.

20. Williams HK, Cannell H, Silvester K, Williams DM. Neurilemmoma of the head and neck. *Br J Oral Maxillofac Surg.* 1993; 31:32.

21. Colin W. Trigeminal intraoral schwannomas. *Compend Cont Ed Gen Dent.* 1990; 11:672.

22. Artzi Z, Taicher S, Nass D. Neurilemmoma of the mental nerve. *J Oral Maxillofac Surg.* 1991; 49:196.

23. Zachariades N, Mezitis M, Vairaktaris D, et al. Benign neurogenic tumors of the oral cavity. *Int J Oral Maxillofac Surg.* 1987; 16:70.

24. Hribernik SJ, Gould AR, Alpert B, Jones JL. Well-circumscribed mass of the lateral floor of the mouth. *J Oral Maxillofac Surg.* 1992; 50:741.

25. Carstens PH, Schrodt GR. Malignant transformation of a benign encapsulated neurilemmoma. *Am J Clin Pathol.* 1969; 51:144.

26. Hatziotis JC, Asprides H. Nerilemmoma (schwannoma) of the oral cavity. *Oral Surg.* 1967; 24:510.

27. Barden E, Pierce HE, Jackson WF. Multiple neurofibromatosis with oral lesion. *Oral Surg.* 1955; 8:263.

28. D'Ambrosio JA, Langlais RP, Young RS. Jaw and skull changes in neurofibromatosis. *Oral Surg Oral Med Oral Pathol.* 1988; 66:391.

29. Yamada N, Uchinuma E, Shioya Y, et al. Plexiform neurofibromatosis in an infant. *Br J Plast Surg.* 1992; 45:175.

30. Kirk JF, Flowers FP, Ramos-Caro FA, Browder JF. Multiple endocrine neoplasia type III: Case report and review. *Pediatr Dermatol.* 1991; 8:124.

31. Irving RM, Parikh A, Coumbe A, Albert DM. Melanotic neuroectodermal tumor of infancy. *J Laryngol Otol.* 1993; 107:1045.

32. Kim YG, Oh JH, Lee SC, Ryu DM. Melanotic neuroectodermal tumor of infancy. *J Oral Maxillofac Surg.* 1996; 54:517.

33. Shah RV, Jambhekar NA, Durgesh N, et al. Melanotic neuroectodermal tumor of infancy: Report of a case with ganglionic differentiation. *J Surg Oncol.* 1994; 55:65.

34. Cutler LS, Chaudhry AP, Topazian R. Melanotic neuroectodermal tumor of infancy: An ultrastructural study, literature review, and reevaluation. *Cancer.* 1981; 48:257.

35. Kershisnik M, Batsakis JG, Mackay B. Pathology consultation–granular cell tumors. *Ann Otol Rhinol Laryngol.* 1994; 103:416.

36. Damm D, Cibull ML, Geissler RH, et al. Investigation into the histogenesis of congenital epulis of the newborn. *Oral Surg Oral Med Oral Pathol.* 1993; 76:205.

37. Mirchandani R, Sciubba JJ, Rabia M. Granular cell lesions of the jaws and oral cavity: A clinicopathologic, immunohistochemical, and ultrastructural study. *J Oral Maxillofac Surg.* 1989; 47:1248.

38. Zuker RM, Buenechea R. Congenital epulis: Review of the literature and case report. *J Oral Maxillofac Surg.* 1993; 51:1040.

39. Al-Qattan MM, Clarke HM. Congenital epulis: Evidence against the intrauterine estrogen stimulus theory. *Ann Plast Surg.* 1994; 33:320.

40. Lack EE, Worsham GF, Callihan MD, et al. Granular cell tumor: A clinicopathologic study of 110 patients. *J Surg Oncol.* 1980; 13:301.

41. Mulliken JB, Glowacki J. Hemangiomas and vascular malformations in infants and children: A classification based on endothelial characteristics. *Plast Reconstr Surg.* 1982; 69:412.

42. Garfinkle TJ, Handler SJ. Hemangiomas of the head and neck in children—a guide to management. *J Otolaryngol.* 1980; 9:439.

43. Edgerton MJ. Treatment of hemangiomas, with special reference to the role of steroid therapy. *Ann Surg.* 1976; 183:517.

44. Stal S, Hamilton S, Spira M. Hemangiomas, lymphangiomas, and vascular malformations of the head and neck. *Otolaryngol Clin North Am.* 1986; 19:769.

45. Mulliken JB, Young AE. *Vascular Birthmarks: Hemangiomas and Malformations.* Philadelphia: WB Saunders; 1988.

46. Kaban LB, Mulliken JB. Vascular anomalies of the maxillofacial region. *J Oral Maxillofac Surg.* 1986; 44:203.

47. Wahrman JE, Honig PJ. Hemangiomas. *Pediatr Rev.* 1994; 15:266.

48. Thwaites MS, Tatum RC. Hemangiomas: Vascular malformations of childhood. Report of a case with literature review. *Quintessence Int.* 1988; 19:841.

49. Fishman SJ, Mulliken JB. Hemangiomas and vascular malformations of infancy and childhood. *Pediatr Clin North Am.* 1993; 40:1177.

50. Krolls SO, Jacoway JR, Alexander WN. Osseous choristomas (osteomas) of intraoral soft tissues. *Oral Surg.* 1971; 32:588.

51. Sookasam M, Philipsen HP. The intra-oral soft tissue osteoma: Report of two cases. *J Dent Assoc Thai.* 1986; 36:229.

52. Chow JM, Skolnik EM. Nonsquamous tumors of the oral cavity. *Otolaryngol Clin North Am.* 1986; 19:573.

53. Cutright DE. Osseous and chondromatous metaplasia caused by dentures. *Oral Surg.* 1972; 34:625.

54. Blum MR, Danford M, Speight PM. Soft tissue chondroma of the cheek. *J Oral Pathol Med.* 1993; 22:334.

55. Kramer S, Gelber RD, Snow GB, et al. Combined radiation therapy and surgery in the management of advanced head and neck cancer: Final report of study 73-03 of the Radiation Therapy Oncology Group. *Head Neck Surg.* 1987; 10:19.

56. Kornblut AD. Clinical evaluation of tumors of the oral cavity. In: Thawley SE, Panje WR, Batsakis JG, Lindberg RD, eds. *Comprehensive Management of Head and Neck Tumors.* Philadelphia: WB Saunders; 1987:469.

57. Scully, C. Oncogenes, tumour suppressors and viruses in oral squamous carcinoma. *J Oral Pathol Med.* 1993; 22:337.

58. Wolf GT, Urba S, Hazuka M. Induction chemotherapy for organ preservation in advanced squamous cell carcinoma of the oral cavity and oropharynx. *Recent Results Cancer Res.* 1995; 134:133.

59. Langford A, Langer R, Lobeck H, et al. Human immunodeficiency virus-associated squamous cell carcinomas of the head and neck presenting as oral and primary intraosseous squamous cell carcinomas. *Quintessence Int.* 1995; 26:635.

60. Jovanovic A, van der Tol IG, Schulten EA. Risk of multiple primary tumors following oral squamous-cell carcinoma. *Int J Cancer.* 1994; 56:320.

61. Shah JP, Lydiatt W. Treatment of cancer of the head and neck. *CA Cancer J Clin.* 1995; 45:352.

62. Mashberg A, Samit A. Early diagnosis of asymptomatic oral and oropharyngeal squamous cancers. *CA Cancer J Clin.* 1996; 45:328.

63. Silverberg E, Boray CC, Squires TS. Cancer statistics. *Cancer.* 1990; 40:9.

64. Jordan RC. Verrucous carcinoma of the mouth. *J Can Dent Assoc.* 1995; 61:797.

65. McCoy JM, Waldron CA. Verrucous carcinoma of the oral cavity. *Oral Surg Oral Med Oral Pathol.* 1981; 52:623.

66. Shroyer KR, Greer RO, Fankhouser CA, et al. Detection of human papillomavirus DNA in oral verrucous carcinoma by polymerase chain reaction. *Mod Pathol.* 1993; 6:669.

67. Murrah VA, Batsakis JG. Proliferative verrucous leukoplakia and verrucous hyperplasia. *Ann Otol Rhinol Laryngol.* 1994; 103:660.

68. Awange DO, Onyango JF. Oral verrucous carcinoma: Report of two cases and review of literature. *East Afr Med J.* 1993; 70:316.

69. Cannon CR, Hayne ST. Concurrent verrucous carcinomas of the lip and buccal mucosa. *South Med J.* 1993; 86:691.

70. Medina JE, Dichtel E, Luna MA. Verrucous squamous carcinomas of the oral cavity: A clinicopathologic study of 104 cases. *Arch Otolaryngol.* 1984; 110:437.

71. Tharp ME II, Shidnia H. Radiotherapy in the treatment of verrucous carcinoma of the head and neck. *Laryngoscope.* 1995; 105:391.

72. Chudrey AP, Vickers RA, Gorlin RJ. Intraoral salivary gland tumors: An analysis of 1,414 cases. *Oral Surg.* 1961; 14:1194.

73. Stuteville OH, Corley RD. Surgical management of tumors of the intraoral minor salivary glands: Report of 80 cases. *Cancer.* 1967; 20:1578.

74. Seifert G. Histopathology of malignant salivary gland tumors. *Oral Oncol Eur J Cancer.* 1992; 28B:49.
75. Hemprich A, Schmidseder R. The adenoid cystic carcinoma: Special aspects of its growth and therapy. *J Craniomaxillofac Surg.* 1988; 16:136.
76. van der Wal JE, Snow GB, Karim ABMF, van der Waal I. Intraoral adenoid cystic carcinoma: The role of postoperative radiotherapy in local control. *Head Neck.* 1989; 11:497.
77. Weber RS, Palmer M, El-Naggar A, et al. Minor salivary gland tumors of the lip and buccal mucosa. *Laryngoscope.* 1989; 99:6.
78. van der Wal JE, Snow GB, van der Waal I. Intraoral adenoid cystic carcinoma: The presence of perineural spread in relation to site, size, local extension, and metastatic spread in 22 cases. *Cancer.* 1990; 66:2031.
79. Clayton JR, Pogrel A, Regezi JA. Simultaneous multifocal polymorphous low-grade adenocarcinoma: Report of two cases. *Oral Surg Oral Med Oral Pathol.* 1995; 80:71.
80. Norberg I, Dardick I. The need for clinical awareness of polymorphous low-grade adenocarcinoma: A review. *J Otolaryngol.* 1992; 21:149.
81. Colmenero CM, Patron M, Burgueno M, Sierra I. Polymorphous low-grade adenocarcinoma of the oral cavity: A report of 14 cases. *J Oral Maxillofac Surg.* 1992; 50:595.
82. Vincent SD, Hammond HL, Finkelstein MW. Clinical and therapeutic features of polymorphous low-grade adenocarcinoma. *Oral Surg Oral Med Oral Pathol.* 1994; 77:41.
83. Evans HL, Batsakis JG. Polymorphous low-grade adenocarcinoma of minor salivary glands: A study of 14 cases of a distinctive neoplasm. *Cancer.* 1984; 53:935.
84. Batsakis JG, Pinkston GR, Luna MA, et al. Adenocarcinoma of the oral cavity: A clinicopathologic study of terminal duct adenocarcinomas. *J Laryngol Otol.* 1983; 97:825.
85. Regezi JA, Lloyd RV, Zarbo RJ, McClatchey KD. Minor salivary gland tumors. A histologic and immunohistochemical study. *Cancer.* 1985; 55:108.
86. Gluckman JL, Barrord J. Nonsquamous cell tumors of the minor salivary glands. *Otolaryngol Clin North Am.* 1986; 19:497.
87. Chaudhry AP, Hampel A, Gorlin RJ. Primary malignant melanoma of the oral cavity: Review of 105 cases. *Cancer.* 1958; 11:923.
88. Hormia M, Vuori EEJ. Mucosal melanoma of the head and neck. *J Laryngol Otol.* 1969; 83:349.
89. Bartowski SB, Panas M, Wilczanska H, et al. Primary malignant melanoma of the oral cavity: A review of 20 cases. *Am J Surg.* 1984; 148:362.
90. Kippax JB, Meyer ER, Gilmore W. Oral melanoma with oral squamous carcinoma: Report of a case. *J Oral Maxillofac Surg.* 1988; 46:620.
91. Peckitt NS, Wood GA. Malignant melanoma of the oral cavity. *Oral Surg Oral Med Oral Pathol.* 1990; 70:161.
92. Eisen D, Voorhees JJ. Oral melanoma and other pigmented lesions of the oral cavity. *J Am Acad Dermatol.* 1991; 24:527.
93. Ficarra G, Berson AM, Silverman S Jr, et al. Kaposi's sarcoma of the oral cavity: A study of 134 patients with a review of the pathogenesis, epidemiology, clinical aspects, and treatment. *Oral Surg Oral Med Oral Pathol.* 1988; 66:543.
94. Greenspan D, Greenspan JS. The oral clinical features of HIV infection. *Gastroenterol Clin North Am.* 1988; 17:535.
95. Scully C, Laskaris G, Pindborg J, et al. Oral manifestations of HIV infection and their management. I. More common lesions. *Oral Surg Oral Med Oral Pathol.* 1991; 71:158.
96. Epstein JB, Siverman S Jr. Head and neck malignancies associated with HIV infection. *Oral Surg Oral Med Oral Pathol.* 1992; 73:193.
97. Regezi JA, MacPhail LA, Daniels TE, et al. Oral Kaposi's sarcoma: A 10-year retrospective histopathologic study. *J Oral Pathol Med.* 1993; 22:292.
98. Ficarra G, Eversol LE. HIV-related tumors of the oral cavity. *Crit Rev Oral Biol Med.* 1994; 5:159.
99. Flaitz CM, Nichols CM, Hicks MJ. An overview of the oral manifestations of AIDS-related Kaposi's sarcoma. *Compendium.* 1995; 16:136.
100. Garrington GE, Scofield HH, Cornyn J, Hooker SP. Osteosarcoma of the jaws: Analysis of 56 cases. *Cancer.* 1967; 20:377.
101. Caron AS, Jahder SI, Strong EW. Osteogenic sarcoma of the facial and cranial bones: A review of 43 cases. *Am J Surg.* 1971; 122:719.
102. deFries HO, Perlin E, Leibel SA. Sarcoma of the mandible. *Arch Otolaryngol.* 1979; 105:358.
103. Mark R, Sercarz JA, Tran L, et al. Osteogenic sarcoma of the head and neck: The UCLA experience. *Arch Otolaryngol Head Neck Surg.* 1991; 117:761.
104. Wanebo HJ, Koness RJ, MacFarlane JK, et al. Head and neck sarcoma: Report of the head and neck sarcoma registry. *Head Neck.* 1992; 14:1.
105. Delgado R, Maafs E, Alferian A, et al. Osteosarcoma of the jaw. *Head Neck.* 1994; 16:246.
106. Calcaterra TC, Wang MB, Sercarz JA. Unusual tumors. In: Meyers E, Suen J., eds. *Cancer of the Head and Neck.* 3rd ed. Philadelphia: WB Saunders; 1996:644.
107. Chaudry AP, Robinovitch MR, Mitchell DF, et al. Chondrogenic tumors of the jaws. *Am J Surg.* 1961; 102:403.
108. Barnes R, Catto M. Chondrosarcoma of bone. *J Bone Joint Surg Br.* 1966; 48:729.
109. Sato K, Nukaga H, Horikoshi T. Chondrosarcoma of the jaws and facial skeleton: A review of the Japanese literature. *J Oral Surg.* 1977; 35:892.
110. Greer RO Jr, Rohrer MD, Young SK. Nonodontogenic tumors: Clinical evaluation and pathology. In: Thawley SE, Panje WR, Batsakis JG, Lindberg RD, eds. *Comprehensive Management of Head and Neck Tumors.* Philadelphia: WB Saunders; 1987: 1510.

III. TREATMENT OF ODONTOGENIC AND BONE-RELATED LESIONS*

- RAINER SCHMELZEISEN
- J. PREIN
- G. JUNDT

The choice of therapeutic procedures for odontogenic tumors depends predominantly on the histology of the lesion. In contrast to many other lesions of the body, head and neck lesions require special consideration concerning preservation of aesthetic and functional aspects in an exposed area.

The most frequent odontogenic lesions are odontogenic cysts. In general, their treatment offers the possibilities of cystostomies and cystectomies.

While malignant odontogenic and nonodontogenic tumors of the jaws must always be treated with adequate radicality and safety margins, benign tumors require decisions whether or not to preserve teeth in contact with the lesion. Additional decisions are to be made on preservation of nerves (i.e., inferior alveolar nerve, infraorbital nerve) or the continuity of the mandible. Large tumors of the maxilla may require classic maxillofacial approaches like the Le Fort I osteotomy.[1]

Lesions in the jaws present with relatively mild and often unspecific symptoms such as swelling, pain, disturbances of sensitivity, and loss of tooth vitality. Very often, these intaosseous lesions are asymptomatic and are detected during routine dental x-ray examinations. Since odontogenic cysts and tumors are not commonly located in areas well visualized by periapical films, panoramic radiographs are recommended in initial patient examination.

Because of the great therapeutic variety (i.e., long-term observation, nonsurgical treatment, enucleation, and radical resection), establishment of a histological diagnosis by biopsy is mandatory. For most odontogenic lesions of limited size, the intraoral route is the preferred approach.[2] Larger lesions, such as those extending into the ascending ramus, are exposed via extraoral approaches. If primary bone-grafting procedures are employed, the extraoral route should be favored, as even the smallest intraoral dehiscence may lead to an infection with loss of the grafted bone.

In edentulous patients or those with small lesions not requiring additional procedures on the teeth, the soft-tissue incision may be performed below the junction of free mucosa with attached gingiva. In dentate patients, marginal incisions often allow for a tighter wound closure. Posterior lesions require incisions at the anterior border of the ascending ramus comparable to the incision in a sagittal split procedure. The lesion is then exposed via the osteotomy of the buccal plate. The removal of the outer cortex should allow exposure of the entire lesion. Circumscribed, encapsulated lesions may be bluntly removed, and softer lesions can be enucleated with an elevator or curette. Endoscopic control may be of

*Based on DÖSAK Registry (German Austrian Swiss Association for the Study of Tumors of the Face and Jaw).

help. Here, a margin of normal bone in all directions can be burred away with round drills for additional safety.

Histologic differentiation of odontogenic lesions may be very difficult, as nonaggressive and aggressive lesions may demonstrate a similar histologic appearance. It is sometimes difficult to differentiate between unicystic ameloblastomas and follicular ameloblastomas or between cementifying fibromas and low-grade osteosarcomas. Therefore, the diagnostic evaluation of odontogenic lesions and the planning of surgical procedures must be interdisciplinary. Histological diagnosis can be made only by an experienced pathologist, with help if necessary from a registry for odontogenic tumors.[3] An open biopsy is mandatory in order to receive sufficient material in both quality and quantity.

Teeth are frequently associated with odontogenic lesions. In general, useful teeth should be retained if they do not compromise the removal of the lesions. The decision for preservation of a tooth is always made with regard to the histology of the lesion and not with regard to the tooth associated with it or with the prosthodontic value of a tooth.

Teeth involved in periapical cysts should be preserved with endodontic fillings and root resections if their stability in the bone can be maintained. Teeth involved with an ameloblastoma generally should be removed. Principally useful teeth should not be removed to gain better access to benign lesions where resection or enucleation would not be compromised by leaving these teeth. Teeth in the proximity of aggressive lesions may be retained if root canal therapy is done first, allowing for radical resection around the roots. Discretion must be used in both the retention and the removal of associated teeth.[4]

ODONTOGENIC LESIONS AND TUMORS—GENERAL REMARKS

Before surgical treatment, precautions should be taken to achieve adequate dental hygiene for preventing infection. In some lesions, it may be advisable to extract teeth in advance to allow for soft-tissue healing. This procedure may facilitate extraoral removal of a lesion without an intraoral perforation, as intraoral dehiscences often occur at the resection margin of the mucosa where the proximity of teeth does not allow for a watertight closure.

In lesions of the maxilla, it may be advisable to prepare a modified splint to keep a soft-tissue flap at the palate in situ or to prevent gauze packing from being dislocated into the oral cavity. After partial mandibular resections, the danger of fractures must be kept in mind. In these cases, reinforcement of the remaining bone with a plate may be advisable.

Table 9–7 presents a comparison of common odontogenic cysts and tumors discussed in the sections that follow.

Follicular and Radicular Cysts

Sensitivity tests of all surrounding teeth or a radiolucency are mandatory in order to detect teeth responsible for radicular cysts. In radicular and follicular cysts of the jaws, cystectomy must be regarded as the therapy of choice. Whether a cystectomy can be performed successfully depends mainly upon the location and the size of the cyst. Complete removal is necessary. If the cyst has contact with the inferior alveolar nerve, dissection must be carried out with great care. In all cysts exceeding the size of periapical lesions, the mucosal incision is performed as a marginal incision in order to avoid placing the suture line over the bony cavity and to avoid soft-tissue breakdown. In radicular cysts, the respective tooth must be extracted. Alternatively, a root resection can be performed. In follicular cysts, generally the impacted tooth is removed. In young patients, a decision made in close cooperation with an orthodontist determines whether the tooth is uncovered and mobilized into the alveolar arch and if its root development justifies its preservation. In selected cases, filling of the bony cavity with autologous bone may be indicated to allow an earlier implant placement. Materials such as hydroxyapatite or tricalcium phosphate should be used with great care.

In 1910, Carl Partsch recommended cystectomy only for small lesions. Larger cysts require a cystostomy if complicated wound healing is expected. Additionally, the dangers of damaging the inferior alveolar nerve or of devitalizing teeth are significantly lower after cystostomy. Marsupialization is also indicated for large lesions that pose a danger of serious bone loss, fractures, or danger to adjacent vital structures.

Parts of bone overlying the resected areas of the cyst are also removed. Opening of the cyst allows for chronic inflammation to subside. During the healing period, the cyst epithelium is replaced by epithelium of the oral mucosa. A mucoperiostal flap can be used to cover the inferior alveolar nerve or the teeth apices. Postoperatively, gauze is applied and changed weekly. After epithelialization of the cavity, an obturator avoids spontaneous closure of the lumen and penetration of foreign materials into the cavity. Large cysts of the mandible are fenestrated into the vestibule (Fig. 9–17 A–C).

Cystostomies are indicated in follicular cysts that originate from a tooth that must be preserved because of orthodontic or prosthodontic considerations. In these cases, the tooth is uncovered within the bone in order to facilitate its spontaneous vertical eruption to the alveolar crest. The decision to preserve teeth within follicular cysts depends on the prosthodontic value of the tooth, the age of the patient, and, especially, the grade of the root development.

TABLE 9–7 SURGICAL TREATMENT OF COMMON ODONTOGENIC CYSTS AND TUMORS

LESION	LOCATION	RADIOGRAPH	CLINICAL PRESENTATION	TREATMENT	RECURRENCE
Dentigerous cyst	Mandible, 3rd molar maxilla canine	Solitary, well-defined radiolucency associated with crown of unerupted tooth	Enlargement of jaw, possible displacement of teeth, intact cortex	Enucleation and curettage	Low
Odontogenic keratocyst	Mandible, 3rd molar/ramus region	Uni- or multilocular radiolucency with smooth or scalloped border	Enlargement of jaw, occasional pain and swelling; basal cell nevus syndrome	Enucleation and curettage	High
Ameloblastoma	Mandible, molar/ascending ramus region	Uni- or multilocular "soapbubble" radiolucency	Slow growth, asymptomatic expansion of jaw. Displacement of teeth, root resorption	Aggressive surgical resection	Recurrence almost certain with incomplete removal
Adenomatoid odontogenic tumor	Maxilla, canine region	Well-defined radiolucency associated with crown of impacted tooth	Asymptomatic, may produce expansion; root resorption	Enucleation and curettage	None
Odontogenic myxoma	Mandible, posterior especially	Mottled or "honeycomb" appearance, uni- or multilocular	Slow growth with bony expansion, possible destruction of cortex, possible displaced teeth, root resorption	Excision and agressive resection	Possible when incompletely removed
Ameloblastic fibroma	Mandible	Uni- or multilocular radiolucency	Slow growth, asymptomatic, possible bone expansion	Enucleation and curettage	Low
Odontoma	Maxilla, mandible	Irregular mass of calcified material surrounded by radiolucent band, may resemble a toothlike structure	Asymptomatic	Enucleation and curettage	Low

Modified according to AAOMS Surgical Update: Odontogenic Cysts and Tumors, Spring 1996 (12).

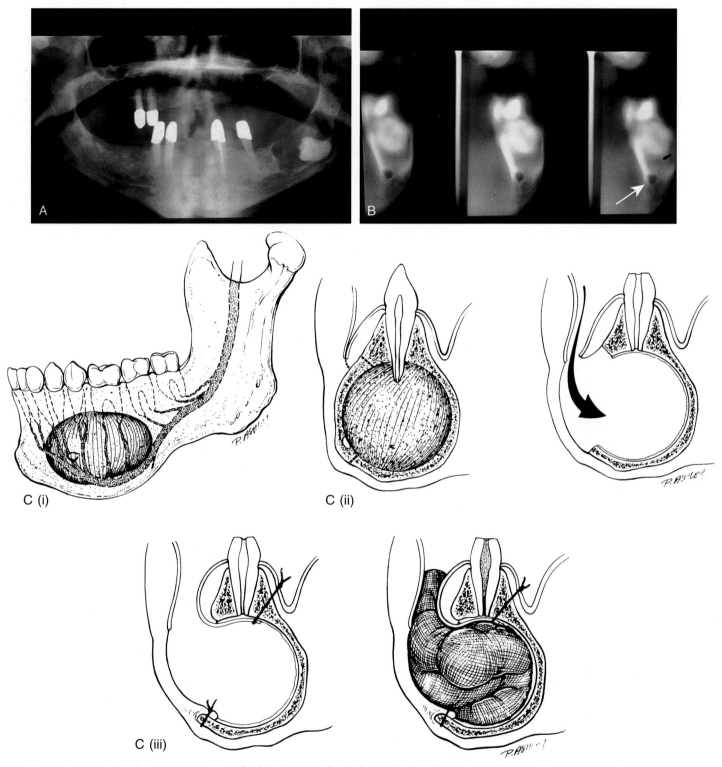

FIGURE 9-17 *A,* Radiologic appearance of a follicular cyst of the left mandible. *B,* The tomography reveals the anatomic relation between the lesion and the inferior alveolar nerve (*arrow*). *C,* Schematic drawings show: (i) cystostomy procedure of a radicular cyst of the body of the mandible, (ii) parts of bone overlying cyst drilled away and lateral aspects of cystic epithelium resected, and (iii) oral mucosa covering parts of the bony cavity and insertion of temporary packing.

Treatment of odontogenic cysts of the maxilla in general does not differ from the treatment of mandibular cysts. Depending on the size, cystostomies and cystectomies must be taken into consideration. Perforations of the nasal cavity and of the palate must be avoided. Therefore, cystostomies are regarded as the treatment of choice in large cysts in order to preserve the mucosal layer of the nasal cavity (Figs. 9–18 *A* and *B*; 9–19 *A–F*).

Follicular cysts protruding into the maxillary sinus are treated by a cystostomy, with the cyst becoming a part of the maxillary sinus. Additionally, a nasoantral opening in the inferior nasal meatus is created (Fig. 9–20).

Odontogenic Keratocyst

Many keratocysts do not cause any pain and are detected during routine dental examination. The mandible is involved in 60% to 80% of the cases (posterior body/ascending ramus). Keratocysts tend to grow in a similar anterior-posterior direction without obvious bone expansion.[5] At the time of detection, they may be extremely large, eventually penetrating into the skull base.[6,7]

Treatment of keratocysts differs significantly from that of other cystic lesions, as the recurrence rate ranges from 5% to 62%.[5] Recurrences have even been described in bone grafts.[8,9] Complete surgical

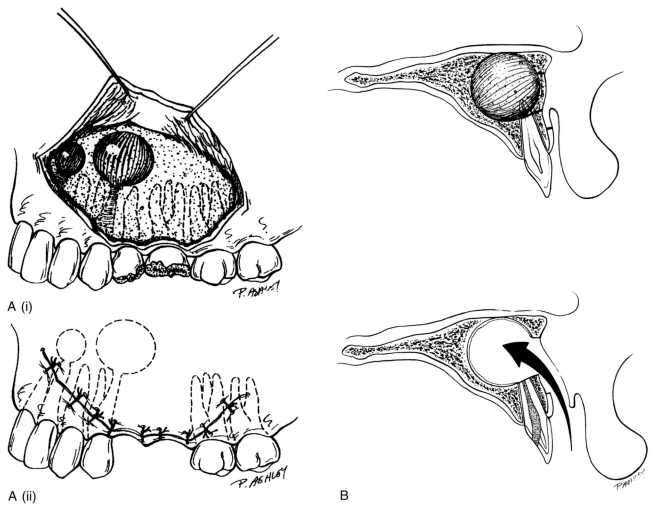

A (i)

A (ii)

B

FIGURE 9–18 *A,* Cystostomy of teeth 12 and 14. (i) A marginal incision combined with adequate wide base of trapezoid flap to provide safe coverage of mucosa over bony cavity. Sutures are never placed over the lumen. (ii) Cyst must be removed completely. Endodontic filling of the avital tooth (the teeth) is performed before or during cystectomy. After removal of radicular cyst, root resection is performed. Retrograde sealing may be performed with thermoelastic filling material or ceramic pins. *B,* Cysts in anterior maxilla are opened toward vestibulum (*arrow*). Perforations to nose should be avoided. Whenever possible, cysts are not fenestrated to nose because of difficulty in cleaning cysts connected to the nasal cavity.

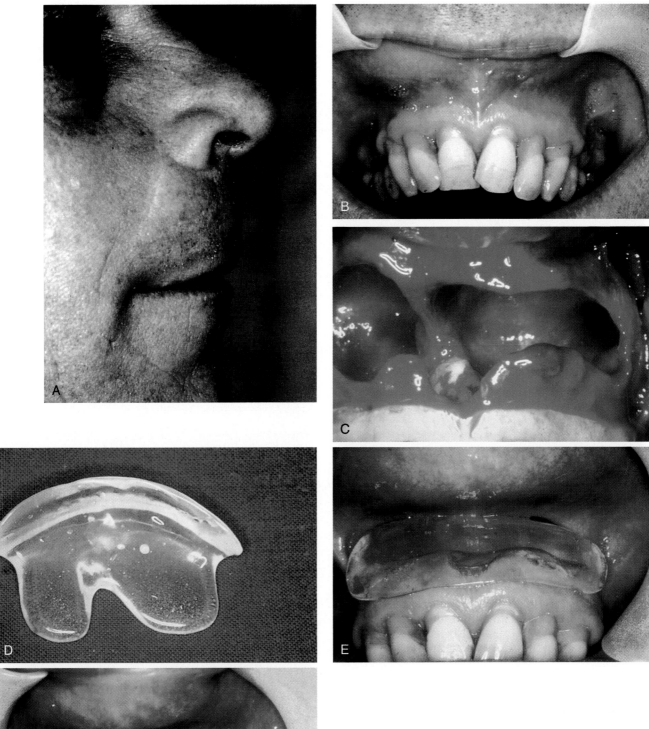

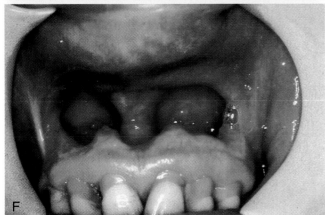

FIGURE 9–19 *A,* Clinical aspect of odontogenic radicular cyst, clinically visible as swelling of upper lip. *B,* Intraoral aspect with prominence of the maxillar vestibular mucosa. Due to large dimension of radicular cyst, the bony nasal floor was eroded. Endodontic fillings of teeth responsible for lesion are performed first. *C,* Intraoperative aspect of cystostomy performed to prevent perforation of nasal floor. *D,* Obturator for temporary occlusion of cystic lumen. *E,* Obturator in place. *F,* Diminishing of obturator volume temporarily decreases size of cyst.

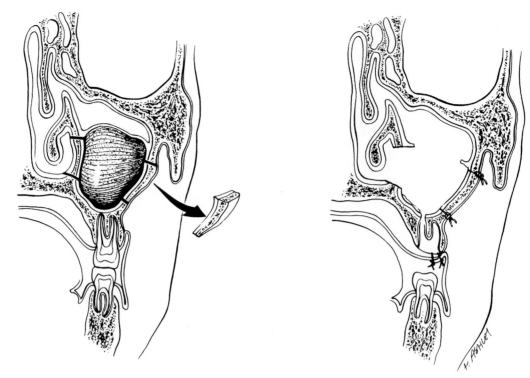

FIGURE 9–20 Cystostomy in the maxillary sinus with lumen of cyst connected to maxillary sinus. Nasoantral window is created in the same operation. Temporarily removed maxillary sinus wall (*arrow, left*) is repaired with resorbable sutures (*right*).

resection is recommended, yet it is important to be aware that the cyst wall is extremely vulnerable and difficult to remove completely. Additional satellite cysts in the wall are potential sources for recurrence. The intraoperative application of chemical cautery agents for the cyst wall, such as Carnoy's solution, facilitates removal. After removal, the bony walls of the cavity should be cleaned with a round drill. Partial or continuity resections of the mandible are indicated in cases of repeated recurrence. Despite the very low risk of malignant transformation, the high recurrence rate justifies a clinical and radiological long-term (5- to 10-year) follow-up.[5,10]

ODONTOGENIC TUMORS AND TUMOR-LIKE LESIONS

Tumors of Odontogenic Eptihelium without Odontogenic Ectomesenchyme

AMELOBLASTOMA

Besides odontoma, ameloblastoma is the most frequent odontogenic tumor. Ameloblastomas may originate from cell rests of the enamel organ, from a developing enamel organ, from the epithelial lining of an odontogenic cyst, or from the basal cells of the oral mucosa.[4] Radiologically, an ameloblastoma may present root resorptions of the teeth, but this sign is not considered pathognomonic for ameloblastoma (Table 9–8). With respect to its clinical behavior, an

TABLE 9 – 8	LESIONS ASSOCIATED WITH TOOTH ROOT RESORPTION ON X-RAYS

Ameloblastoma
Ameloblastic fibroma
Odontogenic myxoma
Adenomatoid odontogenic tumor
Cementoma
Calcifying odontogenic cyst
Odontogenic keratocyst

Ossifying fibroma
Fibrous dysplasia
Desmoplastic fibroma
Eosinophilic granuloma
Giant cell granuloma
Hemangioma
Osteosarcoma
Plasmocytoma

Adapted from Waldron CA, Mustoe TA. Primary intraosseous carcinoma of the mandible with probable origin in an odontogenic cyst. *Oral Surg Oral Med Oral Pathol.* 1989; 67:716–724.

ameloblastoma can be compared with a basal cell carcinoma.[3]

Because the tumor cannot be diagnosed clinically or radiologically with certainty, a biopsy must be performed. Differentiation between conventional ameloblastoma and unicystic ameloblastoma, especially the intraluminal and mural subtypes, is of therapeutic significance. While the intracystic or plexiform variant of unicystic ameloblastoma may be removed by a cystectomy procedure, mural unicystic ameloblastoma (with tumor extension into the wall) requires the same wide surgical en bloc resection as the conventional type of ameloblastoma.[11] However, the diagnosis of the different subtypes of unicystic ameloblastoma can be made only after complete histological evaluation of the resected specimen. If a small ameloblastoma is incidentally found inside a cyst and the external wall of the cyst is not involved or injured during removal, no further treatment is required.[2] Larger lesions are removed by en bloc resection and may require hemimandibulectomy. Postoperative radiotherapy and chemotherapy are contraindicated.[12,13] Long-term follow-up is advisable because of late recurrence even after 10 or more years.

The high rate of recurrence justifies the resection of the involved bone, as the actual margin of the tumor often extends beyond its apparent radiological or clinical margin. As most ameloblastomas are localized within the mandible, especially in the premolar/molar area and in the mandibular angle, radical segmental resection of the involved part via an extraoral approach is mandatory.[14]

In most cases, reconstruction of mandibular continuity is possible with a nonvascularized bone graft from the anterior or posterior iliac crest. The nerve (nerve graft) is positioned laterally to the bone graft to facilitate later implant placement (Fig. 9–21 A–J). Only in patients with large bone defects or if a previous nonvascularized graft has failed are vascularized grafts from the iliac crest, scapula, or fibula indicated. For reconstructions of the angle of the mandible and the ascending ramus including the condyle, fibula grafts can be contoured to match the profile projection of the mandibular angle and provide adequate support of the ascending ramus at the skull base.[15–17]

Possible infiltration of ameloblastoma into the soft tissues must be kept in mind and may also necessitate soft-tissue reconstruction. Rare cases of cervical or pulmonary metastases (malignant ameloblastoma) must be treated surgically.[18,19] Peripheral ameloblastomas arise directly from the surface epithelium or from residues of the dental lamina lying outside the bone and may have a lower recurrence rate than do central ameloblastomas.[20,21]

Only 20% of ameloblastomas are located in the maxilla. Large tumors may obstruct the nasal cavity and cause bleeding.[3] They originate from the canine region and rarely may extend up to the skull base.[22–24] From a clinical perspective, maxillary ameloblastomas seem to be more aggressive. Obviously, this impression is due to the ease with which these tumors penetrate the thin maxillary bone and hide within the maxillary and other paranasal sinuses.[25]

As in the mandible, ameloblastomas require resection of the maxilla with safe margins. With sufficient residual teeth, an obturator may be fixed by conservative prosthodontic procedures. In larger defects, bone grafting may be performed secondarily. Implant insertion into the bone graft allows for prosthodontic rehabilitation. A dental implant at the time of tumor resection is a functionally satisfying alternative in cases with a sufficient residual bony support allowing for an early prosthodontic rehabilitation with an implant-borne prosthesis.

Although a radical resection should be performed, additional external incisions should be avoided if possible. Conventional vestibular incisions provide adequate exposure and allow for a radical resection of the lesion. Larger ameloblastomas, with more cranial extension that are located in the midline, may require a widening of the exposure either by the midfacial degloving technique or a Dieffenbach-Weber-Ferguson incision (Fig. 9–22 A–D). In certain tumor locations, a Le Fort I downfracture technique may provide adequate access to the lesion (Figure 9–23 A and B).[25] Temporary insertion of a petroleum jelly/iodoform gauze prevents excessive scar formation with profile changes in the midface before further reconstructive procedures. Alternatively, a primary reconstruction may be indicated. In any lesions infiltrating the skull base, watertight closure of the skull base with dura repair is indicated before further reconstructive procedures in the midface are undertaken; temporal muscle flaps or myocutaneous grafts may be beneficial in those instances.[26]

SQUAMOUS ODONTOGENIC TUMOR

This tumor consists of islands of well-differentiated squamous epithelium embedded in a fibrous stroma without palisading of peripheral cells. The tumor affects both the mandible and the maxilla equally. Although seen in all age groups, most patients present in the second decade of life. Some of these tumors have a locally aggressive clinical behavior, but it appears that curettage is the treatment of choice.[21]

CALCIFYING EPITHELIAL ODONTOGENIC TUMOR

The calcifying epithelial odontogenic tumor (*Pindborg tumor*) is a locally invasive, benign epithelial neoplasm that affects the mandible in two thirds of cases and shows a prevalence for the molar region.[3] A clear cell variant of the tumor is described. Definitive resection of the mass with tumor-free surgical margins and long-term follow-up is indicated.[27,28]

Text continued on page 495

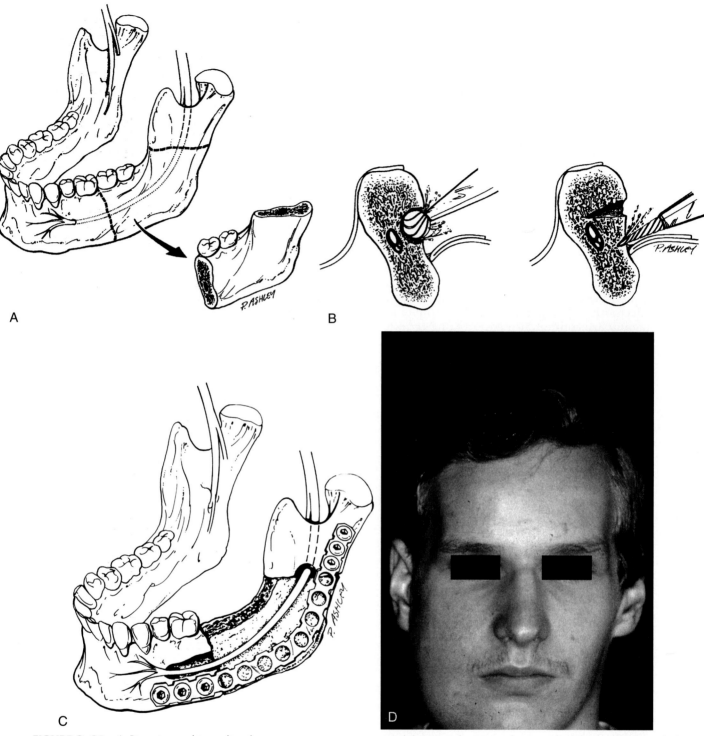

FIGURE 9–21   *A,* Resection and immediate bone reconstruction in patient with benign odontogenic lesion in the left mandible (intended resection shown by dotted line). *B,* Prior to resection, inferior alveolar nerve is freed from bony canal by a round burr or by osteotomy of the vestibular cortical plate. *C,* A reconstruction plate is fixed to the mandible. Screw holes are drilled and plate temporarily fixed. After removal of plate, tumor is resected. Nerve may be removed from tumor in cases of tumor-free frozen sections of nerve sheath. Bone graft is fixed to reconstruction plate, then bone graft is inserted. Nerve is placed laterally to bone graft to allow for later dental implant insertion. *D,* Swelling of right angle of mandible in a 17-year-old patient with histologically proven ameloblastoma.

Illustration continued on opposite page

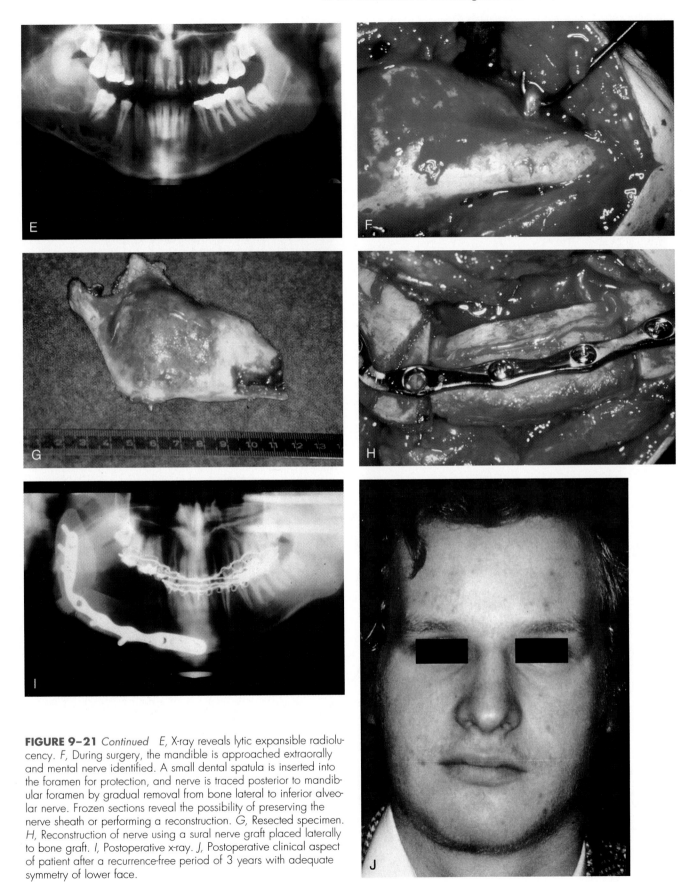

FIGURE 9-21 *Continued   E,* X-ray reveals lytic expansible radiolucency. *F,* During surgery, the mandible is approached extraorally and mental nerve identified. A small dental spatula is inserted into the foramen for protection, and nerve is traced posterior to mandibular foramen by gradual removal from bone lateral to inferior alveolar nerve. Frozen sections reveal the possibility of preserving the nerve sheath or performing a reconstruction. *G,* Resected specimen. *H,* Reconstruction of nerve using a sural nerve graft placed laterally to bone graft. *I,* Postoperative x-ray. *J,* Postoperative clinical aspect of patient after a recurrence-free period of 3 years with adequate symmetry of lower face.

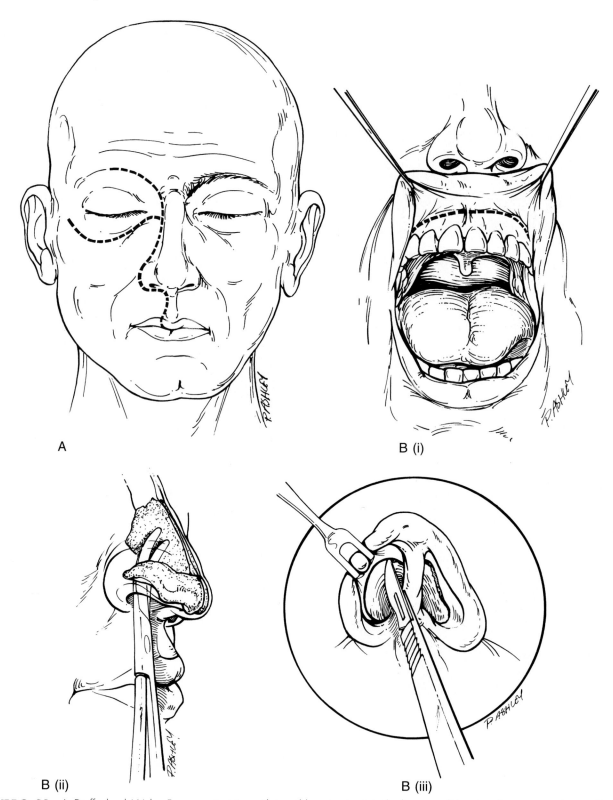

A

B (i)

B (ii)

B (iii)

FIGURE 9–22 *A,* Dieffenbach-Weber-Fergusson incision with possible extension into the lower eyelid or into the upper eyebrow. Cranial extension of the incision is currently usually replaced by a coronal incision. *B,* Midfacial degloving technique is illustrated (i). A full transfixation incision is connected to intercartilaginous, piriform, and nasal floor incisions on both sides (ii, iii)

Illustration continued on opposite page

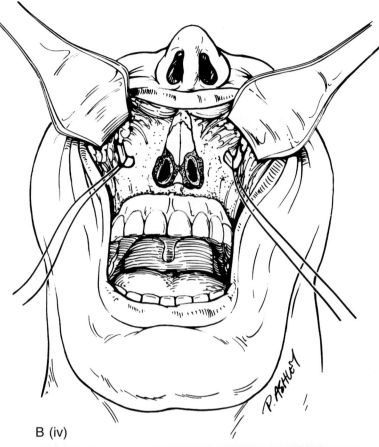

B (iv)

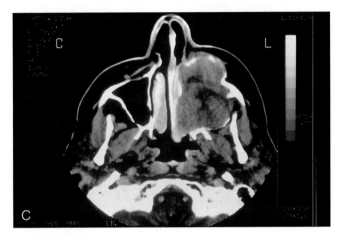

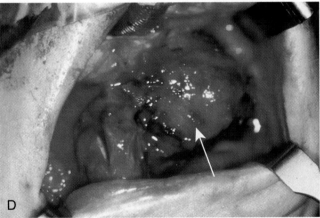

D

FIGURE 9-22 *Continued* A subperiostal dissection is performed and the nasolabial cheek complex retracted over the nasal bridge to the level of the medial canthus (iv). *C*, Radiographic appearance of extensive ameloblastoma of the left midface. *D*, Exposure of the ameloblastoma via midfacial degloving technique. Tumor clearly visible (*arrow*).

ODONTOGENIC CARCINOMAS

Malignant Ameloblastoma/Ameloblastic Carcinoma

Metastasizing (malignant) ameloblastomas exhibit features of typical ameloblastoma but develop distant metastases to lymph nodes or lungs. Ameloblastic carcinomas show atypical, less-differentiated cells within the primary lesion and do not require the proof of metastases for diagnosis.[18] In any case,

radical surgery with safe margins and adequate treatment of the metastasis is necessary.

Ameloblastic carcinomas often demonstrate an aggressive course with destruction of cortical plates of the bone. Wide resection with a margin of safety within the soft tissue is necessary. The resection is combined with a functional neck dissection or submandibular clearance. Resection of bone and soft tissue may necessitate reconstruction with a composite microvascular flap (Fig. 9-24 A–C).

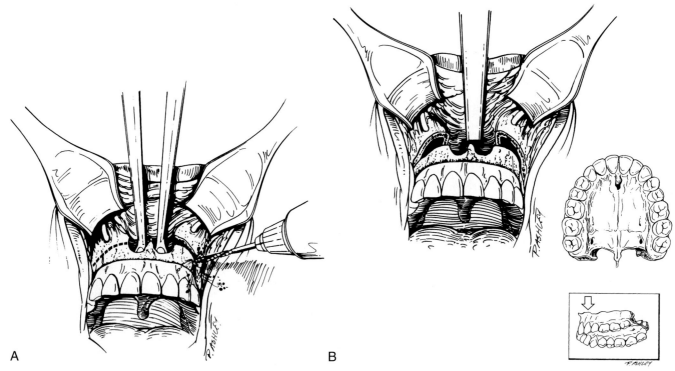

FIGURE 9-23   Le Fort I downfracture technique for access to odontogenic tumors with extension to the skull base. *A*, Osteotomies are made lateral to piriform aperture to pterygomaxillary junction. Nasal septum and lateral nasal walls are osteotomized with a scissel. *B*, The maxilla then can be downfractured.

Primary Intraosseous Carcinoma

Primary intraosseous carcinomas may arise from an odontogenic cyst (residual periapical cyst, dentigerous cyst) or, to a lesser degree, from odontogenic epithelial cell rests. They usually occur in elderly patients. Radical resection of the lesion with adequate margins is mandatory.

Clear Cell Odontogenic Tumor/Carcinoma

This very rare odontogenic tumor seems to be more aggressive than ameloblastoma and originates in both the mandible and maxilla with equal frequency. Most cases are diagnosed in elderly patients. Because of a high recurrence rate and the development of distant metastases, these are designated as clear cell odontogenic carcinomas.[29]

Tumors of Odontogenic Epithelium with Odontogenic Ectomesenchyme, with or without Dental Hard Tissue Formation

AMELOBLASTIC FIBROMA

Ameloblastic fibromas present with strands of epithelial odontogenic cells embedded in a proliferating pulp-like cellular connective tissue. The lesion is usually found in the posterior mandible in children with an equal distribution in both sexes.[3] Ameloblastic fibromas are normally treated by an enucleation; however, recurrences up to 20% are noted. According to reports, 50% of the very rare ameloblastic fibrosarcomas develop after recurrence of ameloblastic fibromas (Fig. 9-25 *A–G*).[30] Therefore, long-term follow-up is mandatory.

AMELOBLASTIC FIBRO-ODONTOMA/ ODONTOAMELOBLASTOMA

The ameloblastic fibro-odontoma shows features of an ameloblastic fibroma, which also contains dentin and enamel. Unlike the ameloblastic fibroma, it is found equally in maxilla and mandible. The lesion does not invade the surrounding bone. The ameloblastic fibro-odontoma should not be treated so radically as an ameloblastoma, as it more closely resembles an odontoma.[31] This lesion separates easily from the bone during curettage or enucleation, which is usually regarded as sufficient.[3] None of the four cases of odontoameloblastoma in the Central Registry of DÖSAK (German-Austrian-Swiss Association for the Study of Tumors of the Face and Jaws) recurred after curettage. It seems questionable whether a differentiation between odontoameloblastoma and

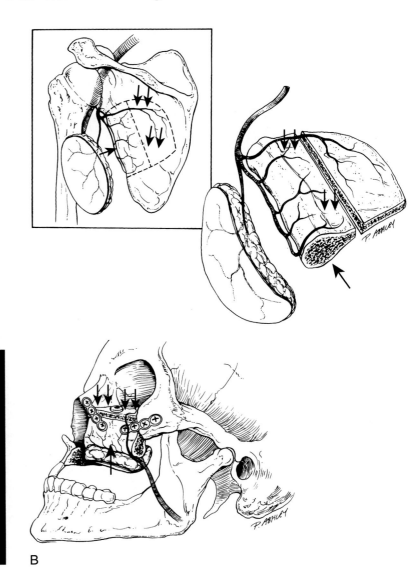

FIGURE 9–24   *A,* Following resection of maxillary malignoma, patient presents with a severe bone and soft-tissue deficit. 3D-CT reveals amount of bony tissue lost; left maxilla, midface, and orbital floor are missing. *B,* Osteocutaneous scapula flap for reconstruction of midface. Thicker lateral border of graft serves for reconstruction of the maxilla including cranial aspects of the alveolar crest (*arrows*). Thinner medial aspect of scapular bone provides orbital support (*double arrows*). Partially de-epithelialized soft-tissue flap is used for soft-tissue augmentation; the cutaneous part of the flap closes an additionally existing intraoral perforating defect.

Illustration continued on following page

fibro-odontoma dentinoma is biologically justified.[32] The very rare ameloblastic fibrosarcoma (ameloblastic sarcoma) requires a local radical resection with an adequate wide surgical approach due to its fast and aggressive growth. Because there is only one report on regional lymph node metastasis, a routinely performed neck dissection is not necessary.[32–34]

ADENOMATOID ODONTOGENIC TUMOR

Although presenting with a different clinical course, adenomatoid odontogenic tumors have long been treated like ameloblastomas. They may mimic a fol-

licular cyst associated with an impacted tooth.[35] As the tumor exhibits an inductive effect on the surrounding mesenchyme (production of dentin-like material), it is separated from ameloblastoma and grouped with odontogenic tumors having both epithelial and ectomesenchymal elements.

The adenomatoid odontogenic tumor most often originates in the maxilla. In contrast to the ameloblastoma, it is usually found in the incisor/canine region. Most cases are associated with an unerupted canine tooth. Therapy differs significantly from that of ameloblastomas and consists of an enucleation of the tumor facilitated by its pseudocapsule.[21,36]

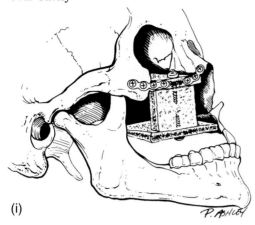

(i)

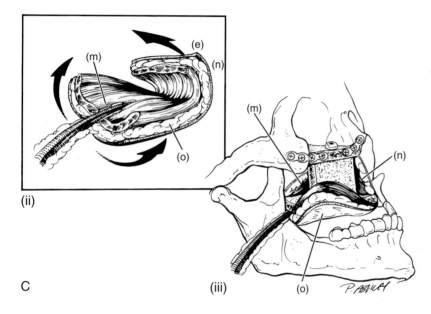

(ii)

C

(iii)

FIGURE 9-24 *Continued* C, In a midface reconstruction in a child with an ossifying fibroma of the maxilla, including the orbital floor and ethmoid, an osteocutaneous scapular flap was not used to avoid growth disturbances in the shoulder area. The facial skeleton (orbital floor, maxillary sinus wall, palate, and alveolar process) were reconstructed with a split iliac crest graft (i); a vascularized latissimus dorsi flap (ii) used for coverage of the ethmoid (e) cells, nasal (n) lining, obturation of maxillary (m) sinus, and reconstruction of aspects of anterior oral mucosa (o).

CALCIFYING ODONTOGENIC CYST/ ODONTOGENIC GHOST CELL TUMOR

The calcifying odontogenic cyst is predominantly found in patients in their second decade of life. Although most lesions represent a cyst, solid forms with formation of dentin-like material and a proliferating and infiltrating ameloblastoma-like component are seen. These lesions are regarded as tumors (odontogenic or dentinogenic ghost cell tumors). Radical resection of solid forms is recommended as the tumors may present with aggressive growth and histologic features, strongly implying malignant potential.[37]

ODONTOMA COMPLEX/COMPOUND

Odontomas are regarded as hamartomas rather than tumors. Therapy of complex and compound odontomas consists of surgical removal and typically has no technical difficulties associated with it. Even in cases of large odontomas, an intraoral approach may

be used.[38] Lesions may recur if incompletely removed at an early stage.[21]

Tumors of Odontogenic Ectomesenchyme with or without included Odontogenic Epithelium

ODONTOGENIC FIBROMA

Odontogenic fibromas consist of cell-rich connective tissue with small islands of odontogenic cells. These very rare lesions are usually sharply demarcated and easily removed by curettage or enucleation.

ODONTOGENIC MYXOMA

Odontogenic myxomas are centrally located and may result in destruction of the bone cortex and resorption of tooth roots. In odontogenic myxomas of the maxilla, prosthodontic rehabilitation after resection of large parts of the palate may be per-

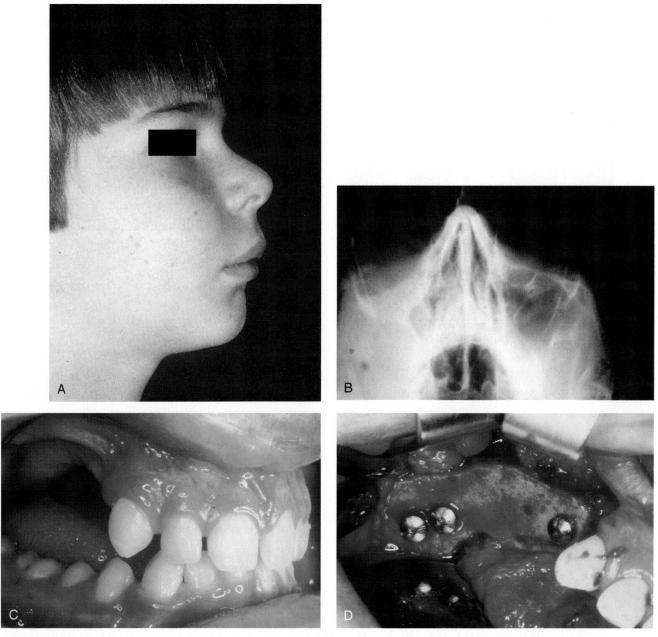

FIGURE 9–25   *A* and *B,* Two views of histologically proven ameloblastic fibroma of the maxilla in a 12-year-old boy. *C,* Intraoperative aspect 4 years after removal of the tumor. *D,* A bone graft from the posterior iliac spine is placed for reconstruction of bony defect and dental implants are inserted.

Illustration continued on following page

formed with insertion of dental implants into the remaining palate.[39] As the odontogenic myxoma demonstrates almost no pseudocapsule and may extend through the bone into the soft tissue without well-defined margins, larger lesions may require extensive resection, including the healthy surrounding bone. Recurrences do occur.

BENIGN CEMENTOBLASTOMA

Benign cementoblastomas most frequently occur at the roots of molars or premolars of the mandible. A complete surgical removal of the tumor is adequate. It may be possible to remove benign cementoblastomas affecting molars without removing the teeth.[40]

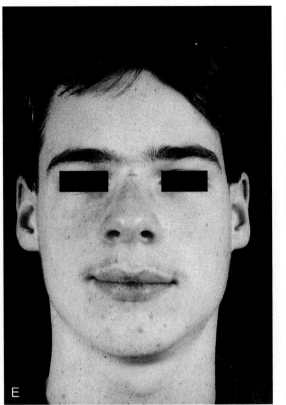

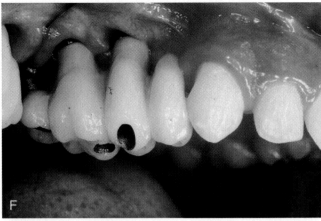

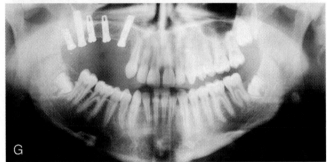

FIGURE 9–25 *Continued*   *E*, Extraoral aspect of the patient after surgery. *F*, Prosthodontic rehabilitation with implant-borne prosthesis. *G*, Radiographic view of patient in 9-25F.

NEOPLASMS AND OTHER BONE-RELATED LESIONS

Benign Fibro-Osseous Lesions

CEMENTO-OSSIFYING FIBROMA/ CEMENTIFYING FIBROMA

Cemento-ossifying fibroma and cementifying fibroma are well-defined neoplasms occurring mostly during the third and fourth decades of life with a female preponderance. Ninety percent of the lesions are located in the mandibular molar area.[41,42] Radiographically, they are well-defined with various degrees of radiopacity depending on the amount of calcified material. Large lesions may demonstrate a typical downward bowing of the mandible.

Enucleation of the tumor is adequate. If not possible because of the dimension of the tumor, modeling osteoma for preservation of the mandibular continuity is sufficient. In all cases, the inferior alveolar nerve should be preserved.[43]

In the maxilla, the therapeutic principles are the same. The size of the tumor determines the reconstructive options. Whereas smaller lesions may be reconstructed by small monocortical bone grafts in combination with implant insertions in the tooth-bearing area, extensive ossifying fibromas that may invade the orbit, the ethmoid cells, and the skull base require more sophisticated procedures.

Non-Neoplastic Bone Lesions

FIBROUS DYSPLASIA

Most cases of fibrous dysplasia are monostotic diseases with the jaws mostly affected at an early age (between 10 and 20 years). Teeth near the slowly growing mass may be dislocated. Radiologically, the typical ground-glass opacification is observed.[41]

Smaller lesions, for example in the mandible, may be surgically resectable. Because many lesions may stop growing in early adulthood, some patients without aesthetic or functional impairments may not require surgery. Larger lesions causing aesthetic or functional impairments require surgical contouring to eliminate disturbing disfiguration (Fig. 9–26 *A–J*). Regrowth may occur with time.

Osteosarcoma arising from a fibrous dysplasia may rarely occur. Radiotherapy of the lesion is contraindicated because of the inherent risk for the development of a postirradiation bone sarcoma.[5]

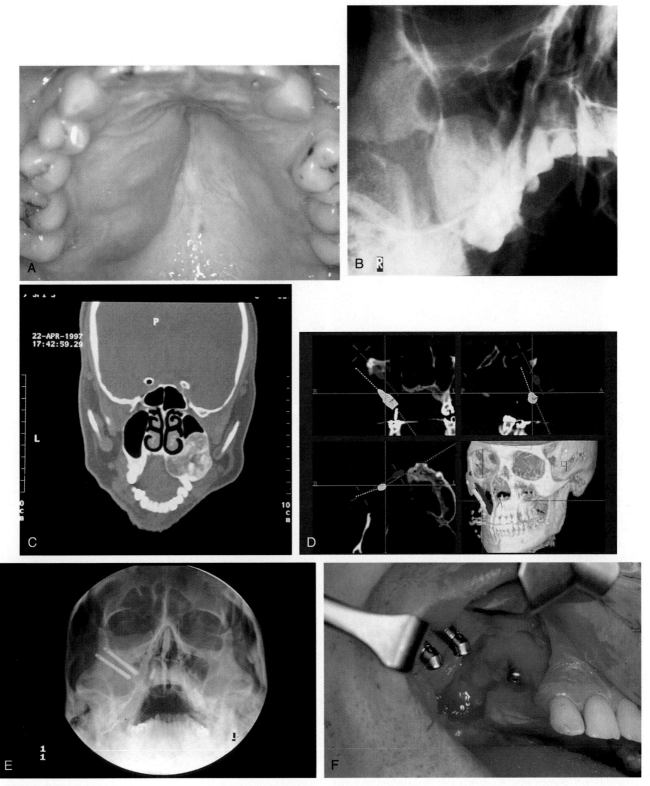

FIGURE 9–26   Ossifying fibroma of the right maxilla. *A*, Clinical impression of tumor volume extending to the midline of the palate. *B*, X-ray demonstrating lesions in the posterior aspect of the right maxilla. *C*, CT scan demonstrating relation to nasal floor. *D*, Planning of insertion of two Cygoma implants (Nobel Biocare, Cologne, Germany) after resection of the process and reconstruction of the defect with an osteocutaneous scapular graft. The navigation process guides the surgeon intraoperatively with an indication of the inclination of implants as well as their distance in bone. *E*, X-ray following insertion of Cygoma implants and conventional implants and anterior maxilla. *F*, Situation after uncovering the two Cygoma implants and the anterior conventional implants before prosthodontic treatment.

Illustration continued on following page

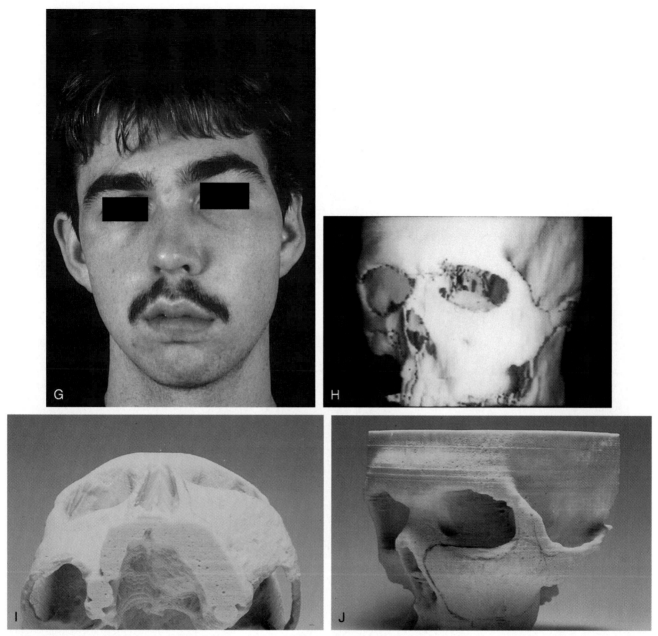

FIGURE 9–26 *Continued* G, Fibrous dysplasia in a 26-year-old male patient. *H*, Preoperative 3D-CT. *I* and *J*, The preoperatively manufactured surgical model allows for exact planning of the amount of bone to be removed.

CEMENTO-OSSEOUS DYSPLASIAS

The radiolucent periapical cemento-osseous dysplasia in the lower anterior periapical region may be mistaken for a periapical infection. However, since teeth are vital, no treatment is required. In patients with focal cemento-osseous dysplasias, long-term observation of the lesion after biopsy is usually adequate.[41]

Florid cemento-osseous dysplasia involves the jaws and may lead to perforations of the mucosa with development of a mild osteomyelititis. Treatment of inflammatory disease is essential and, in asymptomatic patients, close follow-up is adequate.[41]

Other Tumors

MELANOTIC NEUROECTODERMAL TUMOR OF INFANCY

This tumor develops within the first year of life, usually in the maxilla. High urinary levels of vanillylmandelic acid (VMA) are found. These rapidly growing, usually benign, lesions are treated by complete surgical removal and immediate reconstruction (Fig. 9–27 *A–F*). However, recurrences (15%) and malignant transformations have been documented.[44,45]

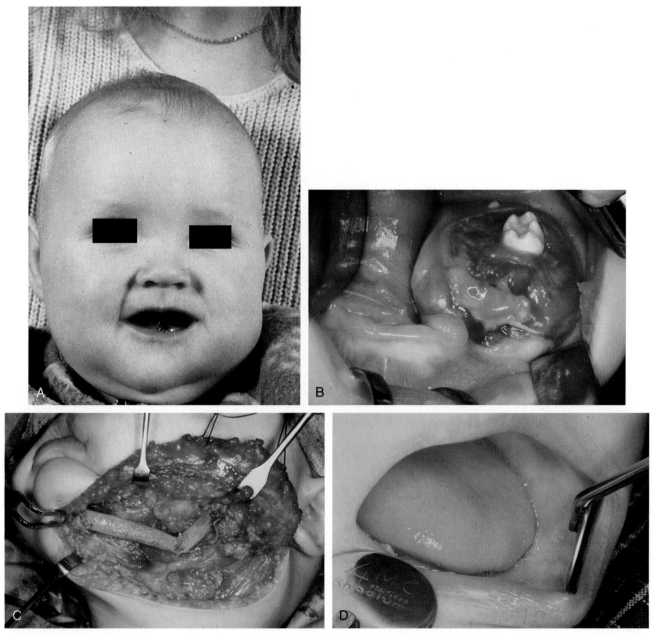

FIGURE 9-27 *A,* Melanotic neuroectodermal tumor of infancy of the left mandible in a 6-month-old child. *B,* Intraoral aspect of the lesion with complete destruction of the mandible. *C,* Extraoral resection of tumor was followed by immediate reconstruction using a rib graft. *D,* Intraoperative/postoperative aspect.

Illustration continued on following page

MALIGNANT BONE LESIONS

Osteosarcoma

After plasmocytoma, osteosarcoma is the most common malignant bone tumor.[46] Forty-one percent of all sarcomas registered in the DÖSAK registry are osteosarcomas.[47] Seven percent of all osteosarcomas are located in the jaws, with an age preponderance in the third decade.[48,49]

Loosening of teeth, paresthesia, and nasal obstruc-

tion may be present. Radiographically, dense sclerotic lesions or mixed sclerotic/radiolucent areas may be found. The periphery of the lesion is ill-defined. A sun-ray appearance in the vicinity of the tumor due to a periosteal reaction may be present. Proper preoperative radiological examination resulting in a more radical surgical procedure may improve the prognosis.[50,51]

The prognosis of maxillary osteosarcoma is worse than that of the mandible.[3,44,52] However, according to the DÖSAK experience, this is due to the fact that tumor-free margins are more easily attainable in

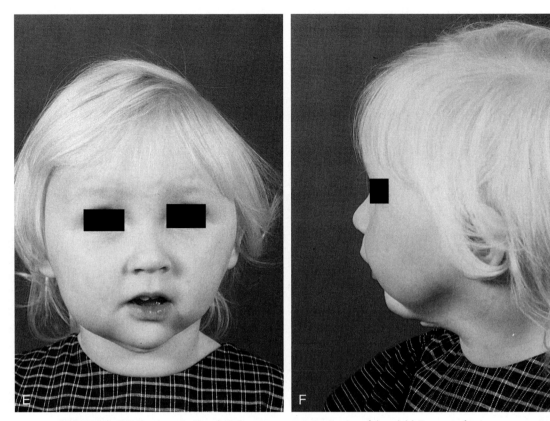

FIGURE 9-27 *Continued   E* and *F*, Postoperative appearance of the child 2 years after surgery.

the mandible than in the maxilla.[41] Metastases from osteosarcomas mainly affect the lung and the skeleton.

As the prognosis and treatment of osteosarcoma is different from that of chondrosarcoma and fibrosarcoma, the histological differentiation between these tumors is important.[53–55] Radical resection of the tumor with wide margins is regarded as the therapy of choice.[56,57] The resection must include bone and the surrounding soft tissue, often necessitating composite microvascular reconstructions, especially in patients treated with preoperative radiation (Fig. 9–28 *A* and *B*).[58] Multimodality therapy in high-grade (grade III) osteosarcoma is favored.[59,60]

Surgery alone may be adequate for small low-grade tumors and negative surgical margins. Patients with incomplete resections or high-grade tumors should receive surgery and radiotherapy.[61] Combined proton and photon radiation therapy may improve the results.[62] On the other hand, no local control was achieved with radiotherapy in patients with incomplete resection.[56] Hence, even repeated resections have to be performed, if possible, since tumor-free margins of resection are crucial for the survival of the patient.

According to DÖSAK experience of 158 osteosarcomas of the jaws, the only variable connected to survival with statistical significance was radical tumor resection regardless of location, histological grade, age, sex, or additional treatment protocols.[41] However, at this time, it is not clear whether neoadjuvant chemotherapy will improve survival in grade III osteosarcoma.

Chondrosarcoma

In the jaws, benign cartilage tumors are exceedingly rare and outnumbered by chondosarcomas. However, chondrosarcomas occur less frequently in the jaws than do osteosarcomas. Pain is a less frequent symptom in chondrosarcoma compared with osteosarcoma.[53,60,63,64] The tumor presents as a painless mass and may cause loosening of the teeth. In children, chondrosarcoma may tend to grow in atypical anatomic sites.[65] Radiographically, the tumor has poorly defined borders and radiolucent areas. Various degrees of calcification may be present.

Radical surgical excision of the tumor is to be regarded as the treatment of choice because the tumor is not sensitive to chemotherapy. Metastases generally occur via the bloodstream as a late and uncommon event. Thus, a neck dissection is indicated only in rare cases.[3,66] High-grade lesions, especially, should be treated aggressively.[60,67] In patients with local recurrences, the median interval from time of first recurrence until death is 25 months.[64] Mesenchymal chondrosarcoma, presenting with sim-

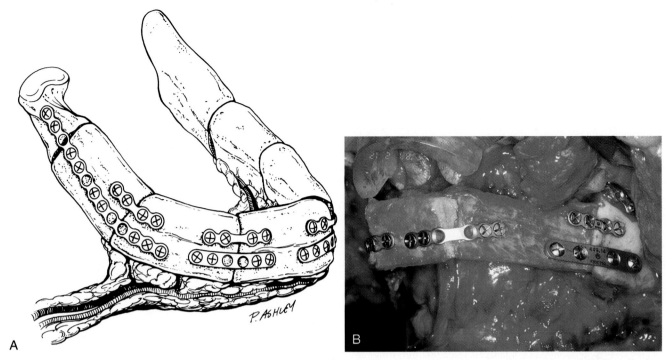

FIGURE 9-28 *A,* Complete mandibulectomy with a vascularized fibula graft. *B,* Intraoperative aspect of a vascularized fibula graft after contouring. Fixation of graft on left side is performed with a 2.4 mm AO plate, anterior osteotomies with 2.0 mm plates.

ilar symptoms as chondrosarcoma, may be treated by wide surgical resection in combination with chemotherapy.

Fibrosarcoma

Fibrosarcoma is less common than osteosarcoma and chondrosarcoma, and the prognosis is usually better.[68] The mandible is affected far more frequently. Fibrosarcoma may develop from pre-existing bony lesions, especially from fibrous dysplasia, ossifying fibromas, and giant cell granulomas. Ionizing radiation is also considered as a possible cause.[69]

Ewing's Sarcoma

Ewing's sarcoma is an uncommon malignancy of the jaws found primarily in children and adolescents.[70] In contrast to many other tumors, the swelling often is combined with pain.[71,72] Paresthesias and loosening of the teeth may be present. Radiographically, the typical "onionskin" periosteal reaction may be found in combination with irregular lytic bone destruction.[41]

The tumor is extremely radiosensitive. The current treatment consists of neoadjuvant chemotherapy with a radical surgical resection as an adjunct to the therapies mentioned, and, if necessary, radiation.[3,72–75] As surgery and radiotherapy alone are unlikely to be curative due to the presence of micrometastases,

multidisciplinary tumor therapy has become increasingly effective in eliminating these cells and in improving local control. In Ewing's sarcoma of the mandible, complete surgical resection may be preferred to irradiation for local control, if surgery can be performed with minimal loss of function and disfigurement.[76,77]

Metastases to the Oral Cavity and Jaws

Metastatic carcinoma is the most common form of cancer involving bone. The vertebrae, ribs, pelvis, and skull are the most frequent sites for metastases. Carcinoma from the lung, breast, thyroid, prostate, and kidney are responsible for the majority of metastases, which are mostly found in the mandible. Metastases in the maxilla are rare.

Although some metastases may be asymptomatic and detected by routine dental x-ray, perioral swelling, for example, may be detected arising from a spontaneous fracture of the mandible. The lesion, most often arising in elderly patients, may also cause a lack of fit of the prosthesis. The usual radiographic sign of a metastasis is a radiolucent defect; in the alveolar region, it may resemble a pericoronal disease.

Although the prognosis of these often already-disseminated diseases is poor, surgical resection of the metastases should be performed to eliminate functional impairment and pain. With regard to histology, age, and general condition of the patient, staged reconstruction techniques have to be applied. In elderly patients, bridging of the defect in the mandible with a reconstruction plate may be adequate.

REFERENCES

1. Alexander R, Weber WD, Theodos LV, Friedman JS. The treatment of large benign maxillary tumors via Le Fort I downfracture: Report of two cases and review of the literature. *J Oral Maxillofac Surg.* 1992; 50:515.
2. Clark WD. Surgical treatment of benign and low-grade malignant lesions of the mandible. In: Bailey BJ, Holt GR, eds. *Surgery of the Mandible.* New York: Thieme; 1987:45.
3. Prein J, Remagen W, Spiessl B, Uehlinger E. *Atlas of Tumors of the Facial Skeleton.* Berlin: Springer Verlag; 1986.
4. Alpert B. Surgical technique in the management of benign cysts and tumors of the jaws. *Oral Maxillofac Surg Clin North Am.* 1991; 3(1):5.
5. Waldron CA. Odontogenic cysts and tumors. In: BW Neville, DD Damm, CM Allen, JE Bouquot, eds. *Oral and Maxillofacial Pathology.* Philadelphia: WB Saunders; 1995:493.
6. Thyne GM, Hunter KM. Primary reconstruction of the mandible with iliac bone and titanium implants following resection of a recurrent odontogenic keratocyst. *NZ Dent J.* 1994; 90:56.
7. Jackson IT, Potparic Z, Fasching M, et al. Penetration of the skull base by dissecting keratocyst. *J Craniomaxillofac Surg.* 1993; 21:319.
8. DeGould MD, Goldberg JS. Recurrence of an odontogenic keratocyst in a bone graft. Report of a case. *Int J Oral Maxillofac Surg.* 1991; 20:9.
9. Worrall SF. Recurrent odontogenic keratocyst within the temporalis muscle. *Br J Oral Maxillofac Surg.* 1992; 30:59.
10. Waldron CA, Mustoe TA. Primary intraosseous carcinoma of the mandible with probable origin in an odotogenic cyst. *Oral Surg Oral Med Oral Pathol.* 1989; 67:716.
11. Ackermann GL, Altini M, Shear M. The unicystic ameloblastoma: A clinicopathological study of 57 cases. *J Oral Pathol.* 1988; 17:541.
12. Reichart PA, Philipsen HP, Sonner S. Ameloblastoma: Biological profile of 3677 cases. *Eur J Cancer B Oral Oncol.* 1995; 31B:86.
13. AAOMS Surgical Update: Odontogenic cysts and tumors. Spring 1996.
14. Pinsolle J, Michelet V, Coustal B, et al. Treatment of ameloblastoma of the jaws. *Arch Otolaryngol Head Neck Surg.* 1995; 121:994.
15. Khanijow VK, Ahmad TS, Lian CB, Jalaludin MA. Mandibular reconstruction: Experience with the free vascularized fibula transfer. *Microsurg.* 1993; 14:375.
16. Yim KK, Wei FC. Fibula osteoseptocutaneous flap for mandible reconstruction. *Microsurg.* 1994; 15:245.
17. Schmelzeisen R, Neukam FW, Shirota T, et al. Postoperative function after implant insertion in vascularized bone grafts in maxilla and mandible. *Plast Reconstr Surg.* 1996; 97:719.
18. Slootweg PJ, Muller H. Malignant ameloblastomas or ameloblastic carcinoma. *Oral Surg Oral Med Oral Pathol.* 1984; 57:168.
19. Sheppard BC, Temeck BK, Taubenberger JK, Pass HI. Pulmonary metastatic disease in ameloblastoma. *Chest.* 1993; 104:1933.
20. Bucci E, Lo Muzio L, Mignogna MD, de Rosa G. Peripheral ameloblastoma: Case report. *Acta Stomatol Belgica.* 1992; 89:267.
21. Kramer IRM, Pindborg JJ, Shear M. *Histological Typing of Odontogenic Tumors.* New York: Springer; 1992.
22. Hell B, Heissler E, Gazounis G, et al. Microsurgical and prosthetic reconstruction of patient with recurrent ameloblastoma extending into the skull base. *Int J Oral Maxillofac Surg.* 1994; 23:90.
23. Sato K, Sudo S, Fukuya Y, Sakuma H. Maxillary ameloblastoma with intracranial invasion—case report. *Neurol Med Chir Tokyo.* 1994; 34:704.
24. Nastri AL, Wiesenfeld D, Radden BG, et al. Maxillary ameloblastoma: A retrospective study of 13 cases. *Br J Oral Maxillofac Surg.* 1995; 33:28.
25. Symingtom OG, Caminiti MF. Le Fort I downfracture approach for the treatment of a posterior maxillary ameloblastoma. *J Canad Dent Assoc.* 1995; 61:1048.
26. Williams RW, Speculand B, Robin PE, Simms M. Second reconstruction of the posterior maxilla with a free latissimus dorsi muscle flap. Case report. *Int J Oral Maxillofac Surg.* 1992; 21:284.
27. Hicks MJ, Flaitz CM, Wong ME, et al. Clear cell variant of calcifying epithelial odontogenic tumor: Case report, review of the literature. *Head Neck.* 1994; 16:272.
28. Basu MK, Matthews JB, Sear AJ, Browne RM. Calcifying epithelial odontogenic tumor: A case showing features of malignancy. *J Oral Pathol.* 1984; 13:310.
29. Waldron CA, Small IA, Silverman H. Clear cell ameloblastoma–an odontogenic carcinoma. *J Oral Maxillofac Surg.* 1985; 43:707.
30. Muller S, Parker DC, Kapadia SB, Budnick SD, Barnes EL. Ameloblastic fibrosarcoma of the jaws: A clinicopathologic and DNA analysis of five cases and review of the literature with discussion of its relationship to ameloblastic fibroma. *Oral Surg Oral Med Oral Pathol.* 1995; 79(4):469.
31. Waechter R, Remagen W, Stoll P. Is it possible to differentiate between odontoameloblastoma and fibro-odontoma? Critical position on basis of 18 cases in DÖSAK list. *Dtsch Zahnärztl Z.* 1991; 46:74.
32. Prein J, Remagen W, Spiessl B, Schafroth U. Ameloblastic fibroma and its sarcomatous transformation. *Path Res Pract.* 1979; 166:123.
33. Chomette G, Auriol M, Gujibert F, Delcourt A. Ameloblastic fibrosarcoma of the jaws. *Path Res Pract.* 1983; 178:40.
34. Howell RM, Burkes EJ. Malignant transformation of ameloblastic fibro-odontoma to ameloblastic fibrosarcoma. *Oral Surg Oral Med Oral Pathol.* 1977; 43:391.
35. Vitkus R, Meltzer JA. Repair of a defect following the removal of a maxillary adenomatoid odontogenic tumor using guided tissue regeneration. A case report. *J Periodontol.* 1996; 67:46.
36. Pantoja R, Delaire J. Une nouvelle observation de tumeur odontogenique adenomatoide. *Rev Stomatol Chir Maxillofac.* 1991; 92:98.
37. Ellis GL, Shmookler, BM. Aggressive (malignant?) epithelial odontogenic ghost cell tumor. *Oral Surg Oral Med Oral Pathol.* 1996; 61:471.
38. Blinder D, Peleg M, Taicher S. Surgical considerations in cases of large mandibular odontomas located in the mandibular angle. *Int J Oral Maxillofac Surg.* 1993; 22:163.
39. Arcuri MR, Tabor MW, Fergason HW, Haganman C. Odontogenic myxoma of the maxillary sinus: A clinical report. *J Prosthet Dent.* 1993; 70:111.
40. Biggs JT, Benenati FW. Surgically treating a benign cementoblastoma while retaining the involved tooth. *J Am Dent Assoc.* 1995; 126:1288.
41. Jundt G, Prein J. Bone tumors and tumor-like lesions in the jaw. Findings of the Basel DÖSAK reference registry. *Mund Kiefer Gesichtschir.* 2000; 4(suppl 1):196.
42. Tasar F, Giray CB, Tasman U, Saysel MY. Ossifying fibroma. A case report. *Turk J Pediat.* 1996; 38(2):265.
43. Kreutziger KL, Weiss LS. Cementifying fibroma: Resection of recurrent mandibular lesion with microsurgical preservation of inferior alveolar nerve and immediate reconstruction. *South Med J.* 1994; 87:653.
44. Kapadia SB, Frisman DM, Hitchcock CL, Ellis GL, Popek EJ. Melanotic neuroectodermal tumor of infancy. Clinicopathological, immunohistochemical, and flow cytometric study. *Am J Surg Pathol.* 1993; 17:566.
45. Pettinato G, Manivel C, d'Amore ESG, Jaszcz W, Gorlin RJ.

Melanotic neuroectodermal tumor of infancy. *Am J Surg Pathol.* 1991; 15(3):233.

46. Greenspan A, Remagen W. *Differential Diagnosis of Tumors and Tumor-Like Lesions of Bones and Joints.* Philadelphia: Lippincott Raven; 1998.

47. Jundt G. Osteosarcoma of the jaws. Statistical report on the recent numbers of the Central Registry of the DÖSAK (German-Austrian-Swiss Association for the Study of Tumors of the Face and Jaws). Personal communication, 1996.

48. Kragh LV, Dahlin DC, Erich JB. Osteogenic sarcoma of the jaws and facial bones. *Am J Surg.* 1958; 96:496.

49. James PL, O'Regan MB, Speight PM. Well-differentiated intra-osseous osteosarcoma in the mandible of a six-year-old child. *J Laryngol Otol.* 1990; 104(4):335.

50. Soderholm AL, Lindqvist C, Teppo L, et al. Bone resection in patients with mandibular sarcoma. *J Craniomaxillofac Surg.* 1988; 16(5):224.

51. Yagan R, Radivoyevitch M, Bellon EM. Involvement of the mandibular canal: Early sign of osteogenic sarcoma of the mandible. *Oral Surg Oral Med Oral Pathol.* 1985; 60(1):56.

52. Garrington GE, Scofield HH, Cornyn J, Hooker SP. Osteogenic sarcoma of the jaws. Analysis of 56 cases. *Cancer.* 1967; 20:377.

53. Jundt G, Remagen W. Knorpelbildende Tumoren des Kiefers. *Verh Dtsch Ges Path.* 1992; 76:372.

54. Wanebo HJ, Koness RJ, MacFarlane JK, et al. Head and neck sarcoma: Report of the Head and Neck Sarcoma Registry. Society of Head and Neck Surgeons Committee on Research. *Head Neck.* 1992; 14(1):1.

55. Dallera P, Bertoni F, Marchetti C, et al. Ameloblastic fibrosarcoma of the jaw: Report of five cases. *J Craniomaxillofac Surg.* 1994; 22(6):349.

56. Hug EB, Fitzek MM, Liebsch NJ, Munzenrider JE. Locally challenging osteo- and chondrogenic tumors of the axial skeleton: Results of combined proton and photon radiation therapy using three-dimensional treatment. *Int J Radiat Oncol Biol Phys.* 1995; 31(3):467.

57. Smeele LE, van der Wal JE, van Diest PJ, et al. Radical surgical treatment in craniofacial osteosarcoma gives excellent survival. A retrospective cohort study of 14 patients. *Eur J Cancer.* 1994; 30B(6):374.

58. Aitasalo K, Virolainen E, Happonen RP. Immediate reconstruction of mandibular defects with revascularized iliac bone grafts after radical surgery for osteosarcoma. *Proceedings of the Finnish Dental Society.* 1990; 86(3–4):149.

59. Herrmann A, Zöller J. Zur Klinik und Therapie des osteogenen Sarkoms im Kieferbereich. *Dtsch Z Mund Kiefer Gesichtschir.* 1990; 14(3):180.

60. Mark RJ, Tran L, Sercarz JA, et al. Chondrosarcoma of the head and neck. The UCLA experience, 1955–1988. *Am J Clin Oncol.* 1993; 16(3):232.

61. Tran LM, Mark R, Meier R, et al. Sarcomas of the head and neck. Prognostic factors and treatment strategies. *Cancer.* 1992; 70(1):169.

62. Panizzoni GA, Gasparini G, Clauser L, et al. Osteosarcoma of the facial bones. *Ann Oncol.* 1992; 3(suppl 2):S47.

63. Anwar R, Ruddy J, Ghosh S, et al. Chondrosarcoma of the maxilla. *J Laryngol Otol.* 1992; 106(1):53.

64. Ruark DS, Schlehaider UK, Shah JP. Chondrosarcomas of the head and neck. *World J Surg.* 1992; 16(5):1010.

65. Chou P, Mehta S, Gonzalez-Crussi F. Chondrosarcoma of the head in children. *Pediat Pathol.* 1990; 10(6):945.

66. Watters GW, Brookes GB. Chondrosarcoma of the temporal bone. *Clin Otolaryngol.* 1995; 20(1):53.

67. Burkey BB, Hoffman HT, Baker SR, et al. Chondrosarcoma of the head and neck. *Laryngoscope.* 1990; 100(12): 1301.

68. Prein J, Remagen W, Spiessl B, Uehlinger E. *Atlas of Tumors of the Facial Skeleton—Odontogenic and Nonodontogenic Tumors.* Berlin: Springer Verlag; 1986.

69. Moloy PJ, Kowal KA, Siegel WM. Fibrosarcoma of the mandible following supravoltage irradiation. Report of a case. *Arch Otolaryngol Head Neck Surg.* 1989; 115(10):1250.

70. Berk R, Heller A, Heller D, et al. Ewing's sarcoma of the mandible: A case report. *Oral Surg Oral Med Oral Pathol Oral Radiol Endod.* 1995; 79(2):159.

71. Som PM, Krespi YP, Hermann G, Shugar JM. Ewing's sarcoma of the mandible. *Ann Otol Rhinol Laryngol.* 1980; 89:20.

72. Mamede RM, Mello FV, Barbieri J. Prognosis of Ewing's sarcoma of the head and neck. *Otolaryngol Head Neck Surg.* 1990; 102(6):650.

73. Cotterill SJ, Ahrens S, Paulussen M, et al. Prognostic factors in Ewing's tumor of bone: Analysis of 975 patients from the European intergroup cooperative Ewing's sarcoma study group. *J Clin Oncol.* 2000; 18:3108.

74. Fiorillo A, Tranfa F, Canale G, et al. Primary Ewing's sarcoma of the maxilla, a rare and curable localization: Report of two new cases, successfully treated by radiotherapy and systemic chemotherapy. *Cancer Letters.* 1996; 103(2):177.

75. Pape H, Laws HJ, Burdach S, et al. Radiotherapy and high-dose chemotherapy in advanced Ewing's tumors. *Strahlenther Onkol.* 1999; 175:484.

76. Jürgens H, Exner U, Gadner H, et al. Multidisciplinary treatment of primary Ewing's sarcoma of bone. *Cancer.* 1988; 61:23.

77. Jürgens H. Interdisziplinäre Therapie des Ewing-Sarkoms Schweiz. *Rundschau Med. (Praxis).* 1995; 84(37):1005.

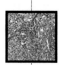

IV. PATHOLOGY OF THE ORAL CAVITY, OROPHARYNX, AND ODONTOGENIC LESIONS

■ LEE J. SLATER

■ SOOK-BIN WOO

Clinicians are familiar with the common conditions affecting the oral and paraoral regions. The surgeon's clinical diagnosis, based on patient examination and imaging studies, is often verified by histopathologic evaluation of an incisional or excisional biopsy. Sometimes, however, microscopic examination of oral tissue specimens results in the diagnosis of an unexpected neoplasm, specific infection, or other condition.

HANDLING OF SPECIMENS

To aid the pathologist in preparing a comprehensive report of surgical pathology findings, laboratories can benefit from a checklist of items to be evaluated in head and neck specimens.[1] Specimens removed from the oral region include:

1. Incisional biopsy of macular lesion
2. Excisional biopsy of a small nodular lesion
3. Excisional biopsy of a large extraosseous mass
4. Incisional biopsy of an intraosseous cystic or solid lesion
5. Excision or resection of an intraosseous lesion

Superficial incisional biopsies—whether taken by a punch, scalpel, or laser—are problematic.[2,3] They yield specimens that are often small, difficult to orient, prone to undesirable tangential sectioning, and may not be representative of the entire lesion. A curled mucosal segment should be sliced ("breadloafed") perpendicular to the long axis of the curl, resulting in C-shaped segments that ensure perpendicular microtome sections through the surface epithelium. Such perpendicular sections give the pathologist more confidence in assessing the presence or absence of invasive carcinoma in a specimen showing intraepithelial neoplasia (dysplasia). The possibility of sampling error should always be considered; if a histologic section reveals dysplasia or "verrucous hyperplasia," then tissue deeper in the paraffin block or tissue adjacent to the biopsy site could potentially show conventional invasive squamous cell carcinoma.

If a small (1.0 cm or smaller) mucosal nodule is excised, the surgeon need not place orientation sutures on the specimen, because if tumor is found to extend to a margin, then the mucosal incision can simply be re-excised. The margins of specimens with small mucosal nodules should be inked to aid the pathologist in assessing whether a margin is positive or not.[4] The inked specimen can be transversely multisected (breadloafed), an effective manner of evaluating margins.

When a circumscribed malignant neoplasm, such as a keratoacanthoma-like squamous cell carcinoma, is excised with a rather narrow rim of normal tissue separating tumor from the inked margin, the pathologist can be reasonably sure that the tumor has been completely excised. However, the completeness of the resection is more difficult to determine for an infiltrative neoplasm showing dispersed small tumor nests; one would be less certain that such a tumor has been completely excised, even though peripheral tumor islands apparently do not extend to the marked margin.[5]

The surgeon should place an orientation tag (suture) on specimens of large extraosseous tumors—a 4.0 cm palatal salivary gland tumor, for example. Such large tumors can be hemisected in the long axis and then transversely multisected (breadloafed) to check margins; this permits estimation of the thickness of normal tissue between the tumor and the surgical margin.[6] However, peripheral vertical sections or oblique sections (Mohs method) are also effective means of assessing the completeness of the resection.[7–9] Ink is usually used to mark the margins, but cornstarch has been used for fatty specimens.[10] Because completely excised tumors have a better prognosis, conscientious evaluation of margins is important.[11,12]

Incisional biopsies of intraosseous lesions, such as odontogenic cysts/tumors or benign fibro-osseous lesions, usually require no special handling. As with all incisional biopsies, sampling error is a potential problem. A preliminary study indicates that an incisional biopsy of a large mandibular cyst at the osseous window often shows histologic features similar to those of endoscopically harvested additional samples of the same cyst.[13] Incisional biopsies of large extraosseous lesions should be deep enough to ensure sampling of representative tissue.

The surgeon can excise mandibular tumors, such as an ameloblastoma or a gingival squamous cell carcinoma that has invaded the mandible, by marginal resection (en bloc resection, resection without continuity defect—preserving the mandibular inferior cortex); segmental resection (with continuity defect); or hemimandibulectomy.[14,15] The mandibular specimen should be fixed overnight in formalin. The size, gross characteristics, and extent of the tumor should be described, and the distance from the tumor to the proximal and distal bony margins should be measured. Mucosal margins can be marked with India ink and processed immediately, but proximal and distal osseous margins require decalcification and therefore delayed assessment. Bony margins should be evaluated for evidence of carcinoma in cancellous bone and perineural or periosteal compartments. To detect potential perineural invasion, the extraosseous proximal segment of the inferior alveolar branch of the mandibular nerve should be sampled.[16,17] If nerve-associated epithelial cords are observed in tissue of the retromolar region medial to the mandibular ramus, the possibilities of Chievitz's organ, a neuroepithelial hamartoma, or odontogenic epithelium should be considered before concluding that perineural carcinoma is present.[18–20] .

The presence and extent of mandibular invasion by a mucosal squamous cell carcinoma can be assessed by using a periosteal elevator (or a #7 dental wax spatula or similar instrument) to separate gingiva or mucoperiosteum from the mandible, and noting the location, size, and shape of the underlying osseous cortical defect.[21,22] The exact location and orientation of sections prepared from this soft-tissue component of the mandibulectomy should be described. This approach can help clarify whether or not a putative primary intraosseous carcinoma or central mucoepidermoid carcinoma located in the retromolar region could possibly have arisen from surface mucosa.

If a band saw is available, the mandible can be cut into transverse segments and again placed in formalin to ensure adequate fixation of the intraosseous component of each segment. If the laboratory is not so equipped, available cutting instruments should be used to breach the cortex, permit fixation of intrabony tumor, and enable sampling of the tumor prior to decalcification of the mandible. Even though decalcification apparently has little effect on tissue immunoreactivity (if heat-induced epitope retrieval is used), undecalcified tissue is preferable for optimal routine staining.[23] The decalcified mandible can then be transversely sectioned with a knife. The inadequacy of curettage in treating ameloblastoma has been demonstrated by using a curette to enucleate the apparently circumscribed tumor from an en bloc resection specimen; subsequent transverse sections prepared from the decalcified specimen often reveal residual tumor islands in mandibular bone some distance from the smooth-walled defect previously occupied by the ameloblastoma.

The principles outlined above for handling mandibular specimens apply also to maxillectomy specimens.[24] See Chapter 6 for a detailed discussion of maxillectomy specimen handling.

The radical neck dissection specimen includes the submandibular gland, sternocleidomastoid muscle, internal jugular vein, spinal accessory nerve, omohyoid muscle, and lymph nodes in the cervical adipose tissue. When surgeons stage a patient with upper aerodigestive tract cancer, they usually identify cervical lymph nodes in five regions or "levels":[25–27]

Level 1   Submandibular and submental
Level 2   Upper jugular
Level 3   Mid-internal jugular
Level 4   Lower internal jugular
Level 5   Posterior triangle

To facilitate clinicopathologic correlation, therefore, the pathologist should segregate lymph nodes from radical neck dissection specimens into these same corresponding groups. In a modified or functional neck dissection, the spinal accessory nerve, internal jugular nerve, and sternocleidomastoid are not included in the specimen. The number of lymph nodes in each group is recorded, and the largest lymph node in each group is measured; gross features of metastatic tumor are described. Numerous fat-free small lymph nodes of similar size can be placed in a single cassette, and representative segments of each large lymph node are sampled. Even if they are apparently grossly uninvolved by tumor, each major structure in the specimen—the sternocleidomastoid muscle, the internal jugular vein, the submandibular gland (and if present, the parotid gland or thyroid gland) should also be histologically sampled.

FROZEN SECTIONS

Frozen sections are used primarily to establish or confirm a histopathologic diagnosis, to assess the completeness of the excision (margins), and to assist in accurate tumor staging.[28–30] Lymphoid and spindle cell neoplasms can be particularly difficult to classify definitively on frozen sections; the pathologist may be able only to categorize the disease process broadly (reactive, benign, or malignant), and in some cases, the diagnosis must be deferred until permanent sections can be evaluated. After the tumor has been excised, the surgeon may elect to sample portions of the surgical bed intraoperatively for evidence of residual tumor. These samples should be tagged with orientation sutures, and the aspect of the specimen representing the new margin should be clearly identified. The surgeon can help minimize the pathologist's potential sampling error by sending frozen section specimens no larger than 2.0 cm.[30] Surgeons should recognize that frozen sections cannot be performed on adipose tissue or cortical bone.[31] However, frozen sections of cancellous bone have been used to evaluate mandibular bony margins.[32] A frozen section intraoperative consultation usually take about 20 minutes to complete.[33]

In tissue sampled from the retromolar trigone area, the organ of Chievitz or odontogenic epithelium should not be misinterpreted as invasive carcinoma.[19,20,34] In addition, pseudocarcinomatous hyperplasia associated with a granular cell tumor or necrotizing sialometaplasia probably represents a greater hazard for misdiagnosis on frozen sections than on permanent sections, particularly if a previous tissue sampling from the site has already established a diagnosis of squamous cell carcinoma.[35–37] To minimize potential misinterpretation of frozen sections, the surgeon should communicate to the pathologist the patient's history of previous malignancies and their therapies; radiation therapy can induce pseudomalignant tissue changes.[38,39]

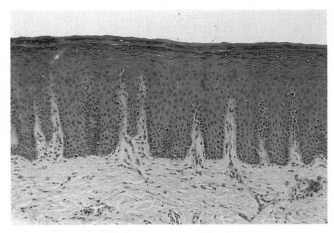

FIGURE 9–29 Normal palate.

SPECIAL STUDIES

When the surgeon believes that direct immunofluorescence studies could be helpful in the evaluation of patients with oral vesiculobullous lesions, paralesional mucosa should be sampled and sent immediately to the immunofluorescence laboratory. Although such specimens reportedly retain immunoreactivity for weeks in Michel's transport medium, one vendor of this medium recommends that the specimen remain in transport medium no longer than 5 days.[40] Keratinocytes demonstrate evidence of cytolysis after 48 hours in Michel's solution.[41]

If the pathologist anticipates that DNA or RNA in situ hybridization studies may be of value in evaluating an intraosseous lesion requiring decalcification, an ethylenediamine tetra-acetic acid (EDTA) containing decalcification solution should be used; it permits more reliable results than does a hydrochloric acid–containing decalcification solution.[42]

NORMAL ANATOMY AND HISTOLOGY OF THE ORAL CAVITY

Oral Mucosa

The oral mucosa consists of the keratinized tissues of the attached gingiva and hard palatal mucosa, nonkeratinized mucosa of the lower labial mucosa (inner lip mucosa), buccal mucosa (inner cheek mucosa), nonattached gingiva (movable gingiva that continues into the maxillary and mandibular sulci), ventral tongue, floor of the mouth, mucosa of the soft palate and tonsillar pillars, and specialized keratinized gustatory mucosa of the dorsum of the tongue.[43]

The keratinized tissues of the attached gingiva and hard palate may be orthokeratinized with a granular cell layer, or may be parakeratinized (Fig. 9–29). The epithelium is three to four times the

thickness of the epidermis of skin. Beneath the epithelium is the lamina propria, composed of fibrous tissue and blood vessels. Since there is no muscularis mucosa, a true submucosa is not present. The mucosa abuts the densely fibrous periosteum of the hard palate or the alveolus of the maxilla and mandible. Mucous glands are present in the lamina propria, particularly in the posterior hard palatal mucosa, with mature fatty tissue being prominent in the anterior hard palatal mucosa. Occasionally, rests of odontogenic epithelium with clear cells are found in the gingiva, the so-called rests of Serres.

The crevicular epithelium is a continuation of the gingival epithelium as it turns inward toward the tooth surface and then toward the root of the tooth. This epithelium is nonkeratinized and often exhibits irregular hyperplasia, leukocyte exocytosis, and microulcerations because of the response of the epithelium to plaque in the gingival crevice. The nonkeratinized mucosas consist of the epithelium with a relatively thick spinous cell layer and the lamina propria (Fig. 9–30). The term "submucosa" is sometimes loosely applied to the deep connective tissue

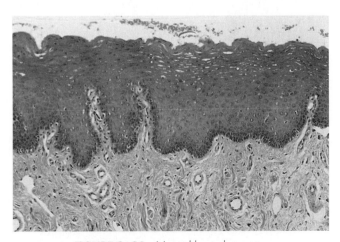

FIGURE 9–30 Normal buccal mucosa.

just above the muscle layer, in which the minor salivary glands are often embedded.

The anterior two thirds of the tongue dorsum is covered by keratinized stratified squamous epithelium specialized to form filiform papillae, pointed projections of keratin often associated with bacterial colonies (Fig. 9–31). In between these are the fungiform papillae, mushroom-shaped elevations of the mucosa that contain taste buds. Separating the anterior two thirds from the posterior one third are eight to twelve circumvallate papillae. These contain many taste buds at their base, and the serous salivary glands of the posterior tongue empty into the crypts surrounding these papillae. The last group of papillae are the foliate papillae located in the posterior lateral tongue in a series of ridges. Each taste bud consists of a barrel-shaped collection of modified epithelial cells extending vertically from the basal lamina to the epithelial surface, opening via a taste pore. They are innervated by terminal nerve twigs from the lamina propria. All the epithelia also contain nonkeratinocytes—melanocytes, Langerhans' cells, Merkel's cells, and lymphocytes.

Teeth

The tooth is composed of enamel, dentin, cementum, and pulp. Enamel is a calcified product laid down by ameloblasts of ectodermal derivation. In its mature form, it is composed of approximately 96% cal-

cified material in the form of hydroxyapatite crystals, 3% water, and 1% organic matrix. In decalcified sections, the small amount of protein matrix appears as hematoxyphilic fragments with a "fish-scale" or "keyhole" configuration. These proteins are known as amelogenins in developing enamel and as enamelins in mature enamel; their amino-acid composition is similar to, but not identical to, keratin.

The dentin forms the bulk of the tooth and is covered by enamel in the crown of the tooth and by cementum in the root. It is composed of 68% inorganic material, 22% organic material (mainly collagen), and 10% water. The odontoblast resides in the pulp and has a long odontoblastic process that extends from the pulp through a tunnel or tubule within the dentin to the dentin–enamel junction. In decalcified sections, the dentin appears as eosinophilic and homogenous with evenly dispersed tubules.

Cementum covers the root of the tooth and is close to bone in its composition and histologic appearance. It is composed of 45% to 50% mineralized material and 50% to 55% organic material. It differs from bone in its lack of haversian systems and blood vessels or nerves within it. It has lacunae, within which reside cementocytes that appear similar to osteocytes; it is deposited incrementally. Periodontal fibers, thick bands of collagen, penetrate the cementum and are attached to the bone of the alveolar process, anchoring the teeth in the jaws.

The pulp is composed of loose connective tissue, neurovascular elements, and the odontoblasts at the periphery. It provides vitality for the tooth as a whole; the neurovascular elements enter the tooth through the apical foramen at the tip of the root.

Minor Salivary Glands

The salivary glands of the labial and buccal mucosa are predominantly mucous with occasional serous units. There are two sites in the mouth where serous minor salivary glands predominate. One is in the posterior tongue, where the serous units are known as the glands of Von Ebner; they secrete into the crypts of the circumvallate and foliate papillae. The other is in the anterior ventral tongue, where they are known as the glands of Blandin-Nuhn.

DEVELOPMENTAL CONDITIONS

Heterotopias

LINGUAL THYROID

Gross Pathology

The lingual thyroid is usually located in the base of the tongue, most often lying between the foramen caecum and the epiglottis; it presents as a fleshy, pink, painless mass.

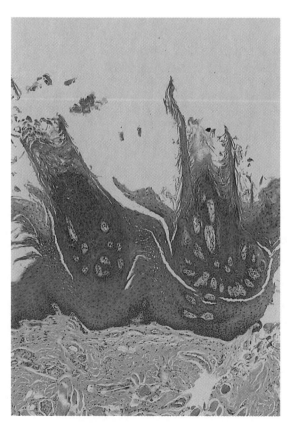

FIGURE 9–31 Normal tongue.

Microscopic Pathology

The lingual thyroid consists of microfollicular, macrofollicular, or fetal adenomatous thyroid gland tissue, with varying degrees of inflammation, cystification, and degeneration (Fig. 9–32).[44,45] Rarely, thyroid follicular lesions (including nodules, adenomas, and carcinomas) may arise in lingual thyroid tissue. If a carcinoma is present, it is usually a thyroid papillary carcinoma.[46]

Clinicopathologic Correlation

Ectopic thyroid tissue may be found anywhere along the normal path of descent of the thyroid gland, from its original anlagal position posterior to the tuberculum impar, to its final pretracheal position. Asymptomatic thyroid tissue has been found in the posterior tongue dorsum in 10% of necropsies.[44] In 70% to 100% of patients, this may be the only existent thyroid tissue.[45] There is a 4:1 female predilection; symptoms such as dysphonia, sore throat, and awareness of a mass in the throat often become evident during adolescence and pregnancy.[45] Radioisotopic imaging typically shows radionuclide activity in the mouth, but not in the neck.

HETEROTOPIC GASTROINTESTINAL AND GLIAL TISSUE

Gross Pathology

Grossly, both types may present as nondescript tongue masses.

Microscopic Pathology

Heterotopic gastroenteric tissue presents as solid or cystic lesions that consist of gastric or colonic mucosa with varying amounts of smooth muscle (Fig. 9–33).[44,47] Heterotopic glial tissue contains glial cells, sometimes with elements of ependyma and choroid plexus.[48,49]

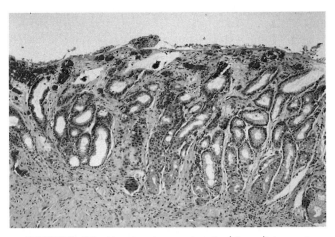

FIGURE 9–33 Heterotopic gastrointestinal tissue lining cyst.

Clinicopathologic Correlation

Heterotopic glial tissue usually presents in infants. Both types of heterotopia likely arise from displaced gastrointestinal and neural elements during embryogenesis.

FORDYCE GRANULES

Fordyce granules (heterotopic sebaceous glands) appear as yellow-white papules on the buccal mucosa and labial mucosa.[50]

Microscopic Pathology

Fordyce granules consist of normal sebaceous glands that often communicate with the surface through a duct. These glands may become hyperplastic with retention of secretions and pseudocyst formation.[51] Adenomas rarely arise.[52]

Clinicopathologic Correlation

Fordyce granules occur in approximately 80% of the population. Because of their high prevalence, many consider them as normal anatomical variations.

OSSEOUS AND CARTILAGINOUS CHORISTOMAS OF THE TONGUE

Gross Pathology

Osseous and cartilaginous choristomas of the tongue generally appear as sessile masses or nodules.

Microscopic Pathology

An osseous choristoma consists of dense lamellar bone with haversian systems, viable osteocytes, and inconspicuous osteoblastic activity. Mature fat may be present, and the lesion is often surrounded by dense fibrous tissue.[44,53] A cartilaginous choristoma consists of a nodule of hyaline cartilage surrounded

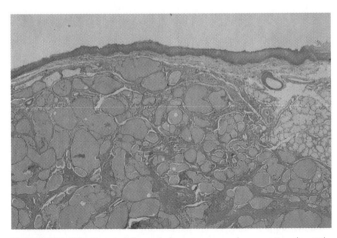

FIGURE 9–32 Lingual thyroid showing normal-appearing thyroid follicles.

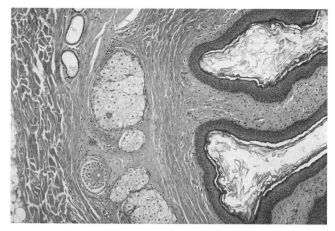

FIGURE 9-34 Dermoid cyst, orthokeratinized, with skin adnexa.

by dense fibrous tissue. Myxoid, primitive-appearing tissue may be present, and chondrocytes are mature without atypia.[44,54]

Clinicopathologic Correlation

Osseous choristomas of the tongue generally occur in adults, in the mid posterior dorsum, just anterior to the circumvallate papillae, with a 4:1 female predilection.[53] Cartilaginous choristomas are less common and tend to occur on the lateral tongue, with the sexes equally affected.[54] Both may result from entrapped pluripotent rests (from brachial cleft mesenchyme) or osseous and cartilaginous metaplasia.[44]

EPIDERMOID/DERMOID/TERATOID CYST

Gross Pathology

Depending on their location in relation to the mylohyoid and geniohyoid, the cyst may present intraorally, or in the submental or submandibular space.[55]

Microscopic Pathology

The epidermoid cyst is sometimes referred to as an epithelial inclusion cyst and is histologically similar to its counterpart on the skin. The cyst is lined by orthokeratinized stratified squamous epithelium with a prominent granular cell layer, with keratinaceous material filling the lumen. The term "dermoid cyst" applies if skin adnexa such as sweat glands, sebaceous glands, and hair follicles are present (Fig. 9–34). If muscle, bone, respiratory and/or gastrointestinal mucosa are also present, the terms "teratoid cyst" or "cystic teratoma" are used.[55]

Clinicopathologic Correlation

These are dysontogenic or developmental cysts of the oral cavity, most often found in the midline of the floor of the mouth or the midline of the ventral tongue. They present as slow-growing, painless, slightly yellowish, soft and doughy masses, with approximately half the patients being younger than 15 years, and an equal sex distribution. They may arise from entrapment of epithelium during fusion of embryonic structures; traumatic implantation of epithelium in utero may be a causative factor.

ORAL LYMPHOEPITHELIAL CYST

Gross Pathology

Generally, oral lymphoepithelial cysts (OLEC) present as soft yellowish masses occurring in the floor of the mouth or the ventral and posterolateral tongue.

Microscopic Pathology

The microscopic appearance is similar to that of the branchial cleft cyst (cervical lymphoepithelial cyst). The cyst is lined by stratified squamous epithelium, often thinly parakeratotic, with lymphocyte exocytosis and desquamation of keratin into the lumen. The epithelium is either completely or partially surrounded by lymphoid tissue that may contain hyperplastic follicles with phagocytic activity (Fig. 9–35). Mucous cells and occasionally respiratory epithelium may also be identified.[56–58]

Clinicopathologic Correlation

OLEC arises in adults (mean age 40 years), with approximately 50% occurring in the floor of the mouth, and most of the remainder in the ventral and posterolateral tongue. One theory suggests that OLEC arises as a result of obstruction of the crypts in oral tonsils, leading to cystic dilatation of the proximal portion of the crypt. Another theory is that OLEC arises from proliferation and cystification of epithelial remnants entrapped within lymphoid ag-

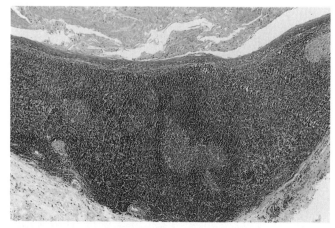

FIGURE 9-35 Oral lymphoepithelial cyst showing squamous lining epithelium with lymphocytic infiltration and lymphoid follicle.

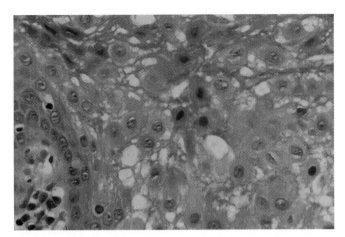

FIGURE 9-36 White sponge nevus with spongiosis with dyskeratosis.

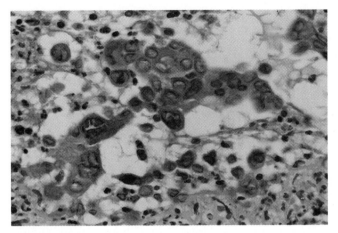

FIGURE 9-37 HSV infection with multinucleated epithelial cells with "ground-glass" and molded nuclei.

gregates similar to the mechanism of the formation of branchial cleft cysts.[56–58]

WHITE SPONGE NEVUS

Gross Pathology

White sponge nevus usually presents as thick, spongy, folded, and boggy-appearing mucosa.

Microscopic Pathology

There is parakeratosis, acanthosis, and dyskeratosis, with prominent spongiosis unassociated with inflammation. Peri- and paranuclear eosinophilic cytoplasmic condensations are characteristic, representing abnormal tonofilament aggregates (Fig. 9–36).[59] Recent investigations have revealed a mutation in differentiation specific keratins in a domain critical for keratin filament stability.[60,61]

Clinicopathologic Correlation

This is an autosomal dominant condition with onset in early childhood. It primarily affects the oral mucous membranes, usually occurring bilaterally on the buccal mucosa, although the alveolar ridge mucosa and tongue may be involved. There may also be involvement of the esophageal, genital, and laryngeal mucosa.[62–64]

INFECTIOUS MUCOSAL CONDITIONS

Herpes Virus Infections

Gross Pathology

Herpes simplex virus (HSV) and cytomegalovirus (CMV) infections present as vesiculobullous and ulcerative lesions, respectively.[65] Infection by Epstein-

Barr virus (EBV) presents in two ways. In infectious mononucleosis, oral ulcers occur on the mucosa, especially in the posterior oral cavity. In oral hairy leukoplakia (most often but not exclusively associated with HIV infection), the EBV infection gives rise to shaggy white lesions on the lateral tongue and other mucosal surfaces.[66]

Histopathology

At the edge of the mucosal HSV ulcer are large multinucleated epithelial cells with "ground-glass" homogenized nuclei, often exhibiting nuclear molding (Fig. 9–37). There may be an accompanying intraepithelial bulla. In CMV infections, the infected cells—usually of fibroblastic, monocytic, or endothelial cell origin—have large nuclei with prominent eosinophilic nucleoli (Fig. 9–38).

Hairy leukoplakia exhibits shaggy parakeratosis and leukoedema (discussed later in this chapter). The EBV-infected epithelial cells have vacuolated cy-

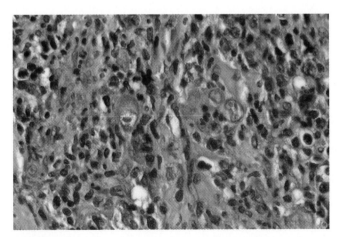

FIGURE 9-38 Cell infected with CMV exhibiting large nuclear inclusion.

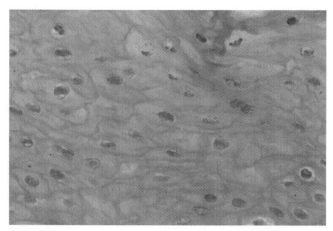

FIGURE 9–39 EBV infection associated with hairy leukoplakia with peripheral condensation of chromatin and large eosinophilic nuclear inclusions.

toplasm and are usually superficially placed, just beneath the keratin. The nuclei show dense central eosinophilic inclusions with condensations of chromatin against the nuclear membrane (Fig. 9–39).[67,68] Candidal hyphae are usually present, unassociated with spongiotic pustules; human papillomavirus, occurs concurrently in 15% to 55% of cases.[69,70]

Special Techniques

In suspected cases of HSV and CMV, immunohistochemical stains may be valuable in the identification of the virus. Herpes-type viruses are seen ultrastructurally in 85% of cases, and EBV is identified in over 80% of cases by in situ hybridization and polymerase chain reaction.[71]

Fungal Infections

CANDIDIASIS

Gross Pathology

The most common fungal infection in the oral cavity is candidiasis. Yellowish-white curdy plaques are typical findings, and the diagnosis is usually made on clinical grounds alone. However, in cases of atrophic candidiasis, which presents with marked mucosal erythema, a biopsy may rule out other inflammatory or neoplastic mucosal disease, such as erythroplakia.

Median rhomboid glossitis is a condition characterized by a raised, nodular, occasionally rhomboidal area of the midline dorsum of the tongue, just anterior to the circumvallate papillae. In symptomatic cases, candida are identified on the biopsy. Some authors believe the area in question to be a

developmental residuum of the tuberculum impar, an embryonic midline structure that failed to retract and is particularly susceptible to candidal infection.[72]

Microscopic Pathology

Candidiasis presents as superficial spongiotic pustules associated with candidal hyphae and a psoriasiform mucositis. In hyperplastic forms, there may be prominent epithelial hyperplasia with reactive atypia. In median rhomboid glossitis, the tongue dorsum exhibits atrophy of the filiform papillae. If the biopsy is taken from the midline, the median raphe may be present, consisting of a densely hyalinized and acellular area beneath the mucosa (Fig. 9–40).[73]

Bacterial Infections

GINGIVAL AND PERIODONTAL INFECTIONS

Gross Pathology

A chronic odontogenic infection may drain via a sinus tract that presents as a nodule on the attached gingiva, known as a "parulis."

Microscopic Pathology

The parulis is an epithelialized nodule of edematous granulation tissue that may be ulcerated. Many acute and chronic inflammatory cells are present. Foamy macrophages may be present and a parulis may sometimes be erroneously diagnosed as a mucocele. Abscesses are often present, and a linear "track" composed of neutrophils may be identified leading from the deep bony aspect to the surface ulcer, through which the abscess drains (Fig. 9–41).

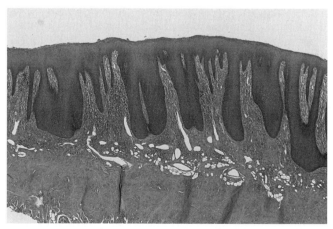

FIGURE 9–40 Median rhomboid glossitis showing psoriasiform mucositis and papillary atrophy of the tongue with median raphe.

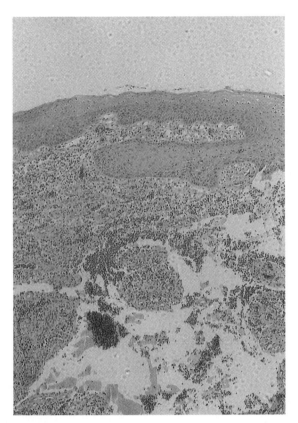

FIGURE 9-41 Parulis consisting of granulation tissue with acute and chronic inflammation and sinus tract.

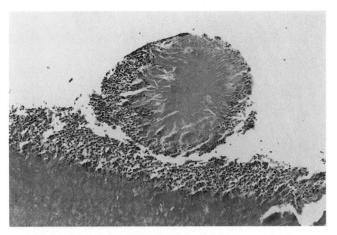

FIGURE 9-42 Actinomycotic colony ("sulfur granule") with radiate periphery associated with many neutrophils.

Clinicopathologic Correlation

These are some of the most common bacterial infections in the mouth. They may present acutely, as gingival, periodontal, dentoalveolar abscesses, or chronically, as chronic periodontal and periapical disease, with progressive bone loss and loosening of the teeth.

ACTINOMYCOSIS

Microscopic Pathology

The organism consists of a clump of gram-positive filaments, often with a surrounding gram-negative, eosinophilic perimeter, almost always surrounded by many neutrophils (Fig. 9-42). Clumps of actinomycetes-like organisms without any evident suppurative reaction most likely represent banal dental calculus and should not be overdiagnosed as actinomycosis.

Clinicopathologic Correlation

Actinomyces is a gram-positive anaerobic organism that may cause cervicofacial actinomycosis, which has several clinical presentations. The most common

form is an acute periapical abscess with associated soft-tissue swelling. The next clinical form is classically described as an indurated board-like swelling of the neck and skin overlying the jaw bones, often with multiple draining sinuses in which "sulfur granules" may be identified. The third and least common clinical form is the one diagnosed incidentally by culture.[74,75] The most common pathogenic species is *A. israelii*. The species *A. naeslundii, A. bovis, A. viscosus,* and *A. odontolyticus* have been implicated in infections with much lower frequency.

INFLAMMATORY MUCOSAL LESIONS

Leukoedema

Gross Pathology

Leukoedema occurs as a milky whiteness of the mucosa that disappears when the mucosa is stretched.

Microscopic Pathology

The mucosa is either thinly parakeratinized or nonkeratinized, and acanthotic. The most superficial keratinocytes often demonstrate loss of nuclei, with cell membranes somewhat collapsed upon one another. Below these is a layer of eosinophilic cells, then a layer of ballooned cells (so-called "intracellular edema") (Fig. 9-43).[76] These changes are seen in biopsies of the linea alba, an area of chronic low-grade injury present bilaterally in the buccal mucosa, adjacent to where the upper and lower teeth meet.

Clinicopathologic Correlation

Leukoedema occurs in 4% to 90% of the population.[77] It may be seen in up to 90% of black patients,

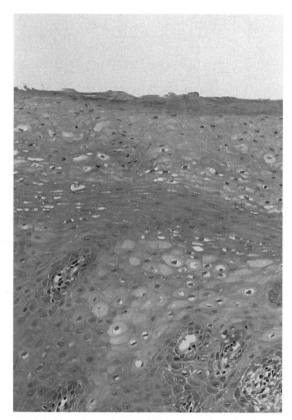

FIGURE 9–43   Leukoedema with superficial degenerated, anucleate cells, middle layer of densely eosinophilic condensed cells, and lower layer of ballooned cells.

probably because the pigmentation of the mucosa allows the overlying whiteness to show up more clearly in contrast. Leukoedema may represent a response to local low-grade noxious stimuli, as it has been associated with the use of tobacco products, chewing coca leaves, and smoking cannabis.[78-80]

Chronic Bite Injury

Gross Pathology

This white mucosal lesion (morsicatio buccarum, morsicatio labiorum, morsicatio linguarum) is painless, rough, shaggy, and white. It has a macerated appearance.

Microscopic Pathology

The epithelium is covered by a thick layer of parakeratin with many superficial fissures and clefts and papillary extensions of keratin rimmed by bacterial colonies, often with concomitant leukoedema (Fig. 9–44).[81,83] Unless ulcers and erosions are present, inflammatory cells are scant.

Clinicopathologic Correlation

This white lesion occurs in a primary and more extensive form, often bilaterally on the buccal mucosa and lateral tongue, because of a chronic habit of chewing the cheek and/or tongue. It is generally painless unless erosions and ulcers occur.[82,83] Occasionally, these changes occur as a secondary and localized finding on chronically traumatized lesions such as fibroma or oral hairy leukoplakia.

Recurrent Aphthous Stomatitis

Gross Pathology

Recurrent aphthous stomatitis appears as an ulcerated lesion with surrounding erythema.

Microscopic Pathology

The mucosa is ulcerated with an overlying fibrin clot. The ulcer base consists of varying amounts of granulation tissue with acute and chronic inflammation. The adjacent epithelium may exhibit reactive atypia and spongiosis. The findings are nonspecific. In patients with Behçet's disease, vasculitis may be present.[84]

Clinicopathologic Correlation

The minor form (less than 1.0 cm in size) afflicts approximately 20% of the population, presenting as recurrent episodes of painful ulcers with surrounding erythema. The ulcers usually heal within 1 to 2 weeks. Aphthous-like ulcers have been associated with systemic conditions such as hematinic deficiencies, Crohn's disease, Behçet's disease, and hypersensitivities to some foods. Major aphthous ulcers are often seen in HIV infection.[85]

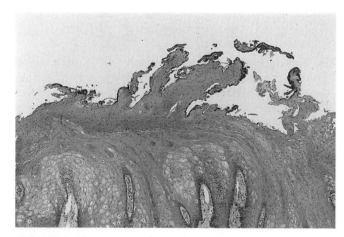

FIGURE 9–44   Hyperparakeratosis with keratotic papillae, fissures, and clefts rimmed by bacteria.

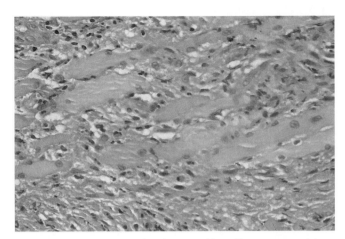

FIGURE 9–45 Mononuclear histiocyte-like infiltrate, eosinophils and muscle degeneration in traumatic ulcerative granuloma.

Traumatic Ulcerative Granuloma

Gross Pathology

As its name implies, these lesions are ulcerated and usually indurated.

Microscopic Pathology

At the ulcer base is abundant granulation tissue containing many acute and chronic inflammatory cells, sometimes forming an obviously exophytic mass. The underlying skeletal muscle exhibits myositis and degeneration; it is associated with a characteristic stromal eosinophilia and a histiocyte-like mononuclear cell infiltrate (Fig. 9–45).[86,87] T cells predominate over B cells. One study showed that the large histiocyte-like cells stained for CD68 while other cells stained for factor XIIIa, a dendritic cell marker. Neither class of cells stained for both.[88] Another study showed that while there were CD68-positive cells in the infiltrate, the large histiocyte-like cells were themselves not stained.[87] Another lesion that may simulate this condition, or even a lymphoma, is the atypical histiocytic granuloma that often contains atypical histiocyte-like cells.[89,90]

Clinicopathologic Correlation

Traumatic ulcerative granuloma presents either as an indurated ulcer of several weeks duration or a rapidly enlarging ulcerated mass that occurs most frequently on the tongue (50% to 75%). It is a condition of adults (mean age 34 years), with men affected from two to five times more frequently than women. Trauma plays an important role, and the term "Riga-Fede disease" has been used for a similar lesion occurring on the ventral tongue of infants and young children as a result of trauma to the tongue from erupting teeth.[86,87]

Lichen Planus/Lichenoid Reactions

Gross Pathology

Four types of lichen planus are recognized:

1. Reticular and/or papular (classic)
2. Atrophic/erosive
3. Bullous
4. Plaque-type

Microscopic Pathology

There is usually hyperpara- or orthokeratosis with variable acanthosis. In erosive forms, the epithelium is thinned. Langerhans' cells are increased in number, and there are variable numbers of apoptotic cells. The basal cells are degenerated, and squamous cells abut the lamina propria that contains a variably intense lymphohistiocytic infiltrate (Fig. 9–46).[91,92] Plasma cells may be prominent in ulcerated lesions. Peri- and paravascular nodular lymphocytic infiltrates may be present (particularly in cinnamon-associated stomatitides).[93] There may be melanin incontinence. In chronic ulcerative stomatitis, which may clinically and histologically resemble oral erosive lichen planus, a speckled nuclear anti-IgG pattern is noted on direct immunofluorescence.[94] If significant papillomatosis is present, a careful evaluation for architectural and cytologic atypia should be undertaken to rule out "lichenoid dysplasia."[95,96]

The lymphocytic infiltrate is primarily a T-cell population (CD4 and CD8 cells), and it is believed that oral lichen planus probably represents a cell-mediated delayed-type hypersensitivity reaction to as yet unidentified antigens and perhaps to a range of antigens. The role of cytokines, integrins, and adhesion molecules in the etiopathogenesis of lichen planus is currently under investigation.[97]

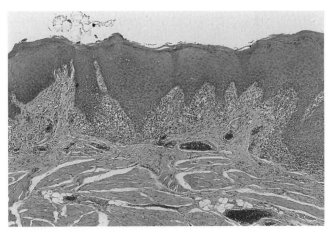

FIGURE 9–46 Lichen planus characterized by parakeratosis, saw-tooth rete ridges, basal cell degeneration, and lymphocytic band.

Clinicopathologic Correlation

Oral lichen planus affects 1% to 2% of the population, with women affected twice as frequently as men; skin lesions may be present in 4% to 44% of cases.[98] While many cases are idiopathic, lichen planus or lichenoid mucositides are also associated with ingestion of certain medications (such as antihypertensive agents) and with contact phenomenon related to dental restorations. In the European literature, hepatitis C and treatment with interferon is associated with the development of lichen planus, possibly related to circulating antibodies to epithelium.[99-101] Patients with autoimmune disorders such as discoid lupus erythematosus and chronic graft-versus-host disease often present with similar lichenoid lesions in the mouth.[102,103]

It appears that the basic etiopathogenesis is a T-cell mediated destruction of the basal epithelial cells, which have surface antigenic alterations.[104] Lichen planus has been associated with a 0.4% to 6.0% rate of malignant transformation to squamous cell carcinoma in both smokers and nonsmokers.[105,106]

Benign Migratory Glossitis/Erythema Migrans

Gross Pathology

Erythema migrans occurs as variably symptomatic, raised, circinate, curvilinear, white lesions that surround erythematous and atrophic areas of the mouth and tongue. The lesions are evanescent and often change in shape during the evolution of the lesion (hence the term "migratory glossitis").[107]

Microscopic Pathology

On the tongue, there is atrophy of the filiform papillae. Psoriasiform mucositis is the primary histologic feature, namely epithelial hyperplasia with thinning of the suprapapillary epithelial plates, neutrophilic exocytosis with spongiotic pustules, edema in the lamina propria, dilatation of papillary vessels, and chronic inflammation (Fig. 9-47).[107] Depending on the stage of evolution of the lesions, the severity of changes varies considerably and may be quite subtle. Stains for candidiasis should be performed and are negative in bona fide lesions of erythema migrans.

Clinicopathologic Correlation

Patients with generalized pustular psoriasis and Reiter's disease may present concurrently with this condition.[108,109] Atopy may be an important predisposing factor.[110]

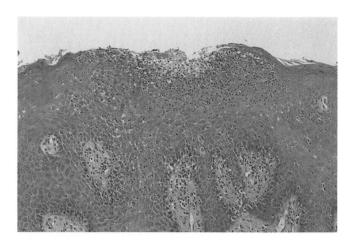

FIGURE 9–47 Psoriasiform mucositis with prominent spongiotic pustulosis in benign migratory glossitis.

Orofacial Granulomatosis

Gross Pathology

The lips are usually swollen and may demonstrate erosions and vesicles.

Microscopic Pathology

There are noncaseating granulomas within the lamina propria that do not contain either organisms using the usual staining techniques or identifiable foreign material (Fig. 9–48).[111,112] There is usually surrounding edema with mild chronic inflammation and dilated lymphatic channels. Serial sections may be necessary to identify granulomas that may be inconspicuous.

Clinicopathologic Correlation

Orofacial granulomatosis is a term used to describe a condition of painless facial and/or lip swelling

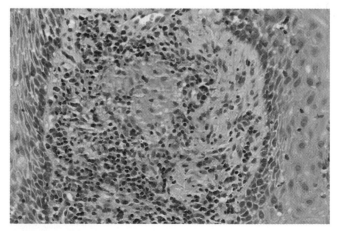

FIGURE 9–48 Non-necrotizing granulomas in orofacial granulomatosis.

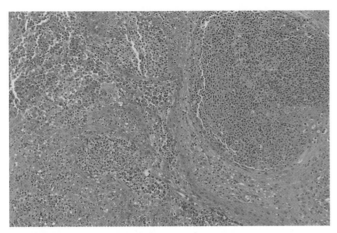

FIGURE 9–49 Pseudoepitheliomatous hyperplasia with mixed inflammatory infiltrate and eosinophilic abscesses in Wegener's granulomatosis.

with gingival hyperplasia caused by a noninfectious granulomatous process. Some investigators use this term to include this condition coexistent with systemic granulomatous disease such as Crohn's disease and sarcoidosis, while others use it to refer to only granulomatous disease of unknown etiology in the orofacial region. Atopy or hypersensitivity reactions to a variety of antigens have been implicated as etiologic factors.[113] The triad of cheilitis granulomatosa, fissured tongue, and VII nerve palsy constitutes the Melkersson-Rosenthal syndrome.

Wegener's Granulomatosis

Gross Pathology

Oral lesions present as ulcers and delayed wound healing. A characteristic feature is reddish-purple, granular, pebbly, "strawberry" gingivitis, often with petechiae.[114–116]

Microscopic Pathology

Lesions are characterized by necrosis, vasculitis, and granuloma formation although the presence of these features depends greatly on specimen adequacy, with the triad present in less than 20% of cases.[117] Fibrinoid necrosis of vessel walls and areas of geographic necrosis may be evident. A mixed inflammatory infiltrate, eosinophilic abscesses, extravasated red blood cells, and pseudoepitheliomatous hyperplasia are often present (Fig. 9–49).[114,115]

Special Stains

The histologic diagnosis of Wegener's granulomatosis is often one of exclusion. Special stains for micro-

organisms—including tissue Gram stain, periodic acid-Schiff (PAS), Gomori methenamine silver (GMS), and acid-fast bacilli (AFB)—are indicated to exclude the presence of an infectious agent.

Clinicopathologic Correlation

In its classic form, Wegener's granulomatosis is characterized by necrotizing granulomatous inflammation of the upper and lower respiratory tract and segmental necrotizing glomerulonephritis.[117] Variants include one that is limited to pulmonary manifestations and a superficial form that presents for protracted periods of time primarily in the upper respiratory tract, mucosa, and skin.[118] Tests should be performed to assess renal function, erythrocyte sedimentation rate, chest and sinus films, and assays for antineutrophil cytoplasmic antibodies, which are present in up to 90% of patients with active otorhinolaryngological disease.[119]

Cheilitis Glandularis

Microscopic Pathology

The salivary glands exhibit dilated excretory ducts with squamous (and sometimes mucous cell) metaplasia that often contains purulent material (Fig. 9–50). There is variable chronic and acute interstitial inflammation with acinar atrophy.[120]

Clinicopathologic Correlation

This uncommon condition of adults causes painful nodular swelling and eversion of the lower lip; it may be related to actinic damage.[121] Purulence may be noted at ductal orifices.

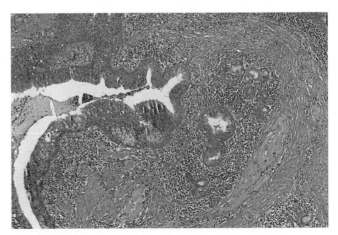

FIGURE 9–50 Ductal dilatation and luminal purulence with surrounding acute and chronic inflammation in cheilitis glandularis.

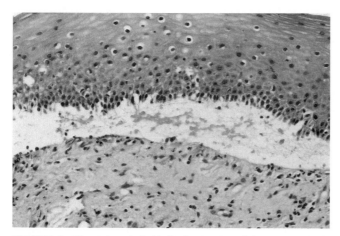

FIGURE 9–51 Subepithelial bulla formation with maintenance of the basal cells in mucous membrane/cicatricial pemphigoid.

Plasma Cell Gingivitis

Microscopic Pathology

The striking feature is sheets of plasma cells in the lamina propria that are polyclonal in nature and do not exhibit atypia. The overlying epithelium is hyperplastic with spongiosis and occasional microcyst and pustule formation.[122] Chronic periodontitis and gingivitis may also exhibit sheets of plasma cells and should be not be confused with plasma cell gingivitis; clinical findings will differentiate between the two.

Clinicopathologic Correlation

This condition is characterized by usually painful, edematous, and markedly erythematous gingival tissue. It was first described in the 1970s, attributed to a hypersensitivity reaction to a component of chewing gum.[123] Some cases, however, are of unknown etiology. The laryngeal mucosa may be involved.[124]

Cicatricial/Mucous Membrane Pemphigoid

Microscopic Pathology

There is subepithelial bulla formation with preservation of the basal cells (Fig. 9–51). Chronic inflammation is present in the lamina propria, which may contain some granulation tissue. Fibrosis is variably present.

Special Techniques

Direct immunofluorescence shows a characteristic linear band at the epithelium-connective interface, with positive staining for anti-IgG and C3.[125] The antigen involved is closely related to BP-230 and BP-180, two antigens found in bullous pemphigoid that localize in the desmosomal plaque and lamina lucida respectively.[126,127]

Clinicopathologic Correlation

This disease mainly affects elderly females who present with oral bullae, often ruptured to form ulcers. The oral mucosa is the most commonly affected site, followed by the eyes and the pharynx.[128,129] Some present primarily with a desquamative gingivitis (painful, red, peeling gingiva), in which case, the lesions may resemble lichen planus, another common oral condition that presents with gingival desquamation.[130] Pemphigus vulgaris may also primarily present as a desquamative gingivitis. Recent research suggests distinguishing mucous membrane pemphigoid from cicatricial pemphigoid, although both have pathogenetic mechanisms similar to bullous pemphigoid, a condition that primarily affects the skin.[97]

Nicotinic Stomatitis

Gross Pathology

The lesion appears as white, thickened mucosa with a cobblestone appearance and multiple red puncta representing the inflamed orifices of the excretory salivary ducts.

Microscopic Pathology

There is squamous metaplasia of the excretory salivary ducts, associated with a sialodochitis (inflammation of the salivary duct). The opening of the duct may exhibit epithelial hyperplasia, and the adjacent mucosa exhibits hyperkeratosis and acanthosis (Fig. 9–52).[131]

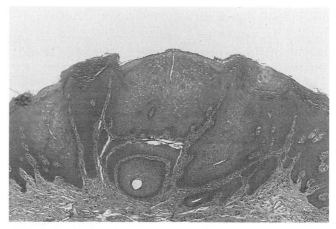

FIGURE 9–52 Squamous metaplasia of excretory ducts and sialodochitis in nicotinic stomatitis.

Clinicopathologic Correlation

Pipe smokers are prone to develop nicotinic stomatitis on the palatal mucosa as a result of heat generated from the pipe.

Smokeless Tobacco Keratosis

Gross Pathology

There is a greyish-white opalescence to the mucosa with faint parallel ridges and grooves. The area where the smokeless tobacco wad (snuff or chewing tobacco) is placed may be lax and stretched, forming a pouch, depending on duration of the habit.

Microscopic Pathology

There is hyperparakeratosis with spires of parakeratin (so-called "chevrons"), mild acanthosis, and usually mild chronic inflammation (Fig. 9–53).[132] The upper one quarter to one third of the spinous cells appear swollen and degenerated, with many anucleate cells—a picture reminiscent of leukoedema. Sometimes a perivascular eosinophilic cuff may be noted. Epithelial dysplasia (see later section in this chapter on leukoplakia) may develop in lesions of leukoplakia after decades of use.[133,134]

Clinicopathologic Correlation

Approximately 13% of patients who use smokeless tobacco will have these lesions.[135] After prolonged and chronic use, an irreversible leukoplakia with attendant risk for carcinoma may develop.[133,136]

Amalgam Tattoo

Gross Pathology

Traumatic implantation of amalgam—a mixture of silver, mercury, and other elements—into the mu-

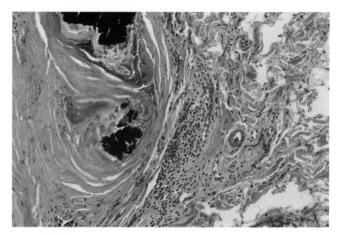

FIGURE 9–54 Coarse and fine granules of amalgam with foreign-body reaction and staining of the basement membrane of blood vessels.

cosa leads to a slate grey or black, painless, discrete macule or even diffuse pigmentation.

Microscopic Pathology

Within the lamina propria are large and small, yellow-brown to black, particulate matter, sometimes associated with a chronic or even granulomatous foreign-body reaction and fibrosis (Fig. 9–54). The fine granules stain the connective tissue fibers (especially the basement membrane of blood vessels and the epithelium), nerve fibers, and the endomysial tissues.[137] If fibers are not stained, another exogenous foreign material such as carbon (from pencil lead) should be considered.

Clinicopathologic Correlation

These may be found in any area of the mouth but are most frequently seen near amalgam restorations on the gingiva, alveolar ridge, and buccal mucosa.[137] Scars from apical surgeries and within tissues from biopsies are also prime sites.

Inflammatory Melanotic Lesions

Gross Pathology

Under this designation, three entities will be discussed: oral melanotic macule, melanoacanthosis, and postinflammatory hyperpigmentation. All present as tan to dark brown painless macules.

Microscopic Pathology

In *oral melanotic macule*, there is increased melanin pigmentation in the basal cells, usually prominent at the tips of the rete ridges, and increased numbers of melanophages in the lamina propria, sometimes associated with incontinent melanin (Fig. 9–55).[138,139]

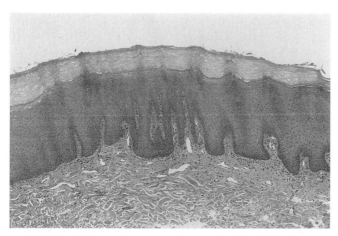

FIGURE 9–53 Coagulative degeneration of superficial epithelium with "chevrons" in smokeless tobacco keratosis.

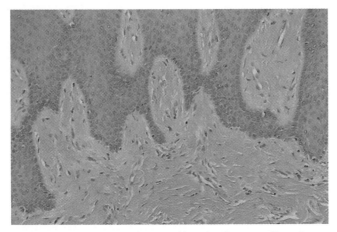

FIGURE 9-55 Hypermelanosis of basal cells especially at the tips of the rete ridges in oral melanotic macule.

There is generally insignificant inflammation, melanocytic hyperplasia, and insignificant epithelial hyperplasia—although this has been disputed.[140] In *melanoacanthosis*, there is epithelial hyperplasia associated with benign hyperplasia of dendritic melanocytes throughout the thickness of the epithelium, basal cell hypermelanosis, increased numbers of melanophages in the lamina propria, variable chronic inflammation, and increased vascularity (Fig. 9-56).[140,141] In *postinflammatory pigmentation*, there is underlying inflammation associated with increased melanin within the basal and suprabasal keratinocytes with incontinent pigment and increased numbers of melanophages in the lamina propria. As was earlier mentioned, this is a common finding in lichenoid reactions where the basal cells have been damaged.

Clinicopathologic Correlation

Oral melanotic macules occur primarily on the vermilion, gingiva, and buccal mucosa of adults. They present as solitary, 1 cm, circumscribed, pigmented lesions that remain constant in size, with the intensity of pigmentation usually unaffected by sunlight.[138] Melanoacanthosis occurs in young black females and presents as a rapidly enlarging, painless macular pigmented area of the buccal mucosa or labial mucosa that resolves over time.[141] This lesion should not be confused with the dermatologic entity of melanoacanthoma that occurs in older men. Postinflammatory hyperpigmentation occurs in dark-skinned individuals at sites of interface damage (as in oral lichen planus or lichenoid reactions). Finally, patients with Albright's or Addison's disease and Peutz-Jeghers syndrome may also present with multifocal macular pigmentation of the lips and oral mucosa.

BENIGN EPITHELIAL/NEVO-MELANOCYTIC PROLIFERATIONS

Papilloma, Verruca Vulgaris, Focal Epithelial Hyperplasia, and Condyloma Acuminatum

Squamous papillomas are warty or exophytic and have a pink or white surface.[142] These can appear similar to the *verruca vulgaris* or the common wart. Oral *condylomas* are similar in appearance to squamous papillomas but tend to be larger. Prime sites include the labial mucosa and soft palate. *Focal epithelial hyperplasia* is a condition characterized by multiple flat, pink-to-white papules on the labial, buccal, and tongue mucosa. It is often seen in the Native American population, mainly in children but also in young adults.[143] It may regress with time.

Microscopic Pathology

The squamous papilloma consists of a papillary proliferation of squamous epithelium usually covered by parakeratin, although a combination of ortho- and parakeratin may be present (Fig. 9-57). Koilocytosis is usually inconspicuous. HPV6 and -11 have been identified in up to 50% of cases.[144,145] The verruca vulgaris usually exhibits axial inclination of the papillary projections, particularly at the periphery; there is hyperorthokeratosis—although about 50% of cases will show a combination of ortho- and parakeratin, prominent coarse keratohyaline granules, and koilocytosis (Fig. 9-58).[142] Verruca vulgaris is also associated with HPV2, -4, -6, -11, and -16.[145]

Condylomas exhibit both exophytic papillary, and sometimes endophytic, epithelial proliferation, forming broad, bulbous rete ridges; koilocytes are usually readily identified (Fig. 9-59). These are generally associated with HPV6, -11, -16, and -18.[146]

In oral focal epithelial hyperplasia, the oral papules exhibit epithelial hyperplasia and koilocytosis

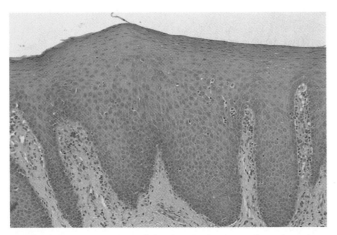

FIGURE 9-56 Presence of dendritic melanocytes throughout the full thickness of the hyperplastic epithelium in melanoacanthosis.

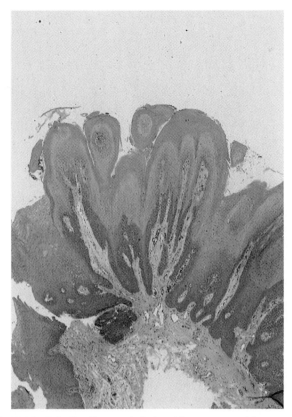

FIGURE 9–57 Papillary epithelial proliferation typical for squamous papilloma.

with mitosoid bodies, which are nuclei exhibiting karyorrhexis (Fig. 9–60).[143,147,148] These lesions are associated with HPV subtypes 13 and 32.

Differential Diagnosis

Foci of dysplastic epithelial changes may occur in these benign epithelial proliferations, but in contrast

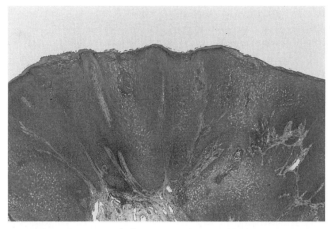

FIGURE 9–59 Large bulbous rete ridges and koilocytosis in condyloma acuminatum.

to squamous cell carcinoma, the dysplastic change is limited in extent; invasive carcinoma is not present. Differentiation from verrucous carcinoma may be problematic, as verrucous carcinomas lack cytologic dysplasia. The downward growth of the rete pegs in verrucous carcinoma is not a feature of these benign epithelial proliferations.

Clinicopathologic Correlation

Squamous papillomas are exophytic papillary squamous proliferations that may be associated with HPV infection. Adults are affected, and the most common sites for oral papillomas are the palate (approximately 20% on the soft palate), tongue, and lips. Verruca vulgaris occur on the lips, tongue, and gingiva, usually from autoinoculation from a skin site such as the fingers.[142] Prime sites for oral condylomas include the labial mucosa and soft palate. Focal epithelial hyperplasia occurs on the labial, buccal, and tongue mucosa.

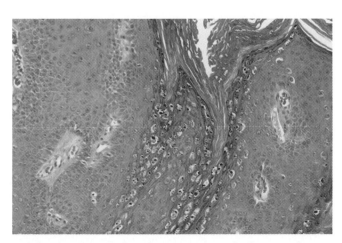

FIGURE 9–58 Hyperkeratosis, coarse keratohyaline granules, and koilocytes in verruca vulgaris.

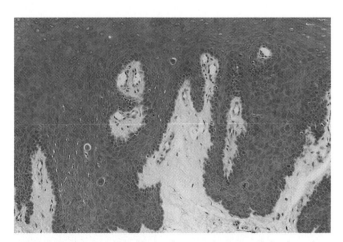

FIGURE 9–60 Epithelial hyperplasia and "mitosoid" bodies of focal epithelial hyperplasia.

Melanocytic Nevi

Oral melanocytic nevi range from fleshy, dome-shaped nodules to pigmented macules and are generally less than 1 cm in size. The most common site is the hard palate, followed by the buccal mucosa.

Microscopic Pathology

The cells of the *intramucosal nevus* are similar to those seen in the skin, both in cytologic features and architectural organization. The more superficial cells tend to be epithelioid and/or cuboidal in a nested configuration and contain the most pigment; occasional multinucleated nevus giant cells are present (Fig. 9–61). The cells themselves have large round nuclei and distinctly outlined pale cytoplasm. Deeper in the lesion, lymphocyte-like nevus cells with scant cytoplasm predominate. In the deepest portions, fibroblast-like nevus cells may be present. In *junctional nevi*, nests of benign nevus cells are present in the lower epithelium; in *compound nevi*, nevus cells are present both in the epithelium and in the lamina propria. There may be concomitant epithelial hyperplasia. In *blue nevi*, spindled and sometimes dendritic pigmented nevus cells are present in the lamina propria (Fig. 9–62).[149]

Differential Diagnosis

The differential diagnosis is primarily with malignant melanoma. The absence of cytologic atypia, asymmetric growth, pagetoid spread, and atypical mitoses assist in differentiating benign nevi from malignant melanoma.

Clinicopathologic Correlation

In one large study of intraoral melanocytic nevi, the most common was the intramucosal nevus, followed by the blue nevus, the compound nevus, and the

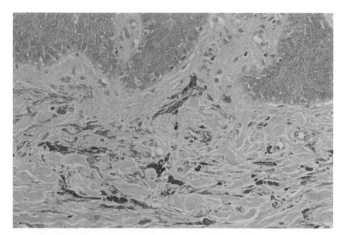

FIGURE 9–62 Dendritic melanocytes in the lamina propria of a blue nevus.

junctional nevus. The first two types comprised 90% of all intraoral nevi.[150]

BENIGN REACTIVE MESENCHYMAL PROLIFERATIONS AND TUMORS

Fibroma and Giant Cell Fibroma

Microscopic Pathology

The tumor consists of a mass of hypocellular fibrous tissue with variable vascularity, with usually mild to absent chronic inflammatory infiltrate, covered by hyperkeratotic squamous epithelium. Ulcerations may be present focally. The epithelium may be thinned, normal, or hyperplastic.

The giant cell fibroma may be multilobular with elongation of the rete ridges, often in a spiky configuration. Giant, stellate-shaped, and multinucleated fibroblasts are prominent, usually just beneath the epithelium (Fig. 9–63).[151,152]

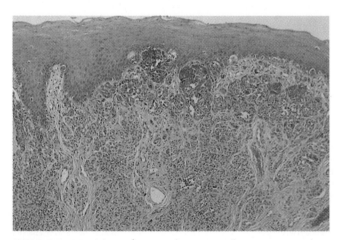

FIGURE 9–61 Nests of nevo-melanocytic cells in intramucosal nevus.

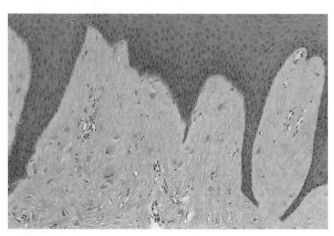

FIGURE 9–63 Spiky epithelial hyperplasia and stellate-shaped giant fibroblasts in giant cell fibroma.

Special Techniques

Ultrastructurally, these giant cells have features of myofibroblasts with microfilaments, dense bodies, and junctional complexes.

Clinicopathologic Correlation

The fibroma is the most common tumor encountered in the oral cavity. It is sometimes referred to as an "irritation" or "bite" fibroma because of its putative etiology. Favored locations are the buccal mucosa along the occlusal plane, the lateral border of the tongue, and the lower labial mucosa.

A variant of the fibroma is the giant cell fibroma, which has a propensity to occur on the gingiva (approximately 50% of cases), palate, and tongue.[151,152] It is often submitted with a clinical impression of papilloma because of the surface papillary configuration.

Gingival Nodules, including Pyogenic Granuloma, Peripheral Giant Cell Tumor, Peripheral Ossifying Fibroma

Nodular gingival proliferations are common and tend to be located on the marginal gingiva, often abutting the teeth. They may be ulcerated, polypoid, or sessile, and they may grow to several centimeters in size. The term "epulis" refers to any growth on the gingiva and does not presume specific etiology or histopathology. Banal fibromas and odontogenic fibromas tend to be flesh-colored, while pyogenic granulomas, peripheral giant cell granulomas, and peripheral ossifying fibromas tend to be vascular and ulcerated.

Pyogenic granulomas of the gingiva consist of lobular proliferations of capillaries and endothelial cells, often associated with surface ulceration and with varying degrees of acute and chronic inflammation. Sometimes referred to as "lobular hemangiomas," these may organize and sclerose, forming densely fibrotic nodules referred to as inflammatory fibrous hyperplasias or fibromas (Fig. 9–64).[153] It is possible that some gingival fibrous hyperplasias develop without a prior pyogenic granuloma phase. The term "granuloma gravidarum" has been used to describe pyogenic granulomas on the gingiva that develop during pregnancy.

The diffuse gingival lesions associated with ingestion of dilantin, essentially fibrous hyperplasias or sclerosing pyogenic granulomas, have been reported in association with elongated "test tube" rete ridges, although this is probably not a specific finding.

The *peripheral ossifying fibroma* consists of a densely cellular proliferation of fibroblasts with associated collagen and with the deposition of spherules or trabeculae of osteoid and/or bone (Fig. 9–65).[154,155] Some of these deposits take the form of calcified spherules akin to cementum, while others form

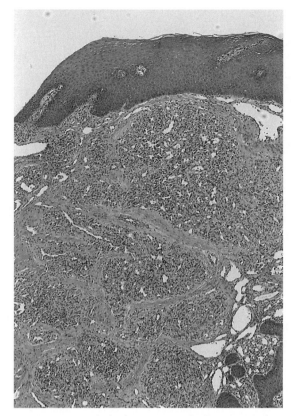

FIGURE 9–64 Lobular hemangioma/pyogenic granuloma.

anastomosing trabeculae of bone. These have also been referred to as "gingival fibromas with osseous metaplasia" or "calcifying fibromas."

The *peripheral giant cell granuloma* consists of a nodular proliferation of osteoclast-like multinucleated giant cells in a vascular stroma with acute and chronic inflammation (Fig. 9–66).[156,157] It is similar to the central giant cell granuloma of the jaw bones, except that in the peripheral lesions, the giant cells tend to be closely packed in sheets and not clustered

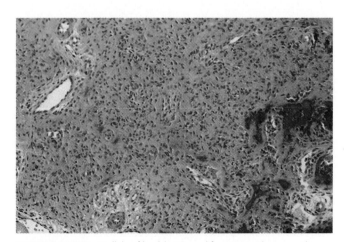

FIGURE 9–65 Cellular fibroblastic proliferation with woven bone and osteoid deposits in peripheral ossifying fibroma.

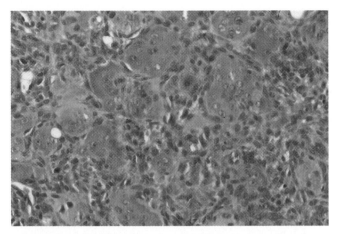

FIGURE 9–66 Multinucleated giant cells in a mononuclear, hemorrhagic stroma in peripheral giant cell fibroma.

as seen in the central lesions. Rarely, these peripheral lesions have been associated with hyperparathyroidism.[158] It is unclear whether such lesions may actually represent central giant cell granulomas that are associated with hyperparathyroidism, breaking through the bony cortex. The peripheral giant cell granuloma may resorb the underlying bone; it has a 10% recurrence rate.

Peripheral odontogenic fibroma is the extraosseous counterpart of the central odontogenic fibroma. It consists of a nonencapsulated proliferation of fibroblast-like cells, often with delicate intervening collagen and varying amounts of odontogenic epithelium (Fig. 9–67).[159,160] The latter is present in strands, cords, and small islands of bland-looking epithelium, sometimes with clear cells, and with a hint of palisading of the basal cell nuclei. Calcified material is often present; this may take several forms: amorphous eosinophilic material ("dentinoid"), cementum-like material, bone, and hematoxyphilic, globular, calcified material that is often encountered within dental follicles.

Diffuse gingival hyperplasia is associated with ingestion of medications such as dilantin, cyclosporine, nifedipine, and other calcium-channel blockers.[162] In many cases of gingival nodules, a combination of pyogenic granuloma, peripheral giant cell granuloma, and peripheral ossifying fibroma are present in various proportions. This is to be expected, as the etiology of all three conditions is local tissue hyperplasia and inflammation in response to local noxious stimuli, most likely from dental plaque.

Denture-Related Injuries

Gross Pathology

Denture-related lesions are exuberant soft-tissue reactions to ill-fitting dentures that chronically irritate the underlying mucosa. The epulis fissuratum, a papulous ridge of tissue found at the edge of a denture in the maxillary or mandibular sulcus, in which the flange of the denture fits, is a lesion usually seen in females; it may be focally ulcerated and have papillary configurations.[161] The clinical entity "papillary hyperplasia of the palate" consists of multiple sessile papillary structures, from 2 to 4 mm in diameter, usually erythematous and clustered in the arch of the palate.[163]

Microscopic Pathology

The epulis fissuratum consists of hyperplasia of fibrous tissue and often epithelium, often in a papillary configuration, sometimes with focal ulceration (Fig. 9–68). Chronic inflammation varies from mild to moderate, and often reactive lymphoid nodules are noted. Salivary glands are present in about 40% of specimens with varying degrees of inflammation.

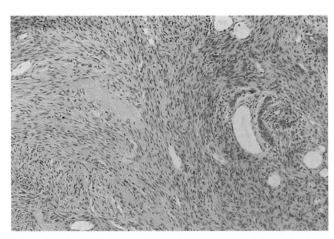

FIGURE 9–67 "Dentinoid" production in a cellular fibroblastic proliferation and cords of odontogenic epithelium in peripheral odontogenic fibroma.

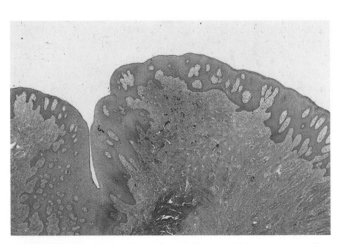

FIGURE 9–68 Hyperplasia of epithelium and fibrous tissue with surface papillomatosis in epulis fissuratum.

In 5% of cases, metaplastic hyaline or fibrocartilage and bone are present.[164] Papillary hyperplasia of the palate reveals the same changes, except that the papillary nature of the specimen is pronounced.[165] Spongiotic pustules may signify concomitant candidal infection. In both types of denture-related hyperplasia, there may be pseudoepitheliomatous hyperplasia.

Verruciform Xanthoma

Gross Pathology

This uncommon condition of the oral mucosa presents in adults as a painless, usually solitary, warty, sessile papule or plaque that is white, pink, or yellowish.

Microscopic Pathology

There is hyperparakeratosis with papillomatosis and characteristic brightly eosinophilic parakeratotic plugs within crypts between the papillary structures. Many large foam cells are present, almost exclusively within the connective tissue papillae, admixed with chronic inflammatory cells. The epithelium is acanthotic, forming uniformly elongated rete ridges that may coalesce at their bases (Fig. 9–69).[166,167]

Special Techniques

The foam cells contain lipid and stain with antibodies against CD68, confirming their histiocyte/macrophage nature.[168] They do not stain for S-100 protein.

Clinicopathologic Correlation

It has been suggested that as the parakeratotic cells in the crypts degenerate, macrophages migrate to

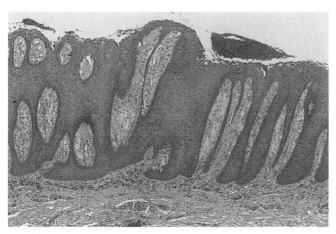

FIGURE 9–69 Papillary epithelial hyperplasia and many foam cells in the lamina propria typical for verruciform xanthoma.

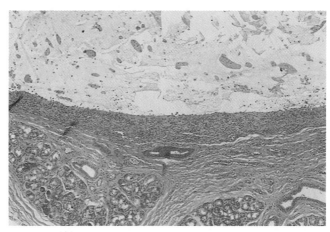

FIGURE 9–70 Pool of mucin surrounded by condensed granulation tissue in mucocele.

the area and ingest the released lipid, becoming xanthomatous.[169] Chronic irritation may be the predisposing factor; this may explain why verruciform xanthomas have been reported coexisting with other inflammatory dermatologic or mucosal conditions.[167,170] Other reports suggest that altered epithelial cell turnover, as is seen in neoplastic epithelial changes, may play an etiopathogenic role.[171] Approximately 75% of lesions occur on the gingiva or palatal mucosa.[166,167] Patients do not have an associated systemic lipidosis.

Mucocele

Gross Pathology

Mucoceles appear as bluish, dome-shaped, sessile, fluid-filled, submucosal masses.

Microscopic Pathology

The mucocele that results from mucus escape contains varying amounts of mucus suspending macrophages and neutrophils, surrounded by a wall of granulation tissue that also contains many muciphages (Fig. 9–70). There is variable inflammation, and a transected feeder duct is sometimes identified.[172] The mucocele that results from distal obstruction presents as a grossly dilated excretory duct lined by low cuboidal/columnar cells, two to five cells thick, often associated with mucous cell, ciliated cell, squamous cell, and/or oncocytic metaplasia (sometimes referred to as salivary duct cyst or reactive oncocytoid cyst) (Fig. 9–71). Papillary epithelial proliferations may be identified, and some of these mucopapillary cysts may be multicystic.[173] The surrounding minor salivary glands exhibit varying degrees of obstruction characterized by dilatation of intralobular ducts, acinar atrophy, interstitial fibrosis, and interstitial inflammation.

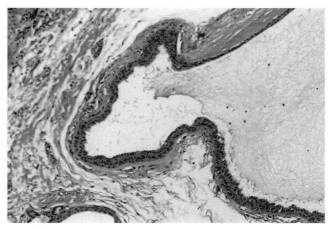

FIGURE 9-71 Dilated duct with oncocytic metaplasia in salivary duct cyst.

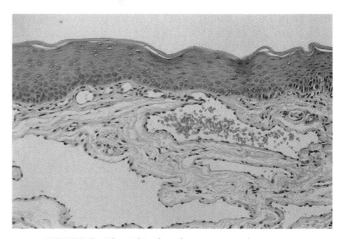

FIGURE 9-72 Dilated and tortuous venules in varix.

Clinicopathologic Correlation

Mucoceles present on the lower labial mucosa, floor of mouth, buccal mucosa, or on any other mucosal surface that normally contains salivary glands and is susceptible to trauma.[172] A mucocele (also called a sialocyst) may occur as a mucus escape phenomenon where severance of an excretory duct causes mucus to spill into the interstitium (a pseudocyst) or as a retention phenomenon where a distal obstruction causes the proximal duct to dilate and fill with mucus (a true cyst).[173] The superficial mucocele occurs on mucosa overlying bone, such as on the palate and retromolar pad, and should not be confused clinically with autoimmune vesiculobullous disorders.[174] The clinical differential diagnosis is mucoepidermoid carcinoma.

Varices (Venous Lakes)

Gross Pathology

Varices are raised, sessile, painless, bluish-purple blebs.

Microscopic Pathology

Within the lamina propria are dilated and tortuous venules that are filled with blood, or occasionally thrombi, in varying degrees of organization (Fig. 9-72).[175] Organizing thrombi at times exhibit intravascular papillary endothelial hyperplasia (Masson's tumor).

Clinicopathologic Correlation

Varices usually occur in adults greater than 30 years of age; 68% of reported cases were found in those over 60 years of age. Sublingual varices are usually bilateral and symmetrical.[176] When presenting as a solitary lesion on the lower labial mucosa or vermil-

ion, they are often referred to as "venous lakes." Thrombosis may be associated with pain.

PREMALIGNANT MUCOSAL DISEASE

Leukoplakia

Leukoplakia, as defined by the World Health Organization (WHO), is a white plaque that does not rub off and cannot be classified as any other known clinical entity. It is therefore a clinical diagnosis of exclusion.

Gross Pathology

Clinical forms include homogenous (thin and thick) type, speckled type (erythroleukoplakia), verrucous, and nodular types.

Microscopic Pathology

Benign cases of leukoplakia exhibit hyperpara- or orthokeratosis, acanthosis, and variable chronic inflammation (Fig. 9-73). Sometimes there is epithelial atrophy. If dysplasia is present, this should be evaluated architecturally and cytologically. Architectural features of dysplasia include bud- or teardrop-shaped rete ridges and an endophytic growth pattern (Fig. 9-74). Cytologic changes are similar to those of dysplastic lesions elsewhere, including basal cell hyperplasia, increased nuclear:cytoplasmic ratio, nuclear enlargement, hyperchromatism, increased mitotic activity, pleomorphism, dyskeratosis, and loss of cohesion.[177,178] The presence of keratinization in deep portions of an otherwise noninvasive dysplastic lesion may be indicative of early invasion, and levels should be obtained. The degree of dysplasia is graded mild, moderate, or severe, depending on whether up to one third, up to two thirds, or more than two thirds of the epithelium is involved

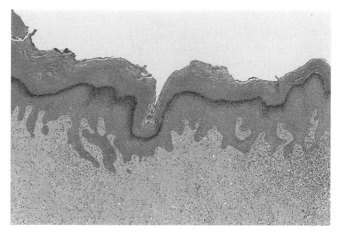

FIGURE 9–73 Hyperothokeratosis and benign epithelial hyperplasia in leukoplakia.

(Fig. 9–75). There is no consistent correlation between the presence of dysplasia of different degrees and the subsequent development of invasive squamous cell carcinoma. In particular, mild dysplasia may be histologically indistinguishable from reversible reactive epithelial atypia. Involvement of salivary ducts by dysplastic cells or carcinoma in situ, especially in floor-of-mouth lesions, results in recurrence rates similar to those of invasive squamous cell carcinoma.[179]

Some lesions also exhibit papillary hyperkeratosis or papillary epithelial hyperplasia. The term "verrucous hyperplasia" has been used occasionally to describe such lesions when these features are well developed.[180] These lesions, especially those exhibiting an endophytic growth pattern, are probably precursors to verrucous carcinoma or papillary squamous cell carcinoma. A band-like lymphocytic infiltrate may also be present in these lesions, which have been called "lichenoid dysplasia."[181]

Proliferative verrucous leukoplakia (PVL) is a form that tends to occur in elderly females. It is a progressive, persistent, and often extensive condition that is associated with tobacco use in only 50% of cases.[182,183] Approximately 57% of patients eventually develop squamous cell carcinoma, while around 30% will develop verrucous carcinoma.

Special Techniques

In one review of the literature, HPV was identified in 18.5% to 30% of cases of epithelial dysplasia, carcinoma in situ, and oral bowenoid papulosis, with 75% of cases involving HPV16 and/or -18.[184] Cases of PVL have been associated with HPV16 in 78% of cases.[185]

Clinicopathologic Correlation

Leukoplakia usually occurs in adult males and has a strong association with cigarette smoking and snuff use.[135,186] Common locations for leukoplakia are the buccal mucosa and gingiva.[187,188] Epithelial dysplasia, carcinoma in situ, or invasive carcinoma are present in 15% to 20% of cases at the time of biopsy, with lesions in the floor of mouth, ventral tongue, and soft palate most likely to show these changes.[177,189] Progression to squamous cell carcinoma over time varies from 16% to 36% in dysplastic lesions and 16% in lesions where epithelial dysplasia was not present in the original biopsy.[177,185]

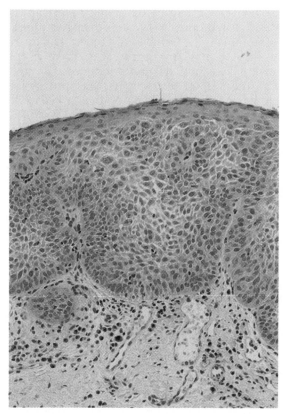

FIGURE 9–75 Severe epithelial dysplasia with dysplastic cells involving more than two thirds of the epithelium.

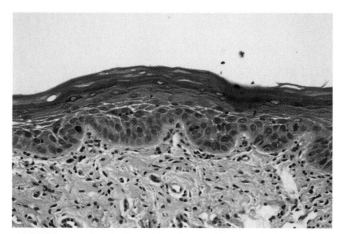

FIGURE 9–74 Moderate epithelial dysplasia exhibiting prominent budding of rete ridges and involvement of half the epithelium.

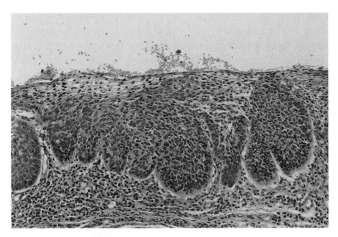

FIGURE 9-76 Carcinoma in situ.

Erythroplakia

Gross Pathology

Like leukoplakia, erythroplakia is a clinical diagnosis. Erythroplakic lesions appear as an erythematous velvety or granular plaque that is usually well circumscribed. Red areas associated with leukoplakia are more usually classified clinically as speckled or erythroleukoplakia.

Microscopic Pathology

Approximately 90% of cases exhibit severe epithelial dysplasia, carcinoma in situ, or invasive squamous cell carcinoma.[190,191] Surface keratin is usually minimally present, and, in benign cases, there is epithelial atrophy so that the underlying vasculature lies close to the surface, causing its red appearance. In carcinoma in situ, dysplastic epithelial cells occupy the full thickness of the epithelium (Fig. 9-76).

Clinicopathologic Correlation

This is a less common precarcinomatous mucosal condition that presents in elderly subjects. Most patients are asymptomatic. Common sites include the floor of mouth, tongue, mandibular gingiva/alveolar mucosa, soft palate/tonsil, and retromolar area.[190,191]

....

MALIGNANT EPITHELIAL PROLIFERATIONS
....

Squamous Cell Carcinoma

Gross Pathology

Clinical presentations for squamous cell carcinoma (SCC) include a nonhealing ulcer with induration, a fungating or rapidly growing mass, or increased nod-

ularity or induration in a pre-existing leukoplakia or erythroplakia.

Microscopic Pathology

The histologic criteria for oral SCC are similar to those used in other body sites. Single cells, as well as islands and cords of atypical squamous cells, infiltrate the stroma. The overlying epithelium may exhibit varying degrees of dyplasia or carcinoma in situ, or it may be histologically benign. Keratin formation may take the form of dyskeratosis and keratin pearl formation, and necrosis may be evident. Different parts of the tumor may vary in degree of differentiation and depth of invasion. As with other sites, SCCs are classified as well, moderately, and poorly differentiated, depending on the amount of keratinization present—although histologic grading may or may not have prognostic significance.[192–194] In general, SCC of the lip tends to be well differentiated (Fig. 9–77), and intraoral ones tend to be moderately to poorly differentiated (Fig. 9–78). HPV has been identified in approximately 26% of oral squamous cell carcinomas, with HPV16 and -18 representing 80% of those cases.[183]

SCC that infiltrates in a pushing fashion with large, cohesive cords and islands of cells has a 60% 5-year survival compared to a 37% survival for tumors that infiltrate in small irregular cords and single islands.[195] These patterns of infiltration also correlate with incidence of lymph node metastases.[196] Tumor thickness and depth of invasion may also correlate with survival and nodal metastases. One study showed that tumors less than 4 mm and those greater than 8 mm had an 8% and 83% metastatic rate, respectively.[196] Other studies have shown that tumors ranging from less than 1.5 mm to less than 5 mm in thickness are less likely to be associated with cervical metastases, treatment failure, or mortality.[193,197,198] The presence of vascular invasion in

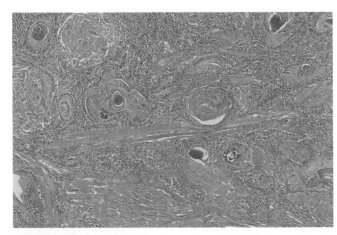

FIGURE 9-77 Well-differentiated squamous cell carcinoma with abundant keratin formation.

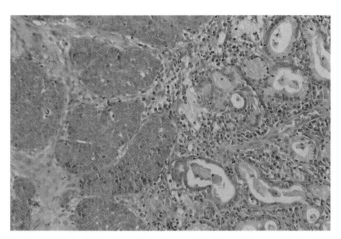

FIGURE 9–78 Poorly differentiated squamous cell carcinoma infiltrating salivary glands.

the tumor correlates with the presence of lymph node metastases.[195,196] Perineural invasion, intralymphatic tumor emboli, and positive margins have also been shown to have prognostic significance.[199–201] The intensity of host response has not been shown to correlate with lymph node metastases.[196]

Clinicopathologic Correlation

SCC of the oral cavity accounts for 90% of all intraoral malignancies and constitutes 3% of all malignancies diagnosed in the United States. Many arise in leukoplakias, erythroplakias, or erythroleukoplakias. Common sites are the tongue, floor or mouth, soft palate, and gingiva. Risk factors include cigarette smoking potentiated by alcohol use, HPV infection, sun damage for lesions on the lower lip, and immunosuppression.[190,202,203] Other, less common, associated inciting factors include the use of smokeless tobacco and betel nut chewing, the latter being popular in parts of Asia. Tobacco-associated leukoplakias are at a lower risk for malignant transformation than idiopathic lesions. The risk of malignant transformation of oral lichen planus to SCC after correction for confounding factors is likely to be in the vicinity of 1% to 2%.[196]

Tumor stage is one of the most important factors in predicting survival.[199] Prophylactic neck dissections in clinically negative necks have shown occult metastasis in 25% of cases.[197] The overall 5-year survival is approximately 50% in whites and 28% in blacks, the latter lower percentage resulting mostly from stage at diagnosis, socioeconomic factors, and access to care.[204] After a primary diagnosis of oral SCC has been established, 14% to 27% of patients subsequently develop a second primary in the upper aerodigestive tract, probably as a result of the phenomenon of field cancerization. The lung and esophagus are other common sites of synchronous or metachronous lesions.[205,206]

Verrucous Carcinoma

Gross Pathology

Verrucous carcinoma is a warty, sessile tumor.

Microscopic Pathology

There is marked exophytic and endophytic papillary epithelial hyperplasia with marked hyperparakeratosis and keratin plugging. The endophytic component takes the form of large, bulbous, frond-like rete ridges that have a broad pushing front. Bone resorption is not uncommon (Fig. 9–79). There is no evidence of single cell infiltration of the stroma; cytologic atypia, if present, is minimal. Separation of the epithelium from the underlying connective tissue is often seen, and a lymphocytic infiltrate is usually identified.[207] If significant atypia is present, a diagnosis of papillary epithelial dysplasia, papillary carcinoma in situ, papillary squamous neoplasm, or papillary squamous cell carcinoma would be more appropriate.[208,209]

Special Techniques

HPV6 and -11 have been identified in 47% and HPV16 and -18 in 35% of cases of verrucous carcinoma in one review.[182]

Differential Diagnosis

The differential diagnosis includes a well-differentiated papillary SCC, which should exhibit significant epithelial atypia; infiltration of the stroma by these atypical cells in islands, cords, or single cells; and deep keratin pearl formation.

A histopathologic entity referred to as "papillary squamous neoplasm" has recently been described.[208,210] It has two patterns: "inverting" if the primary architecture is endophytic and "exophytic,"

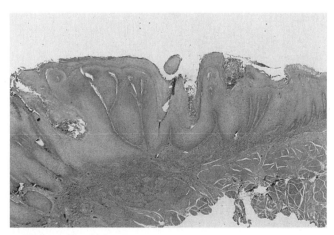

FIGURE 9–79 Verrucous carcinoma with broad fronds of rete ridges and a pushing margin.

similar to condyloma architecture. Cytologic atypia is present in both. This entity shares some similarities with verrucous hyperplasia, a precursor to verrucous carcinoma or papillary squamous cell carcinoma. It may represent one lesion in the histologic spectrum seen in proliferative verrucous leukoplakia (described earlier), but because of its significant atypia, it should not be diagnosed as verrucous carcinoma.

Clinicopathologic Correlation

Verrucous carcinoma is usually seen on the buccal mucosa, alveolar ridge, palate, and/or gingiva of elderly men and women.[207,211,212] Up to 84% of patients smoke or use smokeless tobacco products.[213,214] It is slow-growing and often locally invasive but shows little tendency to metastasize and represents 5% to 10% of the carcinomas of surface origin in the oral cavity. The recurrence rate is up to 67% of cases. Surgery is the favored primary treatment method, with radiation reserved for poor surgical candidates.[215]

Lymph node metastasis is a rare phenomenon, although patients may present with reactive lymphadenopathy. However, "transformation" of verrucous carcinoma to conventional invasive squamous cell carcinoma or coexistence of a small focus of squamous cell carcinoma may lead to lymph node metastasis. Approximately 20% of verrucous carcinoma may contain areas of invasive squamous cell carcinoma, the so-called "hybrid tumors."[214] Earlier theories held that radiation of verrucous carcinoma might have led to anaplastic transformation in approximately 8% of cases; however, more recent studies refute that finding.[216]

Spindle Cell Squamous Carcinoma

Gross Pathology

The tumor generally presents as a polypoid, ulcerated mass.

Microscopic Pathology

The tumor is usually extensively ulcerated. In polypoid tumors, intact epithelium is generally present near the pedicle; this is the area where epithelial dysplasia and/or the conventional invasive squamous cell carcinoma is often noted. Conventional squamous cell carcinoma may be present in only small foci, and there are reports of a "monophasic" spindle cell carcinoma where conventional carcinoma is not present. The striking feature is a malignant bipolar spindle cell proliferation presenting in a fasciculated, myxomatous, or streaming pattern. Larger polygonal cells and squamatoid cells are scattered throughout (Fig. 9–80). The myxomatous variant may contain more pleomorphic and stellate-

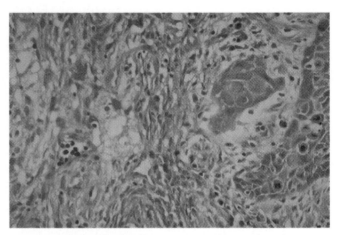

FIGURE 9–80 Spindle cell carcinoma with conventional squamous cell carcinoma.

shaped cells.[217–219] The presence of abundant granulation tissue, usually with a moderately severe inflammatory infiltrate, may make it difficult to distinguish the spindled tumor cells from reactive stromal cells; sometimes a hemangiopericytoma-like pattern may be present. Mitoses are usually abundant and often abnormal. Multinucleated giant tumor cells are common, and osteoid formation may be evident. Metastatic lesions may contain squamous cells and/or malignant spindle cell elements.[217]

Some investigators divide spindle cell carcinoma into superficial or invasive types. The latter invade into the underlying structures, have a strong association with prior radiation, and have higher recurrence, metastatic, and mortality rates.[218]

Special Techniques

The spindle cells stain for keratin and EMA in 50% to 60% of cases, albeit in a spotty pattern. Vimentin is present to varying degrees in the spindle cells in over 90% of cases.[219,220] Keratin and vimentin co-expression within the spindle cells have been demonstrated using double-labelling techniques. In monophasic spindle cell tumors, identification of desmosomes and/or tonofilaments helps to establish the epithelial nature of the spindle cells.[219] Tumor cells lack S-100 protein. In one study with a series of monophasic spindle cell carcinoma without histologic evidence of squamous cell carcinoma, keratin was identified in over half the cases.[219] Smooth muscle actin and desmin have also been identified by immunohistochemical techniques.[221]

Differential Diagnosis

The differential diagnosis includes fibrosarcoma, benign and malignant angioformative tumors such as angiosarcoma and hemangiopericytoma, benign and malignant fibrous histiocytoma, and pseudosarcomatous radiation effect. If large polygonal pleomorphic cells are present, rhabdomyosarcoma is also a consideration. The most helpful single criterion is the identification of invasive squamous cell carcinoma within the tumor.

Clinicopathologic Correlation

This uncommon biphasic tumor occurs in older adults with a mean age in the seventh decade; men are affected two to three times as often as women. The tumor generally presents as a polypoid, ulcerated mass in the lip, posterior tongue, floor of mouth, alveolar ridge/gingiva, larynx, or pyriform sinus.[217–220] A history of prior radiation was noted in approximately 20% to 30% of cases. Recurrence occurs in 25% of cases, and between 36% and 45% of patients develop metastases, usually to lymph nodes, with the lung the most frequent site of distant metastasis. Fifty-five percent of patients die within 2 years, most exhibiting metastatic disease.

Adenoid Squamous Cell Carcinoma

Gross Pathology

This variant of squamous cell carcinoma has similar macroscopic appearances to conventional squamous cell carcinoma.

Microscopic Pathology

Within the conventional squamous cell carcinoma are areas of acantholysis forming gland-like and tubular structures composed of a peripheral single or double layer of cuboidal cells that are atypical; acantholytic and dyskeratotic cells are present within the lumina that may contain eosinophilic material (Fig. 9–81).[222,223] The adjacent skin may exhibit actinic keratosis. Solar elastosis is usually present. Clear cells may be present. Metastatic lesions often maintain their pseudoglandular nature.

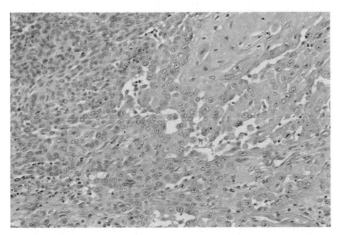

FIGURE 9–81 Adenoid squamous cell carcinoma with acantholysis and pseudoglandular pattern.

Special Techniques

Mucicarmine and alcian blue stains are negative. Immunoreactivity is seen with epithelial markers (e.g., cytokeratin, epithelial membrane antigen).

Differential Diagnosis

Adenoid squamous cell carcinoma may be distinguished from adenocarcinoma, either primary or metastatic, by the association with surface squamous epithelial dysplasia, the acantholytic nature of the pseudoglandular spaces, and the absence of epithelial mucin by histochemistry. Adenoid squamous cell carcinoma may also be mistaken for angiosarcoma. In such instances, immunohistochemical studies for cytokeratin and epithelial membrane antigen are positive in carcinoma, whereas angiosarcoma reacts with endothelial antigens, including CD34 and Factor VIII–related antigen. The presence of significant atypia within the epithelial cells should prevent a diagnosis of pemphigus vulgaris or other inflammatory acantholytic disease.

Clinicopathologic Correlation

Adenoid squamous carcinoma (not to be confused with adenosquamous carcinoma) is also sometimes referred to as pseudoglandular carcinoma. This is a carcinoma of adult and elderly men (mean age in the sixth decade) that occurs primarily on the skin of the head and neck and the vermilion of the lips, including the upper lip. It may originate in the upper portion of the outer root sheath of hair and is probably induced by actinic damage.[222,224,225] Seventy-seven percent of patients were disease-free in a 2-to-72-month follow-up.

Adenosquamous Carcinoma

Gross Pathology

In the oral cavity, adenosquamous carcinoma presents as erythroplakia of the mucosa or as an ulcerated mass.

Microscopic Pathology

Basaloid, squamous, mucous, and undifferentiated cells are organized into the following patterns: carcinoma-in-situ, adenocarcinoma, squamous cell carcinoma, and a pattern suggestive of mucoepidermoid carcinoma.[186] Continuity with the surface epithelium may be observed; central necrosis and occasional acantholysis may be present within large tumor islands and lobules. Perineural invasion was noted in 50% of cases in one series.[226] Metastases to regional lymph nodes may show any or all of the component cells.

Special Techniques

Stains for epithelial mucin, including mucicarmine and periodic acid-Schiff with diastase show intracytoplasmic and/or intraluminal mucin-positive material.

Differential Diagnosis

The most important differential diagnosis is mucoepidermoid carcinoma, with which it shares the presence of squamous cells and mucous cells organized into an adenocarcinoma. The most important difference is that a squamous cell carcinoma with pleomorphic and anaplastic cells is present in an adenosquamous carcinoma and absent in a mucoepidermoid carcinoma—even a high-grade mucoepidermoid carcinoma. Adenoid squamous cell carcinomas, while appearing to have duct-like structures, do not contain mucous cells and do not stain with mucicarmine.

Clinicopathologic Correlation

Adenosquamous carcinoma is an aggressive tumor of the nasal, oral, and laryngeal mucosa, with features of squamous cell carcinoma and mucoepidermoid carcinoma.[226,227] It occurs in older individuals, usually men. Eighty percent of patients develop metastases.

Basaloid Squamous Cell Carcinoma

Gross Pathology

The gross appearance of basaloid squamous cell carcinoma is similar to conventional squamous cell carcinoma and includes the presence of an indurated, exophytic, or fungating mass or a nonhealing ulcer with induration.

Microscopic Pathology

The tumor consists of nests and lobules of packed small basaloid cells with hyperchromatic nuclei, inconspicuous nucleoli, and scanty cytoplasm. Central comedonecrosis of the neoplastic lobules is a characteristic feature, as is the presence of hyalinosis or deposition of basement membrane–like material in and around the neoplastic proliferation (Fig. 9–82). Occasional cribriform areas may be evident. Mitotic figures are usually readily identified and include the presence of atypical forms. The basaloid cell is the dominant cell type. Squamous cell differentiation is usually a minor component and includes foci of abrupt keratinization in the form of keratin pearls or individual cell keratinization, but may also include areas of frank invasive squamous cell carcinoma. The tumor originates from the overlying epithelium,

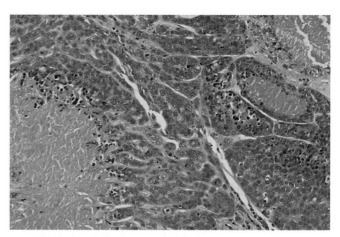

FIGURE 9–82 Basaloid squamous cell carcinoma showing characteristic hyalinosis and comedonecrosis.

which may be dysplastic or exhibit carcinoma in situ.[228,229] Continuity of the basaloid tumor with the overlying epithelium is sometimes seen and supports the origin of this tumor from surface origin.

Special Techniques

Stains for epithelial mucin are negative, although pseudoglandular and microcystic spaces may contain PAS-positive mucinous material. Immunoperoxidase stains are positive for cytokeratin in 100% of cases, EMA in 80% of cases, CEA in 53% of cases, and S-100 protein in 39% of cases.[230] Some authors maintain that S-100 protein positivity is noted only within intratumoral Langerhans' cells; vimentin positivity varies.[231,232] Stains for synaptophysin and chromogranin are negative, as is the stain for muscle-specific actin.

Differential Diagnosis

The differential diagnosis includes adenocarcinoma of salivary gland origin, or even adenoid cystic carcinoma. Neither of these would show frank squamous cell carcinoma. The lack of staining for synaptophysin and chromogranin differentiates this from the rare small-cell carcinoma of salivary gland origin and the Merkel cell carcinoma.[233]

Clinicopathologic Correlation

This is an aggressive variant of squamous cell carcinoma that affects elderly men (median age seventh decade) four times more often than women.[234] It presents primarily in the hypopharynx, supraglottic larynx, base of tongue, and floor of mouth, with smoking and alcohol use being important predisposing factors.[228,229,235] Lymph node metastases were noted in 60% to 80% of cases at the time of diagnosis, and 60% to 80% developed distant metastases, particularly to the lungs.

ODONTOGENIC LESIONS

Odontogenic Cysts

A concise modification of the World Health Organization classification of odontogenic cysts includes two broad categories: inflammatory and developmental (Table 9–9).[236] All gnathic cystic specimens should be evaluated for evidence of odontogenic keratocyst and cystic ameloblastoma before a histopathologic diagnosis is rendered. Periapical and paradental cysts are inflammatory; all other odontogenic cysts are developmental.

Developmental cysts are so named because they are associated with vital teeth and are not induced by inflammation. Because of their tendency to recur following curettage, odontogenic keratocyst and glandular odontogenic cyst are the most important odontogenic cysts.

PERIAPICAL CYST

A periapical cyst (radicular cyst, apical periodontal cyst) or lateral radicular cyst results when trauma or dental caries causes necrosis of the dental pulp, and mediators of inflammation exit the tooth through the apical foramen or lateral canal to cause inflammation and a proliferation of granulation tissue in the surrounding periodontal connective tissue. This inflammation is thought to induce proliferation of epithelial rests of Malassez and cyst formation. Some oral pathologists provide a histopathologic diagnosis of periapical cyst when any evidence of epithelium in a periapical specimen is identified. However, a cyst by definition must have a lumen; therefore, the mere presence of periapical anastomosing squamous epithelial cords is insufficient for

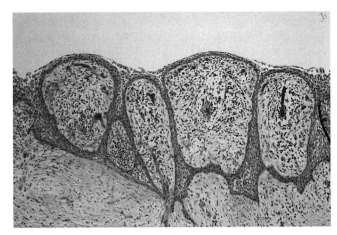

FIGURE 9–83 Periapical cyst. The anastomosing rete processes and chronic inflammation are similar to those in paradental cyst.

an unequivocal diagnosis of periapical cyst. Approximately 15% of periapical lesions are radicular cysts, and these can be true cysts or pocket cysts—that is, a cyst with its lumen confluent with the root canal.[237]

Periapical cysts are lined by thin nonkeratinized stratified squamous epithelium often demonstrating slender interconnecting rete processes, exocytosis of neutrophils, and mural granulation tissue that is subacutely to chronically inflamed (Fig. 9–83). The lining epithelium can occasionally contain mucous cells, intraepithelial curvilinear "hairpin-like" eosinophilic hyaline or Rushton bodies (Fig. 9–84), or evidence of keratinization.[238–242] Squamous odontogenic tumor-like islands of squamous epithelium can sometimes occur in the fibrous wall of the cyst (Fig. 9–85).[243] A periapical cyst associated with a primary (deciduous) molar can mimic an inflamed dentigerous cyst of the underlying permanent premolar.[244–247] If the periapical cyst is not removed when the associated tooth is extracted, the remaining cyst is termed a residual cyst (residual periapical cyst, residual radicular cyst).[248–250]

TABLE 9–9	ODONTOGENIC CYSTS

Inflammatory cysts
  Periapical cyst
  Paradental cyst
Developmental cysts
  Dentigerous cyst
  Odontogenic keratocyst
  Calcifying odontogenic cyst
  Lateral periodontal cyst
  Glandular odontogenic cyst
Nonodontogenic cyst
  Nasopalatine duct cyst
  Nasolabial cyst

From Slater LJ. Fibro-osseous lesions. In: Kelly JPW, ed. *Oral and Maxillofacial Surgery Knowledge Update: Home Study Program.* Rosemont, IL: American Association of Oral and Maxillofacial Surgeons; 1995: PTH/33–47, with permission.

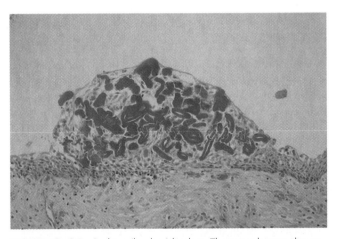

FIGURE 9–84 Rushton (hyaline) bodies. These nonkeratin, linear and globular, intraepithelial, extracellular, proteinaceous deposits become basophilic when they calcify.

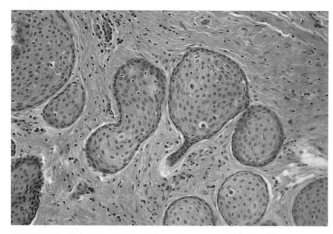

FIGURE 9–85 Squamous odontogenic tumor-like proliferation. Mural epithelial islands demonstrate neither peripheral tall amelo-blastomatous cells nor cytologic atypia.

PARADENTAL CYST

Histologic features of paradental cysts and marked periodontal disease are similar to those of periapical cysts; clinicoradiographic findings are required to distinguish these entities. The paradental cyst (buccal bifurcation cyst, inflammatory paradental cyst, mandibular infected buccal cyst) occurs buccal to a mandibular molar usually within 2 years of its expected eruption.[251] For example, a cyst buccal to the 6-year molar (first molar) usually develops by age 8 years; approximately 35% of first-molar-associated paradental cysts are bilateral.[252] Periodontal inflammation, sometimes associated with deep buccal periodontal pockets, probably induces odontogenic epithelium in the buccal furcation of an erupting vital mandibular molar to proliferate and undergo cystic change.[253,254] This inflammation can also cause proliferative periostitis.[252] A deep periodontal pocket in adults with marked periodontal disease is lined by inflamed sulcular epithelium resembling the lining of a periapical cyst; such a periodontal pocket can extend to surround the tooth apex.

DENTIGEROUS CYST

Gross Pathology

A dentigerous, or follicular, cyst results when fluid accumulates between the enamel and the dental follicle of an unerupted tooth. The cyst is attached to the neck of the tooth, and the crown of the impacted tooth projects into the cyst lumen. Radiographically the dentigerous cyst presents as a pericoronal radiolucency, and large cysts can cause displacement of the affected tooth to the floor of the orbit or inferior border of the mandible.

Microscopic Pathology

Dentigerous cysts are lined by thin nonkeratinized stratified squamous epithelium, often devoid of rete

processes. They exhibit slender cords or small islands of uniform polygonal epithelial cells, "odontogenic epithelium," in mural myxoid fibrous connective tissue (Fig. 9–86). The lining epithelium can display intraepithelial mucous cells or Rushton bodies.[239]

Differential Diagnosis

A small dentigerous cyst often can be differentiated at surgery from a hyperplastic dental follicle, because the latter shows thickening of the myxoid connective tissue that surrounds the normal developing tooth, while the former is found to have a fluid-filled cavity.[255,256] If pericoronal membranous follicular tissue is lined by columnar epithelial cells having eosinophilic cytoplasm (reduced enamel epithelium), the lesion is probably a dental follicle with a thickened hyperplastic connective tissue wall rather than a follicular cyst (Fig. 9–87).

Clinicopathologic Correlation

If radiographs reveal multiple dentigerous cysts, nevoid basal cell carcinoma syndrome or hyperplastic dental follicles associated with a mucopolysaccharidosis should be considered in the differential diagnosis.[257]

Orthokeratinized Dentigerous Cyst

An orthokeratinized dentigerous cyst (the so-called "orthokeratinized variant of odontogenic keratocyst" or "orthokeratinized odontogenic cyst") shows orthokeratosis and a prominent granular layer, and lacks palisaded basal cells. Because this cyst has a low recurrence rate (approximately 2% in one series[258]) and has not been associated with the nevoid

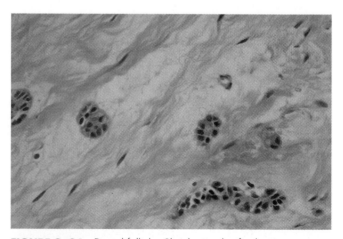

FIGURE 9–86 Dental follicle. Slender cords of odontogenic epithelium composed of small polygonal cells are present in myxoid connective tissue of dental follicular tissue or the wall of the dentigerous cyst. Epithelial rests of Malassez are histologically similar to these epithelial cords.

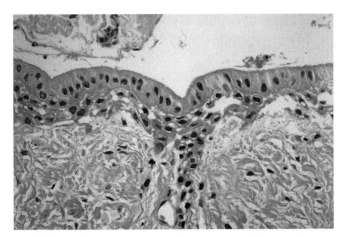

FIGURE 9–87 Reduced enamel epithelium. Slender epithelial cords can bud into the connective tissue from this eosinophilic columnar epithelium.

basal cell carcinoma syndrome, it might more appropriately be considered a variant of dentigerous cyst than of odontogenic keratocyst.[259] Most orthokeratinized cysts are associated with the crown of an impacted tooth; those that are not would appropriately be termed orthokeratinized odontogenic cysts.[260]

ODONTOGENIC KERATOCYST

Odontogenic keratocyst (OKC, also called "primordial cyst" but perhaps more accurately "parakeratinized odontogenic cyst") is the most important jaw cyst due to its tendency to recur following curettage (43% in one study[261]) and its association with the nevoid basal cell carcinoma syndrome (NBCCS, the Gorlin syndrome).[262]

Gross Pathology

Radiographically, OKC presents as a unilocular cyst between or apical to teeth, as a cyst surrounding the crown of an impacted tooth, or as a multilocular cyst, frequently in the posterior mandible. Often it causes less jaw expansion than does ameloblastoma. Gross evidence of luminal yellowish-white pasty or caseous material (desquamated keratin) may be the first clinical indication that a jaw cyst is an OKC.

Microscopic Pathology

This cyst is lined by thin parakeratinized squamous epithelium in which flattened superficial keratinocytes and some luminal desquamated cells retain nuclei. The lining epithelium characteristically has an undulating or corrugated parakeratinized luminal surface, lacks rete processes, and shows basal palisaded columnar cells with hyperchromatic nuclei (Fig. 9–88). Inflamed OKCs may not be readily rec-

ognizable because inflamed portions demonstrate acanthosis with rete ridges and lack surface parakeratin and palisaded basal cells.[263]

Clinicopathologic Correlation

In a young patient presenting with one or more odontogenic keratocysts, the nevoid basal cell carcinoma syndrome (NBCCS) should be considered. Major manifestations of NBCCS include multiple OKCs or multiple basal cell carcinomas occurring at a young age, dyskeratotic palmar pits, macrocephaly, rib anomalies, and dense calcification of the falx cerebri.[264,265] This syndrome is inherited as an autosomal dominant trait; the NBCCS gene, which probably represents a tumor-suppressor gene, has been mapped to chromosome 9q22.3-31.[266,267] The epithelium is more proliferative in OKCs occurring in patients with NBCCS than in those with sporadic OKC. OKC in NBCCS more frequently exhibits diverticula or satellite cysts, mural islands of squamous odontogenic epithelium, or occasional mural ameloblastoma-like proliferations.[268–271]

CALCIFYING ODONTOGENIC CYST

Gross Pathology

Radiographically, calcifying odontogenic cyst (COC, Gorlin cyst) presents as a cyst between tooth roots or as a dentigerous cyst-like lesion; a radiopaque odontoma is associated with approximately 25% of these cysts.[272] Because the soft-tissue portion of odontomas can exhibit focal ghost cell keratinization, a diagnosis of calcifying odontogenic cyst with odontoma should be rendered only if a cyst is present and not merely because ghost cell epithelium is present.[273] Most are intraosseous (central), but extraosseous (peripheral or gingival) lesions sometimes arise.[274,275]

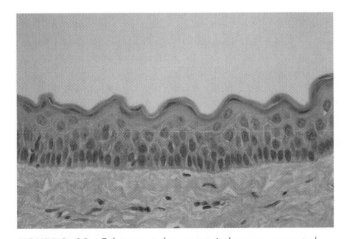

FIGURE 9–88 Odontogenic keratocyst. It shows a corrugated parakeratotic luminal surface and palisaded columnar basal cells with hyperchromatic nuclei.

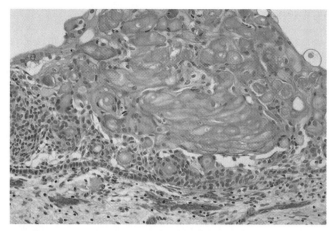

FIGURE 9–89 Calcifying odontogenic cyst with intraepithelial nests of large spinous keratinocytes showing a clear space once occupied by nuclear chromatin (ghost cell keratinization).

Microscopic Pathology

The calcifying odontogenic cyst demonstrates the characteristic histologic finding of ghost cells, which are similar to shadow cells of the cutaneous pilomatrixoma. Epithelium showing ghost cell keratinization displays aggregations of keratinocytes, with each keratinocyte exhibiting abundant eosinophilic cytoplasm and a clear space delimited by a residual nuclear membrane. Dissolution of nuclear chromatin results in pale oval "ghost" in the center of each keratinocyte (Fig. 9–89). Ghost cell keratinization occurs in the lining epithelium, but with epithelial proliferation or cyst disruption, the ghost cells can be found in the connective tissue wall and can induce a multinucleated phagocytic reaction.

Differential Diagnosis

Histologically, COC can resemble cystic ameloblastoma, but a cyst lined by thin epithelium demonstrating basilar ameloblastic cells (i.e., palisaded columnar cells with hyperchromatic nuclei polarized away from the basement membrane with suprabasilar stellate reticulum-like cells) is probably not a cystic ameloblastoma if evidence of ghost cell keratinization is present. However, ameloblastomatous proliferations of unclear prognostic significance and actual solid ameloblastoma can infrequently accompany COC.[276,277] The solid or neoplastic variant of COC is discussed under odontogenic tumors.

LATERAL PERIODONTAL CYST

Gross Pathology

The lateral periodontal cyst (LPC) typically occurs as a 0.5 to 1.0 cm unilocular cyst between the tooth roots in the premolar/canine region of the mandi-

ble.[278] Since LPC is a developmental cyst, the associated teeth are vital, and mural inflammation is usually absent.

Microscopic Pathology

This cyst is lined by thin nonkeratinized epithelium composed of polygonal to flattened or squamous cells. This lining may demonstrate intraepithelial nodular aggregations of polygonal cells with clear cytoplasm (Fig. 9–90), and the connective tissue wall may contain islands of such clear cells or nests of squamous odontogenic epithelium.[279,280]

Clinicopathologic Correlation

The LPC tends not to recur after enucleation. The extraosseous analogue of LPC is typically found in buccal gingiva of the premolar area of the mandible and is termed the gingival cyst of the adult.[281] Multicystic intraosseous LPCs are known as botryoid odontogenic cysts ($\beta o \tau \rho v o$, a cluster of grapes); these multiloculated cysts are larger than LPCs and can recur following curettage.[282,283]

GLANDULAR ODONTOGENIC CYST

Gross Pathology

The glandular odontogenic cyst (GOC, sialo-odontogenic cyst) shares many histologic and clinicoradiographic features with botryoid odontogenic cyst.[284–286] GOC frequently presents as a large multilocular cyst in the anterior mandible.

Microscopic Pathology

Histologic features distinguishing GOC include the presence of surface columnar to cuboidal cells with

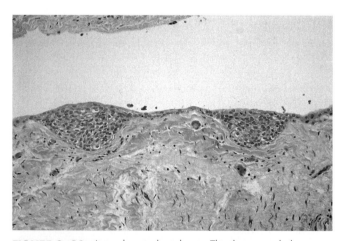

FIGURE 9–90 Lateral periodontal cyst. Thin lining epithelium sometimes shows nodular plaques of polygonal clear cells; mural islands of such clear cells can also be seen.

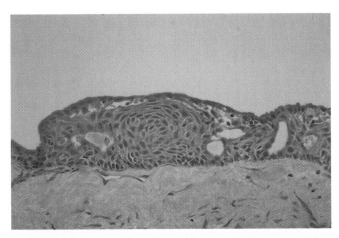

FIGURE 9–91 Glandular odontogenic cyst. Surface eosinophilic cuboidal to columnar cells, intraepithelial ductal lumina, and intraepithelial whorls of keratinocytes are observed.

eosinophilic cytoplasm exhibiting rounded apices; intraepithelial lumina are present in the lining stratified squamous epithelium (Fig. 9–91).[287] Mucous cells (goblet cells) and ciliated cells may be present, but these can occasionally be seen in the lining of any nonkeratinized odontogenic cyst. Intraepithelial nodules of concentrically whorled keratinocytes can be seen in both lateral periodontal cyst and GOC.[288,289]

Clinicopathologic Correlation

Because the GOC can recur following curettage, follow-up is required.[290]

Nonodontogenic Cysts

Discussions of gnathic cysts in the past have usually included "fissural cysts," cysts that putatively arise from epithelium entrapped within the jaw during embryogenesis when two embryonic processes fuse. Since there is presently no evidence for such entrapment, the current WHO classification of jaw cysts has deleted the category of fissural cysts.[236,291,292] Anachronistic "fissural cysts," including the so-called median alveolar, median mandibular, and globulomaxillary cysts, can invariably be classified as odontogenic cysts. The median palatal cyst could theoretically arise from entrapped embryonic palatal medial edge epithelium, but most such cysts likely represent large posteriorly positioned nasopalatine duct cysts.[291]

NASOPALATINE DUCT CYST

The nasopalatine duct cyst (NPDC, incisive canal cyst) typically presents as a 1.0 to 2.0 cm intraosseous cyst of the median anterior maxilla.[293]

Microscopic Pathology

The cyst is lined by thin cuboidal, respiratory, or stratified squamous epithelium, or by a combination of these epithelial types (Fig. 9–92). Contents of the incisive canal (a neurovascular bundle and small islands of hyaline cartilage of nasal septal origin) are frequently curetted with the cyst; salivary gland tissue from nasal floor mucosa may also be present in the cyst specimen.[294,295]

Clinicopathologic Correlation

This cyst is derived from an embryonic duct, which in humans infrequently persists as a patent channel, coursing from a median ostium or two paramedian ostia in the region of a midline palatal gingival papilla, called the incisive papilla, superiorly through the anterior maxilla to ostia in the floor of the nose.[296] Large NPDCs extend posteriorly and superiorly to cause marked palatal and intranasal expansion.[297] The cyst rarely recurs following enucleation. Radiographically, an odontogenic keratocyst can occasionally mimic NPDC.[298]

NASOLABIAL CYST
Gross Pathology

The uncommon nasolabial cyst (nasoalveolar cyst) usually manifests as an approximately 2.0 cm extraosseous cyst anterior to the nasal floor/inferior nasal turbinate causing protrusion of the superior portion of the upper lip, anterosuperior displacement of the nasal ala, and fullness of the mucobuccal fold.[299]

Microscopic Pathology

This cyst typically has a lining of respiratory epithelium, but may additionally exhibit cuboidal to squamous epithelium (Fig. 9–93).[300]

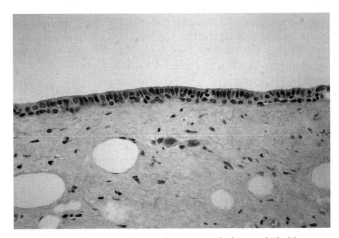

FIGURE 9–92 Nasopalatine duct cyst with thin epithelial lining, which is often composed of cuboidal and columnar cells, but can also be respiratory or squamous epithelium.

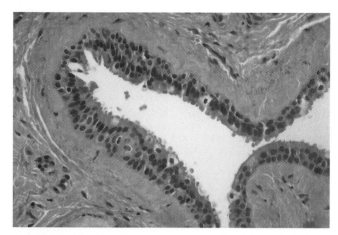

FIGURE 9–93 Nasolabial cyst. It may be lined by epithelium showing apocrine-like, apical, rounded, intraluminal projections.

Clinicopathologic Correlation

Nasolabial cysts probably result from anomalous development of the nasolacrimal duct; a report of familial bilateral nasolabial cysts in patients with nasolacrimal duct aplasia provides some support for this hypothesis.[301] About 75% of these cysts occur in women, and approximately 10% are bilateral.

Odontogenic Tumors

Many odontogenic tumors are associated with unerupted developing teeth. Myxoid connective tissue containing islands of odontogenic epithelium that surrounds an unerupted tooth, termed dental follicular tissue, histologically resembles an odontogenic fibroma; also, button-shaped myxoid tissue subjacent to the crown of an unerupted tooth that has not yet developed roots, called the dental papilla, histologically resembles odontogenic myxoma.[255] Therefore, the possibility of normal or thickened hyperplastic soft tissue associated with normal odontogenesis should be considered before a histologic diagnosis of an odontogenic tumor is rendered. A modification of the World Health Organization classification of odontogenic tumors is set forth in Table 9–10.[236,302]

EPITHELIAL ODONTOGENIC TUMORS

Epithelial odontogenic tumors usually manifest as central (intraosseous) lesions, but they sometimes present as peripheral (gingival, extraosseous) tumors.[303]

AMELOBLASTOMA

Ameloblastoma is the most common odontogenic tumor with the exception of the hamartomatous odontoma.[304]

TABLE 9–10	ODONTOGENIC TUMORS

Epithelial Tumors

Benign
  Ameloblastoma
  Calcifying epithelial odontogenic tumor
  Adenomatoid odontogenic tumor
  Squamous odontogenic tumor
  Epithelial odontogenic ghost cell tumor
Malignant
  Clear cell odontogenic carcinoma
  Odontogenic carcinoma

Mixed Epithelial and Ectomesenchymal Tumors

Benign
  Ameloblastic fibroma
  Ameloblastic fibro-odontoma
  Odontoma
  Odontogenic fibroma
  Granular cell odontogenic firbroma
Malignant
  Ameloblastic fibrosarcoma

Ectomesenchymal

Benign
  Odontogenic myxoma
  Cementoblastoma

Other

Melanotic neuroectodermal tumor

Gross Pathology

An early, small, conventional, intraosseous, solid or multicystic ameloblastoma presents as a unilocular cyst-like radiolucency, but the more advanced lesion manifests as an expansile multiloculated "soap bubble" radiolucent lesion (Fig. 9–94).

Microscopic Pathology

Ameloblastoma somewhat resembles cutaneous basal cell carcinoma; it can demonstrate epithelial islands (termed follicular ameloblastoma), anasto-

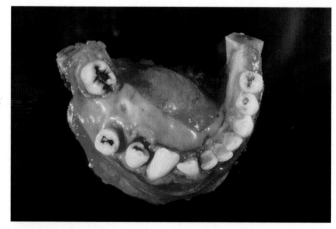

FIGURE 9–94 Ameloblastoma. It expands the right mandibular body and displaces teeth.

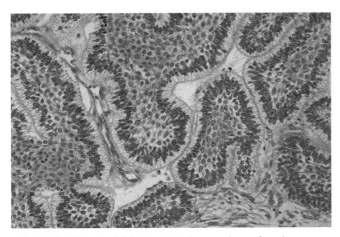

FIGURE 9-95 Ameloblastoma. At the periphery of each tumor island, lined-up columnar cells exhibit hyperchromatic nuclei displaced away from the basement membrane and toward the stellate reticulum by basilar vacuolated clear cytoplasm; this "reverse polarization" is indicative of ameloblastic differentiation.

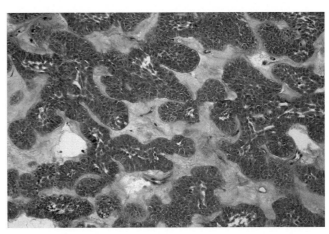

FIGURE 9-97 Maxillary plexiform ameloblastoma with budding and anastomosing cords of basaloid cells creating a pattern mimicking a salivary gland canalicular adenoma.

mosing cords (called plexiform ameloblastoma), or both architectural patterns. The requisite diagnostic cytologic finding is evidence of ameloblastic differentiation: palisaded columnar cells at the periphery of the epithelial islands show hyperchromatic nuclei polarized away from the basement membrane by basilar clear cytoplasmic vacuoles; these cells are said to display "reverse polarization" characteristic of ameloblastic differentiation (Fig. 9–95).[305] The center of the epithelial island frequently shows interconnected dendritic epithelial cells resembling the stellate reticulum of the embryonic dental organ. The neoplastic epithelial cells can resemble epidermal basal cells (basal cell type) or spinous keratinocytes (acanthomatous type), and they can appear ballooned by eosinophilic cytoplasmic granules

(granular cell type) (Fig. 9–96).[306] However, these architectural and cytologic variations apparently have little or no prognostic significance. If a maxillary sinus tumor histologically resembling a minor salivary gland canalicular adenoma is encountered, the more probable diagnosis of plexiform basal cell ameloblastoma should be considered (Fig. 9–97).

Desmoplastic ameloblastoma differs from typical ameloblastoma in that desmoplastic ameloblastoma more frequently presents in the anterior maxilla as a mixed radiolucent/radiopaque lesion radiographically resembling a benign fibro-osseous lesion. It displays islands of epithelium showing only subtle evidence of ameloblastic differentiation widely separated by abundant hypocellular collagenous stroma (Fig. 9–98).[307–309] Conventional ameloblas-

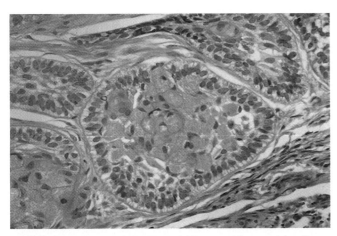

FIGURE 9-96 Granular cell ameloblastoma. The central stellate reticulum area contains cells ballooned with eosinophilic granules; nuclei in these granular cells are eccentrically displaced.

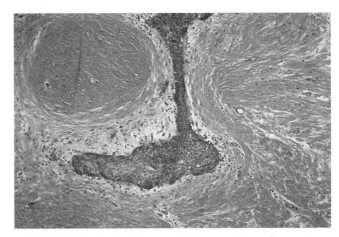

FIGURE 9-98 Desmoplastic ameloblastoma. Dense fibrous connective tissue widely separates epithelial islands showing little evidence of reverse polarization.

toma occurs less frequently (about 15% of cases) in the maxilla than in the mandible.[310]

Differential Diagnosis

An anomalous tooth can form in conjunction with ameloblastoma, a lesion called odontoameloblastoma; however, this occurs exceptionally rarely, and a diagnosis of odontoameloblastoma should be made with great circumspection only after the much more likely ameloblastic fibro-odontoma has been considered.[311,312] Also, if islands of ameloblastic epithelium are widely separated by abundant, cellular, pale, myxoid stroma, then ameloblastic fibroma should be carefully considered before a diagnosis of ameloblastoma is rendered. If an ameloblastoma-like lesion arises in conjunction with a classic odontogenic keratocyst, a diagnosis of proliferative odontogenic keratocyst is more likely than ameloblastoma ex odontogenic keratocyst.[313,314]

UNICYSTIC AMELOBLASTOMA

Gross Pathology

Radiographically, unicystic ameloblastoma (UA, mural ameloblastoma) frequently mimics a dentigerous cyst associated with an unerupted mandibular wisdom tooth (third molar), but it can also resemble a periapical cyst.

Microscopic Pathology

Pathologically, the cyst is lined by epithelium showing requisite ameloblastic differentiation, that is, reverse polarization; islands of follicular ameloblastoma or cords of plexiform ameloblastoma are usually focally present in the connective tissue wall, hence the term mural ameloblastoma, but these are not required for the histologic diagnosis of UA (Fig. 9–99). The suprabasilar epithelium can resemble stellate reticulum.

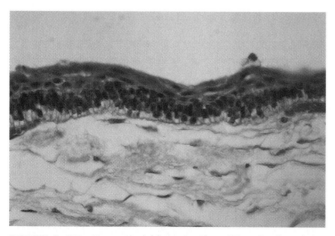

FIGURE 9–99 Cystic ameloblastoma. The tall basal cells with deeply basophilic nuclei showing reverse polarization are indicative of ameloblastoma even in the absence of mural ameloblastomatous islands or cords.

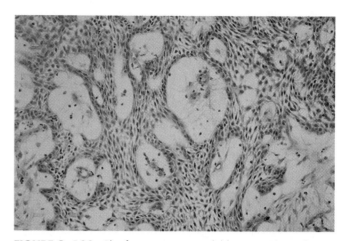

FIGURE 9–100 Plexiform unicystic ameloblastoma. This unilocular cyst exhibits a predominantly intraluminal reticular squamous epithelial proliferation lacking evidence of reverse polarization.

Differential Diagnosis

The plexiform unicystic ameloblastoma (Fig. 9–100) differs from the typical UA in that the plexiform unicystic ameloblastoma demonstrates an intraluminal reticular proliferation consisting of anastomosing cords of squamous epithelium lacking ameloblastic differentiation; it infrequently (in about 18% of cases) shows evidence of mural ameloblastoma, and it has a lower recurrence rate (approximately 10%).[315,316]

Clinicopathologic Correlation

Unicystic ameloblastoma is less likely to recur following curettage than is conventional solid-multicystic ameloblastoma.[317,318] Follow-up is necessary after enucleation, because UA can recur as conventional ameloblastoma.[319,320]

PERIPHERAL AMELOBLASTOMA

Gross Pathology

Peripheral ameloblastoma (PA, extraosseous ameloblastoma) usually presents as a 0.5 to 1.5 cm gingival nodule without radiographic evidence of an intraosseous component.

Microsopic Pathology

PA arises from surface gingival epithelium and frequently shows squamous differentiation (acanthomatous features).

Clinicopathologic Correlation

PA has a low recurrence rate following conservative excision.[321–323] Buccal mucosal tumors histologically

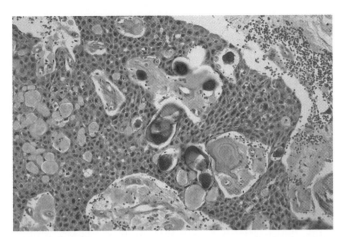

FIGURE 9–101 Calcifying epithelial odontogenic tumor (CEOT) shows squamoid epithelium demonstrating mild nuclear pleomorphism and pale amphophilic globular deposits of amyloid, some of which have calcified.

indistinguishable from ameloblastoma rarely occur.[324,325]

CALCIFYING EPITHELIAL ODONTOGENIC TUMOR

Microscopic Pathology

Histologically, calcifying epithelial odontogenic tumor (CEOT; Pindborg tumor) demonstrates sheets, islands, or cords of polyhedral squamoid cells exhibiting intercellular bridges, often nuclear pleomorphism (i.e., hyperchromatic nuclei showing moderate variation in nuclear size and shape), but little or no evidence of mitotic activity.[326] The presence of amyloid is required to establish the diagnosis of CEOT; globules of hyalinized eosinophilic or amphophilic material are deposited in the epithelium and surrounding collagenous stroma (Fig. 9–101). Some CEOTs demonstrate globular pools of amyloid with little evidence of a residual epithelial component. The amyloid is probably derived from basement membrane components secreted by the tumor cells.[327,328] This amyloid often calcifies to form basophilic, concentrically lamellated, psammomatous calcifications, sometimes called "Liesegang ring calcifications," which can coalesce to form large calcified masses. Calcifications are not necessary for a diagnosis of CEOT, but amyloid must be present.[329]

Differential Diagnosis

The amyloid in CEOT may be helpful in distinguishing it from other tumors in the histologic differential diagnosis which do not typically produce amyloid. These include odontogenic fibroma, primary intraosseous carcinoma, squamous cell carcinoma, or metastatic carcinoma. The Pindborg tumor

rarely shows extensive clear cell change; such tumors can be difficult to distinguish from clear cell odontogenic carcinoma or metastatic clear cell carcinoma.[330]

ADENOMATOID ODONTOGENIC TUMOR

Gross Pathology

Approximately two thirds of adenomatoid odontogenic tumors (AOTs) present in teenaged females as radiographic dentigerous cysts in the anterior maxilla.[331–333]

Microscopic Pathology

Adenomatoid odontogenic tumor is the only odontogenic tumor that histologically routinely demonstrates duct-like or gland-like structures, hence the term "adenomatoid." AOT exhibits three characteristic histologic features: (1) thick fibrous capsule, (2) hypercellular spherical nodules composed of fusiform to epithelioid cells demonstrating scattered microcystic or duct-like spaces lined by simple cuboidal to columnar epithelium, (3) slender cords of spindle-shaped to cuboidal basaloid epithelial cells anastomosing between the spherical nodules (Fig. 9–102). Globules of calcified eosinophilic extracellular matrix give some AOTs a mixed radiopaque and radiolucent radiographic appearance.[334,335] AOT can occasionally display foci histologically indistinguishable from calcifying epithelial odontogenic tumor; this composite tumor, termed "combined epithelial odontogenic tumor," behaves as an AOT; it does not recur following enucleation.[336–338] Epithelium associated with an odontoma can infrequently show adenoid spaces.[339]

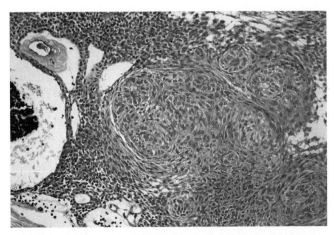

FIGURE 9–102 Adenomatoid odontogenic tumor (AOT) shows slender epithelial cords (*left*) and spherules of fusiform to epithelioid cells containing microcystic lumina lined by cuboidal cells (*right*). These ductal structures are sometimes not readily apparent and must be sought.

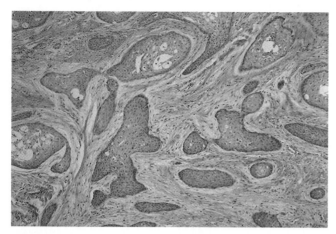

FIGURE 9–103 *Squamous odontogenic tumor (SOT) with "cookie-cutter" shaped islands of bland squamous epithelium lacking peripheral ameloblastic cells and nuclear atypia.*

SQUAMOUS ODONTOGENIC TUMOR

Gross Pathology

The rare squamous odontogenic tumor (SOT) typically presents as a triangular radiolucent lesion between teeth roots in the anterior maxilla or posterior mandible.

Microscopic Pathology

Histologically, this tumor demonstrates oval and characteristic "cookie-cutter" shaped islands of squamous epithelium separated by hypocellular collagenous stroma. The islands are composed of uniform spinous keratinocytes, and cells at the periphery are flattened or cuboidal.

Differential Diagnosis

This tumor can be distinguished from well-differentiated squamous carcinoma by its "cookie cutter" epithelial islands and cells lacking evidence of nuclear pleomorphism and mitotic activity. It can be distinguished from an ameloblastoma showing squamous differentiation (acanthomatous ameloblastoma) because SOT does not display peripheral columnar cells demonstrating reverse polarization (Fig. 9–103). The tumor arises from gingival epithelium or odontogenic epithelium (residual islands of epithelium derived from dental lamina or dental organ present in periodontal tissue).[340] Some squamous islands can show intraepithelial calcification or cystic change. SOT can simultaneously affect several jaw quadrants.[341] The connective tissue wall of odontogenic cysts can exhibit squamous odontogenic tumor-like proliferations; such SOT-like proliferations are incidental findings of no clinical significance.[243,342,343]

Clinicopathologic Correlation

SOT does not recur after surgical excision.

EPITHELIAL ODONTOGENIC GHOST CELL TUMOR

Epithelial odontogenic ghost cell tumor (EOGCT, dentinogenic ghost cell tumor, ghost cell ameloblastoma) is referred to as the rare solid or neoplastic variant of calcifying odontogenic cyst.

Microscopic Pathology

This neoplasm demonstrates features of an ameloblastoma showing squamous differentiation (acanthomatous ameloblastoma), basilar hyperplasia with cytologic atypia (hyperchromatic nuclei and an increased mitotic index), ghost cell keratinization, and sometimes foci of calcified collagenous extracellular matrix (dentinoid).[344,345] The presence of ghost cell keratinization is important; a neoplasm that otherwise might be designated an atypical ameloblastoma or low-grade ameloblastic carcinoma could appropriately be considered an EOGCT if the requisite ghost cell keratinization is observed (Fig. 9–104).

Clinicopathologic Correlation

This tumor can be locally aggressive but apparently has little metastatic potential.[346] Although ghost cell keratinization can be observed in tumors from several anatomic sites including uterus and colon, in gnathic lesions it is limited to calcifying odontogenic cyst and EOGCT.[347] Extraosseous (peripheral) dentinogenic ghost cell tumors are rare.[348]

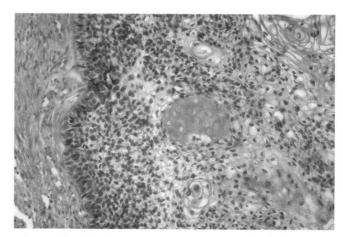

FIGURE 9–104 *Epithelial odontogenic ghost cell tumor (EOGCT). It resembles an ameloblastoma showing cytologic atypia, but is identifiable as an EOGCT because it demonstrates an intraepithelial eosinophilic island of squamous epithelium displaying ghost cell keratinization.*

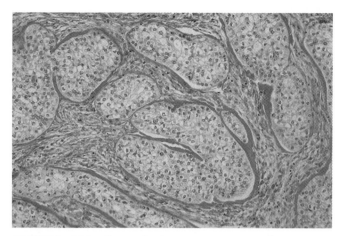

FIGURE 9–105 Clear cell odontogenic carcinoma demonstrating cords or island composed of polygonal epithelial cells showing clear cytoplasm.

CLEAR CELL ODONTOGENIC CARCINOMA

Gross Pathology

The uncommon clear cell odontogenic carcinoma most often occurs as an expansile radiolucent lesion in the anterior mandible of women.

Microscopic Pathology

Histologically, clear cell odontogenic carcinoma displays infiltrative cords or islands of polygonal cells with uniform vesicular to hyperchromatic nuclei and granular eosinophilic cytoplasm; a varying proportion of cells exhibit clear cytoplasm (Fig. 9–105).[349,350] Evidence of nuclear pleomorphism and mitotic activity is usually absent. Some examples show palisaded ameloblastic cells at the periphery of the tumor islands; most do not. Other clear cell epithelial neoplasms should be considered in the histologic differential diagnosis, including metastatic renal cell carcinoma, calcifying epithelial odontogenic tumor (clear cell variant), a salivary gland adenocarcinoma (clear cell adenocarcinoma or clear cell variant of mucoepidermoid carinoma), and clear cell squamous carcinoma.[330,351,352]

Clinicopathologic Correlation

This tumor frequently recurs locally and can show regional or distant metastases.[353–356]

ODONTOGENIC CARCINOMA

Odontogenic carcinoma is a diagnosis of exclusion. Before a carcinoma can be accepted as arising from intraosseous odontogenic epithelium, the following should be considered and excluded: origin from sinonasal mucosa, gingiva, or minor salivary glands (particularly for mandibular angle lesions), as well

as metastasis from a distant primary carcinoma. Some odontogenic carcinomas demonstrate evidence of peripheral palisaded cells exhibiting reverse polarization (ameloblastic differentiation) in addition to the requisite cytologic atypia and mitotic activity; these can be termed ameloblastic carcinomas.[357,358] Ameloblastic carcinomas sometimes show a less-differentiated sarcomatoid spindle cell component (Fig. 9–106).[359,360] Other odontogenic carcinomas resemble squamous cell carcinoma and are called primary intraosseous carcinoma.[361,362] Odontogenic carcinoma can arise in association with an odontogenic cyst, the epithelial lining of which may or may not show evidence of dysplasia (intraepithelial neoplasia).[363,364] Occasionally a histologically benign ameloblastoma can metastasize to the lungs or cervical lymph nodes, and like the gnathic primary tumor, this metastatic tumor also lacks significant cytologic atypia; such tumors are called metastatic ameloblastoma (malignant ameloblastoma).[365–367]

Mixed Epithelial and Ectomesenchymal Tumors

ODONTOGENIC FIBROMA

Odontogenic fibroma is the third most frequent odontogenic tumor (after odontoma and ameloblastoma).[304]

Microscopic Pathology

Histologically, this tumor demonstrates slender islands or strands of odontogenic epithelium devoid of ameloblastic features, widely separated by abundant fibrous connective tissue that varies from densely collagenous to rather myxoid; small calcifications may be present.[368]

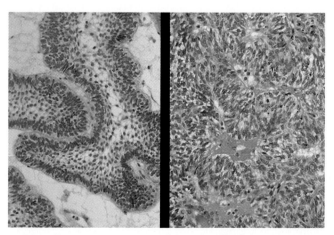

FIGURE 9–106 Ameloblastic carcinoma. Directly contiguous to a proliferative ameloblastoma showing reverse polarization of peripheral columnar cells and central stellate reticulum (*left*) is a hypercellular carcinoma composed of mitotically active fusiform cells (*right*).

Differential Diagnosis

A diagnosis of odontogenic fibroma should not be based exclusively on histologic findings; clinicoradiographic features must also be considered. For example, normal dental follicular tissue and slightly enlarged or markedly enlarged multiple hamartomatous dental follicles can be histologically indistinguishable from odontogenic fibroma (see Fig. 9–86).[255,369,370]

Clinicopathologic Correlation

Odontogenic fibroma is the only odontogenic tumor that presents more frequently as an extraosseous lesion (peripheral) than as an intraosseous lesion (central).[304] Perhaps the gingival fibrous proliferation induces cords of epithelium to bud from surface gingival squamous epithelium.[371] In this regard, it is interesting that many maxillary central odontogenic fibromas show evidence of gingival involvement in the form of a vertical groove or depression of the overlying palatal gingiva.[368,372] The peripheral odontogenic fibroma presents as a gingival nodule and can recur/persist after surgical removal.[373] The central odontogenic fibroma usually appears as a well-circumscribed radiolucency in the anterior maxilla or posterior mandible.[374] It has a low recurrence rate.[368] Central giant cell granuloma-like tissue can be associated with some odontogenic fibromas.[375,376] Since odontogenic fibroma histologically frequently appears poorly circumscribed and infiltrative, metastatic carcinoma should be considered in the histologic differential diagnosis.

GRANULAR CELL ODONTOGENIC FIBROMA

Gross Pathology

The rare granular cell odontogenic fibroma (GCOF, central granular cell odontogenic tumor, granular cell ameloblastic fibroma) appears as a well-circumscribed periapical radiolucency or radiolucency between tooth roots.

Microscopic Pathology

Histologically, this tumor demonstrates sheets of plump histiocytic cells with granular eosinophilic cytoplasm exhibiting scattered slender cords or islands of odontogenic epithelium composed of uniform small polygonal cells (Fig. 9–107). Small calcifications may be present.[377,378]

Differential Diagnosis

The GCOF is readily distinguished from granular cell ameloblastoma; the granular cells in GCOF are stromal histiocytic cells, but in granular cell ameloblastoma they are epithelial cells.

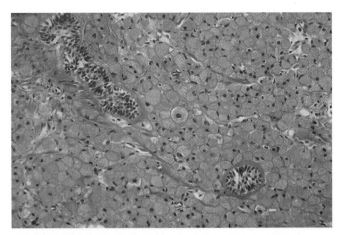

FIGURE 9–107 Granular cell odontogenic fibroma. Slender cords of odontogenic epithelium are widely separated by ballooned stromal cells with abundant granular eosinophilic cytoplasm.

Clinicopathologic Correlation

Granular cell odontogenic fibroma does not recur.

AMELOBLASTIC FIBROMA

Microscopic Pathology

Histologically, ameloblastic fibroma demonstrates slender budding and branching cords of odontogenic epithelium, composed of uniform cuboidal cells two cell layers thick, separated by abundant, cellular, pale, myxoid connective tissue exhibiting stellate fibroblasts with plump oval nuclei (Fig. 9–108).[379,380] The back-to-back epithelial layers composing the cords can "open up" to form islands with central stellate reticulum and peripheral palisaded columnar ameloblastic cells. Such opened-up islands are histologically identical to those seen in follicular ameloblastoma; recognition of the cellular myxoid

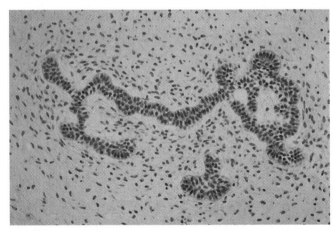

FIGURE 9–108 Ameloblastic fibroma shows slender cords of odontogenic epithelium surrounded by cellular myxoid connective tissue exhibiting plump fibroblasts.

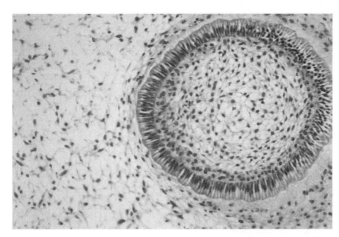

FIGURE 9–109 Ameloblastic fibroma with an "opened-up" epithelial island indistinguishable from that in ameloblastoma; recognition of the surrounding hypercellular myxoid stroma indicative of ameloblastic fibroma is crucial to determining the correct diagnosis.

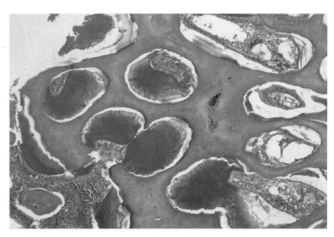

FIGURE 9–110 Complex odontoma. Anastomosing trabeculae of dentin surround and separate oval spaces containing enamel matrix and columnar ameloblastic epithelium.

stroma surrounding the ameloblastomatous islands is essential to avoiding misinterpreting an opened-up ameloblastic fibroma as an ameloblastoma (Fig. 9–109). An ameloblastic fibroma exhibiting foci of eosinophilic collagenous matrix resembling an osseous or dentin-like material has been termed "ameloblastic fibroma with dentinoid" (ameloblastic fibrodentinoma, dentinoma).[381–383] An ameloblastic fibroma associated with a complex odontoma is called an ameloblastic fibro-odontoma, a tumor apparently representing an immature or developing complex odontoma—that is, an odontoma retaining a substantial soft-tissue component.[383,384] While many ameloblastic fibro-odontomas and ameloblastic fibromas occur in young patients as a small tumor associated with an unerupted tooth, these tumors are occasionally 7 cm or larger.[385,386]

ODONTOMA

Odontoma, the most frequent odontogenic tumor, is a hamartoma composed of dental hard tissue including enamel and dentin.[304]

Gross Pathology

Odontomas frequently develop in the dental follicle of an unerupted tooth.[387] Odontomas typically appear either in the anterior jaws as a small mass composed of aggregated anomalous small teeth (compound odontoma) or in the posterior jaws as a large amorphous mass of dental hard tissue (complex odontoma).[388,389]

Microscopic Pathology

Histologically, the complex odontoma (Fig. 9–110) displays interconnecting trabeculae of collagenous matrix that focally show evenly distributed empty tubular spaces (dentinal tubules) indicative of dentin

(Fig. 9–111). The oval spaces between these trabeculae contain decalcified enamel or enamel matrix (Fig. 9–112), a basophilic to amphophilic material resembling fish scales, as well as cords or islands of the columnar ameloblastic epithelium that secrete this enamel matrix. Basophilic concentrically lamellated calcifications ("dysplastic enamel") can sometimes be seen adjacent to the prismatic fish-scale enamel matrix.[390] The compound odontoma is histologically simpler; each small single-rooted tooth composing this tumor demonstrates a dentin body with an enamel cap. As in a normal tooth, a central core of myxoid connective tissue (dental papilla or dental pulp) is found in the dentin body. Odontomas can display small foci of epithelium showing ghost cell keratinization (similar to that seen in calcifying odontogenic cyst) and small foci resembling ameloblastoma or ameloblastic fibroma.[273] If these foci constitute an insignificant proportion of a lesion composed largely of dental hard tissue, the most likely diagnosis remains odontoma.[383]

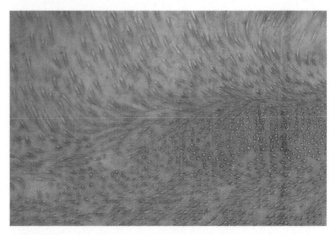

FIGURE 9–111 Dentin in an odontoma. Collagenous matrix exhibits evenly dispersed small dentinal tubules.

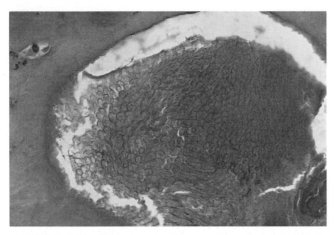

FIGURE 9–112 Prismatic enamel matrix in an odontoma. Decalcified enamel resembles imbricated fish scales.

Clinicopathologic Correlation

Odontomas occasionally erupt through the gingiva.[391] Odontomas can be present in Gardner's syndrome, but gnathic osteomas and impacted teeth are much more reliable indicators of this syndrome.[392]

AMELOBLASTIC FIBROSARCOMA

The rare ameloblastic fibrosarcoma (AFS) architecturally resembles and often arises from ameloblastic fibroma; therefore, it could be considered a sarcoma ex ameloblastic fibroma (Fig. 9–113).[393,394] The ameloblastic epithelial component is usually not mitotically active and can be so well differentiated as to synthesize and secrete enamel matrix. However, the proliferative hypercellular stromal component demonstrates mitotically active plump fibroblastic cells or histiocytic cells forming a neoplasm histologically

resembling fibrosarcoma, malignant fibrous histiocytoma, or hemangiopericytoma.[395] Some cases of AFS recur locally as a sarcoma devoid of an epithelial component.[393,395]

Ectomesenchymal Tumors

ODONTOGENIC MYXOMA

Odontogenic myxoma (myxoma of the jaw) is the third most common odontogenic tumor (after ameloblastoma and odontogenic fibroma), excluding the hamartomatous odontoma.[304]

Gross Pathology

As is true of odontogenic tumors in general, small myxomas present as unilocular cyst-like radiolucencies, but larger expansile myxomas appear radiographically multilocular.[396]

Microscopic Pathology

The grossly translucent slimy myxoma (Greek μυξα, mucus) histologically demonstrates stellate fibroblastic cells widely separated by abundant connective tissue mucus—that is, stroma rich in proteoglycans and glycosaminoglycans that retain much water (Fig. 9–114).[397] Myxoma contains little collagen. A myxoma showing more collagen than usual can be termed a "fibromyxoma." However, the greater the collagen content of a myxoid tumor, the less secure is the diagnosis of myxoma.

Special Techniques

Stromal cells in myxoma are immunoreactive for actin, but they seldom show immunoreactivity for S-100 protein.[398,399]

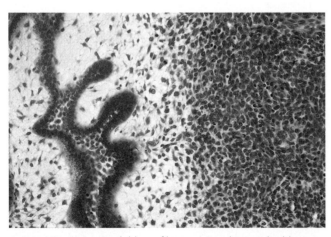

FIGURE 9–113 Ameloblastic fibrosarcoma showing budding cords of ameloblastic epithelium surrounded by a halo of pale myxoid connective tissue (*left*) adjacent to the hypercellular sarcomatous component composed of mitotically active plump stromal cells (*right*).

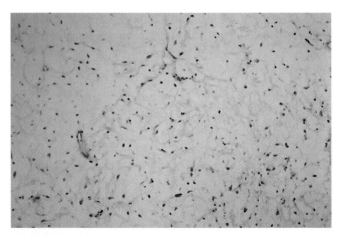

FIGURE 9–114 Odontogenic myxoma showing few cells and scarce collagen fibers widely separated by abundant pale extracellular matrix rich in water-retaining proteoglycans/glycosaminoglycans.

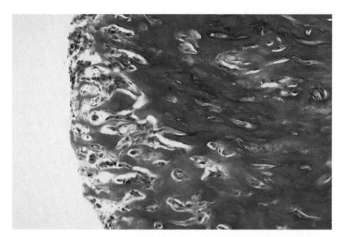

FIGURE 9-115 Cementoblastoma. Polygonal osteoblasts/cementoblasts are observed between radiating osseous trabeculae at the periphery of the bone-like spherule (*left*). Dense osseous tissue toward the center of the lesion (*right*) is often mosaic or pagetoid bone.

Differential Diagnosis

The well-circumscribed, 0.7 cm, button-like, pale, soft-tissue nodule located under the crown of an impacted developing molar lacking root formation is termed the dental papilla; it should not be confused with the histologically identical myxoma.[255] Dental follicular tissue can also mimic myxoma. Myxomas typically lack an epithelial component; if small islands or cords of odontogenic epithelium are observed in myxomatous tissue, the possibilities of dental follicle or odontogenic fibroma should be considered. If a myxomatous tumor shows greater cellularity or vascularity than the typical myxoma, the possibility of a low-grade sarcoma might be considered.[400] Myxomas that expand the anterior maxillary sinus of children can be somewhat more cellular than the classic odontogenic myxoma.[401,402]

CEMENTOBLASTOMA

Cementoblastoma (benign cementoblastoma) is usually included among odontogenic tumors, although it may well represent an osteoblastoma that has fused to the roots of a mandibular molar.[403]

Gross Pathology

Cementoblastoma has a characteristic radiographic presentation: a circumscribed, spherical, radiodense mass with a slender radiolucent band at its periphery resorbs, replaces, and fuses to the apical portion of the associated tooth root. The osteosclerotic mass resembles a snowball attached to a tooth root, often a mandibular molar.[404,405]

Microscopic Pathology

Histologically, cementoblastoma exhibits a core of dense pagetoid bone—that is, hypocellular woven bone displaying a mosaic pattern of intersecting thin basophilic reversal or cement lines, and peripheral radiating osseous trabeculae with intertrabecular osteoblasts or cementoblasts (Fig. 9–115).[406] This osseous tissue (cementum) fuses to radicular dentin.

Differential Diagnosis

Similar pagetoid bone can be seen in Paget's disease of bone, chronic sclerosing osteomyelitis, and florid osseous dysplasia. Focal osseous dysplasia can be quite osteoblastic and histologically resemble osteoblastoma; however, the sclerotic bone of focal osseous dysplasia does not fuse to teeth and does not show radiating osseous trabeculae. Radiographic features can be helpful in distinguishing the poorly circumscribed osteoblastoma-like osteosarcoma from the well-delineated cementoblastoma.[407]

Clinicopathologic Correlation

Up to 38% of cementoblastomas may recur.[408]

MELANOTIC NEUROECTODERMAL TUMOR OF INFANCY

Gross Pathology

Melanotic neuroectodermal tumor of infancy (MNETI, melanotic progonoma, retinal anlage tumor) frequently presents as an intraosseous grey-to-black expansile mass in the anterior maxilla of an infant.[409]

Microscopic Pathology

This tumor demonstrates branching or budding cords or islands separated by moderately cellular collagenous tissue (Fig. 9–116). Some cords are composed of large epithelial cells with vesicular nuclei and cytoplasmic melanin pigment (melanotic epithe-

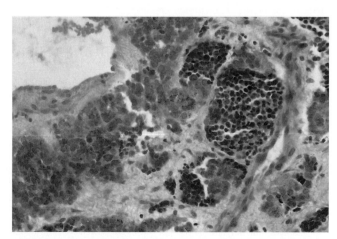

FIGURE 9-116 Melanotic neuroectodermal tumor of infancy. It has two cell types: larger epithelioid cells with granular cytoplasmic melanin pigment (*left*), and small lymphocyte-like neuroblasts (*right*).

lial cells), and other cords are composed of hyperchromatic small round lymphocyte-like cells (neuroblasts). Some islands form "alveolar" structures with a peripheral rim of melanotic epithelial cells surrounding a central space containing discohesive neuroblasts or degenerating cells.

Special Techniques

The melanotic epithelial cells exhibit immunoreactivity for cytokeratin and the melanosomal marker HMB-45. The neuroblasts can additionally display immunoreactivity for synaptophysin.[410,411] The cells usually lack immunoreactivity for S-100 protein. This unusual immunophenotype can be helpful in excluding melanoma.

Ultrastructurally, the melanocytic epithelial cells exhibit premelanosomes, large melanosomes, desmosomes, and tonofilaments; smaller cells can contain membrane-bound dense core granules.[410,412]

MNETI can be multifocal, a factor perhaps contributing to its clinical persistence or recurrence.[413] Gnathic MNETI rarely (in approximately 2% of cases) metastasizes, resulting in fatality.[410]

Benign Fibro-Osseous Lesions

A gnathic fibro-osseous lesion (BFOL) represents a localized proliferation of fibrous connective tissue in which trabecular or globular bone forms. In the past, acellular basophilic globular deposits of calcified collagenous matrix have been termed "cementum." However, cementum is defined as a bone-like substance *attached* to the tooth root, and in this discussion, deposits unattached to tooth structure will be considered bone, whether they are trabecular or globular. Gnathic BFOL cannot be confidently classified based on histologic features alone; clinicoradiographic features are essential for the most appropriate diagnosis. Most gnathic BFOL can be segregated into one of four categories: focal or multifocal osseous dysplasia, ossifying fibroma, fibrous dysplasia, and chronic osteomyelitis (Table 9–11).

TABLE 9–11	BENIGN FIBRO-OSSEOUS LESIONS

Circumscribed Radiographically

Focal osseous dysplasia (focal OD)
   Posterior focal OD
   Anterior focal OD (periapical cemental dysplasia)
   Multifocal OD (florid osseous dysplasia)
Ossifying Fibroma
   Juvenile ossifying fibroma
     Psammomatoid variant
     Trabecular variant
   "Ordinary" ossifying fibroma

Diffuse Radiographically

Fibrous dysplasia

FOCAL OSSEOUS DYSPLASIA

Gross Pathology

Focal osseous dysplasia (focal OD, focal cemento-osseous dysplasia) begins as a circumscribed periapical radiolucent lesion in the mandible that transforms to a mixed radiolucent-radiopaque lesion with increasing ossification.[414] The gross specimen typically consists of numerous small hemorrhagic fragments of tissue; in contrast, the ossifying fibroma usually enucleates as a single large hypovascular mass.

Microscopic Pathology

Histologically, the radiolucent component consists of hypercellular fibrous connective tissue containing slender anastomosing woven bone trabeculae and/or globular ossicles (Fig. 9–117).[415,416] The radiodense component demonstrates broad lobulated hypocellular trabeculae of pagetoid woven bone exhibiting thin basophilic reversal or cement lines with intertrabecular vascular fibrous connective tissue of moderate cellularity. Some lesions have an associated simple (traumatic) bone cyst.[417,418] This condition can affect several areas:

1. The incisor-canine anterior segment of the mandible (anterior focal OD, periapical cemental dysplasia)
2. The premolar-molar posterior segment (posterior focal OD, conventional focal OD)
3. Both anterior and posterior mandibular segments (multifocal OD, florid osseous dysplasia)
4. All three mandibular segments
5. All four posterior jaw quadrants (multifocal OD, florid osseous dysplasia)

Advanced multifocal OD shows large radiographically flocculent, histologically pagetoid osseous

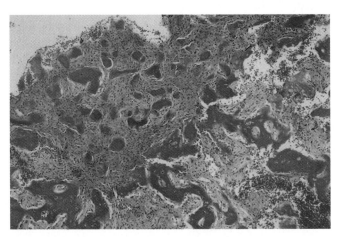

FIGURE 9–117 Focal osseous dysplasia (focal OD). Small acellular globular ossicles surrounded by rather cellular fibrous connective tissue (*upper left*) and slender anastomosing trabeculae of woven bone (*lower right*) are observed. Ossifying fibroma can be histologically indistinguishable from focal OD.

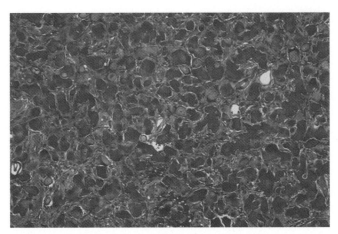

FIGURE 9–118 Psammomatoid juvenile ossifying fibroma showing evenly dispersed small acellular osseous globules ("cementicles") separated by rather cellular fibrous connective tissue.

masses, sometimes with sequestration, bilaterally in the edentulous molar region of the mandible.[419]

Differential Diagnosis

Paget's disease of bone can resemble multifocal OD, but Paget's disease differs in these ways: it arises in older individuals, more often causes facial deformity, affects the maxilla earlier than the mandible, involves nonalveolar basal bone, affects extragnathic bones, is associated with an elevated serum alkaline phosphatase, and infrequently exhibits osseous sequestration.[420]

Clinicopathologic Correlation

Focal osseous dysplasia is the most common BFOL of the jaws.[421–423] It is a non-neoplastic fibro-osseous proliferation disproportionately affecting young adult black females.[424]

OSSIFYING FIBROMA

Ossifying fibroma often presents as a large (approximately 3.8 cm) circumscribed expansile radiolucent lesion; if a smaller circumscribed lesion (perhaps 1.5 cm) showing a prominent central radiodense component is encountered, the possibility of focal osseous dysplasia should be carefully considered before a diagnosis of ossifying fibroma is rendered.[414]

Two categories of ossifying fibroma have been described: juvenile and ordinary. Juvenile ossifying fibroma (juvenile active ossifying fibroma, juvenile aggressive ossifying fibroma) usually affects children or adolescents, and it has a somewhat greater recurrence rate after curettage than ordinary ossifying fibroma.[425] Juvenile ossifying fibroma has two histologic subtypes: the psammomatoid variant and the trabecular variant.

Psammomatoid juvenile ossifying fibroma (psammous desmo-osteoblastoma, juvenile aggressive cemento-

ossifying fibroma) affects the paranasal sinuses more often than the jaws.[426–429] Histologically this tumor demonstrates hypocellular basophilic globular ossicles ("cementum," cementicles) distributed in hypercellular fibrohistiocytic connective tissue (Fig. 9–118). These spherical calcifications have previously been termed cementum, but because these small calcified grains occur in extragnathic lesions, they are probably osseous tissue unrelated to dental cementum and have appropriately been called psammomatoid (sand-like, from the Greek, ψαμμοσ, sand); some are lamellated and resemble meningioma-associated psammoma bodies.[430,431] *Trabecular juvenile ossifying fibroma* affects the jaws more frequently than the paranasal sinuses.[432] Histologically this neoplasm exhibits anastomosing hypercellular collagenous trabeculae showing plump fibroblastic, histiocytic, and osteoblastic cells; these hypercellular collagenous cords calcify and ossify to form anastomosing woven bone trabeculae (Fig. 9–119). Both variants of juvenile ossifying fibroma may display foci of hemorrhage, myxoid change, aggregations of osteoclastic giant cells, and mitotic figures.[433] The differential diagnosis of the trabecular variant might include giant cell granuloma if giant cells are numerous, and well-differentiated osteosarcoma if a permeative radiographic growth pattern or nuclear atypia is observed.[434]

Ordinary ossifying fibroma, a circumscribed fibro-osseous tumor, is a neoplasm of exclusion. This diagnosis should be entertained only in the following situations: if radiographic features of fibrous dysplasia, a poorly circumscribed diffuse lesion, are absent; if clinicoradiographic features and histologic pagetoid bone indicative of focal osseous dysplasia are not present; and if histologic features of psammomatoid or trabecular juvenile ossifying fibroma are

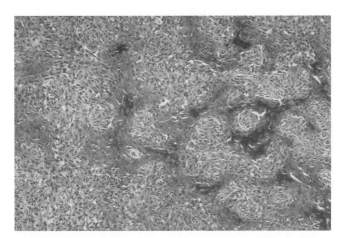

FIGURE 9–119 Trabecular juvenile ossifying fibroma shows anastomosing trabeculae of woven bone surrounded by hypercellular stroma. The osseous trabeculae on the right show greater evidence of calcification (dark eosinophilic areas) than the largely uncalcified trabeculae on the left. From Slater LJ. Fibro-osseous lesions. In: Kelly JPW, ed. *Oral and Maxillofacial Surgery Knowledge Update: Home Study Program*. Rosemont, IL: American Association of Oral and Maxillofacial Surgeons; 1995:PTH/33-47, with permission.

lacking. Ordinary ossifying fibroma enucleates as one piece or several large pieces of hypovascular pale firm tissue. Histologically, ordinary ossifying fibroma demonstrates slender trabeculae of woven bone and/or globular ossicles surrounded by cellular fibrous connective tissue, histologic features quite similar to those of focal osseous dysplasia.[435] A small (1.5 cm) putative "ossifying fibroma" showing pagetoid bone likely represents focal osseous dysplasia.[414,415,422] The simple term "ossifying fibroma" is preferable to "cemento-ossifying fibroma"; globular ossicles ("cementum" or "cementicles") are found in extragnathic bones and are the product of osteoblasts, not heterotopic cementoblasts.[430,436] Cementum and bone are biochemically quite similar; one might reasonably question whether they can be distinguished histologically.[437] Large (8.0 cm) ossifying fibromas, so far reported predominantly in African patients, can occasionally be multiple, and they appear to have a relatively large fibrohistiocytic component and a small osseous component.[438–440]

FIBROUS DYSPLASIA

Gross Pathology

Fibrous dysplasia of the jaw involves the maxilla more often than the mandible and presents as a slowly growing swelling in a child or adolescent. Radiographically, an expansile poorly delineated ground-glass or "peau d'orange" radiodensity exhibits a broad zone of transition between lesional tissue and surrounding uninvolved bone; it shows a blending periphery. The mandibular canal may be superiorly displaced, and a fingerprint pattern, with parallel osseous trabecula forming whorls, may be seen.[441]

Microscopic Pathology

Histologically, nonanastomosing, irregularly shaped, curvilinear woven bone trabeculae lacking osteoblastic rimming are evenly distributed in fibrous connective tissue of moderate cellularity (Fig. 9–120).[439] In older patients, elongated, straight, parallel trabeculae of lamellar bone at the periphery of the lesion often parallel and interconnect with the uninvolved lamellar bone cortex.[416,421]

Differential Diagnosis

Low-grade osteosarcoma can histologically resemble fibrous dysplasia, but fibrous dysplasia typically does not show a permeative growth pattern, nuclear atypia, or an increased mitotic index.[442] Gnathic fibrous dysplasia occasionally undergoes sarcomatous transformation, usually to osteosarcoma.[443,444]

Clinicopathologic Correlation

Fibrous dysplasia is not readily enucleated because lesional bone interconnects with normal bone at the

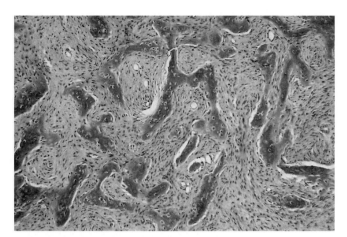

FIGURE 9–120 Fibrous dysplasia showing woven bone trabeculae resembling Chinese characters or Hebrew letters and lacking osteoblastic rimming.

periphery; this contrasts to the readily enucleated ossifying fibroma. Fibrous dysplasia affecting several contiguous bones, such as the maxilla, zygoma, and frontal bones, is termed craniomaxillofacial fibrous dysplasia. If multiple noncontiguous bones are affected, polyostotic fibrous dysplasia (the McCune-Albright syndrome, or Albright syndrome), or the Jaffe-Campanacci syndrome might be considered; these are associated with café au lait skin pigmentation.[445–450]

DIFFUSE SCLEROSING OSTEOMYELITIS OF THE MANDIBLE

Diffuse sclerosing osteomyelitis of the mandible (DSO, chronic recurrent multifocal osteomyelitis, SAPHO syndrome) only superficially resembles fibrous dysplasia, in that it presents as an expansile lesion often affecting the entire hemimandible. Radiographically, it shows diffuse ground-glass opacification.[451–453]

Microscopic Pathology

Histologically, established DSO displays the following: little or no evidence of acute inflammation or osseous sequestration, slender bony trabeculae exhibiting osteoblastic rimming, coarse pagetoid osseous trabeculae showing cement lines indicative of bone turnover, and infrequent small perivascular aggregations of lymphocytes and plasma cells.[454]

Differential Diagnosis

Diffuse sclerosing osteomyelitis differs from fibrous dysplasia in that DSO shows the following: recurrent bouts of mandibular pain and tenderness that can persist for years, intermittent buccal swelling and trismus, "onionskin" periosteal new bone formation, and ill-defined small radiolucent foci. These findings are more suggestive of osteomyelitis than inflamed fibrous dysplasia.

Clinicopathologic Correlation

Patients with DSO should be evaluated for evidence of skin pustules and extragnathic bone or joint involvement, because some cases of DSO represent jaw manifestation of the SAPHO syndrome (synovitis, acne, pustulosis, hyperostosis, osteitis).[455-457]

Benign Jaw Lesions

CENTRAL (INTRAOSSEOUS) GIANT CELL GRANULOMA

Gross Pathology

Central (intraosseous) giant cell granuloma (CGCG, central giant cell lesion) often presents as a unilocular or multilocular expansile radiolucent lesion in the mandible of young women.[458-460]

Microscopic Pathology

Histologically, this lesion demonstrates osteoclastic multinucleated giant cells in a vascular, moderately cellular, fibrohistiocytic stroma exhibiting extravasated red blood cells, foci of myxoid change, and areas of reactive woven bone formation (Fig. 9–121). Stromal histiocytic cells show evidence of mitotic activity.

Differential Diagnosis

The histologic differential diagnosis of CGCG includes several entities. Lesions containing abundant woven bone and scattered aggregations of giant cells share many histologic features with trabecular juvenile ossifying fibroma (JOF), but trabecular JOF has

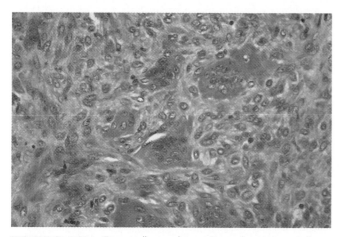

FIGURE 9–121 Giant cell granuloma. Osteoclastic giant cells are associated with sheets of mononuclear histiocytic cells.

characteristic unossified hypercellular fibroblastic/osteoblastic trabeculae not seen in CGCG. Gnathic giant cell granulomas showing gross evidence of cavitation with fibrous septa and histologically displaying pools of red blood cells have been termed aneurysmal bone cysts.[461-463] These latter lesions lack histologic evidence of aneurysms, but instead have pools of extravasated blood.[464]

The brown tumor of hyperparathyroidism is histologically indistinguishable from CGCG, and the presence of multiple gnathic giant cell lesions might be a clue that the patient could have elevated serum levels of parathormone or parathyroid hormone–related peptide.[465] Giant cell granulomas associated with hyperparathyroidism can spontaneously resolve after excision of the parathyroid adenoma.[466] Patients having a Noonan-like syndrome—with attributes of short stature, a webbed neck, and pulmonic stenosis—may also have multiple giant cell lesions of the jaw.[467,468] In several such cases the multiple giant cell lesions were interpreted to be indicative of cherubism.[469] Although subtle differences can be identified using morphometric analysis, giant cell tumor of long bones is histologically similar to CGCG; by convention, jaw lesions are usually termed giant cell granuloma or giant cell lesion, rather than giant cell tumor.[470] Malignant giant cell tumor (giant cell type of malignant fibrous histiocytoma, giant cell osteosarcoma) of the jaw is distinctly uncommon and shows greater cellularity, nuclear atypia, and mitotic activity among the mononuclear cell component than does CGCG.[471] Gnathic giant cell lesions are sometimes associated with Paget's disease of bone, and such lesions can exhibit huge giant cells with nuclei obviously more numerous than those in typical CGCG.[472,473] If a giant cell lesion involving the temporal bone portion of the temporomandibular joint displays islands of chondroid matrix, a diagnosis of chondroblastoma should be considered.[474,475]

Cherubism manifests in children as bilateral expansile multiloculated radiolucent lesions of the posterior mandible. Although the maxilla is often additionally affected, the mandible is invariably affected bilaterally, a pathognomonic radiographic pattern. Rarely, florid nonfamilial cherubism can affect the patient's entire mandible and maxilla.[476] Histologically, cherubism resembles central giant cell granuloma (CGCG), demonstrating areas of osteoclastic giant cells and hemorrhage. Cherubism has relatively broad fibrous histiocytoma-like zones exhibiting interlacing fascicles of plump fibroblastic and histiocytic cells forming a storiform pattern. These areas display little evidence of the reactive changes usually widespread in CGCG; they show relatively few osteoclastic giant cells and little evidence of hemorrhage with hemosiderin pigment, and they lack reactive woven bone (Fig. 9–122).[477] These fibrohistiocytic regions sometimes demonstrate the perivascular collagen deposition reportedly indicative of cherubism.[478] Such fibrohistiocytic areas should

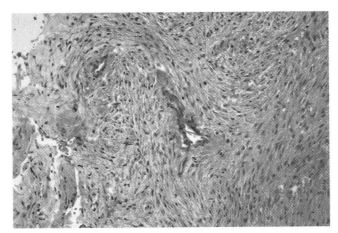

FIGURE 9–122 Cherubism. Fibrohistiocytic stroma lacking giant cells shows perivascular deposition of eosinophilic hyalinized collagen.

prompt the pathologist to consider a diagnosis of cherubism and request radiographic correlation.[479] Cherubism frequently regresses after skeletal maturity is attained.[480,481] Some patients with Noonan's syndrome have cherubism.[482]

Clinicopathologic Correlation

The observed predilection for females is apparently related to factors other than estrogen receptors.[483,484] Approximately 45% of CGCGs recur following curettage.[459,470]

MYOFIBROMA

Gross Pathology

Oral myofibroma typically presents as a circumscribed nodule approximately 2.0 cm in diameter affecting the mandible (intraosseous or parosteal), tongue, or lip/buccal tissues.[485,486]

Microscopic Pathology

Histologically, the tumor demonstrates lobules, each one exhibiting elongated fusiform cells with eosinophilic cytoplasm in a pale basophilic hyaline "chondroid" stroma, separated by hypocellular collagenous septa (Fig. 9–123). Such lobules sometimes surround a central hypercellular hemangiopericytoma-like (HPC-like) zone showing ectatic, crescentic, or branching small blood vessels surrounded by polygonal stromal cells; when present, this zoning is helpful in recognizing myofibroma.[486,487]

Differential Diagnosis

Myofibromas have been misinterpreted as sarcomas because they show mitotic activity among fibroblastic/myofibroblastic cells and because they can infiltrate striated muscle or salivary gland tissue.[485] The fusiform stromal cells of myofibroma display immunoreactivity for smooth muscle actin, but so do those of pseudosarcomatous fasciitis (nodular fasciitis), fibromatosis (desmoid), and infantile fibrosarcoma.[488-492] The histologic findings of lobules and HPC-like zones are therefore more important than immunohistochemistry in distinguishing these entities. When HPC-like areas are observed in a soft-tissue lesion from an infant, the possibility of myofibroma should be considered before diagnosis of infantile hemangiopericytoma is rendered.[493] Inflammatory myofibroblastic tumor might be included in the differential diagnosis of myofibroblastic proliferations having an inflammatory component, and a diagnosis of tumefactive fibroinflammatory lesion might be considered if an inflammatory pseudotumor-like mass shows a sclerotic collagenous component.[494-497]

Clinicopathologic Correlation

Myofibroma is the most common fibrous connective tissue proliferation of infancy and childhood, but it also occurs in adults.[492,498] Multifocal myofibromata (infantile myofibromatosis) involving bones and subcutaneous sites occurs in about 5% of oral myofibroma cases, but disseminated visceral myofibromatosis is quite rare.[485,499] Myofibroma has a low recurrence rate; a recurrence should be re-evaluated for possible reclassification as a sarcoma.[500]

FIBROMATOSIS

Gross Pathology

Fibromatosis (extra-abdominal desmoid fibromatosis, aggressive fibromatosis, juvenile fibromatosis, infantile fibromatosis) of the paraoral area often presents in a child as an approximately 4.0 cm firm paraman-

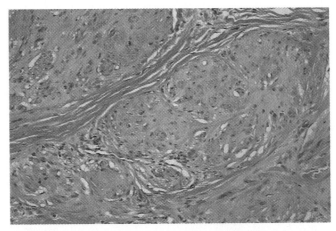

FIGURE 9–123 Myofibroma. Nodules of pale basophilic mucoid or "chondroid" stroma contain strands and bundles of fusiform myofibroblasts with eosinophilic cytoplasm.

dibular mass in the submandibular or submental region.[501] Gross evidence of invasion into bone, usually the mandible, and infiltration of skeletal muscle suggest a malignant process.

Microscopic Pathology

Histologically, this tumor demonstrates benign-appearing broad fascicles of moderately cellular collagenous tissue; the bland stromal cells are fibroblasts and myofibroblasts.[502] Mitotic figures can be seen in more cellular areas, but they are not frequent in fibromatosis (approximately 1 per 10 high power fields).[503] A diffusely hypercellular, mitotically active, infantile fibroblastic proliferation might be more appropriately considered an infantile fibrosarcoma than an infantile fibromatosis.[491,504] While some areas in a fibromatosis can appear myxoid, others show hypocellular collagenous sclerosis. Evaluation of surgical margins, particularly in recurrent lesions, is complicated by the striking resemblance of infiltrative fibromatosis to fibrosis or scar tissue.

Clinicopathologic Correlation

Desmoid tumors associated with Gardner's syndrome occasionally involve the head and neck area, but most are abdominal tumors.[505,506] Desmoplastic fibroma is the term used for an intraosseous desmoid fibromatosis.[507,508] Gnathic desmoplastic fibroma affects the mandible almost exclusively; although lesions occasionally develop in the maxillary sinus, the maxilla is rarely involved.[509,510] Desmoplastic fibroma can arise in patients with tuberous sclerosis.[511]

OSTEOMA

Gross Pathology

Osteoma represents an endosteal circumscribed radiodense lesion or a parosteal, bony-hard, smooth, lobulated, sessile, polypoid, exophytic lesion. The osteoma is less common in gnathic sites than in paranasal sinus or auditory canal sites.

Microscopic Pathology

Histologically, osteoma is composed of mature cortical and/or cancellous lamellar bone.[512]

Differential Diagnosis

Exostoses, occurring on facial alveolar bone, and tori, located on the median hard palate or bilaterally on the premolar region of the lingual cortex of mandibular alveolar bone, are histologically similar to osteomas. They are generally considered developmental abnormalities, not indicative of Gardner's syndrome. Osteoma-like osseous proliferations can occur in edentulous areas of mandibular alveolar bone that have been covered by a metal dental bridge (fixed partial denture), and these have been called subpontic osseous hyperplasia (reactive subpontine exostoses, hyperostoses, subpontic osseous proliferation).[513,514] Iatrogenic peripheral osteoma-like exostoses also can occur at the site of a free gingival graft.[515] It is unclear whether osteomas occurring at a site of muscle attachment ever exhibit a cartilage cap as seen in osteochondroma (osteocartilaginous exostosis).[512,516]

Clinicopathologic Correlation

Gardner's syndrome (familial adenomatous polyposis coli) consists of cutaneous cysts and osteomas as early indicators of premalignant hereditary colonic polyposis.[517] Approximately 10% of patients with this syndrome have supernumerary teeth and/or odontoma formation, and 10% to 20% show multiple unerupted teeth.[518] The osteomatous jaw lesions in Gardner's syndrome range from multiple small mandibular endosteal osteomas resembling dense bone islands (idiopathic osteosclerosis) to multiple large peripheral osteomas.[392,519–521]

LANGERHANS' CELL HISTIOCYTOSIS

Gross Pathology

Langerhans' cell histiocytosis (LCH, histiocytosis X, eosinophilic granuloma of bone) of the oral region arises almost exclusively in bone; disease limited to oral soft tissue is unusual.[522,523] The oral lesions of Langerhans' cell histiocytosis often clinically resemble localized advanced juvenile periodontitis or common periapical inflammatory disease (periapical granuloma).

Microscopic Pathology

Langerhans' cell histiocytosis is characterized by a proliferation of histiocytic cells (Langerhans' cells) showing "coffee-bean" cleaved or lobulated vesicular nuclei, associated with a variable number of eosinophils, neutrophils, lymphocytes, histiocytic cells, and multinucleated giant cells.[524,525] In mucosal sites, this proliferation is usually submucosal in localization.

Special Techniques

Langerhans' cells are S-100 and CD1a immunopositive histiocytic cells. Ultrastructurally, Birbeck granules are observed in the cytoplasm.[526,527]

Differential Diagnosis

Normal Langerhans' cells are dendritic, but Langerhans' cell histiocytes (histiocytosis X cells) are round.[525] The histiocytic cells in extranodal sinus histiocytosis with massive lymphadenopathy (Rosai-Dorfman disease) are S-100 protein positive but are CD1a negative. Further, these usually show emperipolesis, a feature not present in association with Langerhans' cells.

Clinicopathologic Correlation

Histiocytosis X cells show evidence of mitotic activity, with a proliferative fraction of 3% to 24%.[528] The various clinical syndromes/presentations cannot be predicted from histologic features.[529,530] Periapical or periodontal lesions of Langerhans' cell histiocytosis exhibiting few eosinophils and only focal evidence of histiocytosis X cells histologically differ only subtly from periapical or periodontal inflamed granulation tissue; sometimes the correct diagnosis becomes apparent only after histologic evaluation of the recurrent or persistent jaw lesion.

SIMPLE BONE CYST

Gross Pathology

This lesion (also known as traumatic bone cyst, solitary bone cyst, and hemorrhagic bone cyst) often presents in the premolar-molar region of the mandible as a unilocular lesion that "scallops" around and between tooth roots.

Microscopic Pathology

This is not a true cyst because it lacks an epithelial lining. The curetted thin membrane histologically consists simply of fibrous connective tissue with little or no chronic inflammation; a luminal layer of flattened stromal cells is sometimes observed. Some specimens additionally exhibit fragments of benign fibro-osseous tissue showing bone and/or small acellular globular ossicles (cementum); it is unclear whether this fibro-osseous tissue is a reactive/reparative proliferation at the periphery of a simple bone cyst or remnants of a fibro-osseous lesion showing extensive lysis and cavitation. This cementum can also be observed in the fibrous wall of femoral solitary bone cysts.[431] The findings at surgery are important; the pathologist should be reluctant to deem a lesion an "ossifying fibroma" on the basis of tiny fragments of fibro-osseous tissue retrieved from an essentially empty osseous cavity. Simple bone cysts have been reported to occur concurrently with several gnathic osseous lesions, but the most frequent associated condition is focal/multifocal osseous dysplasia.[419,531–533] Surgeons sometimes encounter a multiloculated "empty" cystic cavity in the mandibular angle area; simple bone cysts are infrequently multilocular,[534] and sparse curetted tissue fragments from such an "empty" bone cavity can occasionally reveal histologic evidence of odontogenic keratocyst.

Clinicopathologic Correlation

Simple bone cyst tends to affect two patient populations: adolescent and young adult males, with some trauma-related cases, and middle-aged black females, with many focal/multifocal osseous dysplasia (florid osseous dysplasia) associated cases.[535,536]

Malignant Jaw Lesions

SECONDARY TUMORS

Oral metastatic neoplasms, usually carcinoma metastatic to the mandible, involve the jawbones more frequently than the oral soft tissues. According to data provided by Hirshberg and associates,[537–539] the most common primary site of intraosseous gnathic metastases differs with age: in the first decade neuroblastoma predominates; in the second decade sarcoma predominates (Ewing's sarcoma, osteosarcoma, chondrosarcoma); and in adults carcinoma predominates (breast carcinoma in women and lung carcinoma in men). These data suggest that the most common primary site of oral soft-tissue (extraosseous) metastases in decreasing order of frequency is lung carcinoma, renal cell carcinoma, melanoma, and breast carcinoma.[538] Often histologic features are insufficiently distinctive to unequivocally identify the source of the metastatic carcinoma; in this situation, immunohistochemistry can occasionally be of value. For example, immunoreactivity for thyroglobulin or prostate specific antigen (PSA) might suggest that a primary carcinoma could potentially be found in the thyroid gland or prostate gland, respectively.[540,541] Although PSA is sometimes expressed in nonprostatic neoplasms, such as salivary duct carcinoma, it remains a valuable marker for metastatic prostate carcinoma.[542,543] Other immunohistochemical markers, such as those for breast carcinoma, appear to be less specific and therefore less reliable in identifying the site of the primary tumor.[544,545] Calcifying epithelial odontogenic tumor, an amyloid producing tumor, and odontogenic fibroma would be included in the histologic differential diagnosis of intraosseous metastatic carcinoma. The juxtaoral organ of Chievitz located in the buccal/parapharyngeal region more closely resembles perineural infiltrative well-differentiated squamous cell carcinoma than metastatic carcinoma.[546]

MALIGNANT LYMPHOMA

Oral extranodal malignant lymphoma has been recognized increasingly in severely immunocompromised individuals, particularly patients with human immunodeficiency virus (HIV). These lymphomas often present as palatal, gingival, or retromolar ulcerated swellings, sometimes mimicking periodontal inflammatory disease. Histologically, they frequently represent diffuse immunoblastic large cell lymphomas or Burkitt-like diffuse small noncleaved lymphomas.[547-551] These neoplasms can be multifocal.[552,553] Primary intraosseous lymphoma of the mandible also often histologically displays features of a diffuse large B-cell lymphoma, and those cells showing lobulated nuclei can somewhat resemble Langerhans' cell histiocytes.[554-556] Intraoral low-grade diffuse small B-cell lymphomas with features of mucosa-associated lymphoid tissue (MALT) lymphomas often present in an elderly patient as a swelling of hard palatal mucosa; this lesion should be histologically differentiated from palatal benign follicular lymphoid hyperplasia.[557-559] Before a diagnosis of diffuse large cell lymphoma or Hodgkin's disease of lingual or palatine tonsillar tissue is rendered, the possibility of an Epstein-Barr virus–induced mononucleosis-like lymphoid proliferation should be considered.[560,561] Atypical histiocytic granuloma/eosinophilic ulcer can also mimic extranodal lymphoma; this lesion often presents as a persistent ulcerated nodule of the tongue, and histologically it demonstrates activated T cells, histiocytic cells, and eosinophils.[562-564] While well-differentiated plasma cell myeloma involving the jaws and periodontium is seldom a histopathologic diagnostic problem, blastic myelomas can histologically and immunohistochemically mimic myeloid or lymphoid neoplasms.[565-568]

OSTEOSARCOMA

Osteosarcoma of the jaws, based on data pooled from three studies, can demonstrate predominantly chondroid tissue (47% are chondroblastic osteosarcomas), predominantly osseous tissue (33% are osteoblastic osteosarcomas), or predominantly fibrous connective tissue (20% are fibrosarcomatous osteosarcomas).[569-571] Approximately 30% of gnathic osteosarcomas are histologically low-grade sarcomas (Broders grade 2), and 70% are high grade (45% are Broders grade 3, 25% Broders grade 4). Many pathologists regard a sarcoma showing extensive cartilaginous differentiation as chondroblastic osteosarcoma if it demonstrates only a minute osteoblastic focus. Any jaw lesion containing cartilage should be carefully evaluated for evidence of malignancy. However, before providing a diagnosis of a low-grade parosteal (juxtacortical) osteosarcoma, the possibility of a non-neoplastic periosteal reaction induced by denture trauma should be considered; such lesions exhibit a cartilage cap similar to that seen in osteochondromas.[572-574] A low-grade osteoblastic osteosarcoma can often be distinguished from an osteoblastoma; the sarcoma has radiographic and histologic evidence of a permeative growth pattern, and the osteoblastic cells in the sarcoma show evidence of mitotic activity.[575-579] Low-grade osteosarcoma can occasionally resemble fibrous dysplasia, but the sarcoma displays an infiltrative periphery, cytologic atypia, or mitotic activity.[434,442]

CHONDROSARCOMA

Chondrosarcoma of the jaw often presents as an approximately 4.0 cm mass, firm and pale on cut section, usually composed of rather mature hyaline cartilage; high-grade (grade 3) lesions are uncommon.[580,581] A chondroma-like intraosseous jaw lesion should be evaluated for histologic evidence of chondrosarcoma: relative hypercellularity, multiple cells per lacuna, large chondrocytes, nuclear atypia, and mitotic activity in fibroblastic cells in the myxoid connective tissue at the periphery of cartilaginous lobules. Chondromyxoid fibroma is uncommon in gnathic sites, and radiographic or histologic evidence of malignancy should be absent from lesions so diagnosed; postoperative follow-up should probably be recommended for chondromyxoid fibromas of the jaws. Chondrosarcoma sometimes arises from synovial soft tissue of the temporomandibular joint, but a diagnosis of chondrosarcoma should be rendered only after the possibility of synovial chondromatosis has been carefully considered; both entities can show nuclear atypia.[584-587] Synovial chondromatosis exhibits small cartilaginous nodules rather than sheets of chondroid tissue typical of chondrosarcoma. Chondrosarcoma can arise from synovial chondromatosis.[584] Tophaceous pseudogout of the temporomandibular joint has occasionally been misdiagnosed as chondrosarcoma or chondroblastoma, but the presence of basophilic material with birefringent crystals and multinucleated giant cells is a helpful indicator of pseudogout.[588,589] Mesenchymal chondrosarcoma, a high-grade sarcoma, rarely affects the jaws.[590,591] It histologically demonstrates sheets of undifferentiated small round cells, a hemangiopericytoma-like vasculature, and dispersed islands of cartilage.[592] These undifferentiated cells demonstrate immunoreactivity for CD99 (013, p30/32^{MIC2}, a putative marker for Ewing's sarcoma/peripheral neuroectodermal tumor).[593]

EWING'S SARCOMA

Ewing's sarcoma, which is closely related or identical to the peripheral primitive neuroectodermal tumor (pPNET), is a small round cell malignant neoplasm that occasionally affects the jawbones of children or young adults.[594-599] Histologically, this tumor demonstrates sheets of round cells exhibiting scanty clear cytoplasm containing periodic acid-Schiff (PAS) positive glycogen. If necrosis is extensive, vital tumor cells are present predominantly in perivascular regions. The tumor sometimes exhibits a filigree pattern with anastomosing cords of round cells.[600] Ewing's sarcoma cells show diffuse intense membrane or cytoplasmic immunoreactivity for CD99 (HBA71, 013, p30/32^{MIC2}), as do those of mesenchymal chondrosarcoma and lymphoblastic lymphoma.[601] Other small round cell neoplasms show less intense focal immunoreactivity for CD99, and several spindle cell neoplasms can additionally display CD99 immunoreactivity.[601,602] Evidence of the characteristic reciprocal translocation t(11;22)(q24; q12), often detected by using *EWS/FLI1* fusion transcripts in a reverse transcriptase–polymerase chain reaction assay, can be helpful in confirming the diagnosis of Ewing's sarcoma.[603,604] Small cell osteosarcoma and metastatic neuroblastoma would be included in the histologic differential diagnosis.[537]

Benign Soft-Tissue Tumors

PERIPHERAL NERVE SHEATH TUMORS

A variety of neural tumors (nerve sheath neoplasms) or neural-like lesions can affect oral and paraoral tissues. When encountering a tumor demonstrating lobules of myxoid tissue separated by collagenous septa, the pathologist should consider neurothekeoma, ossifying fibromyxoid tumor, and ectomesenchymal chondromyxoid tumor. The neurothekeoma (nerve sheath myxoma) exhibits variable cellularity and is composed of stellate or spindle cells exhibiting immunoreactivity for S-100 protein.[605,606] Ossifying fibromyxoid tumor (OFT) resembles neurothekeoma histologically and immunohistochemically, but OFT frequently has a peripheral cortex of lamellar bone.[607] Ectomesenchymal chondromyxoid tumor frequently presents as a 1.0 cm nodule on the dorsum of the anterior tongue; histologically it resembles a myoepithelioma, and interconnected stellate tumor cells, in myxoid stroma, typically show immunoreactivity for glial fibrillary acidic protein, cytokeratin, S-100 protein, and smooth muscle actin.[608] The oral palisaded encapsulated neuroma usually presents as a solitary, circumscribed 0.3 palatal or lip nodule exhibiting fascicles of S-100 protein–positive fusiform cells with some interspersed neurofilament protein–positive axons surrounded by an epithelial membrane antigen–positive perineurial capsule.[609,610] Patients with multiple mucosal neuroma syndrome (multiple endocrine neoplasia syndrome, type 2b: MEN 2b) have multiple tongue nodules and thickened nodular lips; these clinical features result from the presence of too many enlarged nerves, many of which are tortuous and nodular.[611,612] At scanning magnification, each neuroma of the MEN 2b syndrome consists of several separate nodules in a pattern resembling plexiform neurilemoma or plexiform neurofibroma.[613–615] However, the neuroma of the MEN 2b syndrome demonstrates fascicles of axons surrounded by a prominent perineurium and therefore more closely resembles a normal nerve than does neurofibroma or neurilemoma (Fig. 9–124).[616] Patients with MEN 2b often demonstrate a mutation of the RET proto-oncogene.[617] The traumatic neuroma shows disordered nerve bundles of varying size separated by moderately abundant hypocellular collagenous tissue.[618,619]

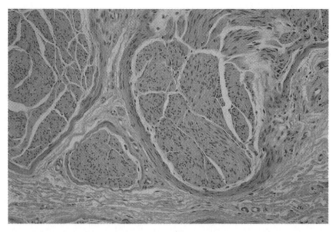

FIGURE 9–124 Mucosal neuroma of MEN 2b syndrome with large nerve bundles surrounded by prominent perineural sheaths.

GRANULAR CELL TUMOR

Oral granular cell tumor often occurs as a superficial pale 0.5 to 1.0 cm nodule on tongue or buccal/lip mucosa. This tumor, thought to be derived from Schwann cells, histologically exhibits sheets of S-100 protein and CD68 immunopositive large cells showing abundant cytoplasm containing eosinophilic granules.[620] Approximately 10% to 20% of these tumors demonstrate marked epithelial hyperplasia (pseudocarcinomatous hyperplasia).[621] Approximately 10% are multifocal, and occasional tumors display collagenous sclerosis.[622,623] Malignant granular cell tumor is quite rare.[624,625]

CONGENITAL EPULIS

Congenital epulis (CE, congenital gingival granular cell tumor) histologically resembles granular cell tumor. Congenital epulis typically presents as a sessile polypoid lesion of the anterior gingiva of female newborn infants.[626] Unlike the granular cell tumor, CE demonstrates prominent arborizing capillaries or venules, often with mild perivascular chronic inflammation (Fig. 9–125). The granular cells in CE lack immunoreactivity for S-100 protein, and while approximately 50% of granular cell tumors exhibit some degree of pseudoepitheliomatous hyperplasia, CE does not show such epithelial hyperplasia.[620,627,628]

VASCULAR NEOPLASMS

Several different angiomatous or vascular lesions can involve the oral region. The rather common *varix* often occurs as a 0.5 to 1.0 cm purple nodule of labial or buccal mucosa.[629] Histologically, the tortuous ectatic vein frequently demonstrates thrombosis,

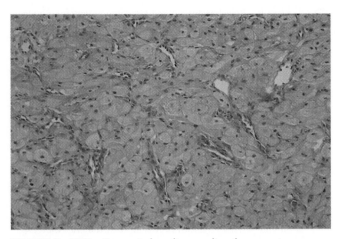

FIGURE 9-125 Congenital epulis revealing the conspicuous arborizing capillaries typical of this lesion.

sometimes with evidence of intravascular papillary endothelial hyperplasia.[630] Cavernous lesions (varix, hemangioma) additionally can show phleboliths, concentrically lamellated collagenous spherules displaying stippled basophilic calcified areas.[631,632] The *caliber-persistent artery* presents as a mucosa-colored or bluish linear papulonodule of upper or lower lip mucosa; most such nodules are pulsatile, but the excised nonpulsatile nodule histologically displays a moderately large, superficially positioned, labial artery.[633,634] *Intramuscular hemangiomas* often involve the masseter muscle, but they can affect other head and neck muscles including those of the lip or tongue; histologically, this tumor often exhibits a cellular or capillary hemangioma extending between striated muscle fibers, but cavernous intramuscular hemangiomas can also be seen.[635,636] Intraosseous (central) "deep" high-flow arteriovenous malformations can cause fatal spontaneous bleeding or postoperative hemorrhage.[637] Although angiograms of such lesions are readily available, the literature has a dearth of information regarding their histologic features; a portion of the vessels in these arteriovenous shunts presumably have a mural smooth-muscle component, as does the low-flow acquired cutaneous papular arteriovenous hemangioma.[638,639]

Intraoral *lymphangiomas* often affect the tongue dorsum as a pebbly translucent bluish plaque. Histologically, this tumor shows endothelium-lined cavernous vascular spaces containing few or no red blood cells, serous fluid, and perhaps luminal aggregations of lymphocytes; a distinctive feature is the close apposition of ectatic lymphatic spaces to surface squamous epithelium with little intervening connective tissue.[640] The cystic hygroma is a large cavernous lymphangiomatous malformation often affecting the neck of a newborn or infant.[641,642]

REFERENCES

1. Min K-W, Houck JR, et al. Protocol for the examination of specimens removed from patients with carcinomas of the upper aerodigestive tract. Carcinomas of the oral cavity including lip and tongue, nasal and paranasal sinuses, pharynx, larynx, salivary glands, hypopharynx, oropharynx, and nasopharynx. *Arch Pathol Lab Med*. 1998; 122:222.
2. Eisen D. The oral mucosal punch biopsy. A report of 140 cases. *Arch Dermatol*. 1992; 128:815.
3. Convissar RA. Laser biopsy artifact [letter]. *Oral Surg Oral Med Oral Pathol*. 1997; 84:458.
4. Paterson DA, Davies JD, McLaren KM. Failure to demonstrate the true resection margins of excised skin tumours: A case for routine marking. *Br J Dermatol*. 1992; 127:119.
5. Seidman JD, Berman JJ, Moore GW. Basal cell carcinoma: Importance of histologic discontinuities in evaluation of resection margins. *Mod Pathol*. 1991; 4:325.
6. Johnson RE, Sigman JD, Funk GF, et al. Quantification of surgical margin shrinkage in the oral cavity. *Head Neck*. 1997; 19:281.
7. Rapini RP. On the definition of Mohs surgery and how it determines appropriate surgical margins [editorial]. *Arch Dermatol*. 1992; 128:673.
8. Rapini RP. Pitfalls of Mohs micrographic surgery. *J Am Acad Dermatol*. 1990; 22:681.
9. Rapini RP. Comparison of methods for checking surgical margins. *J Am Acad Dermatol*. 1990; 23:288.
10. Hunter-Craig C, Lee-McDonagh B, Penman HG. Marking of resection margins. *J Clin Pathol*. 1991; 44:874.
11. Chen TY, Emrich LJ, Driscoll DL. The clinical significance of pathological findings in surgically resected margins of the primary tumor in head and neck carcinoma. *Int J Radiat Oncol Biol Phys*. 1987; 13:833.
12. Ravasz LA, Slootweg PJ, Hordijk GJ, et al. The status of the resection margin as a prognostic factor in the treatment of head and neck carcinoma. *J Craniomaxillofac Surg*. 1991; 19: 314.
13. Garcia-Garcia A, Gandara-Rey JM, Alvarez-Calderon-Prat P. Endoscopy of mandibular cysts after cystotomy: A preliminary report. *J Oral Maxillofac Surg*. 1998; 56:169.
14. Gold L, Upton GW, Marx RE. Standardized surgical terminology for the excision of lesions of bone: An argument for accuracy in reporting. *J Oral Maxillofac Surg*. 1991; 49:1214.
15. Lydiatt DD. Mandibular resection. *Head Neck*. 1995; 17:247.
16. Osguthorpe JD, Abel CG, Lang P, Hochman M. Neurotropic cutaneous tumors of the head and neck. *Arch Otolaryngol Head Neck Surg*. 1997; 123:871.
17. Bagatin M, Orihovac Z, Mohammed AM. Perineural invasion by carcinoma of the lower lip. *J Craniomaxillofac Surg*. 1995; 23:155.
18. Kleiss C, Kleiss E. Über einege morphogenetische Einzelheiten des juxtaoralen (oder Chievitz'schen) Organs beim Menschen. Some morphogenetic aspects of the juxtaoral organ (Chievitz organ) in the human. *Z mikrosk—anat Forsch (Leipzig)*. 1985; 99:59.
19. Tschen JA, Fechner RE. The juxtaoral organ of Chievitz. *Am J Surg Pathol*. 1979; 3:147.
20. Mesa M, Baden E, Grodjesk J, Dolinsky HB. Neuroepithelial hamartoma of the oral cavity. *Oral Surg Oral Med Oral Pathol*. 1994; 78:627.
21. Brown JS, Griffith JF, Phelps PD, Browne RM. A comparison of different imaging modalities and direct inspection after periosteal stripping in predicting the invasion of the mandible by oral squamous cell carcinoma. *Br J Oral Maxillofac Surg*. 1994; 32:347.
22. Brown JS, Browne RM. Factors influencing the patterns of invasion of the mandible by oral squamous cell carcinoma. *Int J Oral Maxillofac Surg*. 1995; 24:417.
23. Arber JM, Arber DA, Jenkins KA, Battifora H. Effect of decalcification and fixation in paraffin-section immunohistochemistry. *Applied Immunohistochem*. 1996; 4:241.

24. Spiro RH, Strong EW, Shah JP. Maxillectomy and its classification. *Head Neck*. 1997; 19:309.
25. Banerjee AR, Alun-Jones T. Neck dissection. Review. *Clin Otolaryngol*. 1995; 20:286.
26. Suen JY, Goepfert H. Standardization of neck dissection nomenclature [editorial]. *Head Neck*. 1987; 10:75.
27. Shah JP, Anderson PE. Evolving role of modifications in neck dissection for oral squamous cell carcinoma. *Br J Oral Maxillofac Surg*. 1995; 33:3.
28. Challis D. Broadsheet number 41: Frozen section and intraoperative diagnosis. *Pathol*. 1997; 29:165.
29. Gandour-Edwards RF, Donald PJ, Wiese DA. Accuracy of intraoperative frozen section diagnosis in head and neck surgery: Experience at a university medical center. *Head Neck*. 1993; 15:33.
30. Gandour-Edwards RF, Donald PJ, Lie JT. Clinical utility of intraoperative frozen section diagnosis in head and neck surgery: A quality assurance perspective. *Head Neck*. 1993; 15:373.
31. Weiss SW, Willis J, Jansen J, et al. Frozen section consultation. Utilization patterns and knowledge base of surgical faculty at a university hospital. *Am J Clin Pathol*. 1995; 104:294.
32. Forrest LA, Schuller DE, Karanfilov B, Lucas JG. Update on intraoperative analysis of mandibular margins. *Am J Otolaryngol*. 1997; 18:396.
33. Novis DA, Zarbo RJ. Interinstitutional comparison of frozen section turnaround time. A College of American Pathologists Q-probe study of 32,868 frozen sections in 700 hospitals. *Arch Pathol Lab Med*. 1997; 121:559.
34. Wysocki GP, Wright BA. Intraneural and perineural epithelial structures. *Head Neck Surg*. 1981; 4:69.
35. van der Wal N, Baak JPA, Schipper NW, van der Waal I. Morphometric study of pseudoepitheliomatous hyperplasia in granular cell tumors of the tongue. *J Oral Pathol Med*. 1989; 18:8.
36. Franchi A, Gallo O, Santucci M. Pathologic Quiz Case 1. *Arch Otolaryngol Head Neck Surg*. 1995; 121:584.
37. Littman CD. Necrotizing sialometaplasia (adenometaplasia) of the trachea. *Histopathol*. 1993; 22:298.
38. Weidner N, Askin FB, Berthrong M, et al. Bizarre (pseudomalignant) granulation-tissue reactions following ionizing-radiation exposure. *Cancer*. 1987; 59:1509.
39. Meehan SA, LeBoit PE. An immunohistochemical analysis of radiation fibroblasts. *J Cutan Pathol*. 1997; 24:309.
40. Vaughn Jones SA, Salas J, McGrath JA, et al. A retrospective analysis of tissue-fixed immunoreactants from skin biopsies maintained in Michel's medium. *Dermatol*. 1994; 189:131.
41. Vaughn Jones SA, Palmer I, Bhogal BS, et al. The use of Michel's transport medium for immunofluorescence and immunoelectron microscopy in autoimmune bullous diseases. *J Cutan Pathol*. 1995; 22:365.
42. Arber JM, Weiss LM, Chang KL, et al. The effect of decalcification on in situ hybridization. *Modern Pathol*. 1997; 10:1009.
43. Ten Cate AR. *Oral Histology*. St. Louis: Mosby; 1994.
44. Chou L, Hansen LS, Daniels TE. Choristomas of the oral cavity. *Oral Surg Oral Med Oral Pathol*. 1991; 72:584.
45. Neinas FW, Gorman CA, Devine KD, Woolner LB. Lingual thyroid: Clinical characteristics of 15 cases. *Ann Intern Med*. 1973; 79:205.
46. Fish J, Moore RM. Ectopic thyroid tissue and ectopic thyroid carcinoma. *Ann Surg*. 1963; 157:212.
47. Lipsett J, Sparnon AL, Byard RW. Embryogenesis of enterocystomas—enteric duplication cysts of the tongue. *Oral Surg Oral Med Oral Pathol*. 1993; 75:626.
48. Bychkov V, Gatti WM, Fresco R. Tumor of the tongue containing heterotopic brain tissue. *Oral Surg Oral Med Oral Pathol*. 1988; 66:71.
49. Strome SE, McClatchey K, Kileny PR, Koopman CFJ. Neonatal choristoma of the tongue containing glial tissue: Diagnosis and surgical considerations. *Int J Pediatr Otorhinolaryngol*. 1995; 33:265.
50. Halperin V, Kolas S, Jefferis KR, et al. Occurrence of fordyce glands, benign migratory glossitis, median rhomboid glossitis, and fissured tongue in 2,478 dental students. *Oral Surg*. 1953; 6:1072.
51. Koutlas IG, Yaholnitsky B. Oral sebaceous retention phenomenon. *J Periodontol*. 1994; 65:186.
52. Ferguson JW, Geary CP, MacAlister AD. Sebaceous cell adenoma. Rare intra-oral occurrence of a tumor which is frequent marker of Torre's syndrome. *Pathol*. 1987; 19:204.
53. Ishikawa K, Mizukoshi T, Notani K, et al. Osseous choristoma of the tongue. *Oral Surg Oral Med Oral Pathol*. 1993; 76:561.
54. Trowbridge M, McCabe B, Resnicek M. Cartilaginous choristoma of the tongue. *Arch Otolaryngol Head Neck Surg*. 1989; 115:627.
55. King RC, Smith BR, Burk JL. Dermoid cyst in the floor of the mouth. *Oral Surg Oral Med Oral Pathol*. 1994; 78:567.
56. Giunta J, Cataldo E. Lymphoepithelial cysts of the oral mucosa. *Oral Surg*. 1973; 35:77.
57. Buchner A, Hansen LS. Lymphoepithelial cysts of the oral cavity. *Oral Surg Oral Med Oral Pathol*. 1980; 50:441.
58. Chaudhry AP, Yamane GM, Scharlock SE, et al. A clinicopathological study of intraoral lymphoepithelial cysts. *J Oral Med*. 1984; 39:79.
59. Morris R, Gansler TS, Rudisil MT, Neville B. White sponge nevus. Diagnosis by light microscopic and ultrastructural cytology. *Acta Cytol*. 1988; 32:357.
60. Rugg EL, McLean WH, Allison WE, et al. A mutation in the mucosal keratin K4 is associated with oral white sponge nevus. *Nat Genet*. 1995; 11:450.
61. Richard G, De-Laurenzi V, Didona B, et al. Keratin 13 point mutation underlies the hereditary mucosal epithelial disorder white sponge nevus. *Nat Genet*. 1995; 11:453.
62. Jorgensen RJ, Levin S. White sponge nevus. *Arch Dermatol*. 1981; 117:73.
63. Nichols GE, Cooper PH, Underwood PB, Greer KE. White sponge nevus. *Obstet Gynecol*. 1990; 76:545.
64. Krajewska IA, Moore L, Brown JH. White sponge nevus presenting in the esophagus—case report and literature review. *Pathol*. 1992; 24:112.
65. Schubert MM. Oral manifestation of viral infections in immunocompromised patients. *Curr Op Dent*. 1991; 1:384.
66. Greenspan D, Greenspan JS. Significance of oral hairy leukoplakia. *Oral Surg Oral Med Oral Pathol*. 1992; 73:151.
67. Sciubba J, Brandsma J, Schwartz M. Hairy leukoplakia. An AIDS-associated opportunistic infection. *Oral Surg Oral Med Oral Pathol*. 1989; 67:404.
68. Fernandez JF, Benito MA, Lizaldez EB, Montanes MA. Oral hairy leukoplakia: A histopathologic study of 32 cases. *Am J Dermatopath*. 1990; 12:571.
69. Eversole LR, Stone CE, Beckman AM. Detection of EBV and HPV DNA sequences in oral "hairy" leukoplakia by in situ hybridization. *J Med Virol*. 1988; 26:217.
70. Ficarra G, Adler-Storthz K, Woods-Francis K, et al. Epstein-Barr virus and human papillomavirus detection in oral hairy leukoplakia and normal oral mucosa of HIV-infected patients. *Int Conf AIDS* (abstr no. M.B. 2290). 1991; 7:254.
71. Felix DH, Jalal H, Cubie HA, et al. Detection of Epstein-Barr virus and human papilloma-virus type 16 in hairy leukoplakia by in situ hybridization and the polymerase chain reaction. *J Oral Pathol Med*. 1993; 22:277.
72. Baughman RA. Median rhomboid glossitis: A developmental anomaly? *Oral Surg*. 1971; 31:56.
73. Wright BA. Median rhomboid glossitis: Not a misnomer. *Oral Surg*. 1978; 46:806.
74. Weir JC, Buck WH. Periapical actinomycosis. *Oral Surg Med Oral Pathol*. 1982; 54:336.
75. Samuels RHA, Martin MV. A clinical and microbiological study of Actinomycetes in oral and cervicofacial lesions. *Br J Oral Maxillofac Surg*. 1988; 26:458.
76. Van-Wyk CW, Ambrosio SC. Leukoedema: Ultrastructural and histochemical observations. *J Oral Pathol*. 1983; 12:319.
77. Martin JL. Leukoedema: A review of the literature. *J Nat Med Assoc*. 1992; 84:938.
78. Hamner JE, Mehta FS, Pindborg JJ, Daftary DK. An epidemiologic and histopathologic study of leukoedema among 50,915 rural Indian villagers. *Oral Surg Oral Med Oral Pathol*. 1971; 32:58.

79. Axell T. Leukoedema—an epidemiologic study with special reference to the influence of tobacco habits. *Community Dent Oral Epidemiol.* 1981; 9:142.

80. Darling MR, Arendorf TM. Effects of cannabis smoking on oral soft tissues. *Community Dent Oral Epidemiol.* 1993; 21:78.

81. Glass LF, Maize JC. Morsicatio buccarum et labiorum (excessive cheek and lip biting). *Am J Dermatopath.* 1991; 13:271.

82. Sewerin I. A clinical and epidemiologic study of morsicatio buccarum/labiorum. *Scand J Dent Res.* 1971; 79:73.

83. Van-Wyk CW, Staz J, Farman AG. The chewing lesion of the cheeks and lips: Its features and prevalence among a selected group of adolescents. *J Dent.* 1977; 5:193.

84. Magro CM, Crowson AN. Cutaneous manifestations of Behcet's disease. *Int J Dermatol.* 1995; 34:159.

85. Woo S, Sonis ST. Recurrent aphthous ulcers: A review of diagnosis and treatment. *J Am Dent Assoc.* 1996; 127:1202.

86. Elzay RP. Traumatic ulcerative granuloma with stromal eosinophilia (Riga-Fede's disease and traumatic eosinophilic granuloma). *Oral Surg.* 1983; 55:497.

87. El-Mofty SK, Wick MR, Miller AS. Eosinophilic ulcer of the oral mucosa. *Oral Surg Oral Med Oral Pathol.* 1993; 75:716.

88. Regezi JA, Zarbo RJ, Daniels TE, Greenspan JS. Oral traumatic granuloma. *Oral Surg Oral Med Oral Pathol.* 1993; 75: 723.

89. Eversole LR, Leider AS, Jacobsen PL, Kidd PM. Atypical histiocytic granuloma. *Cancer.* 1985; 55:1722.

90. Morrison JW, Langston JR, Slater LJ. Atypical histiocytic granuloma. *J Oral Maxillofac Surg.* 1990; 48:630.

91. Scully C, El-Kom M. Lichen planus: Review and update on pathogenesis. *J Oral Pathol.* 1985; 14:431.

92. Jungell P. Oral lichen planus: A review. *Int J Oral Maxillofac Surg.* 1990; 20:129.

93. Miller RL, Gould AR, Bernstein ML. Cinnamon-induced stomatitis venenata. *Oral Surg Oral Med Oral Pathol.* 1992; 73: 708.

94. Beutner EH, Chorzelski TD, Parodi A, et al. Ten cases of chronic ulcerative stomatitis with stratified epithelium-specific antinuclear antibody. *J Am Acad Dermatol.* 1991; 24:781.

95. Krutchkoff DJ, Eisenberg E. Lichenoid dysplasia: A distinct histopathologic entity. *Oral Surg Oral Med Oral Pathol.* 1985; 60:308.

96. Eisenberg E, Krutchkoff DJ. Lichenoid lesions of oral mucosa. *Oral Surg Oral Med Oral Pathol.* 1992; 73:699.

97. Eversole LR. Immunopathology of oral mucosal ulcerative, desquamative, and bullous diseases. *Oral Surg Oral Med Oral Pathol.* 1994; 77:555.

98. Scully C, El-Kom E. Lichen planus: Review and update on pathogenesis. *J Oral Pathol.* 1985; 14:431.

99. Bagan JV, Aquirre JM, Del-Olmo JA, et al. Oral lichen planus and chronic liver disease: A clinical and morphometric study of the oral lesions in relation to transaminase elevation. *Oral Surg Oral Med Oral Pathol.* 1994; 78:337.

100. Cribier B, Garnier C, Laustriat D, Heid E. Lichen planus and hepatitis C virus infection: An epidemiologic study. *J Am Acad Dermatol.* 1994; 31:1070.

101. Lodi G, Olsen I, Piattelli A, et al. Antibodies to epithelial components in oral lichen planus (OLP) associated with hepatitis C (HCV) infection. *J Oral Pathol Med.* 1997; 26:36.

102. Burge SM: Mucosal involvement in systemic and chronic cutaneous lupus erythematosus. *Brit J Dermatol.* 1989; 121: 727.

103. Woo S, Lee SJ, Schubert MM. Graft-vs.-host disease. *Critical Reviews in Oral Biology and Medicine.* 1997; 8:201.

104. Walsh LJ, Savage NW, Ishii T, Seymour GJ. Immunopathogenesis of oral lichen planus. *J Oral Pathol Med.* 1990; 19:389.

105. Holmstrup P, Thorn JJ, Rindum J, Pinborg JJ. Malignant development of lichen planus-affected oral mucosa. *J Oral Pathol.* 1988; 17:219.

106. Barnard NA, Scully C, Eveson JW, et al. Oral cancer development in patients with oral lichen planus. *J Oral Pathol Med.* 1993; 22:421.

107. Marks R, Radden BG. Geographic tongue: A clinico-pathological review. *Australas J Dermatol.* 1981; 22:75.

108. Pogrel MA, Cram D. Intraoral findings in patients with psoriasis with a special reference to ectopic geographic tongue (erythema circinata). *Oral Surg Oral Med Oral Pathol.* 1988; 66:184.

109. Zelickson BD, Muller SA. Generalized pustular psoriasis. *Arch Dermatol.* 1991; 127:1339.

110. Marks R, Czarny D. Geographic tongue: Sensitivity to the enviroment. *Oral Surg.* 1984; 58:156.

111. Worsaae N, Christensen KC, Schiodt M. Melkersson-Rosenthal syndrome and cheilitis granulomatosa. *Oral Surg Oral Med Oral Pathol.* 1982; 54:404.

112. Allen CM, Camisa C, Hamzeh S, Stephens L. Cheilitis granulomatosa: Report of six cases and review of the literature. *J Am Acad Dermatol.* 1990; 23:444.

113. Oliver AJ, Rich AM, Reade PC, et al. Monosodium glutamate-related orofacial granulomatosis. *Oral Surg Oral Med Oral Pathol.* 1991; 71:560.

114. Handlers JP, Waterman J, Abrams AM, Melrose RJ. Oral features of Wegener's granulomatosis. *Arch Otolaryngol.* 1985; 111:267.

115. Allen CM, Camisa C, Salewski C, Weiland JE. Wegener's granulomatosis: Report of three cases with oral lesions. *J Oral Maxillofac Surg.* 1991; 49:294.

116. Napier SS, Allen JA, Irwin CR, McCluskey DR. "Strawberry gums"—a case of Wegener's granulomatosis. *Br Dent J.* 1993; 175:327.

117. Duna GF, Galperin C, Hoffman GS. Wegener's granulomatosis. *Rheum Dis Clin North Am.* 1995; 21:949.

118. Feinberg R. The protracted superficial phenomenon in pathergic (Wegener's) granulomatosis. *Hum Pathol.* 1981; 12:458.

119. Fukase S, Ohta N, Inamura K, et al. Diagnostic specificity of anti-neutrophil cytoplasmic antibodies (ANCA) in otorhinolaryngological diseases. *Acta Otolaryngol (Stockh).* 1994; 51(Suppl): 204.

120. Lederman DA. Suppurative stomatitis glandularis. *Oral Surg Oral Med Oral Pathol.* 1994; 78:319.

121. Swerlick RA, Cooper PH. Cheilitis glandularis: A re-evaluation. *J Am Acad Dermatol.* 1984; 10:466.

122. Sollecito TP, Greenberg MS. Plasma cell gingivitis. *Oral Surg Oral Med Oral Pathol.* 1992; 73:690.

123. Kerr DA, McClatchey KD, Regezi JA. Idiopathic gingivostomatitis. *Oral Surg.* 1971; 32:402.

124. Timms MS, Sloan P. Association of supraglottic and gingival idiopathic plasmacytosis. *Oral Surg Oral Med Oral Pathol.* 1991; 71:451.

125. Laskaris G, Angelopoulos A. Cicatricial pemphigoid: Direct and indirect immunofluorescent studies. *Oral Surg Oral Med Oral Pathol.* 1981; 51:48.

126. Niimi Y, X.J. Z, Bystryn JC. Identification of cicatricial pemphigoid antigens. *Arch Dermatol.* 1992; 128:54.

127. Bernard P, Prost C, Durepaire N, et al. The major cicatricial pemphigoid antigen is a 180-kD protein that shows immunologic cross-reactivities with the bullous pemphigoid antigen. *J Invest Dermatol.* 1992; 99:174.

128. Ahmed AR, Kurgis BS, Rodgers RS. Cicatricial pemphigoid. *J Am Acad Dermatol.* 1991; 24:987.

129. Olsen KD, Rogers RSI. Upper aerodigestive tract manifestations of cicatricial pemphigoid. *Ann Otol Rhinol Laryngol.* 1988; 97:493.

130. Scully C, Carrozzo M, Gandolfo S, Puiatti P, Monteil R. Update on mucous membrane pemphigoid. *Oral Surg Oral Med Oral Pathol Oral Radiol Endodont.* 1999, 88:56.

131. Schwartz DL. Stomatitis nicotina of the palate. *Oral Surg.* 1965; 20:306.

132. Axell T, Mornstad H, Sundstrom B. The relation of the clinical picture to the histopathology of snuff dipper's lesions in a Swedish population. *J Oral Pathol.* 1976; 5:229.

133. Sundstrom B, Mornstad H, Axell T. Oral carcinomas associated with snuff dipping. *J Oral Pathol.* 1982; 11:245.

134. Kaugars GE, Mehailescu WL, Gunsolley JC. Smokeless tobacco use and oral epithelial dysplasia. *Cancer.* 1989; 64:1527.

135. Kaugars GE, Riley WT, Brandt RB, et al. The prevalence of oral lesions on smokeless tobacco users and evaluation of risk factors. *Cancer.* 1992; 70:2579.

136. Winn DM, Blot WJ, Shy CM, et al. Snuff dipping and oral

cancer among women in the southern United States. *N Engl J Med.* 1981; 304:745.

137. Buchner A, Hansen LS. Amalgam pigmentation (amalgam tattoo) of the oral mucosa. A clinicopathologic study of 268 cases. *Oral Surg Oral Med Oral Pathol.* 1980; 49:139.

138. Buchner A, Hansen LS. Melanotic macule of the oral mucosa. A clinicopathologic study of 105 cases. *Oral Surg Oral Med Oral Pathol.* 1979; 48:244.

139. Ho KK, Dervan P, O'Loughlin S, Powell FC. Labial melanotic macule: A clinical, histologic, and ultrastructural study. *J Am Acad Dermatol.* 1993; 28:33.

140. Sexton FM, Maize JC. Melanotic macules and melanoacanthomas of the lip. *Am J Dermatopath.* 1987; 9:438.

141. Tomich CE, Zunt SL. Melanoacanthosis (melanoacanthoma) of the oral mucosa. *J Dermatol Surg Oncol.* 1990; 16:231.

142. Green TL, Eversole LR, Leider AS. Oral and labial verruca vulgaris: Clinical, histologic, and immunohistochemical evaluation. *Oral Surg Oral Med Oral Pathol.* 1986; 62:410.

143. Carlos R, Sedano HO. Multifocal papilloma virus epithelial hyperplasia. *Oral Surg Oral Med Oral Pathol.* 1994; 77:631.

144. Miller CS, White DK, Royse DD. In situ hybridization analysis of human papillomavirus in orofacial lesions using a consensus biotinylated probe. *Am J Dermatopath.* 1993; 15:256.

145. Miller CS. Herpes simplex virus and human papillomavirus infections of the oral cavity. *Seminars in Dermatology.* 1994; 13:108.

146. Zunt SL, Tomich CE. Oral condyloma acuminatum. *J Dermatol Surg Oncol.* 1989; 15:591.

147. Abbey LM, Page DG, Sawyer DR. The clinical and histopathologic features of a series of 464 oral squamous papillomas. *Oral Surg Oral Med Oral Pathol.* 1980; 49:419.

148. Garlick JA, Taichman LB. Human papillomavirus infection of the oral mucosa. *Am J Dermatopath.* 1991; 13:386.

149. Buchner A, Hansen LS. Pigmented nevi of the oral mucosa: A clinicopathologic study of 32 new cases and review of 75 cases from the literature. Part I. A clinicopathologic study of 32 new cases. *Oral Surg Oral Med Oral Pathol.* 1979; 48:131.

150. Buchner A, Hansen LS. Pigmented nevi of the oral mucosa: A clinicopathologic study of 32 new cases and review of 75 cases from the literature. Part II. Analysis of 107 cases. *Oral Surg Oral Med Oral Pathol.* 1980; 49:55.

151. Houston GD. The giant cell fibroma: A review of 464 cases. *Oral Surg Oral Med Oral Pathol.* 1982; 53:582.

152. Savage NW, Monsour PA. Oral fibrous hyperplasias and the giant cell fibroma. *Austral Dent J.* 1985; 30:582.

153. Mills SE, Cooper PH, Fechner RE. Lobular capillary hemangioma: The underlying lesion of pyogenic granuloma: A study of 73 cases from the oral and nasal mucous membranes. *Am J Surg Pathol.* 1980; 4:471.

154. Buchner A, Hansen LS. The histomorphologic spectrum of peripheral ossifying fibroma. *Oral Surg Oral Med Oral Pathol.* 1987; 63:452.

155. Zain RB, Fei YJ. Fibrous lesions of the gingiva: A histopathologic analysis of 204 cases. *Oral Surg Oral Med Oral Pathol.* 1990; 70:466.

156. Giansanti JS, Waldron CA. Peripheral giant cell granuloma: Review of 720 cases. *J Oral Surg.* 1969; 27:787.

157. Katsikeris N, Kakarantza-Angelopoulou E, Angelopoulos AP. Peripheral giant cell granuloma: Clinicopathologic study of 224 new cases and review of 956 reported cases. *Int J Oral Maxillofac Surg.* 1988; 17:94.

158. Parbatani R, Tinsley GF, Danford MH. Primary hyperparathyroidism presenting as a giant-cell epulis. *Oral Surg Oral Med Oral Pathol Oral Radiol Endod.* 1998; 85:282.

159. Kenney JN, Kaugars GE, Abbey LM. Comparison between the peripheral ossifying fibroma and peripheral odontogenic fibroma. *J Oral Maxillofac Surg.* 1989; 47:378.

160. Slabbert H, Altini M. Peripheral odontogenic fibroma: A clinicopathologic study. *Oral Surg Oral Med Oral Pathol.* 1991; 72:86.

161. Buchner A, Begleiter A, Hansen LS. The predominance of epulis fissuratum in females. *Quintessence International.* 1984; 15:699.

162. Butler RT, Kalkwarf KL, Kaldahl WB. Drug-induced gingival hyperplasia: Phenytoin, cyclosporine, and nifedipine. *J Am Dent Assoc.* 1987; 114:56.

163. Bhaskar SN, Beasley JDI, Cutright DE. Inflammatory papillary hyperplasia of the oral mucosa: Report of 341 cases. *J Am Dent Assoc.* 1970; 81:949.

164. Cutright DE. The histopathologic findings in 583 cases of epulis fissuratum. *Oral Surg Oral Med Oral Pathol.* 1974; 37:401.

165. Cutright DE. Morphogenesis of inflammatory papillary hyperplasia. *J Prosthet Dent.* 1975; 33:380.

166. Nowparast B, Howell FV, Rick GM. Verruciform xanthoma. *Oral Surg Oral Med Oral Pathol.* 1981; 51:619.

167. Neville B. The verruciform xanthoma. *Am J Dermatopath.* 1986; 8:247.

168. Mostafa KA, Takata T, Ogawa I, et al. Verruciform xanthoma of the oral mucosa: A clinicopathological study with immunohistochemical findings relating to pathogenesis. *Virch Arch [A].* 1993; 423:243.

169. Zegarelli DJ, Zegarelli-Schmidt EC, Zegarelli EV. Verruciform xanthoma. *Oral Surg Oral Med Oral Pathol.* 1975; 40:246.

170. Miyamoto Y, Nagayama M, Hayashi Y. Verruciform xanthoma occurring within lichen planus. *J Oral Pathol Med.* 1996; 25:188.

171. Drummond JF, White DK, Damm DD, Cramer JR. Verruciform xanthoma within carcinoma in situ. *J Oral Maxillofac Surg.* 1989; 47:398.

172. Cataldo E, Mosadami A. Mucoceles of the oral mucous membranes. *Arch Otolaryngol.* 1970; 91:360.

173. Eversole LR. Oral sialocysts. *Arch Otolaryngol.* 1987; 113:51.

174. Jensen JL. Superficial mucoceles of the oral mucosa. *Am J Dermatopath.* 1990; 12:88.

175. Southam JC, Ettinger RL. A histologic study of sublingual varices. *Oral Surg Oral Med Oral Pathol.* 1974; 38:879.

176. Ettinger RL, Manderson RD. A clinical study of sublingual varices. *Oral Surg Oral Med Oral Pathol.* 1974; 38:540.

177. Lumerman H, Freedman P, Kerpel S. Oral epithelial dysplasia and the development of invasive squamous cell carcinoma. *Oral Surg Oral Med Oral Pathol Oral Radiol Endod.* 1995; 79:321.

178. WHO Collaborating Center for Oral Precancerous Lesions. Definition of leukoplakia and related lesions: An aid to studies on oral precancer. *Oral Surg Oral Med Oral Pathol.* 1978; 46:518.

179. Daley TD, Lovas JG, Peters E, et al. Salivary gland duct involvement in oral epithelial dysplasia and squamous cell carcinoma. *Oral Surg Oral Med Oral Pathol Oral Radiol Endod.* 1996; 81:186.

180. Shear M, Pindborg JJ. Verrucous hyperplasia of the oral mucosa. *Cancer.* 1980; 46:1855.

181. Eisenberg E. Lichen planus and oral cancer: Is there a connection between the two? *J Am Dent Assoc.* 1992; 123:104.

182. Zakrzewska JM, Lopes V, Speight P, Hopper C. Proliferative verrucous leukoplakia: A report of ten cases. *Oral Surg Oral Med Oral Pathol Oral Radiol Endodont.* 1996; 82:396.

183. Silverman S Jr, Gorsky M. Proliferative verrucous leukoplakia: A follow-up study of 54 cases. *Oral Surg Oral Med Oral Pathol Oral Radiol Endodont.* 1997; 84:154.

184. Miller CS. Human papillomavirus expression in oral mucosa, premalignant conditions, and squamous cell carcinoma. *Oral Surg Oral Med Oral Pathol Oral Radiol Endod.* 1996; 82:57.

185. Silverman SJ, Gorsky M, Kaugars G. Leukoplakia, dysplasia, and malignant transformation. *Oral Surg Oral Med Oral Pathol Oral Radiol Endod* [letter]. 1996; 82:117.

186. Axell T. Occurrence of leukoplakia and some other oral white lesions among 20,333 adult Swedish people. *Community Dent Oral Epidemiol.* 1987; 15:46.

187. Silverman S, Gorsky M, Lozada F. Oral leukoplakia and malignant transformation. *Cancer.* 1984; 53:563.

188. Bouquot JE, Gorlin RJ. Leukoplakia, lichen planus, and other oral keratoses in 23,616 white Americans over the age of 35 years. *Oral Surg Oral Med Oral Pathol.* 1986; 61:373.

189. Waldron CA, Shafer WG. Leukoplakia revisited: A clinicopathologic study of 3265 oral leukoplakias. *Cancer.* 1975; 36:1386.

190. Shafer WG, Waldron CA. Erythroplakia of the oral cavity. *Cancer*. 1975; 36:1021.

191. Mashberg A, Samit A. Early diagnosis of asymptomatic oral and oropharyngeal squamous cancers. *CA: Cancer J Clin*. 1995; 45:328.

192. Bryne M, Koppang HS, Lilleng R, et al. New malignancy grading is a better prognostic indicator than Broders' grading in oral squamous cell carcinomas. *J Oral Pathol Med*. 1989; 18:432.

193. Bundgaard T, Bentzen SM, Wildt J, et al. Histopathologic, stereologic, epidemiologic, and clinical parameters in the prognostic evaluation of squamous cell carcinoma of the oral cavity. *Head Neck*. 1996; 18:142.

194. Platz H, Fries R, Hudec M, et al. The prognostic relevance of various factors at the time of the first admission of the patient. *J Maxillofac Surg*. 1983; 11:3.

195. Crissman JD, Liu WY, Gluckman JL, Cummings G. Prognostic value of histopathologic parameters in squamous cell carcinoma of the oropharynx. *Cancer*. 1984; 54:2995.

196. Shingaki S, Suzuki I, Nakajima T, Kawasaki T. Evaluation of histopathologic parameters in predicting cervical lymph node metastasis of oral and oropharyngeal carcinomas. *Oral Surg Oral Med Oral Pathol*. 1988; 66:683.

197. Spiro RH, Huvos AG, Wong GY, et al. Predictive value of tumor thickness in squamous carcinoma confined to the tongue and floor of the mouth. *Am J Surg*. 1986; 152:345.

198. Mohit-Tabatabai MA, Sobel HJ, Rush BF, Mashberg A. Relation of thickness of floor of mouth Stage I and II cancers to regional metastases. *Am J Surg*. 1986; 152:351.

199. Frierson HF, Cooper PH. Prognostic factors in squamous cell carcinoma of the lower lip. *Hum Pathol*. 1986; 17:346.

200. Brown B, Barnes L, Mazariegos J, et al. Prognostic factors in mobile tongue and floor of mouth carcinoma. *Cancer*. 1989; 64:1195.

201. Jones KR, Lodge-Rigal RD, Reddick RL, Tudor GE, Shockley WW. Prognostic factors in the recurrence of state I and II squamous cell cancer of the oral cavity. *Arch Otolaryngol Head Neck Surg*. 1992; 118:483.

202. Curtis RE, Rowlings PA, Deeg J, et al. Solid cancers after bone marrow transplantation. *N Engl J Med*. 1997; 336:897.

203. Johnson NW, Warnakulasuriy S, Tavassoli M. Hereditary and environmental risk factors; clinical and laboratory risk markers for head and neck, especially oral, cancer and precancer. *European Journal of Cancer Prevention*. 1996; 5:5.

204. SEER Cancer Statistics Review 1973–1994. Bethesda, MD: US National Cancer Institute.

205. Tepperman BS, Fitzpatrick PJ. Second respiratory and upper disgestive tract cancers after oral cancer. *Lancet*. 1981; 2:547.

206. Gluckman JL, Crissman JD. Survival rates in 548 patients with multiple neoplasms of the upper aerodigestive tract. *Laryngoscope*. 1983; 93:71.

207. McCoy JM, Waldron CA. Verrucous carcinoma of the oral cavity. *Oral Surg Oral Med Oral Pathol*. 1981; 52:623.

208. Ishimaya A, Eversole LR, Ross DA, et al. Papillary squamous neoplasms of the head and neck. *Laryngoscope*. 1994; 104:1446.

209. Mills SE, Gaffey MJ, Frierson HF Jr. Tumors of the upper aerodigestive tract and ear. *Atlas of Tumor Pathology*, 3rd Series, Fascicle 26, Washington, DC: Armed Forces Institute of Pathology; 2000:85.

210. Crissman JD, Kessis T, Shah KV, et al. Squamous papillary neoplasia of the adult upper aerodigestive tract. *Hum Pathol*. 1988; 19:1387.

211. Ackerman LV. Verrucous carcinoma of the oral cavity. *Surgery*. 1948; 23:670.

212. Shafer WG. Verrucous carcinoma. *Int Dent J*. 1975; 22:451.

213. Kraus FT, Perez-Mesa C. Verrucous carcinoma—clinical and pathologic study of 105 cases involving oral cavity, larynx and genitalia. *Cancer*. 1966; 19:26.

214. Medina JE, Dichtel W, Luna MA. Verrucous-squamous carcinomas of the oral cavity: A clinicopathologic study of 104 cases. *Arch Otolaryngol*. 1984; 110:437.

215. McDonald J, Crissman JD, Gluckman JL. Verrucous carcinoma of the oral cavity. *Head Neck Surg*. 1982; 5:22.

216. Tharp ME, Shidnia H. Radiotherapy in the treatment of ver-

rucous carcinoma of the head and neck. *Laryngoscope*. 1995; 105:391.

217. Ellis GL, Corio RL. Spindle cell carcinoma of the oral cavity. *Oral Surg Oral Med Oral Pathol*. 1980; 50:523.

218. Leventon GS, Evans HL. Sarcomatoid squamous cell carcinoma of the mucous membranes of the head and neck: A clinicopathologic study of 20 cases. *Cancer*. 1981; 48:994.

219. Zarbo RJ, Crissman JD, Venkat H, Weiss MA. Spindle-cell carcinoma of the upper aerodigestive tract mucosa. *Am J Surg Pathol*. 1986; 10:741.

220. Ellis GL, Langloss JM, Heffner DK, Hyams VJ. Spindle-cell carcinoma of the aerodigestive tract. *Am J Surg Pathol*. 1987; 11:335.

221. Nakhleh RE, Zarbo RJ, Ewing S, et al. Myogenic differentiation in spindle cell (sarcomatoid) carcinomas of the upper aerodigestive tract. *Appl Immunohistochemistry*. 1993; 1:58.

222. Jones AC, Freedman PD, Kerpel SM. Oral adenoid squamous cell carcinoma: A report of three cases and review of the literature. *J Oral Maxillofac Surg*. 1993; 51:676.

223. Ferlito A, Devaney KO, Milroy CM, et al. Mucosal adenoid squamous cell carcinoma of the head and neck. *Ann Otol Rhinol Laryngol*. 1996; 105:409.

224. Johnson WC, Helwig EB. Adenoid squamous cell carcinoma (adenoacanthoma). *Cancer*. 1966; 11:1639.

225. Jacoway JR, Nelson JF, Boyers RC. Adenoid squamous-cell carcinoma (adenoacanthoma of the oral labial mucosa). *Oral Surg Oral Med Oral Pathol*. 1971; 32:444.

226. Gerughty RM, Hennigar GR, Brown FM. Adenosquamous carcinoma of the nasal, oral and laryngeal cavities. *Cancer*. 1968; 6:1140.

227. Ferlito A. A pathologic and clinical study of adenosquamous carcinoma of the larynx. Report of four cases and review of the literature. *Acta Otorhinolaryngol Belg*. 1976; 30:380.

228. Wain SL, Kier R, Vollmen RT, Bossen EH. Basaloid-squamous carcinoma of the tongue, hypopharynx, and larynx: Report of 10 cases. *Hum Pathol*. 1986; 17:1158.

229. Luna MA, El-Naggar A, Parichatikanond P, et al. Basaloid squamous carcinoma of the upper aerodigestive tract. *Cancer*. 1990; 66:537.

230. Banks ER, Frierson HF Jr, Mills SE, et al. Basaloid squamous cell carcinoma of the head and neck. *Am J Surg Pathol*. 1992; 16:939.

231. Klijanienko J, El-Naggar A, Ponzio-Prion A, et al. Basaloid squamous carcinoma of the head and neck: Immunohistochemical comparison with adenoid cystic carcinoma and squamous cell carcinoma. *Arch Otolaryngol Head Neck Surg*. 1993; 119:887.

232. Barnes L, MacMillan C, Ferlito A, et al. Basaloid squamous cell carcinoma of the head and neck: Clinicopathological features and differential diagnosis. *Ann Otol Rhinol Laryngol*. 1996; 105:75.

233. Gnepp DR, Ferlito A, Hyams V. Primary anaplastic small cell (oat cell) carcinoma of the larynx: Review of the literature and report of 18 cases. *Cancer*. 1983; 51:1731.

234. Raslan WF, Barnes L, Krause JR, et al. Basaloid squamous cell carcinoma of the head and neck: A clinicopathologic and flow cytometric sudy of 10 new cases with review of the English literature. *Am J Otolaryngol*. 1994; 15:204.

235. Coppola D, Catalano E, Tang C, et al. Basaloid squamous cell carcinoma of floor of mouth. *Cancer*. 1993; 72:2299.

236. Kramer IRH, Pindborg JJ, Shear M. *World Health Organization Histological Typing of Odontogenic Tumours*. 2nd ed. Berlin: Springer-Verlag; 1992.

237. Nair PNR, Pajarola G, Schrieder HE. Types and incidence of human periapical lesions obtained with extracted teeth. *Oral Surg Oral Med Oral Pathol Oral Radiol Endod*. 1996; 81:93.

238. Slabbert H, Shear M, Altini M. Vacuolated cells and mucous metaplasia in the epithelial linings of radicular and residual cysts. *J Oral Pathol Med*. 1995; 24:309.

239. Matthews JB. Hyaline bodies in the walls of odontogenic cysts. In: Brown RM, ed. *Investigative Pathology of the Odontogenic Cysts*. Boca Raton, FL: CRC Press; 1991:191.

240. Philippou S, Rühl GH, Mandelartz E. Scanning electron mi-

croscopic studies and x-ray microanalysis of hyaline bodies in odontogenic cysts. *J Oral Pathol Med.* 1990; 19:447.

241. Browne RM, Matthews JB. Intra-epithelial hyaline bodies in odontogenic cysts: An immunoperoxidase study. *J Oral Pathol.* 1985; 14:422.

242. Antoh M, Hasegawa H, Kawakami T, et al. Hyperkeratosis and atypical proliferation appearing in the lining epithelium of a radicular cyst. Report of a case. *J Craniomaxillofac Surg.* 1993; 21:210.

243. Unal T, Gunel O. Squamous odontogenic tumor-like islands in a radicular cyst. *J Oral Maxillofac Surg.* 1987; 45:346.

244. Mass E, Kaplan I, Hirshberg A. A clinical and histopathological study of radicular cysts associated with primary molars. *J Oral Pathol Med.* 1995; 24:458.

245. Wood RE, Nortjé CJ, Padayachee A, Grotepass F. Radicular cysts of primary teeth mimicking premolar dentigerous cysts: Report of three cases. *ASDC J Dent Child.* 1988; 55:288.

246. Savage NW, Adkins KF, Weir AV, Grundy GE. An histological study of cystic lesions following pulp therapy in deciduous molars. *J Oral Pathol Med.* 1986; 15:209.

247. Benn A, Altini M. Dentigerous cysts of inflammatory origin. A clinicopathologic study. *Oral Surg Oral Med Oral Pathol Oral Radiol Endod.* 1996; 81:203.

248. High AS, Hirschmann PN. Age changes in residual radicular cysts. *J Oral Pathol.* 1986; 15:524.

249. High AS, Hirschmann PN. Symptomatic residual radicular cysts. *J Oral Pathol Med.* 1988; 17:70.

250. Walton RE. The residual radicular cyst: Does it exist? [letter]. *Oral Surg Oral Med Oral Pathol Oral Radiol Endod.* 1996; 82: 471.

251. Vedtofte P, Praetorius F. The inflammatory paradental cyst. *Oral Surg Oral Med Oral Pathol.* 1989; 68:182.

252. Pompura JR, Sándor GKB, Stoneman DW. The buccal bifurcation cyst. A prospective study of treatment outcomes in 44 sites. *Oral Surg Oral Med Oral Pathol Oral Radiol Endod.* 1997; 83:215.

253. Packota GV, Hall JM, Lanigan DT, Cohen MA. Paradental cysts on mandibular first molars in children: Report of five cases. *Dentomaxillofac Radiol.* 1990; 19:126.

254. Wolf J, Hietanen J. The mandibular infected buccal cyst (paradental cyst). A radiographic and histologic study. *Br J Oral Maxillofac Surg.* 1990; 28:322.

255. Kim J, Ellis GL. Dental follicular tissue: Misinterpretation as odontogenic tumors. *J Oral Maxillofac Surg.* 1993; 51:762.

256. Daley TD, Wysocki GP. The small dentigerous cyst. A diagnostic dilemma. *Oral Surg Oral Med Oral Pathol Oral Radiol Endod.* 1995; 79:77.

257. Carr MM, Anderson RD, Clarke KD. Multiple dentigerous cysts in childhood. *J Otolaryngol.* 1996; 25:267.

258. Crowley TE, Kaugars GE, Gunsolley JC. Odontogenic keratocysts: A clinical and histologic comparison of the parakeratin and orthokeratin variants. *J Oral Maxillofac Surg.* 1992; 50:22.

259. Vuhahula E, Nikai H, Ijuhin N, et al. Jaw cysts with orthokeratinization: Analysis of 12 cases. *J Oral Pathol Med.* 1993; 22:35.

260. Li T-J, Kitano M, Chen X-M, et al. Orthokeratinized odontogenic cyst: A clinicopathological and immunohistochemical study of 15 cases. *Histopathol.* 1998; 32:242.

261. Forssell K, Forssell H, Kahnberg K-E. Recurrence of keratocysts. A long-term follow-up study. *Int J Oral Maxillofac Surg.* 1988; 17:25.

262. Gorlin RJ. Nevoid basal-cell carcinoma syndrome. *Medicine.* 1987; 66:98.

263. Rodu B, Tate AL, Martinez MG Jr. The implications of inflammation in odontogenic keratocysts. *J Oral Pathol Med.* 1987; 16:518.

264. Shanley S, Ratcliffe J, Hockey A, et al. Nevoid basal cell carcinoma syndrome: Review of 118 affected individuals. *Am J Med Genet.* 1994; 50:282.

265. Kimonis VE, Goldstein AM, Paskatia B, et al. Clinical manifestations in 105 persons with nevoid basal cell carcinoma syndrome. *Am J Med Genet.* 1997; 69:299.

266. Lench NJ, High AS, Markham AF, et al. Investigation of chromosome 9q22.3-31 DNA marker loss in odontogenic keratocysts. *Oral Oncol Eur J Cancer.* 1996; 32B:202.

267. Wicking C, Gillies S, Smyth I, et al. De novo mutations of the *Patched* gene in nevoid basal cell carcinoma syndrome help to define the clinical phenotype. *Am J Med Genet.* 1997; 73:304.

268. Woolgar JA, Rippin JW, Browne RM. A comparative histological study of odontogenic keratocysts in basal cell naevus syndrome and control patients. *J Oral Pathol.* 1987; 16:75.

269. Woolgar JA, Rippin JW, Browne RM. The odontogenic keratocyst and its occurrence in the nevoid basal cell carcinoma syndrome. *Oral Surg Oral Med Oral Pathol.* 1987; 64:727.

270. Rippin JW, Woolgar JA. The odontogenic keratocyst in BCNS and nonsyndrome patients. In: Browne RM, ed. *Investigative Pathology of the Odontogenic Cysts.* Boca Raton, FL: CRC Press; 1991:211.

271. El Murtadi A, Grehan D, Toner M, McCartan BE. Proliferating cell nuclear antigen staining in syndrome and nonsyndrome odontogenic keratocysts. *Oral Surg Oral Med Oral Pathol Oral Radiol Endod.* 1996; 81:217.

272. Hirshberg A, Kaplan I, Buchner A. Calcifying odontogenic cyst associated with odontoma: A possible separate entity (odontocalcifying odontogenic cyst). *J Oral Maxillofac Surg.* 1994; 52:555.

273. Sedano HO, Pindborg JJ. Ghost cell epithelium in odontomas. *J Oral Pathol.* 1975; 4:27.

274. Buchner A. The central (intraosseous) calcifying odontogenic cyst: An analysis of 215 cases. *J Oral Maxillofac Surg.* 1991; 49:330.

275. Buchner A, Merrell PW, Hansen LS, Leider AS. Peripheral (extraosseous) calcifying odontogenic cyst. *Oral Surg Oral Med Oral Pathol.* 1991; 72:65.

276. Hong SP, Ellis GL, Hartman KS. Calcifying odontogenic cyst. A review of 92 cases with reevaluation of their nature as cysts or neoplasms, the nature of ghost cells, and subclassification. *Oral Surg Oral Med Oral Pathol.* 1991; 72:56.

277. Takeda Y, Suzuki A, Yamamoto H. Histopathologic study of the epithelial components in the connective tissue wall of unilocular type of calcifying odontogenic cyst. *J Oral Pathol Med.* 1990; 19:108.

278. Carter LC, Carney YL, Perez-Pudlewski D. Lateral periodontal cyst. Multifactorial analysis of a previously unreported series. *Oral Surg Oral Med Oral Pathol Oral Radiol Endod.* 1996; 81:210.

279. Wysocki GP, Brannon RB, Gardner DG, Sapp P. Histogenesis of the lateral periodontal cyst and the gingival cyst of the adult. *Oral Surg.* 1980; 50:327.

280. Altini M, Shear M. Lateral periodontal cyst: An update. *J Oral Pathol Med.* 1992; 21:245.

281. Nxumalo TN, Shear M. Gingival cysts in adults. *J Oral Pathol Med.* 1992; 21:309.

282. Kaugars GE. Botryoid odontogenic cyst. *Oral Surg Oral Med Oral Pathol.* 1986; 62:555.

283. Greer RO, Johnson M. Botryoid odontogenic cyst: Clinicopathologic analysis of ten cases with three recurrences. *J Oral Maxillofac Surg.* 1988; 46:574.

284. Machado de Sousa SO, Campos AC, Santiago JL, et al. Botryoid odontogenic cyst: Report of a case with clinical and histogenetic considerations. *Br J Oral Maxillofac Surg.* 1990; 28:275.

285. Heikinheimo K, Happonen R-P, Forssell K, et al. A botryoid odontogenic cyst with multiple recurrences. *Int J Oral Maxillofac Surg.* 1989; 18:10.

286. Semba I, Kitano M, Mimura T, et al. Glandular odontogenic cyst: Analysis of cytokeratin expression and clinicopathological features. *J Oral Pathol Med.* 1994; 23:377.

287. Gardner DG, Kessler HP, Morency R, Schaffner DL. The glandular odontogenic cyst: An apparent entity. *J Oral Pathol.* 1988; 17:359.

288. van Heerden WFP, Raubenheimer EJ, Turner ML. Glandular odontogenic cyst. *Head Neck.* 1992; 14:316.

289. Hussain K, Edmondson HD, Browne RM. Glandular odontogenic cyst. Diagnosis and treatment. *Oral Surg Oral Med Oral Pathol Oral Radiol Endod.* 1995; 79:593.

290. High AS, Main DMG, Khoo SP, et al. The polymorphous odontogenic cyst. *J Oral Pathol Med.* 1996; 25:25.

291. Carette MJM, Ferguson MWJ. The fate of medial edge epithelial cells during palatal fusion in vitro: An analysis by Dil labelling and confocal microscopy. *Development.* 1992; 114: 379.

292. Wysocki GP, Goldblatt LI. The so-called "globulomaxillary cyst" is extinct. *Oral Surg Oral Med Oral Pathol.* 1993; 76:185.

293. Swanson KS, Kaugars GE, Gunsolley JC. Nasopalatine duct cyst: An analysis of 334 cases. *J Oral Maxillofac Surg.* 1991; 49:268.

294. Anneroth G, Hall G, Stuge U. Nasopalatine duct cyst. *Int J Oral Maxillofac Surg.* 1986; 15:572.

295. Bodin I, Isacsson G, Julin P. Cysts of the nasopalatine duct. *Int J Oral Maxillofac Surg.* 1986; 15:696.

296. Chapple IL, Ord RA. Patent nasopalatine ducts: Four case presentations and a review of the literature. *Oral Surg Oral Med Oral Pathol.* 1990; 69:554.

297. Curtin HD, Wolfe P, Gallia L, May M. Unusually large nasopalatine cyst: CT findings. *J Comput Assist Tomogr.* 1984; 8: 139.

298. Neville BW, Damm DD, Brock T. Odontogenic keratocyst of the midline maxillary region. *J Oral Maxillofac Surg.* 1997; 55: 340.

299. Curé JK, Osguthorpe JD, Van Tassel P. MR of nasolabial cysts. *AJNR.* 1996; 17:585.

300. Wesley RK, Scannell, Nathan LE. Nasolabial cyst: Presentation of a case with a review of the literature. *J Oral Maxillofac Surg.* 1984; 42:188.

301. Mindikoglu AN, Erginel A, Cenani A. An unknown syndrome of nose deformity, oxycephaly, aplasia of the nasolacrimal ducts, and symmetrical cyst formation on the upper lip in siblings: Craniorhiny. *Plast Reconstr Surg.* 1991; 88:699.

302. Kramer IRH, Pindborg JJ, Shear M. The WHO histological typing of odontogenic tumours. A commentary on the second edition. *Cancer.* 1992; 70:2988.

303. Buchner A, Sciubba JJ. Peripheral epithelial odontogenic tumors: A review. *Oral Surg Oral Med Oral Pathol.* 1987; 63:688.

304. Daley TD, Wysocki GP, Pringle GA. Relative incidence of odontogenic tumors and oral and jaw cysts in a Canadian population. *Oral Surg Oral Med Oral Pathol.* 1994; 77:276.

305. Vickers RA, Gorlin RJ. Ameloblastoma: Delineation of early histopathologic features of neoplasia. *Cancer.* 1970; 26:699.

306. Hartman KS. Granular-cell ameloblastoma. A survey of twenty cases from the Armed Forces Institute of Pathology. *Oral Surg.* 1974; 38:241.

307. Waldron CA, El-Mofty SK. A histologic study of 116 ameloblastomas with special reference to the desmoplastic variant. *Oral Surg Oral Med Oral Pathol.* 1987; 63:441.

308. Ng KH, Siar CH. Desmoplastic variant of ameloblastoma in Malaysians. *Br J Oral Maxillofac Surg.* 1993; 31:299.

309. Kaffe I, Buchner A, Taicher S. Radiographic features of desmoplastic variant of ameloblastoma. *Oral Surg Oral Med Oral Pathol.* 1993; 76:525.

310. Nastri AL, Wiesenfeld D, Radden BG et al. Maxillary ameloblastoma: A retrospective study of 13 cases. *Br J Oral Maxillofac Surg.* 1995; 33:28.

311. Thompson IOC, Phillips VM, Ferreira R, Housego TG. Odontoameloblastoma: A case report. *Br J Oral Maxillofac Surg.* 1990; 28:347.

312. Raubenheimer EJ, van Heerden WFP, Noffke CEE. Infrequent clinicopathological findings in 108 ameloblastomas. *J Oral Pathol Med.* 1995; 24:227.

313. Siar CH, Ng KH. 'Combined ameloblastoma and odontogenic keratocyst' or keratinizing ameloblastoma. *Br J Oral Maxillofac Surg.* 1993; 31:183.

314. Gardner DG. Some current concepts on the pathology of ameloblastomas. *Oral Surg Oral Med Oral Pathol Oral Radiol Endod.* 1996; 82:660.

315. Gardner DG, Corio RL. Plexiform unicystic ameloblastoma. A variant of ameloblastoma with a low-recurrence rate after nucleation. *Cancer.* 1984; 53:1730.

316. Gardner DG, Corio RL. The relationship of plexiform unicystic ameloblastoma to conventional ameloblastoma. *Oral Surg.* 1983; 56:54.

317. Robinson L, Martinez MG. Unicystic ameloblastoma. A prognostically distinct entity. *Cancer.* 1977; 40:2278.

318. Leider AS, Eversole LR, Barkin ME. Cystic ameloblastoma. A clinicopathologic analysis. *Oral Surg Oral Med Oral Pathol.* 1985; 60:624.

319. Punnia-Moorthy A. An unusual late recurrence of unicystic ameloblastoma. *Br J Oral Maxillofac Surg.* 1989; 27:254.

320. Thompson IOC, Ferreira R, van Wyk CW. Recurrent unicystic ameloblastoma of the maxilla. *Br J Oral Maxillofac Surg.* 1993; 31:180.

321. El-Mofty SK, Gerard NO, Farish SE, Rodu B. Peripheral ameloblastoma: A clinical and histologic study of 11 cases. *J Oral Maxillofac Surg.* 1991; 49:970.

322. Gurol M, Burkes EJ. Peripheral ameloblastoma. *J Periodontol.* 1995; 66:1065.

323. Zhu EX, Okada N, Takagi M. Peripheral ameloblastoma. *J Oral Maxillofac Surg.* 1995; 53:590.

324. Woo S-B, Smith-Williams JE, Sciubba JJ, Lipper S. Peripheral ameloblastoma of the buccal mucosa: Case report and review of the English literature. *Oral Surg Oral Med Oral Pathol.* 1987; 63:78.

325. Shibata T, Kaneko N, Hokazono K, et al. An ameloblastoma-like neoplasm of the buccal mucosa. Report of a case. *Int J Oral Maxillofac Surg.* 1990; 19:203.

326. Fulciniti F, Vetrani A, Zeppa P, et al. Calcifying epithelial odontogenic tumor (Pindborg's tumor) on fine-needle aspiration biopsy smears: a case report. *Diagn Cytopathol.* 1995; 12: 71.

327. El-Mofty S, Swanson P, Liapis H, McKeel D. Nature and origin of amyloid in calcifying epithelial odontogenic tumor (Pindborg tumor) [abstract]. *Oral Surg Oral Med Oral Pathol Oral Radiol Endod.* 1996; 82:208.

328. Pindborg JJ, Vedtofte P, Reibel J, Praetorius F. Calcifying epithelial odontogenic tumor. A review of recent literature and report of a case. *APMIS.* 1991; 23(suppl):152.

329. Takata T, Ogawa I, Miyauchi M, et al. Non-calcifying Pindborg tumor with Langerhans cells. *J Oral Pathol Med.* 1993; 22:378.

330. Hicks JH, Flaitz CM, Wong MEK, et al. Clear cell variant of calcifying epithelial odontogenic tumor: Case report and review of the literature. *Head Neck.* 1994; 16:272.

331. Philipsen HP, Reichart PA, Zhang KH, et al. Adenomatoid odontogenic tumor: Biologic profile based on 499 cases. *J Oral Pathol Med.* 1991; 20:149.

332. Philipsen HP, Samman N, Ormiston IW, et al. Variants of the adenomatoid odontogenic tumor with a note on tumor origin. *J Oral Pathol Med.* 1992; 21:348.

333. Toida M, Hyodo I, Okuda T, Tatematsu N. Adenomatoid odontogenic tumor: Report of two cases and survey of 126 cases in Japan. *J Oral Maxillofac Surg.* 1990; 48:404.

334. El-Labban NG. The nature of the eosinophilic and laminated masses in the adenomatoid odontogenic tumor: A histochemical and ultrastructural study. *J Oral Pathol Med.* 1992; 21:75.

335. Philipsen HP, Reichart PA. The adenomatoid odontogenic tumour: Ultrastructure of tumour cells and non-calcified amorphous masses. *J Oral Pathol Med.* 1996; 25:491.

336. Siar CH, Ng KH. The combined epithelial odontogenic tumour in Malaysians. *Br J Oral Maxillofac Surg.* 1991; 29:106.

337. Montes-Ledesma C, Mosqueda-Taylor A, Romero de León E, et al. Adenomatoid odontogenic tumor with features of calcifying epithelial odontogenic tumor (the so-called combined epithelial odontogenic tumour). Clinico-pathologic report of 12 cases. *Oral Oncol Eur J Cancer.* 1993; 29B:221.

338. Miyake M, Nagahata S, Nishihara J, Ohbayashi Y. Combined adenomatoid odontogenic tumor and calcifying epithelial odontogenic tumor: Report of case and ultrastructural study. *J Oral Maxillofac Surg.* 1996; 54:788.

339. Takeda Y. Duct-like structures in odontogenic epithelium of compound odontoma. *J Oral Pathol Med.* 1991; 20:184.

340. Baden E, Doyle J, Mesa M, et al. Squamous odontogenic

tumor. Report of three cases including the first extraosseous case. *Oral Surg Oral Med Oral Pathol.* 1993; 75:733.

341. Leider AS, Jonker LA, Cook HE. Multicentric familial squamous odontogenic tumor. *Oral Surg Oral Med Oral Pathol.* 1989; 68:175.

342. Wright JM. Squamous odontogenic tumorlike proliferations in odontogenic cysts. *Oral Surg.* 1979; 47:354.

343. Simon JHS, Jensen JL. Squamous odontogenic tumor-like proliferations in periapical cysts. *J Endodont.* 1985; 11:446.

344. Siar CH, Ng KH. Aggressive (malignant?) epithelial odontogenic ghost cell tumour of the maxilla. *J Laryngol Otol.* 1994; 108:269.

345. Badger KV, Gardner DG. The relationship of adamantinomatous craniopharyngioma to ghost cell ameloblastoma of the jaws: A histopathologic and immunohistochemical study. *J Oral Pathol Med.* 1997; 26:349.

346. Stone CH, Gaba AR, Benninger MS, Zarbo RJ. Odontogenic ghost cell tumor: A case report with cytologic findings. *Diagn Cytopathol.* 1998; 18:199.

347. Zámecník M, Michal M. Shadow cell differentiation in tumours of the colon and uterus. *Zentralbl Pathol.* 1994/95; 140: 421.

348. Raubenheimer EJ, van Heerden WFP, Sitzman F, Heymer B. Peripheral dentinogenic ghost cell tumor. *J Oral Pathol Med.* 1992; 21:93.

349. Eversole LR, Duffey DC, Nelson B, Powell NB. Clear cell odontogenic carcinoma. A clinicopathologic analysis. *Arch Otolaryngol Head Neck Surg.* 1995; 121:685.

350. Muramatsu T, Hashimoto S, Inoue T, et al. Clear cell odontogenic carcinoma of the mandible: Histochemical and immunohistochemical observations with a review of the literature. *J Oral Pathol Med.* 1996; 25:516.

351. Eversole LR. On the differential diagnosis of clear cell tumours of the head and neck. *Oral Oncol Eur J Cancer.* 1993; 29B:173.

352. Maiorano E, Altini M, Favia G. Clear cell tumors of the salivary glands, jaws, and oral mucosa. *Semin Diagn Pathol.* 1997; 14:203.

353. Piattelli A, Sesenna E, Trisi P. Clear cell odontogenic carcinoma. Report of a case with lymph node and pulmonary metastases. *Oral Oncol Eur J Cancer.* 1994; 30B:278.

354. Marí A, Escutia E, Carrera M, Pericot J. Clear cell ameloblastoma or odontogenic carcinoma. A case report. *J Craniomaxillofac Surg.* 1995; 23:387.

355. Sadeghi EM, Levin S. Clear cell odontogenic carcinoma of the mandible: Report of a case. *J Oral Maxillofac Surg.* 1995; 53:613.

356. Ferreira de Aguiar MC, Santiago Gomez R, Carvalho Silva E, et al. Clear-cell ameloblastoma (clear-cell odontogenic carcinoma). Report of a case. *Oral Surg Oral Med Oral Pathol Oral Radiol Endod.* 1996; 81:79.

357. Ingram EA, Evans ML, Zitsch RP. Fine-needle aspiration cytology of ameloblastic carcinoma of the maxilla: A rare tumor. *Diagn Cytopathol.* 1996; 14:249.

358. Corio RL, Goldblatt LI, Edwards PA, Hartman KS. Ameloblastic carcinoma: A clinicopathologic study and assessment of eight cases. *Oral Surg Oral Med Oral Pathol.* 1987; 64: 570.

359. Tanaka T, Ohkubo T, Fujitsuka H, et al. Malignant mixed tumor (malignant ameloblastoma and fibrosarcoma) of the maxilla. *Arch Pathol Lab Med.* 1991; 115:84.

360. Nagai N, Takeshita N, Nagatsuka H, et al. Ameloblastic carcinoma: Case report and review. *J Oral Pathol Med.* 1991; 20: 460.

361. Suei Y, Tanimoto K, Taguchi A, Wada T. Primary intraosseous carcinoma: Review of the literature and diagnostic criteria. *J Oral Maxillofac Surg.* 1994; 52:580.

362. Ariji E, Ozeki S, Yonetsu K, et al. Central squamous cell carcinoma of the mandible. Computed tomographic findings. *Oral Surg Oral Med Oral Pathol.* 1994; 77:541.

363. Anand VK, Arrowood JP, Krolls SO. Malignant potential of the odontogenic keratocyst. *Otolaryngol Head Neck Surg.* 1994; 111:124.

364. Yoshida H, Onizawa K, Yusa H. Squamous cell carcinoma arising in association with an odontogenic keratocyst. Report of a case. *J Oral Maxillofac Surg.* 1996; 54:647.

365. Houston G, Davenport W, Keaton W, Harris S. Malignant (metastatic) ameloblastoma: Report of a case. *J Oral Maxillofac Surg.* 1993; 51:1152.

366. Newman L, Howells GL, Coghlan KM, et al. Malignant ameloblastoma revisited. *Br J Oral Maxillofac Surg.* 1995; 33: 47.

367. Witterick IJ, Parikh S, Mancer K, Gullane PJ. Malignant ameloblastoma. *Am J Otolaryngol.* 1996; 17:122.

368. Handlers JP, Abrams AM, Melrose RJ, Danforth R. Central odontogenic fibroma: Clinicopathologic features of 19 cases and review of the literature. *J Oral Maxillofac Surg.* 1991; 49: 46.

369. Lukinmaa P-L, Hietanen J, Anttinen J, Ahonen P. Contiguous enlarged dental follicles with histologic features resembling the WHO type of odontogenic fibroma. *Oral Surg Oral Med Oral Pathol.* 1990; 70:313.

370. Dominguez FV, Pezza V, Keszler A. Fibro-odontogenic dysplasia: Report of two familial cases. *J Oral Maxillofac Surg.* 1995; 53:1115.

371. Weber A, van Heerden WFP, Ligthelm AJ, Raubenheimer EJ. Diffuse peripheral odontogenic fibroma: Report of 3 cases. *J Oral Pathol Med.* 1992; 21:82.

372. Fowler C, Tomich C, Brannon R, Houston G. Central odontogenic fibroma: Clinicopathologic features of 24 cases and review of the literature [abstract]. *Oral Surg Oral Med Oral Pathol Oral Radiol Endod.* 1993; 76:587.

373. Daley TD, Wysocki GP. Peripheral odontogenic fibroma. *Oral Surg Oral Med Oral Pathol.* 1994; 78:329.

374. Kaffe I, Buchner A. Radiologic features of central odontogenic fibroma. *Oral Surg Oral Med Oral Pathol.* 1994; 78:811.

375. Allen CM, Hammond HL, Stimson PG. Central odontogenic fibroma, WHO* type. A report of three cases with an unusual associated giant cell reaction. *Oral Surg Oral Med Oral Pathol.* 1992; 73:62.

376. Odell EW, Lombardi T, Barrett AW, et al. Hybrid central giant cell granuloma and central odontogenic fibroma-like lesions of the jaws. *Histopathol.* 1997; 30:165.

377. Gesek DJ, Adrian JC, Reid EN. Central granular cell odontogenic tumor: A case report including light microscopy, immunohistochemistry, and literature review. *J Oral Maxillofac Surg.* 1995; 53:945.

378. Yih W-Y, Thompson C, Meshul CK, Bartley MH. Central odontogenic granular cell tumor of the jaw: Report of case and immunohistochemical and electron microscopic study. *J Oral Maxillofac Surg.* 1995; 53:453.

379. Becker J, Schuppan D, Philipsen HP, Reichart PA. Ectomesenchyme of ameloblastic fibroma reveals a characteristic distribution of extracellular matrix proteins. *J Oral Pathol Med.* 1992; 21:156.

380. Dallera P, Bertoni F, Marchetti C, et al. Ameloblastic fibroma: A follow-up of six cases. *Int J Oral Maxillofac Surg.* 1996; 25:199.

381. Hansen LS, Ficarra G. Mixed odontogenic tumors: An analysis of 23 new cases. *Head Neck Surg.* 1988; 10:330.

382. Ulmansky M, Bodner L, Praetorius F, Lustmann J. Ameloblastic fibrodentinoma: Report on two new cases. *J Oral Maxillofac Surg.* 1994; 52:980.

383. Philipsen HP, Reichart PA, Praetorius F. Mixed odontogenic tumours and odontomas. Considerations on interrelationship. Review of the literature and presentation of 134 new cases of odontomas. *Oral Oncol.* 1997; 33:86.

384. Slootweg PJ. An analysis of the interrelationship of the mixed odontogenic tumors—ameloblastic fibroma, ameloblastic fibro-odontoma, and the odontomas. *Oral Surg.* 1981; 51:266.

385. Okura M, Nakahara H, Matsuya T. Treatment of ameloblastic fibro-odontoma without removal of the associated impacted permanent tooth: Report of cases. *J Oral Maxillofac Surg.* 1992; 50:1094.

386. Piette EMG, Tideman H, Wu PC. Massive maxillary amelo-

blastic fibro-odontoma. Case report with surgical management. *J Oral Maxillofac Surg.* 1990; 48:526.

387. Morning P. Impacted teeth in relation to odontomas. *Int J Oral Maxillofac Surg.* 1980; 9:81.

388. Kaugars GE, Miller ME, Abbey LM. Odontomas. *Oral Surg Oral Med Oral Pathol.* 1989; 67:172.

389. Blinder D, Peleg M, Taicher S. Surgical considerations in cases of large odontomas located in the mandibular angle. *Int J Oral Maxillofac Surg.* 1993; 22:163.

390. Gardner DG, Dort LC. Dysplastic enamel in odontomas. *Oral Surg.* 1979; 47:238.

391. López-Areal L, Silvestre Donat F, Gil Lozano J. Compound odontoma erupting in the mouth: 4-year follow-up of a clinical case. *J Oral Pathol Med.* 1992; 21:285.

392. Ida M, Nakamura T, Utsunomiya J. Osteomatous changes and tooth abnormalities found in the jaws of patients with adenomatosis coli. *Oral Surg.* 1981; 52:2.

393. Muller S, Parker DC, Kapadia SB, et al. Ameloblastic fibrosarcoma of the jaws. A clinicopathologic and DNA analysis of five cases and review of the literature with discussion of its relationship to ameloblastic fibroma. *Oral Surg Oral Med Oral Pathol Oral Radiol Endod.* 1995; 79:469.

394. Park HR, Shin KB, Sol MY, et al. A highly malignant ameloblastic fibrosarcoma. Report of a case. *Oral Surg Oral Med Oral Pathol Oral Radiol Endod.* 1995; 79:478.

395. Dallera P, Bertoni F, Marchetti C, et al. Ameloblastic fibrosarcoma of the jaws: Report of five cases. *J Craniomaxillofac Surg.* 1994; 22:349.

396. Peltola J, Magnusson B, Happonen R-P, Borrman H. Odontogenic myxoma—a radiographic study of 21 tumours. *Br J Oral Maxillofac Surg.* 1994; 32:298.

397. Kuc IM, Peters, Scott PG. Matrix characterization of odontogenic myxomas [abstract]. *J Oral Pathol Med.* 1996; 25:284.

398. Muzio LL, Nocini P, Favia G, et al. Odontogenic myxoma of the jaws. A clinical, radiologic, immunohistochemical, and ultrastructural study. *Oral Surg Oral Med Oral Pathol Oral Radiol Endod.* 1996; 82:426.

399. Lombardi T, Lock C, Samson J, Odell EW. S100, smooth muscle actin and cytokeratin 19 immunohistochemistry in odontogenic and soft tissue myxomas. *J Clin Pathol.* 1995; 48:759.

400. Mentzel T, Calonje E, Wadden C, et al. Myxofibrosarcoma. clinicopathologic analysis of 75 cases with emphasis on the low-grade variant. *Am J Surg Pathol.* 1996; 20:391.

401. Ang HK, Ramani P, Michaels L. Myxoma of the maxillary antrum in children. *Histopathol.* 1993; 23:361.

402. Heffner DK. Sinonasal myxomas and fibromyxomas in children. *Ear Nose Throat J.* 1993; 72:365.

403. Slootweg PJ. Cementoblastoma and osteoblastoma: A comparison of histologic features. *J Oral Pathol Med.* 1992; 21:385.

404. Ulmansky M, Hjørting-Hansen E, Praetorius F, Haque MF. Benign cementoblastoma. A review and five new cases. *Oral Surg Oral Med Oral Pathol.* 1994; 77:48.

405. MacDonald-Jankowski DS, Wu PC. Cementoblastoma in Hong Kong Chinese. A report of four cases. *Oral Surg Oral Med Oral Pathol.* 1992; 73:760.

406. Jelic JS, Loftus MJ, Miller AS, Cleveland DB. Benign osteoblastoma: Report of an unusual case and analysis of 14 additional cases. *J Oral Maxillofac Surg.* 1993; 51:1033.

407. Bertoni F, Bacchini P, Donati D, et al. Osteoblastoma-like osteosarcoma. The Rizzoli Institute experience. *Modern Pathol.* 1993; 6:707.

408. Fowler C, Brannon R, Carpenter W, Corio R. Cementoblastoma revisited: A clinicopathologic study of 44 cases and a review of the literature [abstract]. *Oral Surg Oral Med Oral Pathol.* 1994; 78:775.

409. Mirich DR, Blaser SI, Harwood-Nash DC, et al. Melanotic neuroectodermal tumor of infancy: Clinical, radiologic, and pathologic findings in five cases. *AJNR.* 1991; 12:689.

410. Pettinato G, Manivel JC, d'Amore ESG, et al. Melanotic neuroectodermal tumor of infancy. A reexamination of a histogenetic problem based on immunohistochemical, flow cyto-

411. Kapadia SB, Frisman DM, Hitchcock CL, et al. Melanotic neuroectodermal tumor of infancy. Clinicopathological, immunohistochemical, and flow cytometric study. *Am J Surg Pathol.* 1993; 17:566.

metric, and ultrastructural study of 10 cases. *Am J Surg Pathol.* 1991; 15:233.

412. Machado de Sousa SA, Soares de Araujo N, Sesso A, Cavalcanti de Araujo V. Immunohistochemical, ultrastructural, and histogenetic considerations in a patient with melanotic neuroectodermal tumor of infancy. *J Oral Maxillofac Surg.* 1992; 50:186.

413. Steinberg B, Shuler C, Wilson S. Melanotic neuroectodermal tumor of infancy: Evidence for multicentricity. *Oral Surg Oral Med Oral Pathol.* 1988; 66:666.

414. Su L, Weathers DR, Waldron CA. Distinguishing features of focal cemento-osseous dysplasia and cemento-ossifying fibromas. II. A clinical and radiological spectrum of 316 cases. *Oral Surg Oral Med Oral Pathol Oral Radiol Endod.* 1997; 84:540.

415. Su L, Weathers DR, Waldron CA. Distinguishing features of focal cemento-osseous dysplasia and cemento-ossifying fibromas I. A histopathologic spectrum of 316 cases. *Oral Surg Oral Med Oral Pathol Oral Radiol Endod.* 1997; 84:301.

416. Slootweg PJ. Maxillofacial fibro-osseous lesions: Classification and differential diagnosis. *Semin Diagn Pathol.* 1996; 13:104.

417. Higuchi Y, Nakamura N, Toshiro H. Clinicopathologic study of cemento-osseous dysplasia producing cysts of the mandible. Report of four cases. *Oral Surg Oral Med Oral Pathol.* 1988; 65:339.

418. Horner K, Forman GH. Atypical simple bone cysts of the jaws. II: A possible association with benign fibro-osseous (cemental) lesions of the jaws. *Clin Radiol.* 1988; 39:59.

419. Melrose RJ, Abrams AM, Mills BG. Florid osseous dysplasia. A clinical-pathologic study of thirty-four cases. *Oral Surg.* 1976; 41:62.

420. Carrillo R, Morales A, Rodriguez-Peralto JL, et al. Benign fibro-osseous lesions in Paget's disease of the jaws. *Oral Surg Oral Med Oral Pathol.* 1991; 71:588.

421. Waldron CA. Fibro-osseous lesions of the jaws. *J Oral Maxillofac Surg.* 1993; 51:828.

422. Summerlin D-J, Tomich CE. Focal cemento-osseous dysplasia: A clinicopathologic study of 221 cases. *Oral Surg Oral Med Oral Pathol.* 1994; 78:611.

423. Melrose RJ. The clinico-pathologic spectrum of cemento-osseous dysplasia. *Oral Maxillofac Surg Clin N Am.* 1997; 9:643.

424. Neville BW, Albenesius RJ. The prevalence of benign fibro-osseous lesions of periodontal ligament origin in black women: A radiographic survey. *Oral Surg Oral Med Oral Pathol.* 1986; 62:340.

425. Terry BC. Aggressive juvenile ossifying fibroma. *Oral Maxillofac Surg Clin N Am.* 1997; 9:751.

426. Störkel S, Wagner W, Makek MS. Psammous desmo-osteoblastoma, ultrastructural and immunohistochemical evidence for an osteogenic histogenesis. *Virch Arch [A].* 1987; 411:561.

427. Bertrand B, Eloy PH, Cornelis JPH, et al. Juvenile aggressive cemento-ossifying fibroma: Case report and review of the literature. *Laryngoscope.* 1993; 103:1385.

428. Wenig BM, Vinh T, Smirniotopoulos JG, et al. Aggressive psammomatoid ossifying fibromas of the sinonasal region. *Cancer.* 1995; 76:1155.

429. Slootweg PJ, Panders AK, Nikkels PGJ. Psammomatoid ossifying fibroma of the paranasal sinuses. An extragnathic variant of cemento-ossifying fibroma. *J Craniomaxillofac Surg.* 1993; 21:294.

430. Sissons HA, Steiner GC, Dorfman HD. Calcified spherules in fibro-osseous lesions of bone. *Arch Pathol Lab Med.* 1993; 117:284.

431. Amling M, Werner, Pösl M, et al. Calcifying solitary bone cyst: Morphological aspects and differential diagnosis of sclerotic bone tumours. *Virch Arch.* 1995; 426:235.

432. Slootweg PJ, Müller H. Juvenile ossifying fibroma. Report of four cases. *J Craniomaxillofac Surg.* 1990; 18:125.

433. Slootweg PJ, Panders AK, Koopmans R, Nikkels PGJ. Juve-

nile ossifying fibroma. An analysis of 33 cases with emphasis on histopathological aspects. *J Oral Pathol Med*. 1994; 23:385.

434. Bertoni F, Bacchini P, Fabbri N, et al. Osteosarcoma. Low-grade intraosseous-type osteosarcoma, histologically resembling parosteal osteosarcoma, fibrous dysplasia, and desmoplastic fibroma. *Cancer*. 1993; 71:338.

435. Slootweg PJ, Müller H. Differential diagnosis of fibro-osseous jaw lesions. A histological investigation on 30 cases. *J Craniomaxillofac Surg*. 1990; 18:210.

436. Povýsil C, Matejovský Z. Fibro-osseous lesion with calcified spherules (cementifying fibromalike lesion) of the tibia. *Ultrastruct Pathol*. 1993; 17:25.

437. Craig RC. Cementum versus bone. An experimental perspective. *Oral Maxillofac Surg Clin N Am*. 1997; 9:581.

438. van Heerden WFP, Raubenheimer EJ, Weir RG, Kreidler J. Giant ossifying fibroma: A clinicopathologic study of 8 tumors. *J Oral Pathol Med*. 1989; 18:506.

439. Eversole LR. Craniofacial fibrous dysplasia and ossifying fibroma. *Oral Maxillofac Surg Clin N Am*. 1997; 9:625.

440. Khanna JN, Andrade NN. Giant ossifying fibroma. Case report on a bimaxillary presentation. *Int J Oral Maxillofac Surg*. 1992; 21:233.

441. Petrikowski CG, Pharoah MJ, Lee L, Grace MGA. Radiographic differentiation of osteosarcoma, osteomyelitis, and fibrous dysplasia of the jaws. *Oral Surg Oral Med Oral Pathol Oral Radiol Endod*. 1995; 80:744.

442. Kurt A-M, Unni K, McLeod RA, Pritchard DJ. Low-grade intraosseous osteosarcoma. *Cancer*. 1990; 65:1418.

443. Ruggieri P, Sim FH, Bond JR, Unni KK. Malignancies in fibrous dysplasia. *Cancer*. 1994; 73:1411.

444. Ebata K, Usami T, Tohnai I, Kaneda T. Chondrosarcoma and osteosarcoma arising in polyostotic fibrous dysplasia. *J Oral Maxillofac Surg*. 1992; 50:761.

445. Triantafillidou K, Antoniades K, Karakasis D, et al. McCune-Albright syndrome. Report of a case. *Oral Surg Oral Med Oral Pathol*. 1993; 75:571.

446. Antoniades K, Karakasis D, Kapetanos G, et al. Chronic idiopathic hyperphosphatasemia. Case report. *Oral Surg Oral Med Oral Pathol*. 1993; 76:200.

447. Mirra JM, Gold RH, Rand F. Disseminated nonossifying fibromas in association with café-au-lait spots (Jaffe-Campanacci syndrome). *Clin Orthop*. 1982; 168:192.

448. Steinmetz JC, Pilon VA, Lee JK. Jaffe-Campanacci syndrome. Case report. *J Pediatr Orthop*. 1988; 8:602.

449. Slootweg PJ. Comparison of giant cell granuloma of the jaw and non-ossifying fibroma. *J Oral Pathol Med*. 1989; 18:128.

450. Rieger E, Kofler R, Borkenstein M, et al. Melanotic macules following Blashko's lines in McCune-Albright syndrome. *Br J Dermatol*. 1994; 130:215.

451. Jacobsson S, Hallén O, Hollender L, et al. Fibro-osseous lesion of the mandible mimicking chronic osteomyelitis. *Oral Surg*. 1975; 40:433.

452. Jacobsson S. Diffuse sclerosing osteomyelitis of the mandible. *Int J Oral Maxillofac Surg*. 1984; 13:363.

453. Suei Y, Taguchi A, Tanimoto K. Radiographic evaluation of possible etiology of diffuse sclerosing osteomyelitis of the mandible. *Oral Surg Oral Med Oral Pathol Oral Radiol Endod*. 1997; 84:571.

454. Reith JD, Bauer TW, Schils JP. Osseous manifestations of SAPHO (Synovitis, Acne, Pustulosis, Hyperostosis, Osteitis) syndrome. *Am J Surg Pathol*. 1996; 20:1368.

455. Kahn MF, Hayem F, Hayem G, Grossin M. Is diffuse sclerosing osteomyelitis of the mandible part of the synovitis, acne, pustulosis, hyperostosis, osteitis (SAPHO) syndrome? Analysis of seven cases. *Oral Surg Oral Med Oral Pathol*. 1994; 78: 594.

456. Suei Y, Tanimoto K, Taguchi A, et al. Possible identity of diffuse sclerosing osteomyelitis and recurrent multifocal osteomyelitis. One entity or two. *Oral Surg Oral Med Oral Pathol Oral Radiol Endod*. 1995; 80:401.

457. Suei Y, Taguchi A, Tanimoto K. Diffuse sclerosing osteomyelitis of the mandible: Its characteristics and possible relationship to synovitis, acne, pustulosis, hyperostosis, osteitis (SAPHO) syndrome. *J Oral Maxillofac Surg*. 1996; 54:1194.

458. Kaffe I, Ardekian L, Taicher S, et al. Radiographic features of central giant cell granuloma of the jaws. *Oral Surg Oral Med Oral Pathol Oral Radiol Endod*. 1996; 81:720.

459. Whitaker SB, Waldron CA. Central giant cell granuloma of the jaws. A clinical, radiologic, and histopathologic study. *Oral Surg Oral Med Oral Pathol*. 1993; 75:199.

460. Tallan EM, Olsen KD, McCaffrey TV, et al. Advanced giant cell granuloma: A twenty-year study. *Otolaryngol Head Neck Surg*. 1994; 110:413.

461. Kershisnik M, Batsakis JG. Pathology consultation: Aneurysmal bone cysts of the jaws. *Ann Otol Rhinol Laryngol*. 1994; 103:164.

462. Matt BH. Aneurysmal bone cyst of the maxilla: Case report and review of the literature. *Int J Pediatr Otorhinolaryngol*. 1993; 25:217.

463. Trent C, Byl FM. Aneurysmal bone cysts of the mandible. *Ann Otol Rhinol Laryngol*. 1993; 102:917.

464. Alles JU, Schulz A. Immunohistochemical markers (endothelial and histiocytic) and ultrastructure of primary aneurysmal bone cysts. *Hum Pathol*. 1986; 17:39.

465. Davis JP, Archer DJ, Fisher C, et al. Multiple recurrent giant cell lesions associated with high circulating levels of parathyroid hormone-related peptide in a young adult. *Br J Oral Maxillofac Surg*. 1991; 29:102.

466. Knezevic G, Uglesic V, Kobler P, et al. Primary hyperparathyroidism: Evaluation of different treatments of jaw lesions based on case reports. *Br J Oral Maxillofac Surg*. 1991; 29:185.

467. van Damme PA, Mooren RECM. Differentiation of multiple giant cell lesions, Noonan-like syndrome, and (occult) hyperparathyroidism. Case report and review of the literature. *Int J Oral Maxillofac Surg*. 1994; 23:32.

468. Betts NJ, Stewart JCB, Fonseca RJ, Scott RF. Multiple central giant cell lesions with a Noonan-like phenotype. *Oral Surg Oral Med Oral Pathol*. 1993; 76:601.

469. Cohen MM, Gorlin RJ. Noonan-like/multiple giant cell lesion syndrome. *Am J Med Genet*. 1991; 40:159.

470. Auclair PL, Cuenin P, Kratochvil FJ, et al. A clinical and histomorphologic comparison of the central giant cell granuloma and the giant cell tumor. *Oral Surg Oral Med Oral Pathol*. 1988; 66:197.

471. Mintz GA, Abrams AM, Carlsen GD, et al. Primary malignant giant cell tumor of the mandible. Report of a case and review of the literature. *Oral Surg*. 1981; 51:164.

472. Hoffman CD, Huntley TA, Wiesenfeld D, et al. Maxillary giant cell tumour associated with Paget's disease of bone. *Int J Oral Maxillofac Surg*. 1994; 23:161.

473. Penfold CN, McCullagh P, Eveson JW, Ramsay A. Giant cell lesions complicating fibroosseous conditions of the jaws. *Int J Oral Maxillofac Surg*. 1993; 22:158.

474. Bertoni F, Unni KK, Beabout JW, et al. Chondroblastoma of the skull and facial bones. *Am J Clin Pathol*. 1987; 88:1.

475. Varvares MA, Cheney ML, Goodman ML. Chondroblastoma of the temporal bone. Case report and literature review. *Ann Otol Rhinol Laryngol*. 1992; 101:763.

476. Ayoub AF, El-Mofty SS. Cherubism: Report of an aggressive case and review of the literature. *J Oral Maxillofac Surg*. 1993; 51:702.

477. Chomette G, Auriol M, Guilbert F, Vaillant JM. Cherubism. Histo-enzymological and ultrastructural study. *Int J Oral Maxillofac Surg*. 1988; 17:219.

478. Hamner JE. The demonstration of perivascular collagen deposition in cherubism. *Oral Surg*. 1969; 27:129.

479. Kaugars GE, Niamtu J, Svirsky JA. Cherubism: Diagnosis, treatment, and comparison with central giant cell granulomas and giant cell tumors. *Oral Surg Oral Med Oral Pathol*. 1992; 73:369.

480. Katz JO, Dunlap CL, Ennis RL. Cherubism: Report of a case showing regression without treatment. *J Oral Maxillofac Surg*. 1992; 50:301.

481. Timosca GC. Le chérubisme: Régression des lésions et régénération osseuse spontanée. *Rev Stomatol Chir Maxillofac*. 1996; 97:172.

482. Dunlap C, Neville B, Vickers RA, et al. The Noonan syn-

drome/cherubism association. *Oral Surg Oral Med Oral Pathol.* 1989; 67:698.

483. Fechner RE, Fitz-Hugh GS, Pope TL Jr. Extraordinary growth of giant cell reparative granuloma during pregnancy. *Arch Otolaryngol.* 1984; 110:116.

484. Whitaker SB, Bouquot JE. Estrogen and progesterone receptor status of central giant cell lesions of the jaws. *Oral Surg Oral Med Oral Pathol.* 1994; 77:641.

485. Foss RD, Ellis GL. Myofibromas and myofibromatosis: A clinicopathologic analysis of 79 cases. *Oral Surg Oral Med Oral Pathol Oral Radiol Endod.* 2000; 89:57.

486. Lingen MW, Mostofi R, Solt DB. Myofibromas of the oral cavity. *Oral Surg Oral Med Oral Pathol Oral Radiol Endod.* 1995; 80:297.

487. Jones AC, Freedman PD, Kerpel SM. Oral myofibromas: A report of 13 cases and review of the literature. *J Oral Maxillofac Surg.* 1994; 52:870.

488. Mentzel T, Fletcher CDM. The emerging role of myofibroblasts in soft tissue neoplasia [editorial]. *Am J Clin Pathol.* 1997; 107:2.

489. Shlomi B, Mintz S, Jossiphov J, Horovitz I. Immunohistochemical analysis of a case of intraoral nodular fasciitis. *J Oral Maxillofac Surg.* 1994; 52:323.

490. Batsakis JG, El-Naggar AK. Pathology consultation: Pseudosarcomatous proliferative lesions of soft tissues. *Ann Otol Rhinol Laryngol.* 1994; 103:578.

491. Coffin CM, Jaszcz W, O'Shea PA, Dehner LP. So-called congenital-infantile fibrosarcoma: Does it exist and what is it? *Pediatr Pathol.* 1994; 14:133.

492. Coffin CM, Dehner LP. Fibroblastic-myofibroblastic tumors in children and adolescents: A clinicopathologic study of 108 examples in 103 patients. *Pediatr Pathol.* 1991; 11:569.

493. Mentzel T, Calonje E, Nascimento AG, Fletcher CDM. Infantile hemangiopericytoma versus infantile myofibromatosis. Study of a series suggesting a continuous spectrum of infantile myofibroblastic lesions. *Am J Surg Pathol.* 1994; 18:922.

494. Chan JKC. Inflammatory pseudotumor: A family of lesions of diverse nature and etiologies. *Adv Anat Pathol.* 1996; 3:156.

495. Shek AWH, Wu PC, Samman N. Inflammatory pseudotumor of the mouth and maxilla. *J Clin Pathol.* 1996; 49:164.

496. Frankenthaler R, Batsakis JG, Suarez PA. Tumefactive fibroinflammatory lesions of the head and neck. *Ann Otol Rhinol Laryngol.* 1993; 102:481.

497. Chan JKC. Inflammatory pseudotumor: A family of lesions of diverse nature and etiologies. *Adv Anat Pathol.* 1996; 3:156.

498. Cooper PH. Fibrous proliferations of infancy and childhood. *J Cutan Pathol.* 1992; 19:257.

499. Coffin CM, Neilson KA, Ingels S, et al. Congenital generalized myofibromatosis: A disseminated angiocentric myofibromatosis. *Pediatr Pathol.* 1995; 15:571.

500. Smith DM, Mahmoud HH, Jenkins JJ, et al. Myofibrosarcoma of the head and neck in children. *Pediatr Pathol Lab Med.* 1995; 15:403.

501. Fowler CB, Hartman KS, Brannon RB. Fibromatosis of the oral and paraoral region. *Oral Surg Oral Med Oral Pathol.* 1994; 77:373.

502. Batsakis JG, Raslan W. Pathology consultation: Extra-abdominal desmoid fibromatosis. *Ann Otol Rhinol Laryngol.* 1994; 103:331.

503. Ayala AG, Ro JY, Goepfert H, et al. Desmoid fibromatosis: A clinicopathologic study of 25 children. *Semin Diagn Pathol.* 1986; 3:138.

504. Bang G, Baardsen R, Gilhuus-Moe O. Infantile fibrosarcoma in the mandible: Case report. *J Oral Pathol Med.* 1989; 18:339.

505. de Silva DC, Wright MF, Stevenson DAJ, et al. Cranial desmoid tumor associated with homozygous inactivation of the adenomatous polyposis coli gene in a 2-year old girl with familial adenomatous polyposis. *Cancer.* 1996; 77:972.

506. Clark SK, Pack K, Pritchard J, Hodgson SV. Familial adenomatous polyposis presenting with childhood desmoids. *Lancet.* 1997; 349:471.

507. Vally I, Altini M. Fibromatoses of the oral and paraoral soft tissues and jaws. Review of the literature and report of 12 new cases. *Oral Surg Oral Med Oral Pathol.* 1990; 69:191.

508. Hopkins KM, Huttula CS, Kahn MA, Albright JE. Desmoplastic fibroma of the mandible: Review and report of two cases. *J Oral Maxillofac Surg.* 1996; 54:1249.

509. Hashimoto K, Mase N, Iwai K, et al. Desmoplastic fibroma of the maxillary sinus. Report of a case and review of the literature. *Oral Surg Oral Med Oral Pathol.* 1991; 72:126.

510. Inwards CY, Unni K, Beabout JW, Sim FH. Desmoplastic fibroma of bone. *Cancer.* 1991; 68:1978.

511. Damm DD, Tomich CE, White DK, et al. Intraosseous fibrous lesions of the jaws. A manifestation of tuberous sclerosis. *Oral Surg Oral Med Oral Pathol Oral Radiol Endod.* 1999; 87:334.

512. Kaplan I, Calderon S, Buchner A. Peripheral osteoma of the mandible: A study of 10 new cases and analysis of the literature. *J Oral Maxillofac Surg.* 1994; 52:467.

513. Ruffin SA, Waldrop TC, Aufdemorte TB. Diagnosis and treatment of subpontic osseous hyperplasia. Report of a case. *Oral Surg Oral Med Oral Pathol.* 1993; 76:68.

514. Morton TH, Natkin E. Hyperostosis and fixed partial denture pontics: Report of 16 patients and review of literature. *J Prosthet Dent.* 1990; 64:539.

515. Otero-Cagide FJ, Singer DL, Hoover JN. Exostosis associated with autogenous gingival grafts: A report of 9 cases. *J Periodontol.* 1996; 67:611.

516. Kurita K, Kawai T, Ikeda N, Kameyama Y. Cancellous osteoma of the mandibular coronoid process: Report of a case. *J Oral Maxillofac Surg.* 1991; 49:753.

517. Narisawa Y, Kohda H. Cutaneous cysts of Gardner's syndrome are similar to follicular stem cells. *J Cutan Pathol.* 1995; 22:115.

518. Søndergaard JO, Bülow S, Jävinen, et al. Dental anomalies in familial adenomatous polyposis coli. *Acta Odontol Scand.* 1987; 45:61.

519. Takeuchi T, Takenoshita Y, Kubo M, Iida M. Natural course of jaw lesions in patients with familial adenomatosis coli (Gardner's syndrome). *Int J Oral Maxillofac Surg.* 1993; 22:226.

520. Thakker N, Davies R, Horner K, et al. The dental phenotype in familial adenomatous polyposis: Diagnostic application of a weighted scoring system for changes on dental panoramic radiographs. *J Med Genet.* 1995; 32:458.

521. Thakker NS, Evans DGR, Horner K, et al. Florid oral manifestations in an atypical adenomatous polyposis family with late presentation of colorectal polyps. *J Oral Pathol Med.* 1996; 25:459.

522. Cleveland DB, Goldberg KM, Greenspan JS, et al. Langerhans' cell histiocytosis. Report of three cases with unusual oral soft tissue involvement. *Oral Surg Oral Med Oral Pathol Oral Radiol Endod.* 1996; 82:541.

523. Kilpatrick SE, Wenger DE, Gilchrist GS, et al. Langerhans' cell histiocytosis (histiocytosis X) of bone. *Cancer.* 1995; 76:2471.

524. Willman CL, Busque L, Griffith BB, et al. Langerhans' cell histiocytosis (histiocytosis X)—A clonal proliferative disease. *N Engl J Med.* 1994; 331:154.

525. Favara B, Jaffe R. The histopathology of Langerhans' cell histiocytosis. *Br J Cancer.* 1994; 70 (suppl XXIII):S17.

526. Emile J-F, Wechsler J, Brousse N, et al. Langerhans' cell histiocytosis. Definitive diagnosis with the use of monoclonal antibody 010 on routinely paraffin-embedded samples. *Am J Surg Pathol.* 1995; 19:636.

527. Lieberman PH, Jones CR, Steinman RM, et al. Langerhans' cell (eosinophilic) granulomatosis. A clinicopathologic study encompassing 50 years. *Am J Surg Pathol.* 1996; 20:519.

528. Hage C, Willman CL, Favara B, Isaacson PG. Langerhans' cell histiocytosis (histiocytosis X): Immunophenotype and growth fraction. *Hum Pathol.* 1993; 24:840.

529. Risdall PJ, Dehner LP, Duray P, et al. Histiocytosis X (Langerhans' cell histiocytosis). Prognostic role of histology. *Arch Pathol Lab Med.* 1983; 107:59.

530. Ben-Ezra J, Bailey A, Azumi N, et al. Malignant histiocytosis X. A distinct clinicopathologic entity. *Cancer.* 1991; 68:1050.

531. Asada Y, Suzuki I, Suzuki M, Fukushinma M. Atypical mul-

tiple benign osteoblastomas accompanied by simple bone cysts. A case report. *J Craniomaxillofac Surg.* 1991; 19:166.

532. Hara H, Ohishi M, Higuchi Y. Fibrous dysplasia of the mandible associated with large solitary bone cyst. *J Oral Maxillofac Surg.* 1990; 48:88.

533. Jones AC, Baughman RA. Multiple idiopathic bone cysts in a patient with osteogenesis inperfecta. *Oral Surg Oral Med Oral Pathol.* 1993; 75:333.

534. Forssell K, Forssell H, Happonen R-P, Neva M. Simple bone cyst. Review of the literature and analysis of 23 cases. *Int J Oral Maxillofac Surg.* 1988; 17:21.

535. Kaugars GE. Traumatic bone cyst. *Oral Surg Oral Med Oral Pathol.* 1987; 63:318.

536. Saito Y, Hoshina Y, Nagamine T, et al. Simple bone cyst. A clinical and histopathologic study of fifteen cases. *Oral Surg Oral Med Oral Pathol.* 1992; 74:487.

537. Hirshberg A, Leibovich P, Buchner A. Metastatic tumors to the jawbones: Analysis of 390 cases. *J Oral Pathol Med.* 1994; 23:337.

538. Hirshberg A, Leibovich P, Buchner A. Metastases to the oral mucosa: Analysis of 157 cases. *J Oral Pathol Med.* 1993; 22: 385.

539. Hirshberg A, Leibovich P, Buchner A. Metastatic tumors to postextraction sites. *J Oral Maxillofac Surg.* 1993; 51:1334.

540. Whitaker B, Robinson K, Hewan-Lowe K, Budnick S. Thyroid metastasis to the oral soft tissues. Case report of a diagnostic dilemma. *J Oral Maxillofac Surg.* 1993; 51:588.

541. Alanen KA, Kuopio T, Koskinen PJ, Nevalainen TJ. Immunohistochemical labelling for prostate specific antigen in non-prostatic tissues. *Pathol Res Pract.* 1996; 192:233.

542. James GK, Pudek M, Berean KW, et al. Salivary duct carcinoma secreting prostate specific antigen. *Am J Clin Pathol.* 1996; 106:242.

543. Zarghami N, Levesque M, D'Costa M, et al. Frequency of expression of prostate-specific antigen mRNA in lung tumors. *Am J Clin Pathol.* 1997; 108:184.

544. Chaubert P, Hurlimann J. Mammary origin of metastases. Immunohistochemical determination. *Arch Pathol Lab Med.* 1992; 116:1181.

545. Kaufmann O, Deidesheimer T, Muehlenberg M, et al. Immunohistochemical differentiation of metastatic breast carcinomas from metastatic adenocarcinomas of other common primary sites. *Histopathol.* 1996; 29:233.

546. Tschen JA, Fechner RE. The juxtaoral organ of Chievitz. *Am J Surg Pathol.* 1979; 3:147.

547. Carbone A, Vaccher E, Barzan L, et al. Head and neck lymphomas associated with human immunodeficiency virus infection. *Arch Otolaryngol Head Neck Surg.* 1995; 121:210.

548. Hicks MJ, Flaitz CM, Nichols CM, et al. Intraoral presentation of anaplastic large cell Ki-1 lymphoma in association with HIV infection. *Oral Surg Oral Med Oral Pathol.* 1993; 76: 73.

549. Groot RH, van Merkesteyn JPR, Bras J. Oral manifestations of non-Hodgkin's lymphoma in HIV-infected patients. *Int J Oral Maxillofac Surg.* 1990; 19:194.

550. Carbone A, Gaidano G, Gloghini A, et al. Morphologic patterns and molecular pathways of AIDS-related head and neck and other systemic lymphomas. *Ann Otol Rhinol Laryngol.* 1996; 105:495.

551. Delecluse HJ, Anagnostopoulos I, Dallenbach F, et al. Plasmablastic lymphomas of the oral cavity: A new entity associated with the human immunodeficiency virus infection. *Blood.* 1997; 89:1413.

552. Piluso S, Di Lollo S, Baroni G, et al. Unusual clinical aspects of oral non-Hodgkin's lymphomas in patients with HIV infection. *Oral Oncol Eur J Cancer.* 1994; 30B:61.

553. Dodd CL, Greenspan D, Heinic GS, et al. Multi-focal oral non-Hodgkin's lymphoma in an AIDS patient. *Br Dent J.* 1993; 175:373.

554. Pileri SA, Montanari M, Falini B, et al. Malignant lymphoma involving the mandible. Clinical, morphologic, and immunohistochemical study of 17 cases. *Am J Surg Pathol.* 1990; 14: 652.

555. Kluin PM, Slootweg PJ, Schuurman HJ, et al. Primary B-cell malignant lymphoma of the maxilla with sarcomatous pattern and multilobated nuclei. *Cancer.* 1984; 54:1598.

556. Pettit CK, Zukerberg LR, Gray MH, et al. Primary lymphoma of bone. A B-cell neoplasm with a high frequency of multilobated cells. *Am J Surg Pathol.* 1990; 14:329.

557. Schaberg SJ, Daliels CA, Loomer L, Addante RR. Clinicopathologic conference. Bilateral hard palate masses. *J Oral Maxillofac Surg.* 1993; 51:1262.

558. Nadimi H. Subclasses of extranodal oral B-cell lymphomas express cIgM, plasmacytoid, and monocytoid differentiation. A study of 10 cases. *Oral Surg Oral Med Oral Pathol.* 1994; 77: 392.

559. Napier SS, Newlands C. Benign lymphoid hyperplasia of the palate: Report of two cases and immunohistochemical profile. *J Oral Pathol Med.* 1990; 19:221.

560. Shin SS, Berry GJ, Weiss LM. Infectious mononucleosis. Diagnosis by in situ hybridization in two cases with atypical features. *Am J Surg Pathol.* 1991; 15:625.

561. Reynolds DJ, Banks RM, Gully ML. New characterization of infectious mononucleosis and a phenotypic comparison with Hodgkin's disease. *Am J Pathol.* 1995; 146:379.

562. El-Mofty SK, Swanson PE, Wick MR, Miller AS. Eosinophilic ulcer of the oral mucosa. Report of 38 cases with immunohistochemical observations. *Oral Surg Oral Med Oral Pathol.* 1993; 75:716.

563. Mezei MM, Tron VA, Stewart WD, Rivers JK. Eosinophilic ulcer of the oral mucosa. *J Am Acad Dermatol.* 1995; 33:734.

564. Morrison JW, Langston JR, Slater LJ. Atypical histiocytic granuloma. Report of a case. *J Oral Maxillofac Surg.* 1990; 48: 630.

565. Tamir R, Pick AI, Calderon S. Plasmacytoma of the mandible: A primary presentation of multiple myeloma. *J Oral Maxillofac Surg.* 1992; 50:408.

566. Ilankovan V, Moos KF, El-Attar A. Intramedullary plasma cell tumours. *Int J Oral Maxillofac Surg.* 1990; 19:323.

567. Petruch UR, Horny H-P, Kaiserling E. Frequent expression of haemopoietic and non-haemopoietic antigens by neoplastic plasma cells: An immunohistochemical study using formalin-fixed, paraffin-embedded tissue. *Histopathol.* 1992; 20:35.

568. Lee S-H, Huang J-J, Pan W-L, Chan C-P. Gingival mass as the primary manifestation of multiple myeloma. Report of two cases. *Oral Surg Oral Med Oral Pathol Oral Radiol Endod.* 1996; 82:75.

569. Bertoni F, Dallera P, Bacchini P, et al. The Istituto Rizzoli-Beretta experience with osteosarcoma of the jaw. *Cancer.* 1991; 68:1555.

570. Clark JL, Unni KK, Dahlin DC, Devine KD. Osteosarcoma of the jaw. *Cancer.* 1983; 51:2311.

571. Delgado R, Maafs E, Alfeiran A, et al. Osteosarcoma of the jaw. *Head Neck.* 1994; 16:246.

572. Millar BG, Browne RM, Flood TR. Juxtacortical osteosarcoma of the jaws. *Br J Oral Maxillofac Surg.* 1990; 28:73.

573. Minic AJ. Periosteal osteosarcoma of the mandible. *Int J Oral Maxillofac Surg.* 1995; 24:226.

574. Daley TD, Damm DD, Wysocki GP, Weir JC. Atypical cartilage in reactive osteocartilagenous metaplasia of traumatized edentulous mandibular ridge. *Oral Surg Oral Med Oral Pathol Oral Radiol Endod.* 1997; 83:26.

575. Peters TED, Oliver DR, McDonald JS. Benign osteoblastoma of the mandible: Report of a case. *J Oral Maxillofac Surg.* 1995; 53:1347.

576. Ataoglu O, Oygur T, Yamalik K, Yucel E. Recurrent osteoblastoma of the mandible. A case report. *J Oral Maxillofac Surg.* 1994; 52:86.

577. Lucas DR, Unni KK, McLeod RA, et al. Osteoblastoma: Clinicopathologic study of 306 cases. *Hum Pathol.* 1994; 25:117.

578. Bertoni F, Bacchini P, Donati D, et al. Osteoblastoma-like osteosarcoma. The Rizzoli Institute experience. *Modern Pathol.* 1993; 6:707

579. Della Rocca C, Huvos AG. Osteoblastoma: Varied histologic presentations with a benign clinical course. An analysis of 55 cases. *Am J Surg Pathol.* 1996; 20:841.

580. Garrington GE, Collett WK. Chondrosarcoma. II. Chondrosarcoma of the jaws: Analysis of 37 cases. *J Oral Pathol Med.* 1988; 17:12.

581. Saito K, Unni KK, Wollan PC, Lund BA. Chondrosarcoma of the jaws and facial bones. *Cancer.* 1995; 76:1550.

582. Miller S, Whitaker SB, Weathers DR. Chondromyxoid fibroma of the mandible. Diagnostic image cytometry findings and review of the literature. *Oral Surg Oral Med Oral Pathol.* 1992; 73:465.

583. Hammad HM, Hammond HL, Kurago ZB, Frank JA. Chondromyxoid fibroma of the jaws. Case report and review of the literature. *Oral Surg Oral Med Oral Pathol Oral Radiol Endod.* 1998; 85:293.

584. Bertoni F, Unni KK, Beabout JW, Sim FH. Chondrosarcoma of the synovium. *Cancer.* 1991; 67:155.

585. Nitzan DW, Marmary Y, Hasson O, Elidan J. Chondrosarcoma arising in the temporomandibular joint: A case report and literature review. *J Oral Maxillofac Surg.* 1993; 51:312.

586. Rosati LA, Stevens C. Synovial chondromatosis of the temporomandibular joint presenting as an intracranial mass. *Arch Otolaryngol Head Neck Surg.* 1990; 116:1334.

587. Nomto M, Nagao K, Numata T, et al. Synovial osteochondromatosis of the temporomandibular joint. *J Laryngol Otol.* 1993; 107:742.

588. Ishida T, Dorfman HD, Bullough PG. Tophaceous pseudogout (tumoral calcium pyrophosphate dihydrate crystal deposition disease). *Hum Pathol.* 1995; 26:587.

589. Dijkgraaf LC, de Bont LGM, Liem RSB. Calcium pyrophosphate dihydrate crystal deposition disease of the temporomandibular joint: Report of a case. *J Oral Maxillofac Surg.* 1992; 50:1003.

590. Crawford JG, Oda D, Egbert M, Myall R. Mesenchymal chondrosarcoma of the maxilla in a child. *J Oral Maxillofac Surg.* 1995; 53:938.

591. Bottrill ID, Wood S, Barrett-Lee P, Howard DJ. Mesenchymal chondrosarcoma of the maxilla. *J Laryngol Otol.* 1994; 108:785.

592. Takahashi K, Sato K, Kanazawa H, et al. Mesenchymal chondrosarcoma of the jaws. Report of a case and review of 41 cases in the literature. *Head Neck.* 1993; 15:459.

593. Granter SR, Renshaw AA, Fletcher CDM, et al. CD99 reactivity in mesenchymal chondrosarcoma. *Hum Pathol.* 1996; 27:1273.

594. Meis-Kindblom JM, Stenman G, Kindblom L-G. Differential diagnosis of small round cell tumors. *Semin Diagn Pathol.* 1996; 13:213.

595. Batsakis JG, El-Naggar AK. Ewing's sarcoma and primitive neuroectodermal tumors: Cytogenetic cynosures seeking a common histogenesis. *Advances in Anatomic Pathol.* 1997; 4:207.

596. Roessner A, Jürgens H. Round cell tumors of bone. *Pathol Res Pract.* 1993; 189:1111.

597. Berk R, Heller A, Heller D, et al. Ewing's sarcoma of the mandible: A case report. *Oral Surg Oral Med Oral Pathol Oral Radiol Endod.* 1995; 79:159.

598. Wood RE, Nortjé CJ, Hesseling P, Grotepass F. Ewing's tumor of the jaw. *Oral Surg Oral Med Oral Pathol.* 1990; 69:120.

599. Wang C-L, Yacobi R, Pharoah M, Thorner P. Ewing's sarcoma: Metastatic tumor to the jaw. *Oral Surg Oral Med Oral Pathol.* 1991; 71:597.

600. Siegal GP, Oliver WR, Reinus WR, et al. Primary Ewing's sarcoma involving the bones of the head and neck. *Cancer.* 1987; 60:2829.

601. Stevenson AJ, Chatten J, Bertoni F, Miettinen M. CD99(p30/32^{MIC2}) neuroectodermal/Ewing's sarcoma antigen as an immunohistochemical marker. Review of more than 600 tumors and the literature experience. *Applied Immunohistochem.* 1994; 2:231.

602. Renshaw AA. 013 (CD99) in spindle cell tumors. Reactivity with hemangiopericytoma, solitary fibrous tumor, synovial sarcoma, and meningioma but rarely with sarcomatoid mesothelioma. *Applied Immunohistochem.* 1995; 3:250.

603. Scotlandi K, Serra M, Manara MC, et al. Immunostaining of the p30/32^{MIC2} antigen and molecular detection of the EWS rearrangements for the diagnosis of Ewing's sarcoma and peripheral neuroectodermal tumor. *Hum Pathol.* 1996; 27:408.

604. Lee CS, Southey MC, Waters K, et al. EWS/FLI-1 transcript detection and MIC2 immunohistochemical staining in the diagnosis of Ewing's sarcoma. *Pediatr Pathol Lab Med.* 1996; 16:379.

605. Katsourakis M, Kapranos N, Papanicolaou SI, Patrikiou A. Nerve-sheath myxoma (neurothekeoma) of the oral cavity: A cases report and review of the literature. *J Oral Maxillofac Surg.* 1996; 54:904.

606. Wang AR, May D, Bourne P, Scott G. PGP9.5—A marker for cellular neurothekeoma. *Am J Surg Pathol.* 1999; 23:1401.

607. Williams SB, Ellis GL, Meis JM, Heffner DK. Ossifying fibromyxoid tumor (of soft parts) of the head and neck: A clinicopathological and immunohistochemical study of nine cases. *J Laryngol Otol.* 1993; 107:75.

608. Smith BC, Ellis GL, Meis-Kindblom JM, Williams SB. Ectomesenchymal chondromyxoid tumor of the anterior tongue. Nineteen cases of a new clinicopathologic entity. *Am J Surg Pathol.* 1995; 19:519.

609. Chauvin PJ, Wysocki GP, Daley TD, Pringle GA. Palisaded encapsulated neuroma of oral mucosa. *Oral Surg Oral Med Oral Pathol.* 1992; 73:71.

610. Magnusson B. Palisaded encapsulated neuroma (solitary circumscribed neuroma) of the oral mucosa. *Oral Surg Oral Med Oral Pathol Oral Radiol Endod.* 1996; 82:302.

611. Ohishi M, Ishii T, Shiratsuchi Y, Tashiro H. Multiple endocrine neoplasia type 3: Three cases with mucosal neuromata. *Br J Oral Maxillofac Surg.* 1990; 28:317.

612. Winkelmann RK, Carney JA. Cutaneous neuropathy in multiple endocrine neoplasia, type 2b. *J Invest Dermatol.* 1982; 79:307.

613. Krolls SO, McGinnis PJ, Quon D. Multinodular versus plexiform neurilemoma of the hard palate. Report of a case. *Oral Surg Oral Med Oral Pathol.* 1994; 77:154.

614. Ishida T, Kuroda M, Motoi T, et al. Phenotypic diversity of neurofibromatosis 2: Association with plexiform schwannoma. *Histopathol.* 1998; 32:264.

615. Geist JR, Gander DL, Stefanac SJ, Oral manifestations of neurofibromatosis types I and II. *Oral Surg Oral Med Oral Pathol.* 1992; 73:376.

616. Sciubba JJ, D'Amico E, Attie JN. The occurrence of multiple endocrine neoplasia type II$_b$, in two children of an affected mother. *J Oral Pathol.* 1987; 16:310.

617. Kahn MA, Cote GJ, Gagel RF. RET protooncogene mutational analysis in multiple endocrine neoplasia syndrome type 2b. Case report and review of the literature. *Oral Surg Oral Med Oral Pathol Oral Radiol Endod.* 1996; 82:288.

618. Sist TC, Greene GW. Traumatic neuroma of the oral cavity. Report of thirty-one cases and review of the literature. *Oral Surg.* 1981; 51:394.

619. Argenyi ZB, Santa-Cruz D, Bromley C. Comparative light-microscopic and immunohistochemical study of traumatic and palisaded encapsulated neuromas of the skin. *Am J Dermatopathol.* 1992; 14:504.

620. Kaiserling E, Ruck P, Xiao J-C. Congenital epulis and granular cell tumor. A histologic and immunohistochemical study. *Oral Surg Oral Med Oral Pathol Oral Radiol Endod.* 1995; 80:687.

621. van der Wal N, Baak JPA, Schipper NW, van der Waal I. Morphometric study of pseudoepitheliomatous hyperplasia in granular cell tumors of the tongue. *J Oral Pathol Med.* 1989; 18:8.

622. Collins BM, Jones AC. Multiple granular cell tumors of the oral cavity: Report of a case and review of the literature. *J Oral Maxillofac Surg.* 1995; 53:707.

623. Garlick JA, Dayan D, Buchner A. A desmoplastic granular cell tumor of the oral cavity: Report of a case. *Br J Oral Maxillofac Surg.* 1992; 30:119.

624. Fanburg-Smith JC, Meis-Kindblom JM, Fante R, Kindblom L-G. Malignant granular cell tumor of soft tissue. Diagnostic criteria and clinicopathologic correlation. *Am J Surg Pathol.* 1998; 22:779.

625. Simsir A, Osborne B, Greenebaum E. Malignant granular cell tumor: A case report and review of the recent literature. *Hum Pathol.* 1996; 27:853.
626. Zuker RM, Buenechea R. Congenital epulis: Review of the literature and case report. *J Oral Maxillofac Surg.* 1993; 51:1040.
627. Filie AC, Lage JM, Azumi N. Immunoreactivity of S100 protein, α-1-antitrypsin, and CD68 in adult and congenital granular cell tumors. *Modern Pathol.* 1996; 9:888.
628. Weir JC, Cade JE, Weinberg R, Green TL. Oral granular cell tumors: Epithelial hyperplasia associated with candida? *J Oral Med.* 1986; 41:38.
629. Weathers DR, Fine RM. Thrombosed varix of the oral cavity. *Arch Dermatol.* 1971; 104:427.
630. Tosios K, Koutlas IG, Papanicolaou SI. Intravascular papillary endothelial hyperplasia: Report of 18 cases and review of the literature. *J Oral Maxillofac Surg.* 1994; 52:1263.
631. Raymond AK, Batsakis JG. Pathology consultation: Angiolithiasis and sialolithiasis in the head and neck. *Ann Otol Rhinol Laryngol.* 1992; 101:455.
632. Sano K, Ogawa A, Inokuchi T, et al. Buccal hemangioma with pheboliths. *Oral Surg Oral Med Oral Pathol.* 1988; 65:151.
633. Lovas JGL, Goodday RHB. Clinical diagnosis of caliber-persistent labial artery of the lower lip. *Oral Surg Oral Med Oral Pathol.* 1993; 76:480.
634. Lovas JGL, Rodu B, Hammond HL, et al. Caliber-persistent labial artery. A common vascular anomaly. *Oral Surg Oral Med Oral Pathol Oral Radiol Endod.* 1998; 86:308.
635. Sund S, Bang G. Intramuscular hemangioma in the oral region: Report of three cases. *Oral Surg Oral Med Oral Pathol.* 1990; 70:765.
636. Rossiter JL, Hendrix RA, Tom LWC, Potsic WP. Intramuscular hemangioma of the head and neck. *Otolaryngol Head Neck Surg.* 1993; 108:18.
637. Lamberg MA, Tasanen A, Jääskeläinen J. Fatality from central hemangioma of the mandible. *J Oral Surg.* 1979; 37:578.
638. Larsen PE, Peterson LJ. A systemic approach to the management of high-flow vascular malformations of the mandible. *J Oral Maxillofac Surg.* 1993; 51:62.
639. Koutlas IG, Jessurun J. Arteriovenous hemangioma: A clinicopathological and immunohistochemical study. *J Cutan Pathol.* 1994; 21:343.
640. Postlethwaite KR. Lymphangiomas of the tongue. *Br J Oral Maxillofac Surg.* 1986; 24:63.
641. Kennedy TL. Cystic hygroma-lymphangioma: a rare and still unclear entity. *Laryngoscope.* 1989; 99(suppl 49, pt. 2):1.
642. de Serres LM, Sie KCY, Richardson MA. Lymphatic malformations of the head and neck. A proposal for staging. *Arch Otolaryngol Head Neck Surg.* 1995; 121:577.

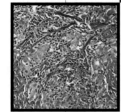

CHAPTER 10

Thyroid Gland

I. CLINICAL CONSIDERATIONS FOR DISEASES OF THE THYROID GLAND

- GEORGE H. PETTI, JR.
- GEORGE D. CHONKICH

SURGICAL ANATOMY

The thyroid gland consists of two lateral lobes connected by an isthmus. It has a bosselated surface, and in approximately 25% of people, a superior extension of the isthmus of thyroid tissue forms a pyramidal lobe. This may become clinically significant if not removed during total thyroidectomy. The gland weighs 15 to 25 g and is one of the most vascular organs that head and neck surgeons encounter.

Blood supply to the thyroid gland is provided by three arteries.

1. The superior thyroid artery, which is usually the first branch of the external carotid artery; in rare instances, it may arise as a branch of the common carotid artery.
2. The inferior thyroid artery, which arises as a branch of the thyrocervical trunk, courses deep to the common carotid artery, and then branches into superior and inferior vessels. This artery is more variable in its course and relations, and is very important in preserving function of the parathyroid glands during thyroid surgery.
3. The thyroidea ima artery, which serves as a replacement or an accessory to the inferior thyroid artery. It may arise from the innominate artery,

from the right common carotid, or directly from the aortic arch. This vessel is present in 5% to 10% of people and is important because it crosses the trachea and may bleed unexpectedly during tracheotomy.

The venous drainage is from the superior, middle, and inferior thyroid veins. The superior and middle thyroid veins drain directly to the internal jugular vein. The inferior thyroid veins may drain to their respective innominate veins, anastomosing freely anterior to the trachea, or they may join a common stem to drain into the left innominate vein.

The lymphatic drainage usually follows the arterial supply. The superior lymphatic vessels drain to the upper deep cervical nodes. The lower lymphatic vessels drain to the lower deep cervical nodes, including supraclavicular, pretracheal, paratracheal, and prelaryngeal nodes. Prelaryngeal and pretracheal nodes, when present, are known as "sentinel nodes or delphian nodes," as they may herald a diagnosis of carcinoma.

In surgery of the thyroid glands, the two recurrent laryngeal nerves (sometimes referred to as the inferior laryngeal nerves) and the superior laryngeal nerves are important. The right recurrent laryngeal nerve arises from the vagus, then loops around the subclavian artery to course in a medial direction to enter the larynx at the inferior border of the cricothyroid muscle. The left recurrent laryngeal nerve arises from the vagus and passes in front of the aortic arch, looping around it and ascending to the lower border of the cricothyroid muscle, where it enters the larynx. The nerves are not necessarily tucked into the tracheoesophageal groove, but they usually run more lateral than this; the right one is more apt to do so. The most common relationship with the inferior thyroid artery shows the right recurrent laryngeal nerve passing between the branches of the artery, and the left recurrent laryngeal nerve posterior to the inferior thyroid artery and its branches. However, these relationships are variable.

The right recurrent laryngeal nerve is most likely to be nonrecurrent. In this case, it is associated with an anomalous origin of the right subclavian artery coursing in a retroesophageal fashion.

Preservation of the recurrent laryngeal nerve is of paramount importance during thyroid surgery. Helpful guides to accomplish this are:

1. Identification of the recurrent laryngeal nerve at the lower pole of the thyroid.
2. Not sacrificing any branches of the nerve, as it may divide outside the larynx.
3. Following the nerve to its entry into the larynx—thyroid tissue should not be clamped around the upper pole until the course of the recurrent laryngeal nerve has been definitively established.

The superior laryngeal nerves arise from the caudal end of the nodose ganglion, pass medially and deep to the external and internal carotid arteries, and divide into a smaller external branch and a larger internal branch. The internal branch supplies sensation and parasympathetic secretomotor function to the mucous glands of the interior larynx. The external branch supplies motor power to the cricothyroid muscle, which tenses the vocal cord. To preserve the external branch during surgery it should be found just medial to the superior thyroid artery as it enters the upper pole of the gland.

PHYSIOLOGY AND TESTING[1,2]

Starting between 70 and 80 days of gestation, the follicular cells of the thyroid acquire the unique ability to accumulate iodide from the serum. The iodide is then oxidized to iodine. The iodine is incorporated into amino acid tyrosine residues in thryoglobulin molecules (probably through thyroid peroxidase) to form monoiodotyrosine, and diiodotyrosine. These couple to form the active hormones thyroxine (T_4) and triiodothyronine (T_3), which in turn form the active hormone thyroglobulin. Thyroglobulin is then hydrolyzed by adenylate cyclase activation, and free T_4 and T_3 are released into the bloodstream. This process takes 10 to 30 minutes after exposure to thyroid-stimulating hormone (TSH) from the pituitary gland. The most active of the hormones is T_3, estimated to be four times as potent as T_4. A major source of T_3 is conversion of T_4 in the liver, the kidney, and the peripheral tissues. Because T_4 is bound strongly to thyroxine-binding globulin, it is eliminated more slowly than T_3; it has a half-life of 6 to 7 days, whereas the half-life of T_3 is 1 day. Degradation and excretion of thyroid hormone is through the liver, the gastrointestinal tract, and the kidney.

The process of iodination of thyroxine can be blocked by drugs such as methimazole and propylthiouracil, which block the action of thyroid peroxidase. Chlorpromazine and lithium inhibit TSH action and can thus decrease thyroid function.

Thyroid gland function is controlled by a hypothalamic–pituitary–thyroid feedback mechanism. Thyrotropin-releasing factor is formed in the hypothalamus. It stimulates the release of TSH from the pituitary, which acts on the thyroid gland to produce T_3 and T_4. As levels of T_3 and T_4 rise in the blood, a negative feedback shuts off TSH. The reverse process occurs as T_3 and T_4 levels drop in the blood (Fig. 10–1).

It is important for the head and neck surgeon evaluating masses in the thyroid gland to know whether the patient is euthyroid. A free T_4 level and a sensitive TSH level are the two most reliable tests of thyroid function status. In the euthyroid state, the

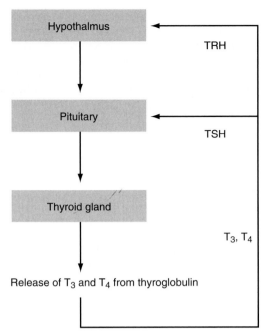

FIGURE 10–1 Algorithm of pituitary thyroid feedback mechanism.

physical examination leads to suspicion of chronic thyroiditis (Hashimoto's thyroiditis), antithyroid microsomal antibody titers should be measured.

In the managed care setting, a cost-effective approach to determine euthyroidism is to order a sensitive TSH (thyrotropin) level.[3] Normal values are 0.4mU/L to 5.5mU/L. When TSH is normal, a clinically euthyroid state is present with rare exceptions. If the TSH (thyrotropin) is high, then a free T_4 and FTI (free thyroid index) are obtained to determine a hypothyroid state. If the TSH is low, free T_4 and FTI assist in diagnosing a subclinical hypothyroid state or an overt state of hypothroidism (Fig. 10–2).

A sensitive TSH alone is appropriate to monitor thyroid hormone replacement postoperatively and post-total thyroidectomy for carcinoma. To follow a patient's progress and treatment for hypothyroidism, TSH (thyrotropin) is not recommended, as the thyrotropin remains high for a prolonged period of time. These patients should have free T_4 or FTI testing, both of which will change quickly with adequate treatment.

EMBRYOLOGY AND MALFORMATIONS

The thyroid gland develops as a median downgrowth of entodermal tissue from the first and second pharyngeal pouches in the region of the base of the tongue (foramen caecum). This downgrowth forms the thyroglossal duct. After descent, the thyroid gland lies inferior to the cricoid cartilage over the upper two or three tracheal rings. During

free T_4 and TSH levels are within normal range. If the patient is thyrotoxic, the free T_4 level is elevated, and the TSH level is decreased. In primary hypothyroidism, the free T_4 level is decreased, and the TSH level is elevated. If both TSH and T_4 levels are low, the patient may have secondary hypothyroidism as a result of pituitary failure or tertiary hypothyroidism due to hypothalamic failure. If the history or the

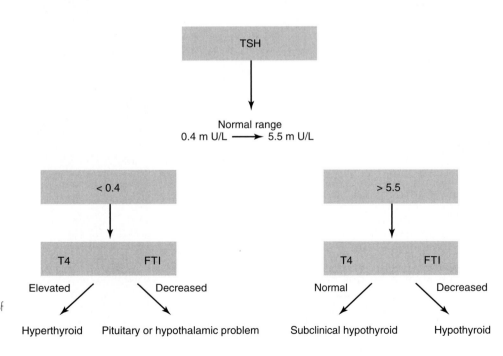

FIGURE 10–2 Algorithm of role of T_4 and FTI in diagnosing hypothyroidism.

migration the follicular cells are joined by the parafollicular cells from the ultimobranchial body.[4] The parafollicular cells are neuroectodermal in origin, are responsible for the development of medullary carcinoma, and are usually concentrated in the posterior superior aspects of the thyroid lobes. The parafollicular and "C" cells produce calcitonin, a serum marker for medullary carcinoma. By the end of the first trimester of pregnancy, this development is complete.

Ectopic thyroid tissue can appear anywhere along this course of development. Patients with arrested descent of the thyroid tissue may present with a mass of tissue at the base of the tongue known as lingual thyroid. Radioactive scanning will confirm the diagnosis of lingual thyroid, and treatment with thyroid hormone is initiated to suppress further increase in glandular size. Surgical removal is reserved for size increases that cause symptoms of respiratory distress or dysphagia.

Lateral neck masses of thyroid tissue are not considered normal, even if their histology is such. They are considered metastatic deposits of thyroid carcinoma, and suitable treatment is administered.[5]

Cysts and fistulas can develop from the thyroglossal duct and can appear anywhere between the base of the tongue and the suprasternal notch. The surgical procedure for treatment of this condition is Sistrunk's operation; this includes removal of the midportion of the hyoid bone and dissection up to, or including, the tissue around the foramen caecum at the base of the tongue.

anaplastic carcinoma is entertained as a diagnosis. Two other causes for a rapidly enlarging thyroid nodule are lymphomatous degeneration of Hashimoto's thyroiditis or hemorrhage into a cyst. If the patient has hypertension, episodic headaches, sweating, palpitation, wheezing (new-onset asthma), or diarrhea, medullary carcinoma and a multiple endocrine neoplasia (MEN) syndrome take priority in diagnosis.

Physical Examination

Vocal cord paralysis or a thyroid nodule associated with cervical adenopathy is considered carcinoma until proven otherwise. Suspicious characteristics of a thyroid nodule being cancerous are: lesions that are hard and fixed, invading surrounding structures, and a nodule greater than 4 cm in size with hard irregular borders.

The trachea and its relative position to the midline must be determined, for if the trachea is deviated, it may be because of substernal extension of the thyroid enlargement, causing compression of the airway (Fig. 10–3). This compression usually progresses slowly, and the patient is not aware of it until after surgery. Patients frequently say, "I feel that a heavy weight has been removed from my neck."

Suspicion is raised that the patient is hyperthyroid when there is a large thyroid, a tremor of the hands,

EVALUATION OF THE PATIENT WITH A THYROID NODULE

Evaluation of the patient with a thyroid nodule consists of history, physical examination, laboratory and x-ray evaluation, and thyroid suppression test.

History

In taking the history, it is important to determine if a patient with a thyroid nodule was given radiation treatments in childhood. If 500 to 2000cgy were given in childhood, the risk of developing cancer 10 to 20 years later is high. If a dose greater than 5000cgy has been given to the thyroid gland, the risk of developing cancer is minimal, as the thyroid has been ablated by this dose of radiation. A family history of thyroid cancer, especially medullary, places the patient at a higher risk for a cancerous nodule. Hoarseness of the voice or dysphagia may herald a paralysis of the recurrent laryngeal nerve or compression-invasion of the aerodigestive tract. If the mass has suddenly increased rapidly in size,

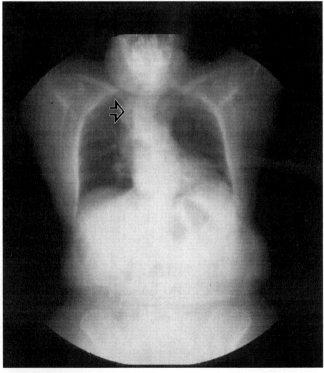

FIGURE 10–3 Elderly patient with lymphoma of the thyroid causing aerodigestive tract compression (*arrow*).

tachycardia, and eye signs. The eye signs that are occasionally seen are:

1. exopthalmos, von Graefe's sign—lid lag, the upper eyelid lags behind the lower lid when looking down.
2. Möbius's sign—a failure of convergence when an object is brought close to the midface.
3. Joffroy's sign—failure to wrinkle the forehead with rapid upper gaze.
4. Stellwag's sign—spasmodic contractions of the upper lid as the patient looks upward.

Dermographia may be present and is a reflection of vasomotor instability. On palpation, you can sometimes feel a thrill or hear a bruit when the patient has a hyperthyroid condition.

Laboratory and X-Ray Evaluation

Serum testing obtaining a TSH level is a cost-effective method to determine euthyroidism (see Fig. 10–2). If there is a suspicion of medullary carcinoma, a serum calcitonin is obtained.

In some cases of medullary carcinoma, CEA (carcinoembryonic antigen) levels may be elevated, usually portending a poor prognosis.

Fine needle biopsy is completed with a 22-gauge needle and a needle biopsy syringe holder.[6–10] This method has a greater than 90% accuracy rate in distinguishing benign from malignant nodules, and has, in our practice, replaced the thyroid I_{123} uptake and scan. If a cyst is aspirated with normal cytology, and the nodule disappears only to return later, it is aspirated again and cytology is obtained. After three such aspirations, a thyroid lobectomy with frozen section is recommended. Fine needle biopsy has its limitations and depends first on obtaining an adequate sample. Small nodules (under 10 mm) are difficult to aspirate. It is also difficult to aspirate a nodule in a short, fat neck. Follicular lesions may be malignant, as vascular and capsular invasion cannot be determined on fine needle specimens.

When the fine needle biopsy is recorded as malignant cells present, or papillary carcinoma, thyroidectomy is recommended. If the fine needle biopsy report is benign, the patient is placed on thyroid replacement and monitored for 3 to 6 months for regression of the nodule. If the nodule increases in size, or does not regress in size during this time frame, surgery is recommended. If the biopsy is of suspicious cytology, an I_{123} uptake and scan is ordered, and if a cold nodule is found, then surgery is recommended. If the nodule is hot on I_{123} scan, a suppression test is done to determine if it is autonomous. If it is autonomous, I_{131} therapy or surgery is recommended. If the nodule is not autonomous, thyroid replacement is begun (Fig. 10–4).

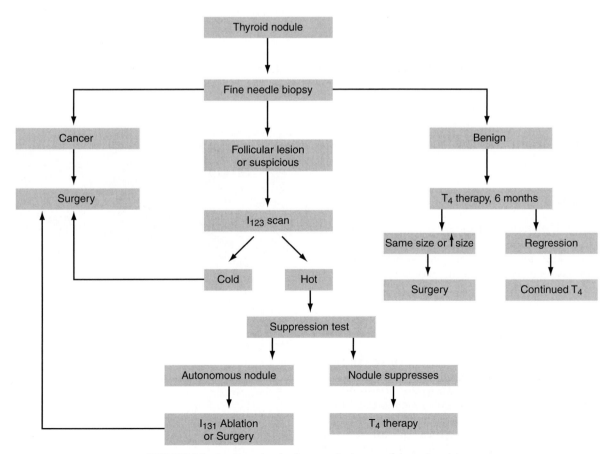

FIGURE 10–4 Algorithm for fine needle biopsy of thyroid nodule.

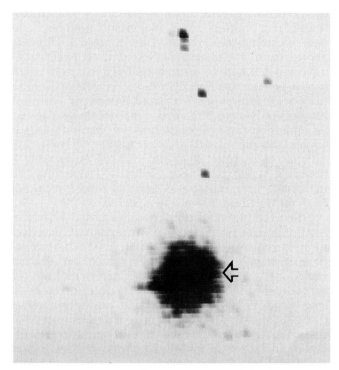

FIGURE 10–5 Patient with an autonomous nodule after attempted suppression with thyroid hormone (*arrow*).

Thyroid Suppression Test[11]

The patient is given cytomel 25 ucmg t.i.d., for 2 to 3 weeks, then an I_{123} scan is repeated while patient is on the medication. If the nodule persists as a hot spot, it is considered autonomous in function (Fig. 10–5). If the nodule does not take up the I_{123}, it is nonautonomous and most likely will continue to respond to thyroid treatment, now using the longer-acting form of thyroid suppression, levothyroxin (Synthroid).

Ultrasound[12]

Ultrasound of the thyroid gland can be obtained for further determination if desired but is not absolutely necessary. The lesion appears as solid, cystic, or mixed in pattern. Solid lesions have a higher incidence of carcinoma.

Radiographs

A chest x-ray that includes visualization of the neck is useful, because it occasionally demonstrates fine speckled calcium deposits within the substance of the thyroid that may represent calcification from psammoma bodies seen in papillary thyroid carcinoma. It may show rim calcification around the nodule, but this is seen in both follicular adenomas

and follicular carcinoma. Deviation of the airway can be substantiated, and the presence of pulmonary metastases can be seen. CT or MRI scans of the neck and mediastinum are helpful in those patients who have large bulky disease, cervical metastases, aerodigestive tract invasion, and those thought to have substernal extension of the thyroid gland.

BENIGN LESIONS OF THE THYROID

Goiters can be solitary nodules or multiple nodules. Nontoxic goiters show no functional disturbance. These are usually related to colloid accumulations. Early on, within the first year of their discovery, TSH levels may be slightly increased as a result of decreased production of T_4 and T_3, resulting in a compensatory increase in TSH by the pituitary gland. The thyroid gland enlarges as a result of this TSH stimulation, and in response to the TSH, the gland produces more T_4 and T_3. TSH levels then come back down within the normal range. Nodular goiters probably arise from repeated cycles of hyperplasia and involution (Fig. 10–6 and 10–7 A and B). As a result, a dominant nodule or a solitary nodule may develop in areas that have become more responsive to TSH, and then may grow more quickly than the adjacent thyroid.[13]

Toxic goiters occur more commonly in iodine-deficient areas and are more common in women over the age of 50 years.[14] The goal of treatment is to make them euthyroid. Thyroid-stimulating immunogloubulins (TSI) are present in the majority of patients with Graves' disease (diffuse toxic goiter).

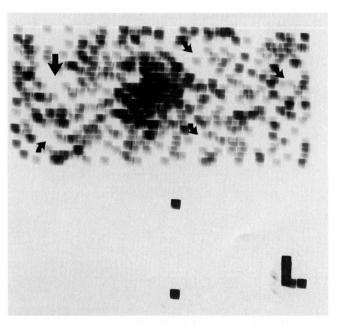

FIGURE 10–6 Patient with multinodular goiter and patchy uptake of I_{123} (*arrows*).

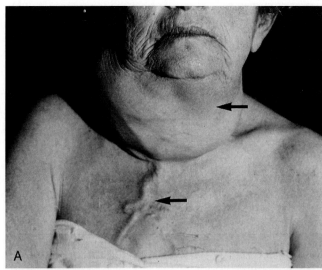

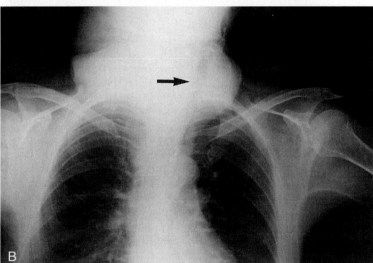

FIGURE 10-7 *A,* Patient with a large goiter and compression of the superior vena cava (*arrows*). *B,* Radiograph displaying a large neck mass with deviation of the trachea (*arrow*).

In Plummer's disease, there are multiple toxic nodules. The nodules in hyperthyroid patients may be autonomous; some may be cold, either from a process of burnout or neoplastic degeneration. Patients with dominant thyroid nodules should have a needle biopsy to better differentiate the pathologic process.

The symptoms of hyperthyroidism include increased nervousness, fatigue, palpation, heat intolerance, tremor, and weight loss.[15] In elderly patients there may be no classic symptomatology—this is called apathetic hyperthyroidism.

Initial blood tests will show low TSH levels and high T_4 levels, although at times T_4 will be normal and T_3 levels will be high—as seen in T3 thyrotoxicosis. On thyroid scan with I_{123}, there will be high uptake and will usually show which nodules are most active (as in Plummer's disease) or if the entire gland is involved (as in Graves' disease). In geographic areas of iodine deficiency, there may be an increased affinity for the gland to take up iodine,

giving a high uptake, but other tests will show that the patient may be euthyroid.

The initial treatment of hyperthyroidism is to start antithyroid medications to make the patient euthyroid. Beta-adrenergic blockers such as propanolol are the cornerstone to treatment and are contraindicated only in patients with asthma, bronchospasm, and congestive failure. The thianamides (PTU methimazole) inhibit the thyroid peroxidase enzyme system, preventing oxidation of trapped iodine, as well as the formation of diiodotyrosine and triiodotyrosine. Agranulocytosis and granulocytopenia are feared complications, so CBC (complete blood count) testing is done in follow-up of these patients. If surgery is in the planned program, as patients become euthyroid, they are prepared with saturated solution of potassium iodide (SSKI) for 10 to 14 days or sodium epodate (ordinarily used for imaging the gall bladder) for 4 to 5 days. These drugs reduce uptake of iodine and inhibit release of thyroid hormone, with resultant decreased vascularity of the

T A B L E 1 0 – 1	BENIGN LESIONS OF THE THYROID

1. Goiter—nontoxic or toxic
2. Adenoma—Follicular—Hürthle cell
3. Thyroid cysts
4. Embryologic—Thyroglossal cysts—Ectopic thyroid
5. Thyroiditis

gland. If surgery is not entertained, then radioactive ablation is carried out. The possible complications of radioactive iodine ablation are development of hypothyroidism, thyroid crisis if the patient is not adequately prepared, leukemia, hyperparathyroidism, and an increased incidence of benign thyroid tumors. Table 10–1 lists benign lesions of the thyroid.

FOLLICULAR ADENOMA[16]

The cytologic diagnosis on many thyroid nodules is recorded as a "follicular process." Follicular adenomas are a common source of thyroid nodules, and malignant potential cannot be determined on needle biopsy. When the clinician's suspicion is heightened, follicular adenomas should be removed by thyroidectomy, for only then can the pathologist diagnose capsular or vascular invasion, the hallmark sign of malignancy (Fig. 10–8).

Clinical parameters suggesting follicular carcinoma rather than adenoma are age of more than 50 years, a nodule greater than 3 cm, and the presence of a history of prior radiation. Thyroid nodules are more common in women than men by a 4-to-1 ratio; however, a nodule in a man is three times more

likely to be malignant. We recommend lobectomy and isthmusectomy as the minimum procedure for follicular neoplasms. If malignancy is entertained, a total thyroidectomy is done.

MALIGNANT LESIONS OF THE THYROID

Carcinoma of the thyroid encompasses a wide range—from slow-growing, well-differentiated neoplasms with a good prognosis to rapidly growing, poorly differentiated tumors with a poor prognosis. Table 10–2 lists these malignant lesions. It is the function of the thyroid surgeon to determine which thyroid cancer is apt to be more aggressive and to apply surgical and medical techniques that provide the patient with the best opportunity for long-term, disease-free survival. When the thyroid is studied carefully at necropsy, approximately 6% of the population have no clinical evidence of thyroid disease but have occult thyroid cancer. It would not be correct, then, for physicians to extrapolate that all thyroid cancers act in a benign nature, and that therapy need not be aggressive. Table 10–3 presents staging for papillary, follicular, medullary, and undifferentiated cancers.

Papillary Carcinoma in Children[17–19]

When radiation therapy was employed for children with benign conditions such as thymic enlargement, tinea capitis, hemangiomas, and acne, 10 to 20 years later they were at increased risk for development of thyroid carcinoma—usually a papillary variety or a mixture of papillary and follicular elements. Pres-

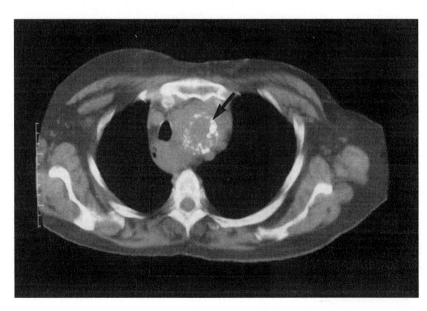

FIGURE 10-8 Patient with a large follicular lesion with a rim of calcification (arrow).

TABLE 10 – 2	MALIGNANT LESIONS OF THE THYROID

1. Papillary carcinoma
2. Follicular carcinoma—Hürthle cell lesions
3. Medullary carcinoma
4. Anaplastic carcinoma
5. Metastatic lesions

ently, radiation exposure of the thyroid in children is a result of treatment of lymphomas of the neck and mediastinum. The cancers that result are usually multifocal and contain lymph node metastases.

The child typically presents with either a neck mass that has not responded to antibiotic therapy or a nodule in the thyroid gland. Hoarseness and dysphagia, secondary to aerodigestive tract invasion heralds aggressive disease that is extensive. The treatment includes a total thyroidectomy and postoperative I_{131} therapy. The pediatric endocrinologist and the nuclear medicine specialist should consult closely; special circumstances may adjust the treatment approach. The child is placed on lifelong thyroid replacement, followed with thyroglobulin and T_4 serum tests, along with chest x-ray and body scans as indicated.

Even with pulmonary metastases, children may survive for decades. Treatment should therefore be initiated with the thought of long-term control. Death, when it occurs from the cancer, is a result of direct tumor invasion or dedifferentiation to an anaplastic carcinoma.

Papillary Carcinoma in Adults[18,20–28]

Approximately 60% to 70% of adult thyroid carcinomas are papillary in nature. Incidence peaks in the third and fourth decades, and is two to three times more frequent in females. (In children, there is a more equal distribution between males and females.)

The most common presenting feature is an asymptomatic neck mass in the thyroid gland. Usually this is an isolated nodule, but it can be present as a dominant nodule in a diffusely enlarged or a multinodular gland. Less than one third of patients have palpable cervical lymph nodes. Less often, there is evidence of local invasion resulting in symptoms of vocal cord paralysis with hoarseness of voice and dysphagia. The nodules may be solid, cystic, or a combination of the two. After preoperative evaluation, as previously discussed, therapy is initiated. There is ongoing controversy regarding the extent of surgery, the indications for radioiodine therapy, and the efficacy and use of thyroid hormone to control tumor recurrence.

Advantages of Total Thyroidectomy

The management of papillary thyroid carcinoma at our institution is initial total thyroidectomy (Table 10–4), evaluation and treatment with radioactive iodine postoperatively, and thyroid replacement therapy with long-term follow-up utilizing serum testing for thyroglobulin, T_4, and TSH. Chest x-rays annually and total body scan on the anniversary of the first year following radioactive iodine therapy are performed and repeated as indicated thereafter.

Experienced head and neck surgeons should perform the surgery to lessen the risks of hypoparathyroidism and vocal cord paralysis. Doing many total thyroidectomies, the surgeon encounters few complications. No parathyroid glands that are normal are sacrificed during surgery. If gland appears to be devascularized, it is biopsy proven to be parathyroid, placed in an iced saline bath, diced, and autotransplanted to a muscle bed at the conclusion of surgery. Patients who have an incidental finding of an occult thyroid carcinoma on final pathology reporting are counseled concerning the advantages and disadvantages of total thyroidectomy. They then decide whether to have further surgery.

TABLE 10 – 3	STAGE GROUPING

Separate stage groupings are recommended for papillary, follicular, medullary, or undifferentiated (anaplastic).

PAPILLARY OR FOLLICULAR

	Under 45 Years	45 Years and Older
Stage I	Any T, Any N, M0	T1, N0, M0
Stage II	Any T, Any N, M1	T2, N0, M0
		T3, N0, M0
Stage III		T4, N0, M0
		Any T, N1, M0
Stage IV		Any T, Any N, M1

MEDULLARY

Stage I	T1	N0	M0
Stage II	T2	N0	M0
	T3	N0	M0
	T4	N0	M0
Stage III	Any T	N1	M0
Stage IV	Any T	Any N	M1

UNDIFFERENTIATED (ANAPLASTIC)

All cases are stage IV.

Stage IV	Any T	Any N	Any M

TABLE 10 – 4	ADVANTAGES OF TOTAL THYROIDECTOMY

1. Removes bilateral multifocal disease.
2. Lessens risk of recurrence.
3. Lessens risk of death from central neck disease.
4. Allows better use of postoperative radioactive I_{131} ablation.
5. Decreases risk of dedifferentiation to anaplastic carcinoma.
6. Allows postoperative follow-up with serum testing of thyroglobulin.

Functional neck dissections are done for palpable disease and when there is a high index of suspicion on CT or MRI scans. Scans are not routinely ordered; instead, their use is reserved for the patient with large, bulky disease, airway compression, substernal extension, palpable neck disease, and recurrent laryngeal nerve paralysis.

Prognosis is related to age (patients 40 years and older), size (greater than 3 cm neoplastic process), and extent (with capsular invasion or angioinvasion or distant metastases having a poor prognosis).[29-31] Nondiploid DNA content in the carcinoma also has a poor outlook and is independent of the aforementioned factors.

Without distant metastases, the overall 5- and 10-year survival rates are 90% and 80%, respectively. With distant metastases the 5- and 10-year survival rates are 35% and 25%, respectively. Cancer mortality from differentiated thyroid cancer is worsened by advancing age and presence of distant metastases in multiple sites (i.e., lung and bone) at the time of first diagnosis of distant metastases.

Follicular Carcinoma

Follicular carcinoma accounts for 15% to 20% of thyroid malignant neoplasms and is often included in the discussion of papillary carcinoma. The diagnostic and therapeutic approaches are similar, but there are important differences that make this tumor a little more aggressive in its nature.

Follicular cancers tend to be encapsulated and can show vascular and capsular invasion (Fig. 10–8). They spread hematologically (and rarely by lymphatic dissemination). They most commonly metastasize to lung and bone. They concentrate I_{131} well and are thus treated with I_{131} postoperatively. Their clinical presentation is similar to papillary carcinoma in that they are slow growing, different in that they are usually solid tumors and that palpable lymph node metastases are less common than in papillary carcinoma. Bone metastases may occur early and may not respond to I_{131} therapy. These may be the symptoms leading to the diagnosis of an occult follicular carcinoma in the thyroid. Another important fact is that metastatic follicular carcinoma may be the cause of thyrotoxicosis.

A follicular carcinoma is differentiated from a follicular adenoma by the presence of capsular invasion and/or vascular invasion.[5,16] The size of the primary is not as important as with papillary carcinoma, because even small occult primaries can produce distant metastases.[31] The important prognostic factors are therefore related to capsular invasion, angioinvasion, and the presence of metastases.[32]

The treatment is total thryoidectomy with postoperative I_{131} ablation of any potential microscopic disease.[33,34] In the treatment of follicular carcinoma, a total thyroidectomy takes a more significant role, because we do not want thyroid tissue in the neck to compete with potential microscopic disease for the uptake of I_{131}.[35] The overall survival rate is lower at 5 and 10 years for follicular carcinoma than it is for papillary cancer. Again, it is noted that patients with aneuploid DNA cancers do more poorly than those with diploid or tetraploid ones.

Variants of Differentiated Thyroid Carcinoma

TALL CELL AND COLUMNAR CELL

Tall cell and columnar cell are subtypes of papillary carcinoma. They are uncommon forms, more aggressive in their growth and metastatic potential.[36-38] They have a higher incidence of extrathyroidal spread and usually occur in older patients. They have been seen in the younger population as well, usually larger at presentation with a tendency for vascular invasion. The treatment of these tumor types is again total thyroidectomy and postoperative I_{131} therapy with closer follow-up than typical papillary carcinoma.[36]

INSULAR

Insular tumors are a solid variant of papillary carcinoma. They are composed of islands of small, uniform, well-differentiated cells that may be confused with medullary carcinoma; however, immunocytochemistry for calcitonin will be negative. Treatment is total thyroidectomy.

HÜRTHLE CELL

Hürthle cell carcinoma is a variant of follicular cancer of the thyroid.[39] In general there is an unreliable correlation between the histologic features of small Hürthle cell carcinoma and its clinical course. The diagnosis of malignancy is determined histopathologically by capsular invasion.[40] When malignant, these tumors have a high incidence of local recurrence, metastases to bone and lung, and increased mortality. They metastasize via the blood stream, and the lesion will rarely respond to I_{131} therapy. Flow cytometry of the nuclear DNA content in Hürthle cell cancer is a significant predictor of outcome.[41] The majority of Hürthle cell cancers that metastasize and cause death are aneuploid tumors.

The treatment is total thyroidectomy for malignant Hürthle cell lesions with regional lymphadenectomy when indicated. For benign Hürthle cell lesions there is ongoing controversy as to whether total or subtotal thyroidectomy is the best choice of treatment.

Coexistent Thyroid Cancer and Hashimoto's Thyroiditis[42,43]

Coexistent cancer in Hashimoto's thyroiditis is present in up to 25% of patients. Lymphomatous degeneration of Hashimoto's thyroiditis and the formation of well-differentiated thyroid carcinoma, or even a squamous cell carcinoma, can arise in the background of a Hashimoto's thyroiditis.[44] The most common differentiated thyroid cancer seen in Hashimoto's thyroiditis is papillary carcinoma. The suspicion of malignancy is enhanced when there is a solitary cold nodule, a suspicious fine needle aspiration biopsy, and failure of a dominant nodule to involute with thyroid hormone therapy.[45] Surgery in the form of either total or subtotal thyroidectomy is recommended for these patients.

Graves' Disease and Thyroid Carcinoma

Prior to 1960 there were few reports in the literature on the coexistence of Graves' disease and thyroid carcinoma. It is believed that the presence of thyroid-stimulating antibodies to the TSH receptor on cells in Graves' disease stimulates growth and function of thyroid tissue to a neoplastic state. The preponderance of carcinomas in Graves' disease are papillary, but follicular carcinoma also occurs in about 25% of cases.[46] The index of suspicion for the presence of carcinoma in Graves' disease is heightened when there is a dominant palpable nodule, when the nodule is cold on thyroid scan, and when the nodule has formed after radiation therapy. Under these circumstances, if cancer is found, it is more often than not a multifocal process, locally invasive. It produces regional metastases and, less often, distant metastases. Treatment includes total thyroidectomy followed by I_{131} therapy.

Medullary Carcinoma

Medullary carcinoma accounts for approximately 5% to 10% of all thyroid cancer. Since its discovery in 1959 by Hazard et al,[47] this tumor has generated a lot of interest by clinicians and research scientists because of its many unique characteristics.

The tumor arises in C cells, so called because they secrete calcitonin, a polypeptide hormone that serves as an excellent plasma tumor marker for medullary thyroid cancer. Embryologically, this is not a true thyroid cancer because the C cells are of neuroectodermal origin from the ultimobranchial body and migrate to the thyroid gland resting, usually, in the posterior superior aspect of the thyroid lobes.[48]

C-cell hyperplasia is a premalignant lesion found in thyroid glands of patients who are afflicted with the hereditary forms of medullary carcinoma. The C cells also have the capacity to secrete CEA (carcinoembryonic antigen), a glycoprotein that, when elevated in association with elevated calcitonin levels, portends a poorer prognosis.[49,50]

The two types of medullary carcinoma found are sporadic and familial.[51] The sporadic variety accounts for 90% of cases, and the familial form represents 10%. The pathology is the same in the two forms, but there are differences as to the age of onset, family history, associated disease processes, and extent of thyroid involvement, as outlined in Table 10–5.

The diagnosis of the familial forms of medullary carcinoma of the thyroid is made early, at a time when there is less disease present. In the sporadic form, because the diagnosis is made at a later age, the disease is usually more advanced (see Table 10–5).

The patient usually presents with a painless, firm, round mass (but a multinodular mass may be present as well) in the substance of the thyroid, most often in the superior aspect of the thyroid lobe. Approximately 15% of patients have palpable lymph nodes in the neck. The disease will spread to the midline neck and superior mediastinum, then usually to the lateral neck. Diarrhea and/or paroxysmal hypertension may on occasion be associated symptoms.[47]

Approximately 10% of patients will have inherited their disease as an autosomal dominant pattern, with half the offspring affected.[49] Screening tests of plasma calcitonin are mandatory in all blood relatives of patients with the diagnosis of medullary carcinoma. Borderline or mildly elevated calcitonin levels in patients with suspected medullary thyroid cancer (MTC) can then be analyzed by one of the most sensitive diagnostic serological tests, the determination of calcitonin after sequential IV administration of calcium gluconate and pentagastrin. Blood samples are obtained before the test, and at 1, 2, 3, and 5 minutes after the administration of the secretagogues. Peak values usually occur at 1 or 2 minutes. Calcitonin is a 32-amino acid polypeptide secreted by the C cells. It decreases osteoclastic activity

TABLE 10–5	MEDULLARY THYROID CARCINOMA	
	SPORADIC FORM	FAMILIAL FORM
Age	Older Age	Younger Age
Family history	No	Yes
Associated diseases	None	Pheochromocytoma Hyperparathyroidism Mucosal neuromas Ganglioneuromas
Thyroid	Usually unilateral involvement	Bilateral involvement

of bones, thus decreasing serum calcium. It also increases the urinary excretion of calcium, phosphorus, sodium, and potassium. Calcitonin increases GI secretion of electrolytes and water in the jejunum and decreases mucosal contact time by an increased rate of movement. Some patients therefore may present with diarrhea. Other hormones that C cells can produce are CEA, ACTH, serotonin, and somatostatin.

Treatment for MTC includes a total thyroidectomy, bilateral paratracheal lymph node dissection, and a superior mediastinal dissection. Radical neck dissection is added to these when there is bulky disease in the midline, when there are multiple positive midline nodes, and when there is palpable, or CT/MRI scan, evidence of lateral neck disease (Fig. 10–9). It is not uncommon to find the recurrent laryngeal nerve involved, and in these cases, the resection would include the removal of the nerve and the diseased tissue around it. Because MTC is neuroectodermal in origin it does not respond to I_{131} treatment. Chemotherapy is of little value at the present time, and radiation therapy is used when there is bulky disease or extrathyroidal extension.

Prognosis is greatly influenced by the initial presentation of the disease. Surgery is the only curative treatment for MTC. When the disease can be encompassed surgically, the 5-year survival rate can be as high as 90% and as low as 40% when cervical nodes are positive. Patients are followed by monitoring calcitonin levels every 4 months, and chest x-rays with further testing when clinical symptoms so indicate.

Multiple Endocrine Neoplasia

The MEN syndrome is a genetically autosomal dominant disorder with high penetrance and protean manifestations. Two subsyndromes, MEN Type 1 (Wermer's) and MEN Type 2 (Sipple's) have been identified.

WERMER'S SYNDROME

This syndrome attacks the parathyroid glands in 85%, the pancreas in 65%, and the pituitary gland in 40% of patients. The thyroid gland can be involved, however—not with medullary carcinoma, but with other thyroid carcinomas. The parathyroid glands display either hyperplasia or an adenoma, and the pancreas is involved with insulinomas or gastrinomas. The pituitary, when involved, most often has a chromophobe adenoma that can produce acromegaly.

SIPPLE'S SYNDROME

MEN Type 2 syndrome is subdivided into Type A and Type B. Some authors are now considering Type B as a separate variety, classifying it as Type 3. The main difference between the two is that in Type B there is no hyperparathyroidism.

Type 2A is characterized by the presence of medullary carcinoma in nearly 100% of patients. Bilateral pheochromocytomas are found in 10% of patients, and hyperparathyroidism is found in approximately 60%. It is important for the head and neck surgeon to remember that the diagnosis and treatment of pheochromocytoma takes precedence over the treatment of the neck disease, in order to avoid a hypertensive crisis that may occur with induction of anesthesia.

Type 2B is characterized by the absence of hyperparathyroidism and the presence of medullary carcinoma and the pheochromocytoma associated with multiple neuromas in the conjunctiva, the lips, and

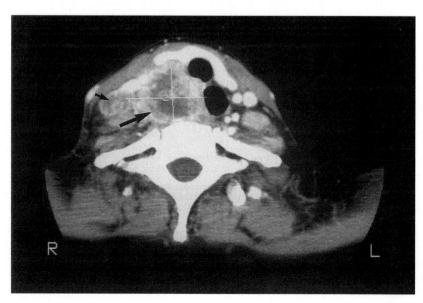

FIGURE 10–9 Patient with a large medullary carcinoma invading the aerodigestive tract, treated with bilateral radical neck dissection and gastric pullup (arrows).

buccal mucosa. Marfanoid habitus without the cardiovascular defects has been reported.

Anaplastic Thyroid Carcinoma

Approximately 10% of thyroid cancers are anaplastic in nature. Males and females are affected equally. Elderly patients in the sixth and seventh decades with rapidly enlarging masses are most suspect for anaplastic carcinoma, but this disease does occur in young patients as well. The tumor, not infrequently, occurs in patients who have had other thyroid neoplasms and have undergone a dedifferentiation process in the thyroid tissue that was not removed.

Clinically, the patient presents with a rapidly enlarging thyroid mass that causes pain, dysphagia, airway distress, hemoptysis, and hoarseness. Preoperative CT or MRI scans are very helpful to determine extent of the disease in the mediastinum and neck.[53]

Surgical extirpation may be difficult, as anaplastic carcinoma invades major structures. Total or near-total excision of all the neoplastic tissue, followed by chemotherapy and radiation therapy, will provide the best option for long-term survival. Long-term survival with this carcinoma can be 1 or 2 years, as most patients succumb to the tumor in a period of months.

The types of anaplastic carcinoma are the very aggressive giant spindle cell variety and those that can be classified as small or large cell lymphomas.[55] Immunohistochemical analysis will often aid in the differentiation of these tumors.[56]

Metastatic Lesions

Metastatic lesions that can present as a thyroid nodule include melanoma, renal cell carcinoma, carcinoma of the lung, carcinoma of the breast, and other carcinomas or sarcomas. While taking the history it is important to query the patient about prior medical conditions that could have been malignant. We have seen melanoma metastasize as long as 35 years after initial treatment. In this case, the patient had forgotten about the skin lesion that had been excised so long ago; it was not until an in-depth discussion of his past medical history that his wife remembered the original event.

COMPLICATIONS OF THYROID SURGERY[57–59]

Wound Complications

These are exceedingly rare, usually related to edema of the flaps and a small hematoma. Infections are unusual unless the operation is being performed on an infected gland. With the use of suction drains, fluid collections that can lead to infections are minimized. When infection does occur, culture and sensitivity tests, wound drainage, and the administration of antibiotics are appropriate treatment.

Hemorrhage

This is probably the most life-threatening complication of thyroid surgery. Its occurrence is unusual when a meticulous technique is adhered to during surgery. The hemorrhage can be either arterial or venous in origin, and it usually occurs immediately after the patient awakens from anesthesia (which is when coughing and straining are most commonly seen) or within the first 8 hours after surgery. The symptoms of neck swelling, stridor, tightness of the neck, and hypoxia are usually present with hemorrhage. It is worthwhile to have a tracheostomy set at the bedside or nearby so the wound can be quickly opened and the bleeding controlled under aseptic conditions. When there is time, the patient should be returned to the operating room, where the wound can be explored while the patient is under anesthesia and in a sterile environment. To avoid hemorrhage, double ties of nonabsorbable sutures are placed on all major arteries and veins during surgery. Postoperatively, the patient is placed in a head-up position, without the application of occlusive dressings (which may obscure the impending crisis). With the use of suction drains (which are not a substitute for careful technique) that are removed when the wound drainage is less than 20 cc over a 24-hour period, serum accumulations are minimized.

Nerve Paralysis

The recurrent laryngeal nerve is the nerve most often injured during thyroid surgery. Cardiothoracic surgery around the aortic arch has replaced thyroid surgery as the most common cause of recurrent laryngeal nerve injury. Unplanned injury to the recurrent laryngeal nerve should occur in approximately 1% or less of patients undergoing thyroid surgery by experienced head and neck surgeons.

Injury to the superior laryngeal nerve is less often recognized and occurs less frequently. The best method of avoiding damage to this nerve and its external branch—which supplies the cricothyroid muscle and causes tensing of the vocal cord—is to isolate the superior pole vessels and individually ligate them as they enter the upper pole of the thyroid gland.

Injury to the recurrent laryngeal nerve can be minimized by identifying the nerve inferiorly and following it superiorly to where it enters the cricothyroid membrane. In this fashion, a right nonrecurrent laryngeal nerve is more easily identified as it crosses either anterior or posterior to the common carotid artery above or below the inferior thyroid artery. Associated with the most common vascular abnormality would be a dorsal origin of the right subclavian artery from the aortic arch. Another surgical principle is not to disturb any branches of the recurrent laryngeal nerve on its way to entering the larynx, as there can often be two or more major divisions of the nerve extralaryngeally that need to be dissected and preserved.

If the nerve is damaged during operation, an immediate end-to-end reanastomosis can be done or the ansa hypoglossi can be anastomosed with the distal end of the severed nerve. When bilateral nerve injury occurs, the patient has marked airway retraction, and tracheotomy is necessary. The long-term management of vocal cord paralysis is with thyroplasty, polytef (Teflon) paste injections, reinnervation procedures, and electrical pacing. (These are not discussed in this chapter.)

At the authors' institution, patients undergoing thyroid surgery also routinely undergo direct laryngoscopy at the conclusion of surgery as the endotracheal tube is removed, in order to document vocal cord mobility. If paralysis is noted a week or so later, it is more likely to be of a temporary nature.

Hypoparathyroidism

During thyroid surgery, the parathyroid glands can be injured, devascularized, or removed. The parathyroids are identified, and the inferior thyroid artery—the major source of nourishment to both the superior and inferior glands—is preserved; its branches are ligated as they enter the substance of the thyroid gland. When clinical conditions do not permit use of this technique, as when so-called midline clean-out is performed for extensive carcinoma, the parathyroids are dissected off the specimen on a back table. A biopsy is then taken to ensure that it is parathyroid tissue, and the parathyroid is autotransplanted.

The incidence of hypoparathyroidism ranges from 1% to 30% in patients undergoing total thyroidectomy, and its occurrence is indirectly proportional to the experience of the surgeon.

The symptoms of hypoparathyroidism include anxiety and paresis, as well as numbness of the fingers, toes, and lips. Chvostek's or Trousseau's sign may be present if the calcium level is low enough. With severe hypocalcemia, carpopedal spasm, laryngeal stridor, convulsions, and death can occur. Treatment should begin before severe symptoms occur. Depending on the degree of damage to the parathyroids, hypocalcemia usually develops within 24 to 72 hours after surgery. Acute treatment is completed with the intravenous use of 10% calcium gluconate, which is stocked in 10 cc vials and contains one gram of calcium per vial. The usual dose used in cases of severe damage is 6 to 12 grams per day

in divided doses every six hours, diluted in 100 cc of saline or dextrose in water and given over a 45-minute period. The patient is started as soon as possible on oral supplements and calciferol (vitamin D), which enchances the absorption of calcium. Daily serum calcium (ionized) determinations are obtained and monitored closely until supplementation is no longer necessary.

Hypothyroidism

Myxedema is expected after all total thyroidectomies, so administration of levothyroxine is begun postoperatively. In older patients, and in patients with a cardiac history, the initial dose is low, with gradual increments every 3 weeks until the lowest dose that will maintain a normal T_4 level and a low TSH blood level is reached. Usually this is 0.12 to 0.15 mg. High doses of levothyroxine are no longer used, because they seem to enhance osteoporosis and demineralization of the skeleton, especially in younger patients.

In the surgical management of hyperthyroidism when less than a total thyroidectomy is performed, the size of the remnant determines function. To avoid recurrent hyperthyroidism and the need for secondary operations or use of radioactive iodine, 1 to 2 gram remnants of thyroid tissue on either side as described by some surgeons may lead to a lesser number of recurrences.

Decreased thyroid function occurs after laryngectomy, partial thyroidectomy, and postoperative radiation. It also occurs in all patients who have been followed for 10 years after radioactive iodine therapy.

The symptoms of hypothyroidism are myriad: intolerance to cold; thickness and dryness of the hair and skin; edema of the face, eyelids, and hands; tendency to be overweight; feeling weak and tired; and sometimes cardiomegaly, bradycardia, and cardiomyopathy. For the otolaryngologist and head and neck surgeon, sleep apnea and obesity hypoventilation syndromes have been associated with hypothyroidism. Serum studies should be obtained to define thyroid function, because patients who are hypothyroid often dramatically improve with thyroid replacement therapy and weight loss. Hearing loss, both conductive and neurosensory, can be seen, and patients may have tinnitus and vertigo. Nasal obstruction secondary to turbinate enlargement can also be seen. Some patients with hypothyroidism have hoarseness of the voice and thickened vocal cords. Two syndromes associated with hypothyroidism that otolaryngologists may encounter are Pendred's syndrome (which is autosomal recessive and associated with goiter and deafness of a neurosensory variety) and Ascher syndrome (an autosomal dominant condition characterized by a nontoxic nodular goiter, blepharochalasis, and a double lip deformity).

POSTOPERATIVE FOLLOW-UP OF PATIENTS UNDERGOING THYROID SURGERY

Follow-up evaluation of patients with differentiated thyroid carcinoma includes monitoring of serum thyroglobulin and TSH levels, total body scans, chest x-rays, and other studies as clinically indicated.

The measurement of serum thyroglobulin is helpful in the detection of recurrent disease in differentiated carcinoma of the thyroid when total thyroidectomy has been the surgical treatment utilized. All patients are placed on levothyroxine postoperatively after ablation with I_{131}—or before if the I_{131} therapy is not going to be used. In this setting the discriminatory value of thyroglobulin measurement is greatest because thyroxine will suppress TSH secretion (thyrotropin). Thyroglobulin is released from normal thyroid in response to TSH stimulation, and when TSH is low one would expect the thyroglobulin to be low. Patients who have low TSH levels and high thyroglobulin levels most likely have recurrent thyroid carcinoma.[60]

REFERENCES

1. Ingbar S. The thyroid gland. In: Williams RH, ed. *Textbook of Endocrinology,* 6th ed. Philadelphia: WB Saunders; 1981:117–247.
2. Nelson JC, Tomei RT. Direct determination of free thyroxin in undiluted serum by equilibrium. *Dialysis/Radioimmunoassay Clin Chem.* 1988; 34:1737–1744.
3. Surks MI, Chopra IS, Nicoloff JT, et al. American Thyroid Association guidelines for use of laboratory tests in thyroid disorders. *JAMA.* 1990; 263:1529–1532.
4. Brown JS, Steener AL. Medullary thyroid carcinoma and the syndromes of MEN. *DM.* 1982; 28:1–37.
5. Schwartz MR. Pathology of the thyroid and parathyroid glands. *Otolaryngol Clin North Am.* 1990; 23:175–212.
6. Hamming JF, Goslings BM, Van Steenis GJ. The value of fine needle aspiration biopsy in patients with nodular thyroid disease divided into groups of suspicious of malignant neoplasms on clinical grounds. *Arch Intern Med.* 1990; 150:113–116.
7. Keller MP, Crabbe MM, Norwood SH. Accuracy and significance of fine needle aspiration and frozen section in determining the extent of thyroid resection, *Surgery.* 1987; 101:632–635.
8. Andersen JB, Webb AJ. Fine needle aspiration biopsy and the diagnosis of thyroid cancer. *Br J Surg.* 1987; 74:292–296.
9. Miller JM, Hamburger JI, Kini SR. The needle biopsy diagnoses of papillary thyroid carcinoma cancer. *Cancer.* 1981; 48:989–993.
10. Von Zuidewijn R. Thyroid surgery: Preoperative tests. *World J Surg.* 1994; 18:505–511.
11. Clark OH. TSH suppression in the management of thyroid nodules and thyroid cancer. *World J Surg.* 1981; 5:39–47.
12. Rosen IB, Wolfish PG, Miskin M. The ultrasound of thyroid masses. *Surg Clinics North Am.* 1979; 51(1):19–33.
13. Studer H, Romelli F. Simple goiter and its variants: Euthyroid and hyperthyroid multinodular goiters. *Endocrine Rev.* 1982; 3:40–61.
14. Seiler CA, Gloser C, Wagner HE. Thyroid gland surgery in an edemic region. *World J Surg.* 1996; 20:593–597.
15. Clark O. *Hyperthyroid: Endocrine Surgery of the Thyroid and Parathyroid Glands.* St. Louis: Mosby; 1985:104–144.
16. Harvey HK. Diagnosis and management of the thyroid nodule. *Otolaryngol Clinics North Am.* 1990; 23:303–333.
17. Bondeson L, Ljungberg O. Occult papillary thyroid carcinoma in the young and aged. *Cancer.* 1984; 53:1790–1793.
18. Zimmerman D, Hay ID, Gough JR, et al. Papillary thyroid carcinoma in children and adults: Long-term following of 1039 patients. *Surgery.* 1988; 104:1157–1166.
19. LoQuaglia MP, Gorbally MT, Heller G, et al. Recurrence and morbidity in differentiated thyroid carcinoma in children. *Surgery.* 1988; 104:1149–1156.
20. Robbins J, Marino M, Norton J, et al. Thyroid cancer: A lethal endocrine neoplasm. *Ann Intern Med.* 1991; 115:133–146.
21. McConahey WM, Hay ID, Woolner CB, et al. Papillary thyroid cancer treated at the Mayo Clinic—1946–1970. Initial manifestations, pathologic findings, therapy and outcome. *Mayo Clin Proc.* 1986; 61:978–996.
22. Noguchi S, Noguchi A, Murakami N. Papillary carcinoma of the thyroid: Developing pattern of metastases. *Cancer.* 1970; 26:1053–1060.
23. Mazzaferri EL, Young RL, Oertel JE, et al. Papillary thyroid carcinoma: The impact of therapy in 576 patients. *Medicine.* 1977; 56:171–195.
24. Noguchi S, Noguchi A, Murakami N. Papillary carcinoma of the thyroid: Value of prophylactic lymph node excision. *Cancer.* 1970; 26:1061–1064.
25. Chonkich GD, Petti G. Treatment of thyroid carcinoma. *Laryngoscope.* 1992; 102:486–491.
26. Rossi RL, Cody B, Silverman ML, et al. Surgically incurable well differentiated thyroid carcinoma—Prognostic factors and results of therapy. *Arch Surg.* 1988; 123:569–574.
27. McHenry C, Lawrence AM, Paloyan E, et al. Improving postoperative recurrence rates for carcinoma of the thyroid gland. *Surg Gynecol Obstet.* 1989; 169:429–434.
28. Donohue JH, Goldfein SD, Miller TR, et al. Do the prognoses of papillary and follicular thyroid carcinoma differ? *Am J Surg.* 1984; 148:168–171.
29. Grant CS, Hay ID, Ryan JJ, et al. Diagnostic and prognostic utility of flow cytometric DNA measurements in follicular thyroid carcinomas. *World J Surg.* 1990; 14:283–290.
30. Beenken S, Guillamondegui O, Shallenberger R, Knapp C, Ritter D, Goepfert H. Prognostic factors in patients dying of well-differentiated thyroid cancer. *Arch Otolaryngol Head Neck Surg.* 1989; 115:326–330.
31. Hay ID. Prognostic factors in thyroid carcinoma. *Thyroid Today.* 1989; 12:1–9.
32. Segal K, Arad A, Lubin E, et al. Follicular carcinoma of the thyroid. *Head Neck.* 1994; 16:533–538.
33. Freitas JE, Gross MD, Ripley S. Radionuclide diagnoses and therapy of thyroid cancer: Current status report. *Semin Nucl Med.* 1985; 15:106–130.
34. Romanna L, Waxman AD, Brachman MB, et al. Treatment rationale in thyroid carcinoma—Effect of scan dose. *Clin Nucl Med.* 1985; 10:687–689.
35. Young RL, Mazzaferri El, Rahe AJ. Pure follicular thyroid carcinoma: Impact of therapy in 214 patients. *J Nucl Med.* 1980; 21:733–737.
36. Hawk WA, Hazard JB. The many appearances of papillary carcinoma of the thyroid. *Cleveland Clin Q.* 1976; 43:207–216.
37. Terpy JH, St. John SA, Karkowski FJ, et al. Tall cell papillary thyroid cancer: Incidence and prognosis. *Am J Surg.* 1994; 168:459–461.
38. Johnson TL, Lloyd RV, Thompson NW, et al. Prognostic implications of the tall cell variant of papillary thyroid carcinoma, *Am J Surg Pathol.* 1998; 12:22–27.
39. Watson RG, Brenan MD, Goellner JR, et al. Invasive Hurthle cell carcinoma of the thyroid: Natural history and management. *Mayo Clin Proc.* 1984; 59:851–855.
40. Davis NL, Gordon M, Robins RE, et al. Clinical parameters predictive of malignancy of thyroid follicular neoplasms. *Am J Surg.* 1991; 161:567–569.
41. McLeod MK, Thompson NW, Hudson JL, et al. Flow cytometric measurements of nuclear DNA and ploidy analysis in

Hurthle cell neoplasms of the thyroid. *Arch Surg.* 1988; 123: 849–854.

42. Eisenberg BL, Hensley SD. Thyroid cancer with coexistent Hashimoto's thyroiditis. *Arch Surg.* 1989; 124:1045–1048.

43. Walker RP, Paloyan EP. The relationship between Hashimoto's thyroiditis, thyroid neoplasia and primary hyperparathyroidism. *Otolaryngol Clin North Am.* 1990; 23:291–302.

44. Chaudhary RK, Barnes EL, Myers EN. Squamous cell cancer arising in Hashimoto's thyroiditis. *Head Neck.* 1994; 16:582–585.

45. Lee KY, Lore JM, Miller PS. Management of the mass in the thyroid. *Adv Otolaryngol Head Neck Surg.* 1987; 1:261–294.

46. Ozaki O, Kunichiko I, Mimura T, et al. Thyroid carcinoma after radioactive iodine therapy for Graves' disease. *World J Surg.* 1994; 18:518–521.

47. Hazard JB, Hawk WA, Crile G. Medullary carcinoma of the thyroid: A clinical pathologic entity. *J Clin Endocrinol Metab.* 1959; 19:152–160.

48. Shapiro MJ. Medullary carcinoma of the thyroid gland. *Laryngoscope.* 1976; 86:1375–1385.

49. Wells S. New approaches to the patient with medullary carcinoma. *Thyroid Today.* 1994; 17:1–9.

50. Kodama T, Okamoto T, Fujimoto Y, et al. C-cell adenoma of the thyroid: A rare, but distinct entity. *Surgery.* 1988; 104:997–1003.

51. Brown JS, Steiner AL. Medullary thyroid carcinoma and the syndromes of MEN. *DM.* 1982; 28:1–37.

52. Block MA. Clinical characteristics distinguishing hereditary from sporadic medullary carcinoma treatment implications. *Arch Surg.* 1980; 115:142–149.

53. Saman NA, Schultz PN, Hickey RC. Medullary thyroid carcinoma: Prognosis of familial vs sporadic disease and the role of radiotherapy. *J Clin Endocrinol Metab.* 1988; 67:801–805.

54. Bakamjian V, Finley RK, Tan RK, et al. Anaplastic carcinoma of the thyroid: A 24 year experience. *Head Neck Surg.* 1995; 17: 41–48.

55. Rogers JD, Lindberg RD, Strattonhill C, et al. Spindle and giant cell carcinoma of the thyroid: A different therapeutic approach. *Cancer.* 1974; 34:1328–1332.

56. Holting T, Moller P, Tschahargone C, et al. Immunohistochemical reclassification of anaplastic carcinoma reveals small and giant cell lymphoma. *World J Surg.* 1990; 14:291–295.

57. Petti GH. Thyroid and parathyroid. In: *Otolaryngology and Head and Neck Surgery.* Meyerhoff W, Rice D, eds. Philadelphia: WB Saunders; 1992:770–791.

58. Wartofsky L. Osteoporosis: A growing concern for the thyroidologist. *Thyroid Today.* 1988; 11:1–11.

59. Falk SA, Birken EA, Baran DT. Temporary postthyroidectomy hypocalcemia. *Arch Otolaryngol Head Neck Surg.* 1988; 114:168–174.

60. Harvey RD, Matheson NA, Grabowski PS, et al. Measurement of serum thyroglobulin is of value in detecting tumor recurrence following treatment of differentiated thyroid carcinoma. *Br J Surg.* 1990; 77:324–326.

II. THYROID GLAND PATHOLOGY

■ KATHLEEN T. MONTONE
■ VIRGINIA A. LIVOLSI

CONGENITAL ABNORMALITIES

Thyroid Development

Embryologic development of the thyroid gland commences in the second to third gestational week and ends by the eleventh week of gestation.[1-3] By 12 weeks, thyroid hormone is being produced by the gland. Glandular growth proceeds without maternal thyroid-associated proteins.[1] The thyroid develops from three pharyngeal bodies, one of which is medial (often referred to as the median anlage) and two others that are located laterally in the neck.

The median anlage develops from an invagination of pharyngeal endoderm located at the base of the tongue in the area of the foramen caecum and between the first two pharyngeal pouches. Develop-

ment occurs in close association with the fetal heart and great vessels.[1] The median anlage is attached to the tongue via the thyroglossal duct. The bilobed median anlage goes through several stages, which include enlargement, lobulation, and bifurcation prior to descent in front of the hyoid bone to its final position in the neck just anterior to the trachea. The gland, once in its final position, enlarges and expands both laterally and caudally. The thyroglossal duct then atrophies.

The development of the thyroid from the lateral anlage is controversial. It is known that the lateral thyroid develops from the branchial pouches. The controversy lies in which branchial pouch is responsible—the caudal end of pouch IV or pouch V.[1,4,5] The question arises whether or not humans have a fifth branchial pouch.[2] Some authors have chosen to use the term "fourth-fifth pouch" to explain the derivation of the lateral thyroid to escape this controversy.[3] Nevertheless, the lateral thyroid is derived from the ultimobranchial body, which arises as an outpouching of the lateral pharynx, but loses its connection to the pharynx after the seventh week of gestation.[1] This solid mass then interacts with the lateral superior areas of the expanding median anlage, and the structures combine to form the gland. The ultimobranchial body gives rise to the calcitonin-secreting parafollicular cell (C cells). It is uncertain whether this structure can differentiate into follicular epithelium. The persistence of the ultimobranchial body, as solid cell nests composed of a collection of stratified epithelial cells with focal cystic change and focal mucin production in close association with parafollicular cells, may be seen in up to 30% of carefully sectioned adult thyroid glands (Fig. 10–10).[3,6,7] Pyriform sinus fistulas are proposed to represent ultimobranchial body remnants or result from altered C-cell migration during thyroid development.[8]

Congenital abnormalities of the thyroid gland may be seen. Most commonly, developmental disorders are secondary to abnormal gland development, although glandular aplasia may be seen.

Thyroid Aplasia

Lack of complete thyroid development is extremely uncommon; however, partial agenesis has been reported. Approximately 100 cases of thyroid hemiaplasia have been reported in the world literature.[9–18] While lack of a thyroid lobe may be due to thyroid asymmetry, unilateral atrophy, inflammatory processes, thyroid maldescent, or surgical manipulation, most cases are believed to be congenital in nature due to lack of development of one of the lobes.[18] The development of thyroid hemiaplasia is believed to be secondary to anomalous bifurcation of the median anlage, and the isthmus is lacking in many reported cases. Interestingly, thyroid agenesis may be familial in nature and has been associated with many thyroid abnormalities—in particular Graves' disease, which has been reported in 30% to 50% of patients with clinical evidence of thyroid hemiaplasia.[12,19] However, the finding of Graves' disease in cases of hemiaplasia may be coincidental since the thyroids of euthyroid patients are not often studied by scinitigraphic studies.

Aberrant Thyroid Rests

Benign thyroid tissue can be identified in many extrathyroidal regions including head and neck and mediastinal sites. The majority of cases of ectopic thyroid tissue can be explained through the embryologic development of the gland. Ectopic tissue results from either lack of tissue resorption along the thyroglossal duct or from disordered migration of the thyroid tissue with inclusions developing in structures that grow in close association with the gland.[1] Failure of descent can be quite serious and can result in the formation of a mass of thyroid tissue in the base of the tongue, the trachea, and the larynx, as well as anywhere along the thyroglossal duct. Rests may be seen anywhere along the migration of the median anlage, as well as the ultimobranchial body complex. Ectopic tissue may be seen in the tongue, esophagus, larynx, and trachea and even within jugular-carotid lymph nodes and soft tissues of the neck.[1,20–38] Because of its close association with the development of the heart and great vessels, ectopic thyroid tissue has been described in close association with the aorta, within the pericardium, and even within the heart itself.[35,38]

Lingual thyroid tissue, although clinically quite rare, is a relatively common microscopic finding at autopsy. While lingual thyroid tissue may be asymptomatic, if the mass is large, serious respiratory distress may occur, especially in infants.[27,28] Histologically, lingual thyroid is characterized by the presence of normal thyroid follicles interdigitating with the skeletal muscle of the tongue. A desmoplastic response (a finding that would be seen in infiltrating carcinoma) should not be seen. Hypothyroidism has been reported as a rare complication in lingual thyroid.[26] Diagnosis of lingual thyroid by fine needle aspiration biopsy has been recently reported.[39] Thyroid tissue may also be ectopic in the trachea and larynx, and masses in these areas may also result in respiratory difficulties.[12,18,19] The most important clinical significance of finding thyroid in these areas is that the tissue may represent the only functioning thyroid in the patient. Appropriate imaging studies are therefore warranted prior to removal in order to avoid acute hypothyroidism in the post-surgical state. Carcinomas may occur in the thyroid in the aberrant locations. This is rare, however, and most reported cases have been poorly doc-

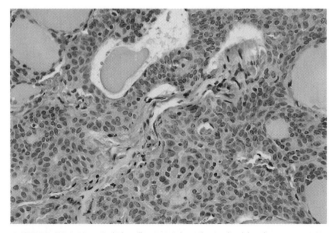

FIGURE 10–10 Solid cell nests (ultimobranchial body remnants) within the thyroid gland. Note the "squamoid" appearance to the nests.

umented, with the exception of carcinoma arising in the thyroglossal duct (discussed later).[28,30]

Solid cell nests may be located within the thyroid gland or even outside the gland in the neck. These nests are believed to be remnants of the ultimobranchial body complex.[3,6,7,40–44] As would be expected, the nests are located in the posterior medial portion of the lateral thyroid lobes. Solid cell nests may be present in one third of carefully sectioned thyroid glands. Histologically, the nests are characterized by the presence of epidermoid-like cells that focally may show lumen or cyst formation. Intermixed with the epidermoid cells are PAS-positive mucinous cells. Immunohistochemical studies have shown that the nests may contain carcinoembryonic antigen and high-molecular-weight cytokeratin.[40,44] In addition, calcitonin immunoreactivity (most likely from the presence of C cells) has been reported.[40,44] It has been proposed that solid cell nests give rise to thyroidal mucoepidermoid carcinomas, but this latter point is controversial.[45–48]

The development of the thyroid gland takes place with other pharyngeal or branchial cleft structures; parathyroid, thymus, and (rarely) salivary gland tissue may be detected within the gland capsule and parenchyma (Fig. 10–11). In addition, these inclusions may give rise to neoplastic lesions in the thyroid.[2,3,41,49] Mesenchymal tissues such as adipose tissue, skeletal muscle, and cartilage may all be seen within the glandular capsule.[49]

Thyroid Inclusions within Lymph Nodes

Neck lymph nodes containing benign-appearing thyroid tissue should be evaluated with caution. Some authors believe that any lymph node with thyroid tissue present within represents metastatic thyroid

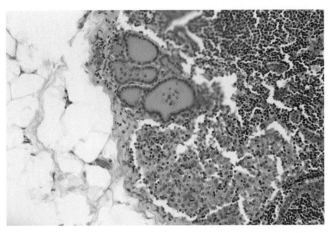

FIGURE 10–12 Benign thyroid inclusion within a capsule of a neck lymph node. Benign thyroid inclusions can be seen in the capsule of medial neck lymph nodes, but thyroid tissue in nodes lateral to the sternocleidomastoid muscle represents metastatic thyroid carcinoma until proved otherwise (H and E stain, original magnification × 33).

carcinoma; however, others believe that lymph nodes medial to the jugular vein may contain benign thyroid inclusions within the capsule (Fig. 10–12).[23–25,36] These inclusions must appear like normal thyroid tissue without nuclear abnormalities, psammoma bodies, or papillary groups in order to be considered benign. While normal thyroid tissue may be present within the lateral neck, particularly in patients with goiter or a previous history of neck surgery.[21,22] There is no dispute, however, that the presence of thyroid tissue—no matter how benign-appearing—within lymph nodes lateral to the internal jugular vein must be considered metastatic papillary thyroid carcinoma.[49]

Thyroglossal Duct Cysts

The developing thyroid maintains its connection to the foramen caecum through the thyroglossal duct. After the gland descends to its final position in the neck, the duct atrophies. However, the duct may persist and become cystic in nature. The development of a cyst may lead to a mass lesion requiring surgical removal. The thyroglossal duct is lined by a thin layer of cuboidal epithelium that may undergo squamous metaplasia, particularly in inflamed cysts. Thyroid tissue is present within the wall of over 60% of cysts (Fig. 10–13).[49]

Malignancies may develop in thyroglossal duct cysts. Interestingly, the tumors arise in association with the thyroid tissue and not the cyst lining. The overwhelming majority of thyroglossal duct carcinomas have been papillary carcinomas.[50–52] Rarely, other thyroid neoplasms have been reported, with the exception of medullary carcinoma, which, as expected, would not develop in this area, considering

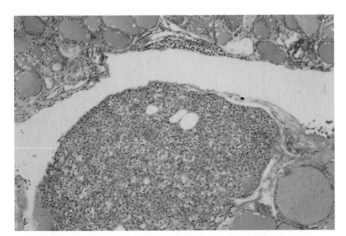

FIGURE 10–11 Histologic section of thyroid indicating the presence of intrathyroidal parathyroid tissue noted as an incidental finding in a patient with papillary thyroid carcinoma (H and E stain, original magnification × 33).

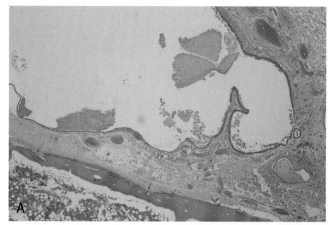

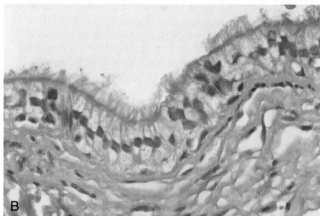

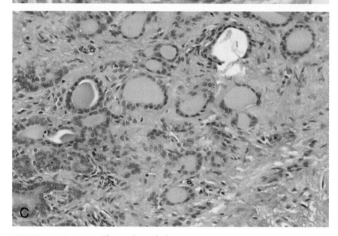

FIGURE 10–13 Thyroglossal duct cyst. *A,* Low-power examination of thyroglossal duct cyst in hyoid bone (H and E stain, original magnification × 6.6). *B,* High-power examination of the cyst wall shows a single layer of ciliated columnar epithelium (H and E stain, original magnification × 198). *C,* Identification of thyroid follicles within the cyst wall (H and E stain, original magnification × 66). Approximately 60% of thyroglossal duct cysts contain thyroid tissue.

the derivation of C cells is from the lateral neck.[49,53] If the diagnosis of papillary carcinoma is made in a thyroglossal duct, the possibility of a metastatic lesion from the thyroid should always be entertained, and the normal thyroid should be evaluated clinically for mass lesions.

ANATOMY OF THE THYROID

Gross Anatomy

Grossly, the adult thyroid gland is an encapsulated bilobed lobulated structure connected in the midline by an isthmus. The normal location of the gland is anterior to the trachea. A pyramidal lobe protruding superiorly from the isthmus may be seen. This lobe is derived from the thyroglossal duct–associated thyroid tissue and is present in approximately 40% of the population.[49] The gland normally weighs approximately 14 to 25 grams; however, the reported weights are extremely variable and depend on gender, activity, hormonal status, individual size, and even iodine intake.[49] The gland is light brown to red in color and of a firm consistency. A thin capsule divides the gland into lobules.

Microscopic Anatomy

Microscopically the thyroid is composed of follicles, each lined by a single layer of thyroglobulin-producing flattened cuboidal cells that surround centrally located colloid (Fig. 10–14). Each follicle is surrounded by basement membrane. A fine capillary network is observed in between follicles. Small collections (three to five cells) of calcitonin-producing, neuroendocrine parafollicular cells (C cells) are situated in the confines of the basement membrane. These cells may be difficult to identify with standard H&E stains but may be readily detected by immunohistochemistry for calcitonin or by the argyrophil reactions that highlight the neuroendocrine granules present in the cytoplasm. While C cells may represent less than 1% of the human adult thyroid, they may occasionally form nodules in older patients. In addition, patients with familial medul-

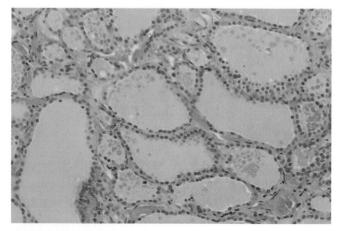

FIGURE 10–14 Histologic examination of normal thyroid showing follicles lined by a single layer of low cuboidal epithelium (H and E stain, original magnification × 66).

lary carcinomas or multiple endocrine neoplasia syndromes may show evidence of C-cell hyperplasia. (See later section on medullary carcinoma.) As mentioned previously, branchial cleft-derived tissues such as parathyroid, thymus, or salivary gland may be identified within the thyroid parenchyma. Solid cell nests as described above can be detected predominantly in the posterior aspects of the lateral lobes. These nests have been described as having a histologic appearance similar to endometrial morules or Walthard rests and are quite common.[49]

PATHOLOGIC EXAMINATION

Frozen Section Analysis

Prior to fine needle aspiration biopsy (FNAB), the most commonly used method for determining the correct surgical approach for a solitary thyroid nodule was frozen section analysis of the nodule. The nodule or the thyroid lobe was surgically removed and sent to the pathologist for evaluation. Depending on the results of the analysis, the surgical approach could be decided. The major problem with frozen section analysis of thyroid nodules is that it has limited utility. Most nodules can be adequately evaluated with FNAB prior to removal, and frozen section usually does not add any more information than determined by the FNAB.

Chen et al[54] analyzed 125 patients with a diagnosis of follicular lesion by FNAB. They observed that 87% of frozen sections were read as "follicular lesion, defer to permanent section." In 5% of cases an incorrect interpretation was given, and in only 3% of cases was the surgery altered as a result of frozen section. This group concluded that frozen section of follicular thyroid lesions provides little useful information for the surgeon. Crowe et al[55] observed that the diagnostic utility of frozen sections was poor for follicular lesions since 65% of the cases determined benign on frozen section were later diagnosed as carcinomas. This group also recommended that frozen sections of follicular lesions be deferred. Rodriguez et al[56] compared the utility of intraoperative frozen sections in patients who had undergone FNAB prior to surgery. They observed that frozen sections were most useful in lesions that were "suspicious" on cytology, but added little to those lesions that were initially called malignant or benign. In a similar study, McHenry et al[57] saw frozen section analysis as useful when the cytology diagnosis was "cellular," but not when the diagnosis was either benign or malignant. Gibb and Pasieka[58] suggest that frozen section is useful when a cytologic diagnosis of "suspicious for malignancy" is rendered, but intraoperative consultation is not necessary when a positive FNAB is obtained. On the other hand, Neale et al[59] insist that frozen section remains the best way to determine the surgical approach for follicular neoplasms. This group identified 40% of patients with follicular carcinoma at the time of frozen section.

The authors believe that frozen section analysis of thyroid lesions is of limited use particularly when a diagnosis of follicular lesion is made by FNAB. In order to differentiate follicular adenomas from carcinomas, careful examination of the lesional capsule is required, and this cannot be studied by FNAB or frozen section (Fig. 10–15). Frozen section analysis can be useful when the diagnosis of typical papillary carcinoma is in question and the surgeon has not performed a previous FNAB of the lesion. If the lesion is a papillary carcinoma, the surgeon can complete the thyroidectomy at the time of initial surgery. In addition, if FNAB is suspicious for follicular variant of papillary carcinoma, frozen section analysis may aid in diagnosis if nuclear changes, sclerosis, and/or psammoma bodies are identified (see Fig. 10–15).[60]

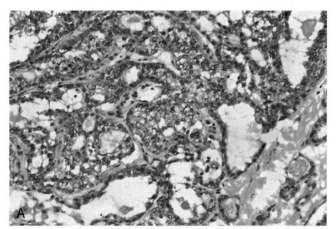

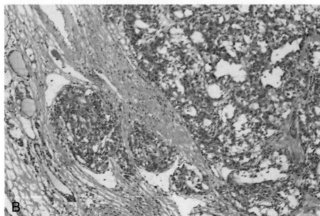

FIGURE 10–15 *A,* Original frozen section material showing a follicular neoplasm with nuclear features consistent with follicular variant of papillary carcinoma (H and E stain, original magnification × 132) *B,* Examination of this frozen section showed capsular and vascular invasion and could be interpreted as malignant (H and E stain, original magnification × 132). Frozen sections of thyroid follicular neoplasms often need to be deferred because diagnostic criteria are often not present or interpretable on frozen section.

Fine-Needle Aspiration Biopsy

Fine-needle aspiration biopsy (FNAB) has become an extremely useful screening procedure for evaluating the solitary thyroid nodule.[61–68] Other indications for thyroid FNAB include evaluation of diffuse goiter, screening for familial carcinomas, and drainage of colloid cysts.[61] This procedure is advantageous because it can be performed routinely in the physician's office at the patient's initial presentation, is widely accepted by patients, is cost-effective, has little if any morbidity, and in the long run has led to a decrease in the number of unnecessary thyroid surgeries. Several studies now indicate that FNAB has a better sensitivity, specificity, and accuracy for evaluating thyroid nodules than do ultrasound imaging and scintigraphy.[61,62] These studies are difficult to compare, however, because diagnostic criteria vary significantly among different groups, particularly in how investigators categorize patients with indeterminate or suspicious diagnoses. Nevertheless, most studies have found FNAB to be useful.

According to Rosai et al,[69] most cytology reports are placed into one of three diagnostic groups: probable benign nodule, follicular neoplasm/Hürthle cell lesion, or papillary carcinoma. The latter two would require surgery for definitive diagnosis and therapy, while the first category could be initially treated without surgical intervention. Reports of other benign and malignant disease entities have also been reported by fine needle aspiration and will not be detailed here.

While there are advantages of FNAB, there are disadvantages to the FNAB procedure:[70,71]

1. A negative or benign diagnosis by FNAB may need to be confirmed if the suspicion for malignancy is high, as in patients with a family history of MEN 2/medullary carcinoma, rapid growth of the lesion, involvement of surrounding structures, enlarged regional nodes, and evidence of distant metastases.
2. Aspiration of cystic lesions may lead to false negative diagnoses because papillary carcinomas may sometimes be cystic. If the appropriate cell types are not obtained in the cyst fluid, a correct diagnosis will not be made.[72]
3. A diagnosis of follicular or Hürthle cell carcinoma cannot be made by FNAB because these diagnoses rely predominantly on the presence of capsular and/or vascular invasion.
4. An inadequate specimen should not be interpreted as a negative specimen and should be repeated.
5. FNAB can alter the histologic appearance of the lesion, once resected, and these alterations can lead to misdiagnosis if these changes are not recognized by the pathologist. FNAB can result in lesional hemorrhage, sclerosis, necrosis, calcification, infarction (particularly in Hürthle cell lesions), papillary endothelial hyperplasia (the differential that includes the rare angiosarcoma), and entrapment of lesional cells in the lesional capsule.[73–78] These artifacts can be worrisome and should be interpreted with caution if the history involves FNAB. LiVolsi and Merino[78] coined the phrase "WHAFFT" ("worrisome histologic alteration following fine needle aspiration of the thyroid") and described several of these features that may be seen post-FNAB. The most worrisome features include pseudocapsular and pseudovascular invasion. FNAB can result in distortion of the capsule of a follicular lesion resulting in entrapment of lesional cells. This should not be misinterpreted as true capsular invasion. True invasion tends to bud or mushroom perpendicularly through the capsule, while pseudocapsular invasion is linear to the capsule. Capsular invasion may be difficult to ascertain in lesions that have undergone FNAB. The number of areas of invasion, the histologic appearance of the invasion, and invasion away from the area of the needle tract are all useful means for distinguishing true invasion from pseudoinvasion. FNAB can also result in the presence of lesional cells within vascular spaces. This finding should also be interpreted with caution, and true vascular invasion should be diagnosed only if the tumor cells are attached to the vessel wall or associated with thrombus formation. It should also be mentioned that post-FNAB artifact can interfere with frozen section interpretation, leading to overdiagnosis of pseudoinvasive foci as malignant (Fig. 10–16).
6. False-positive results may be obtained when aspirating hot nodules because these nodules may be hypercellular and show cytologic atypia; a diagnosis of follicular neoplasm may be given, necessitating surgical removal.
7. FNABs that contain normal thyroid tissue may be misinterpreted as microfollicular lesions and may promote unnecessary surgery.[79]

While there are disadvantages to FNAB, the advantages far outweigh them. The disadvantages are important mainly from the standpoint of the pathologist in order to avoid overcalling a lesion as a malignancy and therefore prohibiting unnecessary surgery.

Specimen Handling

Gross examination of the thyroid should be thorough prior to sectioning for histologic analysis. Examination should include weighing and measuring the gland, including measurement of each lobe, the isthmus, pyramidal lobe if present, and any nodules. The gland should be thoroughly analyzed for the presence of any parathyroid glands or lymph nodes that may have been removed with the surgery. In order to retain the orientation of the capsule, the external surface should be marked with ink. The gland should then be serially sectioned and any lesions described and appropriately measured. The

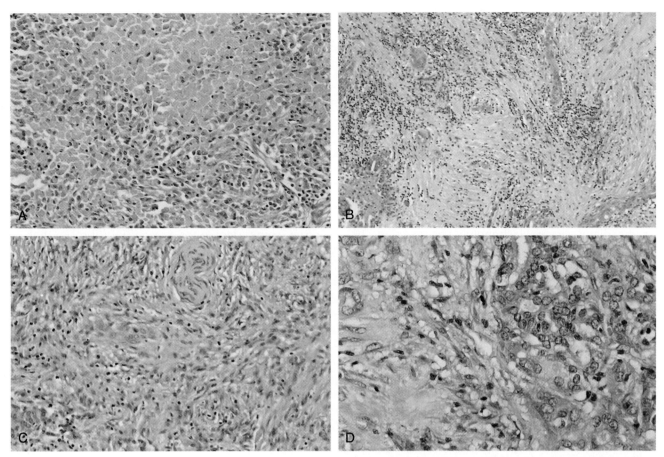

FIGURE 10–16 Fine needle aspiration biopsy of thyroid lesions may result in histologic alteration of the thyroid nodule. *A,* A common feature post-FNAB is lesional necrosis. This can be so extensive that the entire lesion appears necrotic (H and E stain, original magnification × 66). *B,* Low-power examination of this thyroid lesion that has previously undergone FNAB shows extensive fibrosis, inflammation, and entrapped thyroid follicles. The entrapped follicles should not be misinterpreted as carcinoma (H and E stain, original magnification × 33). *C,* This needled lesion shows a cellular response resembling that seen in nodular fasciitis (H and E stain, original magnification × 132). *D,* Clear cell nuclear change may be evident in thyroid follicular epithelium entrapped within and surrounding an FNAB site (H and E stain, original magnification × 132).

number of histologic sections examined appears to vary. For a distinct nodule at least one section per centimeter of lesion with the surrounding capsule should be taken. However, in large lesions, this may generate an excess number of histologic sections. In these cases, approximately 10 sections total is recommended, since this should suffice to identify significant capsular invasion if present.[80] Diagnostic reporting of malignant thyroid lesions should include tumor type, tumor extent, lymph node involvement, and margins.

AUTOIMMUNE THYROIDITIS

Classic Chronic Lymphocytic Thyroiditis (Hashimoto's Disease)

Classically, chronic lymphocytic thyroiditis is often referred to as Hashimoto's disease, an autoimmune thyroid disorder associated with hypothyroidism

and a distinctive histologic appearance. Some authors prefer to use the descriptive term "chronic lymphocytic thyroiditis with oxyphilic cells" for this entity because of the prominent Hürthle cell change that is characteristically seen in the thyroids from these individuals. Patients often demonstrate a variety of antibodies targeting thyroid- and nonthyroid-related proteins. Hashimoto's disease is seen most commonly in females who present with clinical hypothyroidism and goiter. Occasionally patients may present hyperthyroidism or show normal thyroid function.

Gross Pathology

Grossly, the gland is firm and symmetrically enlarged with weights ranging from 25 to 250 grams.[49,81] The glandular parenchyma takes on a tan-yellow color and has a "fish flesh" appearance because of the prominence of lymphocytes. Fibrosis in between the lobules may be grossly evident and may result in accentuation of the lobular architecture of the gland. The changes are diffuse, although nodule formation may occur.

Microscopic Pathology

Microscopically, the thyroid gland is diffusely infiltrated by a mononuclear cell infiltrate composed of lymphocytes, plasma cells, and immunoblasts.[49,81] This infiltrate is seen in the stroma in between the follicles and may even overrun existing follicles. Germinal center formation with evidence of tingible body macrophages is common. The thyroid follicles are often small, atrophic, and devoid of colloid. Hürthle cell metaplasia is often present, and some consider this to be one of the most important criteria for the diagnosis of Hashimoto's disease (Fig. 10–17). The Hürthle cells may show significant atypia with hyperchromatic nuclei, nuclear enlargement, and pleomorphism. In addition, the follicular cell nuclei may show clearing and focal overlapping. A diagnosis of papillary carcinoma may be enter-

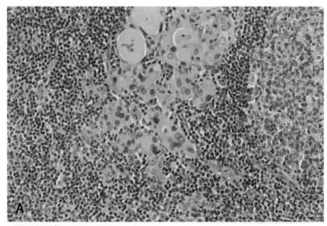

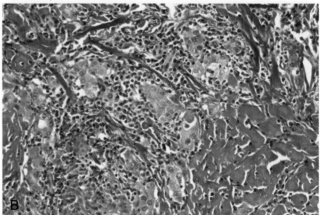

FIGURE 10–17 *A,* Photomicrograph of chronic thyroiditis with oxyphilic cells (Hashimoto's disease) showing lymphoplasmacytic reaction with germinal center formation and Hürthle cell metaplasia (H and E stain, original magnification × 66). *B,* Dense keloidal fibrosis, Hürthle cell change, and lymphocytic infiltrate are characteristically evident in fibrosing Hashimoto's disease (Trichrome stain, original magnification × 66).

tained, but the changes in Hashimoto's disease are multifocal, diffuse, and usually associated with inflammation. LiVolsi[49] has suggested that this nuclear change may reflect possible cytokine effect. Berho and Suster[82] analyzed thyroids from 12 patients with Hashimoto's thyroiditis and observed scattered multifocal follicular lesions with optically clear nuclei, intranuclear cytoplasmic inclusions, and occasional nuclear grooves, all features similar to the nuclear changes seen in papillary carcinoma. They state that when these nuclear changes are seen, they should be interpreted in the context of the case in order to prevent overdiagnosis of papillary carcinoma. Squamous metaplasia may be seen but is more prominent in the fibrous variant (discussed later). There is often some degree of interstitial fibrosis that can vary from focal to extensive.

The lymphocytic infiltrate is composed of B and T cells. Interestingly there is almost a 1:1 ratio of B to T cells (predominantly suppressor T cells).[49] This contrasts with the peripheral circulation, which normally shows a T-cell predominance (predominantly helper T cells). The B cells within the thyroid have a tendency to be of the IgG-kappa subclass.[83–85] Monocytoid B cells, a cell type often seen in autoimmune states, may be part of the B-cell infiltrate. Studies have revealed that apoptosis is likely to play a role in thyroid injury in Hashimoto's thyroiditis.[86]

The classic diagnosis of Hashimoto's thyroiditis involves the presence of:

1. Lymphoplasmacytic infiltrate with germinal center formation
2. Oxyphilic cell metaplasia
3. Atrophic thyroid follicles
4. Fibrosis

Infiltration alone of the thyroid by lymphocytes is not sufficient to make the diagnosis of autoimmune thyroiditis. Recently, Mizukami et al[87] developed a classification scheme for chronic lymphocytic thyroiditis. They studied over 600 cases and divided them into four groups:

1. Chronic thyroiditis, oxyphilic: This group refers to what has been classically called Hashimoto's thyroiditis, and most patients in this group are hypothyroid. Histologically, there is a diffuse lymphoplasmacytic infiltrate associated with Hürthle cell change and fibrosis.
2. Chronic thyroiditis, mixed: This group shows a lymphocytic infiltrate that is less than classic oxyphilic type and is associated with either normal follicles, hyperplastic follicles, or Hürthle cell change. Fibrosis is minimal. This histology may be associated with normo-, hyper-, or hypothyroidism.
3. Chronic thyroiditis, hyperplastic: These glands show hyperplasia of the follicular epithelium with only a focal lymphocytic infiltrate. The overwhelming majority of patients are hyperthyroid.

4. Chronic thyroiditis, focal: This group is characterized by only a focal mononuclear cell infiltrate and most patients are normothyroid.

This classification will be valuable for categorizing patients with chronic inflammatory cell infiltrates involving the thyroid, and it indicates that lymphocytic infiltration alone is not sufficient for a diagnosis of autoimmune thyroiditis.

Electron Microscopy

Ultrastructural examination of thyroid tissue from patients with Hashimoto's thyroiditis shows classic Hürthle cells containing a large number of mitochondria as well as poorly formed Golgi and decreased endoplasmic reticulum.[49] In addition, hyperplastic cells with Golgi, dilated endoplasmic reticulum, and normal mitochondria may also be observed. Studies have revealed electron-dense deposits along the basement of follicles, leading to speculation that these represent immune deposits.[88] This has been confirmed by immuno-EM studies that have detected IgG and complement in the follicular basement membranes.[89]

HASHIMOTO'S DISEASE AND RISK OF THYROID NEOPLASIA

It is well known that patients with autoimmune diseases have an increased risk for cancer development. Hashimoto's thyroiditis is no exception. Easily the most common malignancy encountered in patients with Hashimoto's disease is malignant lymphoma. In fact, almost all patients with primary thyroid lymphoma have a history of lymphocytic thyroiditis.[90–92] Chan et al[93] described a peculiar variant of mucoepidermoid carcinoma associated with prominent eosinophilia and sclerosis in patients with fibrosing Hashimoto's disease. An increased risk for plasmacytomas has also been suggested in patients with Hashimoto's disease.[94–97]

VARIANTS OF HASHIMOTO'S THYROIDITIS

Fibrosing Variant and Differential Diagnosis

The fibrosing variant of Hashimoto's thyroiditis represents about 10% of all cases of Hashimoto's disease.[83,98] This variant classically affects elderly patients. Grossly, the gland is enlarged and firm. Sectioning reveals a yellow to tan color and extensive fibrosis. Histologically, the atrophic gland is replaced by dense keloidal fibrosis that often contains a plasma cell infiltrate; however, the lobular architecture of the gland remains intact. The keloidal fibrosis surrounds areas of residual atrophic thyroid showing features of classic Hashimoto's disease (see Fig. 10–17). Extensive squamous metaplasia resembling morular metaplasia of the endometrium is often prominent and may actually represent hyperpla-

sia of ultimobranchial body rests. The fibrosing reaction is confined to the thyroid and does not involve the surrounding tissues. This latter finding is an extremely important point because it helps differentiate this variant of Hashimoto's from Riedel's disease.

Fibrous Atrophy of the Thyroid. Fibrous atrophy of the thyroid results from longstanding idiopathic myxedema. The gland typically weighs less than 5 grams and is not really recognizable as thyroid tissue. Histologically, the gland looks quite similar to that seen in the fibrosing variant of Hashimoto's disease. Knowledge of the clinical scenario is necessary to differentiate the two lesions on a histologic basis.

Riedel's Thyroiditis (Riedel's Disease, Riedel's Struma). While Riedel's disease has been considered a form of thyroiditis, the disease actually involves the thyroid (as well as other structures in the neck).[99–101] Riedel's disease is extremely rare and shows a female predominance. The majority of patients present with an enlarging painless goiter and difficulty in breathing. Because of the firm consistency and fixation to surrounding structures, the lesion is often clinically considered to be carcinoma. Riedel's disease can be confined to the neck but also may be associated with fibrosing lesions in other sites such as the mediastinum, retroperitoneum, and retroorbital areas.

Classically, Riedel's is characterized by infiltration of the thyroid and surrounding tissues including soft tissues, blood vessels, and nerves by a rock-hard tumor mass, which in some descriptions has the consistency of wood.[83,99–101] The surgeon often reports difficulty removing the gland and may not observe a recognizable tissue plane for dissection. Histologically, the lesion is characterized by dense fibrosis that is often keloidal and is associated with a lymphoplasmacytic infiltrate.[99–101] This fibrous tissue typically grows beyond the thyroid capsule to involve surrounding nerves, soft tissues, and blood vessels and has a growth pattern similar to that seen in fibromatoses. Total encasement of the parathyroids may be seen. A prominent feature is the presence of a phlebitis which is characterized by intimal hyperplasia, medial disruption, and thrombosis.[102] All of the microscopic findings are similar to those encountered in retroperitoneal fibrosis.[103,104]

The most difficult lesion from which to distinguish Riedel's disease is the fibrosing variant of Hashimoto's disease. Most importantly, Riedel's disease extends outside the thyroid while the fibrosing variant of Hashimoto's is confined to the gland. In addition, Riedel's disease shows a predominance of IgA lambda–light chain producing cells, while Hashimoto's characteristically is an IgG kappa–light chain predominant disease.[83] Riedel's is proposed to be autoimmune in origin, although this has yet to be proven.

Chronic Radiation Changes in the Thyroid. The thyroid gland may show findings similar to the fibros-

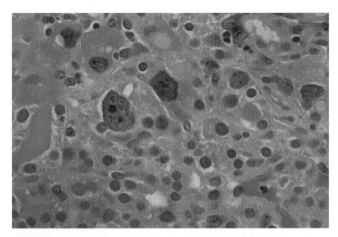

FIGURE 10–18 *Random follicular cell atypia in thyroid status post-radiation therapy (H and E stain, original magnification × 132).*

ing variant of Hashimoto's disease months to years after radiation to the neck, with the exception that nuclear atypia in the follicular cells and stromal cells may be more prominent following radiation, and vessels following radiation often show intimal thickening and medial sclerosis. These findings are typical to those seen with radiation damage in other sites. LiVolsi[49] outlines several changes encountered in the thyroid following radiation exposure (Fig. 10–18).

Hashitoxicosis

Occasionally, patients may present with the classic clinical symptoms of Graves' disease, but histologic examination of the thyroid shows changes of Hashimoto's disease. This disease entity which is often referred to as "Hashitoxicosis" or "hyperthyroiditis" is quite interesting and supports the possibility of an important relationship between these two autoimmune disorders.[105]

Juvenile Form of Chronic Lymphocytic Thyroiditis

In this variant, which occurs in young individuals, a lymphocytic infiltrate is prominent; however, Hürthle cells and glandular atrophy are not prominent.[106] Hyperplasia may be seen, and patients may have symptoms of Graves' disease. The disease is similar to what the Mayo Clinic has classified under "Hashitoxicosis."[105]

Graves' Disease (Diffuse Toxic Goiter)

This autoimmune-related thyroid disease is a common cause of hyperthyroidism in females. The disease results from antibodies that stimulate the TSH receptor, in turn stimulating the follicular epithelium to produce thyroid hormones. The disease is sys-

temic and affects the eyes and skin in addition to the thyroid. As with most other entities involving the thyroid, Graves' disease is seen predominantly in females. The possibility that cellular adhesion molecules play a role in the pathogenesis of Graves' disease has recently been proposed.[107]

Gross Pathology

Grossly the thyroid gland is symmetrically enlarged. Weights usually range from 50 to 150 grams. Sectioning through the gland reveals a deep red "meaty" thyroid tissue.

Microscopic Pathology

Microscopic examination reveals marked follicular hyperplasia. The follicles are usually devoid of colloid (in the untreated case) and lined by columnar cells with pale cytoplasm and large nuclei. If colloid is present within the follicles there is often scalloping along the edges of the colloid toward the epithelial surface. Due to constant stimulation of the gland by TSH-like antibodies, the follicular epithelium undergoes hypertrophy and hyperplasia to the detriment of the normal follicular architecture; the glandular tissue then forms papillary infoldings.[108] Even though these papillae may be occasionally associated with focal nuclear clearing (which is not as prominent as that seen in typical papillary carcinoma or even in Hashimoto's disease) and, rarely, psammoma bodies, these are not true papillae and should not be confused with papillary carcinoma, particularly since the changes are diffuse and not associated with sclerosis (Fig. 10–19).[109] In the stroma, a lymphocytic infiltrate with germinal centers is present. Both B and T cells make up this infiltrate. In contrast to Hashimoto's disease, helper T cells predominate.[110,111] Plasma cells are not a feature.

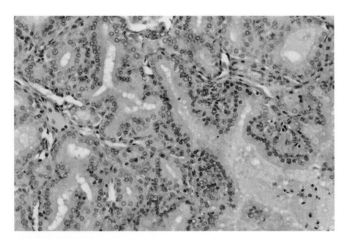

FIGURE 10–19 *Graves' disease (diffuse toxic goiter) showing diffuse follicular hyperplasia with pseudopapillae formation (H and E stain, original magnification × 132).*

Treatment with radioiodine often causes involution. The gland may revert to relatively normal architecture and then undergo atrophy and fibrosis. Significant cellular atypia may be noted in the remaining follicular epithelium.

GRAVES' DISEASE AND THE RISK OF THYROID NEOPLASIA

It remains controversial whether there is an increased risk of carcinoma developing in thyroids of patients with Graves' disease. Recent studies state papillary carcinoma occurs in approximately 2% to 4% of patients with Graves'.[112] This incidence is not significantly different from the incidence in the general population.

Other Hyperthyroid States

Occasionally, hyperthyroidism may be seen in patients with clinical evidence of nodular goiter. In these patients the histology is similar to that seen in Graves' disease; however, the changes are seen within nodules, not diffusely present throughout the gland. Hyperthyroidism may be seen rarely in patients with typical follicular adenomas or carcinomas. Other hyperthyroid states are rare and can be related to disorders affecting the pituitary/hypothalamus, gestational trophoblastic diseases, subacute thyroiditis, and struma ovarii as well as other disorders.

Acute Thyroiditis

Acute thyroiditis is extremely rare and most commonly results from involvement of the gland by infectious pathogens. The disease is thus usually encountered in immunosuppressed patients or in otherwise healthy patients following trauma to the gland. Clinically, patients present with painful enlargement of the gland. Grossly, the gland appears normal but may be soft or show distinct abscess formation. Microscopically, areas of acute inflammation and necrosis are present. A variety of pathogens including bacteria, fungi, viruses, and parasites may be seen (Fig. 10–20).[113–115] In addition, acute thyroiditis can be seen in the thyroid after recent exposure to radiation.

Granulomatous Thyroiditis

This entity may also be referred to as non-suppurative thyroiditis, subacute thyroiditis, or de Quervain's disease. Subacute thyroiditis is a rare entity that most commonly presents in females. A genetic predisposition has been proposed, and the disease has been associated with HLA Bw35.[116,117] In general, the granulomatous reaction is believed to result

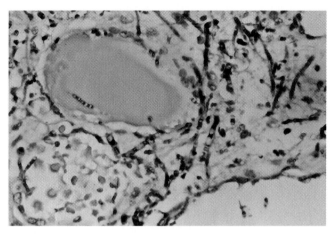

FIGURE 10–20 Acute thyroiditis secondary to *Aspergillus* at autopsy of an immunosuppressed transplant recipient with disseminated *Aspergillus fumigatus*. Organisms are highlighted by an in situ hybridization assay for *Aspergillus* rRNA (original magnification × 132).

from a systemic viral infection.[118,119] Most patients present with systemic findings such as fever, weakness, elevated erythrocyte sedimentation rate, abnormal thyroid function tests, and a painful neck mass (although pain may be absent). If a mass lesion in observed, biopsy is often necessary to rule out malignancy.

Grossly, the thyroid is asymmetrically enlarged and firm to palpation. Sectioning often reveals white nodules that may grossly resemble carcinoma.[81] The histologic appearance varies with the stage of the disease process. In the initial stages, the follicular epithelium degenerates, and thyroglobulin may leak into the circulation. Neutrophils followed by mononuclear cells, including lymphocytes and histiocytes, infiltrate the gland. A giant cell reaction ensues (Fig. 10–21). The giant cells most likely represent histiocytes;[81] however, the possibility that they represent a

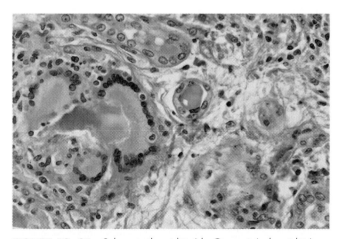

FIGURE 10–21 Subacute thyroiditis (de Quervain's thyroiditis). Note the granulomatous reaction with giant cell formation (H and E stain, original magnification × 132).

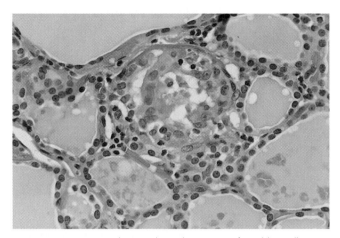

FIGURE 10–22 "Palpation thyroiditis" is manifested by collections of histiocytes and giant cells within the thyroid parenchymal. These changes are usually seen in surgically removed thyroids and most likely result from vigorous palpation. (H and E stain, original magnification × 132).

viral cytopathic effect in follicular epithelial cells has been proposed.[118,119] Following the inflammatory stage, fibrosis occurs. It may be focal or diffuse.

Palpation Thyroiditis

"Palpation thyroiditis" is a term used to refer to the histologic changes seen in the thyroid following minor trauma.[120] The majority of cases are observed in glands resected for other thyroid abnormalities and most likely result from physical examination of the gland. Histologically, the lesion is characterized by the presence of small groups of follicles showing focal replacement of the epithelium by mononuclear cells, predominantly histiocytes (Fig. 10–22). Focal hemorrhage and hemosiderin deposition may be seen. The lesions most likely regress. The differential diagnosis includes ultimobranchial body remnant and C-cell hyperplasia.

Other Causes of Granulomatous Thyroiditis

There are numerous other causes of granulomatous diseases in the thyroid including infections, malignancies, vasculitis, trauma, hypersensitivity, foreign material, or idiopathic (sarcoidosis). Please see for review of granulomatous disease in the thyroid. LiVolsi[49] gives a detailed outline of granulomatous thyroid diseases in a recent monograph.

THYROID NEOPLASMS

The thyroid gland may be involved by a variety of tumors, benign or malignant. By far, the majority of thyroid neoplasms are benign. While malignancies of the thyroid gland are fairly uncommon, they are of great interest because of their genetic predisposition, their association with external factors such as radiation, and their detection by minimally invasive procedures such as fine needle aspiration biopsy.

Papillary Thyroid Carcinoma

Papillary carcinoma is the most common thyroid gland malignancy, representing approximately 80% to 90% of all thyroid carcinomas. Despite being the most common thyroid carcinoma, papillary carcinoma is rare and constitutes approximately 1% of all malignancies diagnosed in the United States. However, the incidence appears to be much higher in autopsy studies where occult tumors (papillary microcarcinomas, discussed later) may be seen. The mortality rate for this lesion is extremely low. Papillary carcinoma is of interest because of its good prognosis despite a high incidence of intraglandular and lymph node metastases, its association with radiation exposure, and particular variants that behave in a highly aggressive fashion. This section will detail the pathologic aspects of the usual type of papillary carcinoma as well as many of the variants of this tumor.

Risk Factors

The etiology of papillary carcinoma is not completely understood, and most cases do not have a specific etiology; however, specific risk factors have been identified. Environmental, familial, racial, and genetic influences have been proposed.

Environmental. The development of papillary carcinoma in animals and humans has been associated with excess of iodine in the diet.[121–123] This increased incidence was noticed after the administration of iodine into areas where goiter was endemic.[121,122,124] In addition, a decrease in follicular carcinomas was also identified in these areas. Several dietary factors and chemical agents have been implicated in papillary carcinoma, but these have yet to be proven as etiologic risk factors for disease development.[125–130]

External Radiation. Exposure to radiation (either therapeutically or accidentally), particularly in childhood, is a known risk factor for papillary carcinoma development. The average time from exposure to tumor development is classically reported as 20 years; however, times for development have been reported within a few years after major nuclear facility accidents such as encountered in Chernobyl.

The accident in Chernobyl precipitated a significant rise in childhood papillary carcinomas in Belarus and Ukraine.[131,132] This increased risk was evident just 4 years after the accident that released significantly high amounts of I_{131} and short-lived radioiodines into the atmosphere. The amount of radioactive iodine released was far greater than any other nuclear accident in history. Interestingly, the therapeutic doses of I_{131} used for the treatment of thyroid malignancies or hyperthyroid states such as Graves' disease is not associated with increased risk of thyroid carcinomas. The majority of thyroid carcinomas encountered following the disaster in Chernobyl are papillary carcinomas, and many of them have been aggressive lesions, with over 50% showing extracapsular extension. In a recent study, Nikiforov et al[132] observed that many of the patients who developed thyroid carcinoma after the Chernobyl accident were under 1 year of age at the time of exposure. A decreasing incidence with increasing age at the time of the accident was noted in this study. This group also noted what they termed "micropapillary hyperplasia," the possible precursor to papillary carcinoma development.

Autoimmune Disease. Papillary carcinoma may also arise in association with autoimmune thyroid disease, although a statistically significant association has yet to be shown.[69]

Genetic Syndromes. Papillary carcinoma may arise in association with several genetic syndromes. Interestingly, associations with familial polyposis syndromes (Gardner's syndrome) and Cowden's syndrome have been reported.[133-137] While many of these lesions have been described as papillary carcinomas, recent reports have shown that these tumors have an unusual histology with cribriform and solid spindle cell lesions.[133] The association of papillary thyroid cancer with other familial syndromes awaits further study. In addition, the carcinomas reported in Cowden's syndrome are poorly documented and may be hyperplasias misinterpreted as carcinomas.

Gross Pathology

Grossly, papillary carcinomas are variable. Typical papillary carcinomas are usually clinically palpable and may be located anywhere within the gland. By definition, these lesions are larger than 1 cm, averaging in size between 2 and 3 cm, and may or may not have a capsule. Sectioning of the lesion reveals a tumor that is invasive, firm, and usually white in appearance. Calcifications are common and may be extensive, necessitating decalcification prior to histologic examination. Extensive sclerosis can be seen, and sometimes the lesion appears to be a scar. Cystic change may be apparent, but papillary carcinomas are rarely completely cystic without solid areas. Hemorrhage can be present, but necrosis should alert the pathologist to the possibility of a higher grade lesion.

Microscopic Pathology

Histologically, the usual type of papillary carcinoma is characterized by a papillary proliferation of thyroid epithelium associated with distinct nuclear changes (Fig. 10–23). The papillae are true papillae, consisting of a central fibrovascular core most com-

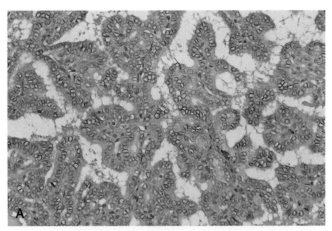
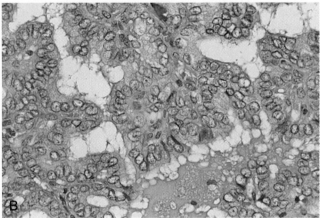

FIGURE 10–23 *A,* Usual type papillary thyroid carcinoma showing true papillae formation. Papillae are often arranged in a haphazard formation (H and E stain, original magnification × 66). *B,* Higher power shows typical nuclear change with nuclear enlargement, clearing, overlap, and grooves (H and E stain, original magnification × 132).

monly lined by a single layer of tumor cells. The most notable feature of papillary carcinoma is the nuclear changes. The nuclei of the tumor cells have been described as clear, pale, ground-glass, or even "Orphan Annie eyed."[49,69,138-143] The nuclear envelopes may be quite prominent. The nuclei are larger than normal follicular nuclei and often overlap one another. Occasional nucleoli may be evident. Close examination of the nuclei often reveals nuclear grooves and intranuclear inclusions.[49,69,139-145] Nuclear grooves are seen in almost all carcinomas, but taken alone are not diagnostic of this lesion, since many benign and malignant conditions may also have grooved nuclei (although usually to a lesser degree than seen in papillary carcinoma). Scopa et al[145] observed grooved nuclei in a variety of thyroid adenomas and carcinomas as well as in Hashimoto's thyroiditis, adenomatous hyperplasia, and diffuse hyperplasia. Most lesions showed fewer grooves than papillary carcinomas, but some lesions did show numerous grooves. Mitotic activity is often

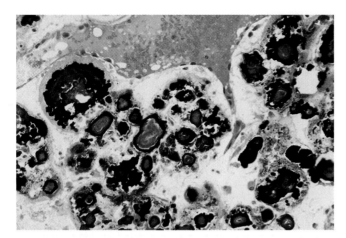

FIGURE 10-24 Numerous calcifications and psammoma bodies adjacent to a cystic papillary carcinoma (H and E stain, original magnification × 66).

minimal, although a high mitotic activity may be evident in more aggressive lesions and in the vicinity of a previous FNAB. The classic nuclear changes are seen in the majority of papillary carcinomas. Nuclear clearing, however, may be evident in benign conditions such as autoimmune thyroiditis (particularly Hashimoto's disease), although the other nuclear features, such as nuclear overlap and prominent nuclear envelopes, are often not fully developed in these benign conditions.

Psammomatous calcifications are a characteristic finding in papillary carcinoma and are present in about one half of the cases (Fig. 10-24).[49,69,139-143,146] These calcifications most likely represent the remnants of infarcted papillae. The psammoma body characteristically has a lamellated appearance and is found within the papillae or the surrounding stroma, but not within neoplastic follicles. It is critical that these calcifications be distinguished from the dystrophic calcifications seen so often in a variety of benign thyroid entities, which are not lamellated and are often large and irregular. Psammoma bodies are characteristic of papillary carcinoma. The presence of these calcifications within normal thyroid or within lymph nodes should alert the pathologist to search for a papillary carcinoma close by. While psammoma bodies may be seen in Graves' disease and Hashimoto's thyroiditis, if psammoma bodies are seen in these lesions, the tissue should be examined with caution in order to not miss an underlying carcinoma.[147,148]

Another prominent feature of papillary carcinoma is dense fibrosis.[49,69,139-143] Sclerosis can be so prominent, in fact, that the underlying carcinoma cells may be difficult to discern. Scarring within the thyroid should be carefully evaluated, since papillary carcinomas may undergo regressive changes. Other features that may be seen in papillary carcinoma include a lymphocytic infiltrate, follicular differentiation, squamous metaplasia, and solid areas. The le-

sions have become extensively cystic. In addition, cystic metastases to lymph nodes may be seen. Care must be taken not to misinterpret these lesions as branchial cleft cysts (Fig. 10-25). The lesion characteristically invades into the lymphatics. Extensive intraglandular spread throughout the lymphatics is a common finding and invokes the appearance of multiple small primaries within the gland. Lymph node metastases are very common and are seen in over 50% of patients at the time of tumor diagnosis.[49,69,139-143] Despite their presence, lymph node metastases do not usually alter the disease prognosis. Distant metastases to lung and bone have been described and are seen in about 5% of cases.[49,69,139-143]

Differential Diagnosis

The differential diagnosis of papillary carcinoma includes papillary hyperplasia, papillary hyperplastic nodule, and the papillary variant of medullary carcinoma. These differentials can be very difficult to distinguish from one another. Papillary hyperplasia is most commonly seen in Graves' disease. Due to overstimulation by TSH-like antibodies, the glandular epithelium undergoes hypertrophy and hyper-

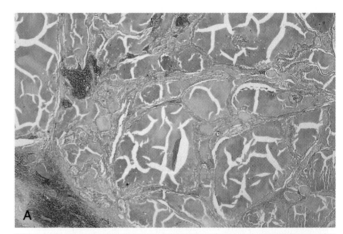

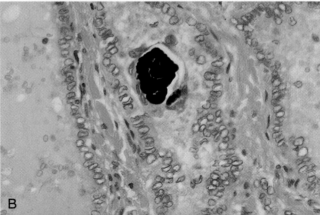

FIGURE 10-25 *A,* Low-power view of papillary cystic thyroid carcinoma. *B,* High-power examination must be undertaken to reveal the presence of typical papillary carcinoma nuclei.

plasia to the detriment of the normal follicular architecture, and the cells begin to form papillary infoldings. The papillae are differentiated from papillary carcinoma by the absence of a fibrovascular core. In addition, the papillary changes are usually diffusely present throughout the gland. The nuclei, while they may be enlarged, do not usually overlap and show the classic clearing seen in papillary carcinoma. Papillary hyperplasia may be evident within a follicular nodule. These nodules have a tendency to occur in children and young adults and consist of a well-circumscribed, encapsulated, partially cystic nodule associated with a papillary proliferation of follicular epithelium without the characteristic nuclear changes or psammoma bodies (Fig. 10–26). The papillary groups are usually avascular and edematous. In addition, LiVolsi[149] describes the papillae in these hyperplastic nodules as directed toward the nodules' center, a finding distinguishable from the haphazard arrangement of the papillae in papillary carcinoma. The papillary variant of medullary carcinoma is rare; it can be distinguished from

papillary carcinoma by the absence of characteristic nuclear changes and the presence of calcitonin by immunohistochemistry.

Ultrastructure

Ultrastructural examination of papillary carcinoma nuclei often shows dispersed chromatin and numerous folds in the nuclear membrane that often lack nuclear pores.[49,69,150,151] Microvilli are often present on the apical surfaces of the cells. Numerous lysosomes, mitochondria, and filaments are observed in the cytoplasm. Keratohyaline granules can be seen in areas of squamous metaplasia.

Immunohistochemistry

Almost 100% of papillary carcinomas show diffuse staining for thyroglobulin.[152] Most lesions stain for low-molecular-weight cytokeratins (CAM5.2) and may stain for high-molecular-weight cytokeratins (AE1/3).[153–157] High-molecular-weight cytokeratins are not typically present in thyroid epithelium. Their presence in papillary carcinoma may be useful for distinguishing this lesion from follicular lesions and papillary hyperplasia, with the exception of Hashimoto's thyroiditis, which can also react with antibodies to high-molecular-weight cytokeratins.[156]

Flow Cytometry/Chromosomal Studies

By flow cytometric analysis, most papillary carcinomas show diploid cell populations, although aneuploidy may be seen in approximately 20% of cases.[158–162] By univariate analysis, aneuploidy has been associated with a poor prognosis; however, multivariate analysis has shown that ploidy is not an independent prognostic variable. Distant metastases have been reported in many aneuploid papillary carcinomas, while only a small percentage of diploid tumors metastasize distantly.[158,159,162] However, most of the tumors in these studies have been associated with other variables that would place their tumors into a poorer prognosis category.

Karyotypic analysis has shown that tumors usually show no chromosomal abnormalities, although Jenkins et al[163] and Antonini et al[164] have shown abnormalities involving the long arm of chromosome 10 (which is interestingly the location of the ret proto-oncogene).

Prognostic Variables

All in all, the prognosis of papillary carcinoma is excellent, with a mortality rate of approximately 5%. Several clinical and pathologic prognostic indicators have been identified for papillary carcinoma.[49,69,139–143,149,165–176] Hay[168] described several of these variables and developed the mnemonic AGES, standing for age, grade (histologic), extent of tumor, and size of tumor. These four indicators appear to

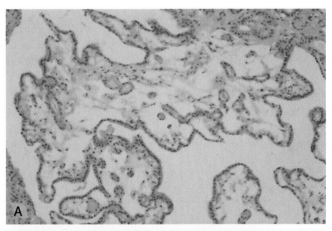

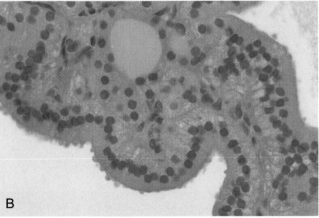

FIGURE 10–26 *A,* Low-power examination of a papillary hyperplastic nodule showing papillae with central edema. These are not true papillae (H and E stain, original magnification × 33). *B,* Higher power examination of a papillary group shows small round regular nuclei without nuclear clearing, enlargement, or significant overlap (H and E stain, original magnification × 100).

be the most important for determining patient outcome. Patients greater than age 50 have a poorer outlook than younger patients. In addition, papillary carcinoma in children and young adults is associated with a good outcome even in the presence of lymph node or distant metastases. Papillary carcinomas are usually considered to be low cytologic grade or well-differentiated tumors. If areas of dedifferentiation are observed, the prognosis is poorer. As would be expected, larger lesions behave in a more aggressive fashion, although small lesions may also do poorly. Gross, but not microscopic, extracapsular extension is also a poor prognostic sign. Carcangiu et al[141,142] describe variables associated with improved prognosis. These include encapsulation, growth with pushing borders, and cystic changes. Matsubayashi et al[177] indicate that the presence of a lymphocytic infiltrate surrounding or within the tumor is associated with a reduced incidence of recurrence and possibly a better prognosis. Pilotti[175] recently observed that patients with poorly differentiated forms of papillary thyroid carcinoma (tall cell, columnar cell, mixed tall cell–columnar cell) were more likely to have tumor recurrence and recurrence-related deaths.

Several studies employing Cox regression analysis to determine independent prognostic variables in papillary thyroid carcinoma are currently available. In a recent multivariate analysis study, Morena-Egea et al[178] observed that independent prognostic factors for patient survival included tumor size, extrathyroidal extension, and histopathologic subtype. Noguchi et al[176] observed different prognostic factors for men and women in a study evaluating more than 2100 patients. Factors important for predicting survival in men included age and the presence or absence of gross nodal metastases. Factors in women included these same two factors plus tumor size and the number of structures adhered to the gland. Based on these factors, this group divided patients into three prognostic groups (excellent, intermediate, poor).

Papillary Microcarcinoma and Variants

According to the WHO classification, papillary microcarcinoma is a term used for papillary carcinomas measuring 1 cm or less.[179] Use of the term "occult" is discouraged since this terminology does not indicate the lesional size. Other terms that have been used for these lesions include: occult sclerosing carcinoma, occult papillary carcinoma, and nonencapsulated sclerosing tumor. These lesions are commonly observed as incidental findings at autopsy or thyroidectomy for benign diseases and have been described in 4% to 36% of carefully evaluated autopsies.[180–190] In a recent study, Fink et al[190] identified papillary microcarcinoma in up to 24% of thyroids

removed for diseases other than follicular-derived carcinoma. This group also found that these incidental lesions were more commonly identified in males, a finding in contrast to clinically significant papillary carcinoma.

The fact that many micropapillary carcinomas are silent does not mean they have not developed the ability to metastasize both to lymph nodes and distantly.[191–198] These small carcinomas have been divided into two groups: *minute*, which refers to tumors less than 5 mm in diameter, and *tiny*, which refers to lesions between 5 and 10 mm in diameter.[186,199–201] Tiny lesions have a higher incidence of both lymph node metastases and extrathyroidal extension, although minute lesions may also metastasize. Distant metastases to bone, lung, and pericardium have been reported. Chan[143] uses the term "occult carcinoma" to describe those patients who present with metastases and are subsequently found to have a thyroid tumor. He then uses the term "latent papillary carcinoma" to refer to those patients identified as having carcinoma incidentally in thyroidectomy specimens or at autopsy.

Grossly, papillary microcarcinomas appear as small, white, sclerotic nodules that are usually present in the subcapsular area. Histologically, the lesions most often have a follicular architecture, but show typical papillary carcinoma nuclei (Fig. 10–27). Sclerosis may be dense.

FOLLICULAR VARIANT

The follicular variant of papillary carcinoma was initially described by Linsday.[202] It was then redescribed by Chen and Rosai,[140,143] after which it became recognized as a distinctive variant of this cancer.[202–208] It is difficult to ascertain the incidence of this neoplasm, because many cases have been (and are still being) classified as follicular carcino-

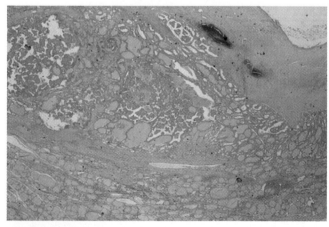

FIGURE 10–27 Occult sclerosing papillary carcinoma (papillary microcarcinoma), low-power view showing papillary growth, sclerosis, and a thick fibrous capsule with calcification (H and E stain, original magnification × 6.6).

mas despite the classic nuclear changes of papillary carcinoma that should be present to entertain this diagnosis.[208] These nonencapsulated lesions are characterized histologically by a predominant follicular pattern associated with the nuclear changes seen in papillary carcinomas (Fig. 10–28). The follicles vary from small to large (macrofollicular variant) and may show scalloping of the colloid; however, hyperthyroidism is not a feature.[209] Psammoma bodies, a desmoplastic response, and a prominent lymphoid reaction may be seen. These lesions may be multicentric and often show lymph node metastases that are papillary in configuration.[69,203,204] Lymphatic as well as vascular invasion may be identified.

The follicular variant of papillary carcinoma may be quite difficult to diagnose. The differential diagnosis includes adenomatous nodule, follicular adenoma, and follicular carcinoma. The identification of the classic nuclear changes—as well as sclerosis, psammoma bodies, and a lymphocytic reaction—lead to a diagnosis of follicular variant of papillary carcinoma. In addition, immunohistochemical staining with cytokeratins is similar to classic papillary carcinoma and differs from follicular carcinoma. The follicular variant of papillary carcinoma is often difficult to distinguish from true follicular neoplasms. Vascular and capsular invasion indicate malignancy, but it may still be difficult to determine if the lesion is papillary or follicular. Rosai and colleagues[69] propose that, when a lesion is clearly malignant but cannot be classified as follicular or papillary, it should be referred to as well-differentiated thyroid carcinoma, not otherwise specified. This same group also proposed a three-category schematic for follicular lesions:

1. Follicular variant of papillary carcinoma: Follicular lesions containing a small, easily recognized focus of papillary carcinoma, arising in what appears to be a hyperplastic nodule. Close inspection reveals diffuse papillary carcinoma nuclei.
2. Follicular variant of papillary carcinoma arising in follicular adenoma: Focus of papillary carcinoma within a follicular nodule without classic nuclear change. These lesions are extremely rare.
3. Follicular adenoma: Follicular neoplasm with some focal nuclear clearing but no other features of papillary carcinoma.

DIFFUSE FOLLICULAR VARIANT/ ENCAPSULATED FOLLICULAR VARIANT

Sobrinho-Simoes et al[210] reported a rare lesion (with only eight reported cases), which they referred to as the diffuse follicular variant. Patients, who are usually female, present with a diffuse bilateral goiter and may be associated with hyperthyroidism. The gland is so diffusely replaced by the follicular variant of papillary carcinoma that a distinct mass lesion may not be seen. Of the eight patients in the study, most had lymph node and distant metastases. Two patients died of disease, while the remaining six responded to radioactive iodine therapy. While this variant appears to be aggressive, more cases must be examined to make any conclusions about this rare subtype. On the other hand, the encapsulated form of the follicular variant usually has an even better outlook than the usual follicular variant of papillary carcinoma.

TALL CELL VARIANT

This variant of papillary carcinoma was first described in 1976 by Hawk and Hazard.[184] Approximately 10% of papillary carcinomas fall into this category.[49,69,140,143,211–215] These lesions are classically more aggressive than usual type papillary carcinoma and occur in higher age groups.[49,69,140,143,211–215] As with typical papillary carcinoma, the tumor is more common in women than men. Grossly, the lesions are large, often measuring more than 6 cm in greatest dimension. Histologically, the lesion is characterized by extensive papillae formation and the pres-

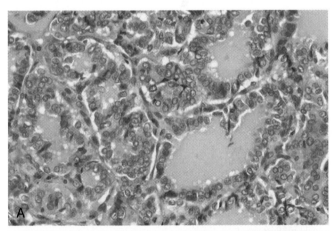

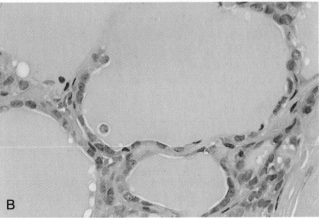

FIGURE 10–28 A, Follicular variant of papillary carcinoma characterized by the neoplastic follicle lined by typical papillary carcinoma nuclei (H and E stain, original magnification × 132). B, Nuclear changes may not be evident in lymph node metastases from these tumors (H and E stain, original magnification × 132).

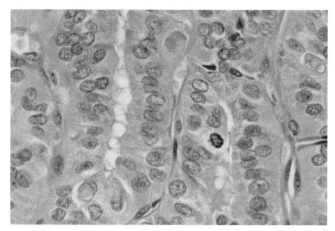

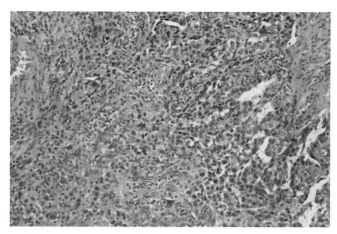

FIGURE 10–29 Tall cell variant of papillary carcinoma is characterized by typical papillary carcinoma nuclei. The cells are twice as tall as they are wide and often are referred to as "pink cells." Mitotic activity is often identified. (H and E stain, original magnification × 198).

FIGURE 10–31 Tall cell variant of papillary carcinoma with poorly differentiated thyroid carcinoma arising within (H and E stain, original magnification × 25).

ence of cells twice as tall as they are wide (Figs. 10–29 and 10–30). These cells should comprise at least 30% of the lesional cells. The cells characteristically demonstrate typical papillary carcinoma nuclei and have moderate amounts of eosinophilic cytoplasm. In fact, these tumors are often referred to as "pink cell" variant of papillary carcinoma.[49,69,140] Mitotic figures are quite common. The tumor often extends beyond the confines of the thyroid to involve surrounding structures, and vascular as well as lymphatic invasion is often seen. By electron microscopy, numerous mitochondria are seen in the tumor cell's cytoplasm, but the lesional cells do not appear to be Hürthle cells. LiVolsi[212] has observed these tumors in thyroids with chronic lymphocytic thy-

roiditis. Bronner and LiVolsi[216] also observed that these lesions may be associated with spindle cell squamous carcinoma (Fig. 10–31).

Flint et al[215] and Stern et al[217] performed flow cytometry studies on tall cell variants and compared them to typical papillary carcinoma. No significant differences were noted between the two tumor types. While the nuclear features are those of papillary carcinoma, and the nuclear content by flow cytometry has shown no significant differences between typical papillary carcinoma and tall cell variant, the clinical behavior of these lesions is more aggressive than that seen in typical papillary carcinoma. The poor outlook seen in tall cell variant may be due to the fact that these lesions are associated with poor prognostic variables (older age, extra thyroidal extension, distant metastases, and high mitotic rate).

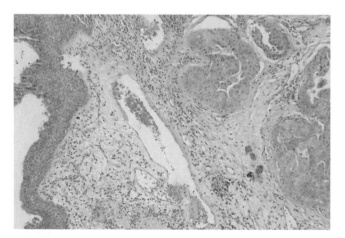

FIGURE 10–30 Low-power examination of vocal cord being infiltrated by tall cell variant of papillary carcinoma. In this case, the carcinoma extended up to and ulcerated the laryngeal mucosa and was initially diagnosed on biopsy as "adenocarcinoma." Radial laryngectomy showed a thyroid primary (H and E stain, original magnification × 33).

COLUMNAR CELL VARIANT

Columnar cell carcinoma is rare, with less than 10 cases reported in the literature. It was initially described in 1986 by Evans.[218] While this tumor is uncommon, recognizing it is important because of its unusually aggressive behavior for a papillary neoplasm.[49,69,140,143,212,218–223] The columnar cell variant is characterized by its aggressiveness, propensity to occur in males, and distinctive histologic appearance.

Grossly, the tumors are often large, measuring greater than 6 cm in greatest dimension. Hui et al[221] reported a tumor diagnosed by fine needle aspiration biopsy, however, that was only 1.5 cm. The tumor may extend outside the thyroid to involve surrounding structures and regional lymph nodes. Histologically, columnar cell carcinoma is characterized by a predominantly papillary growth pattern (some lesions may show only focal papillary growth), although a microfollicular pattern and poorly differentiated areas may be focally evident in some lesions (Fig. 10–32). The papillae are lined by tall stratified columnar cells that do not show the typical nuclear features of usual type papillary carcinomas (although Gaertner, et al[220] recently described a case of columnar cell carcinoma with typical papillary carcinoma nuclear features). In turn, the nuclei are often basally oriented, elongated, and hyperchromatic with a punctate chromatin pattern. Cytoplasm is often scant, but when present is usually clear with vacuolar change. In fact, the cytologic features seen in columnar cell carcinoma have been equated to those seen in early secretory endometrium.[49] While the tumors are predominantly papillary, areas of solid growth, microacini, organoid and cribriform growth patterns, and squamous metaplasia have been reported. Mitotic figures are often present. Psammoma bodies are not usually evident but have been described.[219] The tumor often invades the thyroid capsule and extends into surrounding tissues. Widespread dissemination has been reported with distant metastases to bones, lung, mediastinum, and adrenal. Immunohistochemistry reveals positivity for thyroglobulin and cytokeratin (AE1/3) but negativity for calcitonin and chromogranin. The tumor is highly aggressive, with early metastases and death within less than 10 years of diagnosis.

The histologic appearances of columnar cell carcinoma are quite distinct, and, despite its rarity, a diagnosis can be readily made if all the distinctive features are present. The lesion should not be confused with the tall cell variant, which is present more often in women, is histologically distinct with the presence of cells which are twice as tall as they are wide, and has eosinophilic cytoplasm. Despite aggressive behavior, the lesions are less aggressive than columnar cell carcinoma. Despite these differences between the two tumors, tumors with mixed tall cell and columnar cell features have been described.[224] Some medullary carcinomas have clear

cell features. A calcitonin stain will be useful in those cases, however. Another important differential diagnosis is metastatic clear cell renal carcinoma, which may be distinguished from columnar cell carcinoma by immunohistochemical staining for thyroglobulin.

The classification of columnar cell carcinoma is controversial. The marked papillary architecture of this neoplasm has often placed this tumor as a variant of a papillary carcinoma. However, many of the features seen with this lesion conflict with that placement. These include its propensity for blood-borne over lymph node metastases, its presence predominantly in males, and its aggressive behavior, with most patients experiencing recurrence or death due to disease. While the classification of this neoplasm may be in question, this is a highly aggressive tumor that should be recognized and not confused with typical papillary carcinomas. Despite controversy, the columnar cell carcinoma has been classified as a variant of papillary carcinoma in the WHO classification scheme.[179] The rarity of this neoplasm has precluded detailed evaluation of prognostic factors and disease etiology. An encapsulated form of columnar cell thyroid neoplasms with a more favorable outcome has recently been reported by Evans.[225]

DIFFUSE SCLEROSIS VARIANT

The diffuse sclerosis variant was originally described in 1985 by Vickery and colleagues.[226] Since then, there have been several reports on the histopathology and clinical aspects of this papillary carcinoma variant.[49,69,140,143,149,227–234] Diffuse sclerosing variant is quite rare. In a series of 121 differentiated thyroid carcinomas, Moreno-Egea et al[232] found only four examples of this lesion representing approximately 3.3% of thyroid papillary carcinomas. This lesion often affects children and young adults and tends to behave in a more aggressive fashion than typical papillary carcinomas, although mortality is limited. Approximately 10% of the thyroid carcinomas arising in children following the nuclear accident in Chernobyl have been the diffuse sclerosis subtype.[235] Clinically, patients may present with bilateral diffuse goiter, often delaying diagnosis. Tumors are more commonly seen in women. Hyperthyroidism has been reported. The disease is often difficult to diagnose clinically because of the diffuse nature of the illness, and FNAB and frozen section analysis may result in false negative results. Grossly, the thyroid is described as firm with a gritty texture. A solitary mass lesion may be observed in more than 50% of cases. Vickery et al[226] identified specific morphologic criteria for inclusion in this distinct subtype of papillary carcinoma. Histologically, the lesions are composed of a papillary proliferation associated with solid areas that have often been referred to as squamous metaplasia and have been described as resembling morular metaplasia of the endometrium. The

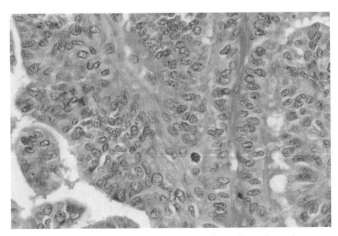

FIGURE 10–32 Columnar cell variant of papillary thyroid carcinoma showing elongated nuclei, pseudostratification, and mitotic activity. Areas reminiscent of "early secretory" endometrium may also be seen in these aggressive tumors (H and E stain, original magnification × 100).

solid areas may represent more than half of the lesion. The tumor diffusely infiltrates the thyroid gland in a pattern suggesting extensive lymphatic infiltration by the tumor. Dense sclerosis, psammoma bodies, and lymphocytic infiltration are prominent features. The nuclear features are those of typical papillary carcinoma. While the lesions often show extension beyond the thyroid capsule, distant and lymph node metastases, and a decreased disease-free survival when compared to typical papillary carcinoma, mortality is reported to be low.

SOLID VARIANT

Papillary carcinomas often exhibit solid growth. Usually this growth pattern is focal, comprising less than 25% of the tumor. The prognosis of tumors with focal solid change is the same as usual type papillary carcinomas. Solid variant of papillary carcinoma should be diagnosed only when the solid pattern is seen in the majority (>50%) of the neoplasm (Fig. 10–33).[49,69,140,143,149] These lesions are more common in children.[131,132,227] More than 30% of

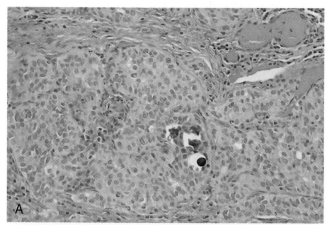

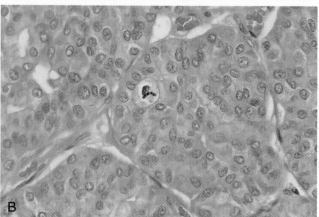

FIGURE 10–33 *A,* Low-power examination of solid variant of papillary carcinoma showing solid cell growth and psammoma bodies (H and E stain, original magnification × 66). *B,* Higher power examination shows nuclear features of papillary carcinoma and mitotic activity (H and E stain, original magnification × 132).

papillary carcinomas diagnosed in patients following the nuclear accident at Chernobyl have been of this subtype.[235] Histologically, classic papillary carcinoma nuclei are seen. Most importantly, this variant must not be overdiagnosed as more aggressive lesions such as insular carcinomas or anaplastic carcinomas. The prognosis of these lesions is controversial, with some studies reporting survival similar to the usual type papillary carcinoma and others reporting aggressiveness (particularly in children).[236]

ENCAPSULATED VARIANT

The encapsulated variant of papillary thyroid carcinoma comprises approximately 10% of all thyroid papillary carcinomas[49,69,140,143,237,238] This lesion is characterized by the gross appearance of an adenoma and the histologic appearance of an encapsulated papillary neoplasm. The lesion displays classic papillary carcinoma nuclear features and may or may not invade into the surrounding capsule. This subtype seems to have an improved outlook compared to regular papillary cancers, although lesions may metastasize to lymph nodes. Since this lesion often shows minimal (if any) capsular invasion, the major differential diagnosis is with papillary hyperplasia; however, the lesional architecture as well as the cytology of the lesional cells should be useful for determining the correct diagnosis.

OTHER VARIANTS

A number of other variants of papillary carcinoma have been described. These include oncocytic (Hürthle cell) variant, clear cell variant, papillary carcinoma with lipomatous stroma, papillary carcinoma with fasciitis-like stroma, papillary carcinoma with fibromatosis-like stroma, myxoid variant, and cribriform variant.[49,69,149,237–247] Too little information is available on these subtypes at the current time.

FOLLICULAR THYROID LESIONS

Follicular Adenoma

A follicular adenoma is an encapsulated neoplasm composed of a collection of follicular epithelium, which usually shows a uniform architecture. These lesions arise in approximately 3% to 4% of the general population and are approximately five times more common than follicular carcinomas, an entity from which they must be distinguished.[69] Most lesions are solitary and arise in normal glands. Patients may present with hyperthyroidism (toxic adenoma); however, this is an uncommon presentation.[248,249] Adenomas are an extremely common cause for a solitary thyroid nodule; therefore, FNAB is often performed prior to removal. Unfortunately, FNAB is often unrewarding, failing to distinguish carcinomas from adenomas, so surgical removal is necessary for careful capsular examination.

Gross Pathology

Grossly, adenomas are usually circumscribed, encapsulated lesions. The capsule is often thin and regularly shaped. Lesions often measure approximately 1 to 3 cm, although larger lesions may be seen.[69] The tumors vary in color from grey to white to tan and may show hemorrhage, fibrosis, calcification, and cyst formation.

Microscopic Pathology

Microscopically, follicular adenomas show a variety of patterns (trabecular, microfollicular, macrofollicular, normofollicular); however, these different patterns behave in a similar fashion (Fig. 10–34). While there is considerable variability, the lesions classically show uniformity throughout. The lesions have a thin capsule, contrasting to the thick capsules commonly seen in carcinoma.[250] Mitotic activity is generally low, but proliferation may be brisk surrounding an area of trauma such as an FNAB. The presence of mitotic activity in the absence of trauma should be interpreted with caution, and the possibility of carcinoma should be considered. Variation in nuclear size may be evident along with bizarre atypical cells. Follicular adenomas can undergo a myxoid or cystic degeneration. Recent and old hemorrhage may be evident. Calcification and ossification are seen in older lesions. Necrosis is not a common feature in the absence of a history of previous FNAB. Papillary hyperplasia, which must be distinguished from papillary carcinoma, can be identified. Occasionally follicular adenomas may contain fat (adenolipoma) or cartilage (adenochondroma).[251,252] Adenomas composed predominantly of signet-ring cells have been reported. While these lesions may appear histologically alarming, they behave in a benign fashion.[49]

The most important aspect of histologic evaluation is to rule out malignancy. The capsule must be carefully examined for invasion and for the presence of vascular invasion.

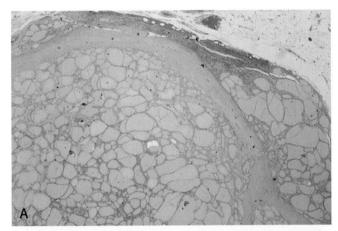

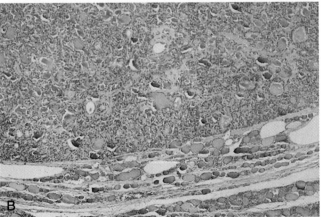

FIGURE 10–34 *A,* Low-power examination of follicular adenoma showing a thick fibrous capsule. No capsular or vascular invasion was seen in this lesion (H and E stain, original magnification × 6.6). *B,* Compared to the follicular adenoma, an adenomatous follicular nodule has a capsule that is thin or incomplete (H and E stain, original magnification × 10).

Immunohistochemistry

Follicular adenomas stain similarly to follicular epithelium with antibodies against thyroglobulin, low-molecular-weight cytokeratins (8 and 18), and vimentin, but show no reactivity with antibodies for high-molecular-weight cytokeratins.[153–155,157,158,253]

Special Studies

By flow cytometry, 25% of follicular adenomas are aneuploid; however, this finding does not correlate with malignant behavior.[254–257] It has been suggested that some adenomas may represent in situ carcinomas, but this has yet to be proven. In addition, adenomas may show cytogenetic abnormalities.[258]

Differential Diagnosis

Follicular adenomas may be difficult to differentiate from adenomatous follicular nodules and follicular carcinomas. Meissner[259] has described features to aid in differentiating adenomas from adenomatous nodules. Adenomatous nodules are usually multiple and circumscribed but not (or only partially) encapsulated (see Fig. 10–34). Adenomas are usually distinct from, and are seen to compress, the surrounding thyroid. The most important differential diagnosis, however, is between follicular carcinoma and follicular adenoma. This differential can be extremely difficult and careful examination of the capsule for true capsular and vascular invasion is necessary. Adenomas may show entrapment of the epithelium within the capsule, particularly after fine needle aspiration, adding to the difficulty. While the presence of mitotic activity and necrosis may suggest malignancy, these features are not diagnostic of carcinoma.

Variants of Follicular Adenomas

HYALINIZING TRABECULAR ADENOMA

This lesion, derived from follicular epithelium, is sometimes referred to as paraganglioma-like adenoma of the thyroid (PLAT). It is characterized by a distinctive microscopic appearance.[260–266] Grossly, the lesions resemble typical adenomas, but microscopically show a distinctive pattern of nests of cells in a trabecular arrangement surrounded by dense hyaline material (Fig. 10–35). The appearance in some areas has been compared to that of paragangliomas; however, this lesion is follicular in origin.[260] The nuclei are round or oval, often exhibiting nuclear grooves and pseudoinclusions. Occasional psammoma bodies have been reported.[264,265] In fact, some authors have considered this lesion to represent a variant of papillary carcinoma; however, to

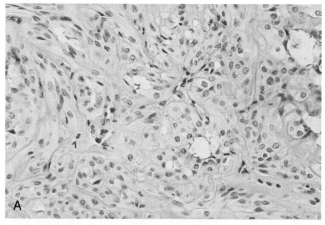

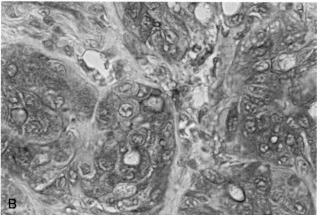

FIGURE 10–35 A, Paraganglioma-like adenoma of the thyroid (hyalinizing trabecular adenoma) showing nests of cells embedded in a dense hyalinized stroma (H and E stain, original magnification × 50). B, These lesions are positive for thyroglobulin and negative for calcitonin (Thyroglobulin immunostain, hematoxylin counterstain, original magnification × 100).

date most reported lesions have behaved in a benign fashion.[264,265] Using FNAB, the lesion may be extremely difficult to distinguish from papillary carcinoma.[266]

By immunohistochemistry, the lesional cells are positive for thyroglobulin and negative for calcitonin—an indication of follicular origin; however, neuroendocrine differentiation has been suggested by the identification of neuron specific enolase, chromogranin A, neurotensin, and B endorphin.[69,260,263] The hyaline material appears to be composed of basement membrane. An association with chronic lymphocytic thyroiditis has been reported.[265]

ATYPICAL FOLLICULAR ADENOMA

In 1954, Hazard and Kenyon[267] proposed the term "atypical follicular adenoma" to describe follicular lesions that appear to have atypical features but do not show the characteristic vascular and capsular invasion that is diagnostic of follicular carcinoma. Worrisome features include necrosis, infarction, increased cellularity, and mitoses—all in the absence of a history of FNAB. These lesions should be examined carefully to rule out capsular and vascular invasion. While these lesions show some atypical features, follow-up reveals that they behave in a benign fashion.[267,268]

Follicular Carcinoma

By definition, follicular carcinoma of the thyroid is a malignancy derived from the follicular epithelium that cannot be assigned to any other category of thyroid gland malignancy. The tumor represents approximately 5% of all thyroid malignancies; however, the incidence increases in areas of endemic goiter and iodine deficiency.[121–124] The actual worldwide incidence of the tumor is unknown, because many cases of the follicular variant of papillary carcinoma may be placed into the follicular carcinoma category.[208] With improved diagnostic criteria, however, true follicular carcinoma is being diagnosed less frequently, as more cases of follicular variant of papillary carcinoma, atypical follicular adenomas, and "insular-type" carcinomas are identified and as populations in endemic goiter regions receive iodine supplements.[208] As with most other thyroid cancers, follicular carcinoma is seen predominantly in females; patients are usually older than patients with papillary carcinoma. Risk factors for development include iodine deficiency, advanced age, female sex, radiation exposure (although to a lesser degree than papillary carcinoma), and patients with dyshormonogenesis.[69,80,269–271]

Follicular carcinoma is divided into two subtypes based on the level of invasiveness: minimally invasive (encapsulated) follicular carcinoma and widely invasive follicular carcinoma.

Minimally Invasive Follicular Carcinoma

Gross Pathology. Grossly, these tumors are quite similar to follicular adenomas except for the possibility of a thicker lesional capsule in carcinomas. The tumors vary considerably in size and may show hemorrhage and cyst formation like adenomas.

Microscopic Pathology. Minimally invasive follicular carcinoma may be difficult to diagnose histologically. Cytologically and architecturally, minimally invasive follicular carcinoma is not dissimilar from follicular adenoma. Carcinomas have a tendency to be more cellular and have more mitotic activity than adenomas; however, the diagnosis of carcinoma can only be made by careful examination of the lesional capsule in order to determine the presence or absence of capsular and vascular invasion. Because careful capsular examination is necessary for disease diagnosis, minimally invasive follicular carcinoma cannot be diagnosed by FNAB.

The actual definition of capsular invasion is controversial, making the diagnosis of carcinoma even harder. Some authors suggest that invasion into the capsule is sufficient for a diagnosis of carcinoma, while others suggest that the lesion must invade through the capsule to be considered malignant.[49,207,208,272,273] Still others believe that the diagnosis of carcinoma should be made only in the presence of vascular invasion.[49] True capsular invasion occurs in a pushing fashion, in which a focus of tumor invades into the capsule perpendicular to the capsule itself. After penetration, the lesion then can spread between the capsular collagen fibers. The capsule is disrupted in this area and may mount a fibroblastic response. On the other hand, nests of lesional cells may become entrapped in the capsule and not actually represent invasion. In these cases a desmoplastic response is really not evident. Obviously extensive "entrapment" of glands should be studied with caution in order not to a miss a diagnosis of carcinoma. Entrapment of epithelium in the capsule of a follicular lesion is quite common after FNAB.[78] In these cases, some authors believe that the presence of vascular invasion is the only actual way to make a definitive diagnosis of carcinoma.

Vascular invasion may also be difficult to diagnose. Vascular invasion within the lesion itself is not considered to be prognostically important. Invasion of vessels in or just beyond the capsule is necessary in order to make a diagnosis of vascular invasion. Vascular invasion may be difficult to assess because epithelium entrapped within the capsule often has artifactual clefting surrounding the group. In true vascular invasion, the tumor cells usually form a polyp, which is located subendothelially and invades into the vascular lumen. The presence of tumor cells within vascular spaces alone is not diagnostic of true vascular invasion and should be interpreted with caution, as the cells may actually represent artifact from surgery or from sectioning the specimen. The tumor cells often form a tumor thrombus covered by endothelial cells. This thrombus may or may not be attached to the vessel wall. The difficulty of determining vascular invasion may be circumvented by the use of immunohistochemistry for vessel-related antigens such as Factor VIII, CD34, CD31, or *Ulex europaeus.* However, these stains (particularly Factor VIII) are often negative for unknown reasons even when true vascular invasion is present.[49,274]

The authors prefer to use the term "minimally" invasive follicular carcinoma to describe those tumors with histologic evidence of capsular invasion only. These patients usually do well following surgical excision. However, patients with vascular invasion have a definitive risk for disease recurrence, metastases, and death from tumor. These lesions should be separated from the minimally invasive category and perhaps be placed into a separate category termed "angioinvasive" follicular carcinoma.

Since vascular and capsular invasion may be only focal in these lesions, the pathologist must adequately sample the lesion. While some authors have recommended limited sampling of follicular lesions, Kahn and Perzin[272] state that the entire capsule with the adjacent tumor must be studied. In some large lesions, this may not be practical and Fransilla[80] recommends that 10 blocks are likely not to miss a carcinoma since large lesions would be more likely to have areas of invasion.

Immunohistochemistry. Immunohistochemically, follicular carcinomas are similar to follicular adenomas and normal follicular epithelium (discussed earlier). In poorly differentiated areas, immunostaining for thyroglobulin may be diminished compared to normal follicular epithelium.

Prognosis. Follicular carcinomas most commonly spread through vascular channels in contrast to papillary carcinomas, which predominantly spread by lymphatics. Metastases to lung, bone, brain, and liver may be identified, as well as more obscure locations such as the heart and sinonasal tract.[49,69,80,275–277] Metastatic disease may be seen 20 years or more after primary diagnosis (Fig. 10–36). In addition, metastatic disease, particularly to bone, may be the initial presentation of tumor. Local recurrence and lymph node metastases are rare.

The prognosis of minimally invasive follicular carcinoma is quite good, with some studies approaching 100% survival.[270,278–281] The presence of distant metastases, metastasis to multiple sites, and patient age greater than 50 years are considered to be the most important poor prognostic factors.[280] In addition, tumor size greater than 4 cm, marked vascular invasion, the presence of extracapsular extension, and poorly differentiated areas are also important prognostic factors. Brennan et al[270] found a 5-year survival of less than 50% if two or more of these indicators were present in their patients; survival rate was almost 100% in patients without any of the aforementioned variables. Use of the AGES scheme commonly used for papillary carcinomas is useful

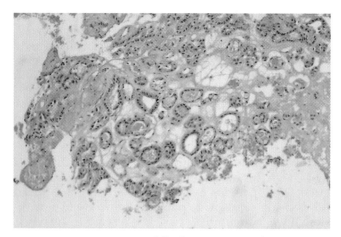

FIGURE 10-36 *Metastatic follicular carcinoma to femur 20 years after primary diagnosis. Note the well-differentiated follicles (H and E stain, original magnification × 132).*

for predicting outcome in follicular carcinomas as well. By multivariate analysis of over 220 patients with follicular carcinoma, Shaha[282] has recently found that adverse independent prognostic indicators were age greater than 45 years, extrathyroidal extension, distant metastases, and tumor size greater than 4 cm.

Differential Diagnosis. The differential diagnosis of minimally invasive follicular carcinoma includes follicular adenoma, a dominant nodular in a goiter, and the follicular variant of papillary carcinoma. As explained previously, minimally invasive follicular carcinoma may be difficult to differentiate from a follicular adenoma. The presence of capsular and/or vascular invasion is necessary to establish a carcinoma diagnosis. In cases where mitoses and cellularity are noted, but there is no capsular/vascular invasion, a diagnosis of atypical adenoma may be made. These lesions behave most often like a benign adenoma.

Special Studies. One of the biggest questions that arises in examination of a follicular nodule is whether or not the lesion is benign or malignant. Unfortunately, to date, DNA ploidy and cytogenetic studies have not been useful for distinguishing adenomas from carcinomas.[254-256,283] Adenomas and carcinomas may both be aneuploid and show cytogenetic aberrations. However, the presence of aneuploid cell populations in follicular carcinoma has been associated with a poorer prognosis than diploid tumors.[254-256,280,283]

Widely Invasive Follicular Carcinoma

Widely invasive follicular carcinoma refers to follicular carcinoma that is clinically and surgically carcinoma. There is no question histopathologically that the lesion is malignant, and the pathologist must decide whether to classify the lesion in the follicular carcinoma category or into a more aggressive group such as insular carcinoma. Most patients develop metastatic disease, and there is a 20% to 50% mortality rate.[207]

Hürthle Cell Lesions[49,69,283,284]

The term Hürthle cell is a misnomer, since the cells that Hürthle was describing in 1894 were most likely C cells.[49] In 1898, Askanazy described these oncocytic cells.[49] However, the term Hürthle cell is still widely used to describe the cells that Askanazy actually described. These cells are derived from follicular epithelium since they are capable of synthesizing thyroglobulin. Hürthle cells are characteristically large with small hyperchromatic nuclei, distinct cell borders, and abundant granular cytoplasm. The cytoplasm is pink on H&E stain and under electron microscopy contains numerous mitochondria. Hürthle cells are believed to represent a common metaplastic change in damaged follicular epithelium, and they can be seen scattered throughout the thyroid gland in a variety of conditions such as nodular goiter and following radiation or chemotherapy. In addition, the cells may be seen with normal aging. However, they are most characteristic of chronic lymphocytic thyroiditis (Hashimoto's disease), where they are often found in groups and may form dominant nodules. Most importantly, Hürthle cells may form non-neoplastic and neoplastic nodules.

Adenomas composed predominantly of Hürthle cells occur and are most often referred to as Hürthle cell adenoma. These lesions may also be referred to as oncocytoma, oncocytic adenoma, and follicular adenoma-oxyphilic cell type. Hürthle cell adenomas most commonly occur in women with an 8:1 female-to-male ratio.[69] Carcinomas composed almost entirely of Hürthle cells also occur and comprise about 20% of all follicular carcinomas and about 2% of all thyroid malignancies.[69] Since these Hürthle cell carcinomas are derived from follicular cells, they are often categorized with follicular carcinomas. The WHO classification now refers to these lesions as follicular carcinoma, oxyphilic cell type.[179] However, the term Hürthle cell carcinoma is used in this discussion. Lesions occur more commonly in females than males (ratio 2:1).

Gross Pathology

Grossly, Hürthle cell lesions are usually circumscribed and often encapsulated. The lesions are brown or mahogany in color and range in size from 1 to several cm. An important aspect of gross examination is that Hürthle cell lesions may spontaneously infarct. This finding does not indicate malignancy, because both benign and malignant lesions can infarct and, rarely, spontaneously regress. Infarction may also be evident following FNAB. Adenomas and carcinomas have similar gross appearances, although carcinomas may more commonly show necrosis, hemorrhage, and scarring.

Microscopic Pathology

By definition, Hürthle cell lesions are composed of greater than 75% Hürthle cells.[49,69] Histologically, adenomas and carcinomas are quite similar. Tumors usually grow in a follicular pattern (micro- or macrofollicular), although in areas the growth may become more solid and trabecular in nature. These latter two growth patterns are seen more frequently in carcinomas.[69] Pseudopapillae formation may be identified. Cytologically both lesions are similar and can be difficult to distinguish from one another. The oncocytic cells usually show uniform nuclei; however, enlarged atypical hyperchromatic cells are often present. The presence of these cells does not correlate with malignant behavior. Calcifications that may be confused with psammoma bodies may be seen; however, these do not have the characteristic lamellated appearance and are usually present in inspissated colloid produced by the tumor.[69] Features more common in malignant tumors include increased nuclear/cytoplasmic ratio, the presence of columnar (instead of polygonal) cells, and increased mitotic rate. However, malignancy cannot be diagnosed without identification of capsular and/or vascular invasion (Figs. 10–37 and 10–38).[69]

Unlike follicular carcinomas, Hürthle cell carcinoma metastasizes via vascular and lymphatic routes. Distant metastases may be seen in lungs, bone, and liver. Survival rates are about 50% to 60% at 5 years.[49,69,284,285]

Immunohistochemistry

By immunohistochemistry, these lesions are positive for thyroglobulin.[286–288] The presence of CEA has been described by Johnson et al,[286] although not substantiated in other studies.[284,288] Abu-Alfa et al[287]

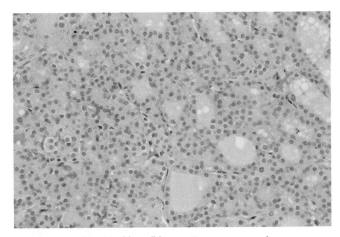

FIGURE 10–38 Hürthle cell lesion. Benignity or malignancy cannot be determined in this lesion without full examination of the capsule.

studied Hürthle cell lesions for S-100 protein and saw intense staining in benign and malignant lesions. Staining for HMB-45 was absent in all of these cases. Interestingly, they found that oncocytic tumors arising in other organ systems (kidney, parathyroid, and parotid) were negative for S-100 and HMB-45.

Electron Microscopy

Ultrastructurally, Hürthle cell lesions demonstrate the presence of numerous mitochondria.[69,288] These mitochondria may be normal but often varying in size and shape. Nesland, et al[288] describe the tendency of oncocytic neoplasms to show the presence of smooth-surfaced cells interspersed with cells containing surface microvilli.

Special Studies

DNA analysis through flow cytometry has been widely applied to Hürthle cell tumors.[285,289–292] Like follicular adenomas, Hürthle cell adenomas may show aneuploid cell populations; however, this finding does not correlate with aggressive behavior. While flow cytometric analysis may not aid in the distinction between benign and malignant Hürthle cell tumors, it may be important for the determining prognosis in malignant tumors. Aneuploid carcinomas are more likely to behave in an aggressive fashion.[285,290]

MEDULLARY CARCINOMA AND VARIANTS

Medullary carcinoma is a malignant tumor derived from the calcitonin-producing parafollicular cells (C cells). This tumor is interesting and important be-

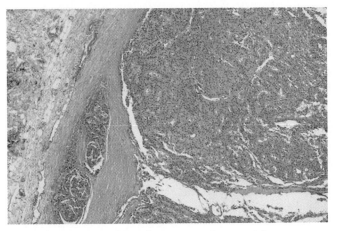

FIGURE 10–37 Hürthle cell carcinoma showing definitive capsular and vascular invasion. (H and E stain, original magnification × 50).

cause of its aggressiveness compared to follicular and papillary carcinomas, its close association with familial syndromes including MEN types 2A and 2B, and its association with a precursor (C-cell hyperplasia) in familial cases that may be detected prior to tumor development.[293–296] Medullary carcinomas account for less than 10% of all thyroid malignancies.

Gross Pathology

In general, medullary carcinomas vary significantly in size. In fact, lesions may be so small that they are not appreciated on gross examination. Medullary carcinomas are usually soft, circumscribed, unencapsulated lesions that are typically tan/pink in color.[49,69] Calcification and fibrosis may be evident. Lesions can be bilateral, particularly in familial cases. In addition, the lesions may also be firm yellow to white in color and diffusely infiltrate the gland. This latter gross appearance is more common in familial cases.[49,69]

Microscopic Pathology[49,69,293,295]

Microscopically, medullary carcinomas can exhibit a variety of histopathologic patterns and often mimic other types of thyroid gland tumors. Most commonly, the lesions exhibit a nested, trabecular, or solid growth pattern invading the surrounding thyroid tissues (Fig. 10–39). In addition, the lesions may exhibit a follicular or papillary growth pattern. The cells are round or spindle-shaped and contain nuclei with a "salt and pepper" chromatin pattern and inconspicuous nucleoli. There is often variation in nuclear size. Mitotic activity is generally low, but may be high in poorly differentiated lesions. The tumor cells often demonstrate eosinophilic cytoplasm on hematoxylin and eosin stain. Intra- and extracellular mucin droplets may be seen by mucicarmine stain. Necrosis and hemorrhage are not common in small lesions but can be extensive in larger lesions. Calcification and even an occasional psammoma body may be evident; however, the presence of psammoma bodies should alert the pathologist to the possibility of papillary carcinoma.

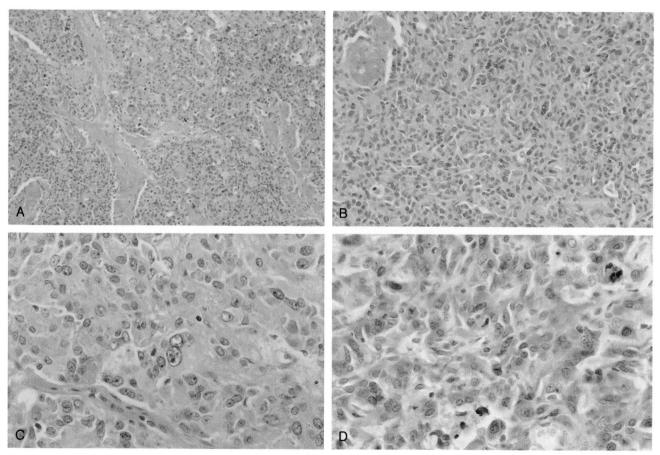

FIGURE 10–39 A, Low-power view of medullary carcinoma showing nests of cells surrounded by amyloid stroma (H and E stain, original magnification × 33). B, Medullary carcinoma showing spindle cells (H and E stain, original magnification × 66). C, Higher power view of medullary carcinoma with random nuclear atypia (H and E stain, original magnification × 132). D, Calcitonin immunostain in medullary carcinoma (Hematoxylin counterstain, original magnification × 132).

Immunohistochemical staining may be necessary to differentiate between the two lesions.

One of the characteristic features of medullary carcinoma is the presence of amyloid stroma between the nests of tumor cells. The amyloid protein in seen in almost 80% of cases and may be so abundant as to resemble amyloid goiter.[49] The amyloid is similar to other types of amyloid in that it is Congored positive and exhibits the classic apple-green birefringence. Medullary carcinoma amyloid is most likely derived from precalcitonin and is often highlighted by immunohistochemical staining for calcitonin. Significant sclerosis resembling amyloid may also be evident. Stromal calcification, particularly in areas of amyloid deposition, can be seen.

Medullary carcinoma may spread by both lymphatic and vascular routes. Over 15% of patients may present with distal metastases to lung, liver, bone, and even adrenal.[49,69,293,295]

Medullary Carcinoma Variants

One of the characteristics of medullary carcinoma is the variation in histologic appearance that may be seen. Some of these variants are discussed in the following sections.

PAPILLARY VARIANT

Medullary carcinoma may show papillary histology, which can be in the form of pseudopapillae or true papillae. The pseudopapillary variant of medullary carcinoma is more common and is most likely due to artifact where tumor cells separate from the surrounding tumor stroma, making the lesion appear to be forming papillary groups.[69] The true papillary variant is extremely rare and must be differentiated from classical papillary carcinoma of the thyroid.[297]

FOLLICULAR VARIANT

Medullary carcinomas may exhibit a follicular, tubular, or glandular growth pattern.[69,297] These lesions may be confused with entrapped normal follicles. In the latter situation, the follicles are located at the periphery of the lesion and stain with antibodies against thyroglobulin.

ENCAPSULATED VARIANT

Medullary carcinomas are most commonly unencapsulated, but they may have a capsule.[298,299] These often resemble hyalinizing trabecular adenomas and may resemble an intrathyroidal paraganglioma; however, the lesions express calcitonin. Some authors prefer to refer to encapsulated C-cell lesions as adenomas.[300] The literature describing these lesions is quite rare, however, so the term carcinoma should be used to describe these lesions until analysis detailing clinical behavior becomes available.

SMALL CELL VARIANT

Small cell variants of medullary carcinoma have been described. These tumors resemble the intermediate cell variant of small cell lung cancer.[49,69,295] These lesions rarely show amyloid, are often extensively necrotic, and have an aggressive course. These lesions are often negative for calcitonin, but often display immunoreactivity for CEA. The possibility of a lung lesion involving the thyroid should always be excluded.

GIANT CELL VARIANT

Many medullary carcinomas contain areas of giant cell formation; however, these areas are usually focal. Kakudo et al[301] described the giant cell variant of medullary carcinoma, characterized by the presence of large atypical anaplastic cells intermixed with areas of typical medullary carcinoma. The giant cell variant should be differentiated from anaplastic carcinomas.[301–303] This differentiation is important because the giant cell variant of medullary carcinoma has an overall better prognosis than anaplastic carcinoma.

CLEAR CELL VARIANT

Landon and Ordonez[304] describe a variant of medullary carcinoma composed predominantly of cells with clear cytoplasm. By immunohistochemistry, the tumors are positive for calcitonin and negative for thyroglobulin. Stains for mucin and glycogen are negative in the tumor cells. The lesion should be differentiated from follicular carcinoma with clear cell cytoplasm and from metastatic clear cell carcinoma of the kidney, which not uncommonly involves the thyroid gland.

OTHER VARIANTS

Rare cases of oncocytic, hyalinizing trabecular adenoma-like, and squamous variants of medullary carcinoma have been described.[305] Calcitonin and CEA immunoreactivity are often necessary to establish these rare variants as medullary carcinoma.

MIXED MEDULLARY AND FOLLICULAR DERIVED CARCINOMAS

Mixed medullary-follicular carcinomas, in which there is a dual population of cells both by immunohistochemistry (calcitonin and thyroglobulin immunoreactivity) and ultrastructurally, have been described but are considered distinctly rare and should be diagnosed with caution.[306–310] These lesions must be differentiated from the follicular variant of medullary carcinoma and from medullary carcinoma with entrapped normal thyroid. Thyroglobulin immunostaining alone in a typical medullary carcinoma cannot be used to determine dual differentiation, since the tumor cells may have picked up surrounding thyroglobulin secreted from normal follicular cells. Mixed medullary-papillary carcinoma has also been described, but again, only rarely.

Familial versus Sporadic Medullary Carcinoma/C-Cell Hyperplasia

Medullary carcinoma may arise sporadically or may show a familial pattern. Familial cases represent approximately 20% of all cases. Familial medullary carcinoma can occur alone or may be associated with MEN 2A (Medullary carcinoma, pheochromocytoma, parathyroid hyperplasia, adrenal medullary hyperplasia, C-cell hyperplasia) or MEN 2B (medullary carcinoma, pheochromocytoma, skeletal abnormalities, mucosal neuromas, gastrointestinal ganglioneuromas, adrenal medullary hyperplasia, C-cell hyperplasia).[49,69,293] In general, sporadic and familial medullary carcinomas are quite similar to each other; however, there are some differences. Familial carcinomas often occur at a younger age and can be associated with other abnormalities as listed previously. Sporadic medullary carcinomas are often unilateral, while familial cases are most often bilateral.

Familial medullary carcinomas are often associated with hyperplasia of C cells in the surrounding gland.[69,311–314] These areas of hyperplasia are believed to be precursors of medullary carcinoma. Thyroids removed from patients with a family history of medullary carcinoma should be scrutinized for C-cell hyperplasia and C-cell nodules even if no carcinoma is evident.

C-cell hyperplasia is most prominent in the middle third of the lateral lobes of the gland. Normally, C cells occur singly or in small groups of three to five cells. What actually constitutes C-cell hyperplasia is controversial. Definitions ranging from greater than 50 C cells per low-power field, to greater than 40 C cells/cm², to greater than 50 C cells per 3 low-power fields have been used to define hyperplasia.[69,313,315] Using these definitions, C-cell hyperplasia is not confined just to patients with familial medullary carcinoma or MEN 2 syndromes (primary or neoplastic C-cell hyperplasia) and may be seen in patients with hyperparathyroidism and chronic hypercalcemia, as well as in patients with Hashimoto's disease, and even in the thyroid tissue adjacent to nonmedullary carcinomas (secondary or physiologic C-cell hyperplasia).[313,316–318] To that end, the terminology of C-cell hyperplasia has become very confusing. Perry et al[313] noted several differences between primary and secondary C-cell hyperplasia.

First of all, in secondary C-cell hyperplasia, the C cells are not clearly evident in H&E staining since the cells are bland and difficult to separate from normal follicular cells. Immunohistochemical staining and quantitative analysis is necessary for diagnosis. On the other hand, neoplastic C-cell hyperplasia is readily observed in H&E stained sections since the cells are large and often atypical and share many features with medullary carcinomas. In this scenario, the actual number of cells is probably of no significance. Their mere presence, regardless of their number, is most likely significant enough for diagnosing C-cell hyperplasia. Komminoth et al[314] observed phenotypic differences between primary and secondary C-cell hyperplasia in that polysialic acid is produced by medullary carcinomas and associated primary C-cell hyperplasia, but not by secondary hyperplastic C cells (discussed later) (Fig. 10–40).

As noted earlier, medullary carcinoma and C-cell hyperplasia constitute the spectrum of endocrine pathologies that may be encountered in MEN 2A and 2B syndromes. Detection of these syndromes has re-

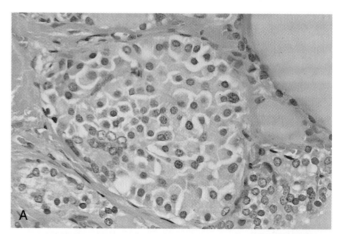

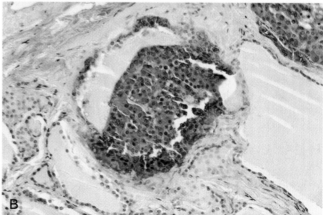

FIGURE 10–40 *A,* Nodule of C cells in patient with MEN 2B syndrome (H and E stain, original magnification × 132). *B,* Calcitonin immunostain in C-cell hyperplasia (Hematoxylin counterstain, original magnification × 66).

cently become feasible since the gene for this disease is located on the long arm of chromosome 10.[319,320]

Histochemistry

Up to 40% of medullary carcinomas contain mucin. In the majority of cases the mucin is extracellular; however, intracytoplasmic mucin can be seen in almost 15% of cases.[321] As was mentioned previously, almost 80% of medullary carcinomas produce an amyloid stroma that can be demonstrated by Congored or Cresyl-violet staining. Rarely, medullary carcinoma cells form melanin pigment and premelanosomes; which can be shown by ultrastructural examination.[322] The significance of the presence of melanin pigment is unknown.

Immunohistochemistry

The majority of medullary carcinomas express calcitonin and calcitonin gene–related peptide protein and/or mRNA.[323–325] Staining is usually seen in the majority of tumor cells, although focal positivity may be noted. Carcinoembryonic antigen is often expressed.[323] Numerous other peptides have been shown to be produced by these tumors.[49,69,326,327] These include: somatostatin, bombesin, synaptophysin, ACTH, beta endorphin, HCG, substance P, vasoactive intestinal peptide, glucagon, gastrin, insulin, and serotonin as well as numerous others. Other neuroendocrine markers that may be seen in these tumors include neuron specific enolase, chromogranin, synaptophysin, and histaminase.

Low-molecular-weight (but not high-molecular-weight) cytokeratins are often seen in medullary carcinomas.[323–327] Most medullary carcinomas express CEA, and this oncofetal protein is often elevated in the serum of these patients.[323–327] Studies have shown that, while poorly differentiated lesions may show decreased calcitonin production, CEA production often remain unchanged. Komminoth et al[314] studied the expression of polysialic acid (a post-translation modification of neural cell adhesion molecule) in medullary carcinomas and found immunoreactivity in medullary but not in other thyroid tumors. In addition, they observed that primary C-cell hyperplasia reacted with this antibody; however, in secondary C-cell hyperplasia and in normal C cells, reactivity was not observed. This group suggested that this protein may be a marker for medullary carcinoma and help to distinguish primary from secondary C-cell hyperplasia.

Electron Microscopy

Ultrastructural examination of medullary carcinomas often reveals the presence of neurosecretory granules ranging in size from 100 to 350 nm.[69] Fewer of these granules appear than are seen in normal and in hyperplastic C cells which explains why immuno-reactivity for calcitonin is often present to a lesser degree in carcinoma than in normal C cells. The carcinoma cells tend to show prominent Golgi and rough endoplasmic reticulum, which indicate active protein synthesis. Within the tumor stroma, amyloid fibers may be seen.

Differential Diagnosis

As has been indicated, medullary carcinoma can resemble almost any type of benign or malignant thyroid neoplasm. When the criteria for the diagnosis of a specific thyroid malignancy cannot be perfectly met, it may be necessary to study the lesion by immunohistochemistry for calcitonin and thyroglobulin. This may aid in determining the histogenesis of the tumor. The differentiation between follicular-derived lesions and medullary carcinoma is important, as medullary carcinomas have a worse prognosis and can be hereditary.

Prognosis

The 5-year survival for medullary carcinoma is approximately 60%. The prognosis of medullary carcinoma is worse than either papillary or follicular carcinomas but better than anaplastic thyroid carcinomas. Several studies have analyzed prognostic factors in this tumor.[294,328,329] Disease stage appears to be the most important prognostic indicator. Age less than 40 years and female sex are considered to be good prognostic factors. Other prognostic factors have included tumor type, the presence of amyloid, pleomorphism, necrosis, and mitoses. Lesions with extensive necrosis, mitoses, pleomorphism, and small cell histology are associated with a poor prognosis. Tumors with little pleomorphism, and possibly extensive amyloid deposition, are associated with a better outcome.

POORLY DIFFERENTIATED CARCINOMA (INSULAR CARCINOMA)

In 1984, Carangiu and Rosai[332] described what they termed "poorly differentiated thyroid carcinoma," which they believe was first described by Langhans in 1907. They used the term "insular" carcinoma to describe the growth pattern of this follicular-derived neoplasm, distinctive because of its survival rate in between well-differentiated thyroid carcinomas and anaplastic carcinoma.[69,137,330–335] The incidence of this rare tumor appears to vary with geographic location: an institution in Italy reports an incidence of 4% to 5% of all thyroid tumors, while in the United States this tumor is less common.[335] Affected individuals are usually elderly, older than patients with well-differentiated thyroid lesions. Although this lesion is described as a separate entity in some series, the WHO committee continues to classify this tumor as a subtype of follicular carcinoma.[179]

Gross Pathology

Grossly, the lesions are large, with most measuring greater than 5 cm in maximum dimension, and are usually grey-white in color with multifocal necrosis. The tumors are not circumscribed or encapsulated and often invade into the surrounding thyroid tissue and even into perithyroid tissues.

Microscopic Pathology

Histologically, insular carcinoma is characterized by the presence of solid nests (insulae) of tumor cells separated by a loose connective tissue network (Fig. 10–41). The tumor characteristically has a carcinoid-like growth pattern and has been said to resemble pancreatic islets. The cells are usually small and contain round nuclei and scant cytoplasm. While solid nests and trabeculae predominate, follicles that re-

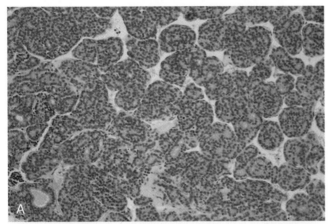

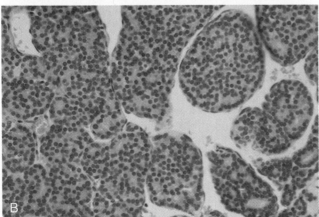

FIGURE 10–41 *A,* Low-power view of insular carcinoma showing nest of cells with a "carcinoid-like" growth pattern (H and E stain, original magnification × 25). *B,* Higher power of insular carcinoma showing a nested neoplasm composed of small round cells that focally form microacini (H and E stain, original magnification × 100).

sult in a cribriform architecture may also be seen. Necrosis, vascular invasion, and mitotic activity are often identified. By immunohistochemistry, the tumor cells are positive for thyroglobulin and are negative for calcitonin.

Because of the nested microscopic appearance, this lesion may be confused with medullary carcinoma or other neuroendocrine neoplasms. In some series these lesions may have been diagnosed as a subtype of anaplastic carcinoma. However, the clinical behavior is less aggressive than the latter tumor.

These lesions are aggressive and often spread by lymphatic and vascular routes. Metastases are most commonly seen in lymph node, lung, and bone. The mortality rate is between that of well-differentiated tumors and anaplastic tumors. Burman et al[137] thoroughly reviewed the literature on all cases of insular carcinoma, finding it more likely to metastasize distantly. More patients with insular carcinoma die of or with the disease than well-differentiated thyroid carcinomas.

A recent study reported that insular differentiation may be seen focally in lesions otherwise classified as papillary or follicular carcinomas.[336] In this study, the outcome was not influenced by the presence of the insular component.

ANAPLASTIC CARCINOMA (UNDIFFERENTIATED CARCINOMA)

Anaplastic carcinoma constitutes a group of high-grade thyroid neoplasms characterized by undifferentiated histology and a highly aggressive course, with death most commonly seen within 3 months of diagnosis.[49,69,333,337–342] Other terms for this high-grade malignancy include undifferentiated, dedifferentiated, or sarcomatoid. Rosai et al[69,323] and others[49,343] believe that the term dedifferentiated is a more correct term to describe this neoplasm since many cases actually arise from a pre-existing lower grade tumor. Special studies reveal that these tumors are epithelial derived.

Anaplastic carcinoma is seen predominantly in elderly females (age >60 years), although disease has been reported in young individuals. However, the diagnosis of anaplastic carcinoma in patients under 40 years should be made with caution. Approximately 10% of malignant thyroid tumors are anaplastic carcinomas. Most patients present with a rapidly enlarging neck mass that can compress surrounding structures, resulting in dyspnea and dysphagia. Patients may present with distant metastases and metastases to neck lymph nodes. The risk factors for development are largely unknown, although tumor incidence appears to increase in patients receiving neck radiation and in areas of iodine deficiency.[344,345] About 80% of patients have a long history of goiter.[49,69]

Aldinger[338] described 84 cases of anaplastic carcinomas, noting that the tumor may arise in different clinical scenarios. Along with a history of goiter, anaplastic carcinomas have also been described in patients with history of low-grade carcinoma, as an unexpected finding in thyroids removed for other reasons, and in a large proportion of patients without any known thyroid disease. Rarely, patients may present with metastatic disease of unknown primary and are found at autopsy to have a primary thyroid carcinoma.

Gross Pathology

Grossly these lesions are characterized by the presence of a large, white-tan, invasive mass involving the thyroid and perithyroidal tissues often associated with extensive hemorrhage and necrosis. Because of the extent of involvement of the surrounding structures, surgical resection is often not feasible.

Microscopic Pathology

The microscopic appearance of anaplastic carcinoma is quite variable, and several patterns are identified (Figs. 10–42 and 10–43).[49,69,333,336,338,340] The majority of cases consist of giant and/or spindle cells, although up to 30% of cases may show clear epithelial differentiation described as "squamoid." Most cases show a variety of cell types. Classically, the tumor is composed of bizarre mitotically atypical cells. The tumor typically invades into and between follicles, resulting in extensive tissue destruction. Necrosis is often extensive, and the lesion may be almost completely necrotic. Rosai et al[69] describe the necrosis as often palisading, with appearance similar to that of glioblastoma multiforme. The histologic appearance confirms the gross impression that the tumor is widely invasive and often involves surrounding soft tissue structures. Vascular invasion is often prominent and may explain the extensive necrosis often present in these lesions. In fact, the tumor often replaces the media of medium-sized vessels, which may help differentiate the lesion from sarcoma.[69] Inflammatory cells may be seen in the lesions, and in some cases inflammation is marked, masking the tumor cells. Occasionally, mesenchymal components may be seen.

The cases with clear epithelial differentiation often take on the appearance of large cell undifferentiated carcinoma seen in other organs such as lung or cervix. In this subtype, the cells are cohesive and form nests. While "squamoid" differentiation may be noted, keratinization is uncommon, and these lesions should not be regarded as squamous cell carcinomas. Glandular differentiation is not evident.

The spindle cell tumors or the "sarcoma-like" pattern is characterized by the proliferation of atypical spindle cells that can take on the appearance of high-grade sarcoma such as fibrosarcoma, malignant fibrous histiocytoma, and even rhabdomyosarcoma.

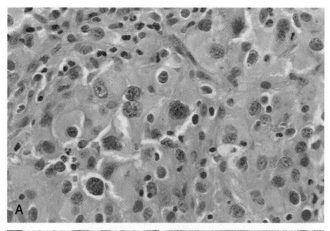

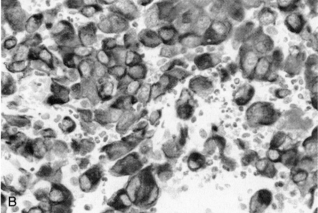

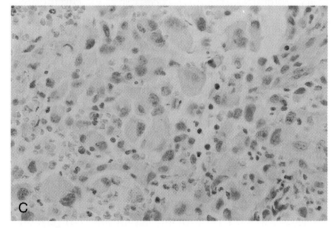

FIGURE 10–42 *A,* Anaplastic carcinoma (undifferentiated carcinoma) of the thyroid showing large atypical pleomorphic cells. *B,* These cells are positive for cytokeratin. *C,* These cells are often negative for thyroglobulin. (Both are original magnifications × 132.)

The appearances in areas may resemble a vascular tumor such as malignant hemangiopericytoma and even angiosarcoma. Most of the spindle-cell tumors are associated with giant cell formation, and tumors composed predominantly of "osteoclast-like" giant cells can also be seen. These cells are believed to be stromal or histiocytic in origin, lack definite epithelial differentiation by special studies, and have been

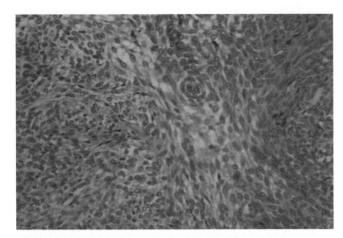

FIGURE 10-43 Anaplastic carcinoma (undifferentiated carcinoma) composed predominantly of spindle cells (H and E stain, original magnification × 50).

described in tumors in other organs such as breast and pancreas.[346] Wan et al[347] recently described a "paucicellular variant" of anaplastic carcinoma characterized by the presence of hypocellular fibrous tissue with calcifications and epithelial marker–positive atypical cells. The distinction from Riedel's, which has an overall good prognosis, must be made.

In many cases, anaplastic carcinoma is associated with the history of prior well-differentiated (papillary, follicular, or Hürthle cell) thyroid carcinomas. In fact, transition zones between anaplastic foci and well-differentiated tumors have been described.[49,69,333,343] The diagnosis of anaplastic carcinoma may be made several years after the diagnosis of a low-grade carcinoma, or the two may coexist. The probability of transformation of a low-grade lesion to undifferentiated carcinoma is most likely less than 2%, however.[69]

Immunohistochemistry

The majority of undifferentiated carcinomas express high-molecular-weight and/or low-molecular-weight cytokeratins.[348-350] Reactivity is most prominent in those cases with prominent "squamoid" differentiation. Staining is more variable in the giant cell and spindle cell variants and is seen in isolated cells and small groups of tumor cells. Staining with antibodies against thyroglobulin has led to conflicting results. Some studies have seen no reactivity with undifferentiated carcinomas, while others have reported some degree of reactivity. The cases in which thyroglobulin staining is evident may be due to trapping of residual follicular epithelium or from uptake of the protein by the tumor cells.

Electron Microscopy

On ultrastructural exam, anaplastic carcinomas are epithelial in nature. Sometimes, however, the tumor may be so undifferentiated that the phenotype cannot be determined.

RARE THYROID TUMORS

Squamous Lesions

Many thyroid lesions can undergo squamous metaplasia. These include benign and malignant conditions such as Hashimoto's disease (particularly the fibrosing variant) and papillary carcinoma (particularly the diffuse sclerosis variant). Squamous cell carcinomas, adenosquamous carcinomas, and mucoepidermoid carcinomas rarely present as primary thyroid malignancies.

Squamous Cell Carcinoma

Primary thyroid squamous cell carcinoma does occur; however, this lesion is extremely rare, comprising less than 1% of all thyroid malignancies.[351-354] Metastasis or direct extension from a primary head and neck area must always be considered when pure squamous carcinoma is encountered in the thyroid. These lesions occur in elderly patients who often have a longstanding history of goiter. Patients may present with systemic symptoms and signs such as hypercalcemia, elevated white count, and fever. Histologically, the lesion resembles classic squamous carcinoma in other organs and may range anywhere from well to poorly differentiated. The tumors lack thyroglobulin by immunohistochemistry. Metastasis to lung, nodes, liver, and mediastinum have been reported.

Some authors prefer to classify these lesions among anaplastic carcinomas because the prognosis is similar (rapid course with most deaths in less than 3 months). Others prefer to place these lesions into a separate category. The pathogenesis is unclear, but these tumors possibly arise in areas of squamous metaplasia, although Harada et al[351] saw no evidence for squamous metaplasia in 19 cases of primary thyroid squamous carcinoma. An association with external radiation has been considered.

Mucoepidermoid Carcinoma

Mucoepidermoid carcinomas are rare malignancies that may arise within the thyroid gland.[45-49,93,355-359] To date, fewer than 40 cases have been reported in the literature. These lesions characteristically have an excellent prognosis once resected. Thyroid mucoepidermoid carcinomas occur more frequently in females, who often present with a painless mass in the neck. Grossly, the lesions are usually smaller than 4 cm and are often cystic and solid. Microscopically, sheets of squamoid cells in association with mucus cells are present. The histologic appearance is similar to intermediate- or high-gland mucoepidermoid carcinomas arising in salivary gland tissue. Chronic lymphocytic thyroiditis may be seen in the surrounding gland. A focal papillary carcinoma component may be identified. In fact, papillary carcinoma and mucoepidermoid carcinoma have several features in common, including dense sclerosis, psammoma bodies, and the propensity for lymph node metastasis. It is believed that mucoepidermoid carcinoma of the thyroid may actually arise from papillary carcinoma.[48,356] By immunohistochemistry most thyroid mucoepidermoid carcinomas are positive for cytokeratin and thyroglobulin and negative for neuroendocrine markers. Extracapsular extension can be seen, and the lesions can metastasize to lymph nodes and rarely to distant sites; however, death from disease has not been reported.

The pathogenesis of thyroid mucoepidermoid carcinoma remains obscure. The initial theories suggested that these lesions arose from solid cell nests. More recent theories propose that they arise from the thyroid follicular epithelium, particularly from squamous metaplasia which is common in lymphocytic thyroiditis.[45–47,93,360] Wenig et al[47] reported immunoreactivity for thyroglobulin and polyclonal CEA but not monoclonal CEA or neuroendocrine markers, suggesting that these tumors do not arise from solid cell nests.

Chan et al[93] described a variant of mucoepidermoid that they termed sclerosing mucoepidermoid carcinoma with eosinophilia. This rare tumor is a low-grade malignancy that has been described solely in patients with fibrosing Hashimoto's thyroiditis. This lesion shows distinctive areas of mucoepidermoid carcinoma in association with a dense fibrous stroma and a prominent inflammatory reaction consisting of eosinophils. The tumors may show vascular invasion, perineural invasion, extracapsular extension, and lymph node metastases, but distant metastases and death have not been reported to date.

Sarcomas

Primary sarcomas of the thyroid gland do occur but are extremely rare.[49,69,361] In many cases, lesions that histologically resemble sarcoma are actually anaplastic carcinomas with a prominent spindle cell component. However, there are cases in which malignant mesenchymal tumors are observed in the gland. Primary liposarcomas, fibrosarcomas, leiomyosarcomas, chondrosarcomas, osteosarcomas, and angiosarcomas may be seen.[49,69] The most distinctive of these lesions is angiosarcoma; the tumor arises in a specific geographic location—the mountainous areas of central Europe—where it may represent greater than 15% of all malignant thyroid lesions (Fig. 10–44).[361]

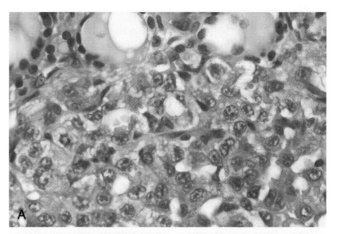

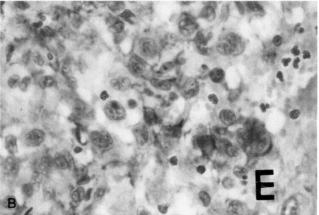

FIGURE 10–44 *A,* Epithelioid angiosarcoma arising within the thyroid. These lesions are rare and should be confirmed with endothelial markers. *B,* Factor VIII immunostaining in this case.

Malignant Lymphoma[49,69,362–366]

The thyroid may be involved by malignant lymphoma that can be either primary or secondary. Primary lymphomas of the thyroid are extremely rare, comprising less than 5% of all lymphomas arising in extranodal sites and approximately 1% to 3% of all thyroid malignancies. Primary lymphomas usually arise in glands affected by autoimmune chronic lymphocytic thyroiditis (Hashimoto's disease); however, the development of lymphoma in these patients is rare, and chronic lymphocytic thyroiditis should in no way be considered a premalignant state. The pathogenesis of primary thyroid lymphoma remains unknown.

As with most thyroid neoplasms, lymphoma is most commonly seen in females. Disease is most common in elderly individuals. Most patients present with an enlarged thyroid that is quite firm.

Gross Pathology

Grossly, primary thyroid lymphoma usually presents as a solid homogeneous mass and takes on the classic "fish flesh" appearance of lymphomas in other sites. The lesions are often ill-defined and may invade into the surrounding thyroid tissue. Necrosis and hemorrhage are not prominent features.

Microscopic Pathology

The histopathology of thyroid lymphoma depends on the histologic subtype of lymphoma (Fig. 10–45). The majority of lymphomas are non-Hodgkin's lymphomas, although primary Hodgkin's disease and plasmacytomas have been reported.[94-97,362-367] As mentioned earlier, most primary lymphomas are associated with autoimmune thyroid disease, and—as in most cases of lymphomas arising in autoimmune disease—thyroid lymphomas are predominantly large cell B-cell neoplasms or immunoblastic lymphomas (70% to 80%). Intermediate-grade as well as low-grade lymphomas have also been reported.[49,69]

The lesions characteristically grow between and within thyroid follicles and are often associated with dense fibrosis that may result in the formation of

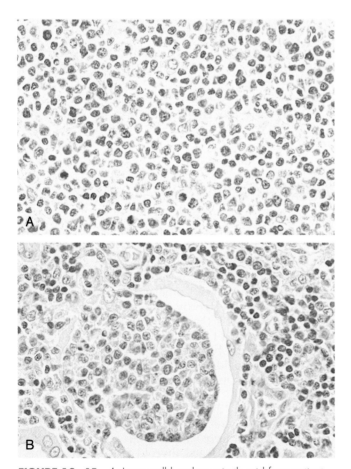

FIGURE 10–45 *A,* Large cell lymphoma in thyroid from patient with history of chronic lymphocytic thyroiditis (H and E stain, original magnification × 50). *B,* Lymphoepithelial lesions are characteristic of lymphoma in the thyroid (H and E stain, original magnification × 100).

nests of cells resembling carcinoma. Thyroid lymphomas are usually diffuse but may be nodular. Plasmacytic differentiation is common. The tumor cells often grow along the walls of blood vessels and involve the intimal layer. At the periphery of the lesion, vascular proliferation may be evident. Cytologically, the cells are large, predominantly noncleaved, with large nuclei that often contain prominent nucleoli.

In 1985, Anscombe and Wright[365] proposed that thyroid lymphomas be classified as tumors arising in association with mucosa associated lymphoid tissues (MALT). They listed similarities between thyroid lymphomas and "MALTomas" arising in other sites: they often form lymphoepithelial lesions, show plasmacytic differentiation, and are predominantly localized to the thyroid. Rare cases have been associated with EBV.[368,369]

Immunohistochemically, most thyroid lymphomas react with B-cell markers.[49] Some may show light chain restriction on paraffin sections, however this is best detected by flow cytometry or frozen section immunostaining. Immunohistochemical staining for *p53* and *BCL-2* fails to distinguish between florid lymphoma-like thyroiditis and primary thyroid lymphoma.[370]

Tumors often grow to involve the entire thyroid gland and may then spread into perithyroid tissues and regional lymph nodes. The majority of patients present with stage I disease, and the prognosis is excellent in these patients. The prognosis is poorer for advanced-stage lesions. Interestingly, patients with primary thyroid lymphoma have a propensity to develop gastrointestinal lymphomas, particularly after therapy.[49] Mutations in the *p53* genetic locus have not been seen.[371]

Metastatic Lesions

It is not uncommon for the thyroid to be involved by direct extension of tumors from elsewhere in the neck, such as the larynx, trachea, and esophagus. The majority of these tumors are squamous carcinomas that have invaded through the laryngeal cartilages to involve the thyroid parenchyma. It should be reiterated that squamous cell carcinomas arising in the thyroid gland are extremely rare. If a squamous carcinoma is observed in the thyroid, the possibility of secondary involvement by an adjacent carcinoma should be considered.

Metastatic lesions are quite commonly seen at postmortem examination.[372] However, patients with metastatic lesions may initially present with thyroid abnormalities. The most common malignancies to metastasize to the thyroid include malignant melanoma and carcinoma, especially carcinomas of the lung, colon, breast, and kidney.[69,372] When these lesions present as a "primary" thyroid mass, it is the role of the pathologist to establish that the lesion is a metastatic tumor so the primary site can be dis-

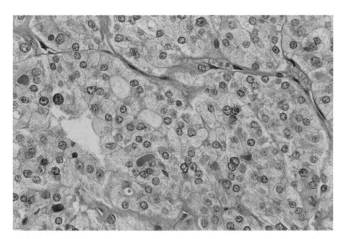

FIGURE 10-46 Metastatic renal cell carcinoma to the thyroid. Clear cell medullary carcinoma is in the differential diagnosis of this lesion. Calcitonin immunoreactivity was not seen in this lesion. (H and E stain, original magnification × 132).

covered. Metastases may involve benign or malignant primary thyroid lesions. The possibility that any lesion considered metastatic may still actually represent a rare form of primary thyroid carcinoma should always be considered, and the appropriate stains should be performed prior to diagnosis.

The most important metastatic lesion to recognize is renal cell carcinoma, clear cell type (Fig. 10–46).[373] Primary thyroid neoplasms including medullary and follicular carcinomas may have clear cell features, and the distinction between these tumors and a metastatic renal cell carcinoma is therefore critical. Metastatic clear cell renal cell cancer is often multifocal, extremely vascular, and contains cells with clear cytoplasm that are devoid of glycogen. While the histopathologic findings may suggest a metastatic kidney cancer, the absence of thyroglobulin in the tumor cells is a clear-cut aid in establishing the diagnosis. The presence of focal thyroglobulin, though, may be seen as a result of absorption of this marker by the tumor cells following disruption of the normal thyroid epithelium.

REFERENCES

1. Hoyes AD, Kershaw DR. Anatomy and development of the thyroid gland. *Ear, Nose Throat J.* 1985; 64:318.
2. Weller GL. Development of the thyroid, parathyroid, and thymus glands in man. *Contrib Embryol Carneg Inst.* 1933; 141:93.
3. Sugiyama S. The embryology of the human thyroid including ultimobranchial body and others related. *Adv Anat Embryol Cell Biol.* 1971; 44:1.
4. Ohri AK, Ohri SK, Sing MP. Evidence for thyroid development from the fourth branchial pouch. *J Laryngol Otol.* 1994; 108(1):71.
5. Williams ED, Toyn CE, Harach HR. The ultimobranchial gland and congenital thyroid abnormalities in man. *J Pathol.* 1989; 159(2):135.
6. Harach HR. Solid cell nests of the thyroid: An anatomic survey and immunohistochemical study for the presence of thyroglobulin. *Acta Anat.* 1985; 122:249.
7. Harach HR. Solid cell nests of the thyroid. *J Pathol.* 1988; 155:191.
8. Himi T, Kataura A. Distribution of C cells in the thyroid gland with pyriform sinus fistula. *Otolaryngol Head Neck Surg.* 1995; 112:268.
9. Ozaki O, Ito K, Mimura-Takashi M, et al. Hemiaplasia of the thyroid associated with Graves' disease: Report of three cases and a review of the literature. *Surg Today.* 1994; 24:164.
10. Hamburger JI, Hamburger SW. Thyroidal hemiagenesis: Report of a case and comment on clinical ramifications. *Arch Surg.* 1970; 100:319.
11. Harada T, Nishikawa Y, Ito K. Aplasia of one thyroid lobe. *Am J Surg.* 1972; 124:617.
12. Rosenberg T, Gilboa Y. Familial thyroid ectopy and hemiagenesis. *Arch Dis Child.* 1980; 55:639.
13. Greening WP, Sarker SK, Osborne MP. Hemiagenesis of the thyroid gland. *Br J Surg.* 1980; 67:446.
14. Melnick JC, Stembrowski PE. Thyroid hemiagenesis (hockey stick sign): A review of the literature and a report of four cases. *J Clin Endocrinol Metab.* 1981; 52:247.
15. Friedman A, Bauman A. Hemiagenesis of the thyroid. *South Med J.* 1979; 72:927.
16. Mortimer PS, Tomlinson JW, Rosenthal FD. Hemiaplasia of the thyroid with thyrotoxicosis. *J Clin Endocrinol Metab.* 1981; 52:152.
17. Piera J, Garriga J, Calabuig R, Bargallo D. Thyroidal hemiagenesis. *Am J Surg.* 1986; 151:419.
18. Orti E, Castells S, Qazi QH, Inamdar S. Familial thyroid disease: Lingual thyroid in two siblings and hypoplasia of a thyroid lobe in a third. *J Pediatr.* 1971; 78:675.
19. Kaplan M, Kauli R, Raviv U, et al. Hypothyroidism due to ectopy in siblings. *Am J Dis Child.* 1977; 131:1264.
20. Kaplan M, Kauli R, Lubin E, et al. Ectopic thyroid gland. *J Pediatr.* 1978; 92:205.
21. Rubenfeld S, Joseph UA. Ectopic thyroid in the right carotid triangle. *Arch Otolaryngol Head Neck Surg.* 1988; 114:913.
22. Moses DC, Thompson NW, Nishiyama RH, Sisson JC. Ectopic thyroid tissue in the neck. *Cancer.* 1976; 38:361.
23. Butler JJ, Tulinius H, Ibanez ML, et al. Significance of thyroid tissue in lymph nodes associated with carcinoma of the head, neck or lung. *Cancer.* 1967; 20:103.
24. Ibrahim NB, Milewski PJ, Gillett R, Temple JG. Benign thyroid inclusions within cervical lymphnodes. *Aust NZ J Surg.* 1981; 51:188.
25. Meyer JS, Steinberg LS. Microscopically benign thyroid follicles in cervical lymph nodes. *Cancer.* 1969; 24:302.
26. Borgoni F, Liberatori E, Giambagli M, et al. Lingual thyroid and hypothyroidism: Report of a case in a middle aged woman. *Panminerva Med.* 1994; 36:95.
27. Jain SN. Lingual thyroid. *Int Surg.* 1969; 52:320.
28. Nienas FW, Gorman CA, Devine KD, et al. Lingual thyroid: Clinical characteristics of 15 cases. *Ann Intern Med.* 1973; 79:205.
29. Bone RC, Biller HF, Irwin TM. Intralaryngotracheal thyroid. *Ann Otol.* 1972; 81:424.
30. Fish J, Moore RM. Ectopic thyroid tissue and ectopic thyroid carcinoma. *Ann Surg.* 1963; 157:212.
31. Spears RP, Wei JP. Nonmalignant ectopic thyroid tissue. *Am Surg.* 1993; 59(2):133.
32. Parham DM. Laterally situated neck cysts derived from the embryologic remnants of thyroid development. *Histopathology.* 12(1):95, 1988.
33. Walling AD. Ectopic thyroid tissue. *Am Fam Phys.* 1987; 36(3):147.
34. Chanin LR, Greenberg LM. Pediatric upper airway obstruction due to ectopic thyroid: Classification and case reports. *Laryngoscope.* 1988; 98(4):422.
35. Schemin RJ, Marsh JD, Schoen FJ. Benign intracardiac thyroid mass causing right ventricular outflow obstruction. *Am J Cardiol.* 1985; 56:828.
36. Roth L. Inclusions of nonneoplastic thyroid tissue within cervical lymph nodes. *Cancer.* 1965; 18:105.
37. Richardson GM, Assor D. Thyroid tissue within the larynx. *Laryngoscope.* 1971; 81:120.

38. Porqueddu M, Antona C, Polvani G, et al. Ectopic thyroid tissue in the ventricular outflow tract: Embryologic implications. *Cardiology.* 1995; 86(6):524.

39. Kumar PV, Akbari HM, Arjmand F. Lingual thyroid diagnosed by fine needle aspiration cytology. *Acta Cytol.* 1996; 40:387.

40. Autelitano F, Santeusanio G, Di Tondo U, et al. Immunohistochemical study of solid cell nests of the thyroid gland found from an autopsy study. *Cancer.* 1987; 59:477.

41. Carpenter GR, Emery JL. Inclusions in the human thyroid. *J Anat.* 1976; 122:77.

42. Yamaoka Y. Solid cell nests (SCN) in the human thyroid gland. *Acta Pathol Jpn.* 1973, 23:493.

43. Wolfe HF, Voeckel EF, Tashijan AH. Distribution of calcitonin-containing cells in the normal adult human thyroid gland. *J Clin Endocrinol Metab.* 1974; 41:1076.

44. Harach HR, Vujanic GM, Jasani B. Ultimobranchial body nests in human fetal thyroid: An autopsy, histological, and immunohistochemical study in relation to solid cell nests and mucoepidermoid carcinoma of the thyroid. *J Pathol.* 1993; 169(4):465–469.

45. Harach HR. A study on the relationship between solid cell nests and mucoepidermoid carcinoma of the thyroid. *Histopathology.* 1985; 9:195.

46. Harach HR, Day ES, de Strizic NA. Mucoepidermoid carcinoma of the thyroid. *Medicina (B Aires).* 1986; 146:213.

47. Wenig BM, Adair CF, Heffess CS. Primary mucoepidermoid carcinoma of the thyroid gland: A report of six cases and a review of the literature of a follicular-epithelial derived tumor. *Hum Pathol.* 1995; 26:1099.

48. Viciana MJ, Galera-Davidson H, Martin-Lacauc I, Segure DI, Loizage JM. Papillary carcinoma of the thyroid with mucoepidermoid differentiation. *Arch Pathol Lab Med.* 1996; 120: 397.

49. LiVolsi VA. *Surgical Pathology of the Thyroid.* Philadelphia: WB Saunders, 1990; Major Problems in Pathology Series; vol 22.

50. Kimberly B, Cohen J, Posalsky I. Papillary thyroid carcinoma within a thyroglossal duct cyst. *Arch Otolaryol Head Neck Surg.* 1987; 113:206.

51. Kristensen S, Juul A, Moesner J. Thyroglossal cyst carcinoma. *J Laryngol Otol.* 1984; 98:1277.

52. Villet WT, Kemp CB. Thyroglossal duct carcinoma. *S Afr Med J.* 1981; 60:795.

53. Nussbaum M, Buchwald RP, Ribner A, et al. Anaplastic carcinoma arising from median ectopic thyroid (thyroglossal duct remnants). *Cancer.* 1981; 48:2724.

54. Chen H, Nicol TL, Udelsman R. Follicular lesions of the thyroid. Does frozen section evaluation alter operative management? *Ann Surg.* 1995; 222:101.

55. Crowe PJ, Chetty R, Dent DM. Thyroid frozen section: Flawed but helpful. *Aust NZ J Surg.* 1993; 63:275.

56. Rodriguez JM, Parrilla P, Sola J, et al. Comparison between preoperative cytology and intraoperative frozen-section biopsy in the diagnosis of thyroid nodules. *Br J Surg.* 1994; 81: 1151.

57. McHenry CR, Rosen IB, Walfish PG, Bedard Y. Influence of fine-needle aspiration biopsy and frozen section examination on the management of thyroid cancer. *Am J Surg.* 1993; 166: 353.

58. Gibbs GK, Pasieka JL. Assessing the need for frozen sections: Still a valuable tool in thyroid surgery. *Surgery.* 1995; 118: 1005.

59. Neale ML, Delbridge L, Reeve TS, Poole AG. The value of frozen section examination in planning surgery for follicular thyroid neoplasms *Aust NZ J Surg.* 1993; 63:610.

60. Bronner MP, Hamilton R, LiVolsi VA. Frozen section analysis of thyroid follicular lesions. *Endocrine Pathol.* 1994; 5:154.

61. Atkinson BF. Fine needle aspiration of the thyroid. *Monogr Pathol.* 1993; 35:166.

62. Jones AJ, Aitman TJ, Edmonds CJ, et al. Comparison of fine needle aspiration cytology, radioisotopic and ultrasound scanning in the management of thyroid nodules. *Postgrad Med.* 1990; 66:914.

63. Aggrawal SK, Jayaranm G, Kakar A, et al. Fine needle aspiration in cytologic diagnosis of the solitary cold thyroid nodule. Comparison with ultrasonography radionuclide perfusion study and xeroradiography. *Acta Cytol.* 1989; 33:41.

64. Cristallini EG, Bolis GB. Fine needle aspiration biopsy in the preoperative diagnosis of solitary thyroid nodules. *Appl Pathol.* 1989; 7:149.

65. Dwarakanathan AA, Ryan WG, Staren ED, Martiano M, Economou SG. Fine needle aspiration biopsy of the thyroid. Diagnostic accuracy when performing a moderate number of such procedures. *Arch Intern Med.* 1989; 149:2007.

66. Hamburger JI. Fine needle diagnosis of thyroid nodules: Perspective. *Thyroidology* 1988; 1:21.

67. Kendall CH. Fine needle aspiration of thyroid nodules: Three years experience. *Clin Pathol.* 1989; 42:23.

68. LaRosa GL, Belfiore A, Giuffrida D, et al. Evaluation of the fine needle aspiration biopsy in the preoperative selection of cold thyroid nodules. *Cancer.* 1991; 67:2137.

69. Rosai J, Carcangiu ML, DeLellis. *Tumors of the Thyroid Gland.* Atlas of Tumor Pathology; series 3, fascicle 5. Washington, DC: Armed Forces Institute of Pathology; 1993.

70. Hall TL, Layfield LJ, Phillippe A, Rosenthal DL. Sources of diagnostic error in fine needle aspiration of the thyroid. *Cancer.* 1989; 63:718.

71. Caraway NP, Sneige N, Samaan NA. Diagnostic pitfalls in thyroid fine-needle aspiration: A review of 394 cases. *Diagn Cytopathol.* 1993; 9:345.

72. Muller N, Cooperberg PL, Suen KCH, Thoroson SC. Needle aspiration biopsy in cystic papillary carcinoma of the thyroid. *Am J Pathol.* 1985; 144:251.

73. Alejo M, Matias-Cruiu X, delas Heras-Duran P. Infarction of a papillary thyroid carcinoma after fine needle aspiration. *Acta Cytol.* 1991; 35:478.

74. Axiotis, Merino MJ, Ain K, Norton JA. Papillary endothelial hyperplasia in the thyroid following fine needle aspiration. *Arch Pathol Lab Med.* 1991; 115:240.

75. Keyhani-Rofagha S, Kooner DS, Keyhani M, O'Toole RV. Necrosis of a Hurthle cell tumor of the thyroid following fine needle aspiration. *Acta Cytol.* 1990; 34:805.

76. Kini SR, Miller JM, Abrash MP, Gaba A, Johnson T. Post fine needle aspiration biopsy infarction in thyroid nodules. *Lab Invest.* 1988; 58:48a. Abstract.

77. Layfield LJ, Lones MA. Necrosis in thyroid nodules after fine needle aspiration biopsy. Report of two cases. *Acta Cytol.* 1991; 35:427.

78. Livolsi VA, Merino M. Worrisome histologic artifacts following fine needle aspiration of the thyroid (WHAFFT). *Pathol Annu.* 1994; 29:99.

79. Mowschenson PM, Hodin RA, Wang HH, Upton M, Silen W. Fine-needle aspiration of normal thyroid tissue may result in the misdiagnosis of microfollicular lesions. *Surgery.* 1994; 116:1006.

80. Franssila KO, Ackerman LV, Brown CL, Hedinger CE. Follicular carcinoma. *Semin Diagn Pathol.* 1985; 2:101.

81. Volpe R. The pathology of thyroiditis. *Hum Pathol.* 1978; 9: 429.

82. Berho M, Suster S. Clear nuclear changes in Hashimoto's thyroiditis: A clinicopathologic study of 12 cases. *Ann Clin Lab Sci.* 1995; 25:513.

83. Harach HR, Williams ED. Fibrous thyroiditis—An immunopathological study. *Histopathology.* 1983; 7:739.

84. Knecht H, Saremaslani P, Hedinger C. Immunohistological findings in Hashimoto's thyroiditis, focal lymphocytic thyroiditis and thyroiditis of de Quervain. *Virch Arch [A]* 1981; 393:215.

85. Yagi Y. Electron microscopy and immunohistochemical studies in Hashimoto's thyroiditis. *Acta Pathol Jpn.* 1981; 31:611.

86. Kotani T, Aratake Y, Hirai K, et al. Apoptosis in thyroid tissue from patients with Hashimoto's thyroiditis. *Autoimmunity.* 1995; 20:231.

87. Mizukami Y, Michigishi T, Kawato M, et al. Chronic thyroiditis: Thyroid function and histologic correlations in 601 cases. *Hum Pathol.* 1992; 23:980.

88. Kalderon AE, Bogaars HA, Diamond I. Ultrastructural alterations of the follicular basement membrane in Hashimoto's thyroiditis. *Am J Med.* 1973; 55:485.

89. Pfaltz M, Hedinger CE. Abnormal basement membrane structures in autoimmune thyroid disease. *Lab Invest.* 1986; 55:531.

90. Williams ED. Malignant lymphoma of the thyroid. *Clin Endocrinol Metab.* 1981; 10:83.

91. Holm LE, Blomgren H, Lowhagen T. Cancer risks in patients with chronic lymphocytic thyroiditis. *N Engl J Med.* 1985; 312:601.

92. Kato I, Tajima K, Suchi T, et al. Chronic lymphocytic thyroiditis as a risk factor of B-cell lymphoma in the thyroid gland. *Jpn J Cancer Res.* 1984; 53:2515.

93. Chan JK, Albores-Saavedra J, Battifora H, Carcangiu ML, Rosai J. Sclerosing mucoepidermoid carcinoma of the thyroid with eosinophilia. A distinctive low-grade malignancy arising from the metaplastic follicles of Hashimoto's thyroiditis. *Am J Surg Pathol.* 1991; 15:438.

94. Aozasa K, Inoue A, Yoshimura H, et al. Plasmacytoma of the thyroid gland. *Cancer.* 1986; 58:105.

95. Rubin J, Johnson JT, Killeen R, Barnes L. Extramedullary plasmacytoma of the thyroid associated with a serum monoclonal gammopathy. *Arch Otolaryngol Head Neck Surg.* 1990; 116:855.

96. Ohshima M, Momiyama T, Souda S, et al. Primary plasmacytoma of the thyroid: A case report and comparative literature study between Western nations and Japan. *Pathol Int.* 1994; 44:645.

97. Kovacs CS, Mant MJ, Nguyen GK, Ginsberg J. Plasma cell lesions of the thyroid: Report of a case of solitary plasmacytoma and a review of the literature. *Thyroid.* 1994; 4:65.

98. Katz SM, Vickery AL. The fibrous variant of Hashimoto's thyroiditis. *Hum Pathol.* 1974; 5:161.

99. Katsikas D, Shorthouse AJ, Taylor S. Riedel's thyroiditis. *Br J Surg.* 1976; 63:929.

100. Schwaegerle SM, Bauer TW, Esselstyn CB, et al. Riedel's thyroiditis. *Am J Clin Pathol.* 1988; 90:715.

101. Woolner LB, McConanahey WM, Beahrs OH. Invasive fibrous thyroiditis (Riedel's struma). *J Clin Endocrinol Metab.* 1957; 17:201.

102. Meijer S, Hausman R. Occlusive phlebitis, a diagnostic feature in Riedel's thyroiditis. *Virch Arch [A]* 1978; 377:339.

103. Mitchinson MJ. Retroperitoneal fibrosis revisited. *Arch Pathol Lab Med.* 1986; 110:784.

104. Wold LE, Weiland LH. Tumefactive fibro-inflammatory lesions of the head and neck. *Am J Surg Pathol.* 1983; 7:477.

105. Fatourechi V, McConahey WM, Woolner LB. Hyperthyroidism associated with histologic Hashimoto's thyroiditis. *Mayo Clin Proc.* 1971; 46:682.

106. Rallison ML, Dobyns BM, et al. Occurrence and natural history of chronic lymphocytic thyroiditis in childhood. *J Pediatr.* 1975; 86:675.

107. Nakashimi M, Eguchi K, Ida H, et al. The expression of adhesion molecules in thyroid glands from patients with Graves' disease. *Thyroid.* 1994; 4:119.

108. Spjut HJ, Warren WD, Akerman LV. Clinical-pathologic study of 76 cases of recurrent Graves' disease, toxic (nonexophthalmic) goiter, and non-toxic goiter. *Am J Clin Pathol.* 1957; 27:367.

109. Patchefsky AS, Hoch WS. Psammoma bodies in diffuse toxic goiter. *Am J Clin Pathol.* 1972; 57:551.

110. Tezuka H, Eguchi K, Fukuda T, et al. Natural killer and natural killer−like cell activity of peripheral blood and intrathyroidal mononuclear cells from patients with Graves' disease. *J Clin Endocrinol Metab.* 1988; 66:702.

111. Okita N, How J, et al. Suppressor T lymphocytes dysfunction in Graves' disease: Role of the H-2 histamine receptor-bearing suppressor T lymphocytes. *J Clin Endocrinol Metab.* 1981; 53:1002.

112. Ozaki O, Ito K, Kobayashi K, et al. Thyroid carcinoma in Graves' disease. *World J Surg.* 1990; 14:437.

113. Berger SA, Zonsein J, Villamena P, Mittman N. Infectious disease of the thyroid gland. *Rev Infect Dis.* 1983; 5:108.

114. Frank TS, LiVolsi VA, Connor AM. Cytomegalovirus infection of the thyroid in immunocompromised adults. *Yale J Biol Med.* 1987; 60:1.

115. Jeng LB, Lin JD, Chen MF. Acute suppurative thyroiditis: A ten year review in a Taiwanese hospital. *Scan J Infect Dis.* 1994; 26:297.

116. Nyulassy S, Hnilica P, Buc M, et al. Subacute (de Quervain's) thyroiditis: Association with HLA-Bw35 antigen and abnormalities of the complement system, immunoglobulins and other serum proteins. *J Clin Endocrinol Metab.* 1977; 45: 270.

117. Goto H, Uno H, Tamai H, et al. Genetic analysis of subacute (de Quervain's) thyroiditis. *Tissue Antigens.* 1985; 26:110.

118. Satoh M. Virus-like particles in the follicular epithelium of the thyroid from a patient with subacute thyroiditis (de Quervain). *Acta Pathol Jpn.* 1975; 25:499.

119. Stancekova M, Stancek D, Ciampor F, et al. Morphological, cytological and biological observations on viruses isolated from patients with subacute thyroiditis of de Quervain. *Acta Virol.* 1976; 20:183.

120. Carney JA, Moore SB, Northcut RC, et al. Palpation thyroiditis (multifocal granulomatous thyroiditis). *Am J Clin Pathol.* 1975; 64:639.

121. Harach HR, Escalante DA, Onativia A, et al. Thyroid carcinoma and thyroiditis in an endemic goitre region before and after iodine prophylaxis. *Acta Endocrinol.* 1985; 108:55.

122. Williams ED, Doniach I, Bjarnason O, Michie W. Thyroid carcinoma in an iodide rich area. *Cancer.* 1977; 39:215.

123. Kolnel LN, Hankin JH, Wilkens LR, et al. An epidemiologic study of thyroid cancer in Hawaii. *Cancer Causes Control.* 1990; 1:223.

124. Hofstatder F. Frequency and morphology of malignant tumours of the thyroid before and after the introduction of iodine prophylaxis. *Virch Pathol Anat.* 1980; 385:263.

125. Glattre E, Haldorsen T, Berg JP, et al. Norwegian case control study testing the hypothesis that seafood increases the risk of thyroid cancer. *Cancer Causes Control.* 1993; 4:11.

126. Glattre E, Thomassen Y, Thoresen SO, et al. Prediagnostic serum selenium in a case control study of thyroid cancer. *Int J Epidemiol.* 1989; 18:45.

127. Pesatori AC, Consonni D, Tironi A, et al. Cancer in a young population in a dioxin contaminated area. *Int J Epidemiol.* 1993; 22:1010.

128. Grimalt JO, Sunyer J, Moreno V, et al. Risk excess of soft tissue sarcoma and thyroid cancer in a community exposed to airborne organochlorinated compound mixtures with a high hexachlorobenzene content. *Int J Cancer.* 1994; 56:200.

129. Franceschi S, Talamini R, Fassina A, et al. Diet and epithelial cancer of the thyroid gland. *Tumori.* 1993; 76:331.

130. Zimmerman LM, Shubik P. Experimental production of thyroid tumors by alternating hyperplasia and involution. *J Clin Endocrinol Metab.* 1954; 14:1367.

131. Becker DV, Robbins J, Beebe GW, et al. Childhood thyroid cancer following the Chernobyl accident: A status report. *Endocrinol Metab Clin North Am.* 1996; 25:197.

132. Nikiforov Y, Gnepp DR, Fagin JA. Thyroid lesions in children and adolescents after the Chernobyl disaster: Implications for the study of radiation tumorigenesis. *J Clin Endocrinol Metab.* 1996; 81:9.

133. Harach HR, Williams GT, Williams ED. Familial adenomatous polyposis associated thyroid carcinoma: A distinct type of follicular cell neoplasm. *Histopathology.* 1994; 25:549.

134. Bell B, Mazzaferri EL. Familial adenomatous polyposis (Gardner's syndrome) and thyroid carcinoma: A report of a case and review of the literature. *Digest Dis Sci.* 1993; 38:185.

135. Haibach H, Burman TW, Carlson HE. Multiple hamartoma syndrome (Cowden's disease) associated with renal cell carcinoma and primary neuroendocrine carcinoma of the skin (Merkel cell carcinoma). *Am J Clin Pathol.* 1992; 97:705.

136. Plail RO, Bussey HJ, Glazer G, et al. Adenomatous polyposis: An association with carcinoma of the thyroid. *Br J Surg.* 1987; 74:377.

137. Burman KD, Ringel MD, Wartofsky I. Unusual types of thyroid neoplasms. *Endocrinol Metab Clin North Am.* 1996; 25:49.

138. Hapke MR, Dehner LP. The optically clear nucleus: A reliable sign of papillary carcinoma of the thyroid? *Am J Surg Pathol.* 1979; 3:31.

139. Rosai J, Zampi G, Carcangiu M. Papillary carcinoma of the thyroid. *Am J Surg Pathol.* 1983; 7:809.

140. Rosai J. Papillary carcinoma. *Monogr Pathol.* 1993; 35:138.

141. Carcangiu ML, Zampi G, Pupi A, et al. Papillary carcinoma of the thyroid. A clinicopathologic study of 244 cases treated at the University of Florence, Italy. *Cancer.* 1985; 55:805.

142. Carcangiu ML, Zampi G, Rosai J. Papillary thyroid carcinoma: A study of its many morphologic expressions and clinical correlates. *Pathol Annu.* 1985; 20(p1):1.

143. Chan JKC. Papillary carcinoma of the thyroid: Classical and variants. *Histol Histopathol.* 1990; 5:241.

144. Chan JKC, Saw D. The grooved nucleus: A useful diagnostic criterion of papillary carcinoma of the thyroid. *Am J Surg Pathol.* 1986; 10:672.

145. Scopa CD, Melachrinou M, Saradopoulou C, Merino MJ. The significance of the grooved nucleus in thyroid lesions. *Mod Pathol.* 1993; 6:691.

146. Johannessen JV, Sobrinho-Simoes M. The origin and significance of thyroid psammoma bodies. *Lab Invest.* 1980; 43:287.

147. Patchefsky AS, Hoch WS. Psammoma bodies in diffuse toxic goiter. *Am J Clin Pathol.* 1972; 57:551.

148. Dugan JM, Atkinson BF, Avitabile A, et al. Psammoma bodies in fine needle aspirate of the thyroid in lymphocytic thyroiditis. *Acta Cytol.* 1987; 31:330.

149. LiVolsi VA. Papillary neoplasms of the thyroid: Pathologic and prognostic features. *Am J Clin Pathol.* 1992; 97:426.

150. Gould VE, Gould NS, Benditt EP. Ultrastructural aspects of papillary and sclerosing carcinoma of the thyroid. *Cancer.* 1972; 29:1613.

151. Beaumont A, Ben Othman S, Fragu P. The fine structure of papillary carcinoma of the thyroid. *Histopathology.* 1981; 5:377.

152. Harach HR, Franssila KO. Thyroglobulin immunostaining in follicular thyroid carcinoma. *Histopathology.* 1988; 13:43.

153. Raphael SJ, Apel RL, Asa RL. Brief report: Detection of high molecular weight cytokeratins in neoplastic and non-neoplastic thyroid tissues using microwave antigen retrieval. *Mod Pathol.* 1995; 8:870.

154. Raphael SJ, McKeown-Eyssen G, Asa SL. High molecular weight cytokeratin and cytokeratin 19 in the diagnosis of thyroid tumors. *Mod Pathol.* 1994; 7:295.

155. Buley ID, Gatter KC, Heryet A, Mason DY. Expression of intermediate filament proteins in normal and diseased thyroid glands. *J Clin Pathol.* 1987; 40:136.

156. Henzen-Logmans SC, Mullink H, Ramaekers FC, Tadema T, Meijer CJ. Expression of cytokeratins and vimentin in epithelial cells of normal and pathologic thyroid tissue. *Virch Arch [A].* 1987; 410:347.

157. Schelfout LJ, Van Muijen GN, Fleuren GJ. Expression of cytokeratin 19 distinguishes papillary thyroid carcinoma from follicular carcinomas and follicular thyroid adenoma. *Am J Clin Pathol.* 1989; 92:179.

158. Cohn K, Backdahl M, Forsslund G, et al. Prognostic value of nuclear DNA content in papillary thyroid carcinoma. *World J Surg.* 1984; 8:474.

159. Joensuu H, Klemi P, Eerola E, Tuominen J. Influence of cellular DNA content on survival in differentiated thyroid cancer. *Cancer.* 1986; 58:2462.

160. Johannessen JV, Sobrinho-Simoes M, Tangen KO, Lindmo T. A flow cytometric DNA analysis of papillary thyroid carcinoma. *Lab Invest.* 1981; 45:336.

161. Kraemer B, Srigley JR, et al. DNA flow cytometry of thyroid neoplasms. *Arch Otolaryngol.* 1985; 111:34.

162. Backdahl M. *Nuclear DNA Content and Prognosis in Papillary, Follicular, and Medullary Carcinomas of the Thyroid.* Stockholm, Sweden; Karolinska Medical Institute; 1985. Thesis.

163. Antonini P, Venaut AM, Linares G, et al. Translocation (7:10) (q35q21) in a differentiated papillary carcinoma of the thyroid. *Cancer Genet Cytogenet.* 1989; 41:139.

164. Jenkins RB, Hay ID, Herath JF, et al. Frequent occurrence of cytogenetic abnormalities in sporadic nonmedullary carcinoma. *Cancer.* 1990; 66:1213.

165. Russel MA, Gilbert EF, Jaeschke WF. Prognostic features of thyroid carcinoma: A long-term follow-up of 68 cases. *Cancer.* 1975; 36:553.

166. Torres J, Volpato RD, Power EG, et al. Thyroid cancer: Survival in 148 cases followed for 10 years or more. *Cancer.* 1985; 56:2298.

167. Simpson WJ, McKinney SE, Carruthers JS, et al. Papillary and follicular thyroid cancer: Prognostic factors in 1578 patients. *Am J Med.* 1987; 83:479.

168. Hay ID. Papillary thyroid carcinoma. *Endocrinol Metab Clin North Am.* 1990; 19:545.

169. Tubiana M, Schlumberger M, Rougier P, et al. Long-term results and prognostic factors in patients with differentiated thyroid carcinoma. *Cancer.* 1985; 56:2298.

170. Har-El G, Sidi J, Kahan E, et al. Thyroid cancer in patients 70 years of age or older. *Ann Otol Rhinol Laryngol.* 1987; 96:403.

171. Ibanez ML, Russell WO, Albores-Saavedra J, et al. Thyroid carcinomas: Biologic behavior and mortality. Postmortem findings in 42 cases including 27 in which disease was fatal. *Cancer.* 1966; 19:1039.

172. Forquet A, Asselain B, Joly J. Cancer of the thyroid: A multidimensional analysis of prognostic factors. *Ann Endocrinol.* 1983; 44:121.

173. Cody HS, Shah JP. Locally invasive well differentiated thyroid cancers: 22 years experience at Memorial Sloan-Kettering Cancer Center. *Am J Surg.* 1981; 142:480.

174. Ruegemer JJ, Hay ID, Bergstralh EJ, et al. Distant metastases in differentiated thyroid carcinoma: A multivariate analysis of prognostic variables. *J Clin Endocrinol.* 1988; 67:501.

175. Pilotti S, Collini P, Manzari A, Marubini E, Rilke F. Poorly differentiated forms of papillary thyroid carcinoma: Distinctive entities or morphologic patterns. *Semin Diagn Pathol.* 1995; 12:249.

176. Noguchi S, Murakami N, Kawamoto H. Classification of papillary carcinoma of the thyroid based on prognosis. *World J Surg.* 1994; 18:522.

177. Matsubayashi S, Kawai K, Matsumoto Y, et al. The correlation between thyroid carcinoma and lymphocytic infiltration in the thyroid gland. *J Clin Endocrinol Metab.* 1995; 80:3421.

178. Moreno-Egea A, Rodriguez-Gonzales JM, Sola-Perez J, Soria-Cogollos T, Parrilla-Paricio P. Multivariate analysis of histopathlogical features as prognostic factors in patients with papillary thyroid carcinoma. *Br J Surg.* 1995; 82:1092.

179. Hedinger CE, Williams ED, Sobin LH. Histological typing of thyroid tumors. In: Hedinger CE, ed. *International Histological Classification of Tumours,* vol 11, 2nd ed. Berlin: Springer Verlag; 1988.

180. Arellano L, Ibaarra A. Occult carcinoma of the thyroid gland. *Pathol Res Pract.* 1984; 179:88.

181. Bocker W, Schroder S, Dralle H. Minimal thyroid neoplasia. *Rec Results Cancer Res.* 1988; 106:131.

182. Gikas PW, Labow SS, DiGiulio W, Finger JE. Occult metastasis from occult papillary carcinoma of the thyroid. *Cancer.* 1967; 20:2100.

183. Harach HR, Franssila KO, Wasenius VM. Occult papillary carcinoma of the thyroid: A "normal" finding in Finland. A systematic autopsy study. *Cancer.* 1985; 56:531.

184. Hawk WA, Hazard JB. The many appearances of papillary carcinoma. *Clev Clin Q.* 1976; 43:207.

185. Lang W, Borrusch H, Bauer L. Occult carcinomas of the thyroid. Evaluation of 1,200 sequential autopsies. *Am J Clin Pathol.* 1988; 90:72.

186. Naruse T, Koike A, Kanemitsu T, Kato K. Minimal thyroid carcinoma: A report of nine cases discovered by cervical lymph node metastases. *Jpn J Surg.* 1984; 14:118.

187. Sampson RJ, Woolner LB, Bahn RC, et al. Occult thyroid carcinoma in Olmstead County, Minnesota. Prevalence at autopsy compared with that in Hiroshima and Nagasaki Japan. *Cancer.* 1974; 34:2072.

188. Yamamoto Y, Maeda T, Izumi K, Otsuka H. Occult papillary carcinoma of the thyroid: A study of 408 autopsy cases. *Cancer.* 1990; 65:1173.

189. Komorowski RA, Hanson GA. Occult thyroid pathology in the young adult: An autopsy study of 138 patients without clinical thyroid disease. *Hum Pathol.* 1988; 19:689.

190. Fink A, Tomlinson G, Freeman J, Rosen IB, Asa SL. Occult micropapillary carcinoma associated with benign follicular thyroid disease and unrelated thyroid neoplasms. *Mod Pathol.* 1996; 9:816.

191. Sampson RJ, Oka H, Key CR, et al. Metastases from occult thyroid carcinoma. An autopsy study from Hiroshima and Nagasaki Japan. *Cancer.* 1970; 25:803.

192. Pasakoy N, Ozturk H, Demircan A, Artvinl M. Occult papillary carcinoma of the thyroid presenting as an intratracheal tumor. *Euro J Surg Oncol.* 1994; 20:694.

193. Janic-Zguricas M, Jankovic R. Occult papillary carcinoma of the thyroid gland revisited by cancer pericarditis. *Pathol Res Pract.* 1986; 181:761.

194. Chen KTK. Minute (less than 1 mm) occult papillary thyroid carcinoma with metastasis. *Am J Clin Pathol.* 1989; 91:746.

195. Lloyd RV, Beierwaltes WH. Occult sclerosing carcinoma of the thyroid: Potential for aggressive biologic behavior. *South Med J.* 1983; 76:437.

196. Patchefsky AS, Keller IB, Mansfield CM. Solitary vertebral column metastasis from occult sclerosing carcinoma of the thyroid gland. *Am J Clin Pathol.* 1970; 53:596.

197. Laskin W, James L. Occult papillary carcinoma of the thyroid with pulmonary metastasis. *Hum Pathol.* 1983; 13:83.

198. Strate SM, Lee EL, Childres JH. Occult papillary carcinoma of the thyroid with distant metastases. *Cancer.* 1984; 54:1093.

199. Kasai N, Sakamoto A. New subgrouping of small thyroid carcinoma. *Cancer.* 1987; 60:1767.

200. Yamashita H, Nakayam I, Noguchi S, et al. Minute carcinoma of the thyroid and its development to advanced carcinoma. *Acta Pathol Jpn.* 1985; 35:781.

201. Yamashita H, Nakayama I, Noguchi S, et al. Thyroid carcinoma in benign thyroid diseases: An analysis from minute carcinoma. *Acta Pathol Jpn.* 1985; 35:781.

202. Linsday S. *Carcinoma of the Thyroid Gland.* Springfield IL: Charles C Thomas; 1960.

203. Chen KTK, Rosai J. Follicular variant of thyroid papillary carcinoma. A clinicopathologic study of six cases. *Am J Surg Pathol.* 1977; 1:123.

204. Rosai J, Zampi G, Carangiu ML. Papillary carcinoma of the thyroid. A discussion of its several morphologic expressions with particular emphasis on the follicular variant. *Am J Surg Pathol.* 1983; 76:809.

205. Tielens ET, Sherman SI, Hruban RH, et al. Follicular variant of papillary thyroid carcinoma: A clinicopathologic study. *Cancer.* 1994; 73:424.

206. Mizukami Y, Noguchi M, Michigishi T, et al. Papillary thyroid carcinoma in Kanazawa, Japan: Prognostic significance of histological subtypes. *Histopathology.* 1992; 20:243.

207. LiVolsi VA: Current concepts in follicular tumors of the thyroid. *Monogr Pathol.* 1993; 35:118.

208. LiVolsi VA, Asa SL. The demise of follicular carcinoma of the thyroid gland. *Thyroid.* 1994; 4:233.

209. Albores-Saavedra J, Gould E, Vardaman C, Vuitch F. The macrofollicular variant of papillary thyroid carcinoma: A study of 17 cases. *Hum Pathol.* 1991; 22:1195.

210. Sobrinho-Simoes M, Soares J, Carneiro F, et al. Diffuse follicular variant of papillary carcinoma of the thyroid: Report of eight cases of a distinct aggressive type of thyroid tumor. *Surg Pathol.* 1990; 3:189.

211. Hicks MJ, Batsakis JG. Tall cell carcinoma of the thyroid gland. *Ann Otol Rhinol Laryngol.* 1993; 102:402.

212. LiVolsi VA. Unusual variants of papillary thyroid carcinoma. *Adv Endocrin Metab.* 1995; 6:39.

213. Moreno-Egea A, Rodriguez Gonzalez JM, Sola Perez J, et al. Prognostic value of the tall cell variety of papillary cancer of the thyroid. *Eur J Surg Oncol.* 1993; 19:517–521.

214. Johnston TL, Lloyd RV, Thompson NW, et al. Prognostic implications of tall cell variant of papillary thyroid carcinoma. *Am J Surg Pathol.* 1988; 12:22.

215. Flint A, Davenport RD, Lloyd RV. The tall cell variant of papillary carcinoma of the thyroid gland. *Arch Pathol Lab Med.* 1991; 115:196.

216. Bronner MP, LiVolsi VA. Spindle cell squamous carcinoma of the thyroid arising in association with tall cell carcinoma. *Mod Pathol.* 1991; 4:637.

217. Stern Y, Medelia O, Feinmesser M, et al. Nuclear DNA content of the tall cell variant of papillary carcinoma of the thyroid gland. *Ann Otol Rhinol Laryngol.* 1996; 105:713.

218. Evans HL. Columnar cell carcinoma of the thyroid: A report of two cases of an aggressive variant of thyroid carcinoma. *Am J Clin Pathol.* 1986; 85:77.

219. Berends D, Mouthaan PJ. Columnar cell carcinoma of the thyroid. *Histopathology.* 1992; 20:360.

220. Gaertner EM, Davidson M, Wenig B. The columnar cell variant of thyroid papillary carcinoma: Case report and discussion of an unusually aggressive thyroid papillary carcinoma. *Am J Surg Pathol.* 1995; 19:940.

221. Hui PK, Chan JKC, Cheung PSY, et al. Columnar cell carcinoma of the thyroid. Fine needle aspiration findings in a case. *Acta Cytol.* 1990; 34:355.

222. Mizukami Y, Nonomura A, Michighishi T, et al. Columnar cell carcinoma of the thyroid: A case report and review of the literature. *Hum Pathol.* 1994; 25:1098.

223. Sobrinho-Simoes M, Nesland JM, Johannessen JV. Columnar cell carcinoma: Another variant of poorly differentiated carcinoma of the thyroid. *Am J Clin Pathol.* 1988; 89:264.

224. Akslen LA, Varaug JE. Thyroid carcinoma with mixed tall-cell and columnar-cell features. *Am J Clin Pathol.* 1990; 94: 442.

225. Evans HL. Encapsulated columnar cell neoplasms of the thyroid: A report of four cases suggesting a favorable prognosis. *Am J Surg Pathol.* 1996; 20:1205.

226. Vickery AL, Carcangiu M, Johannessen JV, Sobrinho-Simoes M. Papillary carcinoma. *Semin Diagn Pathol.* 1985; 2:90.

227. Chan JKC, Tsui MS, Tse CH. Diffuse sclerosing variant of papillary carcinoma of the thyroid: A histological and immunohistochemical study of three cases. *Histopathology.* 1987; 11: 191.

228. Carcangiu ML, Bianchi S. Diffuse sclerosis variant of papillary carcinoma: Clinicopathologic study of 15 cases. *Am J Surg Pathol.* 1989; 13:1041.

229. Fujimoto Y, Obara T, Ito Y, et al. Diffuse sclerosing variant of papillary carcinoma of the thyroid. *Cancer.* 1990; 66:2306.

230. Gomez-Morales M, Alvaro T, Munoz M, et al. Diffuse sclerosing papillary carcinoma of the thyroid gland: Immunohistochemical analysis of the local host immune response. *Histopathology.* 1991; 18:427.

231. Hayashi Y, Sasao T, Takeichi N, et al. Diffuse sclerosing variant of papillary carcinoma of the thyroid: A histopathological study of four cases. *Acta Pathol Jpn.* 1990; 40:193.

232. Moreno-Egea A, Rodriguez Gonzalez JM, Sola Perez J, Soria T, Parilla Paricio P. Clinicopathological study of the diffuse sclerosing variety of papillary cancer of the thyroid. Presentation of 4 new cases and review of the literature. *Eur J Surg Oncol.* 1994; 20:7.

233. Soares J, Limbert E, Sobrinho-Simoes M. Diffuse sclerosing variant of papillary thyroid carcinoma: A clinicopathologic study of ten cases. *Pathol Res Pract.* 1989; 185:200.

234. Schroder S, Bay V, Dumke K, et al. Diffuse sclerosing variant of papillary thyroid carcinoma: s100 protein immunocytochemistry and prognosis. *Virch Arch [A].* 1990; 416:367.

235. Furmanchuk AW, Averkin JI, Egloff B, et al. Pathomorphological findings in thyroid cancers of children from the republic of Belarus: A study of 86 cases occurring between 1986 (post Chernobyl) and 1991. *Histopathology.* 1992; 21:401.

236. Peters SB, Chatten J, LiVolsi VA. Pediatric papillary thyroid carcinoma. *Mod Pathol.* 1994; 7:55. Abstract.

237. Evans HL. Encapsulated papillary neoplasms of the thyroid: A study of 14 cases followed for a minimum of 10 years. *Am J Surg Pathol.* 1987; 11:592.

238. Schroder S, Bocker W, Dralle H, et al. The encapsulated papillary carcinoma of the thyroid: A morphologic subtype of the papillary thyroid carcinoma. *Cancer*. 1984; 54:90.

239. Bisi H, Longatto Filho A, Asat de Camargo RY, Fernandes VSO. Thyroid papillary carcinoma lipomatous type: Report of two cases. *Pathologica*. 1993; 85:761.

240. Gnepp DR, Orgorzalek JM, Heffess CS. Fat-containing lesion of the thyroid gland. *Am J Surg Pathol*. 1989; 13:605.

241. Bruno J, Ciancia EM, Pingitore R. Thyroid papillary adenocarcinoma: Lipomatous type. *Virch Arch [A]*. 1989; 414: 371.

242. Chan JKC, Rosai J. Papillary carcinoma of the thyroid with exuberant fasciitis like stroma: Report of three cases. *Am J Clin Pathol*. 1991; 95:309.

243. Chan JKC, Loo KT. Cribriform variant of papillary thyroid carcinoma. *Arch Pathol Lab Med*. 1990; 114:622.

244. Mizukami Y, Kuruyama H, Kitagawa T, et al. Papillary carcinoma of the thyroid with fibromatosis-like stroma: A case report and review of the literature. *Mod Pathol*. 1995; 8:366.

245. Ostrowski MA, Moffat FL, Asa SL, Rostein LE, Chamberlain D. Myxomatous change in papillary carcinoma of the thyroid. *Surg Pathol*. 1989; 2:249.

246. Vestfrid MA. Papillary carcinoma of the thyroid gland with lipomatous stroma: Report of a peculiar histologic type of thyroid tumour. *Histopathology*. 1986; 10:97.

247. Beckner ME, Heffess CS, Oertel JE. Oxyphilic papillary thyroid carcinomas. *Am J Clin Pathol*. 1995; 103:280.

248. Hamburger JI. The autonomously functioning thyroid adenoma. *N Engl J Med*. 1983; 309:1312.

249. Pamke TW, Croxson MS, et al. Triiodothyroninine secreting (toxic) adenoma of the thyroid gland. *Cancer*. 1978; 41:528.

250. Evans HL. Follicular neoplasms of the thyroid. A study of 44 cases followed for a minimum of 10 years with emphasis on differential diagnosis. *Cancer*. 1984; 54:535.

251. DeRienzo D, Truong L. Thyroid neoplasms containing mature fat: A report of two cases and review of the literature. *Mod Pathol*. 1989; 2:506.

252. Visona A, Pea M, Bozzola L, Stracca-Pansa V, Meli S. Follicular adenoma of the thyroid gland with extensive chondroid metaplasia. *Histopathology*. 1991; 18:278.

253. Wilson NW, Pameakian H, Richardson TC, et al. Epithelial markers in thyroid carcinoma. An immunoperoxidase study. *Histopathology*. 1986; 10:815.

254. Greenabaum E, Koss LG, Elequin F, Silver CE. The diagnostic value of flow cytometric DNA measurements in follicular tumors of the thyroid gland. *Cancer*. 1985; 56:2011.

255. Hicks DG, LiVolsi VA, Neidich JA, Puck JM, Kant JA. Clonal analysis of solitary follicular nodules in the thyroid. *Am J Pathol*. 1990; 137:553.

256. Hostetter AL, Frankelsson J, Wingren SO, Enestrom S, Nordenskjold B. A comparative study of DNA cytometry methods for benign and malignant thyroid tissue. *Am J Clin Pathol*. 1988; 89:760.

257. Joensuu H, Klemi P, Eerola E. DNA aneuploidy in follicular adenomas of the thyroid gland. *Am J Pathol*. 1987; 124:373.

258. Antonini P, Venuat AM, Linares G, et al. Cytogenetic abnormalities in thyroid adenomas. *Cancer Genet Cytogenet*. 1991; 52:157.

259. Meissner WA. Surgical pathology. In Sedgwick CE, ed. *Surgery of the Thyroid Gland*. Philadelphia: WB Saunders; 1974: 24.

260. Bronner MP, LiVolsi VA, Jennings TA. PLAT: Paraganglioma-like adenomas of the thyroid. *Surg Pathol*. 1988; 1:383.

261. Carney JA, Ryan J, Goellner JR. Hyalinizing trabecular adenoma of the thyroid gland. *Am J Surg Pathol*. 1987; 11:583.

262. Chan JK, Tse CC, Chiu HS. Hyalinizing trabecular adenoma-like lesion in multinodular goiter. *Histopathology*. 1990; 16: 611.

263. Katoh R, Jasani B, Williams ED. Hyalinizing trabecular adenoma of the thyroid: A report of three cases with immunohistochemical and ultrastructural studies. *Histopathology*. 1989; 15:211.

264. Sambade C, Franssila K, Cameselle-Teijeiro J, Nesland J, Sobrinho-Simoes M. Hyalinizing trabecular adenoma: A misnomer for a peculiar tumor of the thyroid gland. *Endocrinol Pathol*. 1991; 2:83.

265. Chetty R, Beydoun R, LiVolsi VA. Paraganglioma-like (hyalinizing trabecular) adenoma of the thyroid. *Pathology*. 1994; 26:429.

266. Goellner JR, Carney JA. Cytologic features of fine needle aspirates of hyalinizing trabecular adenoma of the thyroid. *Am J Clin Pathol*. 1989; 91:115.

267. Hazard JB, Kenyon R. Atypical adenoma of the thyroid. *Arch Pathol*. 1954; 58:554.

268. Lang W, Georgii G, et al. The differentiation of atypical adenomas and encapsulated follicular carcinomas in the thyroid gland. *Virch Arch [A]*. 1980; 385:125.

269. Grebe SKG, Hay ID. Follicular thyroid cancer. *Endocrinol Metab Clin North Am*. 1995; 24:761.

270. Brennan MD, Bergstralh EJ, van Heerden JA, McConahey WM. Follicular thyroid cancer treated at the Mayo Clinic, 1946 through 1970: Initial manifestations, pathologic findings, therapy and outcome. *Mayo Clin Proc*. 1991; 66:11.

271. Cooper DS, Schneyer CR. Follicular and Hurthle cell carcinoma of the thyroid. *Endocrinol Metab Clin North Am*. 1990; 19:577.

272. Kahn N, Perzin KH. Follicular carcinoma of the thyroid: An evaluation of the histologic criteria used for diagnosis. *Pathol Annu*. 1983; 18(p1):221.

273. Yamashina M. Follicular neoplasms of the thyroid. Total circumferential evaluation of the fibrous capsule. *Am J Surg Pathol*. 1992; 16:392.

274. Harach HR, Jasani B, Williams ED. Factor VIII as a marker of endothelial cells in follicular carcinoma of the thyroid. *J Clin Pathol*. 1983; 36:1050.

275. Yamasoba T, Kikuchi S, Sagasawa M, Higo R, Sasaki T. Occult follicular carcinoma metastasizing to the sinonasal tract. *J Otorhinol Laryngol Rel Spec*. 1994; 56:239.

276. Clare-Salzer MJ, Van Herle AJ, Varki NM, Tillisch J. Endocardial metastases of follicular thyroid carcinoma: A case report and review of the literature. *Eur J Surg Oncol*. 1991; 17:219.

277. Cumberworth VL, Ohri A, Morrissey G, Stirling R. Late sinonasal metastasis from follicular thyroid carcinoma. *J Laryngol Otol*. 1994; 108:1010.

278. Lang W, Choritz H, Hundeshagen H. Risk factors in follicular thyroid carcinomas. A retrospective follow-up study covering a 14 year period with emphasis on morphologic findings. *Am J Surg Pathol*. 1986; 10:246.

279. Crile G, Pontius KI, Hawk WA. Factors influencing the survival of patients with follicular carcinoma of the thyroid gland. *Surg Gynecol Obstet*. 1985; 160:409.

280. Hruban RH, Huvos AG, Traganos F, et al. Follicular neoplasms of the thyroid in men older than 50 years of age. A DNA flow cytometric study. *Am J Clin Pathol*. 1990; 94:527.

281. Schroder S, Pfannschmidt N, Dralle H, Arps H, Bocker W. The encapsulated follicular carcinoma of the thyroid. *Virch Arch [A]*. 1984; 402:259.

282. Shaha AR, Loree TR, Shah JP. Prognostic factors and risk group analysis in follicular carcinoma of the thyroid. *Surgery*. 1995; 18:1131.

283. Cusick EL, Ewen SWB, Krukowski ZH, Matheson NA. DNA aneuploidy in follicular thyroid neoplasia. *Br J Surg*. 1991; 78:94.

284. Bronner MP, LiVolsi VA. Oxyphilic (Askanazy/Hurthle cell) tumors of the thyroid: Microscopic features predict biologic behavior. *Surg Pathol*. 1988; 1:137.

285. Rainwater LM, Farrow GM, Hay ID, Lieber MM. Oncocytic tumours of the salivary gland, kidney, and thyroid. *Br J Cancer*. 1986; 53:799.

286. Johnson TL, Lloyd RV, Burney RE, Thompson NW. Hurthle cell thyroid tumors: An immunohistochemical study. *Cancer*. 1987; 59:107.

287. Abu-Alfa AK, Straus FH II, Montag AG. An immunohistochemical study of thyroid Hurthle cells and their neoplasms: The roles of S-100 and HMB-45 proteins. *Mod Pathol*. 1994; 7: 529.

288. Nesland JM, Sobrinho-Simoes MA, Holm R, Sambade MC, Johannessen JV. Hurthle-cell lesions of the thyroid: A combined study using transmission electron microscopy, scanning electron microscopy, and immunocytochemistry. *Ultrastruct Pathol.* 1985; 8:269.

289. Wallin G, Backdahl M, Lundell G, Auer G, Lowhagen T. Nuclear DNA content and prognosis in Hurthle cell tumors of the thyroid gland. *Acta Chir Scand.* 1988; 154:501.

290. Bronner MP, Clevenger CV, Edmonds PR, et al. Flow cytometric analysis of DNA content in Hurthle cell adenomas and carcinomas of the thyroid. *Am J Clin Pathol.* 1988; 89:764.

291. El Naggar AK, Batsakis JG, Luna MA, Hickey RC. Hurthle cell tumors of the thyroid: A flow cytometric DNA analysis. *Arch Otolaryngol Head Neck Surg.* 1988; 114:520.

292. McLeod MK, Thompson NW, Hudson JW, et al. Flow cytometric measurements of nuclear DNA and ploidy analysis in Hurthle cell neoplasms of the thyroid. *Arch Surg.* 1988; 123:849.

293. DeLellis RA. The pathology of medullary thyroid carcinoma and its precursors. *Monogr Pathol.* 1993; 35:72.

294. Saad MF, Ordonez NG, Rashid RK, et al. Medullary carcinoma of the thyroid. A study of the clinical features and prognostic factors in 161 patients. *Medicine (Baltimore).* 1984; 63:319.

295. Albores-Saavedra J, LiVolsi, VA, Williams ED. Medullary carcinoma. *Semin Diagn Pathol.* 1985; 2:137.

296. Uribe M, Fenoglio-Preiser CM, Grimes M, Feind C. Medullary carcinoma of the thyroid gland. Clinical, pathological, and immunohistochemical features with review of the literature. *Am J Surg Pathol.* 1985; 9:577.

297. Sambade C, Baldaque-Faria A, Cardoso-Oliveira M, Sobrinho-Somões M. Follicular and papillary variants of medullary carcinoma of the thyroid. *Pathol Res Pract.* 1984; 98:184.

298. Huss LJ, Mendelsohn G. Medullary carcinoma of the thyroid gland: An encapsulated variant resembling the hyalinizing trabecular (paraganglioma-like) adenoma of thyroid. *Mod Pathol.* 1990; 3:581.

299. Driman D, Murray D, Kovacs K. Encapsulated medullary carcinoma of the thyroid. A morphological study including immunocytochemistry, electron microscopy, flow cytometry and in situ hybridization. *Am J Surg Pathol.* 1991; 15:1089.

300. Kodama T, Okamoto T, Fujimoto Y, et al. C-cell adenoma of the thyroid. A rare but distinct clinical entity. *Surgery.* 1988; 104:997.

301. Kakudo K, Miyauchi A, Ogihara T, et al. Medullary carcinoma of the thyroid. Giant cell type. *Arch Pathol Lab Med.* 1978; 102:445.

302. Mendelsohn G, Baylin SB, Bigner SH, Wells SA, Eggleston JC. Anaplastic variants of medullary thyroid carcinoma. A light microscopic and immunohistochemical study. *Am J Surg Pathol.* 1980; 4:333.

303. Martinelli G, Bazzocchi F, Govoni E, Santini D. Anaplastic type of medullary thyroid carcinoma. An ultrastructural and immunohistochemical study. *Virch Arch [A].* 1983; 400:61.

304. Landon G, Ordonez NG. Clear cell variant of medullary carcinoma of the thyroid. *Hum Pathol.* 1985; 16:844.

305. Dominguez-Malagon H, Delgado-Chavez R, Torres-Najera M, Gould E, Albores-Saavedra J. Oxyphil and squamous variants of medullary thyroid carcinoma. *Cancer.* 1989; 63:1183.

306. Pfaltz M, Hedinger CE, Muhlethaler JP. Mixed medullary and follicular carcinoma of the thyroid. *Virch Arch [A].* 1983; 400:53.

307. Sobrinho-Simoes M. Mixed medullary and follicular carcinoma of the thyroid. *Histopathology.* 1993; 23:287.

308. Albores-Saavedra J, De la Mora TG, De la Torre-Rendon F, Gould E. Mixed medullary papillary carcinoma of the thyroid: A previously unrecognized variant of thyroid carcinoma. *Hum Pathol.* 1990; 21:1151.

309. Hales M, Rosenau W, Okerlund MD, Galante M. Carcinoma of the thyroid with a mixed medullary and follicular pattern: Morphological, immunohistochemical, and clinical laboratory studies. *Cancer.* 1982; 50:1352.

310. Holm R, Sobrinho-Simões M, Nesland JM, Johannesson JV.

311. Wolfe H J, Melvin KE, Cervi-Skinner, et al. C-cell hyperplasia preceding medullary thyroid carcinoma. *N Engl J Med.* 1973; 289:437.

312. Albores-Saavedra J. C-cell hyperplasia. *Am J Surg Pathol.* 1989; 13:987.

313. Perry A, Molberg K, Albores-Saavedra J. Physiologic versus neoplastic C-cell hyperplasia of the thyroid: Separation of distinct histologic and biologic entities. *Cancer.* 1996; 17:750.

314. Komminoth P, Roth J, Saremasiani P, et al. Polysialic acid of the neural cell adhesion molecule in the human thyroid: A marker for medullary carcinoma and primary C-cell hyperplasia. An immunohistochemical study on 79 thyroid lesions. *Am J Surg Pathol.* 1994; 18:399.

315. Guyetant S, Wion-Barbot N, Rousselet MC, et al. C-cell hyperplasia associated with chronic lymphocytic thyroiditis: A retrospective quantitative study of 112 cases. *Hum Pathol.* 1994; 25:514.

316. Albores-Saavedra J, Monforte H, Nadji M, Morales AR. C-cell hyperplasia in thyroid tissue adjacent to follicular cell tumors. *Hum Pathol.* 1988; 19:795.

317. Chan JKC, Tse CH. Solid cell nest-associated C-cells; another possible explanation for C-cell hyperplasia adjacent to follicular cell tumors. *Hum Pathol.* 1989; 20:498.

318. Biddinger PW, Brennan MF, Rosen PP. Symptomatic C-cell hyperplasia associated with chronic lymphocytic thyroiditis. *Am J Surg Pathol.* 1991; 15:599.

319. Simpson NE, Kidd KK, Goodfellow PJ, et al. Assignment of multiple endocrine neoplasia type 2A to chromosome 10 by linkage. *Nature.* 1987; 328:528.

320. Grieco M, Santoro M, Berlingieri MT, et al. PTC is a novel re-arranged form of the ret proto-oncogene and is frequently detected in vivo in human thyroid papillary carcinoma. *Cell.* 1990; 60:557.

321. Zaatari GS, Saigo PE, Huvos AG. Mucin production in medullary carcinoma of the thyroid. *Arch Pathol Lab Med.* 1983; 107:70.

322. Marcus JN, Dise CA, LiVolsi VA. Melanin production in a medullary thyroid carcinoma. *Cancer.* 1982; 49:2518.

323. DeLellis RA, Rule AH, Spiler F, et al. Calcitonin and carcinoembryonic antigen as tumor markers in medullary thyroid carcinoma. *Am J Clin Pathol.* 1978; 70:587.

324. Holm R, Sobrinho-Simões M, Nesland JM, Gould VE, Johannessen JV. Medullary carcinoma of the thyroid gland: An immunocytochemical study. *Ultrastruct Pathol.* 1985; 8:25.

325. Sikri KL, Varndell IM, Hamid QA, et al. Medullary carcinoma of the thyroid. An immunocytochemical and histochemical study of 25 cases using eight separate markers. *Cancer.* 1985; 56:2481.

326. Matsubayashi S, Yanaihara C, Ohkubo M, et al. Gastrin-releasing peptide immunoreactivity in medullary thyroid carcinoma. *Cancer.* 1984; 53:2472.

327. Roth KA, Bensch KG, Hoffman AR. Characterization of opioid peptides in human thyroid medullary carcinoma. *Cancer.* 1987; 59:1594.

328. Bergholm V, Adami H-O, Auer G, et al. Histopathologic characteristics and nuclear DNA content as prognostic factors in medullary thyroid carcinoma. *Cancer.* 1989; 64:135.

329. Schroder S, Bocker W, Baisch H, et al. Prognostic factors in medullary thyroid carcinoma. Survival in relation to age, sex, stage, histology, immunocytochemistry, and DNA content. *Cancer.* 1988; 61:806.

330. Carcangiu ML, Zampi G, Rosai J. Poorly differentiated (insular) thyroid carcinoma. *Am J Surg Pathol.* 1984; 8:655.

331. Flynn SD, Forman BH, Stewart AF, Kinder BK. Poorly differentiated ("insular") carcinoma of the thyroid gland: An aggressive subset of differentiated thyroid neoplasms. *Surgery.* 1988; 104:963.

332. Bal C, Padhy AK, Panda S, Kumar L, Basu AK. "Insular" carcinoma of the thyroid. A subset of anaplastic thyroid malignancy with a less aggressive clinical course. *Clin Nucl Med.* 1993; 18:1056.

333. Rosai J, Saxen EA, Woolner L. Undifferentiated and poorly differentiated carcinoma. *Semin Diagn Pathol.* 1985; 2:123.

334. Kileen RM, Barnes L, Watson CG, et al. Poorly differentiated ("insular") thyroid carcinoma. Report of two cases and review of the literature. *Arch Otolaryngol Head Neck Surg.* 1990; 116:1082.

335. Papotti M, Botto Micca F, Favero A, et al. Poorly differentiated thyroid carcinomas with primordial cell component: A group of aggressive lesions sharing insular, trabecular and solid patterns. *Am J Surg Pathol.* 1993; 17:291.

336. Ashfaq R, Vuitch F, Delgado R, et al. Papillary and follicular thyroid carcinomas with an insular component. *Cancer.* 1994; 73:416.

337. Carcangiu ML, Steeper T, Zampi G, Rosai J. Anaplastic thyroid carcinoma. A study of 70 cases. *Am J Clin Pathol.* 1985; 83:135.

338. Aldinger KA, Samaan NA, Ibanez M, Hill CS Jr. Anaplastic carcinoma of the thyroid: A review of 84 cases of spindle and giant cell carcinoma of the thyroid. *Cancer.* 1978; 41: 2267.

339. Hadar T, Mor C, Shvero J, et al. Anaplastic carcinoma of the thyroid. *Eur J Surg Oncol.* 1993; 19:511.

340. Lampertico P. Anaplastic (sarcomatoid) carcinoma of the thyroid gland. *Semin Diagn Pathol.* 1993; 10:159.

341. Nicolosi A, Addis E, Massidda B, et al. Anaplastic carcinoma of the thyroid: Our experience. *Minerva Chir.* 1992; 47:1161.

342. Venkatesh YS, Ordonez NG, Schultz PN, et al. Anaplastic carcinoma of the thyroid. A clinicopathologic study of 121 cases. *Cancer.* 1990; 66:321.

343. Spires JR, Schwartz MR, Miller RH. Anaplastic thyroid carcinoma, association with differentiated thyroid cancer. *Arch. Otolaryngol Head Neck Surg.* 1988; 114:40.

344. Getaz EP, Shimaoka K, Rao U. Anaplastic carcinoma of the thyroid following external irradiation. *Cancer.* 1979; 43:2248.

345. Kapp DS, LiVolsi VA, Sanders MM. Anaplastic carcinoma following well differentiated thyroid cancer: Etiologic considerations. *Yale J Biol Med.* 1982; 55:521.

346. Gaffey MJ, Lack EE, Christ ML, Weiss LM. Anaplastic thyroid carcinoma with osteoclast-like giant cells. A clinicopathologic, immunohistochemical, and ultrastructural study. *Am J Surg Pathol.* 1991; 15:160.

347. Wan SK, Chan JK, Tang SK. Paucicellular variant of anaplastic thyroid carcinoma. A mimic of Riedel's thyroiditis. *Am J Clin Pathol.* 1996; 105:388.

348. LiVolsi VA, Brooks JJ, Arendash-Durand B. Anaplastic thyroid tumors. Immunohistology. *Am J Clin Pathol.* 1987; 87: 434.

349. Ordonez NG, el Naggar AK, Hickey RC, et al. Anaplastic thyroid carcinoma. Immunohistochemical study of 32 cases. *Am J Clin Pathol.* 1991; 96:15.

350. Hurlimann J, Gardiol D, Scazziga B. Immunohistology of anaplastic thyroid carcinoma. A study of 43 cases. *Histopathology.* 1987; 11:567.

351. Harada T, Shimaoka K, Yakumaru K, et al. Squamous cell carcinoma of the thyroid gland-transition from adenocarcinoma. *J Surg Oncol.* 1982; 19:36.

352. Budd DC, Fink DL, Rashti MY, et al. Squamous cell carcinoma of the thyroid. *J Med Soc NJ.* 1982; 79:838.

353. Harada T, Shimaok K, Katagari M, et al. Rarity of squamous cell carcinoma of the thyroid: Autopsy review. *World J Surg.* 1994; 18:542.

354. Kasantikul V, Manseeri S, Panichabhong V, Lerdlum S. Adenosquamous carcinoma of the thyroid: A case report and review of the literature. *J Med Assoc Thailand.* 1995; 78:197.

355. Katoh R, Sugai T, Ono S, et al. Mucoepidermoid carcinoma of the thyroid gland. *Cancer.* 1990; 65:2020.

356. Miranda RN, Myrint MA, Gnepp DR. Composite follicular variant of papillary carcinoma and mucoepidermoid carcinoma of the thyroid. Report of a case and review of the literature. *Am J Surg Pathol.* 1995; 19:1209.

357. Franssila KO, Harach HR, Wasenius VM. Mucoepidermoid carcinoma of the thyroid. *Histopathology.* 1984; 8:847.

358. Rhatigan RM, Roque JL, Bucher RL. Mucoepidermoid carcinoma of the thyroid gland. *Cancer.* 1977; 39:210.

359. Mizukami Y, Matsubara F, Hashimoto T, et al. Primary mucoepidermoid carcinoma in the thyroid gland. *Cancer.* 1984; 53:1741.

360. Vollenweider I, Hedinger C. Solid cell nests in Hashimoto's thyroiditis. *Virch Arch [A].* 1988; 412:357.

361. Tanda F, Massarelli G, Bosincu L, Cossu U. Angiosarcoma of the thyroid: A light, electron microscopic and immunological study. *Hum Pathol.* 1988; 19:742.

362. Brownlie BE, Fitzharris BM, Abdelaal AG, et al. Primary thyroid lymphoma: Clinical features, treatment, and outcome. A report of 8 cases. *NZ Med J.* 1994; 107:301.

363. Devine RM, Edis AJ, Banks PM. Primary lymphoma of the thyroid: A review of the Mayo Clinic experience through 1978. *World J Surg.* 1981; 5:33.

364. Hahn JS, Chung HC, Min YH, et al. Primary lymphoma of the thyroid. *Yonsei Med J.* 1995; 36:315.

365. Anscombe AM, Wright DH. Primary malignant lymphoma of the thyroid—A tumour of mucosa-associated lymphoid tissue: Review of seventy-six cases. *Histopathology.* 1985; 9:81.

366. Aozasa K, Inoue A, Tajima K, et al. Malignant lymphomas of the thyroid gland. Analysis of 79 patients with emphasis on histologic prognostic factors. *Cancer.* 1986; 58:100.

367. Feigin GA, Buss DH, Paschal B, Woodruff RD, Myers RT. Hodgkin's disease manifested as a thyroid nodule. *Hum Pathol.* 1982; 13:774.

368. Tomita Y, Ohsawa M, Kannu H, Matsuzuka F, Kuma K, Aozasa K. Sporadic activation of Epstein-Barr virus in thyroid lymphoma. *Leukemia Lymphoma.* 1995; 19:129.

369. Takahashi K, Kashima K, Daa T, et al. Contribution of Epstein-Barr virus to development of malignant lymphoma of the thyroid. *Pathol. Int.* 1995; 45:366.

370. Chetty R, O'Leary JJ, Biddolph SC, Gatter KC. Immunohistochemical detection of p53 and bcl-2 proteins in Hashimoto's thyroiditis and primary thyroid lymphoma. *J Clin Pathol.* 1995; 48:239.

371. Iyota K, Takeda K, Matsuzuka F, et al. Absence of p53 mutations in Japanese patients with thyroid lymphoma. *J Endocrinol Invest.* 1994; 17:775.

372. Czech JM, Lichter TR, Carney JA, van Heerden JA. Neoplasms metastatic to the thyroid gland. *Surg Gynecol Obstet.* 1982; 155:503.

373. Green LK, Ro JY, Mackay B, Ayala AG, Luna MA. Renal cell carcinoma metastatic to the thyroid. *Cancer.* 1989; 63:1810.

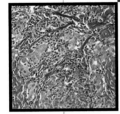

CHAPTER 11

Parathyroid

I. DISEASES OF THE PARATHYROID GLAND

- ■ GEORGE D. CHONKICH
- ■ GEORGE H. PETTI, JR.

SURGICAL ANATOMY

Generally, there are four parathyroid glands situated in close proximity to the thyroid gland; however, in 2% to 8% of patients there can be as few as three glands or as many as six glands.[1] Each gland weighs 35 to 60 mg and is about the size and shape of a lentil bean.[2] The usual size is 3 to 6 mm in length, 2 to 4 mm in width, and 0.5 to 2 mm thick, with an average dimension of $5 \times 3 \times 1$ mm (Fig. 11–1). The glands are usually yellow-tan to orange-tan, depending on the amount of fat, degree of vascular congestion, and number of oxyphilic cells. The amount of fat present in a parathyroid gland varies with the patient's age and body habitus.

The blood supply to the inferior and superior parathyroid glands is generally derived from the distal branches of the inferior thyroid artery. Occasionally, the superior parathyroid glands receive their blood supply from the superior thyroid artery. The parathyroid glands may be closely adherent to the thyroid capsule; however, as shown by Halstead,[3] the blood supply comes only from the parathyroid artery branches (Fig. 11–2). This is helpful to remember when attempting to locate a parathyroid gland that may be atrophic, or in an ectopic location.

EMBRYOLOGY AND MALFORMATION

The parathyroid glands form from the third and fourth branchial pouches (Fig. 11–3). The third pouch also forms the thymus gland, so the third pouch parathyroid glands migrate inferiorly with the thymus gland to their usual location at the level of the lower pole of the thyroid gland.[3] The fourth pouch parathyroid glands normally descend to a position on the posterior capsule of the thyroid lobe at the level of the cricothyroid junction.[1] Parathyroid glands have been found as high as the internal carotid artery, and as low as the aortopulmonary window, anterior or posterior to the aortic arch (Fig. 11–4). The number of parathyroid glands may vary from three to five or more. Eighty percent of people have four glands, 13% to 15% have five or more glands, and 5% have only three glands.[4]

Edis et al[5] found that 10% of parathyroid glands were located in the thymus, 1% were intrathyroidal, 1% were within the carotid sheath, and 0.5% were undescended at the level of the carotid bulb. Aberrant parathyroid glands occur in 15% to 20% of patients (Fig. 11–5).[6] Surgeons must have a thorough

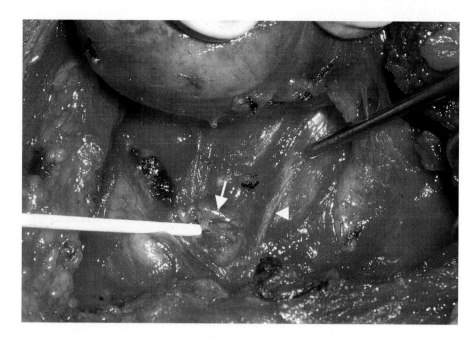

FIGURE 11–1 Intraoperative view of the normal parathyroid gland *(long arrow)* with a recurrent laryngeal nerve evident in the tracheoesophageal groove *(arrowhead).*

knowledge of parathyroid embryology in order to locate ectopic glands (Table 11–1).[7]

PHYSIOLOGY AND PATHOPHYSIOLOGY

The primary function of the parathyroid glands is to maintain calcium and phosphorus homeostasis. Calcium is important for the formation of intracellular ground substance, teeth, and bone. At the cellular level, calcium affects neuromuscular irritability, muscle contractility, and cardiac rhythmicity. It is pumped from the extracellular to the intracellular level, circulating in the extracellular compartment in three forms. Forty-seven percent of calcium is ionized in its free and active form; 47% is bound to albumin and globulin, with levels fluctuating according to the serum protein level; and 6% is bound to anions, such as bicarbonate, phosphate, and citrate. There is slightly more than 1 kg of calcium in the average 70-kg male. It is absorbed primarily

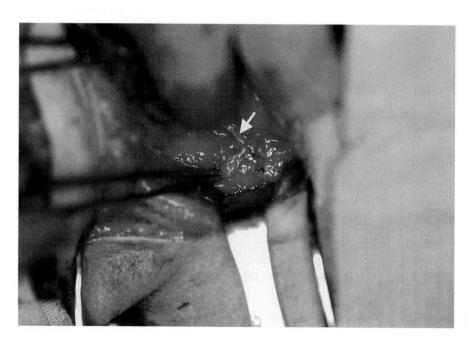

FIGURE 11–2 Intraoperative view of a normal parathyroid gland with its blood supply derived from a terminal branch of the inferior thyroid artery *(arrow).*

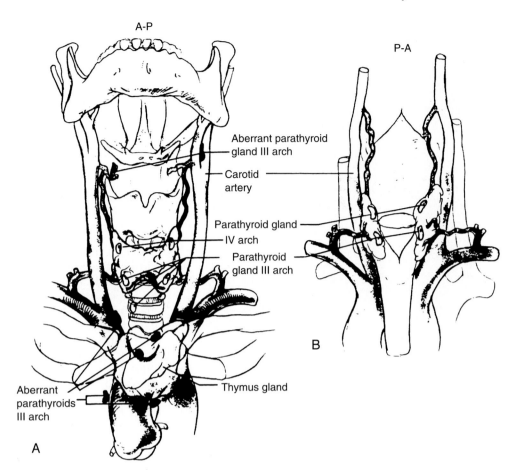

A-P

Aberrant parathyroid
gland III arch

Carotid
artery

Parathyroid gland

IV arch

Parathyroid
gland III arch

Aberrant
parathyroids
III arch

Thymus gland

P-A

B

A

FIGURE 11–3 Diagram showing the normal location of the parathyroid gland and aberrant locations. *A,* Anteroposterior view. *B,* Posteroanterior view. From Petti GH. Parathyroid disease and surgery. In: Bailey BJ, ed. *Head and Neck Surgery—Otolaryngology. Vol 1.* Philadelphia: JB Lippincott; 1993:1248, with permission.

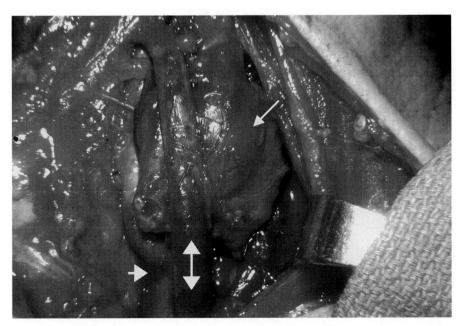

FIGURE 11–4 Photograph of a large parathyroid adenoma located at the carotid bifurcation. The double arrow indicates the internal jugular vein. The short arrow shows the carotid artery bifurcation. The long arrow points to the parathyroid adenoma.

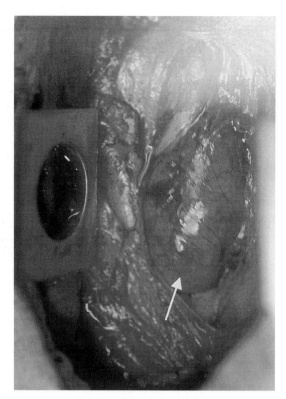

FIGURE 11-5 Mediastinal gland depicted on MRI. An operative view through a median sternotomy shows a large parathyroid adenoma in the anterior mediastinum (arrow).

TABLE 11-1	ABERRANT LOCATION OF PARATHYROID GLANDS

Superior Parathyroid Glands (4th Pouch)
Posterior mediastinum
Retroesophageal, prevertebral
Tracheoesophageal groove
Intrathyroidal

Inferior Parathyroid Glands (3rd Pouch)
Anterior mediastinum
Thymus
Aortopulmonary window
Carotid bifurcation

Adapted from Petti GH. Endocrinology. In: Bailey BJ, ed. *Head and Neck Surgery—Otolaryngology.* Vol. 1. Philadelphia: JB Lippincott; 1993: 140.

from the duodenum and upper jejunum, and it exists in four forms: 1 kg is stable in bone, 4 g are exchangeable in bone, 11 g exist as intracellular calcium, and 1 g represents extracellular fluid.[7]

When serum calcium levels fall, the parathyroid glands release parathyroid hormone (PTH), which results in the following changes:[8]

1. Increased osteoclastic activity leading to bone resorption and release of calcium
2. Increased resorption of calcium at the renal tubular cell
3. Increased absorption of calcium from the intestine
4. Stimulation of renal-1 hydroxylase, which allows 1-hydroxylation of vitamin D in the kidney

Parathyroid hormone acts directly on bone and kidney and indirectly on the intestines by promoting the formation of vitamin D. Vitamin D is produced by exposure to sunlight or by dietary intake. The inactive form of vitamin D is transported to the liver, where it is converted to 25-hydroxyvitamin D_2. This form of vitamin D_2 is then transported to the kidney, where the enzyme renal-1 hydroxylase, at the proximal tubule level, converts it to 1, 25 dihydroxyvitamin D_3. The active form of vitamin D increases the absorption of calcium and phosphorus from the small intestine, and increases calcium mobilization from bone (Fig. 11–6). Parathyroid hormone is a peptide composed of 84 amino acids with an active amino terminal and an inactive carboxyl terminal. PTH is secreted in response to low levels of ionized calcium and a high phosphate level.[8] Calcitonin is a 32–amino acid peptide that influences calcium homeostasis by suppressing osteoclastic activity in bone and decreasing the amount of calcium available to the extracellular space.[7]

BENIGN LESIONS

Primary Hyperparathyroidism

Primary hyperparathyroidism is the leading cause of hypercalcemia in the United States and the second most common cause of this condition, after malignant disease, in hospitalized patients. With the increased routine use of the chemistry profile, most cases of hypercalcemia are now diagnosed in patients who are asymptomatic.

Epidemiology

Mundy et al[9] estimated the annual incidence of primary hyperparathyroidism to be 25 cases per 100,000 population. With increasing age, the incidence increases to 200 cases per 100,000 population in females, and 1 per 100,000 in males.[10] Primary hyperparathyroidism is caused by adenoma in 85% of cases and by hyperplasia in the remaining 15% (Fig. 11–7).

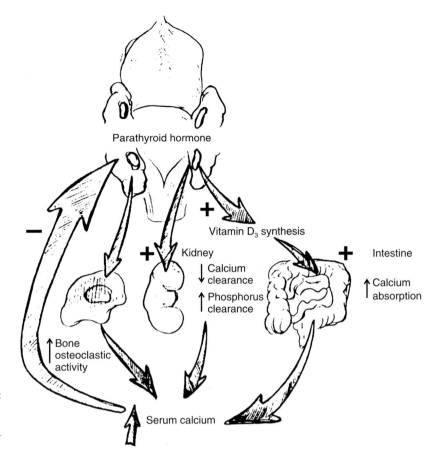

FIGURE 11-6 Diagram outlining the physiologic effects of parathyroid hormone on bone, kidney, and small intestine. From Petti GH. Endocrinology. In: Bailey BJ ed. *Head and Neck Surgery—Otolaryngology.* Vol. 1. Philadelphia: JB Lippincott; 1993:140, with permission.

Etiology

Some cases of primary hyperparathyroidism are inherited as familial hyperparathyroidism or as multiple endocrine neoplasia (MEN), types 1 and 2. In these cases, the usual finding is four-gland hyperplasia. Ninety percent of the cases of primary hyperparathyroidism are sporadic in origin (no known cause). Neonatal primary hyperparathyroidism is genetically transmitted as an autosomal dominant condition.[11] It is frequently seen in children whose parents have benign familial hypocalciuric hypercalcemia.[12] Primary

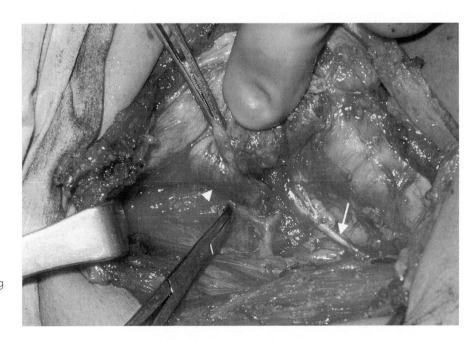

FIGURE 11-7 Photograph of a superior parathyroid adenoma *(arrowhead)* showing a branch of the inferior thyroid artery *(clamp)* and the adjacent recurrent laryngeal nerve *(long arrow).*

hyperparathyroidism may also be caused by exposure to low-dose therapeutic radiation.[13] Other possible causes of primary hyperparathyroidism include chronic excessive stimulation of the parathyroid glands with the use of chronic administration of furosemide and prolonged intake of a phosphate-rich, calcium-poor diet.[14,15] Primary hyperparathyroidism is known to be most common in postmenopausal women owing to metabolic changes and osteoporosis.[16] Primary hyperparathyroidism occasionally occurs with other conditions that may cause hypercalcemia, such as thyrotoxicosis, sarcoidosis, Paget's disease, milk alkali syndrome, and cancer.[17]

Clinical Presentation

Primary hyperparathyroidism can involve many body systems, and the symptoms may be nonspecific. In the authors' series of patients with primary hyperparathyroidism treated at Loma Linda University Medical Center, the following incidence of symptoms was reported:

Fatigue, 40%

Musculoskeletal complaints, 20%

Gastrointestinal complaints, 20%

Renal stones, 10%

Renal failure, 15%

Hypertension, 10%

Hyperparathyroidism may also occur as part of MEN syndromes. Common symptoms include polydipsia, nephrocalcinosis, bone and joint pain, constipation, anorexia, nausea, hypertension, depression, lethargy, pancreatitis, and band keratopathy.[1]

Advanced disease may be manifested as osteitis fibrosa cystica, which appears on x-ray studies as a moth-eaten appearance of the skull and subperiosteal resorption of the middle phalanges.[1] There may also be true bone cysts, so-called brown tumors, seen on x-ray films in patients with advanced disease.

Normocalcemic Hyperparathyroidism. Normocalcemic hyperparathyroidism is an uncommon presentation. Patients with symptomatic nephrolithiasis and hypercalciuria are most often suspected as having normocalcemic hyperparathyroidism. In these patients, the following conditions can occur: hypoalbuminemia, pancreatitis, renal failure; increased phosphate intake, vitamin D deficiency, hypomagnesemia, or lab error.[18-21] All of the aforementioned conditions are associated with a low or normal serum calcium level.

The correct diagnosis can be established by evaluating the patient's clinical findings, along with determining the serum albumin, blood urea nitrogen (BUN), creatinine, amylase, vitamin D, and magnesium levels. If all of these values are normal, a 24-hour urine calcium study should be obtained. If the urine calcium level is greater than 250 to 300 mg in 24 hours, a differential diagnosis of hyperparathyroidism, absorption hypercalciuria, or renal hypercalciuria should be considered. A PTH level can then help to differentiate between these three possible causes. If the PTH is low, absorption hypercalciuria is the cause.[22] If it is elevated, the elevation may be secondary to compensation of the parathyroid gland for a renal loss of calcium (renal hypercalciuria).[23] In these patients, the use of thiazide diuretics will correct the excessive loss of renal calcium. If a patient with normocalcemic hyperparathyroidism is treated with a thiazide diuretic, the PTH level and the urinary calcium level remain elevated and the serum calcium level increases.[24]

Nichols et al[24] described a phosphate deprivation test that can help to differentiate patients with normocalcemic hyperparathyroidism from those with idiopathic hypercalciuria.[24] Those patients whose serum calcium level increases above normal, or those who have persistent hypercalciuria usually have hyperparathyroidism.

Diagnosis

The evaluation of a patient with hypercalcemia should include an awareness by the physician of the multiple causes, other than primary hyperparathyroidism, for this condition (Table 11–2).[25] The preoperative evaluation should include an evaluation for a family history of MEN or hyperparathyroid-

T A B L E 11 – 2	**CAUSES OF HYPERCALCEMIA**

1. Primary hyperparathyroidism (most common cause)
2. Malignant disease (second most common cause; related to metastatic bone disease from carcinoma of the breast, lung, kidney, and prostate)
3. Other endocrine disorders
   Hyperthyroidism
   Adrenal insufficiency
   Pheochromocytoma
   VIPoma
4. Vitamin D toxicity
5. Granulomatous diseases
   Sarcoidosis
   Tuberculosis
   Histoplasmosis
   Coccidiomycosis
   Leprosy
6. Lymphomas (with ectopic production of 1,25-dihydroxyvitamin D)
7. Drugs
   Thiazide diuretics
   Lithium
   Estrogen/anti-estrogens
   Milk alkali syndrome
   Vitamin A (toxicity)
8. Immobilization
9. Acute and chronic renal disease
10. Benign familial hypocalciuric hypercalcemia

Adapted from Petti GH. Endocrinology. In: Bailey BJ, ed. *Head and Neck Surgery—Otolaryngology.* Vol. 1. Philadelphia: JB Lippincott; 1993: 140.

ism, a history of low-dose radiation exposure, or chronic use of diuretics, such as Lasix (furosemide).

The physical examination does not usually reveal any neck masses. However, a marfanoid habitus, mucosal and cutaneous neuromas, thyroid masses, or the presence of hypertension may indicate the possibility of MEN syndrome, which requires a more extensive work-up, and involves ruling out pheochromocytoma, pituitary tumor, and medullary thyroid carcinoma.[8]

An elevated serum calcium level should prompt at least three laboratory tests for serum calcium concentrations. Simultaneous serum protein levels should be obtained because 80% to 85% of nonionized calcium is bound to albumin. For each gram per deciliter that the serum albumin is reduced, one needs to increase the total serum calcium by 0.8 mg/dL.[8] PTH concentrations are elevated in primary hyperparathyroidism. A new assay, immunoradiometric assay (IRMA)–PTH, uses antibodies against the C terminal and the N terminal of the parathyroid horomone, and is quite specific for parathyroid hormone. This assay can differentiate true parathyroid hormone from the parathryoid hormone–like peptides secreted by individuals with hypercalcemia associated with malignant disease.

An elevated alkaline phosphate level in the absence of liver disease indicates overt bone disease. Postoperatively, these patients exhibit a bone hunger for calcium, and temporary calcium supplementation is frequently needed. Serum phosphorus levels are usually low in cases of primary hyperparathyroidism. If elevated, the patient probably has renal failure or an excess intake of phosphorus. Serum chloride levels may be elevated because PTH decreases the resorption of bicarbonate in the kidney, resulting in an increased resorption of chloride and a mild hyperchloremic renal tubular acidosis.[8] BUN and serum creatinine testing is used to evaluate renal function.

Radiologic Evaluation

Radiographic films of the phalanges, skull, or extremities, looking for soft tissue calcification, are not routinely obtained. There is disagreement regarding the need for preoperative localization tests in the patient undergoing an initial surgical exploration for primary hyperparathyroidism. Those who favor preoperative localization tests prior to the time of the first operation believe that, if accurate, these tests can decrease operating room time, length of hospital stay, and the potential morbidity of hypoparathyroidism by directing the surgeon to the offending gland.[26]

Localization techniques include technetium-thallium parathyroid scanning, ultrasonography, computed tomography (CT) scans, magnetic resonance imaging (MRI), arteriography, and venography with selected venous catheterization for parathyroid hormone levels (Fig. 11–8). The technetium-thallium scan is the least expensive of these, and in the au-

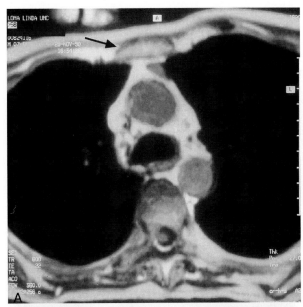

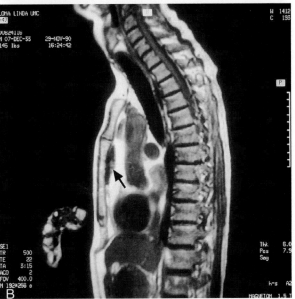

FIGURE 11–8 *A,* Anteroposterior view of an anterior mediastinal adenoma demonstrated on MRI *(arrow). B,* Lateral view of an anterior mediastinal adenoma *(arrow).*

thors' institution it has proven accurate in 85% to 90% of cases (Fig. 11–9).[26] The scan's accuracy is decreased to 35% in patients with hyperplasia, and false-positive results may be attained in patients with associated thyroid disease. The scan also may not localize small glands, and its accuracy decreases in patients who are receiving suppressive thyroid medication. Recently, sestamibi scans have been used in place of the technetium-thallium scan; however, there is no consensus yet as to any advantage the former test may have over the technetium-thallium scan.[27]

Ultrasonography is not able to penetrate air or bone, and is also unable to locate small parathyroid

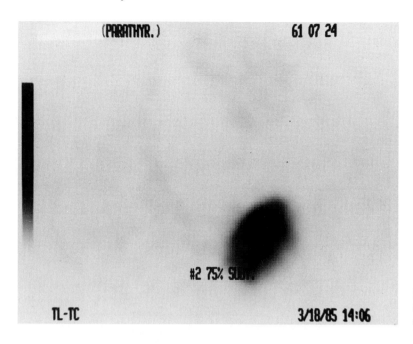

(PARATHYR.)   61 07 24

#2 75% SUB

TL-TC   3/18/85 14:06

FIGURE 11-9 Parathyroid technetium-thallium subtraction scan demonstrating a left inferior parathyroid adenoma.

glands.²⁸ CT scans cannot identify glands measuring less than 1 cm in diameter, or glands that are intimately associated with the thyroid gland.²⁹

Selective venography is time-consuming, technically demanding, and expensive. It should only be used in patients requiring reoperation for hypercalcemia (Fig. 11–10). If, during previous operations,

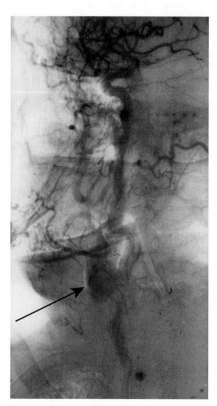

FIGURE 11-10 Selective venography demonstrating a large parathyroid adenoma (arrow) at the carotid bifurcation.

the thyroid vein were ligated, the test may be nonlocalizing.

Treatment

The treatment of primary hyperparathyroidism is surgical exploration of the neck with parathyroidectomy. In the hands of an experienced surgeon, the initial operation should be curative in 95% of cases. Most authors believe that asymptomatic primary hyperparathyroidism may not require surgical treatment.³⁰⁻³² A large proportion of patients with asymptomatic hyperparathyroidism do not show any evidence of worsening hypercalcemia or bone or renal disease, although the potential for this to occur is still being investigated. Most surgeons believe that any patient with a serum calcium level of greater than 1 mg/dL above the normal level should undergo surgical exploration. Some authors have stated that patients who are asymptomatic with only mildly elevated calcium levels (less than 11.5 mg/dL) would also benefit from parathyroidectomy.³³,³⁴

The incidence of hyperparathyroidism is 0.2% to 0.5% of the population, and 100,000 cases are diagnosed each year in the United States. Because many of the patients who are diagnosed with hyperparathyroidism have minimal or no symptoms, there is disagreement among physicians as to the need for parathyroidectomy in all of these patients. This problem was addressed at the National Institute of Health (NIH) Consensus Development Conference convened on October 29, 1990.³⁵ The conference participants addressed three questions:

1. Are there patients with asymptomatic parathyroidism who can be safely monitored?
2. If they do not undergo surgery, how should asymptomatic patients be monitored?

3. What are the indications for surgery in patients with asymptomatic hyperparathyroidism?

The following are the criteria established by the conference participants for proceeding with surgery in these patients:

1. A serum calcium level of greater than 11.5 mg/dL
2. A history of life-threatening hypercalcemia
3. Reduced renal function; creatinine clearance values decreased by 30%
4. Radiologic evidence of kidney stones or nephrocalcinosis
5. A 24-hour urine calcium level greater than 400 mg
6. A reduction in bone density of greater than two standard deviations below normal for age-, gender-, and race-matched normal subjects
7. Patients in whom medical surveillance is not desirable or advisable

Surgery was also indicated in patients who requested it, those unwilling to comply with medical management, those whose coexisting illness might complicate management, and patients younger than 50 years of age because no study has monitored a large series of such patients for several decades. If medical follow-up evaluation is elected, a serum calcium and creatinine level should be assessed every 6 months for 3 years, along with blood pressure measurements and creatinine clearance testing. Every 2 years, the patient should undergo a 24-hour urine test for calcium excretion, as well as bone densitometry.[36-38]

According to Rao et al,[32] the proportion of patients eventually requiring surgery may be less than 30%. Scholz and associates[34] evaluated 147 patients with minimal hyperparathyroidism for a period of 10 years. Thirty-eight patients underwent parathyroidectomy, 35 died, 13 were lost to follow-up, and 61 patients remained unoperated. In the unoperated group, 38 had persistent disease, 13 had an indeterminate status, and 10 refused follow-up studies. Parathyroidectomy was performed in 50% of the patients alive and available for follow-up studies. The likelihood of a patient with a calcium concentration of less than 11 mg/dL requiring parathyroidectomy is slight; only one patient in the series reported by Scholz et al[34] underwent surgery. Most authors who have recommended observation of affected patients have not monitored their patients for a long enough period or have not had enough patients undergo the necessary follow-up studies to determine whether or not surgery was needed. Still other authors believe that true asymptomatic hyperparathyroidism is unusual. Many of the vague symptoms reported do not correlate with the degree of hypercalcemia; however, fatigue, bone pain, and weight loss have been found to correlate with the degree of hypercalcemia.[27] In a small study of 13 patients treated surgically, 6 of whom had asymptomatic hyperparathyroidism and 7 of whom had symptomatic hyperparathyroidism, Kaplan et al[33] noted that the outcome in the asymptomatic group was similar to that of the symptomatic group. That is, serum calcium and PTH levels returned to normal, bone density improved, and urinary calciuria decreased in all patients. In three of these six patients, renal function also improved. Clark et al[39] have noted that certain conditions occur more frequently in patients with primary hyperparathyroidism, including osteopenia, hypertension, nephrolithiasis, gout, decreased renal function, peptic ulcer disease, osteitis fibrosa cystica, and pancreatitis. Scholz and co-workers[34] reported that 81% of the patients in their series who were referred with symptoms improved after parathyroidectomy. In the study of 250 patients conducted by Uden et al,[40] more than 92% of the patients were symptomatic. Of these, the older patients (47%) were more likely to have hypertension than the younger patients (28%), whereas the younger patients (31%) were more likely to have nephrolithiasis than the older patients (12%). In both groups, 82% of the patients reported an improvement in symptoms postoperatively.[40] Several studies have found a decreased survival rate in patients with asymptomatic hyperparathyroidism.[41-44] The increased death rate in these patients was primarily attributable to cancer and cardiovascular disease.

The surgical approach is similar to that used in performing a thyroidectomy. Many surgeons believe that all four parathyroid glands must be identified. However, with the use of more accurate localization tests, some surgeons advocate unilateral exploration with the identification of the enlarged gland, and biopsy of one normal gland.

Unilateral Surgical Exploration. In a series of 371 patients undergoing surgery over a 15-year period, Worsey et al[45] performed unilateral exploration in 125 patients. Of these, 122 patients had a single adenoma, two patients had parathyroid carcinoma, and one patient had an unrecognized hyperplasia. In the 246 patients who had bilateral exploration, four had a double adenoma and four had parathyroid carcinoma. The authors concluded that unilateral exploration was safe and effective in selected cases.

Other authors have demonstrated a reduction in operating time from 3.0 to 2.5 hours when preoperative localization was used. This savings in time, however, must be weighed against the additional cost of preoperative localization techniques.[46] Many surgeons believe that all four glands need to be identified in every case.[47] Duh et al[48] attempted to resolve this controversy by using a mathematical model. These researchers concluded that only 41% of the patients treated by the unilateral approach actually undergo unilateral exploration. They believe that the probability of missing a tumor on the unexplored side of the neck parallels the prevalence of multiple adenomas.[48] Thompson and associates[49] noted an 8% incidence of double adenoma; these researchers strongly advocate routine bilateral exploration.

In patients with diffuse hyperplasia either 3.5 glands are resected or a total parathyroidectomy is performed, with autotransplantation of approximately 40 mg of parathyroid tissue. Parathyroid autotransplantation was first reported almost 100 years ago by Halstead[50] to be possible in dogs. In 1929, Catell[51] recommended autotransplantation of parathyroid glands removed during thyroidectomy. Wells et al[52] suggested autotransplantation in the following four clinical situations:

1. Primary parathyroid hyperplasia
2. Secondary parathyroid hyperplasia in patients requiring dialysis
3. When surgical reexploration is indicated for persistent or recurrent hyperparathyroidism
4. When total thyroidectomy is performed for carcinoma

The technique involves saving the equivalent of one parathyroid gland (40 mg), cutting the gland into multiple 1- to 3-mm slices, and then transplanting these slices into three to four muscle pockets, with 5 to 10 pieces being placed in each muscle pocket (Fig. 11–11).[53] Other researchers advocate inserting approximately 20 1- to 3-mm pieces in individual muscle pockets.[54] In patients with parathyroid hyperplasia, the autografts are placed in the brachioradialis muscle of the forearm. In patients undergoing total thyroidectomy, the transplanted tissue can be placed in the sternomastoid muscle, thereby avoiding any additional incisions. The pockets are closed with nonabsorbable sutures or surgical clips. In patients undergoing total or subtotal parathyroidectomy, any parathyroid gland that is devascularized should be autotransplanted. It usually takes about 6 weeks for the graft to function, and

the success rate is reported to be more than 85%. Patients should not have blood drawn from the arm with the autografts, nor should a blood pressure cuff be placed on that arm. If the calcium levels drop below 7 mg/dL, the patient should be given intravenous calcium gluconate and vitamin D, and then switched to oral calcium supplements after several days. In performing parathyroid surgery, it is advisable for the surgeon to remember that the inferior parathyroid glands are most variable in location, but are usually within 1 to 2 cm of the inferior thyroid artery. It is also important for the surgeon to realize that a small percentage of adenomas are located intrathyroidally, in which case thyroid lobectomy may be needed to locate the missing parathyroid gland. The superior parathyroid glands are more constant in location, being generally located on the posterior aspect of the thyroid lobe, at a point where the recurrent laryngeal nerve passes deep to the cricothyroid muscle.

No parathyroid gland that appears normal should be removed unless a biopsy shows it to be hyperplastic. The parathyroid glands contain a variable amount of fat, and with surgical manipulation, will turn a deep red-brown color. If the blood supply to the gland is interrupted, the gland will turn a blue-black color. In this case, it should be removed and diced for autotransplantation to the neck or forearm muscles (Fig. 11–12). It is important to remember that the incidence of double adenoma can be as high as 20% for patients older than 60 years of age. In considering hyperplasia, the size of the individual glands can be quite variable.

Cryopreservation of removed parathyroid tissue will allow for autotransplantation in the event that the patient's hypoparathyroidism persists postoperatively. The ability to cryopreserve parathyroid tissue

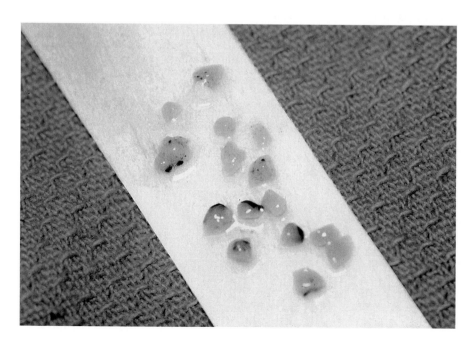

FIGURE 11–11 Photograph of a parathyroid gland that has been diced into small pieces in preparation for autotransplantation.

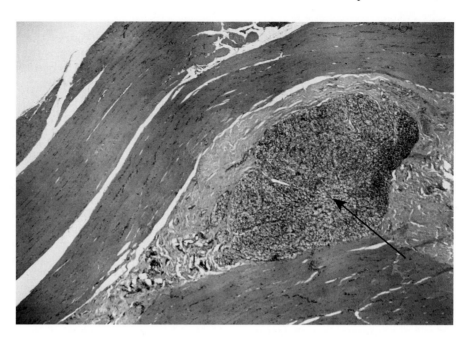

FIGURE 11-12 Photograph demonstrating a functioning parathyroid gland (arrow) transplanted into the forearm muscle.

for later use has been a very beneficial advance in the treatment of diffuse parathyroid hyperplasia. In the event that the autotransplantation is unsuccessful, it is wise to take any parathyroid tissue that is not placed in muscle pockets and cryopreserve the fragments for possible later use. Cryopreservation is particularly helpful in patients undergoing reoperation for diffuse hyperplasia or thyroid carcinoma. The technique of cryopreservation has been well described by Wells et al,[55] and it is the same technique used by our immunology laboratory at Loma Linda University Medical Center. Three to four 1- to 3-mm slices of parathyroid tissue are placed in individual vials containing a chilled solution of 10% dimethyl sulfoxide (DMSO), 10% pooled human serum, and 80% tissue culture medium RPMI-1640. The vials are then placed in an alcohol freezing bath kept at a temperature of $-80°$ C. The vials are then moved the next day to a liquid nitrogen storage tank and kept at $-200°$ C.

At the time of thawing, the vial is immediately placed in a 37° C water bath and gently agitated until the last ice crystals disappear. The vials are emptied, and the removed parathyroid tissue is washed three times in chilled RPMI-1640 tissue culture medium containing 20% pooled human serum to remove the DMSO, which is toxic at room temperature.[55] Tissue that has been cryopreserved for as long as 18 months has been known to function after transplantation.[56]

Prognosis

The cure rate in primary hyperparathyroidism is approximately 95%; in the remaining 5% of patients, recurrent hyperparathyroidism develops. The patients with recurrent disease require preoperative localization studies, and there is an increased risk of recurrent laryngeal nerve injury and hypoparathyroidism in this group. Surgical complications include postoperative hemorrhage, seroma, temporary hypocalcemia (20% to 30%), and vocal cord paralysis (<1%). If the patient develops symptomatic hypocalcemia postoperatively, they should be treated temporarily with intravenous calcium gluconate and then switched to oral calcium supplements for a period of several weeks.

Secondary Hyperparathyroidism

Secondary hyperparathyroidism occurs as a result of chronic renal disease or malabsorption. The common denominator is hypocalcemia, which stimulates parathyroid hormone secretion and results in varying degrees of parathyroid gland hyperplasia. Most patients with secondary hyperparathyroidism respond to medical management, whereas 5% to 10% of the affected patients require surgical treatment. Successful renal transplantation will usually correct the secondary hyperparathyroidism.[57] The other factors involved in the development of secondary hyperparathyroidism include phosphate retention and hyperphosphatemia, altered vitamin D metabolism, impaired PTH degradation, skeletal resistance to the hypercalcemic action of PTH, and, finally, magnesium retention.

The medical treatment of secondary hyperparathyroidism includes a low-phosphate diet, administration of phosphate binders with meals, oral calcium supplementation, and vitamin D supplementation. Parathyroidectomy is recommended for patients with secondary hyperparathyroidism who have complications, such as severe pruritis, extensive soft tissue calcification, calciphylaxis, bone pain, spontaneous bone fractures, psychoneurologic disorders, and serum calcium levels greater than 11 mg/dL.[57] Patients who are compliant and willing to take their medications should undergo subtotal parathyroidectomy. Total parathyroidectomy with forearm autotransplantation is advised in patients who are noncompliant, patients with recurrent or persistent hyperparathyroidism, and patients who have fewer than four hyperplastic glands identified at surgery.[58]

Tertiary Hyperparathyroidism

Tertiary hyperparathyroidism occurs if PTH production is autonomous in patients with normal or low serum calcium levels. The condition is seen in some patients who have undergone successful renal transplantation.[25] Several substances, such as prostaglandins, transforming growth factor, interleukin-1, and lymphotoxin, can increase serum calcium levels by increasing osteoclastic activity or by secreting amino acids similar to PTH. With increasing age, the rise in PTH is thought to be attributable to alterations in renal function, decreased calcium absorption, and some degree of target organ resistance to the action of PTH.

Parathyroid Cysts

Parathyroid cysts are uncommon and generally are not clinically significant. They occur as solitary, palpable neck masses and are usually nonfunctional. Up until 1968, only 56 cases had been reported in the literature.[59] The cysts occur, with equal sex distribution, in patients 30 to 50 years of age. Symptoms can arise secondary to tracheal deviation, which is characterized by respiratory obstruction or hoarseness, or secondary to recurrent laryngeal nerve compression. The cysts are usually located near the lower pole of the thyroid lobe, pushing it forward. They have an avascular covering, can be shelled out easily, are unilocular, and are usually hormonally inactive, with the average size approaching 4 cm. The epithelial lining consists of a single layer of flattened cuboidal or columnar epithelium covered by a thin layer of connective tissue. In order to establish the diagnosis, parathyroid cells must be identified in the cyst wall.

MALIGNANT LESIONS

Parathyroid Carcinoma

Parathyroid carcinoma is a rare cause of hyperparathyroidism, occurring in 0.5% to 1% of cases.[60] This diagnosis is usually not established prior to surgical exploration and microscopic examination of the removed tissue. A high index of suspicion is warranted when there is a palpable neck mass, when the preoperative calcium level is excessively high, when there is marked fibrous tissue reaction around the parathyroid gland, and when the high serum calcium level persists after surgery. According to Holmes et al,[61] only 5% of patients with primary hyperparathyroidism have a palpable neck mass, whereas 50% of those with parathyroid carcinoma have a palpable mass. In contrast to patients with benign primary hyperparathyroidism, 70% of patients with parathyroid carcinoma have a calcium level of greater than 14 mg/dL, elevated alkaline phosphatase levels, and bone disease. Also in this population, there is a greater than 50% incidence of renal disease, anemia, palpable neck mass, and recurrent hyperparathyroidism.

The best opportunity for cure is at the time of the first operation. Findings at surgery may include adherence of the mass to the strap muscles, to fibrofatty tissue, and to the thyroid gland. Instead of a smooth, glistening capsule, there is a thick, fibrous capsule that is greyish-white. Surgical treatment should include removal of the parathyroid gland, unilateral thyroid lobectomy, and skeletonization of the tracheoesophageal groove with excision of the paratracheal lymph nodes, keeping the tumor mass intact. A radical neck dissection is only done in cases in which there are palpable neck nodes. The surgeon must identify all four glands because parathyroid carcinoma can occur with other parathyroid abnormalities, and in patients with familial hyperparathyroidism.

The local recurrence rate is 30%, with distant metastasis to the lung, liver, and bone occurring in 25% to 30%. Recurrence of hypercalcemia usually presents within 2 years; local spread accounts for 60% of these recurrences, whereas distant spread is responsible for 40%. There is a 50% 5-year survival rate, with most patients with recurrent disease dying of metabolic complications related to the hypercalcemia. Radiation therapy and chemotherapy have not proven to be useful in the treatment of parathyroid carcinoma.

REFERENCES

1. Rice DH. Surgery of the parathyroid glands. *Otolaryngol Clin North Am.* 1996; 29:693.
2. DeLellis RA. Tumors of the parathyroid gland. In: *Atlas of Tumor Pathology,* 3rd Series, Fascicle 6. Washington, DC: Armed Forces Institute of Pathology; 1993:1.
3. Halstead WS, Evans HM. The parathyroid glandules: Their blood supply and their preservation in operations of the thyroid gland. *Ann Surg.* 1907; 46:489.
4. Akerstrom G, Malmaeus J, Bergstrom R. Surgical anatomy of human parathyroid glands. *Surgery.* 1984; 95:14.
5. Edis AJ, Purnell DC, von Heerden JA. The undescended parathymus: An occasional cause of failed neck exploration for hyperparathyroidism. *Ann Surg.* 1979; 190:64.
6. Meakins JL, Milne CA, Hollomby DJ, et al. Total parathyroid-

ectomy; parathyroid hormone levels and supernumerary glands in hemodialysis patients. *Clin Invest Med.* 1984; 7:21.

7. Petti GH. Endocrinology. In: Bailey BJ, ed. *Head and Neck Surgery—Otolaryngology.* Vol. 1. Philadelphia: JB Lippincott; 1993:140.

8. Petti GH. Hyperparathyroidism. *Otolaryngol Clin North Am.* 1990; 23:339.

9. Mundy GR, Cove DH, Fishen R. Primary hyperparathyroidism: Changes in the pattern of clinical presentation. *Lancet.* 1980; 1:13.

10. Broadus AE. Mineral metabolism. In: Felig P, Baxter JD, Broadus AE, eds. *Endocrinology and Metabolism.* New York: McGraw-Hill; 1984:1019.

11. Spiegel AM, et al. Neonatal primary hyperparathyroidism with autosomal dominant inheritance. *J Pediatr.* 1977; 90:269.

12. Marx SJ, Attie MF, Spiegel AM, et al. An association between neonatal severe primary hyperparathyroidism and familial hypercalciuria in 300 patients. *N Engl J Med.* 1982; 306:257.

13. Prinz RA, Paloyan E, Lawrence AM, et al. Radiation associated hyperparathyroidism: A new syndrome. *Surgery.* 1977; 82:296.

14. Venkataraman PS, Boykung KH, Tsang RC, et al. Secondary hyperparathyroidism and bone disease in infants receiving long term furosemide therapy. *Am J Dis Child.* 1983; 137:1157.

15. Krook L. On the etiology of primary parathyroid hyperplasia. *Rev Cancer Biol.* 1965; 24:63.

16. Mueller H. Sex, age and hyperparathyroidism. *Lancet.* 1969; 1:449.

17. Pyrah LN, Hodgkinson A, Anderson CK. Primary hyperparathyroidism. *Br J Surg.* 1966; 53:16.

18. Clark OH. *Endocrine Surgery of the Thyroid and Parathyroid Gland.* St. Louis: Mosby; 1985:202.

19. Cholst IN, Steinberg SF, Tropper PJ, et al. The influence of hypermagnesemia on serum calcium and parathyroid hormone levels in human subjects. *N Engl J Med.* 1984; 310; 1221.

20. Coburn JW, Popovtzer MM, Massry SG, et al. The physiochemical state and renal handling of divalent ions in chronic renal failure. *Arch Intern Med.* 1969; 124:302.

21. Mather HG. Hyperparathyroidism with normal serum calcium. *Br Med J.* 1953; 2:424.

22. Reiner M, Sigurdsson G, Nunziata V, et al. Abnormal calcium metabolism in normocalcemic sarcoidosis. *Br Med J.* 1976; 2: 1473.

23. Yendt ER, Quay GF, Garcia DA. The use of thiazides in the prevention of renal calculi. *Can Med Assoc J.* 1970; 102:614.

24. Nichols G Jr, Flanagan B. Normocalcemic hyperparathyroidism. *Trans Assoc Am Phys.* 1967; 80:314.

25. Petti GH. Parathyroid disease and surgery. In Bailey BJ, ed. *Head and Neck Surgery—Otolaryngology.* Vol. 1. Philadelphia: JB Lippincott; 1993:1248.

26. Voorman GS, Petti GH, Chonkich GD, et al. The pitfalls of technetium Tc 99mm-thallium 201, pararthyroid scanning. *Arch Otolaryngol Head Neck Surg.* 1988; 114:993.

27. Shaha, AR, Sarkar S, Strashun A, et al. Sestambi scan for preoperative localization in primary hyperparathyroidism. *Head Neck Surg.* 1997; 19:87.

28. Davidson J, Noyek A, Gottesman I, et al. The parathyroid adenoma: An imaging surgical perspective. *J Otolaryngol.* 1988; 17(6):282.

29. Carmalt HL, Gillett DJ, Chen J, et al. Perspective comparison of radionuclide ultrasound and computed tomography and the preoperative localization of parathyroid glands. *World J Surg.* 1988; 12:830.

30. Bilezikian JP, Silverberg SJ, Shane E, et al. Characterization and evaluation of asymptomatic primary hyperparathyroidism. *J Bone Mineral Res.* 1981; 6(suppl 2): 585.

31. Parfitt AM, Rao DS, Kleerehoper M. Asymptomatic primary hyperparathyroidism discovered by multichannel biochemical screening: Clinical course and considerations bearing on the need for surgical intervention. *J Bone Mineral Res* 1991; 6(suppl 2): 583.

32. Rao DS, Wilson RJ, Kleerehoper M. Lack of biochemical progression or continuation of accelerated bone loss in mild

33. asymptomatic primary hyperparathyroidism: Evidence for biphasic disease course. *J Clin Endocrinol Metab.* 1988; 67:1294.

33. Kaplan RA, Snyder WH, Stewart A, et al. Metabolic effects of parathyroidectomy in asymptomatic primary hyperparathyroidism. *J Clin Endocrinol Metab.* 1976; 41:415.

34. Scholz DA, Purnell DC. Asymptomatic primary hyperparathyroidism: A 10 year prospective study. *Mayo Clinic Proc.* 1981; 56:473.

35. Consensus Development Conference Statement. *J Bone Mineral Res.* 1991; 6:59.

36. Sampson J, Hoff WV, Bicknell EJ. The conservative management of primary hyperparathyroidism. *QJ Med.* 1987; 65:1009.

37. Mitlak BH, Dale M, Potts JT, et al. Asymptomatic primary hyperparathyroidism. *J Bone Mineral Res.* 1991; 6:103.

38. Posen S, Clifton BP, Reeve TS, et al. Is parathyroidectomy of benefit in primary hyperparathyroidism? *Medicine* (Baltimore). 1985; 54:241.

39. Clark OH, Wilkes W, Siperstein AE, Duh QY. Diagnosis and management of asymptomatic hyperparathyroidism: Safety, efficacy and deficiencies in our knowledge. *J Bone Mineral Res.* 1991; 6:135.

40. Uden P, Chan A, Duh QY, et al. Primary hyperparathyroidism in younger and older patients: Symptoms and outcome of surgery. *World J Surg.* 1992; 16:791.

41. Reinhoff WF Jr. The surgical treatment of hyperparathyroidism with a report on 27 cases. *Ann Surg.* 1980; 131:917.

42. Hedbeck G, Tisell LE, Bengtssen BA, Hedman I, Oden A. Premature deaths in patients operated on for primary hyperparathyroidism. *World J Surg.* 1990; 14:829.

43. Hedbeck G, Oden A, Tisell L. The influence of surgery on the risk of death in patients with hyperparathyroidism. *World J Surg.* 1991; 15:399.

44. Palmer M, Adami HO, Bergstrom R, Jakobsson S, Aberstrom G, Ljunghall S. Survival and renal function in untreated hypercalcemia: A population-based cohort study with 14 years of follow-up. *Lancet.* 1987; 1:59.

45. Worsey MJ, Catty E, Watson CG. Success of unilateral neck exploration for sporadic primary hyperparathyroidism. *Surgery.* 1993; 114:1024.

46. Casas AT, Burke GJ, Sathyanarayana, et al. Prospective comparison of technetium 99m - sestambi/iodine-123 radionuclide scan versus high resolution ultrasonography for the preoperative localization of abnormal parathyroid glands in patients with previously unoperated primary hyperparathyroidism. *Am J Surg.* 1993; 166:369.

47. Shaha AR, La Rosa CA, Jaffe BM. Parathyroid localization prior to primary exploration. *Am J Surg.* 1993; 166:289.

48. Duh QY, Uden P, Clark OH. Unilateral neck exploration for primary hyperparathyroidism: Analysis of a controversy using a mathematical model. *World J Surg.* 1992; 16:654.

49. Thompson NW, Eckhauser FE, Harness JK. The anatomy of primary hyperparathyroidism. *Surgery.* 1992; 92:814.

50. Halstead WS. Auto and isotransplantation in dogs of the parathyroid glandules. *J Exp Med.* 1908; 11:175.

51. Catell RB. Parathyroid autotransplantation: A report of autografts of parathyroid glands removed during thyroidectomy. *Am J Surg.* 1929; 7:4.

52. Wells SA, Striver JA, Bolman RM, et al. Transplantation of the parathyroid glands, clinical and experimental results. *Surg Clin North Am.* 1978; 58:391.

53. Katz AD. Parathyroid autotransplantation in patients with parathyroid disease and total thyroidectomy. *Am J Surg.* 1981; 142:490.

54. Wells SA, Ross AJ, Cole JD, et al. Transplantation of the parathyroid gland: Current status. *Surg Clin North Am.* 1979; 59:167.

55. Wells SA, Gunnells JC, Guttman RA, et al. The successful transplantation of frozen parathyroid tissue in MEN. *Surgery* (St. Louis). 1977; 81:86.

56. Brennan MF, Brown EM, Spiegel AM, et al. Autotransplantation of cryopreserved tissue in MEN. *Ann Surg.* 1979; 189: 139.

57. Clark OH. Seconday and tertiary hyperparathyroidism. In: Najouon JS, Delaney JP, eds. *Endocrine Surgery.* New York: Symposia Specialists, Inc., Publications; 1980:239.
58. Dubose C, Drueke T. Comparison of subtotal parathyroidectomy with total parathyroidectomy and autotransplantation. In: Kaplan EL, ed. *Surgery of the Thyroid and Parathyroid Glands.* Edinburgh: Churchill-Livingstone; 1983:253.
59. Haid SP, Method HL, Beal JM. Parathyroid cysts: Report of two cases and a review of the literature. *Arch Surg.* 1967; 94: 421.
60. Mashburn M, Chonkich GD, Petti GH Jr, et al. Parathyroid carcinoma: Two new cases. Laryngoscope. 1987; 97(2):215.
61. Holmes EC, Minton, DL, Ketcham AS. Parathyroid carcinoma: A collective review. *Am Surg.* 1909; 169:631.

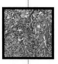

II. PATHOLOGY OF THE PARATHYROID GLAND

■ S C O T T   D .   N E L S O N

HANDLING OF SPECIMENS AND FROZEN SECTIONS

When any organ system is examined, close communication between the pathologist and the clinician is essential. In the diagnosis and treatment of lesions of the parathyroid gland, this seems especially true. Benign and malignant lesions share many characteristics, both clinically and pathologically. Any of these lesions may even mimic normal glands in some circumstances.

Most, if not all, pathologists likely feel most comfortable examining formalin-fixed permanent sections of tissue and prefer this method to the examination of frozen sections. The reasons for this include the comparatively inferior quality and artifact distortions inherent in frozen section preparations. Also, the luxury of examining a permanent section in an unhurried manner affords more careful consideration. Indeed, frozen sections are sometimes thought of as "quick and dirty" by the pathologist. The pathologist greatly appreciates and respects the surgeon who understands both the utility and the limitations of frozen section analysis, and requests

such analyses judiciously and appropriately. The surgical exploration of the neck in a patient with hyperparathyroidism is definitely an instance when frozen section examination is an appropriate and necessary tool. Working together, the surgeon and pathologist emergently make decisions that dictate the course of surgery in the patient who is anesthetized on the table.

Frozen Sections

Ideally, the frozen section laboratory is located in very close proximity to the operating room. This facilitates prompt processing of specimens and accurate communication between the pathologist and surgeon. It is helpful if the pathologist is present in the operating room to view the gross anatomy in the surgical field.

Regarding specimens, the pathologist needs to know exactly what he is looking at. There can be no question as to the anatomic location and designation of the specimens. The pathologist and surgeon need to use the same designation and numbering system on the specimen container, frozen section request form, and frozen section report.[1] The pathologist must keep an accurate frozen section report because many specimens may be examined concurrently or sequentially during a single case.

The surgeon must clearly inform the pathologist about the appearance of the glands in situ. Such information must include the size of the gland in relation to other glands and the relationship of the gland to other structures.[2] If a biopsy specimen of a gland is submitted, the surgeon should inform the pathologist of the approximate percentage of whole gland that the sample represents.[1]

Upon arrival in the frozen section laboratory, the specimen should be freed from adherent fat, measured, weighed, and described grossly before being processed for frozen section. If relative density measurements (discussed in a section that follows) have not yet been performed and are desired, this is the time to do them. The pathologist should have in mind the average size and weight of a normal parathyroid gland. Average size is 3 to 6 mm in length, 2 to 4 mm in width, and 0.5 to 2 mm in thickness. The average weight per gland is approximately 30 to 55 mg.[3–6] Usually, the surgeon excises the largest parathyroid gland first and submits it in its entirety.[1]

After weights and measurements have been obtained and recorded, the gland should be prepared for frozen section. A representative section, which ideally includes the capsule and extends through the hilum, is obtained, and a frozen section is mounted, stained, and coverslipped. It is helpful if the surgeon marks the vascular hilus with a suture to increase the likelihood of encountering a rim of normal tissue.[2] At the time of frozen section preparation, additional sections should be prepared and left unstained for examination by fat stain. Also at this time, touch preparations and smears may be made and stained with hematoxylin-eosin (H&E) stain at the frozen section bench, or stained with cytologic stains. If adequate tissue is available, a portion should be frozen at −70° for molecular studies.[7] A small piece may be placed in glutaraldehyde for electron microscopic studies if warranted.

The first responsibility of the pathologist is to identify the tissue brought from the operating room. Fragments of putative parathyroid may turn out to be thyroid tissue, lymph node, skeletal muscle, fat, or nerve. Once identified as parathyroid, ideally, the search continues until all parathyroids are identified by the surgeon.

Once a gland or piece of tissue is identified as parathyroid, a determination must be made as to whether the glandular tissue is normal or in a hyperfunctional state. On sections stained with H&E, glands in a hyperfunctional state usually exhibit a proliferation of chief cells with decreased or no intercellular or parenchymal fat. Of course, it must be remembered that the amount of fat in a normal parathyroid gland is highly variable. Even within the same individual, the amounts of fat in different

glands, and within the same gland, may vary. The amount of fat varies with constitution factor, diet, age, and other factors. Abu-jawdeh[4] makes the useful observation that, "in normal glands the stromal fat appears to 'compress' the surrounding parenchyma, while in hyperplastic or adenomatous glands the fat cells appear scattered among the parenchymal cells." Keeping these factors in mind, in most cases, a normal gland will have an appreciable component of adipocytes, whereas a hyperfunctional gland will have a small or absent population of adipocytes.[8,9]

If the first gland submitted is the largest and the only abnormally enlarged gland and, on histologic examination, shows a proliferation of chief cells, decreased adipocytes, a rim of normal or compressed parathyroid, and nuclear pleomorphism, a putative diagnosis of adenoma may be made. An additional gland, or biopsy studies of at least one additional normal-appearing gland, should be obtained. If this gland is histologically normal or suppressed (not hyperfunctional), then the diagnosis of adenoma is essentially confirmed.[1]

Conversely, if more than one gland is enlarged, the most likely diagnosis is hyperplasia. Usually, all of the glands will be enlarged in hyperplasia, although the enlargement is often asymmetrical. Occasionally, one hyperplastic gland will be quite large in comparison to the remaining glands, which are grossly normal in appearance. Upon histologic examination, however, these normal-appearing glands are found to be hyperfunctional, thus confirming the hyperplastic nature of the large pseudoadenomatous gland.[1,10]

Fat Staining

As mentioned previously, both adenoma and hyperplasia may present with a single enlarged gland, in which case biopsy study of a second gland is necessary to verify the diagnosis. In the case of adenomas, which are usually singular, biopsy examination of an additional gland usually reveals normal, non-hyperfunctioning tissue. Conversely, in hyperplasia, the additional gland usually shows evidence of hyperplasia as well, even if the additional gland is normal in size. One of the criteria used to differentiate a hyperfunctioning gland from a normal gland is the amount of stromal fat. If an entire gland is obtained for examination and a complete cross section is available, this determination may not be difficult. However, after the single, enlarged gland is removed, the surgeon may provide the pathologist with a small biopsy specimen of an additional gland, that is not with an entire gland. Using stromal fat as a criterion to differentiate normal from hyperfunctional glands may not be possible with small biopsy specimens. In fact, it may be confusing. Stromal fat content in normal glands may be quite variable between individuals, within different glands in the same individual, and within different regions within the same gland.[4,7,8,11] This may be true in hyperplastic glands as well.[9]

The amount of intracytoplasmic fat (as opposed to parenchymal fat, or adipocytes) varies with the functional state of the chief cell. A decreased or absent intracytoplasmic lipid content correlates with increased secretory activity, or a hyperfunctional state. Normal and suppressed parathyroid glands show an abundance of intracytoplasmic fat (Fig. 11–13) when compared to hyperfunctioning glands, which show little or no intracytoplasmic lipid vacuoles (Fig. 11–14).[9,12,13] The amount of intracytoplasmic lipid in the chief cells is not related to the presence or absence of stromal fat in the particular area of the biopsy.[13] Additionally, there are no apparent differences in intra-parenchymal fat content with regard to sex, age, or degree of preoperative hypercalcemia.[9] This knowledge may be useful to the pathologist in determining whether a band of compact parathyroid parenchyma is composed of hyperfunctioning chief cells or of normal or suppressed chief cells with few or no accompanying adipocytes.[13]

In examining presumably normal parathyroid glands that have been sampled subsequent to a single, prominent gland being removed, visualization of intraparenchymal fat may be of great help in the intraoperative distinction between adenoma (single-gland disease) and hyperplasia, at least in classical four-gland disease.[9]

It should be noted that frozen section analysis of intracytoplasmic fat is but one tool to be used in the assessment of parathyroid disease, and it must be used in conjunction with considerations of other factors and techniques. It is a useful technique, but yields accurate results in only approximately 80% of cases.[1]

In a study of 191 hypercalcemic patients with hyperparathyroidism who underwent surgical treat-

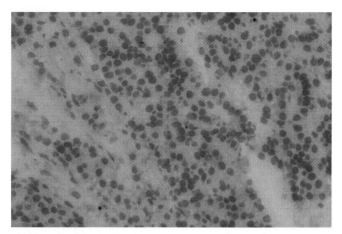

FIGURE 11–14 Frozen section of a hyperfunctioning parathyroid gland demonstrating markedly decreased intracytoplasmic fat (oil red O stain, × 200).

ment, Bondeson et al[9] found that the use of intraoperative frozen section staining for fat was a very valuable tool in reliably discriminating between adenoma and hyperplasia. This method involves frozen section analysis of two complete glands, not just biopsy studies of presumably normal glands. One slide is stained with H&E stain, and another is air-dried and stained for fat with a modified oil red O stain. Sudan IV stain may also be used, but oil red O stain yields better results. After staining, the chief cells are examined for staining of intracytoplasmic fat droplets. Cells are considered functionally inactive if they contain fat droplets; they are considered hyperfunctional if they lack stainable droplets.[9]

A diagnosis of adenoma is confirmed when a second gland (or third or fourth gland, if submitted) is determined to be normal. To be considered normal, the gland must be within standard limits for weight and dimension, and must demonstrate intracytoplasmic fat (without areas absent of intracytoplasmic fat). Bondeson et al[9] did not take into account the amount of stromal fat because of the possible marked variation. Using this method, most adenomas are found not to contain significant amounts of intracytoplasmic lipid, although at close examination, very small amounts may frequently be seen. Additionally, approximately 10% of adenomas may contain more substantial amounts of diffusely distributed lipid vacuoles. However, when compared with the amount of fat present in normal glands, the amount of fat in this group of adenomas is substantially less. Using this method of fat staining, a rim of normal parathyroid tissue may be identified in up to 80% of cases. This rim will have a fat distribution similar to that of the normal or suppressed glands.

Chief cells in a lipoadenoma have a decreased amount of intracytoplasmic lipid. In contrast, the surrounding normal gland has abundant, regularly distributed, intracytoplasmic fat.[9]

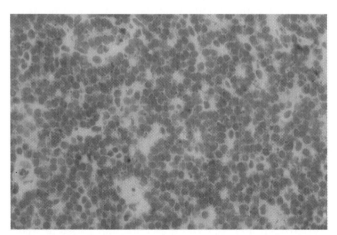

FIGURE 11–13 Frozen section of a normal parathyroid gland showing abundant intracytoplasmic fat (oil red O stain, × 200).

In hyperplasia, two or more glands examined microscopically will display absent or significantly reduced intracytoplasmic fat. Depending on the architecture of the pathologic gland, the distribution of fat-depleted chief cells may be diffuse or nodular. In the nodular type, internodular areas may have significant amounts of intraparenchymal fat. The intracytoplasmic content of fat may vary widely among hyperplastic glands from the same patient. Oxyphilic nodules are considered to be equivocal and so are not considered in the diagnosis, as they may be present in both normal and hyperfunctional glands, and the fat pattern is similar in both.[9]

Two cases of water-clear cell hyperplasia examined by Bondeson et al[9] demonstrated no intracytoplasmic fat. Similarly, in glands removed from patients with secondary hyperplasia, fat was absent. The amount of intracytoplasmic fat in glands from patients with tertiary hyperplasia varied. In a case of parathyroid carcinoma, the parenchymal cells contained no intracytoplasmic fat, whereas the accompanying normal glands contained regularly distributed, intraparenchymal lipid droplets.[9]

Thus, in a typical case, when a single enlarged gland is identified, this gland, along with a normal-appearing gland, is submitted for frozen section evaluation, including an intracytoplasmic fat stain. If the large gland shows evidence of hyperfunction and the normal-appearing gland appears inactive (as suggested by the presence of intracytoplasmic fat), the enlarged gland is considered to be an adenoma. If both of the removed glands show evidence of hyperfunction (decreased or absent intracytoplasmic fat), the likely diagnosis is hyperplasia.[9]

Density Gradient Measurement

One manifestation of the fact that normal and suppressed parathyroid glands contain relatively more stromal and intracytoplasmic fat is that these glands are less dense than hyperfunctioning glands. In other words, the increased proportion of parenchymal tissue to fat in hyperfunctioning glands makes them more dense than normal and suppressed glands. A test that may be performed in the operating room at the time of surgery or in the frozen section laboratory makes use of this fact to help differentiate hyperfunctioning glands from normal glands, and adenomas from hyperplasia. This test involves cleaning the presumptive adenoma of extraglandular fat and placing it in a solution of 25% mannitol. The adenoma will float in this solution. Isotonic saline is then added and mixed into the solution until the gland sinks. A second, presumably normal gland is then similarly stripped of fat and placed in the solution. Because of its relative lesser density, the normal gland should float, thus adding a piece of confirmatory information to the diagnosis of adenoma. If, on the other hand, the second piece sinks as well, showing an equal density to the enlarged gland, the most likely diagnosis is hyperplasia.[14] The glands may then be processed for frozen section analysis.

NORMAL PARATHYROID GLANDS

The parathyroid glands are usually paired organs, with two superior glands and two inferior glands arising from the third and fourth branchial pouches, hence the reference to the glands as parathyroid III and IV, respectively. The thymus also arises from the third branchial pouch, and as it migrates caudad to the mediastinum, parathyroid III migrates along with it. At some point during the migration, the parathyroid III separates from the thymus. This relatively long migratory course accounts for the varied locations in which parathyroid III, or the inferior parathyroid glands, may be found. Parathyroid IV, or the superior parathyroid glands, migrate with the fourth branchial pouch and assume a more constant location near the intersection of the recurrent laryngeal nerve and the medial thyroid artery.[4,15]

Besides the usual location in the neck, parathyroid glands may be present in less common positions, including the upper neck at a level as high as the hyoid bone, the capsule of the thyroid, the soft tissue of the jaw, the mediastinum, and within the vagus nerve.[4,7,16,17] In one study, parathyroid glands were present in 22% of 58 fetal thyroid glands obtained from autopsy material.[18] Approximately 15% of these were located in the subcapsular tissue, and 7% were located in the parenchyma of the thyroid gland. Parathyroid glands may also be found in the periesophageal tissue. (The author recently saw a case in which a "bump" was seen in the esophagus during upper endoscopy and an endoscopic biopsy was performed. A frozen section was then performed, revealing a normal parathyroid gland.)

Small rests of cells in the soft tissue outside of the glands proper, known as parathyromatosis, may occur anywhere along the course of parathyroid migration. These rests may become hyperplastic in patients with hyperparathyroidism.[19]

Gross Anatomy

Most individuals have four parathyroid glands. In a study by Wang,[3] approximately 97% of postmortem subjects were found to have four parathyroid glands, 2% had three glands, and less than 1% had more than four parathyroid glands. As few as 2 glands and as many as 12 glands may be present.[11,20] Complete absence of parathyroid glands may occur as part of the rare DiGeorge syndrome, in which the third and fourth branchial pouches fail to form.[7]

The parathyroid glands are usually oval to lentiform in shape, being somewhat flattened with round or tapered edges. The color is yellow or tan to red-tan. A more intense red coloration may occur secondary to surgical manipulation. The consistency is malleable but not friable.[3,4] Although bilobed and multilobed glands may occasionally be seen, bulbous projections are usually suggestive of a pathologic gland.[7,21]

In the assessment of parathyroid disease, the weight of the glands, both individually and in total, is an important parameter. For this reason, each gland must be carefully weighed before frozen section preparation or fixation in formalin.

The weight of the parathyroid glands is not constant, but changes with age and other health and disease factors. After birth, a progressive increase in the weight of the parathyroids occurs; the increase then ceases in the third or fourth decade. At this point in time, the average weight of a parathyroid gland is approximately 31 mg in men and 30 mg in women.[5] Total glandular weight is approximately 120 ± 3.5 mg in men and 142 ± 5.2 mg in women.[21] For practical purposes, most pathologists consider an individual parathyroid gland weight of greater than 40 to 50 mg to be abnormal for upper glands, and a weight of 60 mg to be abnormal for lower glands. Although this number is useful in frozen section analysis, it must be remembered that glandular weights in excess of 60 mg, and even in the 70- to 90-mg range, have been recorded in patients without evidence of parathyroid disease.[22–24] In adults, the percentage of the glandular weight represented by parenchymal tissue, or parenchymal weight, is estimated to be 74% of total glandular weight.[23]

Microscopic Anatomy

The thin capsule surrounding the parathyroid glands is fibrous in nature and is perforated by arteries and veins at the vascular pole. A vascular plexus develops from these larger vessels, penetrating along fibrous septa into the parenchyma to form a rich vascular network of arterioles, capillaries, and venules. Indeed, the vascular network is seen to abut every chief cell. With age, the perivascular stroma becomes thicker and increases in collagen, eventually forming fibrous septa that divide the parenchyma into vague lobules.[4] Two lymphatic plexuses service the glands, and portions may share structures with the lymphatic system of the thyroid.[25]

External to the capsule of the parathyroid is usually the fibroadipose tissue of the neck, or thymic tissue.[4] Thyroid tissue is present in cases of intrathyroidal parathyroid.[18]

In the adult parathyroid, adipocytes are intermingled among the parenchymal cells. The collections of adipocytes appear to compress the parenchymal cells.[4] In childhood and up until puberty, the amount of stromal fat is minimal. The amount of stromal fat increases around the time of puberty, starting in the perivascular and septal areas and extending into the parenchyma. This increase in stromal fat continues until the fourth to fifth decades, when the adipocytes constitute approximately 30% to 50% of the gland (Fig. 11–15).[8] Some studies have found that the average amount of stromal fat is less than was previously thought, in the range of 20%.[26] After the fourth or fifth decade, the amount of fat decreases. Women tend to have a higher percentage of stromal fat than men. The amount and distribution of stromal fat between individuals of the same sex and same age may be quite variable. Additionally, this variability may be seen between glands from the same individual, and even within a single gland. The amount of stromal fat is affected by constitutional factors, including nutritional state, chronic disease, and malignant disease. Genetic factors play a role as well.[4]

As mentioned, a lobular pattern is imposed on the adult gland by the fibrovascular septa that extend from the capsule into the parenchyma. Cells may be arranged in a variety of patterns, including solid, compact masses; anastomosing columns; trabeculae of varying thicknesses; and pseudofollicular or gland-like structures containing eosinophilic, colloid-like material. These gland-like structures increase in number with age.[8]

The cells that make up the parathyroid parenchyma are of two types: chief cells and oxyphil cells. The chief cell is recognized under the light microscope by its round shape, amphophilic cytoplasm, and centrally placed nuclei. Cell boundaries are indistinct, and the typical cell measures between 8 and 12 μm. The nucleus is small and round with distinct nuclear borders and, rarely, a small nucleolus (Fig. 11–16).[4] Chief cells may be present in an active or inactive form. The inactive chief cell may be identified by the cleared out or vacuolated appearance of the cytoplasm, which corresponds to intracytoplasmic lipid, glycogen, and lysosomes.[4,27] The func-

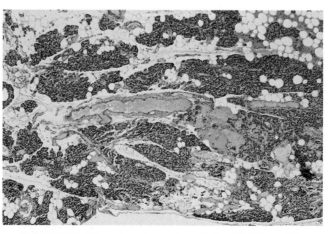

FIGURE 11–15 Normal parathyroid gland (H&E, × 40).

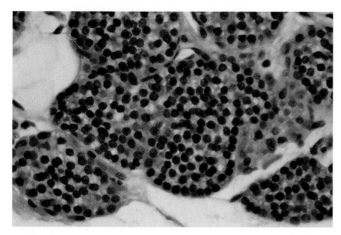

FIGURE 11–16 Appearance of chief cells in a normal parathyroid gland (H&E, × 400).

tional activity of the chief cells is inversely related to the amount of intracytoplasmic fat. Nonsecretory or suppressed glands contain intracytoplasmic fat droplets, which can be demonstrated by modified oil red O staining of frozen sections of glands.[4,9] Approximately 80% of the chief cells in adult parathyroids contain intracytoplasmic fat and are in the nonsecretory phase.[12,28]

The oxyphil cell is thought to represent a modification of the chief cell. Although not common in the glands of children, oxyphil cells increase in number with age.[4,8] These cells may be distributed diffusely as single cells, or as sheets or nodules of cells.[4,21] Large clusters may be recognized on gross examination. Oxyphil cells are considered to be nonfunctional. They are larger than chief cells, measuring 12 to 20 μm in diameter. Cell boundaries are distinct, and the nucleus is dark and pyknotic in appearance. The most recognizable feature is the eosinophilic granular cytoplasm, which is abundant.[4] Cells referred to as transitional oxyphil cells are smaller and less brightly eosinophilic than mature oxyphil cells.[7] Both transitional and mature oxyphil cells contain only very small amounts of intracytoplasmic fat.[29]

Upon staining with periodic acid–Schiff (PAS) stain, most chief cells are seen to have glycogen in their cytoplasm. Oxyphil cells also stain positively, but to a lesser degree.[7]

Immunohistochemistry

Parathyroid tissue, in both normal and neoplastic glands, may be recognized by immunohistochemical staining methods using antibodies against parathormone. Both formalin-fixed and frozen section material may be used. Markers found in neuroendocrine cells are also present in parathyroids. In chief cells, chromogranin A is demonstrable in varying intensities depending on functional activity; in oxyphil cells it is absent. Neuron-specific enolase (NSE) is present in both normal and neoplastic parathyroid

tissue.[30] Low-molecular-weight keratins, including keratins 8, 18, and 19, are expressed in normal and neoplastic parathyroid glands. These keratins are expressed in both chief and oxyphil cells. High-molecular-weight keratins, typically found in stratified epithelia, are not present in parathyroid parenchymal cells. Vimentin proteins are also not present in parenchymal cells.[31] It should be noted that, like normal glands, hyperfunctioning glands demonstrate variable reactivity for parathormone, chromogranin, synaptophysin, and NSE.[30]

Detection of mRNA by in situ hybridization methods may be more sensitive than immunohistochemistry in detecting parathormone, especially in cells that produce but do not store much parathyroid hormone.[30]

Ultrastructure

Being an endocrine organ, the parathyroid gland shares many ultrastructural properties with other hormone-producing glands that have a more or less well-developed assortment of organelles necessary for the manufacture, packaging, storage, transportation, and release of product.[32] Well-formed basal lamina are present, separating the parenchymal cells from the interstitial space, which contains collagen bundles and elastic fibers. Capillaries abut every chief cell, and the capillary lining cells exhibit fenestrations similar to those seen in other endocrine organs.[4,29]

The ultrastructural characteristics of the chief cell vary with its functional state.[27] In the resting phase, the plasma membranes are rather straight and simple and are connected to adjacent cells by desmosomes.[7] With increased levels of functional activity, the plasma membranes become much more complex and demonstrate interdigitations.[33]

The endoplasmic reticulum is granular and is usually located in a perinuclear location. In the resting phase, it is rather small and inconspicuous, as are the Golgi apparatus and secretory granules. As activity increases, the granular endoplasmic reticulum takes on a stacked appearance and increases in prominence. The Golgi apparatus also increases in size, and increased numbers of vesicles, vacuoles, and presecretory granules are evident.[4,7]

In the resting or inactive phase, cytoplasmic accumulations of glycogen and large lipid bodies are present. These lipid bodies correspond to the intracytoplasmic fat demonstrated on frozen section preparations stained for fat. The accumulations of glycogen and lipid are the best indicators of the resting or functionally supressed cell. In the normal parathyroid gland, approximately 80% of the chief cells are in the resting phase. In prepubertal glands, about one half that number are in the resting phase.[4,7] The number of lipid bodies in suppressed glands in the presence of adenomas may be equal to or greater than that found in normal parathyroid glands.[4,33]

Mitochondria in chief cells are moderate in number and rather randomly distributed.[7] Oxyphil cells are characterized by large numbers of mitochondria, which virtually fill their cytoplasm. The mitochondria may be much larger than normal, and bizarre in shape. Other organelles, including Golgi apparatus and endoplasmic reticulum, as well as secretory granules and lipid bodies, are fewer in number than in chief cells.[4,7]

PARATHYROID CYSTS

As with normal parathyroid glands and adenomas, parathyroid cysts may occur anywhere from the superior portion of the neck to within the mediastinum. Cysts occur in approximately 4% of patients undergoing parathyroid operations.[34] As would be expected, these cysts occur much more commonly in the cervical region than in the mediastinum. Parathyroid cysts may be functional or nonfunctional with regard to parathyroid hormone, and patients may present with parathyroid crisis. Functioning cysts are thought to arise from adenomas or hyperplastic glands. Coalescence of microcysts that are often seen in parathyroids may play a role.[34,35] Nonfunctioning cysts may arise during development.[7] Such cysts have been known to occur along with other developmental anomalies.[36] Some cysts contain elements of both parathyroid and thymic tissue and are designated as third pharyngeal pouch cysts. Parathyroid cysts tend to occur in adults, and although some studies have suggested a female predominance, more recent studies show a nearly equal sex ratio.[34,36,37] Functional parathyroid cysts may present with hypercalcemia and its manifestations, including renal calculi. Although most cysts present as asymptomatic masses, close proximity of the cysts to the adjacent cervical and mediastinal structures may result in a mass effect, such as tracheal deviation, hoarseness, dysphagia, or respiratory distress.[37]

Gross Pathology

Parathyroid cysts generally measure 1 to 10 cm in diameter, with a mean diameter of 4 cm.[34] The cyst walls are thin, translucent, and whitish, and may contain a small amount of orange-colored tissue.[36] Cyst fluid is usually watery and either clear or straw-colored, but it may be serosanguinous, amber, cloudy green, opalescent, or brown (Fig. 11–17).[7,36,37]

Microscopic Pathology

The cyst wall may be thin or thickened, and is usually composed of rather hypercellular collagen, often with attached adipose tissue. Nests of parathyroid may appear trapped within this lining. The lining cells are often cuboidal and arranged in a single layer. This layer may blend with multilayered ex-

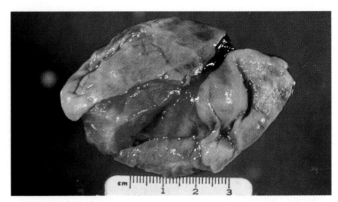

FIGURE 11–17   Gross appearance of a parathyroid cyst.

panses or acinar arrangements of cells with intraluminal colloid.[36] The cellular component may include any of the cell types normally found in the parathyroid. Typically, the cells have the appearance of chief cells. If significant scarring has occurred, it may not be possible to identify residual parathyroid tissue.[7] The cystic space may be filled with lightly eosinophilic fluid, or it may contain other components, including eosinophilic debris, red blood cells, hemosiderin, macrophages, and cholesterol clefts (Fig. 11–18). Lymphoid tissue may also be present.

Differential Diagnosis

Clinically, the differential diagnosis includes all those cystic lesions that may present in the cervical region, including thyroid adenoma, branchial cleft cyst, and thyroglossal duct cyst, as well as the many cystic lesions that may occur in the mediastinum, such as lymphangiomas, meningoceles, and thymic, pericardial, pleural, pancreatic, thoracic duct, cervical, mediastinal, hydatid, teratomatous, and foregut cysts.[37] Identification of the typical parathyroid epi-

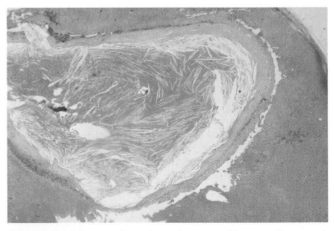

FIGURE 11–18   Parathyroid cyst showing a fibrous wall surrounding the cyst contents, including eosinophilic debris, hemosiderin, and cholesterol clefts (H&E, × 12.5).

thelial cells, namely the chief cells, is key to recognizing that these cystic structures are, in fact, of parathyroid origin. Staining of cytoplasmic glycogen within chief cells may be helpful. Absence of a stratified squamous epithelium helps to rule out branchial cleft cyst. Positive immunohistochemical tests for thyroglobulin or calcitonin in lesions of thyroid origin may be useful when these lesions are included in the differential diagnosis. Immunohistochemical positivity may be demonstrated by chief cells, but this reaction may be quite faint and variable.[7] Cyst fluid, obtained by fine-needle aspiration biopsy performed prior to or at the time of surgery, should be sent for evaluation of the parathyroid hormone (PTH) level because increased levels are virtually diagnostic of a parathyroid cyst.[37]

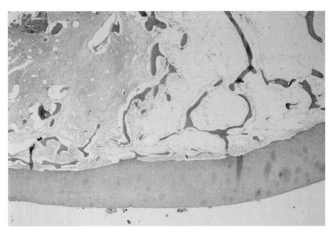

FIGURE 11-20 Severe osteopenia and fibrosis of the marrow in the femoral head of a patient with hyperparathyroidism (same patient as in Figure 11-7) (H&E, × 12.5).

PRIMARY HYPERPARATHYROIDISM

The term primary hyperparathyroidism refers to an abnormal increase in parathyroid hormone production caused by hyperplasia, adenoma, or carcinoma of the parathyroid glands. Typically, hypercalcemia is a feature of primary hyperparathyroidism, and soft tissue deposition of calcium is commonly seen (Fig. 11-19). Normocalcemic hyperparathyroidism has also been known to occur.[7] The metabolic consequences of hyperparathyroidism include the well-known effects on the skeletal system, which include diffuse osteopenia (Fig. 11-20), osteitis fibrosa cystica, and the so-called "brown tumors," or osteitis fibrosa cystica generalisata (Von Recklinghausen's disease) (Fig. 11-21). The designation of "brown tumor" is a reflection of the gross appearance of the lesion. Histologically, the giant cell–rich lesion of hyperparathyroidism and the giant cell tumors of other diseases may be indistinguishable on gross and histologic examination. Mirra[38] has observed that when a giant cell tumor is associated with hy-

percalcemia and hypophosphatemia, it should be considered a brown tumor of hyperparathyroidism. Full-blown von Recklinghausen's disease is now seldom seen.

Parathyroid Adenoma

Parathyroid adenoma is the most common cause of primary hyperparathyroidism, comprising approximately 80% of all cases. As with other lesions of the parathyroid glands, these benign neoplasms can be found in typical locations in the neck, as well as within the parenchyma and capsule of the thyroid and in the mediastinum.[7,17] Other less common sites include the pericardium, periesophageal tissue, the soft tissue about the jaw, and the vagus nerve.[7,16] Most parathyroid adenomas are present within a single, enlarged gland, and the remaining parathyroids are usually of normal size. Multiple adenomas

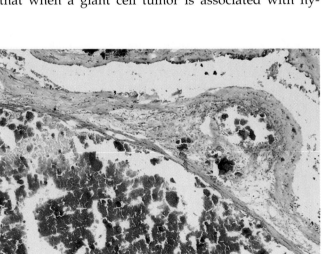

FIGURE 11-19 Deposition of calcium in the soft tissues in a patient with hyperparathyroidism (H&E, × 25).

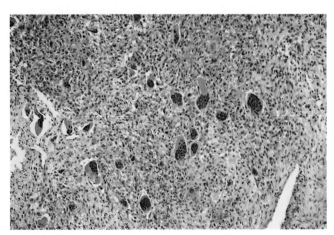

FIGURE 11-21 Giant cell–rich lesion, or "brown tumor" of hyperparathyroidism (H&E, × 100).

causing primary hyperparathyroidism have been proposed, but their existence remains a controversial issue.[39] Some concede that multiple adenomas may exist, but that many such cases "probably represent asymmetric or pseudoadenomatous hyperplasia."[7] Attie and associates[40] have described 33 cases of multiple adenomas, both synchronous and metachronous. They cite previous similar studies and give compelling examples and results.[39,40] What is not controversial is that parathyroid adenomas occur in female patients much more frequently than in male patients, at a ratio of approximately 3:1.[7,40] Adenomas can occur at any age, but tend to occur in adults, with most presenting in the fourth decade of life.[7]

The term adenoma implies a clonal proliferation of cells. Early research suggested that adenomas were polyclonal and would, therefore, be more correctly thought of as localized chief cell hyperplasia.[41,42] More recent studies, utilizing more reliable molecular biological methods, have confirmed, however, that adenomas are, in fact, monoclonal proliferations.[43,46]

Gross Pathology

Parathyroid adenomas vary greatly in size. Microadenomas may occupy only a portion of an otherwise normal-appearing gland, and may have a diameter as small as 5 mm. Such lesions may not be noticed on gross examination and may be discovered only microscopically.[47] Adenomas most commonly present in the lower glands.[1] Most adenomas are noticeably larger than normal parathyroid glands, measuring more than 1.5 cm at largest diameter, and most weigh between 1 and 5 g. Abnormal glands weighing more than 100 g have been reported.[48] In one study, in patients with severe skeletal manifestations, the average weight of the adenoma was 10 g.[21] Most adenomas are oval in shape, but the shape may be quite varied and asymmetric. Large adenomas may have their shape altered by surrounding structures, such as arteries. Such lesions may be bilobed or multilobed (Fig. 11–22). The adenoma may have completely effaced the host gland, or it may be

seen as a protuberance extending from the host gland.[40] A rim of normal parathyroid tissue may be present, usually in the hilar region.[7] In general, parathyroid adenomas are encapsulated by a thin, transparent membrane, and are usually easily separated from surrounding fatty tissue, if present. Microadenomas may lack such a capsule.

Glands taken from previously explored necks may be adherent to scar tissue and so may be less easily delineated. The adenoma is soft, but is often firmer than the normal parathyroid. Adenomas tend to be darker than the tan color seen in the normal parathyroid, and may be orange-brown in appearance.[7,40] An exception to this description is the lipoadenoma, which is quite soft and yellow-tan. These lesions tend to be larger than conventional adenomas.[49] Adenomas are often cystic, and indeed, many functioning parathyroid cysts represent adenomas with cystic degeneration.[37] The cysts may vary greatly in size and may contain fluid that ranges in color from clear to brown.[7]

Variants of adenoma are known to exist and, although rare, have been well documented. As with other adenomas, they are associated with hyperparathyroidism. The variant of adenoma known as the oncocytic adenoma may be indistinguishable from conventional adenoma on gross examination. Oncocytic adenomas are usually brown, tan, or orange and are soft. Lipoadenomas are soft, fatty, encapsulated masses of varying sizes. DeLellis[7] has reported weights ranging from 0.5 to 420 g.

Microscopic Pathology

On microscopic examination, the typical parathyroid adenoma appears as a hypercellular collection of chief cells arranged in a sheet-like pattern, usually with other patterns present as well (Fig. 11–23). Cord-like arrangements are commonly seen, as are small tubular profiles. These tubules may contain

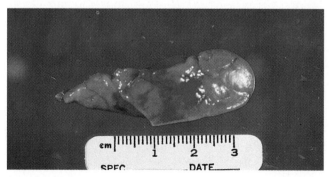

FIGURE 11–22 Gross appearance of a parathyroid adenoma. Note the glistening capsule and lobulated appearance.

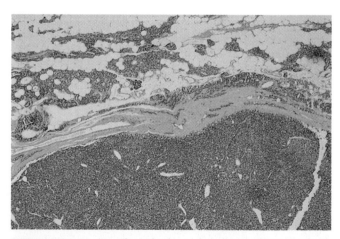

FIGURE 11–23 Parathyroid adenoma showing a sheet-like proliferation of cells with virtually no parenchymal fat. A rim of normal gland is visible at top (H&E, × 25).

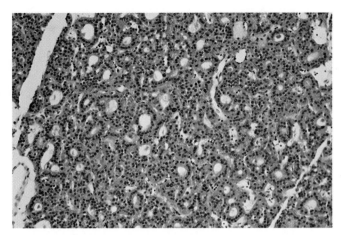

FIGURE 11-24 Adenoma with follicular architecture. Note the oxyphilic nature of the cytoplasm in this example (H&E, × 100).

lightly eosinophilic material, and may bear a close resemblance to small follicles seen in the thyroid gland (Fig. 11–24). Palisading of tumor cells around blood vessels may also be evident (Fig. 11–25).[7]

A rim of residual, compressed, or normal parathyroid gland may be present, usually in the hilar region. Absence of such a rim does not preclude the diagnosis of adenoma, however. Some investigators have found that this often-described feature is present in about 50% of cases, and is most likely to be present if the adenoma is small.[1,7] Bondeson et al,[9] in studies involving analysis of fat-stained frozen sections, found such a rim to be present 80% of the time.[9] Cells within the rim of normal tissue tend to be smaller than the neoplastic cells, and tend to have more abundant and coarsely dispersed parenchymal fat when compared with the adenoma.[9]

In general, adenomas are devoid of fat, or at least have much less stromal fat than do normal and hyperplastic parathyroid glands.[1,50] Based on analyses of frozen sections stained for fat, most adenomas display absent or markedly decreased amounts of intracytoplasmic fat.[9] It should be remembered, however, that adenomas may contain some, or even abundant, stromal fat.[7] At the extreme are lipoadenomas, which contain abundant stromal fat as a principal component.[51,52] The chief cells of lipoadenomas contain little intracytoplasmic fat compared to the surrounding normal gland.[9] On the other hand, the rim of host gland may be compressed or atrophic and may contain little or no stromal fat. Upon examination of fat-stained frozen sections, the rim of normal tissue is seen to contain significant intracytoplasmic lipid, as would be expected.[9] Depending on constitutional and other factors, nonadenomatous, nonhyperplastic parathyroid glands may have very little visible stromal fat as well.[6]

Cystic structures are often present in adenomas. Some adenomas may degenerate to the point where only cystic structures are evident. Usually, cystic structures are lined by chief cells that have a cuboidal appearance.[36] The capsule of these cysts may be thickened and may contain trapped nests of chief cells. Calcification and even ossification may be present within the thickened capsule.[7] Other degenerative changes may be present, including cholesterol clefts, giant cells, and deposits of hemosiderin (Fig. 11–26).

As mentioned previously, adenomas frequently contain small glandular structures. These small, tubular structures often contain pink material that resembles colloid. It is no wonder that these structures are easily mistaken for thyroid gland or a thyroid neoplasm. Such follicular structures may be a minor or major component, even comprising the entire adenoma.[7] These structures and their contents will stain negatively for immunohistochemical markers characteristic of thyroid. The intraluminal material of adenomas and normal parathyroids may demonstrate properties of amyloid upon staining with Congo red.[53] True papillary structures in parathyroid adenomas are rare, and may be mistaken for papillary carcinoma of the thyroid, especially if fine-needle aspiration is the diagnostic method.[54]

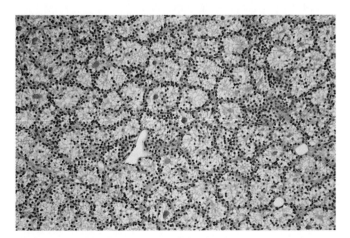

FIGURE 11-25 Adenoma with follicular architecture and prominent vascular palisading of cells (H&E, × 100).

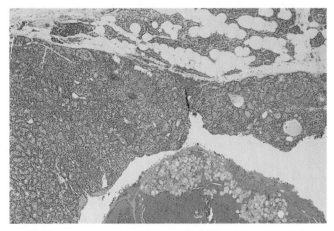

FIGURE 11-26 Cystic adenoma containing hemorrhage and foam cells. Note the rim of normal gland at the top (H&E, × 40).

Typically, adenomas are composed of compactly arranged, polygonal chief cells. Oncocytic cells and transitional chief cells may also be seen, and often, a mixture of these component cells is present.[7] As mentioned previously, individual chief cells in adenomas are larger than their counterparts in normal glands. The nucleus is centrally located and hyperchromatic, and nuclear borders are distinct. A single, small nucleolus may be present. Cytoplasm is lightly eosinophilic and may be vacuolated. Intercellular boundaries are usually indistinct. Within an adenoma, there may be focal aggregates or nodules of cells with similar morphologic characteristics. Nodules of cells containing large amounts of glycogen-containing, clear cytoplasm may be obvious. These cells may have more distinct cytoplasmic boundaries. Other aggregates of smaller cells with scanty, eosinophilic cytoplasm may be less evident.[7]

Most parathyroid adenomas are composed of a rather monotonous and bland cell population with little nuclear pleomorphism. However, pleomorphic nuclei may be present in approximately 25% of adenomas, and even a striking degree of pleomorphism in the absence of other features of malignant disease does not qualify a lesion as being malignant.[7] Pleomorphic nuclei may be diffusely scattered throughout the adenoma, or may occur focally (Figs. 11–27 and 11–28).[21] Binucleate forms may be present as well, a feature that is not typically seen in hyperplasia.[55]

Although nuclear pleomorphism alone may be present in an adenoma without necessarily raising serious suspicions of malignant disease, an adenoma with significant mitotic activity is cause for concern. Occasional mitotic figures may be present in an adenoma that behaves in a typically benign fashion. San-Juan et al[56] found that 42% of adenomas studied displayed mitotic activity. Snover and Foucar[57] described mitoses in 71% of the adenomas in their series. Of these, 59% contained less than 1 mitotic fig-

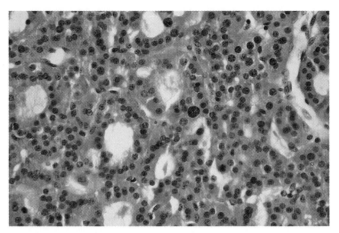

FIGURE 11–28 Oxyphilic adenoma exhibiting a follicular pattern and pleomorphic nuclei (H&E, × 250).

ure per 10 high-power fields (HPFs), and 12% contained more than 1 mitotic figure per 10 HPFs. The most mitotically active adenoma contained four mitoses per HPF. Of special concern are cases in which more than one mitotic figure is present per HPF. Such individuals must be examined carefully for other criteria of malignancy, and must be monitored closely to rule out the possibility of carcinoma. It is recommended that adenomas with more than 1 mitotic figure per 10 HPFs be designated as atypical adenomas.[56]

As the name implies, those lesions known as oncocytic adenomas are encapsulated neoplasms composed of cells containing a moderate to large amount of eosinophilic cytoplasm. The cells may be arranged in sheets, broad bands, trabecular patterns, or acinar patterns. Nuclei are small and hyperchromatic, and pleomorphic and multinucleate forms may be present.[7] Parenchymal fat is reduced compared to that in a normal gland. Transitional oxyphil cells and rare chief cells may be scattered throughout the lesion.[58] A rim of normal parathyroid tissue may be present. Oncocytic adenomas represent approximately 3% of all parathyroid adenomas.[59]

Lipoadenomas are composed of a parenchyma dominated by adipose tissue with a distinct lobular pattern. These lobules contain arborizing cords of chief cells and scattered oncocytic cells.[7] As with other adenomas, they are encapsulated. There is usually no significant inflammatory component or nuclear pleomorphism.[49]

Immunohistochemistry

As in normal parathyroid glands, the chief cells of parathyroid adenoma show positive reactivity for low-molecular-weight keratin, PTH, chromogranin A, synaptophysin, and NSE.[30] Staining for chromogranin B has been reported to virtually always yield

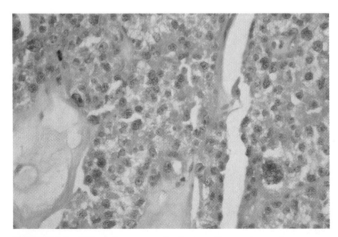

FIGURE 11–27 Adenoma with pleomorphic nuclei and a mitotic figure (*top left*) (H&E, × 250).

negative results.[60] Although normal parathyroid cells are not reactive to antibodies against proliferating cells—namely, proliferating cell nuclear antigen (PCNA) and Ki-67—neoplastic cells are reactive. Nodular areas show the most intense reactivity.[61]

In most cases, oncocytic adenomas have low endocrine function. Hyperparathyroidism caused by functioning oncocytic adenomas has been reported to be cured by surgical resection.[58,59,62] McGregor[58] demonstrated, by radioimmunoassay, the ability of oncocytic adenoma cells to synthesize proparathormone and parathormone, although at lower levels than normal parathyroid glands.

Adenomas studied by flow cytometry reveal a high proportion of tetraploid cells, and a lesser component of aneuploid cells.[46]

Ultrastructure

Ultrastructural examination of parathyroid adenomas has revealed that the chief cells display evidence of a hyperfunctional state. Plasmalemmal membranes are complex and interdigitated, Golgi regions are enlarged, and granular endoplasmic reticulum is increased.[63] Mitochondria show a greater degree of pleomorphism than normal chief cells.[7] In cases of one-gland disease, Cinti et al[63] also observed ribosomal lamellar complexes, annulate lamellae, groups of centrioles, intracytoplasmic lumina with microvilli, and nuclear inclusions. Annulate lamellae and intracytoplasmic microlumina had, at one time, been suggested as markers for adenomas.[64] These structures have also been identified in cases of chief cell hyperplasia. A clear ultrastructural marker for adenoma has not been identified to date.[63]

Primary Parathyroid Hyperplasia

Primary hyperplasia of the parathyroid glands defines a condition in which the absolute mass of the parathyroid glands is increased. This increased mass is the result of the proliferation of chief cells, transitional cells, oncocytic cells, and the so-called water-clear cells. Parathyroid secretion remains abnormally elevated without a known stimulus.

Chief cell hyperplasia is much more common than water-clear cell hyperplasia. Of 85 cases of primary hyperplasia, Castleman et al[65] found that 66 (78%) were attributable to chief cell hyperplasia, whereas 19 (22%) were caused by hyperplasia of the water-clear cell type. More recently, Tominaga et al[66] found that, of 109 cases of nonfamilial parathyroid hyperplasia, 100 (92%) were of the chief cell type, whereas 9 (8%) were of the water-clear cell type. This illustrates the fact that, for unknown reasons, the incidence of water-clear cell hyperplasia is decreasing with time, and is now an infrequent occur-

rence. Interestingly, water-clear cell hyperplasia was the first type to be described.[67]

PRIMARY CHIEF CELL HYPERPLASIA

Gross Pathology

In classic cases of chief cell hyperplasia, all four glands are enlarged. In a series of 54 cases of chief cell hyperplasia reported by Castleman et al,[65] the total weight of glandular tissue removed in each case was found to be greater than the weight of four normal glands. The weight ranged from 150 mg to 10 g. Fifty-four percent weighed less than 1 g.[65]

Pathologists and surgeons consider it a fortunate circumstance when they are able to identify four enlarged glands to confirm a diagnosis of parathyroid hyperplasia. Unfortunately, cases are not always so clear-cut, and the hyperplasia is frequently asymmetric. Tominaga and co-workers[66] reported that, of 100 patients with chief cell hyperplasia, 11 had a single parathyroid of increased weight, 44 patients had two enlarged glands, 28 had three enlarged glands, and only 7 had enlargement of all four glands. Three patients had normal-sized glands on gross examination, although histologically, the glands appeared hyperplastic. Likewise, Bondeson et al[9] reported that, in cases in which two glands were enlarged and hyperplastic, each and every additional gland, even if normal in weight and appearance, had some distinct evidence of hyperactivity.

On cut section, the parenchyma is dark tan to tan-red in appearance. This is in contrast to the normal gland, which is lighter in color owing to the presence of stromal fat.[68] Although not common, cysts may be present and will contain clear to tan fluid.[67] Hyperplastic glands may appear swollen and homogeneous, or they may have a nodular appearance, corresponding to diffuse and nodular histologic appearances, respectively. Of the largest glands, nodular, hyperplastic glands occur considerably more frequently than the diffuse type.[66] As with adenomas, hyperplastic glands may be asymmetric.

Hyperplastic glands of the water-clear cell type tend to be larger than those of the chief cell type. Castleman et al[65] found that, although only 18% of chief cell type hyperplastic glands weighed more than 5 g and none weighed more than 10 g, 79% of glands of the water-clear cell type weighed in excess of 5 g, and 47% weighed more than 10 g.[65] Total weight of glandular tissue from water-clear hyperplasia in the series reported by Tominaga et al[68] ranged from 950 mg to 38 g.[66]

Microscopic Pathology

With low-power microscopy, two patterns of hyperplasia are classically recognized. These include diffuse hyperplasia and nodular hyperplasia. The diffuse type displays a uniform proliferation of chief

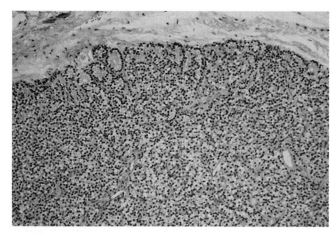

FIGURE 11–29 Parathyroid hyperplasia, diffuse type. Note the absence of stromal fat (H&E, × 100).

cells throughout the gland (Fig. 11–29). In the nodular type, distinct aggregates of cells are seen within the tissue of the parathyroid parenchyma. Fibrous septa may separate the nodules (Fig. 11–30).[66] Which type is more common is debatable. Black[48] divided hyperplastic glands into three groups having approximately the same frequency of occurrence. These groups included "classic" or diffuse type, "pseudoadenomatous" or nodular, and "occult," representing those glands that were normal to the eye of the surgeon but displayed microscopic hyperplasia and were associated with clinical hyperparathyroidism.[48] In the experience of DeLellis,[7] the nodular type of chief cell hyperplasia is most common. Tominaga and associates[66] observed that essentially diffuse hyperplasia was approximately five times more common than predominantly nodular hyperplasia in glands that were excised or that underwent biopsy study. Five percent of glands were essentially

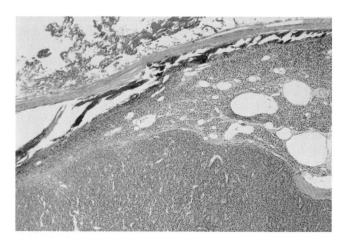

FIGURE 11–30 Parathyroid hyperplasia of the nodular type showing fibrous bands separating the nodules. Note the oxyphilic change in one of the nodules, as well as the peripheral calcification (H&E, × 40).

normal on histologic examination, but had increased weight.

Higher-power microscopy reveals that the expansion of the mass of the hyperplastic gland is due to a proliferation of rather monotonous chief cells that may appear larger than normal chief cells. Admixed oncocytic and transitional cells are present.[21] Mitotic figures may occasionally be seen in chief cell hyperplasia of the primary or secondary type, and in hyperplasia associated with multiple endocrine neoplasia 2A (MEN 2A) syndrome.[57] Although mild nuclear atypia and anisochromism may be present, marked nuclear atypia is generally not seen and is more suggestive of adenoma.[7]

In the diffuse type of hyperplasia, the cells are usually arranged in a solid pattern.[66] Like adenomas, cells may also be arranged in cords or glandular structures. Areas of nodularity may be present within a predominantly diffuse hyperplasia.[7] As a rule, there is a marked reduction in parenchymal fat with a more or less even distribution. Very minimal or no intercellular fat may be present.[1] It must be noted, however, that marked variations in the amount of stromal fat exist, and the amount and distribution of fat may be similar or even more abundant than that in normal glands.[66] Abundant stromal fat in a small biopsy specimen from an enlarged gland may lead to an erroneous frozen section diagnosis of normal parathyroid.[7] Bruining and van Houten,[69] in a series of 615 patients with primary hyperplasia, found that hyperplastic glands with relatively abundant fat were of normal or moderately enlarged size, whereas markedly enlarged glands tended to have a much reduced fat content. Frozen section staining for fat demonstrates that the parenchymal cells in most cases of hyperplasia contain markedly decreased or absent intracytoplasmic lipid.[9]

Nodular architecture in parathyroid hyperplasia may be prominent, particularly in the early course of the disease.[7] Such glands usually contain less than five nodules measuring only a few millimeters in size or smaller. The nodules are usually composed of either chief cells or oncocytic cells or, less commonly, a mixture of both types.[66] The nodular aggregates are usually devoid of stromal fat cells. The tissue between and adjacent to the nodules displays stromal fat cells.[7] These areas may be misinterpreted as a rim of normal tissue associated with an adenoma. Serial sections reveal that this represents a "pseudo-rim," that is, a direct connection, or gradual interface, between this tissue and the hyperplastic nodule.[65] Fat stains are useful in this situation, as a rim of true normal or suppressed tissue would show an abundance of parenchymal fat, whereas a hyperplastic gland would usually show a very small amount, if any.[7]

Mitotic figures may be present in hyperplasia. Indeed, Snover and Foucar[57] found mitotic figures to be present in 80% of cases. Twenty percent of cases exhibited no mitotic activity, 60% exhibited less than

1 mitosis per 10 HPFs, and 20% demonstrated more than 1 mitosis per 10 HPFs. One patient with MEN 2 demonstrated 5 mitoses per 10 HPFs.

Parathyromatosis refers to the presence of multiple collections of hyperplastic chief cells in the soft tissues of the neck and mediastinum. These rests most commonly result from spillage of cells during parathyroid surgery. They may also be present in necks that have not been operated on. These aggregates probably represent rests of parathyroid tissue left behind during embryologic development.[1] These aggregates become stimulated in patients with primary chief cell hyperplasia. These lesions are significant in that they may cause persistent or recurrent hyperparathyroidism in treated patients.[7]

Immunohistochemistry

Both normal and hyperfunctioning parathyroid glands display varying degrees of immunoreactivity for parathormone. Also present is staining for NSE; keratins 8, 18, and 19; chromogranin; and synaptophysin.[30,31] These positive results may be present in normal, hyperplastic, adenomatous, and malignant glands. Immunohistochemical staining for parathormone may be of help in distinguishing parathyroid tissue from other tissue, such as thyroid, that may simulate parathyroid tissue. This may be especially useful in evaluating metastatic disease. It must be remembered, however, that ectopically produced parathormone may be produced by nonparathyroid neoplasms.[30]

Ultrastructure

Hyperplastic chief cells show the ultrastructural correlates of hyperfunction, namely, hypertrophic Golgi apparatuses, abundant granular endoplasmic reticulum, scanty intracytoplasmic lipid, and complex and elongated interdigitations of the plasma membranes.[21,33,63,64] Cinti et al[63] also identified annulate lamellae and intracytoplasmic microlumina in patients with hyperplasia. Further, Cinti and co-workers[63] found that, in patients with primary hyperparathyroidism, glands that appeared normal on gross and light microscopic examination displayed distinct features of secretory activity when examined by electron microscopy, strongly suggesting that the correct diagnosis was hyperplasia.

CLEAR CELL HYPERPLASIA

As mentioned, the incidence of clear cell hyperplasia appears to be decreasing with time. On gross, microscopic, and ultrastructural evaluations, hyperplastic parathyroids of the clear cell type display characteristics that are both common to and divergent from chief cell hyperplasia. In most cases of clear cell hyperplasia, all four glands are enlarged, and there may be marked variations in the size of affected glands in a single case. The upper glands are usually larger than the lower glands.[7] The glands tend to attain a larger size than in chief cell hyperplasia. In a series of 19 cases, 79% weighed more than 5 g, and 47% weighed in excess of 10 g.[65] The shape of the glands is also variable and tends to be irregular, with projections extending into the surrounding tissue. On cut section, the glands are red-brown to brown, and may show cystic change, hemorrhage, and fibrosis.[7]

At low power, the hyperplastic gland displays a diffuse pattern of involvement with no apparent stromal fat. Cells may be arranged in tubular structures. Cystic structures containing proteinaceous fluid may be present. At medium power, the abundant clear cytoplasm within the polyhedral cells is apparent. Groups of cells are bordered by small blood vessels that are accentuated by the tendency of the nuclei to be polarized to the portion of the cell adjacent to the vessels (Fig. 11–31). Nuclei may be slightly hyperchromatic and have an eccentrically placed, small nucleolus. Multinucleated cells may be present, as may scattered cells with enlarged, pleomorphic, and hyperchromatic nuclei. In addition to displaying enlarged nuclei, these scattered cells usually contain ample clear cytoplasm.[7,65] Oncocytic cells are not present, and admixed small chief cells are rare. At higher power, it becomes evident that the cytoplasm is composed of thin wisps of cytoplasmic material and variable numbers of multiple small vacuoles measuring 0.2 to 0.8 μm in diameter. Large cells contain numerous vacuoles, whereas smaller cells may contain few.[65] Moderate amounts of glycogen are present within these cells, but staining for neutral fats yields negative results.[7]

Ultrastructural examination reveals vacuoles that appear empty except for the presence of small, electron-dense cores resembling those seen in secretory granules. Also present may be membrane-limited secretory granules; these may also be evident in normal, adenomatous, and hyperplastic chief cells.[65] The vacuoles are thought to be derived from the Golgi vesicles. On the basis of electron microscopic

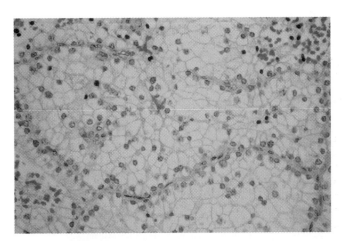

FIGURE 11-31   Clear cell hyperplasia.

evidence, Roth[70] has postulated that water-clear cells are derived from chief cells, and that the two types of hyperplasia are variations of the same disease.

LIPOHYPERPLASIA

Strauss et al[71] have described lipohyperplasia, a variant of hyperplasia, in five patients with hyperparathyroidism. All of the patients were women with four-gland enlargement. The average size of the glands was approximately 100 to 200 g, with the largest gland weighing 820 g. Histologically, the glands displayed an admixture of parathyroid parenchymal cells and mature-appearing fat cells at a ratio of approximately 1:1. The glands were thinly encapsulated and contained focal myxoid stroma. Removal of 3.5 glands resulted in a euparathyroid state.

PARATHYROID CARCINOMA

Parathyroid carcinoma is the cause of approximately 4% of all cases of primary hyperparathyroidism. In more than 80% of patients, the disease presents in the third to sixth decades of life, with the average age being 44 years. The male:female ratio is approximately 1:1.[72,73] This malignant tumor usually manifests with severe, symptomatic hypercalcemia. A palpable neck mass is present in up to one third of patients.[74] Parathyroid carcinomas tend to grow rather slowly, and metastases occur late in the disease. Rare cases of nonfunctioning parathyroid carcinoma have been reported.[73,75] Extremely rare cases of parathyroid carcinoma have been documented in the setting of familial hyperparathyroidism.[76,77] Streeten and co-workers[76] reported four family members in two generations with hyperparathyroidism, including two with carcinoma and two with atypical adenomas that may represent early carcinoma. Rare cases of parathyroid carcinoma have also been seen in association with parathyroid adenoma, hyperplasia, and MEN type 1.[78-81]

Gross Pathology

Often, the surgeon may suspect carcinoma on the basis of the lesion's intraoperative appearance, noting that the tumor is firm and adherent to adjacent structures (Fig. 11–32).[82] Because of this, an en bloc resection may be performed instead of simple removal of the gland. Parathyroid carcinoma may be encapsulated as well, in a manner indistinguishable from adenoma.[7] The mass is round to oval and has a firm consistency. The cut surface is grey-tan to white. The tumor may appear lobulated owing to dense bands of fibrosis. In their series of 70 cases, Schantz and Castleman[72] found the average weight to be 12 g, with a range of 0.8 to 42.4 g. In another series, the average weight was reported to be 6.7 g.[74]

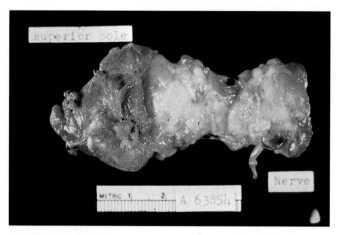

FIGURE 11–32 Gross appearance of a parathyroid carcinoma. Note the white fibrotic cut surface and adherence to the adjacent nerve. Courtesy of Dr. Karl H. Perzin, Columbia University College of Physicians and Surgeons, New York.

Microscopic Pathology

Microscopic features that suggest malignant disease include thick, fibrous bands; increased mitotic activity; and capsular, perineural, and blood vessel invasion (Figs. 11–33 and 11–34). All of these features may not be found in any one individual, but often, several are present. Schantz and Castleman[72] found that the mitotic count was the most important criteria, as discussed later.

Upon low-power examination, the tumor has a vaguely lobulated appearance owing to prominent, hypocellular, fibrous bands that course through the tumor, separating the parenchymal elements into compartments. Schantz and Castleman[72] found this feature to be present in 90% of cases. In some cases, a thickened, partial or complete capsule was continuous with the fibrous bands. It should be remembered, however, that adenomas may also contain such fibrous bands and thickened capsules.[7]

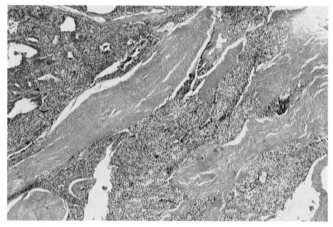

FIGURE 11–33 Parathyroid carcinoma that has been separated into compartments by dense, fibrous bands (H&E, × 25).

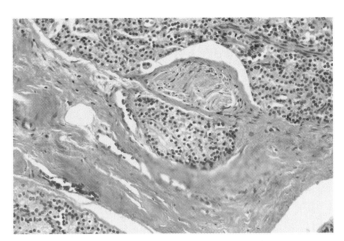

FIGURE 11-34 Perineural invasion by parathyroid carcinoma (H&E, × 100).

Mitotic activity may, of course, be present in carcinomas, but it may also be present in adenomas and hyperplastic glands. Care must be taken to count only true mitotic figures in parenchymal cells, and not pyknotic nuclei or endothelial mitoses.[72] Mitotic counts of 1 per 10 HPFs are supportive of a diagnosis of malignant disease when other criteria point to this diagnosis. However, benign lesions may also display such a mitotic rate.[56] In one study of mitotic rates in benign and malignant parathyroid lesions, no benign lesions exhibited more than four mitotic figures per HPF.[57] By contrast, mitotic figures in carcinoma may be quite numerous, numbering more than 10 mitoses per HPF.[83]

A thickened capsule, either complete or partial, is usually present and may extend into the fibrous bands within the tumor. The fibrosis may also extend into adjacent structures within the neck, including the connective tissue, thyroid, skeletal muscle, and nerves.[7,83] Capsular invasion is noted in approximately 70% of cases.[72] The invasive component is composed of tongues of cells insinuating themselves between collagenous strands of the capsule.[7]

The parenchymal component of the tumor is composed of chief cells arranged in sheets, trabeculae, and lobules of tumor surrounded by fibrous bands.[72] Schantz and Castleman[72] found a trabecular arrangement of cells to be a useful criterion for malignant disease, but van Heerden et al[84] found this to be the least useful of the criteria. Nuclear palisading may be present.[7] Individual tumor cells generally contain nuclei that are not particularly pleomorphic, although the cells are larger than in normal glands. Parathyroid carcinomas with an anaplastic appearance and pleomorphic nuclei, prominent nucleoli, and clumped nucleoplasm may occur.[38,72] However, nuclear pleomorphism is not a reliable criterion of malignancy in this case; in fact, such features are more likely to be associated with an adenoma.[72] The cytoplasm of cells in parathyroid carcinoma is generally granular and clear or eosinophilic.[7] Scattered groups of oncocytic cells may be present as well.[83] The oncocytic cell type may predominate; hence, these tumors have been called oncocytic variants of parathyroid carcinoma.[85]

The possibility of a mucinous variant of parathyroid carcinoma also exists. Edelson et al[86] reported a case of a 67-year-old patient who, in previous years, had undergone resection of a mass that was diagnosed as a mucinous thyroid carcinoma. The patient was subsequently reported to have lung metastases, hypercalcemia, and an increased serum PTH level. Removal of the lung metastases resulted in resolution of the hypercalcemia. Histologic analysis of the lung metastases was similar to that of the original resection from the thyroid, demonstrating cords of adenocarcinoma cells surrounded by and floating in mucin that tested positive for mucicarmine, PAS with diastase, and alcian blue. This tumor showed immunohistochemical positivity for parathyroid hormone and negativity for thyroid markers. Northern blot hybridization of total RNA confirmed the presence of messenger RNA for PTH, but not for PTHrP. Other criteria were not completely characteristic of parathyroid carcinoma, and the evidence is not definitive at this time.[86]

Vascular invasion is a feature in more than 10% of the cases.[72] This is most likely to be observed in areas where the capsule is quite thick. In parathyroid carcinomas, true vascular invasion requires that a portion of the intravascular component be attached to the vessel wall, as benign endocrine tumors may exhibit intravascular collections of glandular cells. When this criterion is met, such vascular invasion is virtually diagnostic of malignant disease.[7]

Ultrastructurally, the plasma membranes demonstrate complex interdigitations with the membranes of adjacent cells. Ring forms and parallel stacks of rough endoplasmic reticulum (RER) with transition to annulate lamellae are noted, in addition to a close spatial relationship between the RER and mitochondria. Golgi regions are well developed.[83,87] Secretory granules may be plentiful, although extrusion of granules has not been reported.[83,88] Desmosomes may be plentiful or rare.[83,87] Regular components of the cytoplasm include glycogen particles, lipid material, and lysosomes. Intramitochondrial small, dense bodies and myelin figures may be present. Increased numbers of mitochondria are present in oncocytic cells.[83] Occasionally, intracytoplasmic lumina may be present.[7]

Mallette[46] reviewed studies reporting the usefulness of DNA quantitation by flow cytometry in parathyroid lesions. It appears that, even though several studies show that a significant proportion of carcinomas are aneuploid, the incidence of aneuploidy in adenomas is frequent enough that a classification as benign or malignant based on this parameter is not reliable.[46] Likewise, the nuclear DNA content of the tumor cannot at this point be used reliably to differentiate benign from malignant lesions. However, it may be, as has been suggested by Irvin et al,[89] that aneuploidy in a known or presumed carcinoma may be a predictor of poor prognostic behavior.

Differential Diagnosis

Parathyroid adenoma and carcinoma share many characteristics. Both present with hyperparathyroidism, although the associated hypercalcemia and related symptoms are more severe with malignant disease. Nonfunctioning variants of both lesions are known to exist. Each may present with a solitary, enlarged parathyroid gland. A palpable neck mass is present in approximately one third of patients with parathyroid carcinoma.

Of course, metastatic spread of disease is diagnostic of malignant disease. Although metastasis to regional lymph nodes may be present, metastatic disease is not usually a finding at initial presentation. Metastasis is reported to occur in approximately 30% of patients during the course of their disease.[1,90]

Both adenoma and carcinoma may display mitotic activity. In the absence of other features of malignant disease, tumors with less than 1 mitotic figure per 10 HPFs should be considered to be benign. Glands that display more than 1 mitosis per 10 HPFs represent either atypical adenoma, which should be monitored closely, or carcinoma.[56] Tumors with more than 4 mitoses per 10 HPFs should be considered to be carcinoma until proven otherwise.[57]

Vascular invasion by carcinoma is a specific sign of malignant disease, but it is infrequently seen. True vascular invasion requires attachment of tumor cells to the vascular wall. This is important to remember, as pseudovascular invasion may occur in approximately 5% of adenomas.[56] Additionally, it has been pointed out that only vascular invasion, which occurs external to the capsule of the neoplasm, is significant in terms of malignancy.[1]

Although cellular and nuclear pleomorphism may occur in carcinoma, it is more likely to be indicative of adenoma.[72] A thickened capsule is a nonspecific sign; however, extension of the parathyroid tissue into the surrounding structures in a previously undisturbed surgical bed suggests malignant disease. It should be remembered, however, that adenomas that have undergone degenerative changes may be adherent to adjacent structures.[1]

Capsular invasion by parenchymal cells is another finding that is consistent with malignant disease. Adenomas and parathyroid cysts may display nests of cells within the capsule. However, these small clusters of cells differ in appearance from the more substantial, tongue-like projections of tumor cells in carcinoma.[7]

Carcinomas of thyroid origin may be misdiagnosed as parathyroid carcinoma.[75,86] These tumors should react positively to thyroid-specific immuno-

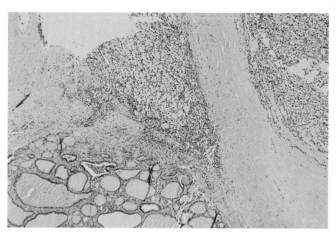

FIGURE 11–35 Metastatic renal cell carcinoma of the thyroid in a patient with hypercalcemia and an adjacent parathyroid adenoma. The patient had a known history of renal cell carcinoma and subsequently presented with a neck mass (H&E, × 40).

histochemical markers, including thyroglobulin and, possibly, calcitonin. By contrast, parathyroid carcinomas will react negatively to these markers and positively for parathyroid hormone.

Additionally, metastatic tumors to the thyroid, lung, and other sites may be mistaken for parathyroid carcinoma, especially in patients with hypercalcemia. Immunohistochemical methods may be helpful in establishing the correct diagnosis in this circumstance as well (Fig. 11–35).

Electron microscopic studies of parathyroid tumors causing primary hyperparathyroidism reveal evidence of activity in the cells of adenomatous, hyperplastic, and carcinomatous lesions. Normal glands show features of inactivity or suppression.[12,63] The utility of electron microscopy in differentiating between benign and malignant parathyroid neoplasms has not been definitively demonstrated, however. Likewise, although molecular biological techniques have elucidated many of the features of lesions responsible for primary hyperparathyroidism, the overlapping characteristics of benign and malignant lesions have thus far precluded definitive differentiation.[91]

Distinguishing between parathyroid adenoma and carcinoma may be very difficult, if not impossible. Patients who do not have sufficient findings to warrant a diagnosis of malignant disease may, at times, be so diagnosed only when there is a recurrent lesion in the neck.[1,90]

SECONDARY HYPERPARATHYROIDISM

Conditions in which serum calcium levels are decreased may result in compensatory hyperfunction of the parathyroid glands. The most common such state is chronic renal failure, and the effects on the parathyroid glands are especially evident when the patient undergoes dialysis. Vitamin D deficiency secondary to a poor diet or intestinal malabsorption is another common cause. Pseudohypoparathyroidism, in which there is a subnormal response to parathormone at the receptor level, also results in increased production of parathormone. In these states, there is an adaptive increase in the function and size of the parathyroids in response to a stimulus; this has been termed "secondary parathyroid hyperplasia."[7,92] By contrast, in primary hyperparathyroidism, the increase in function and size is autonomous.

Gross Pathology

The size of parathyroid glands in secondary hyperparathyroidism is variable, especially with long-standing disease. In a study of 200 cases, Roth[92] found weights ranging from 120 to 6000 mg. The size of the glands was found to be inversely related to the serum calcium level, and positively correlated with the serum phosporus level. Unlike primary hyperparathyroidism, the lower glands tend to be larger than the upper glands. The consistency of the glands is firmer than in normal glands.

Microscopic Pathology

In the early course of the disease, when glandular weights are not significantly increased, the most noticeable changes are decreased numbers of parenchymal fat cells and their replacement by chief cells. This relative increase in the number of chief cells occurs in a rather uniform manner throughout the gland. The cells are usually arranged in sheets, but trabecular and more rarely, glandular patterns may also be present, as is seen in primary hyperfunctioning states. Focal nodular aggregates of cells, usually oxyphil or transitional cells, may occur.[92]

In the larger glands of more advanced disease, there is an increased tendency toward nodularity. These nodules may be composed of chief cells or oxyphil cells, and may or may not be divided by fibrous septa.[92] Fibrosis, hemorrhage, chronic inflammation, and formation of cystic structures may be evident.[7]

The chief cells in secondary hyperparathyroidism display features considered to be characteristic of chronic stimulation. The cell has a vacuolated cytoplasm and discrete cell membranes.[92] These cells are rich in glycogen, and the intracytoplasmic lipid content is decreased.[7] The cell measures 6 to 8 μm in diameter, and the eccentrically placed nucleus is pyknotic in appearance. The vacuous cytoplasm does not contain the many small wisps of eosinophilic cytoplasm that characterize the cells of water-clear cell hyperplasia.

Increased numbers of oxyphil and transitional cells may be present. In patients with chronic renal disease, rare cells or groups of cells with a distinct epithelioid appearance may be noted.[92]

As reported by Harlow et al,[93] aneuploid cells may also be present in secondary hyperparathyroidism. In their study, 22% of the glands removed from five patients demonstrated an aneuploid population.

Ultrastructure

Ultrastructural studies confirm the presence of chief, oxyphil, and transitional cells. The chief cells display electron-transparent cytoplasm with numerous ribosomes and dispersed or aggregated, granular endoplasmic reticulum. Mitochondria are aggregated in the region of the Golgi apparatus. Nuclear chromatin is evenly distributed, and the nuclear envelope is prominent. A basement membrane is present and separates the cell from the extracellular environment. Interestingly, the plasma membranes are rather straight and simple, with rare desmosomes.[92]

TERTIARY HYPERPARATHYROIDISM

The term tertiary hyperparathyroidism refers to the development of autonomous hyperparathyroidism arising in the setting of a continuous stimulus causing secondary hyperparathyroidism.[94] Chronic renal disease and malabsorption syndromes may provide the stimulus necessary for the establishment of this sequence of events. With this condition, production of parathyroid hormone cannot be suppressed by the infusion of calcium.[95] In the case of tertiary hyperparathyroidism occurring in the setting of chronic renal failure, which is by far the most common presentation, the pathologic features simulate those of hyperplasia. In patients with malabsorption syndromes or vitamin D–resistant rickets, the pathologic changes take on an adenomatous appearance.[96,97]

Clearly, a thorough history and clinical correlation are absolutely necessary in the diagnosis of tertiary hyperparathyoidism. Without such information, it may be impossible to distinguish tertiary hyperparathyroidism from the primary type.

Gross Pathology

Harach and Jasani[98] have reported that glands from patients with tertiary hyperparathyroidism weigh 34 to 40 times the maximum weight of normal parathyroid glands, with the individual mean weight of excised parathyroid tissue ranging from 0.1 to 9.05 g, and combined mean weights ranging from 3.01 to 12.43 g. They also found that superior glands tended to be larger than the inferior glands. As with other hyperfunctioning parathyroid states, pathologic glands may be found anywhere within the migratory path of the third and fourth branchial pouches. Lossef and co-workers[99] reported on a female patient with tertiary hyperparathyroidism who, in addition to a normal complement of hyperplastic glands in the neck, had three discrete hyperplastic glands in the anterior mediastinum.

The glands are round to oval in shape and, on cut section, display diffuse to nodular enlargement. These nodules may be well or poorly defined and range from dark brown to grey to bluish in color. Macrocyst and microcyst formation, calcification, fibrosis, and hemosiderin deposition may also be present.[7,98]

Microscopic Pathology

The microscopic appearance of the glands may be quite varied, and either a diffuse or nodular pattern may be apparent. Harach and Jasani[98] found that 84% of the glands displayed nodular changes. Another study found a nodular pattern in 66% of cases and a diffuse pattern in the remainder.[97] These nodules are usually multiple and vary in shape and size, containing a mix of parenchymal cell types. Most of the nodules are sharply demarcated from the surrounding stroma, but a subtle blending of the areas may also be present.[98] True adenomas rarely occur in patients with tertiary hyperparathyroidism.[7]

The constituent cells grow in many patterns, including nests, trabeculae, solid sheets, glands, and palisading arrangements. Glandular structures may contain colloid-like material, some of which may have the staining properties of amyloid.[98]

The appearance of the chief cells is also quite variable with respect to intensity of staining, size of cells, and nuclear pleomorphism. Oxyphil and transitional cells are abundant and are either diffusely arranged or aggregated into nodules. Multinucleated chief or oxyphil cells may be noted.

Fibrosis, calcification, cystic changes, hemorrhage, infarction, cholesterol granulomas, and chronic inflammation may be present. Fibrosis may present as a pseudoinfiltrating pattern simulating carcinoma. Parenchymal fat cells may be present within diffuse areas, as well as within nodules.[98]

It should be noted that areas indistinguishable from normal tissue may be present in more than 50% of the glands.[98] Immunohistochemical staining for parathyroid hormone, as well as staining for argyrophilia, yields variable results ranging from weak to strong and diffuse to patchy reactivity.[98]

MULTIPLE ENDOCRINE NEOPLASIA SYNDROMES

The syndromes associated with MEN include a group of rare inherited disorders that characteristically involve defined sets of endocrine glands, dispersed neuroendocrine cells, and sometimes, neural elements. These syndromes are categorized as types 1, 2A (or 2), and 2B (or 3). Parathyroid glands are involved in these syndromes with variable frequency according to type, demonstrating hyperplastic or adenomatous changes.[100] In fact, approximately 20% of cases of primary chief cell hyperplasia occur in the setting of one of the MEN syndromes.[7] Parathyroid involvement is commonly seen in types 1 and 2A, but rarely in type 2B.

MEN type 1, or Wermer's syndrome, consists of parathyroid hyperplasia/adenoma along with involvement of the anterior pituitary and pancreatic islets. Also present may be gastrointestinal carcinoids, adrenocortical adenomas, and thyroid follicular neoplasms. Parathyroid involvement in this phenotype is common, occurring in approximately 90% of cases.[7,100]

In MEN type 2A, proliferative lesions of the thyroid C cells (medullary carcinoma) and adrenal medulla (pheochromocytoma) accompany parathyroid hyperplasia/adenoma. Involvement of the parathyroids is less common in this type than in type 1, with an approximate incidence of 30% to 40%.[7,100]

MEN type 2B includes features of type 2A along with ocular and mucocutaneous changes, ganglioneuromatosis of the gastrointestinal tract, and skeletal tissue abnormalities. The parathyroid glands are rarely involved in MEN type 2B.[100]

Besides the defined sets of tissue involvement set forth by the classic MEN phenotypes, other combinations may occur and additional tissues may be involved in the mixed MEN syndromes. Parathyroid gland involvement may be a part of these constellations as well. Other conditions that may accompany parathyroid and other classic components of MEN syndromes in these mixed MEN syndromes include neurofibromas, eosinophilic pituitary adenomas, adrenocortical adenomas, bronchial carcinoids, chemodectomas, bronchogenic small cell carcinomas, gastroduodenal gastrin cell hyperplasia, gastric leiomyomas, gastric carcinoids, multicentric papillary thyroid carcinoma, and carotid body tumors.[100–105]

The most common underlying parathyroid pathology associated with MEN syndromes is diffuse and nodular hyperplasia. Thus, the presence of diffuse and nodular hyperplasia should raise the possibility of a MEN syndrome.[100]

MALIGNANCY-ASSOCIATED HYPERCALCEMIA

One of the most common endocrine manifestations of malignant disease is hypercalcemia. Of course, carcinoma of the parathyroid gland results in hypercalcemia, but other nonparathyroid malignant lesions resulting in hypercalcemia are much more common.[106] In fact, the most common cause of hypercalcemia in the general population is malignant disease.[107] Although a parathyroid substance has been identified in malignant diseases associated with elevated serum calcium levels, it appears that parathyroid hormone production by nonparathyroid tumors is not the responsible mediator in most cases. Prostaglandins may play a role.[107,108] The most common causes of malignancy-associated hypercalcemia are breast carcinoma and squamous carcinoma of the lung, both of which are common cancers. Pancreatic, ovarian, renal, and transitional cell carcinomas are other relatively common, solid tumors that may be complicated by elevated serum calcium levels. Not all common carcinomas result in hypercalcemia, as is evidenced by the fact that colon and uterocervical carcinomas are only rarely a cause of increased calcium levels. Uncommon carcinomas that are commonly accompanied by elevated serum calcium levels include cholangiocarcinoma and lesions induced by vasoactive intestinal polypeptide.[108] In pediatric patients, Wilms' tumor and rhabdomyosarcoma may be associated with the syndrome.[7]

Hematologic malignant diseases may be associated with hypercalcemia. The most common such tumor is myeloma. Others include Burkitt's lymphoma, and adult T-cell lymphoma.[108]

CONCLUSION

A review of the literature and some practical experience in examining parathyroid pathology confirm that, in most cases, a straightforward diagnosis can be made. In addition to the standard examination of H&E–stained sections, technical aids, such as frozen section fat staining, are helpful at the time of surgery to determine the functional status of the gland in question. To arrive at a correct diagnosis, adequate clinical information is an essential provision. Using these elements, the pathologist and surgeon are usually able to conclude, in a particular case, whether the most appropriate diagnosis is adenoma, hyperplasia, or carcinoma.

Although immunohistochemical methods and electron microscopy can be useful in demonstrating a hyperfunctional state, a "marker" for malignant disease has not yet been identified. Even when discriminating between adenoma and hyperplasia, the distinction is not always clear. Mention in the literature of certain concepts, such as localized hyperplasia and multiple adenomas, illustrates this point.[39–42] Clearly, additional investigation is needed to clarify the nature of these lesions.

REFERENCES

1. LiVolsi VA, Hamilton R. Intraoperative assessment of parathyroid gland pathology. A common view from the surgeon and pathologist. *Am J Clin Pathol.* 1994; 102:365.
2. Grimelius L, Åkerström G, Bondeson L, et al. The role of the pathologist in diagnosis and surgical decision making in hyperparathyroidism. *World J Surg.* 1991; 15:698.
3. Wang CA. The anatomic basis of parathyroid surgery. *Ann Surg.* 1976; 183:271.
4. Abu-jawdeh GM, Roth SI. Parathyroid glands. In: Sternberg SS, ed. *Histology for Pathologists.* New York: Raven Press; 1992: 311.
5. Dufour DR, Wilkerson SY. Factors related to parathyroid weight in normal persons. *Arch Pathol Lab Med.* 1983; 107:167.
6. Defour DR, Wilkerson SY. The normal parathyroid revisited: Percentage of stromal fat. *Hum Pathol.* 1982; 13:717.
7. DeLellis RA. *Tumors of the Parathyroid Gland.* 3rd series, fascicle 6. Washington DC: Armed Forces Institute of Pathology; 1993.
8. Saffros RO, Rhatigan RM, Urgulu S. The normal parathyroid and the borderline with early hyperplasia: A light microscopic study. *Histopathology.* 1984; 8:407.
9. Bondeson AG, Bondeson L, Ljunberg O, Tibblin S. Fat staining in parathyroid disease—Diagnostic value and impact on surgical strategy. *Hum Pathol.* 1985; 16:1255.
10. Roth SI, Wang CA, Potts JT. The team approach to primary hyperparathyroidism. *Hum Pathol.* 1975; 6:645.
11. Åkerström G, Malmaeus J, Bergstrom R. Surgical anatomy of human parathyroid glands. *Surgery.* 1984; 95:14.
12. Black WC. Correlative light and electron microscopy in primary hyperparathyroidism. *Arch Pathol.* 1969; 88:225.
13. Roth SI, Gallagher MJ. The rapid identification of "normal" parathyroid glands by the presence of intracellular fat. *Am J Pathol.* 976; 84:521.
14. Wang CA, Reider SV. A density test for the intraoperative differentiation of parathyroid hyperplasia from neoplasia. *Ann Surg.* 1978; 187:63.
15. Gilmore JR. The embryology of the parathyroid glands, the thymus, and certain associated rudiments. *J Pathol Bacteriol.* 1937; 45:507.
16. Reiling RE, Cady B, Clerkin EP. Aberrant parathyroid adenoma within the vagus nerve. *Lahey Clin Bull.* 1972; 25:158.
17. Speigel AM, Marx SJ, Doppman JL, et al. Intrathyroidal parathyroid adenoma or hyperplasia. *JAMA.* 1975; 234:1029.
18. Harach HR, Vujanic GM. Intrathyroidal parathyroid. *Pediatric Pathol.* 1993;13:71.
19. Reddick RL, Costa JC, Marx SJ. Parathyroid hyperplasia and parathyromatosis. *Lancet.* 1977; 1:549.
20. Alveryd A. Parathyroid glands in thyroid surgery. *Acta Chir Scand.* 1968; 389(suppl):1.
21. Castleman B. *Tumor of the Parathyroid Gland.* 2nd series, fascicle 14. Washington, DC: Armed Forces Institute of Pathology; 1974.
22. Grimelius L, Åkerström G, Johansson H, et al. The parathyroid glands. In: Kovacs K, Asa S, eds. *Functional Endocrine Pathology.* Vol 1. Boston: Blackwell Scientific; 1990:375.
23. Grimelius L, Åkerström G, Johansson H, Bergstrom R. Anatomy and histopathology of human parathyroid glands. *Pathol Annu.* 1981; 16(pt 2):1.
24. Ghandur-Mnaymneh L, Cassady J, Hajianpour MA, et al. The parathyroid gland in health and disease. *Am J Pathol.* 1986; 125:292.
25. Balashev VN, Ignashkina MS. Lymphatic system of parathyroid glands in man. *Probl Endokrinol Gormonoterapii.* 1964; 10: 52.
26. Dekker A, Dunsford HA, Geyer SJ. The normal parathyroid gland at autopsy: The significance of stromal fat in adult patients. *J Pathol.* 1979; 128:127.
27. Roth SI, Capen CC. Ultrastructure and functional correlations of the parathyroid glands. *Int Rev Exp Pathol.* 1974; 161:13.
28. Roth SI. The parathyroid gland. In: Silverberg SG, DeLellis RA, Frable WJ, eds. *Principles and Practice of Surgical Pathology.* 3rd ed. New York: Churchill Livingstone; 1997:2709.
29. Alpern HD, Roth SI, Olson JE. Intracellular lipid droplets in functioning transitional parathyroid oxyphil adenomas. A caveat. *Arch Surg.* 1990; 125:410.
30. Chaiwun B, Cote RJ, Taylor CR. Diffuse neuroendocrine and endocrine systems. In: Taylor CR, Cote RJ, eds. *Immunomicroscopy: A Diagnostic Tool for the Surgical Pathologist.* 2nd ed. Philadelphia: WB Saunders; 1994:163.

31. Miettenen M, Clark R, Lehto VP, et al. Intermediate-filaments proteins in parathyroid glands and parathyroid adenomas. *Arch Pathol Lab Med*. 1985; 109:986.
32. Battifora HA. Ultrastructure of endocrine neoplasms. *Ann Clin Lab Sci*. 1979; 9:164.
33. Cinti S, Sbarbati A, Morrini M, et al. Parathyroid glands in primary hyperparathyroidism: An ultrastructural morphometric study of 25 cases. *J Pathol*. 1992; 167:283.
34. Calandra DB, Shah KH, Prinz RA, et al. Parathyroid cysts: A report of eleven cases including two associated with hyperparathyroid crisis. *Surgery*. 1983; 94:887.
35. Fields TW, Staley CJ. Functioning parathyroid cysts. *Arch Surg*. 1961; 82:937.
36. Fisher RF, Gruhn J. Parathyroid cysts. *Cancer*. 1957; 1:57.
37. Downey RJ, Cerfolia RJ, Deschamps C, et al. Mediastinal parathyroid cysts. *Mayo Clin Proc*. 1995; 70:946.
38. Mirra JM. *Bone Tumors*. Philadelphia: Lea and Febiger; 1989: 1795.
39. Harness JK, Ramsburg SR, Nishiyama RH, Thompson NW. Multiple adenomas of the parathyroids: Do they exist? *Arch Surg*. 1979; 114:468.
40. Attie JN, Bock G, Auguste LJ. Multiple adenomas: Report of thirty-three cases. *Surgery*. 1990; 108:1015.
41. Jackson CE, Cerny JC, Block MA, Fialko PF. Probable clonal origin of aldosteronomas versus multcellular origin of parathyroid adenomas. *Surgery*. 1982; 92:875.
42. Fialko PJ, Jackson CE, Block MA, Greenawald KA. Multicellular origin of parathyroid "adenomas." *N Engl J Med*. 1977; 297:696.
43. Shinzaburo N, Motomura K, Inaji H, et al. Clonal analysis of parathyroid adenomas by means of the polymerase chain reaction. *Cancer Lett*. 1994; 78:93.
44. Arnold A, Staunton CE, Kim HG, Gaz RD, Kronenberg HM. Monoclonality and abnormal parathyroid hormone genes in parathyroid adenomas. *N Engl J Med*. 1988; 318:658.
45. Friedman E, Sakaguchi K, Bale AE, et al. Clonality of parathyroid tumors in familial multiple endocrine neoplasia type I. *N Engl J Med*. 1989; 321:1057.
46. Mallette LE. DNA quantitation in the study of parathyroid lesions. A review. *Am J Clin Pathol*. 1992; 98:305.
47. Rasbach DA, Monchik JM, Geelhoed GW, Harrison TS. Solitary parathyroid microadenoma. *Surgery*. 1984; 96:1092.
48. Black WC. The differential diagnosis of parathyroid adenoma and chief cell hyperplasia. *Am J Clin Pathol*. 1968; 49:761–775.
49. Geelhoed GW. Parathyroid adenolipoma: Clinical and morphologic features. *Surgery*. 1982; 92:806.
50. Black WC, Utley JR. The differential diagnosis of parathyroid adenoma and chief cell hyperplasia. *Am J Clin Pathol*. 1968; 49:761.
51. Geelhoed GW. Parathyroid adenolipoma: Clinical and morphologic features. *Surgery*. 1982; 92:806.
52. Abul-Haj SK, Conklin H, Hewitt WC. Functional lipoadenoma of the parathyroid gland. Report of a case. *N Engl J Med*. 1962; 266:121.
53. Anderson TJ, Ewen SW. Amyloid in normal and pathological parathyroid glands. *J Clin Pathol*. 1974; 27:656.
54. Friedman M, Shimaoka K, Lopez AC, Shedd DP. Parathyroid adenoma diagnosed as papillary carcinoma of the thyroid on needle aspiration smears. *Acta Cytol*. 1983; 27:337.
55. DeLellis RA. The endocrine system. In: Cotran RS, Kumar V, Collins T, eds. *Robbins Pathologic Basis of Disease*. 6th ed. Philadelphia: WB Saunders; 1999:1121.
56. San-Juan J, Monteaguda C, Fraker D, et al. Significance of mitotic activity and other morphologic parameters in parathyroid adenomas, and their correlation with clinical behavior, *Am J Clin Pathol*. 1989; 92:523. Abstract.
57. Snover DC, Foucar K. Mitotic activity in benign parathyroid disease. *Am J Clin Pathol*. 1981; 75:345.
58. McGregor DH, Lotuaco LG, Rao MS, Chu LLH. Functioning oxyphil adenoma of parathyroid gland, an ultrastructural and biochemical study. *Am J Pathol*. 1978; 92:691.
59. Wolpert HR, Vickery AL Jr, Wang CA. Functioning oxyphil cell adenomas of the parathyroid gland. A study of 15 cases. *Am J Surg Pathol*. 1989; 13:500.
60. Schmidt KW, Hittmair A, Ladurner D, et al. Chromogranin A and B in parathyroid tissue of cases of primary hyperparathyroidism: An immunohistochemical study. *Virch Arch [Cell Pathol]*. 1991; 418:295.
61. Massimo L, Lipman J, Cukor B, et al. Nodular foci in parathyroid adenomas and hyperplasias: An immunohistochemical analysis of proliferative activity. *Hum Pathol*. 1994; 25:1050.
62. Selzman HM, Fechner RE. Oxyphil adenoma and primary hyperparathyroidism: Clinical and ultrastructural observations. *JAMA*. 1967; 199:359.
63. Cinti S, Colussi G, Minola E, Dickersin GR. Parathyroid glands in primary hyperparathyroidism: An ultrastructural study of 50 cases. *Hum Pathol*. 1986; 17:1036.
64. Cinti S, Sbarbati, A. Ultrastructure of human parathyroid cells in health and disease. *Microsc Res Tech*. 1995; 32:164.
65. Castleman B, Schantz A, Roth S. Parathyroid hyperplasia in primary hyperparathyroidism. *Cancer*. 1976; 38:1668.
66. Tominaga Y, Grimelius L, Johansson H, et al. Histological and clinical features of nonfamilial primary parathyroid hyperplasia. *Pathol Res Pract*. 1992; 188:115.
67. Albright F, Bloomberg E, Castleman B, Churchill EB. Hyperparathyroidism due to diffuse hyperplasia of all parathyroid glands rather than an adenoma of one. Clinical studies on three such cases. *Arch Intern Med*. 1934; 54:315.
68. Passman JM. Changing concepts of parathyroid pathology in primary hyperparathyroidism. *Lab Med*. 1976; 7:7.
69. Bruining HA, van Houten H, Juttman JR, et al. Results of operative treatment of 615 patients with primary hyperparathyroidism. *World J Surg*. 1981; 5:85.
70. Roth SI. The ultrastructure of primary water-clear cell hyperplasia of the parathyroid glands. *Am J Pathol*. 1970; 61:233.
71. Strauss FH, Kaplan EL, Nishiyama RH, Bigos ST. Five cases of parathyroid lipohyperplasia. *Surgery*. 1983; 94:901.
72. Schantz A, Castleman B. Parathyroid carcinoma. A study of 70 cases. *Cancer*. 1973; 31:600.
73. Anderson BJ, Samaan NA, Vassilopoulou-Sellin R, et al. Parathyroid carcinoma: Features and difficulties in diagnosis and management. *Surgery*. 1983; 94:906.
74. Wang CA, Gaz RD. Natural history of parathyroid carcinoma. Diagnosis, treatment and results. *Am J Surg*. 1985; 149:522.
75. Ordonez NG, Samaan NA, Ibanez ML, Hickey RC. Immunoperoxidase study of uncommon parathyroid tumors. Report of 2 cases of nonfunctioning parathyroid carcinoma and one intrathyroid parathyroid tumor-producing amyloid. *Am J Surg Pathol*. 1985; 7:535.
76. Streeten EA, Weinstein LS, Norton JA, et al. Studies in a kindred with parathyroid carcinoma. *J Clin Endocrinol Metab*. 1992; 75:362.
77. Mallette LE, Bilezikian JP, Ketcham AS, Aurbach GD. Parathyroid carcinoma in familial hyperparathyroidism. *Am J Med*. 1974; 57:642.
78. Dinnen JS, Greenwood RH, Jones JH, et al. Parathyroid carcinoma in familial hyperparathyroidism. *J Clin Pathol*. 1977; 30: 966.
79. Cope O. Hyperparathyroidism: Diagnosis and management. *Am J Surg*. 1960; 99:394.
80. Golden A, Canary JL, Kerwin DM. Concurrence of hyperplasia and neoplasia of the parathyroid glands. *Am J Med*. 1960; 38:562.
81. Kramer WH. Association of parathyroid hyperplasia with neoplasia. *Am J Clin Pathol*. 1970; 53:275.
82. Jarman WT, Myers RT, Marshall RB. Carcinoma of the parathyroid. *Arch Surg*. 1978; 113:123.
83. Holck S, Pedersen NT. Carcinoma of the parathyroid gland. A light and electron microscopic study. *Acta Path Microbiol Scand Sect*. 1981; 89:297.
84. van Heerden J, Weiland L, ReMine et al. Cancer of the parathyroid gland. *Arch Surg*. 1979; 114:475.
85. Obara T, Fujimoto Y, Yamaguchi K. Parathyroid carcinoma of the oyphil cell type. A report of two cases, light and electron microscopic study. *Cancer*. 1985; 5:1482.
86. Edelson GW, Kleerekoper M, Talpos GB, et al. Mucin-producing parathyroid carcinoma. *Bone*. 1992; 13:7.
87. Faccini JM. The ultrastructure of parathyroid glands removed

from patients with primary hyperparathyroidism: A report of 40 cases, including four carcinomata. *J Pathol.* 1970; 102:186.

88. Murayama T, Kawake K, Tagami M. A case of parathyroid carcinoma concurred with hyperplasia: An electron microscopic study. *J Urol.* 1977; 118:126.

89. Irvin GL III, Taupier MA, Block NL, et al. DNA patterns in parathyroid disease predict postoperative parathyroid hormone secretion. *Surgery.* 1988; 104:1115.

90. Schantz A, Castleman B. Parathyroid carcinoma: A study of 70 cases. *Cancer.* 1973; 31:600.

91. Backdahl M, Howe JR, Lairmore TC, Wells SA. The molecular biology of parathyroid disease. *World J Surg.* 1991; 15:756.

92. Roth SI, Marshall RB. Pathology and ultrastructure of the human parathyroid glands in chronic renal failure. *Arch Intern Med.* 1969; 124:397.

93. Harlow S, Roth SI, Bauer K, Marshall RB. Flow cytometric DNA analysis of normal and pathological parathyroid glands. *Mod Pathol.* 1991; 4:310.

94. St Goar WT. Case records of the Massachusetts General Hospital. *N Engl J Med.* 1963; 268:943.

95. Davies DR, Dent CE, Watson L. Tertiary hyperparathyroidism. *Br Med J.* 1968; 3:395.

96. Smith JF. Parathyroid adenomas associated with the malabsorption syndrome and chronic renal disease. *J Clin Pathol.* 1970; 23:362.

97. Krause MW, Hedinger CE. Pathologic study of parathyroid glands in tertiary hyperparathyroidism. *Hum Pathol.* 1985; 16:772.

98. Harach HR, Jasani B. Parathyroid hyperplasia in tertiary hyperparathyroidism: A pathological and immunohistochemical reappraisal. *Histopathology.* 1992; 21:513.

99. Lossef SV, Zeissman HA, Alijani MR, et al. Multiple hyperfunctioning mediastinal parathyroid glands in a patient with tertiary hyperparathyroidism. *Am J Roentgenol.* 1993; 161:285.

100. DeLellis RA, Yogeshwar D, Tischler AS, et al. Multiple endocrine neoplasia (MEN) syndromes: Cellular origins and interrelationships. *Int Rev Exp Pathol.* 1986; 28:163.

101. Rode J, Dhillon AP, Cotton PB, et al. Carcinoid tumour of stomach and primary hyperparathyroidism: A new association. *J Clin Pathol.* 1987; 40:546.

102. Berg B, Biörkland A, Grimelius L, et al. A new pattern of multiple endocrine adenomatosis: Chemodectoma, bronchial carcinoid, GH-producing pituitary adenoma, and hyperplasia of the parathyroid glands, and antral and duodenal gastrin cells. *Acta Med Scand.* 1976; 200:321.

103. Hansen OP, Hansen M, Hansen H, Rose B. Multiple endocrine adenomatosis of mixed type. *Acta Med Scand.* 1976; 200: 327.

104. Larraza-Hernandez O, Alvores-Saavedra J, Benavides G, et al. Multiple endocrine neoplasia: Pituitary adenoma, multicentric papillary thyroid carcinoma, bilateral carotid body paraganglioma, parathyroid hyperplasia, gastric leiomyoma, and systemic amyloidosis. *Am J Clin Pathol.* 1981; 78:527.

105. Benson L, Ljunghall S, Åkerström G, Öberg K. Hyperparathyroidism presenting as the first lesion in multiple endocrine neoplasia type 1. *Am J Med.* 1987; 82:731.

106. Mundy GR, Cove DH, Fisken R. Primary hyperparathyroidism: Changes in the pattern of clinical presentation. *Lancet.* 1980; 1:1317.

107. Besarab A, Caro JF. Mechanisms of hypercalcemia in malignancy. *Cancer.* 1978; 41:2276.

108. Mundy GR, Ibbotson KJ, D'Souza SM, et al. The hypercalcemia of cancer: Clinical implications and pathogenic mechanisms. *N Eng J Med.* 1984; 310:1718.

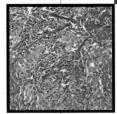

CHAPTER 12

Ear and Temporal Bone

I. CLINICAL CONSIDERATIONS FOR NON-NEOPLASTIC LESIONS OF THE EAR AND TEMPORAL BONE

■ EDWARD L. APPLEBAUM

■ BRIAN E. DUFF

KELOIDS

Keloids result from an abnormal process where dense connective tissue is overproduced while a cutaneous wound is healing. The term keloid is derived from the Greek *chele*, meaning "crab claw," describing the tendency for these lesions to extend well beyond the original site of injury. The earlobe is the most common site of keloids in the head and neck, primarily due to the practice of ear piercing. Keloids appear as shiny, smooth, globular fibrous growths on one or both sides of the lobule. Presenting signs and symptoms include the obvious cosmetic deformity, pruritis, and, rarely, pain or paresthesia.[1]

The precise cause of keloids is unknown, but genetic transmission by both autosomal dominant and autosomal recessive routes has been proposed, and multiple HLA associations have been discovered.[2-4] The high incidence (4.5% to 16%) in black and His-

panic populations may correlate with the increased melanin content of the dermis compared to that of whites.[5]

Unlike hypertrophic scars, keloids do not regress and tend to recur after attempts at excision. Since the 1800s a multitude of therapeutic regimens has been implemented with widely varying success rates. A majority of the studies on treatment outcome are limited by small patient numbers; inadequate, indeterminate, or absent follow-up; and ill-defined measures of response.

Intralesional steroids alone provide response rates of 50% to 100% with recurrence rates of 5% to 50% at 5 years.[6,7]

Surgical excision alone yields recurrence rates of 45% to 100%.[8,9] When surgery is followed by steroid injection or radiation therapy, recurrence rates are consistently below 50%.[10-13] Carbon dioxide laser vaporization produces 39% to 92% recurrence rates when used as a single modality and 25% to 74% recurrence rates in combination with postoperative steroid injections.[14-16] Results of Argon and Nd:YAG vaporization are comparable, with 45% to 93% and 53% to 100% recurrence rates, respectively.[15]

Cryotherapy alone has been shown to produce complete flattening and no recurrence in 51% to 74% of cases.[17-19] With the addition of injectable steroids, this response rate increases to 84%.[20]

External-beam radiation therapy alone has shown response rates of 16% to 94%.[10,21] Occlusive pressure dressings with and without hydration have shown 75% to 100% improvement in over one half of patients.[22] Silicone sheeting worn over keloids produced minimal improved responses compared to controls.[23] Intralesional injection of interferon has shown reduction in size of 50% or less, and response appears to be limited to the area treated.[24,25]

AURICULAR PSEUDOCYST

Pseudocysts of the auricle are uncommon lesions that present as asymptomatic swellings of the helix and antihelix. They are occasionally bilateral.[26] Most individuals affected are young, healthy adult males, though any age group, any race, and either sex may be affected.

These lesions arise over a period of weeks to years as painless swellings of the cartilage without overlying ulceration or erythema. Though they may arise anywhere on the auricle, the scaphoid fossa (80%) is the most common site.[27]

Engel,[28] the first to describe auricular pseudocysts in the English literature, believed that these lesions were secondary to repeated minor trauma. He attributed them to the habit of sleeping on hard pillows, though he could not substantiate his claim. Others have also proposed these lesions as traumatic in origin, citing the wearing of motorcycle helmets, stereo headphones, or the Italian birthday custom of having one's auricle pulled.[29,30] Despite these theories, in only one documented case has there been a history of preceding trauma.[31]

Current thought is that pseudocysts may arise within a potential plane left during embryonic fusion of the auriclar hillocks. Ischemic necrosis of the cartilage or the abnormal release of lysosomal enzymes by chondrocytes may also be cofactors.[26,32] Though various etiologies have been proposed, the cause remains unknown—hence the alternate name of benign idiopathic cystic chondromalacia. The short list of differential diagnoses includes relapsing polychondritis, subperichondrial hematoma, and chondrodermatitis nodularis chronica helicis.

In addition to the obvious cosmetic concerns, long-standing lesions may result in deformity of the ear. Several treatments have been described with the common goal of complete eradication without distortion of the underlying cartilage framework. Steroid injection alone has been unsuccessful and may result in cartilage deformity. Incision and drainage or curettage has shown variable success. Needle aspiration alone results in rapid reaccumulation of fluid but, when combined with bolster suture compression, no recurrences were seen with long-term follow-up.[33] Equal success is reported with removal of the anterior wall of the pseudocyst and application of a sclerosing agent (1% tincture of iodine) to the residual posterior wall.[34]

CHONDRODERMATITIS NODULARIS CHRONICA HELICIS

First described by Winkler,[35] chondrodermatitis nodularis chronica helicis is an inflammatory disorder characterized by painful nodules of the external ear. These lesions are seen most commonly on the helix and antihelix but may arise at any site on the auricle. They typically present as round, reddish, tender areas less than 5 mm in diameter. The etiology is unknown, although cold injury, actinic damage, local trauma, and degenerative change with pressure necrosis have been proposed. The exposed location, relative vascular deficiency, and absence of a subcutaneous fat layer render the superior helical rim susceptible to injury. Patients typically present in their sixth decade, and a male predominance has been noted. Even gentle manipulation may precipitate excruciating pain, which eventually prompts patients to seek treatment.

Though there is no malignant potential, differentiating these lesions from basal cell carcinoma and squamous cell carcinoma frequently requires biopsy. Treatment strategies have included wedge excision,[36] cartilage excision alone,[37] curettage, CO_2 laser vaporization,[38] external beam radiation, radium implants, and intralesional steroids.[39] A minority of lesions may respond to steroid injection, but most require surgical intervention. Cure rates vary with thoroughness of removal.

RELAPSING POLYCHONDRITIS

Relapsing polychondritis is a rare disorder of unknown etiology first described in 1923 by Jaksch-Wartenhorst.[40] It is characterized by recurrent, destructive, inflammatory lesions involving cartilaginous structures, with the auricle being most commonly affected. Multiple sites may be involved, including the nose, larynx, trachea, inner ear, articular cartilage, eye, cardiovascular system, and skin. Pearson et al[41] was the first to note the episodic nature of attacks over months to years and termed it relapsing polychondritis.

The current diagnostic criteria are defined by three or more of the following:[42,43]

1. recurrent chondritis of both auricles

2. nonerosive inflammatory arthritis
3. chondritis of nasal cartilages
4. ocular inflammation, including conjunctivitis, keratitis, scleritis/episcleritis, and/or uveitis
5. chrondritis of the upper respiratory tract involving the larynx and/or tracheal cartilages
6. cochlear and/or vestibular damage manifested by sensorineural hearing loss, tinnitus, and/or vertigo

Diagnosis may be confirmed by one or more of the aforelisted criteria with histological confirmation or by chondritis in two or more separate anatomical locations with response to steroids and/or dapsone.

Relapsing polychondritis occurs primarily in whites, with other ethnic groups rarely reported in the literature. No gender or familial predilection has been reported, with the single exception of a pregnant woman with relapsing polychondritis who delivered a child affected at birth.[43] Symptoms occur most frequently between the age of 40 and 60 years, with a mean of 44 years. The cause remains unknown, though it is generally believed to be an autoimmune disorder, since corticosteroids reduce the inflammatory response. Antibodies to cartilage have never been identified, but the discovery of elevated concentrations of circulating antibodies to type II collagen has provided support for the immune-mediated hypothesis.[44]

There appear to be two subsets of patients with relapsing polychondritis: those with chronic indolent disease and those with fulminant disease. In the chronic indolent group, symptoms can last from days to weeks and may resolve spontaneously if left untreated. Among those with fulminant disease, serious morbidity and mortality can occur due to airway collapse with respiratory obstruction or large-vessel involvement.

Ninety percent of all patients eventually develop auricular involvement, though it is the initial manifestation in only 25%. Auricular chondritis is typically bilateral but may be unilateral and sudden in onset. The pinnae become erythematous and tender to palpation with a notable sparing of the lobule. The diagnosis is straightforward only for patients with the classic findings of bilateral auricular disease. Other, less common, otologic manifestations include otitis media with effusion due to involvement of the eustachian tube cartilage and cochleovestibular symptoms.[45] Hearing loss, presumably due to internal auditory arteritis, may be sensorineural or mixed, unilateral or bilateral, sudden or progressive over weeks. Vestibular symptoms can range from mild dysequilibrium to vertigo with nausea and vomiting.

Arthropathy is the second most common finding (25% to 80%), and any joint may be affected. Due to the migratory nature of symptoms and presence of an inflammatory effusion, isolated joint involvement may be difficult to distinguish from rheumatoid arthritis. Ocular involvement can present as inflammation of any structure including the lids or adnexae

and, as with arthropathy, without other manifestations there is little evidence to isolate the diagnosis of relapsing polychondritis.

Nasal involvement presents as acute, painful swelling of the nasal dorsum with occasional epistaxis and/or a sensation of fullness. If left untreated, quadrangular or lateral cartilage destruction may result in a saddle-nose deformity. Repair of collapsed nasal cartilage has been reported, but controversy exists regarding the timing of surgical reconstruction in view of the relapsing nature of the disease process. Damiani and Levine[43] propose that cosmetic surgery be deferred until the disease process is quiescent for several years, reasoning that surgery itself may act as a trigger for reactivation and that disease recurrence with subsequent collapse might be assessed as a surgical failure.

Airway involvement eventually occurs in over one half of patients. Many fatal cases of fulminant disease are due to upper airway involvement, as acute inflammation of the larynx or trachea can lead to rapid obstruction. Chronic disease may result in cicatricial stenosis or obstructive lung disease. Laryngotracheal reconstruction has been reported but should be considered only after prolonged quiescence.[46] Twenty-five percent of relapsing polychondritis patients develop cardiovascular involvement, but only 10% display clinical symptoms. Any vessel can be affected with resultant morbidity based on the individual end organ. Aortic dissection and coronary valve insufficiency represent the highest risks for life-threatening complications.

Laboratory findings are nonspecific and include normochromic, normocytic anemia, mild leukocytosis, and an elevated erythrocyte sedimentation rate that is used as a marker for response to therapy.

Corticosteroids are the mainstay of treatment. Dapsone may be used as an alternative, with immunosuppressive medications as supplemental therapy in recalcitrant cases. Steroids are typically given for several weeks with a slow tapering off to prevent the occasional relapse seen with a rapid reduction in dosage. Patients are occasionally unable to discontinue medication without exacerbation of symptoms.

ANGIOLYMPHOID HYPERPLASIA WITH EOSINOPHILIA

Angiolymphoid hyperplasia with eosinophilia is a rare, benign, vascular proliferative disorder that presents as single or multiple red-brown papules and nodules in the dermis or subcutaneous tissues. The most frequent site of occurrence is the head and neck region, especially the periauricular area. Patients tend to be middle-aged to elderly women who classically present with pruritic, friable, raised lesions that may bleed profusely after minor trauma. Lesions may be painful or, less commonly, present

TABLE 12–1	CLINICAL DIFFERENCES BETWEEN KIMURA'S DISEASE AND ANGIOLYMPHOID HYPERPLASIA WITH EOSINOPHILIA	
FEATURES	**KIMURA'S DISEASE**	**ALHE**
Sex	Male (85%) > Female	Female (70%) > Male
Peak incidence	2nd–3rd decade	3rd–4th decade
Head and neck site	Postaural, scalp	Periauricular, forehead
Lymphadenopathy	Common	Rare if <2 cm
Peripheral eosinophilia	>50%	<25%
Mean duration of symptoms	9.6 years	2–2.5 years
Origin	Subcutaneous	Subcutaneous and dermal

ALHE, angiolymphoid hyperplasia with eosinophilia

as an asymptomatic mass. Secondary infections are prone to occur, particularly when the external auditory canal is involved.

This disease was first described in the English literature by Wells and Whimster[47] in 1969; they termed the condition subcutaneous angiolymphoid hyperplasia with eosinophilia. Merhregan and Shapiro[48] first coined the term angiolymphoid hyperplasia with eosinophilia after proving that lesions showing subcutaneous or dermal involvement were variations of the same disease entity. Pseudonyms have included pseudopyogenic granuloma, inflammatory angiomatous nodules, histiocytoid hemangioma, and epithelioid hemangioendothelioma.

The etiology of this disease is unknown. Proposed mechanisms include infection,[49] allergy,[49,50] immune-mediated,[51] endocrine,[49] inflammation,[52] and an atypical proliferation of endothelial cells resembling a true vascular neoplasm.[53,54] Reactive lymphadenopathy is seen in less than 15% of patients, but is more common with lesions greater than 2 cm. Peripheral eosinophilia is a variable feature, noted in less than 20% of patients.[55]

The differential diagnosis includes cutaneous malignancy, granuloma faciale, lymphocytoma, eosinophilic granuloma, lymphoma, pyogenic granuloma, angiomatous lymphoid hematoma, and Kimura's disease. Since its original description there has been a great deal of discussion about the association between angiolymphoid hyperplasia with eosinophilia and Kimura's disease, since the two conditions were once thought to represent opposite ends along a single disease spectrum.[48,55,56] In 1987, a study by Urabe et al[57] first outlined the multiple clinical and pathological differences between the two conditions resulting in their current classification as distinct disease entities (Table 12–1).

Histological evaluation is mandatory. In a study of 116 patients with angiolymphoid hyperplasia with eosinophilia, only one was assigned the correct diagnosis prior to biopsy.[53] Differentiating these lesions from malignancy is critical, because angiosarcoma remains one of the most common clinical misdiagnoses.

The natural history of this disease process is of a slowly progressive lesion(s) that may have been present for months to years before prompting medical attention. Spontaneous remission has been reported, but the severity of symptoms usually mandates intervention.[58–60] Local recurrence is common following incomplete excision; surgical resection resulting in uninvolved margins is the treatment of choice.[52,60,61] Alternative surgical methods such as electrodesiccation with curettage and cryotherapy result in frequent recurrence due to the inability to confirm clear margins.[62] Carbon dioxide laser vaporization has proven curative, but abundant granulation tissue in the healing wound may result in a prolonged recovery.[56,63] Irradiation has also proven effective, but debate lingers regarding its use for treatment of a benign lesion.[52]

Medical regimens including intralesional or systemic steroids have been used frequently with some success in treating symptoms but have not proven to be curative. An investigational protocol of intralesional vincristine, bleomycin, and fluorouracil has proven to be of no value.[62] Surgical resection with pathological confirmation of clear margins and skin graft coverage of the resulting defect remains the most reliable treatment option.

INFECTIOUS AND INFLAMMATORY LESIONS OF THE EXTERNAL AUDITORY CANAL (EXTERNAL OTITIS)

The lining of the external auditory canal is richly vascularized and protects the surface epithelium from invading organisms. There is a constant lateral movement of keratin debris from the tympanic membrane to the external meatus. Chance of opportunistic infection is reduced by the bacteriostatic and fungistatic properties of cerumen and is further inhibited by the acidic milieu produced by the apocrine glands. Breakdown of these protective mechanisms is required for external otitis to develop.[64]

Several factors are known to predispose an individual to external otitis. These include high ambient temperature and humidity, trauma, bacterial contamination, allergy, and anatomic narrowing of the canal. Retained keratin debris acts as an ideal culture medium in a humid microenvironment. Extended contact between wet keratin and the canal skin results in tissue maceration and creates a portal of entry for pathogenic bacteria.[65]

During the early stages of external otitis, most patients complain of pruritus or fullness, and attempts to scratch only serve to further macerate the canal skin. Otalgia begins as the canal epithelium becomes more edematous and erythematous. Manipulation of the tragus or auricle elicits exquisite pain due to the tight connection to the canal skin. Conductive hearing loss may occur as edema occludes the lumen. Otorrhea is less common and may initially present as a thin serous drainage. Cellulitis of the auricle suggests a severe infection, and consideration of systemic therapy is warranted when it develops. The presence of yellow, grey, or black debris with hyphae signals a fungal pathogen (otomycosis).

Pseudomonas aeruginosa and *Staphylococcus aureus* are responsible for most bacterial infections. Treatment is directed at these organisms and cultures are usually deferred unless there is a lack of prompt response. Topical agents usually contain a combination of aminoglycoside, steroids, and propylene glycol buffered to an acidic pH. If canal edema prohibits free passage of the drops, a wick may be inserted until the edema resolves. As the lumen diameter increases, gentle removal of all keratin debris and cerumen may be performed. The vast majority of infections can be managed with topical therapy alone, and oral agents such as ciprofloxacin should be reserved only for severe infections.

Candida albicans and *Aspergillus* species account for most cases of otomycosis. Specific risk factors for fungal infection include prolonged use of antibiotic ear drops and diabetes or other immune deficiency conditions. Treatment is cleansing of the canal and topical antifungal agents. Systemic therapy is rarely required except in the severely immunocompromised patient.[66]

Chronic external otitis represents a low-grade infection in combination with long-term changes in the lining of the canal. Epithelial atrophy, repeated trauma, and contact dermatitis all predispose the canal skin to a smoldering bacterial infection. Patients complain of pruritus or discomfort, and long-standing involvement may result in a markedly thickened appearance to the canal lining. Therapy combines topical antimicrobials and steroids with meticulous aural hygiene. Canaloplasty and split-thickness skin grafting is reserved for recalcitrant cases.[67]

Furunculosis is an isolated abscess of a hair follicle most often caused by staphylococcal infection.[68] Symptoms are similar to acute external otitis, and

treatment in the early stages is aimed at symptomatic relief combined with systemic antibiotics. In later stages, when the abscess begins to point, the lesion should be incised and drained under the microscope followed by topical antibiotics.[65]

NECROTIZING (MALIGNANT) EXTERNAL OTITIS

Necrotizing, or "malignant" external otitis is an aggressive, invasive osteomyelitis of the temporal bone. The disease most commonly affects elderly diabetics, though any immunocompromised individual is at increased risk. At present, it is not known if this infection represents a severe progress of acute external otitis or whether the two disease entities are fundamentally dissimilar. Symptoms of severe pain, otorrhea, and the presence of granulation tissue in the external auditory canal that does not respond promptly to antibiotic drops and aural hygiene should alert the clinician to suspect necrotizing external otitis. If not treated early and aggressively, this disease can progress to osteomyelitis of the skull base, which even today carries a high risk for mortality.

Necrotizing external otitis begins with disruption of skin integrity by moisture or trauma followed by inoculation of an opportunistic pathogen. *Pseudomonas aeruginosa*, a gram-negative bacillus not normally found in the external auditory canal, is the most common pathogen, with other bacteria or fungi occasionally reported. Chandler[69], who coined the term "malignant external otitis," believed that diabetic microangiopathy in combination with the necrotizing vasculitis produced by the *Pseudomonas* bacterium resulted in impaired circulation. Poor antibiotic and inflammatory cell penetration then permitted the extensive spread of the infection through the soft tissues with attendant morbidity and mortality.

Patients with necrotizing external otitis typically have stable vital signs and are afebrile. Granulation tissue located at the osseocartilaginous junction of the external canal may be helpful in differentiating this from acute external otitis. Periparotid swelling, trismus, and facial paralysis may be seen in severe cases. Measurement of the erythrocyte sedimentation rate, a nonspecific marker of inflammation, can be helpful in differentiating necrotizing external otitis from acute external otitis and carcinoma, the two entities most commonly included in the differential diagnosis. The erythrocyte sedimentation rate can also be used as a marker for response to therapy but may remain elevated long after evidence of clinical improvement is observed in long-standing cases.[70]

Radiographic evaluation with computerized tomographic scan provides good visualization of bone destruction and soft tissue changes in 80% of cases.[71] Radionuclide imaging techniques such as technetium bone scan may demonstrate increased uptake early in the disease weeks before changes are evident on CT.[72]

The infectious process spreads primarily via vascular and fascial planes. Sigmoid sinus thrombophlebitis and cranial nerve deficits signal skull base extension. Death may occur from intracranial complications, aspiration pneumonia, cardiac decompensation, or multiple organ failure. Mortality rates over 50% were common before the widespread use of modern antibiotic regimens.

Biopsy of granulation tissue is often required to rule out malignancy, and cultures should be sent to determine the pathogen. Injection of local anesthetic agents or debridement under general anesthesia may be required. The use of quinolone antibiotics and third-generation cephalosporins have radically changed the outcome for patients with necrotizing external otitis so that mortality rates below 10% are now common. Disease recurrence or subclinical extension may occur weeks after resolution of pain and external canal findings. As a general rule, treatment should be continued for 2 weeks after resolution of otalgia and granulation tissue. Gallium scan imaging is used to confirm complete eradication of the osteomyelitis. Temporal bone resection, a mainstay of therapy prior to the advent of modern antimicrobial agents, is now considered only for recalcitrant disease.

KERATOSIS OBTURANS

Keratosis obturans is an obstructing plug of desquamated keratin debris in the external auditory canal. Patients typically present with sudden onset of severe otalgia and conductive hearing loss due to mechanical obstruction of the external canal.[73] Keratosis obturans is frequently bilateral (up to 90%) and is more common in individuals aged 20 years or younger.[74]

Because of an association with sinusitis and bronchiectasis, Morrison[75] believed the condition was due to a sympathetic nervous system reflex affecting the cerumen glands, which, in turn, caused a hyperemia of the canal skin and keratin plugs to develop. An alternate theory contends that a combination of epithelial cell overproduction, faulty migration, and inability of the canal to clean itself is the probable cause.[76]

On examination, the medial external canal is filled by a tenacious keratin plug that, upon removal, reveals an inflamed epithelium and circumferential widening of the bony canal. The tympanic membrane is usually spared and has been described as remaining to "stand out in relief" following reabsorption of the proximal bony canal.[77]

Treatment consists of frequent aural hygiene and steroid-containing topical medications to reduce the inflammation. General anesthesia may be required because of the exquisite pain elicited in removing the keratin plug. Schucknecht[78] and Paparella and Goycoolea[79] have advocated canaloplasty with split-thickness skin grafting of the external canal in refractory cases.

EXOSTOSES

Exostoses are broad-based outgrowths of bone arising from the wall of the external auditory canal. They are usually bilateral, often multiple, and tend to remain asymptomatic until they reach a size sufficient to interfere with the normal egress of cerumen and exfoliated skin. The most common presentation is recurrent external otitis followed by aural fullness, hearing loss, and tinnitus.

Exostoses are most common among individuals with an extensive history of cold water exposure, such as surfers or divers, with the highest incidence being found in Australia and New Zealand.[80] Schucknecht[81] and others have proposed a mechanism of "refrigeration periosteitis" with subsequent growth of dense bony lamellae as a reaction to each cold exposure.

Should accumulation of debris occur, conservative management consists of an emollient such as mineral oil to soften the debris with gentle suction, using the surgical microscope if necessary.[82] Steroid creams may lessen the rate of desquamation and prevent further buildup. External otitis should be managed with microscopic debridement and antibiotic drops.

Surgery is reserved for recalcitrant or recurrent problems. A thorough knowledge of temporal bone anatomy is mandatory to prevent injury to the glenoid capsule, facial nerve, and tympanic membrane. Sensorineural hearing loss may occur if the surgeon's drill inadvertently contacts an intact ossicular chain. Preservation of the canal skin overlying the exostoses limits the amount of exposed surface area and risk of granulation tissue formation with subsequent stenosis. Meticulous postoperative aural hygiene is required until epithelialization is complete.

OTITIS MEDIA

Otitis media is the most common reason for pediatric visits to physicians' offices. Ninety percent of all children have at least one episode of acute otitis media by age 7 years, and over 40% have more than three episodes.[83] Combined direct and indirect costs of treatment for otitis media exceed $3.5 billion each year in the United States alone.[84] It is universally acknowledged that otitis media represents a major health problem.

Acute otitis media is defined as fluid present in the middle ear accompanied by a sign of acute illness. Otitis media with effusion is the presence of middle ear fluid without signs or symptoms of acute infection. Chronic otitis media is defined as continuous otorrhea through a tympanic membrane perforation or tympanostomy tube for 2 months or more.

Eustachian tube dysfunction is central to most theories on pathogenesis of acute otitis media. Allergy or upper respiratory tract infection results in mucosal edema, decreased mucociliary clearance, stasis of secretions, eustachian tube obstruction, secondary bacterial or viral ascension, and proliferation. As gas within the middle ear is absorbed, negative pressure results in effusion that provides a fertile culture medium for potential pathogens.

The pathophysiologic effects of microbial contamination of the normally sterile middle ear are mediated by a complex chain of pro-inflammatory cytokines. Leukocyte margination, adhesion, migration from the bloodstream, and activation is thereby facilitated. Microbial killing is accomplished via phagocytosis coupled with degranulation of toxic free radicals and proteolytic enzymes.

While most episodes of acute otitis media resolve without serious sequelae, persistent effusion with conductive hearing loss, middle ear scarring, and ossicular bone resorption may lead to chronic changes.[85]

A number of risk factors for recurrent otitis media have been identified. Male gender, young age (6 to 24 months), attendance at day-care facility, passive cigarette smoke inhalation, allergy, and immunodeficiency have been proven to increase the chance of acute infection.[86] A racial predilection has been noted in Native Americans, Eskimos, and certain African village populations.[87] Children with cleft palate and other craniofacial anomalies are at increased risk secondary to eustachian tube dysfunction.

Common bacterial pathogens in acute otitis media include *Streptococcus pneumoniae*, *Haemophilus influenzae*, and *Branhamella catarrhalis*. In a recent review of the literature, viral isolates were identified in 17% of middle ear effusions.[88]

Children with acute otitis media may present with fever, pain, irritability, ear tugging, feeding difficulties (fussiness, anorexia), or sleep disturbance. Diagnosis is confirmed by pneumatic otoscopic findings of an immobile, bulging, opaque, or erythematous tympanic membrane. A flat tympanogram (type B, no impedance peak) is suggestive of fluid in the middle ear.

Standard treatment for acute otitis media is systemic antimicrobial therapy. Oral steroids have been shown to have a short-term benefit in the treatment of otitis media with effusion, but long-term effectiveness remains unproven.[89] Surgery is reserved for medical management failures and includes myringotomy with or without tube insertion and adenoidectomy. Chronic otitis media is treated surgically with tympanoplasty and possible mastoidectomy.

Complications occur when the inflammatory process extends beyond the mucoperiosteum of the middle ear and mastoid. These are classified as intratemporal, extratemporal, and intracranial complications. Intratemporal complications include anatomic disruption of the tympanic membrane or ossicular chain, labyrinthitis, facial paralysis, coalescent mastoiditis, and spread to the petrous apex. Extratemporal spread is most often seen as formation of a subperiosteal abscess over the mastoid cortex. Intracranial complications include meningitis, abscess formation, sigmoid sinus thrombophlebitis, and otitic hydrocephalus.

AURAL POLYP

Aural polyps are inflammatory lesions representing an irritative response to chronic otitis media with or without cholesteatoma. Other causes such as mycobacterial infection and Langerhans' cell histiocytosis are considerably less common. Retained ventilating tubes should always be considered in children with a history of prior tympanostomy.[90] Patients typically complain of otorrhea while otalgia, hearing loss, and otorrhagia occur less frequently. Polyps are usually found in the proximal external auditory canal and may be large enough to obscure the tympanic membrane.

Topical antimicrobials are the first line of treatment with polypectomy reserved for medical management failures. It is important to determine the presence of cholesteatoma, retained ventilating tube, or other important disease processes because of the likelihood that more extensive operative intervention will be required. Audiometry is helpful in identifying conductive hearing loss, a strong predictor of cholesteatoma.[90] A CT scan finding of bone erosion in the lateral epitympanum (scutum) correlates highly with a diagnosis of cholesteatoma, and CT may also prove useful in identifying a retained foreign body. In a series of 60 patients, Williams et al[91] were able to eradicate the otorrhea in 58% with polypectomy and routine aural toilet. Of those patients who failed this regimen, 94% were found to have underlying cholesteatoma at the time of surgical exploration.

CHOLESTEATOMA/KERATOMA

The term "cholesteatoma" was originally proposed to describe pearl-like tumors of keratin often associated with cholesterol crystals in the middle ear cavity.[92] Since then, cholesteatoma and cholesterol granuloma have been defined as two separate pathological entities. The more accurate term of "keratoma" will be used here to describe the true cholesteatoma, a cystic structure lined by keratinizing stratified squamous epithelium within the middle ear or other pneumatized portion of the temporal bone.

Keratoma may be categorized as either congenital or acquired. Congenital keratoma is defined as a whitish keratin-filled mass behind an intact tympanic membrane in patients with no history of otorrhea, perforation, or prior ear surgery.[93] Prior bouts of otitis media are not grounds for exclusion, according to some authorities.[94] This rare lesion is classically described as an isolated mass in the anterosuperior mesotympanum, yet may be found anywhere within the pneumatized portions of the temporal bone. Among the various theories of origin, the persistence of an embryonic cell rest appears to have gained widest acceptance.[95]

Acquired keratoma may be either primary or secondary, depending upon whether or not there is a history of otitis media. Primary acquired keratoma is described as originating from a retraction pocket in either the pars flacida or pars tensa in patients with no history of prior infection. Secondary acquired keratomas arise in the pars tensa and are associated with perforations in ears with a history of infection.

Theories of acquired keratoma formation include squamous epithelium implantation, through surgery or trauma, invasion through a perforation margin, metaplasia of native middle ear cuboidal epithelium due to chronic infection, and tympanic membrane invagination secondary to eustachian tube dysfunction with retraction pocket formation.[96] Negative pressure (up to 600 mg H_2O) develops when middle ear ventilation is disrupted.[97] Retraction of the tympanic membrane may occur with its invagination eventually forming the sac wall of the keratoma. Obstruction of the epitympanum or mastoid by the keratoma, granulation tissue, or fibrosis may perpetuate negative pressure even if eustachian tube function returns to normal.[97]

Keratomas spread via two mechanisms: (1) gradual expansion of the intact cyst surface and (2) epithelial migration at the leading edge of the cyst margin. Cystic expansion occurs by filling of the available pneumatized space in the temporal bone, aided by negative pressure as described, and internal desquamation. Epithelial migration occurs at the margin of perforations or by ulceration of the epithelial layer of an existing keratoma.

The danger of keratomas lies in their ability to destroy bone. Pyogenic osteitis may develop when inadequate, self-cleansing, epithelial migration results in accumulation of keratin debris. Trapping of moisture and proliferation in bacteria may, in turn, cause ulceration of the epithelial layer and granulation tissue formation. Resultant bone destruction is enhanced by proteolytic enzymes produced within the cyst lining.[98]

Patients classically present with symptoms of (conductive) hearing loss, chronic infection, or both. Aural and intracranial complications secondary to keratoma are relatively rare. In order of decreasing frequency, these include sensorineural hearing loss, labyrinthine fistula, extradural abscess, labyrinthitis (serous or suppurative), facial paralysis, meningitis, brain abscess, sigmoid sinus thrombosis, and subperiosteal abscess.[97]

Keratoma may be managed via one of two general approaches. The first is concerned with the removal of keratin debris in an effort to prevent the continued growth of the cyst and thereby minimize bone destruction. This may be accomplished in an office setting with suction and gentle manipulation if the entire extent of the cyst can be seen. If this is not possible, then wide operative marsupialization with preservation of the medial cyst wall is performed to allow continued office management. The second, and usually preferable, approach is total removal of the keratoma. The advantage to this method is elimination of the risk for continued enzymatic bony destruction by an intact medial cyst wall. Regardless of the method of treatment, long-term surveillance for residual or recurrent disease is mandatory.

EOSINOPHILIC GRANULOMA

Eosinophilic granuloma is a localized form of Langerhans' cell histiocytosis, a benign proliferation of histiocytes capable of producing a mass of infiltrating tissue. The stimulus for proliferation is unknown. Proposed theories have included metabolic, genetic, infectious, and neoplastic causes.[99,100] Eosinophilic granuloma is the least aggressive manifestation of Langerhans' cell histiocytosis and carries an excellent prognosis (Table 12–2). Patients typically present in childhood (50% before age 5 years) or as young adults (75% before age 20 years), but lesions may occur at any age.[101]

TABLE 12–2	MANIFESTATIONS OF LANGERHANS' CELL HISTIOCYTOSIS		
	EOSINOPHILIC GRANULOMA	HAND-SCHÜLLER-CHRISTIAN DISEASE	LETTERER-SIWE DISEASE
Age at Onset	Children >5 years old	Children 1–5 years old	Children 0–3 years old
Disease Involvement	Unifocal	Multifocal	Multiple organ systems
	long bone, skull	bone, skin, viscera, and brain	constitutional symptoms, liver, spleen, lymphatic, lung, and bone marrow
Prognosis	Excellent	Good	Poor

Eosinophilic granuloma is typically characterized by lytic lesions of a single bone but is occasionally multifocal, and soft tissue may be affected. The most frequently affected areas are the skull, long bones, ribs, vertebrae, pelvis, maxilla, and mandible. Dull pain or swelling are the usual presenting signs with bone involvement.[102]

Otologic involvement in Langerhans' cell histiocytosis has been reported in 15% to 76% of patients and may be the sole presenting symptom in 5% to 25% of patients.[103–105] Isolated mastoid lesions are most commonly reported, but any site within the temporal bone may be affected. Patients classically present with postaural swelling, erosion of the posterior wall of the external canal, or both. Otorrhea is due to secondary infection with granulation tissue formation.

Conductive hearing loss may result from external canal, tympanic membrane, middle ear, or ossicular involvement. Sensorineural hearing loss secondary to bony labyrinth destruction is now exceedingly uncommon and found only in advanced disease. Facial nerve involvement has been reported in less than 3% of patients and is more often due to brainstem or CNS involvement than intratemporal nerve compression or destruction.[106]

Local therapy consisting of excision, curettage, or biopsy alone is indicated for unifocal disease that can be surgically accessed with minimal morbidity. For more extensive, progressive, or persistent disease, low-dose irradiation is the proven treatment of choice for temporal bone involvement. Chemotherapy is given in combination with radiation for disseminated disease.

ROSAI-DORFMAN DISEASE (SINUS HISTIOCYTOSIS WITH MASSIVE LYMPHADENOPATHY)

Rosai-Dorfman disease, also known as sinus histiocytosis with massive lymphadenopathy, is a rare reactive histiocytic proliferative disorder of unknown etiology.[107] Patients typically are young adults (average age of 20.6 years) who present with markedly enlarged lymph nodes.[108] Nearly 40% of cases develop extranodal sites of involvement, and any organ system can be affected. Rosai-Dorfman disease occasionally occurs in the absence of lymph node involvement.

These lesions usually have a self-limited course and, in most instances, can be safely observed after biopsy confirmation. Fatalities have been reported when vital structures become involved or when associated immunologic abnormalities such as autoimmune hemolytic anemia or polyclonal gammopathy occur.[109] In such instances surgery and/or chemotherapy may be required.

CHORISTOMA

A choristoma is a growth of histologically normal tissue in an ectopic location. Taylor and Martin[110] provided the first description of a rare choristoma of the middle ear in 1961, and to date 18 cases have been described in the English-language literature. A majority of these cases were of salivary gland origin with single examples each of neural and sebaceous tissue described.[111,112] These lesions are composed of congenital rests of tissue and have little or no potential for further growth. A single case of malignant transformation to adenoid cystic carcinoma has been proposed.[113]

Patients have ranged in age from 5 to 52 years with a slight male predilection (1.3 : 1). Most patients present with a long-standing conductive hearing loss and middle ear mass evident on otoscopic examination. Because of the frequent association of these lesions with anomalies of the incus, stapes superstructure, and tympanic facial nerve, a developmental error in second branchial arch formation prior to the fourth intrauterine month has been proposed.[114] This theory holds that ectopic tissue becomes trapped in the middle ear as the tympanic ring fuses with the squamous and mastoid portions of the temporal bone. In the single case of neural choristoma, the authors propose that the neural tissue was displaced through Hyrtl's fissure before its closure during development.[111]

Choristomas range in size from 5 mm to lesions filling the entire middle ear and mastoid antrum. Only one case of bilateral choristoma has been described.[115] Because of the rarity of these lesions, choristoma is seldom considered in the differential diagnosis until biopsy confirms it. Adherence to a dehiscent facial nerve precludes removal, as both temporary and permanent facial palsy have been described after biopsy.[110,116–118] Most authors have deferred ossiculoplasty (with normal contralateral hearing), stating that the severity of the ossicular anomalies reduces the likelihood of successful reconstruction, although three of the five reported attempts have resulted in hearing gain.[114,116,119–121]

With little chance for continued growth, significant risk of facial nerve injury, and limited potential for ossicular chain reconstruction, the surgeon should consider biopsy and observation as an alternative to excision.

REFERENCES

1. Berman B, Bieley HC. Keloids. *J Am Acad Dermatol*. 1995; 33: 117–123.
2. Omo-Dare P. Genetic studies on keloids. *J Natl Med Assoc*. 1975; 67:428–432.
3. Castagnoli C, Perveccio D, Stella M, et al. The HLA-DR beta 16 allogenotype constitutes a risk factor for hypertrophic scarring. *Hum Immunol*. 1990; 29:229–232.
4. Castagnoli C, Stella M, Magliacani G, et al. Anomalous expression of HLA class II molecules on keratinocytes and

fibroblasts in hypertrophic scars consequent to thermal injury. *Clin Exp Immunol.* 1990; 82:350–354.

5. Alhady SM, Sivanan TK. Keloids in various races: A review of 175 cases. *Plast Reconstr Surg.* 1969; 44:564–566.

6. Griffith BH, Monroe CW, McKinney P. A follow-up study on the treatment of keloids with triamcinolone acetonide. *Plast Reconstr Surg.* 1970; 46:145–150.

7. Kiil J. Keloids treated with topical injections of triamcinolone acetonide (Kenalog), immediate and long-term results. *Scand J Plast Reconstr Surg.* 1977; 11:169–172.

8. Kosman B, Krikelair GF, Ju MC, et al. The surgical treatment of keloids. *Plast Reconstr Surg.* 1961; 27:335–358.

9. Lawrence WT. In search of the optimal treatment of keloids: A report of a series and a review of the literature. *Ann Plast Surg.* 1991; 27:164–178.

10. Escarmant P, Zihmermann S, Amar A, et al. The treatment of 783 keloid scars by iridium 192 interstitial irradiation after surgical excision. *Int J Radiat Oncol Biol Phys.* 1993; 26:245–257.

11. Sallstrom K-O. Treatment of keloids with surgical excision and postoperative x-ray radiation. *Scand J Plast Surg.* 1992; 45:371–373.

12. Tang YW. Intra and postoperative steroid injections for keloids and hypertrophic scars. *Br J Plast Surg.* 1992; 45:371–373.

13. Stucker FJ, Shaw GY. An approach to management of keloids. *Arch Otolaryngol Head Neck Surg.* 1992; 188:63–67.

14. Apfelberg DB. Failure of carbon dioxide laser excision of keloids. *Lasers Surg Med.* 1989; 9:382–388.

15. Henderson DL, Cromwell TA, Mes LG. Argon and CO_2 laser treatment of hypertrophic and keloid scars. *Lasers Surg Med.* 1984; 3:271–277.

16. Norris JCE. The effect of carbon dioxide laser surgery on the recurrence of keloids. *Plast Reconstr Surg.* 1991; 87:44–49.

17. Muti E, Ponzio E. Cryotherapy in the treatment of keloids. *Ann Plast Surg.* 1983; 3:227–232.

18. Rusciani L, Rossi G, Bono RX. Use of cryotherapy in the treatment of keloids. *J Dermatol Surg Oncol.* 1993; 19:529–534.

19. Zouboulis CC, Blume V, Buttmer P, et al. Outcomes of cryosurgery in keloids and hypertrophic scars: A prospective consecutive trial of case series. *Arch Dermatol.* 1993; 129:1146–1151.

20. Ceilley RI, Barin RW. The combined use of cryosurgery and intralesional injections of suspension of fluorinated adrenocorticosteroids for reducing keloids and hypertrophic scars. *J Dermatol Surg Oncol.* 1979; 5:54.

21. Jacobsson F. The treatment of keloids at Radium-hemmet, 1921–1941. *Acta Radiol.* 1948; 29:251–267.

22. Sawada Y, Sone K. Hydration and occlusion treatment for hypertrophic scars and keloids. *Br J Plast Surg.* 1992; 45:599–603.

23. Gold MH. Topical silicone gel sheeting in the treatment of hypertrophic scars and keloids. *J Dermatol Surg Oncol.* 1993; 19:912–916.

24. Larrabee WF Jr, East CA, Jaffe HS, et al. Intralesional interferon gamma treatment for keloids and hypertrophic scars. *Arch Otolaryngol Head Neck Surg.* 1990; 116:1159–1162.

25. Granstein RD, Rook A. Flotte TJ. Controlled trial of intralesional recombinant interferon gamma in the treatment of keloidal scarring. *Arch Dermatol.* 1990; 126:1295–1302.

26. Lazar RH, Heffner DK, Huges GB, Hyams VK. Pseudocyst of the auricle: a review of 21 cases. *Otolaryngol Head Neck Surg* 1986; 94:360–361.

27. Kontis TC, Goldstone A, Brown M, Paull G. Pathological quiz: Auricular pseudocyst. *Arch Otolaryngol Head Neck Surg.* 1992; 118:1128–1130.

28. Engel D. Pseudocysts of the auricle in Chinese. *Arch Otolaryngol.* 1966; 85:29–34.

29. Glamb R, Kim R. Pseudocyst of the auricle. *J Amer Acad Dermatol.* 1984; 11:58–63.

30. Borroni G, Brazzeli V, Merlino M. Pseudocyst of the auricle. A birthday ear pull. *Br J Dermatol.* 1991; 125:292–294.

31. Grabski WJ, Salasche SJ, McCollough ML, Angeloni VL.

32. Saunders MW, Jones NS, Balsitis M. Bilateral auricular pseudocyst: A case report and discussion. *J Laryngol Otol.* 1993; 107:39–41.

33. Ophir D, Marshak G. Needle aspiration and pressure sutures for auricular pseudocyst. *Plast Reconstr Surg.* 1991; 87:783–784.

34. Choi S, Lam K, Chan K, Ghadially FN, Ng ASM. Endochondral pseudocysts of the auricle in Chinese. *Arch Otolaryngol.* 1984; 110:792–796.

35. Winkler M. Knotchen-Erkrankung am Helix. *Arch Derm Syph.* 1915; 121:278–285.

36. Kitchens GG. Auricular wedge resection and reconstruction. *Ear Nose Throat.* 1989; 68:673–683.

37. Lawrence CM. The treatment of chondrodermatitis nodularis with cartilage removal alone. *Arch Dermatol.* 1991; 127:530–535.

38. Karam F, Bauman T. Carbon dioxide laser treatment for chondrodermatitis nodularis chronica helicis. *Ear Nose Throat.* 1988; 67:757–763.

39. Wade TR. Chondrodermatitis nodularis chronica helicis. *Cutis.* 1978; 24:406–409.

40. Jaksch-Wartenhorst R. Polychondropathia. *Arch Int Med.* 1923; 6:93–97.

41. Pearson CM, Klene HM, Newcomer VD. Relapsing polychondritis. *N Eng J Med.* 1960; 263:51–58.

42. McAdam LP, O'Hanlon MA, Bluestone R, Pearson CM. Relapsing polychondritis: Prospective study of 23 patients and a review of the literature. *Medicine* (Baltimore). 1976; 55:193–215.

43. Damiani JM, Levine JL. Relapsing polychondritis—report of ten cases. *Laryngoscope* 1979; 89:929–946.

44. Flodart JM, Shigeto A. Antibodies to type II collagen in relapsing polychondritis. *N Eng J Med.* 1978; 299:1203–1207.

45. Cody DTR, Sones DA. Relapsing polychondritis: Audiovestibular manifestations. *Laryngoscope.* 1971; 81:1208–1222.

46. Irani BS, Martin-Hirsch DP, Clark D, Hand DW, Vize CE, Black J. Relapsing polychondritis—a study of four cases. *J Laryngol Otol.* 1992; 106:891–914.

47. Wells GC, Whimster IW. Subcutaneous angiolymphoid hyperplasia with eosinophilia. *Br J Dermatol.* 1969; 81:1–15.

48. Mehregan AH, Shapiro L. Angiolymphoid hyperplasia with eosinophilia. *Arch Dermatol.* 1971; 103:50–57.

49. Moy R, Luftman D, Nguyen Q, et al. Estrogen receptors and the response to sex hormones in angiolymphoid hyperplasia with eosinophilia. *Arch Dermatol.* 1992; 128:825–828.

50. Razquin S, Mayayo E, Citores M, et al. Angiolymphoid hyperplasia with eosinophilia of the tongue: Report of a case and review of the literature. *Hum Pathol.* 1991; 22:837–839.

51. Grimwood R, Swinehart J, Aeling J. Angiolymphoid hyperplasia with eosinophilia. *Arch Dermatol.* 1979; 115:205–207.

52. Barnes L, Koss W, Nieland ML. Angiolymphoid hyperplasia with eosinophilia: A disease that may be confused with malignancy. *Head Neck.* 1980; 2:425–434.

53. Googe PB, Harris NL, Mihm MC Jr. Kimura's disease and angiolymphoid hyperplasia with eosinophilia: Two distinct histopathological entities. *J Cutan Pathol.* 1987; 14:263–271.

54. Olsen TG, Helwig EB. Angiolymphoid hyperplasia with eosinophilia: A clinicopathologic study of 116 patients. *J Am Acad Dermatol.* 1985; 12:781–796.

55. Henry PG, Burnett JW. Angiolymphoid hyperplasia with eosinophilia. *Arch Dermatol.* 1978; 114:1168–1172.

56. Thompson JW, Colman M, Williamson C, Ward PH. Angiolymphoid hyperplasia with eosinophilia of the external ear canal. *Arch Otolaryngol.* 1981; 107:316–320.

57. Urabe A, Tsuneyushi H, Enjoji M. Epithelioid hemangioma versus Kimura's disease. A comparative clinicopathologic study. *Am J Surg Pathol.* 1987; 11:758–766.

58. Vallis RC, Davies DG. Angiolymphoid hyperplasia of the head and neck. *J Laryngol Otol.* 1988; 102:100–101.

59. Johnson WC. Pathology of cutaneous vascular tumors. *Int J Dermatol.* 1976; 15:239–270.

60. DelGaudio JM, Myers MW, Telian SA. Angiolymphoid hy-

perplasia with eosinophilia involving the external auditory canal. *Otolaryngol Head Neck Surg.* 1994; 111:669–673.

61. Murty GE, Cox NH. Angiolymphoid hyperplasia with eosinophilia: An uncommon tumor of the external auditory canal. *Ear Nose Throat J.* 1990; 69:102–107.

62. Baum DW, Sams WM, Monheit GD. Angiolymphoid hyperplasia with eosinophilia. The disease and a comparison of treatment modalities. *J Dermatol Surg Oncol.* 1982; 8:966–970.

63. Hobbs ER, Bailin PL, Ratz JL, Yarbrough CL. Treatment of angiolymphoid hyperplasia of the external auditory canal with carbon dioxide laser. *J Am Acad Dermatol.* 1988; 19:345–349.

64. Johnson A, Hawke M. The nonauditory physiology of the external ear canal. In: Jahn A, Sanros-Saceni J, eds. *Physiology of the Ear.* New York: Raven Press; 1988:345.

65. Jahn AJ, Hawke M. Infections of the external ear. In: Cummings CW, Harker LA, eds. *Otolaryngology–Head and Neck Surgery.* 2nd ed. St. Louis: Mosby; 1993:2788.

66. Lucent FE. Fungal infections of the external ear. *Otolaryngol Clin.* 1993; 26(6):995–1006.

67. Paparella MM, Kurkjian JM. Surgical treatment for chronic stenosing external otitis. *Laryngoscope.* 1966; 76:232–234.

68. Schuknecht HF. *Pathology of the Ear.* Philadelphia: Lea & Febiger; 1993:191.

69. Chandler J. Malignant external otitis. *Laryngoscope.* 1968; 78: 1257–1294.

70. Evans I, Richards S. Malignant (necrotizing) otitis externa. *J Laryngol Otol.* 1973; 87:13–20.

71. Fritz P, Reiden K, Lenarz T, et al. Radiological evaluation of temporal bone disease: High resolution computed tomography versus conventional x-ray diagnosis. *Br J Radiol.* 1989; 63:107–113.

72. Grobman LR, Ganz W. *Malignant External Otitis.* St. Louis: Mosby; 1993:355–372.

73. Piepergerdes JC, Kramer BM, Behnke EE. Keratosis obturans and external auditory canal cholesteatoma. *Laryngoscope.* 1980; 90:383–391.

74. Black J, Clayton RG. Wax keratosis in children's ears. *Br Med J.* 1958; 2:673–675.

75. Morrison AW. Keratosis obturans. *J Laryngol Otol.* 1956; 70: 317–321.

76. Paparella M, Shumrick D. In: *Otolaryngology.* Vol 2. 2nd ed. Philadelphia: WB Saunders; 1980:1393.

77. Bunting WP. Ear canal cholesteatoma and bone absorption. *Trans Am Acad Ophthalmol Otolaryngol.* 1968; 72:161–172.

78. Schucknecht HF. *Pathology of the Ear.* 2nd ed. Philadelphia, Pa: Lea & Febiger; 1993.

79. Paparella MM, Goycoolea MV. Canalplasty for chronic intractable external otitis and keratosis obturans. *Otolaryngol Head Neck Surg.* 1981; 89:400–443.

80. Fisher EW, McManus TC. Surgery for external auditory canal exostoses and osteomata. *J Laryngol Otol.* 1994; 108:106–110.

81. Schuknecht HF. Exostoses of the external auditory canal. In: *Pathology of the Ear.* Philadelphia: Lea & Febiger; 1993:398–399.

82. Graham MD, Kemink JL. Osteomas and exostoses of the external auditory canal—medical and surgical management. *J Otolaryngol.* 1982; 11:101–106.

83. Klein JO, Teele DW, Rosner BA, et al. Epidemiology of acute otitis media in Boston children from birth to seven years of age: In: Lim DJ, Bludstone CD, Klein JO, Nelson JD, eds. *Recent Advances in Otitis Media.* Philadelphia: BC Decker; 1988:14.

84. Stool SE, Field MJ. The impact of otitis media. *Pediatr Inf Dis J.* 1989; 8:S11.

85. Saez-Llorens X. Pathogenesis of acute otitis media. *Pediatr Inf Dis J.* 1994; 13:1035–1038.

86. Daly K. Risk factors for otitis media sequelae and chronicity. *Ann Otol Rhinol Laryngol.* 1994; 103:S39–S42.

87. Klein JO. Otitis media. *Clin Inf Dis.* 1994; 19:823–833.

88. Ruuskanen O, Heikkinen T. Viral bacterial interaction in acute otitis media: Increasing evidence for clinical significance. *Pediatr Infect Dis J.* 1994; 13:S23–S26.

89. Schwartz RH, Puglese J, Schwartz DM. Use of a short course of prednisone for treating middle ear effusion: A double-blind crossover study. *Ann Otol Rhinol Laryngol.* 1980; 89:296.

90. Gliklich RE, Cunningham MJ, Eavey RD. The cause of aural polyps in children. *Arch Otolaryngol Head Neck Surg.* 1993; 119:669–671.

91. Williams SR, Robinson PJ, Brightwell AP. Management of the inflammaotry aural polyp. *J Laryngol Otol.* 1989; 103: 1040–1042.

92. Muller J. *Uber den feinerm Bau und die Fromen der Kranhaften Geschwulst.* Berlin: G. Reimer; 1838:50.

93. Derlacki EL, Clemis JD. Congenital cholesteatoma of the middle ear and mastoid. *Ann Otol Rhinol Laryngol.* 1968; 78: 1050–1078.

94. Levinson MJ, Michaels L, Parisier SC. Congenital cholesteatomas of the middle ear in children: origins and management. *Otolaryngol Clin North Am.* 1989; 22:941–954.

95. Friedberg J. Congenital cholesteatoma. *Laryngoscope.* 1994; 104(suppl):62.

96. Broekart D. The problem of middle ear cholesteatoma: Etiology, genesis and pathobiology: A review. *Acta Oto rhinolaryngol Belg.* 1991; 45:355–367.

97. Neely JG. Treatment of uncomplicated aural cholesteatoma (keratoma). Self-instructional Package (Si-Pac) from the American Academy of Otolaryngology. 1977.

98. Abramson M. Collagenolytic activity in middle ear cholesteatoma. *Ann Otol Rhinol Laryngol.* 1969; 94:76–95.

99. Nolph MB, Luiin GA. Histiocytosis X. *Otolaryngol Clin North Amer.* 1982; 15:635–648.

100. Groopman JE, Golde DW. The histiocytic disorders: A pathophysiologic analysis. *Ann Intern Med.* 1981; 94:95.

101. Slater JN, Swarm OJ. Eosinophilic granuloma of bone. *Med Pediatric Oncol.* 1980; 8:151–164.

102. Cunningham MJ, Curtin HD, Jaffe R, Stool DE. Otologic manifestations of Langerhans' cell histiocytosis. *Arch Otolaryngol Head Neck Surg.* 1989; 115:807–813.

103. Goldsmith AJ, Myssiorek D, Valderrama E, Patel M. Unifocal Langerhans' cell histiocytosis (eosinophilic granuloma) of the petrous apex. *Arch Otolaryngol Head Neck Surg.* 1993; 119: 113–116.

104. McCaffrey TV, McDonald TJ. Histiocytosis X of the ear and temporal bone. *Laryngoscope.* 1979; 89:1735–1742.

105. Smoler J, Rivera-Camascho R, Viva-Mejia G, Levy-Pinto S. Otolaryngologic manifestations of histiocytosis X. *Laryngoscope.* 1972; 81:1903–1911.

106. Tos M. Facial palsy in Hand-Schuller-Christian's disease. *Arch Otolaryngol.* 1969; 90:563–567.

107. Rosai J, Dorfman RF. Sinus histiocytosis with massive lymphadenopathy, a newly recognized benign clincopathological entity. *Arch Pathol.* 1969; 87:63–70.

108. Tsang WYW, Chan JKC, Ho WK, et al. Extranodal Rosai-Dorfman disease: An uncommon cause of persistent nodule in the ear. *J Laryngol Otol.* 1992; 106:249–251.

109. Foucar E, Rosai J, Dorfman R. Sinus histiocytosis with massive lymphadenopathy (Rosai-Dorfman disease). Review of the entity. *Sem Diagnost Pathol.* 1990; 7:19–73.

110. Taylor GD, Martin HF. Salivary gland tissue in the middle ear. *Arch of Otolaryngol.* 1961; 3:651–653.

111. Gulya AJ, Glasscock ME III, Pensak ML. Neural choristoma of the middle ear. *Otolaryngol Head Neck Surg.* 1987; 97:52–56.

112. Nelson EG, Kratz RC. Sebaceous choristoma of the middle ear. *Otolaryngol Head Neck Surg.* 1993; 108:372–373.

113. Cannon CR, McLean WC. Adenoid cystic carcinoma of the middle ear and temporal bone. *Otolaryngol Head Neck Surg.* 1983; 91:96–99.

114. Abadir W, Pease W. Salivary gland choristoma of the middle ear. *J Laryngol Otol.* 1978; 92:247–252.

115. Peron DL, Schucknecht HF. Congenital cholesteatoma with other anomalies. *Arch Otolaryngol.* 1975; 101:498–505.

116. Bruner RC. Salivary gland choristoma of the middle ear: A case report. *Arch Otolaryngol.* 1970; 91:303.

117. Hociota D, Ataman T. A case of salivary gland choristoma of the middle ear. *J Laryngol Otol.* 1975; 89:1065–1068.

118. Kartush JM, Graham MD. Salivary gland choristoma of the middle ear: A case report and review of the literature. *Laryngoscope.* 1984; 94:228–230.
119. Noguera JT, Hoarse FR. Congenital ossicular defects with a normal auditory canal: Its surgical treatment. *Eye, Ear, Nose, Throat Mon.* 1964; 43:37–39.
120. Kley HA. Monomorphous tubular salivary gland adenoma of the middle ear. *Laryngol Rhinol.* 1979; 58:65–67.
121. Saeger KL, Gruskin P, Carberry JN. Salivary gland choristoma of the middle ear. *Arch Pathol Lab Med.* 1982; 106:39–40.

II. CLINICAL CONSIDERATIONS FOR NEOPLASMS OF THE EAR AND TEMPORAL BONE

■ JAMES E. SAUNDERS

■ B. HILL BRITTON

■ JESUS E. MEDINA

The pathological variability of tumors in the ear and temporal bone is immense; however, clinical presentation and treatment for many of these entities is similar. The clinical course and management may depend as much on the location of the tumor as on the pathology. Nonetheless, variations in pathology may affect the management or prognosis. As a detailed discussion of all possible pathologies in this region is beyond the scope of this chapter, we will discuss the clinical presentation, evaluation, management, and prognosis of the major clinical entities.

Neoplasms of the ear can be divided into two categories based on their location: lesions of the external ear and lesions of the deep temporal bone, including the middle ear, mastoid, jugular foramen, internal auditory canal, and petrous apex. There is obviously a great deal of overlap between these two categories. Lesions that begin in the external canal may also involve the middle ear and mastoid. Likewise, lesions in the mastoid or middle ear may erode into the external auditory canal (EAC). Because of the complex anatomy of the ear, the location of a tumor may have more bearing on its management and prognosis than the pathology of the lesion. For example, a hemangioma or meningioma of the middle ear is managed differently than a similar lesion in the internal auditory canal.

CLINICAL EVALUATION AND IMAGING

Along with physical examination, patients suspected of having a neoplasm of the ear should have a detailed history taken. Historical features of importance include the presence of pain, discharge, bleeding, hearing loss, tinnitus, facial weakness or spasm, swallowing or voice problems, sun exposure, and progression of symptoms. Chronic aural discharge from a neoplasm is often misdiagnosed as chronic otitis media. The examiner should be particularly suspicious of a tumor when there is pain involved or when the condition does not respond to therapy. Physical examination of the ear includes a careful inspection of the pinna and examination of the external auditory canal and tympanic membrane with a binocular microscope. Middle ear tumors can usually be identified through the tympanic membrane and should be evaluated for pulsations and Brown's sign (blanching of a middle ear mass with insufflation). A detailed head and neck examination is mandatory, with special attention given to cranial nerve function (include vocal cord mobility) and cervical adenopathy. A complete hearing examination, including pure tone audiometry and speech discrimination, is required in all patients. Tympanometry, acoustic reflex testing, auditory brainstem response testing (ABR), and vestibular function tests may also be helpful.

Although the specific radiographic features of each pathological entity will be discussed in more detail, a few general comments about temporal bone imaging are worthwhile. The basic mainstays of the radiographic evaluation of temporal bone lesions are high-resolution computerized tomography (CT) and magnetic resonance imaging with gadolinium enhancement (MRI/Gd).[1] Arteriography may also be helpful in assessing the vascularity of a lesion or for preoperative embolization. In general, lesions of the EAC, middle ear, and mastoid are best evaluated with a high resolution CT scan including both coronal and axial sections. Since a major clinical question in these lesions is bone erosion, these images should be formatted to demonstrate bone detail (Fig. 12–1). The location and extent of bony erosion will help with the diagnosis of the lesion and in planning a surgical procedure (e.g., an infiltrative lesion of the EAC). Iodine contrast enhancement may also help to demonstrate the vascularity of a lesion.

MRI/Gd is the procedure of choice when the lesion involves the intracranial structures. It is extremely useful in evaluating lesions of the internal auditory canal and petrous apex. Although the gadolinium-enhanced MRI imaging technique is a sensitive and useful screening examination, a complete study of a lesion in this area should also include nonenhanced T1 weighted images as well as T2

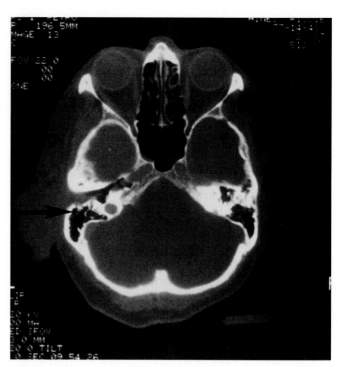

FIGURE 12–1 Axial CT scan showing erosion of the left temporal bone by a basal cell carcinoma.

weighted images. Subtle differences on these various scanning techniques will help the clinician to identify unusual lesions in this area.

Finally, it is extremely important to note that CT and MRI are complementary studies. While the CT scan shows the intricate details of the bony anatomy, it does not adequately demonstrate the soft tissue structures. On the other hand, MRI scans show exquisite details of the soft tissues but fail to demonstrate the bony anatomy. The use of both of these technologies may be quite helpful in making an accurate diagnosis and planning appropriate treatment for a temporal bone tumor.

EXTERNAL AUDITORY CANAL AND PINNA

Anatomy and Surgical Approaches

The pinna, or auricle, consists of an irregular cartilaginous structure covered by skin. The helix, the C-shaped cartilage, defines the outer perimeter of the pinna. The concha is a deep bowl-shaped cartilage, surrounded superiorly and posteriorly by the antihelix, a C-shaped cartilage extending more or less parallel to the helix. The antihelix parallels the helix and begins superiorly with two crura divided by the triangular fossa and ends inferiorly in the antitragus. The meatus of the EAC lies between the anterior tragus and the antitragus.

The EAC is a blind-end canal approximately 25 mm in length. The lateral half of the canal is composed primarily of a trough-shaped cartilage and a dense fibrous tissue forming the superior portion of the lateral canal. The medial half of the EAC is a bony tunnel through the temporal bone ending at the tympanic membrane and angular ligament. The canal is variably tortuous with a convex surface anteriorly and a concave surface posteriorly. The temporomandibular joint creates an anterior bulge in the EAC that may obscure the direct visualization of the anterior portion of the tympanic membrane. The skin of the EAC has a variable amount of subcutaneous tissue that is much thicker in the lateral end of the canal. The skin of the medial EAC is thin, compared to the lateral canal. Numerous sebaceous glands, ceruminous glands, and hair are also found in the lateral end of the EAC.

The arterial supply of the external ear is primarily through the posterior, auricular, and superficial temporal arteries. Venous drainage from the external ear is through the temporal vein and the posterior auricular vein, which in turn may drain through the external jugular or the transverse sinus via a mastoid emissary vein. Lymphatic drainage of the external ear usually drains to the upper jugulodigastric nodes or anteriorly through the parotid nodes. Lesions of the posterior helix and medial surface of the pinna may drain to retroauricular nodes and the posterior nodes of the neck. There are two important communications between the anterior surface of the EAC and the parotid region. Small fissures in the anterior EAC (fissures of Santorini) and a non-ossified area of the tympanic bone (foramen of Huschke) offer an opportunity for direct communication between the EAC and the parotid gland.[2]

Because of its complex external anatomy, surgical reconstruction of the pinna presents a particular challenge. If possible, lesions of the helix should be resected in a way that limits the amount of cupping or notching of the helical rim. Approximately 1 cm of helical rim may be excised without creating a significant cosmetic deformity; however, when larger areas must be excised, a portion of the more medial pinna and conchal bowl should also be resected. Advancement flaps or a composite skin-cartilage graft from the opposite ear may be used to reconstruct large defects of the pinna.[3] When complete surgical removal of the pinna is necessary, a prosthetic ear, carefully crafted to match the opposite ear, may give the best cosmetic results.

Primary excision of EAC lesions ("sleeve resections") may be reconstructed with a split-thickness skin graft with a Merocel sponge to stent the EAC and avoid stenosis. Traditionally, lateral temporal bone resection (LTR) implies any procedure that involves resection of a portion of the bony EAC leaving the inner ear intact, while subtotal temporal bone resection and total temporal bone resection include resection of the labyrinth (Fig. 12–2).[4] Unfortunately, this terminology often groups together a variety of procedures with very different indications and clinical consequences. We prefer to divide LTR into four basic types depending upon the status of

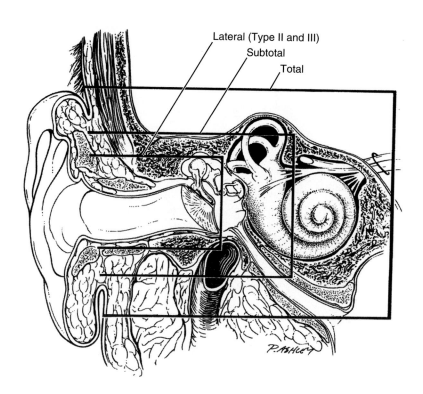

FIGURE 12–2 Margins of total, subtotal, and lateral (Type II and III) temporal bone resections.

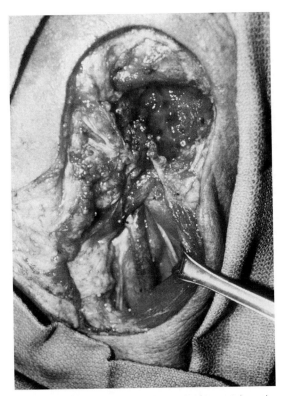

FIGURE 12-3 Intraoperative photograph of Type II lateral temporal bone resection showing the complete removal of the tympanic bone, tympanic membrane, and external auditory canal with preservation of the facial nerve.

the facial nerve and the extent of bone resected.[5] Type I is a resection of the EAC, leaving the tympanic membrane intact. Type II and III LTR include: (1) a mastoidectomy including extensive dissection of the zygomatic arch, mastoid tip, and facial recess, thus completely outlining the bony EAC; (2) separation of the incudostapedial joint and division of the tensor tympani; (3) outfracture of the EAC with gentle pressure; and (4) en bloc resection of the tumor along with the malleus, incus, and tympanic membrane (Fig. 12–3). In the Type II LTR the dissection is lateral to the facial nerve, whereas the facial nerve is sacrificed in a Type III LTR. In a Type IV resection, only the mastoid tip and the inferior temporal bone are removed. The lateral temporal bone resection can be extended to remove a portion of the temporomandibular joint, the middle fossa plate (tegmen), and posterior fossa dura. A subtotal temporal bone resection involves all of the above steps with the added dissection of the labyrinth and cochlea through a labyrinthectomy. Total temporal bone resection includes resection of the internal auditory canal with preservation of the carotid artery and trigeminal nerve (Fig. 12–4). If necessary, the facial nerve can be reconstructed using a cable graft technique. Reconstruction after extensive surgical resection may employ temporalis muscle flaps, myocutaneous flaps from regional sources, or free myocutaneous flaps, with or without cocommitant nerve grafts.

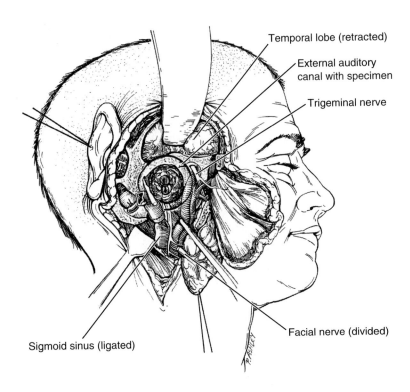

Temporal lobe (retracted)

External auditory canal with specimen

Trigeminal nerve

Facial nerve (divided)

Sigmoid sinus (ligated)

FIGURE 12-4 Total temporal bone resection with dissection to the petrous apex exposing the geniculate ganglion and carotid artery. The facial nerve and jugular vein are sacrificed.

Benign Tumors

ADENOMATOUS TUMORS

Adenomatous tumors of the external ear are rare lesions that arise from the ceruminous and sebaceous glands in the cartilaginous portion of the EAC. Several different pathological entities have been collectively referred to as "ceruminomas," but this term has been abandoned.[6-8] Typically, these tumors obstruct the EAC with symptoms of conductive hearing loss, fullness, or pain. Obstruction of the EAC also prevents the externalization of skin and wax, which may contribute to these symptoms. Clinically, they appear as smooth skin-covered tumors that are either sessile or polypoid. It is important to differentiate polypoid lesions clinically from polyps arising from the middle ear. If a probe can be passed completely around the polyp at its base, it originates from the EAC and not from the middle ear. CT scans are helpful to rule out bone erosion, which would signify a more destructive, possibly malignant, lesion. It may be otherwise difficult to clinically distinguish benign adenomas from adenocarcinoma or adenoid cystic carcinoma. Local excision may be accomplished by a polypectomy or a resection of the underlying EAC skin. Larger tumors may require a sleeve resection. Recurrent benign tumors are probably the result of incomplete resection. In general, the prognosis of these benign lesions is very good.

KERATOACANTHOMA

Keratoacanthoma is a benign lesion that clinically resembles a squamous cell carcinoma. The clinical course of this lesion is quite different, though, in that it undergoes a rapid growth over a period of weeks to months. It is a globular tumor with a central ulceration with a core of keratin debris. After its rapid growth phase, this lesion typically involutes. Biopsy is indicated if the diagnosis is uncertain; curettage may be helpful. Local excision may be necessary for cosmesis if a significant scar remains after involution.[9]

NEVI

Benign nevi of the external ear are relatively common. They are usually intradermal, but all varieties of nevi are encountered in this location. These lesions can usually be differentiated from melanoma by clinical examination. Excisional biopsy is indicated, however, if the diagnosis is not clear. Some patients prefer to have these lesions removed for cosmetic reasons.

OSTEOMAS AND EXOSTOSES

Solitary osteomas of the EAC are relatively uncommon lesions. They are pedunculated lesions that typically occur in the lateral half of the osseous canal. They should be differentiated from diffuse exostoses—more common, broad-based hyperostotic lesions of the tympanic bone. These bilateral lesions are believed to be related to cold water exposure and may lead to complete canal stenosis. The less common solitary osteomas are unilateral and do not appear to be related to water exposure. Smaller osteomas, which are medial to the isthmus and occur near the notch of Rivinus, may be rarely encountered. These are usually multiple broad-based lesions and do not typically require treatment.

Osteomas may occur at any stage in life and may be more common in males. Symptoms are intermittent obstruction of the ear. Often these lesions are noted at routine examinations. Although the bony lesions in the EAC may be seen on CT scans, radiographic imaging is rarely necessary to make the diagnosis. Osteomas should be removed in most cases. A hook can usually be passed medial to the base of the tumor and a chisel used to gently loosen the lesion. In those unusual cases where the lesion extends medial to the isthmus or along a suture line, it is usually advisable to use a drill at the base of the lesion and to enlarge the isthmus before attempting to remove the tumor. Malignant degeneration is extremely rare, and recurrences have not been reported.[10]

Malignant Tumors

The most common malignant tumor to affect the auricle is basal cell carcinoma; squamous cell carcinomas are much more likely to involve the deeper structures of the EAC.[11,12] Extensive surgical procedures and lateral temporal bone resections are, therefore, most commonly done for squamous cell carcinoma. Approximately 5% to 10% of cutaneous malignancies involve the ear, accounting for about 60,000 cases each year.[13] The relatively thin skin of the auricle with its limited subcutaneous tissue is particularly susceptible to deep invasion of these cancers. The tissue planes formed by the embryologic hillocks may create a barrier to extension of disease within the pinna but also provide pathways for deep extension. Lesions of the pre- or postauricular skin often extend to deeper structures, while lesions of the helix typically extend around the external ear and involve deep structures only late in the course of the disease. Both basal and squamous cell carcinoma are associated with sun exposure and often are preceded by severe actinic changes in the skin. Aggressive treatment of early actinic changes in the skin and sun protection may therefore avert malignant degeneration.[13]

BASAL CELL CARCINOMA

Basal cell carcinomas typically begin as indurated nodules that eventually ulcerate, leaving an indurated raised edge. They are locally invasive malignant lesions that rarely metastasize to regional lymph nodes or distant sites and usually do not extend into the EAC. Most authors agree that the ratio of basal cell carcinoma to squamous cell carcinoma of the external ear is similar to other cutaneous structures in the body.[13]

Because of their external location, basal cell carcinomas are often diagnosed early. They may be painful, although more commonly the patient or physician will notice the raised ulcerative lesion before other symptoms develop (Fig. 12–5). Wide local excision is the best treatment, and Mohs's surgery, with concurrent intraoperative assessment of surgical margins, is quite helpful in insuring complete resection.[11,14] Local treatments of cryosurgery and/or curettage may be used for small basal cell carcinomas but should not be used for larger tumors. The role of radiation therapy has been debated, but most clinicians feel that this treatment modality should be reserved for unresectable disease.[9]

After establishing the diagnosis, the surgeon must decide whether or not to resect the underlying cartilage and how best to reconstruct the external ear. The cartilage should always be resected if the perichondrium is invaded. Nodular basal cell carcinoma that does not grossly involve the perichondrium can usually be resected without removing cartilage, but basosquamous and morphea types should be treated more aggressively. A variety of advancement flaps of the auricle are available to aid in cosmetic recon-

struction. When complete excision of the external ear is required, a prosthetic ear may be secured with glue or with osseointegrated magnets.

Cure rates of over 90% have been reported using Mohs's surgical technique. In general, treatment failures of basal cell carcinoma of the ear are due to local recurrence. The recurrence rate from primary excision is higher in cases of morphea type in which there is extensive subcutaneous spread of disease. When extensive basal cell carcinoma does involve the EAC, the local recurrence rate is higher than squamous cell carcinomas in this area.[14]

SQUAMOUS CELL CARCINOMA

Overall, squamous cell carcinoma is less common than basal cell carcinoma in the ear. Only 15% of malignant tumors of the external ear are squamous cell carcinomas; however, they make up nearly 80% of advanced tumors in this area. Squamous cell carcinomas tend to have a more destructive growth pattern and are more likely to involve the EAC. Symptoms often include pain, bleeding from the ear, obstruction of the EAC, or conductive hearing loss. Regional metastases are relatively common, with reported incidence from 6% to 20% at the time of original diagnosis.[13]

Surgical treatment of squamous cell carcinoma in the external ear should be based on a careful assessment of the extent of the disease, including a high-resolution CT scan to assess bone involvement. Le-

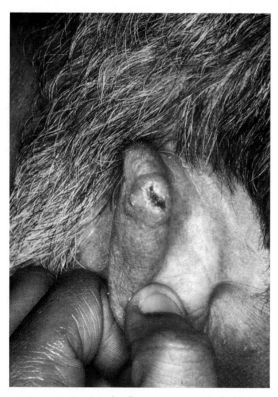

FIGURE 12–5 Basal cell carcinoma on the helical rim.

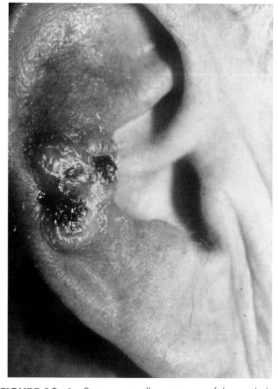

FIGURE 12–6 Squamous cell carcinoma of the antihelix.

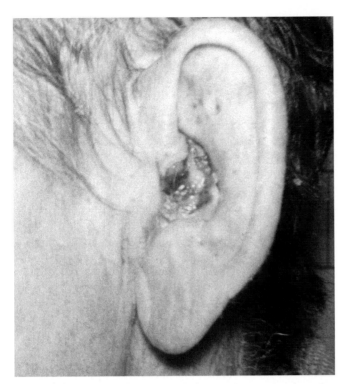

FIGURE 12-7 Squamous cell carcinoma with extension through the conchal cartilage and into the EAC.

sions of the auricle or external meatus that are limited to skin may be treated with primary excision and careful assessment of the surgical margins (Fig. 12–6). Squamous cell carcinoma involving the EAC meatus should be treated aggressively (Fig. 12–7). There is very little subcutaneous tissue in this area, and bone erosion is common. Most lesions that extend into the EAC also involve the tympanic membrane. Crabtree et al[15] recognized that en bloc resection of carcinoma was more effective than limited procedures. They also noted that the postoperative morbidity and mortality were much higher with extensive procedures (subtotal and total TBR) with little apparent difference in cure. Postoperative radiation should be given for the majority of squamous

cell carcinomas requiring temporal bone resection.[11,12,16] Other authors have advocated radiation therapy as a primary treatment, citing an approximate 30% overall 5-year control rate.[11,17] With combined therapy, 5-year survival rates are over 50% for tumors confined to the EAC and roughly 30% for advanced disease.[4,16]

Although a uniform staging system has not been adopted, several have been proposed. Arriaga et al[18] proposed a staging system based on clinical factors appearing to influence outcome[16,19] (Table 12–3). Facial nerve involvement is a poor prognosticator and may be present in up to 35% of patients with extensive disease. Other factors that appear to affect survival are middle ear involvement and dural involvement. Although some authors have suggested that tumor differentiation and size (greater than 3 cm) affect survival, others have not found an independent correlation between these factors and survival. Because of the relatively high incidence of cervical metastases, radical neck dissection with parotidectomy is usually recommended; however, radical neck dissection itself does not appear to improve survival.[18]

MELANOMA

Overall malignant melanoma is the third most common tumor in the external ear but is second only to basal cell carcinoma in malignancies of the pinna (Fig. 12–8). Approximately 5% of all cutaneous melanomas and 7% to 15% of head and neck melanomas originate from the ear.[20–23] Because of the scarcity of subcutaneous tissue, complex anatomical subdivisions, and abundant lymphatic drainage, malignant melanomas of the ear have the poorest prognosis of any site in the head and neck area.[23,24] As with other locations, clinical staging is dependent upon the tumor thickness and the level of invasion. Wide local excision with generous surgical margins is considered the only appropriate treatment for malignant melanoma. Malignant melanomas rarely extend into the EAC.[20] When melanoma does extend down into the osseous EAC, a lateral temporal bone resection is usually the treatment of choice.

TABLE 12 – 3	**TNM STAGING SYSTEM PROPOSED FOR EAC MALIGNANCY**	
T1	Tumor limited to EAC; no bone erosion or soft tissue extension	T1, N0, M0 Stage I
T2	Limited bone erosion (not full thickness); <0.5 cm of soft tissue extension	T2, N0, M0 Stage II
T3	Full thickness bone erosion with <0.5 cm soft tissue extension, or tumor with middle ear, mastoid involvement, or facial paralysis	T3, N0, M0 Stage III
T4	Tumor eroding cochlea, petrous apex, medial wall of middle ear, carotid canal, jugular foramen or dura, or >0.5 cm of soft tissue extension	T4, N0, M0 Stage IV
N	Any adenopathy places patient at advanced stage (T1, N1 = Stage III; T2-4, N1 = Stage IV)	
M	Any distant metastasis	Stage IV

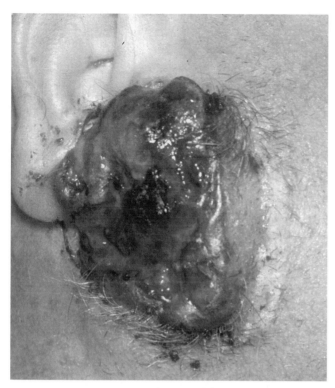

FIGURE 12-8 Large melanoma of the preauricular skin.

The role of elective neck dissection in melanoma of the ear is still somewhat controversial. Pack et al[20] reported a high incidence of regional metastasis (33%) at the time of initial presentation, while disseminated disease was found in fewer than 5% of patients. Based on these observations, a prophylactic lymph node dissection is often recommended. A statistical difference in survival has not been shown, however, for those patients who received prophylactic lymph node dissection. Most authors agree that auricular lesions with depth less than 0.75 mm do not require elective neck dissection, although it should be considered for lesions thicker than 0.75 mm. Palpable nodes in the parotid should be removed with a total parotidectomy with facial nerve preservation, and a superficial parotidectomy should be performed during prophylactic neck dissection[13,21] Five-year survival rates from malignant melanoma in the ear range from 22% to 31%. Rapid dissemination of disease is evident in that 25% of patients die within one year of diagnosis.[25]

ADENOCARCINOMA

Adenocarcinoma of the external ear is extremely rare in the auricle but accounts for nearly 10% of tumors in the EAC and nearly 5% of advanced malignancies.[11,14] These tumors arise from the ceruminous glands and sebaceous glands at the external meatus.[6] These tumors typically undergo rapid growth and the most common clinical sign is obstruction of the EAC. Bone erosion does not appear to be as common in adenocarcinomas as it is with squamous cell carcinomas, but a high-resolution CT scan is still advised. Treatment of adenocarcinoma of the EAC is similar to the treatment for squamous cell carcinoma at this site, except that adenocarcinomas do not appear to be as radiosensitive.[26] Lesions that are lateral at the meatus to the canal may be treated with wide local excision, whereas deeper lesions usually require bone removal with a temporal bone resection. There is a high rate of recurrence following conservative surgical treatment even with postoperative radiation therapy. Hicks[6] pointed out the unpredictable, aggressive, and unrelenting behavior of these lesions and recommended that the lymph nodes in the parotid and jugular digastric area be sampled at the time of surgery. Late recurrences and intracranial extension have been reported several years after the original treatment. Five-year survival rates are not known.

ADENOID CYSTIC CARCINOMA

Adenoid cystic carcinoma presents a special problem for the head and neck surgeon because of its tendency for perineural invasion and distant metastasis that may occur many years after original treatment. Adenoid cystic carcinoma may arise from the ceruminous glands in the EAC. Conley and Schuller[27] reported a 9.8% incidence of adenoid cystic carcinoma in their series of 61 patients with EAC malignancy over a 25-year period. The presenting symptom was usually a painful mass in the EAC.[6] The gross appearance of the tumor is relatively benign and unfortunately often leads to inadequate treatment. Excisional biopsy with examination of permanent sections is necessary since the characteristic histological architecture may not be recognizable on frozen section. A CT scan of the EAC may help to identify bone erosion or invasion into the deep structures of the temporal bone.

These tumors are slow-growing, and distant metastases to lung, kidney, and brain may occur very late in the disease, as long as 30 years after the initial treatment. Aggressive management is imperative with careful examination of tumor margins and special attention to neural tissues, especially the facial nerve. Inadequate treatment with sleeve resections or local excisions often results in recurrences. Wide en bloc resection of the entire ear canal with a lateral temporal bone resection followed by postoperative radiation is often indicated. If the lesion is confined to the EAC, the facial nerve may be preserved. For lesions that extend beyond boundaries of the external canal into the middle ear and temporal bone, sacrificing the facial nerve with cable grafting should be considered. Regional metastasis is uncommon; therefore, elective dissection of a clinically negative neck is indicated only when there is extensive disease.[6]

MIDDLE EAR AND DEEP TEMPORAL BONE

Anatomy and Surgical Approaches

Although the tympanic membrane serves as a clear-cut anatomic division between the middle ear and the external ear, this structure provides very little barrier to the growth of tumors. As can be seen from the preceding discussion, tumors that arise in the EAC often require surgical approaches that extend well beyond the confines of the EAC and into the deeper structures of the temporal bone. In general, the major structures within the middle ear are the tympanic membrane, the middle ear ossicles (malleus, incus, and stapes), and the chorda tympani nerve. The eustachian tube enters anteriorly, and neoplasms may therefore extend through this orifice toward the nasopharynx or from the nasopharynx to the ear. The tensor tympani muscle passes along the medial wall of the eustachian tube and turns at the cochleariform process to insert on the malleus. The facial nerve leaves the geniculate ganglion and runs just superior to the cochleariform process and oval window. The facial nerve then makes its second bend or genu to descend and exit the mastoid at the stylomastoid foramen. The stapedius muscle, which arises medial to the facial nerve, extends anteriorly from the pyramidal eminence to insert on the stapes. These muscles, the stapedius and tensor tympani, are the only striated muscles within the temporal bone itself and are the site of origin for temporal bone rhabdomyosarcoma. The sinus tympani, a space that lies just medial to the pyramidal eminence and facial nerve, is one of the most difficult spaces in the temporal bone to access surgically. The carotid artery and the jugular bulb lie just inferior to the hypotympanum. The jugular foramen extends from the jugular bulb through the skull base and is divided into pars nervosa—which transmits the ninth, tenth, and twelfth cranial nerves—and the pars vascularis, which receives venous drainage from the sigmoid and petrosal sinuses. The tegmen is the roof of the middle ear and mastoid that meets the posterior fossa dura and sigmoid sinus at the sinodural angle.[2]

The inner ear is divided into the cochlear structures and the vestibular labyrinth. The basal turn of the cochlea forms the promontory of the medial wall of the middle ear. The cochlea turns anteriorly and inferiorly to form its two-and-a-half turns. The vestibular portion of the inner ear is divided into three semicircular canals (lateral, superior, and posterior) and two otolith organs (saccule and utricle). The saccule and utricle lie in the large central vestibule of the inner ear. The internal auditory canal forms the medial wall of the vestibule and contains the cochlear nerve, facial nerve, and both divisions of the vestibular nerve (superior and inferior). The pet-rous apex refers to that portion of the temporal bone that extends anteriorly from the otic capsule to the clivus. Pneumatization of the petrous portion of the temporal bone is variable, and tumors may originate in this area.[2]

Small tumors in the middle ear may be approached directly through a tympanoplasty or a tympanomastoidectomy. A facial recess approach allows wide access to the middle ear without removing the EAC wall, through the potential space between the facial nerve and chorda tympani or (in an extended approach) the tympanic membrane annulus. Otologic endoscopes may also provide access to areas that cannot otherwise be directly visualized (e.g., the sinus tympani).[28]

Tumors of jugular foramen or mastoid that extend anteriorly may require transposition of the facial nerve. Fisch[29] described a series of infratemporal fossa approaches in which the facial nerve is dissected out of the facial canal from the geniculate ganglion down to the stylomastoid foramen. A cuff of tissue is left on the stylomastoid foramen, and the facial nerve is transposed anteriorly. The EAC wall can then be taken down completely, providing broad access to the jugular foramen and carotid artery. Ligation of the sigmoid sinus and the jugular vein allows complete resection of tumors that extend all the way from the posterior fossa dura down to the deep structures of the neck (Fig. 12–9). This approach can be further enhanced by anterior extension and dissection of tumor to the carotid and foramen ovale (Type B infratemporal fossa approach).[29]

Tumors of the inner ear may be approached through a translabyrinthine or transcochlear approach. These surgical procedures are done through the mastoid cavity and involve complete removal of the vestibular labyrinth (translabyrinthine) or both the vestibular and cochlear structures (transcochlear). Tumors of the internal auditory canal may be approached through translabyrinthine, transcochlear, suboccipital, or middle fossa approaches (Fig. 12–10). The choice of a surgical approach to these tumors depends upon the patient's age, hearing status, and the size of the tumor.[30]

Relatively small tumors that extend into the lateral segment of the internal auditory canal with good hearing are best approached through the middle fossa. The middle fossa craniotomy is an extradural approach that allows full exposure to the distal internal auditory canal and identification of the facial nerve in the lateral end of the EAC where it is not displaced by tumor.[31] Its disadvantages include limited exposure of the cerebellopontine angle, which makes resection of a large tumor difficult through this approach. In general, tumors greater than 3 cm are not considered good candidates for hearing preservation, and the middle fossa surgery is not recommended for patients over 65 years of age. A suboccipital or retrosigmoid approach can be used for any size tumor, and acceptable hearing

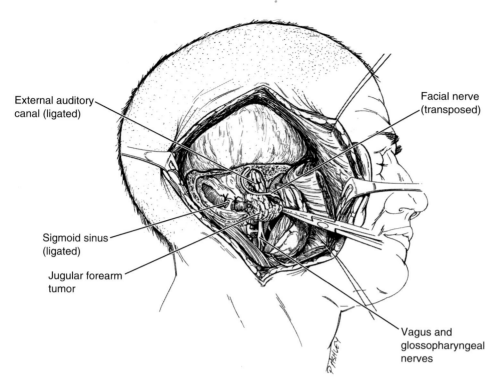

External auditory
canal (ligated)

Facial nerve
(transposed)

Sigmoid sinus
(ligated)

Jugular forearm
tumor

Vagus and
glossopharyngeal
nerves

FIGURE 12–9 Infratemporal fossa approach for a large glomus jugulare (paraganglioma) tumor. The facial nerve has been transposed anteriorly out of the fallopian canal.

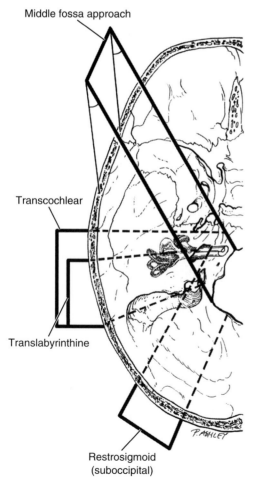

Middle fossa approach

Transcochlear

Translabyrinthine

Restrosigmoid
(suboccipital)

FIGURE 12–10 View of the posterior fossa and temporal bone from above showing the various approaches to the cerebellopontine angle (CPA).

preservation rates can be attained with relatively small tumors that are limited to the cerebellopontine angle or medial internal auditory canal. Advantages of a suboccipital craniotomy include rapid exposure of the entire cerebellopontine angle. The primary disadvantage of a suboccipital craniotomy is limited exposure of the distal internal auditory canal. Large tumors (greater than 3 cm) and tumors in which there is significant preoperative loss of hearing are best managed through a translabyrinthine approach. The facial nerve can be identified in the distal portion of the internal auditory canal by the vertical crest that separates the facial nerve and superior vestibular nerves (Bill's bar). Transcochlear procedures are usually reserved for extensive lesions that extend anteriorly along the medial surface of the petrous apex.

Benign Tumors

PARAGANGLIOMAS (GLOMUS TUMORS)

In 1941, Guild[32] described neurovascular structures in the temporal bone and called them glomus bodies. In 1945, Rosenwasser[33] described a series of tumors of the temporal bone derived from these structures. Although histologically inaccurate and clinically nondescript, the term "glomus tumor" has remained firmly entrenched in the literature to this day. Glomus tumors are actually paragangliomas. Their clinical manifestations depend primarily on their site of origin and extension. Clinically, glomus tumors are divided into two types: glomus tympanicum and glomus jugulare.[34] The former are usually limited to the middle ear, whereas the latter may extend from the jugular

TABLE 12-4	CLASSIFICATION OF GLOMUS TUMORS			
	JACKSON/GLASSCOCK		DE LA CRUZ	
FISCH	Glomus Tympanicum	Glomus Jugulare	Type/Location	Surgical Approach
Type A: Limited to middle ear	Type I: Small mass of tympanic cavity	Type I: Small mass of the tympanic cavity, jugular bulb, and mastoid	Tympanic	Transcanal
Type B: Limited to tympanomastoid without infralabyrinthine involvement	Type II: Complete involvement of the tympanic cavity	Type II: Extension under the IAC with or without intracranial extension	Tympanomastoid	Mastoid-extended facial recess
Type C: Infralabyrinthine involvement and petrous apex extension	Type III: Complete involvement of tympanic cavity, extension into the mastoid	Type III: Extension to the petrous apex, with or without intracranial extension	Jugular bulb	Mastoid-neck (possible facial nerve rerouting)[a]
Type D1: Less than 2 cm of intracranial extension	Type IV: Complete involvement of tympanic cavity, extension into the mastoid and through the tympanic membrane, or into carotid canal	Type IV: Extension beyond the petrous apex (clivus or infratemporal fossa) with or without intracranial extension	Carotid artery	Infratemporal fossa
Type D2: More than 2 cm of intracranial extension			Transdural	Infratemporal fossa/intracranial

[a] Described as transtemporal approach in text.

foramen to the neck or intracranially. The majority (85%) of glomus jugulare and glomus tympanicum tumors arise from the hypotympanum. Approximately 12% of tumors arise from Jacobson's plexus on the promontory, and an additional 3% arise from Arnold's nerve.[26] The two clinical entities are distinguished by their route of extension and spread of the tumor from their site of origin. House and Glasscock[35] were the first to emphasize the clinical significance of these clinical subtypes.

There are numerous classification schemes for glomus tumors. Fisch[29] divided tumors into four basic subgroups, depending upon the extent of tumor growth. Jackson et al[36] emphasized the clinical difference between glomus jugulare and glomus tympanicum tumors and devised a classification scheme based on these two basic subtypes. Salvivelli and De la Cruz[37] later devised a simplified classification scheme based on the recommended surgical approach (Table 12–4).

Paragangliomas are most common in white females. Multicentric tumors, including associated carotid body tumors, occur in 3% to 10% and bilaterally in approximately 1% to 2% of patients.[34,38] There is a familial tendency in some patients, and approximately 33% of familial tumors are multicentric. Approximately 1% of paragangliomas actively secrete catecholamines. These tumors may endocrinologically resemble pheochromocytomas and require pharmacological suppression prior to surgery.[39,40]

Approximately 90% of patients with glomus tympanicum tumors are women.[38] These tumors may occur at any age, from 20 to 70 years, but over 50% of patients are older than 50 years. The typical symptoms of a glomus tympanicum tumor are conductive hearing loss and pulsatile tinnitus. Fullness and pain are relatively uncommon (18%), and cranial neuropathies only occur with very extensive lesions. Clinically, the tumors appear as a hypervascular mass that is usually low in the tympanic membrane or resting on the promontory (Fig. 12–11). Insufflation of the

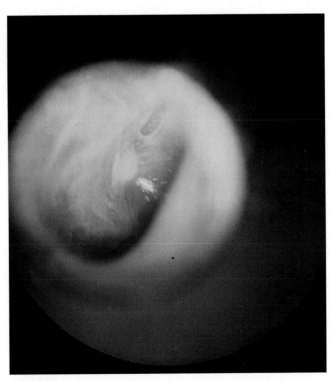

FIGURE 12-11 Otoscopic view of a small glomus tympanicum (paraganglioma).

tympanic membrane may result in a blanching of the underlying mass (Brown's sign). Biopsy through a myringotomy incision is strongly discouraged, as it may result in brisk bleeding or the inadvertent biopsy of an abhorrent carotid artery or high jugular bulb. The general rule of management is resection of the tumor through the EAC or via an intact canal wall mastoidectomy with an extended facial recess. Most tumors require the latter, and a transcanal approach is advisable only if the margins of the tumors can be visualized in a full 360 degrees. Rarely, the canal wall must be removed for adequate resection of a glomus tympanicum tumor. Arteriography is rarely necessary, and embolization is not required. A defocused CO_2 laser or Nd:YAG laser may be helpful in minimizing blood loss.[41] A complete resection of a tympanicum tumor is possible over 90% of the time, and recurrence rates after successful surgery are low (less than 5% of patients).[38] Hearing can be preserved in the majority of cases, and ossicular continuity can be maintained in roughly 50% of patients.[38]

The most common symptoms of glomus jugulare tumors are also conductive hearing loss and pulsatile tinnitus. A middle ear mass can be seen in the majority of cases. Cranial neuropathies are much more common, however, with these tumors. Facial palsy was noted to be the most common cranial neuropathy in early clinical series; however, a recent report indicated a preoperative facial palsy in only 12% of 52 patients and a complete paralysis in only one patient.[42] This discrepancy may be due to earlier diagnosis in the latter series. The frequency of other cranial neuropathies does not appear to have changed that much—with weakness of the vagus nerve in 34%, glossopharyngeal nerve in 23%, spinal accessory nerve in 18%, and hypoglossal nerve in 20% of patients. Intracranial extension occurs in nearly 30% of patients.[42]

The preoperative evaluation of a suspected glomus jugulare tumor includes a CT scan with and without iodine contrast (Fig. 12–12). Although MRI/Gd scans may be helpful to assess soft tissue extension, particularly intracranially or into the neck, they are not adequate alone for preoperative planning. MRI/Gd scans may also be helpful in assessing the degree of involvement of the carotid artery. Conventional arteriography is usually performed as a preoperative study with planned embolization, but may also be helpful if the diagnosis is unclear. Embolization of glomus jugulare tumors has drastically reduced surgical blood loss and should be done within 48 hours of a planned surgery; otherwise, there is a potential for recanalization and revascularization of the tumor. Finally, the preoperative evaluation of patients with a suspected glomus jugulare tumor should include a urine and serum analysis for catecholamines.[43]

The appropriate surgery for glomus jugulare tumors depends upon the extent of the tumor. Tumors that are limited to the jugular bulb and that involve

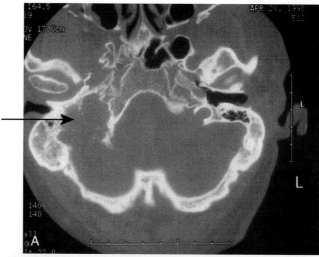

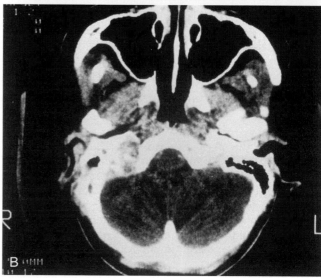

FIGURE 12–12   Axial CT scans of large glomus jugulare (paraganglioma) tumors. *A,* High-resolution scan with bone detail showing erosion of bone surrounding the jugular bulb extending to the carotid canal. *B,* Similar scan with intravenous iodine contrast. Note the enhancement of the vascular glomus tumor in the right temporal bone.

the internal carotid artery below the tympanic facial nerve may be approached through a transtemporal extended facial recess approach.[44] Hearing may be preserved in approximately 93% of these cases, and the recurrence rate after a successful transtemporal surgery is less than 10%.[44] Unfortunately, very few glomus jugulare tumors meet these criteria. A Type A infratemporal fossa approach is recommended for larger tumors that involve the internal carotid artery above the tympanic segment, extend into the neck, or extend intracranially.[29,42] This approach requires closure of the EAC with a postoperative conductive hearing loss. A total hearing loss is usually associated with cochlear invasion and occurs 5% to 10% of the time. Lower cranial nerve palsies following sur-

TABLE 12–5	HOUSE-BRACKMANN FACIAL NERVE GRADING SYSTEM	
GRADE	DESCRIPTION	CHARACTERISTICS
I	Normal	Normal
II	Mild dysfunction	Slight weakness
III	Moderate dysfunction	Obvious—complete eye closure
IV	Moderately severe dysfunction	Obvious—incomplete eye closure
V	Severe dysfunction	Barely perceptible motion
VI	Total paralysis	No movement

Adapted from House JW, Brackmann DE. Facial nerve grading system. *Otolaryngol Head Neck Surg.* 1985; 93(2):146.

gery occur in more than 50% of cases, and vocal cord augmentation is required in approximately one third of patients. Cerebrospinal fluid leak occurs only rarely. The recurrence rate after successful surgery is approximately 3%. The facial nerve is anteriorly transposed during an infratemporal fossa approach in order to allow adequate access to the carotid artery. In a series of 52 cases, the nerve was transposed intact in 45 cases (87%) and transsected in seven patients (13%). The majority of patients (73%) had good facial nerve results (House-Brackmann Grade I or II/ VI [Table 12–5]) following surgery.

Radiation therapy is an alternative treatment for large glomus jugulare tumors.[45,46] Adequate radiation treatment requires a dose of greater than 4000 rads, whereas lower doses are associated with unacceptably high recurrence rates (25%). Brackmann[47] found a vascular fibrosis with persistent tumor cells in pathological specimens of patients whose glomus tumors had been treated with radiation. The effect of radiation on these tumors, therefore, appears to be through fibrosis of the vascular channels supplying the tumor. These tumors can be removed using current skull-base surgery techniques with minimal mortality and acceptable morbidity; therefore, radiation therapy is currently advised only for elderly patients or patients who are not good surgical candidates. Radiation therapy is almost never indicated for a glomus tympanicum tumor.

SALIVARY GLAND CHORISTOMAS

Salivary gland tissue may present in the middle ear as either a growth of normal tissue (choristoma) or a salivary neoplasia.[47] Choristomas are extremely rare tumors, related to a second branchial arch dysgenesis. There is often an associated congenital abnormality of the facial nerve, oval window, stapes, and incus.[48] The symptoms of these tumors are typically conductive hearing loss, aural fullness, and—occasionally—an associated sensorineural hearing loss.[49] Preoperative CT scanning is advised to identify any dehiscence of the facial nerve.

The surgery for these lesions is somewhat controversial. Pedunculated lesions can be safely resected; however, large broad-based lesions should not be resected because of a very likely adherence to the facial nerve.[47,49] Kartush[49] reported an adherence to the facial nerve in 10 out of 12 patients with a 25% postoperative facial nerve palsy. Once the relationship with the facial nerve is established, a biopsy is necessary to rule out a salivary gland malignancy.[48]

PRIMARY ADENOMAS

Primary adenomas of the middle ear usually present as a hypovascular, noninvasive mass in the middle ear.[26,50–52] Typical symptoms are hearing loss, tinnitus, and fullness; tumors may occur at any age. These tumors may extend into the mesotympanum or into the EAC, thus somewhat confusing their site of origin. Differential diagnosis includes a plasmacytoma, ceruminoma, or paraganglioma.[52] The majority of these can be removed through an exploratory tympanotomy or by an extended facial recess approach. Recurrence is rare after simple excision of the tumor.[26] Bone destruction, pain, facial weakness, and chronic otorrhea are extremely rare in these tumors and suggest an underlying malignancy.[50]

ENDOLYMPHATIC SAC TUMORS

A special subtype of adenomatous tumor of the temporal bone is a papillary tumor appearing to arise from the endolymphatic sac.[53,54] These tumors are often associated with extensive temporal destruction. Papillary endolymphatic sac tumors are aggressive tumors that have extensive local spread and bone destruction. Because of the extensive nature of these tumors at the time of diagnosis, their site of origin may be obscure. Although some authors have classified these tumors with middle ear adenomas,[55] it is clear that they represent a distinct entity.[54] These tumors have been considered by some as low-grade malignancies.[56] There appears to be an association with von Hippel-Lindau syndrome in some cases.

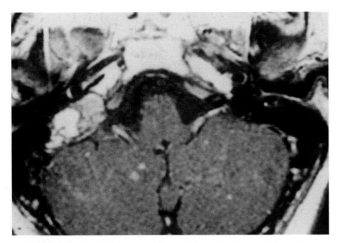

FIGURE 12-13 MRI scan with gadolinium of an endolymphatic sac tumor.

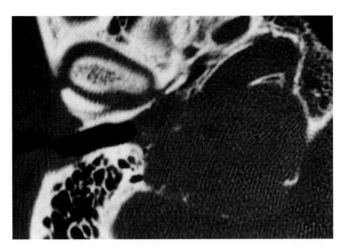

FIGURE 12-14 Axial CT scan of jugular foramen schwannoma. Note the relatively smooth margins of bone erosion.

The destructive lesion may be seen on both CT and MRI scans (Fig. 12–13). Surgery with complete resection is the recommended treatment, and prognosis is very good even in the face of intracranial extension. There does not appear to be a role for adjuvant radiation or chemotherapy treatment.

TERATOMAS AND DERMOIDS

Teratomas are true tumors of embryonic tissue that form well-defined tissues. Dermoid tumors, on the other hand, are hamartomas—not true neoplasms. Both tumors are relatively rare in the temporal bone and may present as chronic otitis media or conductive hearing loss in young adults. They are adequately treated with mastoidectomy and extended facial recess approach.[57,58]

JUGULAR FORAMEN SCHWANNOMAS

Any of the cranial nerves in the par nervosa of the jugular foramen (cranial nerves IX, X, and XI) may develop a schwannoma (often clinically referred to as neuroma). Symptoms relate to their location within the jugular foramen with palsies of cranial nerves IX, X, and XI. The typical radiographic picture with these tumors is an enlarged jugular foramen. Unlike glomus jugulare tumors, neuromas in the jugular foramen typically produce a smooth bony margin (Fig. 12–14). The surgical approach for a neuroma is similar to glomus jugulare tumors (Type A infratemporal fossa approach). These are rare, with less than 100 cases reported in the literature. Lower cranial nerve dysfunction is common.[59]

VESTIBULAR SCHWANNOMA

By far the most common tumor in the internal auditory canal and cerebellopontine angle is a vestibular schwannoma. Like glomus tumors, vestibular schwannomas are more commonly referred to by an imprecise name—"acoustic neuroma." Since these tumors arise from the Schwann cells of the vestibular nerve, not the acoustic (cochlear) nerve, the term vestibular schwannoma is more appropriate. The term acoustic neuroma, however, is widely used by clinicians to describe this tumor. Approximately 90% of tumors in the internal auditory canal and cerebellopontine angle are vestibular schwannomas.[60] The tumors usually originate at the myelin-glial junction within the internal auditory canal (Fig. 12–15). As the tumor grows, it fills the canal and extends into the cerebellopontine angle. The tumors may arise from either superior or inferior nerve, and there appears to be an equal distribution between the two nerves. The characteristic clinical symptoms of hearing loss and tinnitus are the result of compression of the cochlear division of the nerve. Slow tumor growth within the vestibular nerve allows the vestibular system time to compensate for the loss of vestibular function, so vertigo and disequilibrium are not major clinical factors. Facial paralysis is also

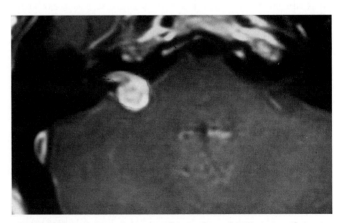

FIGURE 12-15 Gadolinium-enhanced axial MRI scans of a small vestibular schwannoma (acoustic neuroma) within the left internal auditory canal.

rare, although the facial nerve is usually displaced anteriorly by the tumor.[61]

The characteristic symptoms of vestibular schwannomas are gradual hearing loss (77% to 95%), with poor speech discrimination that is out of proportion with the degree of hearing loss. Sudden hearing loss occurs in approximately 15% of patients with acoustic neuromas, and nearly 25% of patients with acoustic neuromas have had sudden fluctuations in hearing during their clinical course.[62] On the other hand, only 3% of patients who have a sudden sensorineural hearing loss will have an acoustic neuroma.[63] Unilateral tinnitus is the second most common symptom (53% to 70%), followed by disequilibrium (48%). True vertigo is a presenting symptom in less than one fourth of patients. It should be emphasized that nearly 25% of patients will present with some unusual symptom complex, and therefore a clinical suspicion should remain high for any unilateral otologic symptom. Trigeminal symptoms, cerebellar dysfunction, and headache are more common with larger tumors.[62] Lower cranial nerve palsies and increased intracranial pressure are quite rare.

If early signs of tumor growth within the internal auditory canal are ignored or not recognized, the tumor may grow out of the internal auditory canal and into the cerebellopontine angle. Considerable tumor growth may be possible before the secondary symptoms of trigeminal nerve dysfunction, cerebellar dysfunction, or headache ultimately result in the diagnosis. There is often a latent period of 1.5 to 2 years before the tumor is recognized. One study has cited a delay between the onset of symptoms and the diagnosis of acoustic neuroma of approximately 3.6 years.[64] Large cerebellopontine angle tumors are associated with a much higher morbidity; a cost-effective diagnostic strategy, therefore, should be based primarily on the patient's history with a high index of suspicion.[61,64]

MRI/Gd is considered the gold standard of vestibular schwannoma diagnosis. The sensitivity of this imaging modality is over 99%, and the specificity is also extremely high. The false-positive findings with MRI/Gd scans are higher for exceptionally small lesions.[65] False-positive results may be associated with neuritis of the vestibulocochlear nerves, and dural enhancement alone within the internal auditory canal should not be misinterpreted as a tumor.

The second diagnostic modality for vestibular schwannoma is an auditory brainstem response (ABR) test. Brachmann and Gherini[60] looked at various parameters of ABR and found that the wave V intra-aural latency difference of greater than 0.2 ms was the most reliable indicator of a vestibular schwannoma. Using this criteria, the sensitivity rate is considered to be greater than 90% for all tumors. With smaller tumors, however, the sensitivity of ABR falls significantly.[66,67] The specificity of the test is also wanting, with a specificity of 70% or less.[68]

Perhaps the greatest limitation to ABR testing is the inability to use it when there is sensorineural hearing loss greater than 70 to 80 dB at 4000 Hz.

A carefully taken history with some assessment as to the risk of the patient for a vestibular schwannoma should be the first step in any diagnostic strategy. The diagnosis should be considered in any patient who has a unilateral otologic symptom. The next step in evaluation should be an audiogram to assess any asymmetry of the hearing loss and speech discrimination. Acoustic reflex testing may also be quite helpful in assessing the risk of a given patient. Patients who are thought to have low risk of a tumor may be evaluated with an auditory brainstem response test or with frequent serial audiograms. Patients with history and audiometric findings highly suggestive of an acoustic neuroma should be evaluated with an MRI/Gd scan. An MRI/Gd scan is also recommended for patients under 65 who have a moderate risk of developing a tumor. This is based primarily on the fact that these patients would theoretically be candidates for hearing preservation surgery if a tumor were identified at an early stage. Patients over 65 years of age with a moderate risk of a tumor can be evaluated with an auditory brainstem response, provided adequate follow-up audiometry is feasible.

Once diagnosed, the management of a vestibular schwannoma depends primarily upon the patient's age, tumor size, and the status of their preoperative hearing. Vestibular schwannomas are slow-growing tumors. Although growth rates are variable, most tumors grow less than 2 mm per year.[69] Therefore, older patients may not require any treatment. The standard of care for most patients with vestibular schwannomas is microsurgical resection. The surgical approach is based primarily upon whether or not hearing is to be preserved. In general, hearing preservation is rare for tumors over 2.5 to 3 cm in diameter, and patients over 65 years of age do not tolerate hearing preservation procedures as well as do younger patients. The options for hearing preservation include a suboccipital (retrosigmoid) approach or a middle fossa (supratemporal) approach. Hearing preservation is possible with middle fossa craniotomy, with over 70% for tumors less than 3 cm in size[31] as opposed to a 44% hearing preservation rate with a suboccipital approach.[70] Tumor size, auditory brainstem response characteristics, and speech discrimination are factors that influence hearing preservation.

When hearing preservation is not a realistic goal, the best approach is a translabyrinthine approach. The advantages of this approach are minimal dural retraction, wide exposure of the internal auditory canal and cerebellopontine angle, and identification of the facial nerve in the distal portion of the internal auditory canal. The primary disadvantage is the complete loss of hearing on the operated side. Facial nerve results following translabyrinthine surgery are very good, with over 90% of patients having a

Grade I-II/VI function (House-Brackmann scale) regardless of tumor size. CSF leak is a rare complication (less than 5%) following translabyrinthine surgery. The surgical treatment of vestibular schwannoma has been greatly enhanced by the use of intraoperative facial nerve monitoring.[71] Cochlear nerve monitoring also appears to improve hearing preservation rates in appropriate cases.[72]

Stereotactic radiation therapy is an option for patients who are not surgical candidates or who refuse surgery. This technique consists of a single treatment session with a precise delivery of a high dose of radiation to the tumor. There is minimal hospitalization and very little discomfort from the procedure. The primary goal of stereotactic radiation is the reduction or stabilization of tumor growth, which is possible in approximately 85% of cases.[73,74] Unfortunately, the long-term consequences of radiation therapy may not be evident for months or even years following the procedure. Furthermore, radiation treatment to the internal auditory canal and cerebellopontine angle complicate subsequent surgery to remove a tumor that did not respond to treatment.[75] A long-term study of stereotactic radiation reported a hearing preservation rate of approximately 26%, facial palsy in approximately 15%, and trigeminal neuropathy in 18% of patients following treatment.[73] Better control rates, but slightly higher morbidity, have been reported in recent studies.[74] Unfortunately, there is not enough data on long-term results with this alternative treatment modality.

Bilateral vestibular schwannomas occur in neurofibromatosis type 2 (NF2), a hereditary disease that presents a particular challenge for the neurotologist. Clinical features of NF2 include bilateral vestibular schwannomas, meningiomas, juvenile cataracts, cafe au lait spots, and interdigital freckling. The cutaneous neurofibromas characteristic of neurofibromatosis type 1 (von Recklinghausen's disease) are unusual in patients with NF2. Patients with NF2 are typically younger than other vestibular schwannoma patients, the tumors are more difficult to remove, and hearing preservation rates are not as good.[76] Hearing preservation in patients with bilateral tumors presents a challenging clinical problem.[77] Some options for these patients include decompression of the internal auditory canal without attempting removal of the tumor or early removal of a small tumor with hearing preservation.[76,78] Finally, auditory sensation can be restored to patients after the resection of large tumors with an auditory brainstem implant.[77]

MENINGIOMAS

Meningiomas account for approximately 14% of all intracranial tumors and between 3% and 13% of tumors in the cerebellopontine angle. Approximately 10% of all intracranial meningiomas are located in the cerebellopontine angle. Meningiomas affect

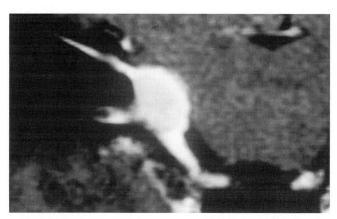

FIGURE 12-16 Axial MRI scan with gadolinium of right CPA meningioma.

females more often than males. Like vestibular schwannomas, hearing loss and tinnitus are common symptoms, but the progression of the symptoms tends to be more rapid in meningiomas, and other cranial nerve symptoms are more common. Generally, meningiomas will have better hearing and ABR results than do vestibular schwannomas (Fig. 12–16).[60,79,80]

The radiographic features of meningiomas are more variable than those of acoustic neuromas. Typically, they are off-center from the internal auditory canal and adjacent to the petrous bone with a hyperostosis of the adjacent bone on CT scan. Intratumoral calcium may be seen on CT with some histologic types. Meningiomas enhance with gadolinium but may have a more variable appearance on nonenhanced images, presumably due to differences in tumor histology or vascularity.[81,82]

Meningiomas may extend into the middle ear from the internal auditory canal or may originate in the middle ear.[26] These tumors are thought to arise from arachnoid granulations present in the middle ear as embryologic rests. They are extremely rare tumors occurring almost exclusively in females. The typical symptom in these patients is hearing loss, but they may also complain of pain, facial palsy, or chronic otorrhea. Clinically, the tumors do not appear as vascular as a paraganglioma, but this distinction may be difficult. Complete resection is usually possible with good prognosis. Unlike intracranial meningiomas, the histological subclass does not appear to be predictive of clinical behavior.

FACIAL NERVE SCHWANNOMAS

Facial nerve schwannomas may occur anywhere along the length of the facial nerve. The geniculate ganglion is the most common site, and multiple segments of the nerve are involved in 80% of cases. Hearing loss is present in nearly 70% of patients. A slowly progressive facial nerve paralysis occurs in slightly less than half of patients, and a facial twitch may be present in almost 20%. It is estimated that 5% of patients with total facial paralysis have an underlying tumor. Any patient who has paralysis persistent for more than 6 months should therefore have an MRI/Gd scan.[83–86] Because a facial nerve schwannoma may present in the middle ear with conductive hearing loss, it is strongly recommended that an unidentified middle ear mass not be biopsied without preoperative imaging to assess the status and location of the facial nerve. An enlargement of the fallopian canal can usually be seen on a high resolution CT scan.[87] MRI/Gd may also be useful to demonstrate enhancement of the facial nerve that extends through the temporal bone even without significant enlargement of the bony fallopian canal.[88]

It is generally recommended that patients with severe palsy or paralysis due to a facial nerve schwannoma have the tumor resected as early as possible. Doing so may prevent degeneration of the facial nucleus in the brain.[84] Resection of the tumor with rerouting and reanastomosis of the nerve is possible if there is less than 1 cm of resected nerve. Otherwise a cable graft may be used to re-establish facial nerve continuity. Small tumors in patients who have minimal facial nerve dysfunction may be observed.

HEMANGIOMAS

Hemangiomas in the temporal bone are often associated with the facial nerve.[89] These are most commonly seen at the geniculate ganglion or internal auditory canal, but may occur in the middle ear or along the descending facial nerve. Tumors within the internal auditory canal usually present with sensorineural hearing loss. Although facial palsy is more common in these patients, these symptoms may otherwise be difficult to distinguish from a vestibular schwannoma. Tumors arising from the geniculate ganglion usually present with facial nerve palsy. On CT scans these tumors may have intratumoral calcium and have thus been called "ossifying hemangiomas."[90] They are usually hyperintense on nonenhanced T1 and T2 weighted MRI images.[91] The most common surgical approaches to these tumors are a middle fossa or translabyrinthine craniotomy. Tumors arising within the geniculate ganglion often require grafting of the facial nerve.

Hemangiomas and hemangiopericytomas rarely occur as isolated middle ear tumors.[92,93] They present as a vascular mass that does not appear as pulsatile as a glomus tumor. CT scanning with intravenous contrast is the imaging study of choice, and angiography may not demonstrate the typical "tumor blush." Most of these tumors can be resected through a mastoidectomy with exposure through the facial recess (Fig. 12–17). Because of the possible association with the facial nerve, a dehiscent fallopian canal should be anticipated.

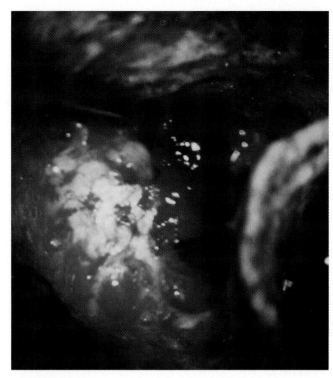

FIGURE 12–17 Intraoperative photograph of right temporal bone hemangioma in the middle ear and mastoid approached through an extended facial recess approach. The tumor appeared to arise from a dehiscent area in the descending fallopian canal.

EPIDERMOID TUMORS

Epidermoid tumors or primary cholesteatomas of the cerebellopontine angle account for 2% to 3% of tumors within this region. Clinically, these patients present with hearing loss and poor discrimination. Because of the irritative effects on the facial nerve, facial nerve hemispasm is not uncommon. Radiographically these tumors have irregular margins and are less dense than brain on CT scans. The MRI characteristics are a lesion which has a brighter signal on T2 than T1 weighted images. Because of the epidermoid matrix, complete removal of these tumors is a necessity, and recurrence rates are relatively high.[94]

LIPOMAS

Lipomas of the internal auditory canal and CPA account for a very small proportion of tumors in this location (less than 0.2%). Unlike lipomas elsewhere in the body, these tumors are typically nonencapsulated and densely adherent to the surrounding structures, particularly the cochlear nerve and facial nerve. Attempts to preserve hearing with small lipomas in the internal auditory canal are almost always unsatisfactory. Lipomas have unique MRI features with an intense signal on T1 even without gadolin-

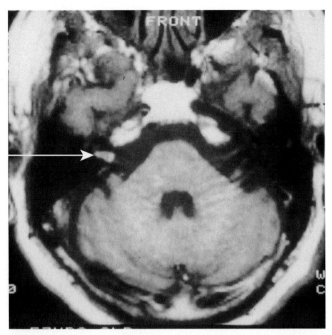

FIGURE 12-18 Axial MRI scan *without* gadolinium demonstrating a right internal auditory canal lipoma. There was very little signal change with gadolinium infusion.

ium contrast (Fig. 12–18) and a very low-signal intensity on T2 weighted images.[95]

CHORDOMA

Chordomas account for a very small percentage of tumors in the cerebellopontine angle and petrous apex. These are benign neoplasms arising from the notochord remnant. Clinically, the patient may present with visual problems and fronto-orbital headaches; cranial nerve palsies are relatively common. Bone erosion is usually seen on CT scan.

CHOLESTEROL GRANULOMA

A cholesterol granuloma is a cyst that can occur within any of the pneumatized spaces of the temporal bone. It may occur in the petrous apex and result in otalgia, dizziness, and hearing loss, as well as diplopia and trigeminal symptoms. Radiographically these lesions present with a smooth bone erosion and an otherwise well-pneumatized temporal bone. On MRI scans both T1 and T2 weighted signals are elevated. Complete resection of these lesions is not necessary, and decompression can be accomplished through an infralabyrinthine approach.[96]

Malignant Tumors

SQUAMOUS CELL CARCINOMA

Squamous cell carcinoma is the most common malignant tumor within the middle ear. Many studies, however, include tumors that arise from the EAC.

Michael and Wells[97] reported 28 cases of squamous cell carcinoma that appeared to arise from within the middle ear. The average age of these patients was 64 years, with a range of ages from 34 to 80 years. The most common symptoms in these patients were pain and chronic aural drainage. A chronically inflamed mucosa may lead to the development of these cancers, since there is no squamous tissue intrinsic in the middle ear. Standard therapy is subtotal temporal bone resection (petrosectomy) or radical mastoidectomy with postoperative radiation therapy, with a 5-year survival rate of 31% to 48%. Primary radiation alone may provide a slightly lower survival rate (22% to 36%), but these treatment modalities have not been compared in a controlled study.

RHABDOMYOSARCOMA

Rhabdomyosarcoma is the most common malignant tumor of the temporal bone in children. It arises from the middle ear, and the most common symptoms are discharge, bleeding, pain, and hearing loss. The Intergroup Rhabdomyosarcoma Study developed a classification scheme based primarily on the resectability of the disease and the presence of metastasis.[98] The histological subtypes of temporal bone rhabdomyosarcoma do not appear to influence prognosis. Distant metastases are present in 14% of patients at the time of diagnosis, with the most common site being the lungs. Spread to the regional lymph nodes is relatively common in the head and neck (5% to 20%), but is rare for middle ear tumors. Temporal bone rhabdomyosarcomas tend to follow the facial nerve and extend intracranially. Death is usually due to meningeal spread or metastasis.[99,100]

The current treatment for patients with rhabdomyosarcoma is surgical resection if possible, although wide surgical margins are deemed unnecessary, and a temporal bone resection is generally not indicated. The mainstay of treatment is radiation therapy with greater than 4500 rads and chemotherapy with vincristine, actinomycin-D, and Cytoxan. Survival from tumors at parameningeal sites is less than 50% at 7 years, and these results are poorer than rhabdomyosarcomas from other locations.[98,99]

PRIMARY ADENOCARCINOMA

Primary adenocarcinoma of the middle ear is a rare tumor that presents with rapid growth and massive bone destruction. It is most commonly seen in middle-aged males. Prognosis is very poor even with radical surgery and radiation therapy. In general, adenocarcinomas of the middle ear are less sensitive to radiation than squamous cell tumors. High-grade adenosquamous types are the most common.[100]

TEMPORAL BONE METASTASIS

The majority of metastatic lesions to the temporal bone appear within the middle ear. These tumors

TABLE 12-6	METASTATIC TUMORS TO THE TEMPORAL BONE (DISTANT PRIMARY SITES OF 103 CASES)
PRIMARY SITE AND/OR NEOPLASTIC CLASSIFICATION	**NUMBER OF CASES**
Breast carcinoma	18
Lung carcinoma	12
Renal adenocarcinoma	10
Stomach carcinoma	8
Larynx carcinoma	5
Melanoma	5
Prostate carcinoma	4
Thyroid carcinoma	4
Pharyngeal carcinoma	4
Cervical and uterine carcinoma	4
Miscellaneous	29

Adapted from Hill BA, Kohut RI. Metastatic andenocarcinoma of the temporal bone. *Arch Otolaryngol* 1976; 102:568.

often present at multiple sites with rapid growth, and progression of symptoms is the rule. The primary site of a large series of metastatic temporal bone tumors is shown in Table 12–6.[101]

CHONDROSARCOMA

Chondrosarcoma is an extremely rare malignant tumor of the petrous apex accounting for less than 0.1 % of cerebellopontine angle tumors. It is a malignant lesion located more laterally than the benign chordoma. Typical appearance on a CT is massive bone destruction (Fig. 12–19). Cochleovestibular symptoms in these patients are relatively rare.[102]

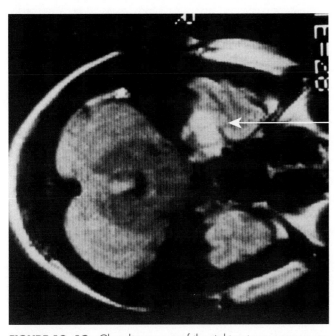

FIGURE 12–19 Chondosarcoma of the right petrous apex on an enhanced axial MRI scan.

REFERENCES

1. Valvassori GE. Imaging studies of the temporal bone. In: Bailey BJ, ed. *Head and Neck Surgery—Otolaryngology.* Vol. 2. Philadelphia: Lippincott; 1993:1518.
2. Donaldson JA, Duckert LG, Lambert PM, Rubel EW. *Surgical Anatomy of the Temporal Bone.* New York: Raven Press; 1994.
3. Paparilla MM, Meyerhoff WL, Morris MS, da Costa S. Surgery of the external ear. In: Paparilla MM, ed. *Otolaryngology.* Philadelphia: WB Saunders; 1991:1259.
4. Kuhel WI, Hume CR, Selesnick SH. Cancer of the external auditory canal and temporal bone. *Otolaryngol Clin North Am.* 1996; 29(5):827.
5. Medina JE, Park AO, Neely JG, et al. Lateral temporal bone resections. *Am J Surg.* 1990; 160:427.
6. Hicks GW. Tumors arising from the glandular structures of the external auditory canal. *Laryngoscope.* 1983; 93:326.
7. Mansour P, George MK, Pahor AL. Ceruminous gland tumors: A reappraisal. *J Laryngol Otol.* 1992; 106:727.
8. Mills RG, Douglas-Jones T, Williams RG. Ceruminoma: A defunct diagnosis. *J Laryngol Otol.* 1995; 109:180.
9. Ludman H. *Mawson's Diseases of the Ear.* Chicago: Yearbook Medical Publishers; 1988.
10. Sheehy JL. Diffuse exostoses and osteomata of the external auditory canal: A report of 100 operations. *Otolaryngol Head Neck Surg.* 1982; 90:337.
11. Lederman M. Malignant tumors of the ear. *J Laryngol Otol.* 1965; 79:85.
12. Lewis JS. Cancer of the ear. *CA Cancer J Clin.* 1987; 37:78.
13. Estrem SA, Renner GJ. Special problems associated with cutaneous carcinoma of the ear. *Otolaryngol Clin North Am.* 1993; 26:231.
14. Niparko JK, Swanson NA, Baker SR et al. Local control of auricular, periauricular, and external canal cutaneous malignancies with Mohs surgery. *Laryngoscope.* 1990; 100:1047.
15. Crabtree JA, Britton BH, Pierce MK. Carcinoma of the external auditory canal. Meeting of the Western Section, American Laryngological, Rhinological and Otological Society, Inc., Newport Beach, CA, January 25, 1975.
16. Austin JR, Stewart KL, Fawzi N. Squamous cell carcinoma of the external auditory canal: Therapeutic prognosis based on a proposed staging system. *Arch Otolaryngol Head Neck Surg.* 1994; 120:1228.
17. Birzgalis AR, Keith AO, Farrington WT. Radiotherapy in the treatment of middle ear and mastoid carcinoma. *Clin Otolaryngol.* 1992; 17:113.
18. Arriaga M, Hirsch BE, Kammerer DB et al. Squamous cell carcinoma of the external auditory meatus (canal). *Otolaryngol Head Neck Surg.* 1989; 101:330.
19. Arriaga M, Cartin H, Hirsch BE, Takahashi H, Kammerer DB: Staging proposal for external auditory meatus carcinoma based on preoperative clinical examination and CT findings. *Ann Otol Rhinol Laryngol.* 1990; 99:714.
20. Pack GT, Conley J, Oropeza R. Melanoma of the external ear. *Arch Otolaryngol.* 1970; 92:106.
21. Byers RM, Smith JL, Russel N, Rosenberg V. Malignant melanoma of the external ear. *Am J Surg.* 1980; 140:518.
22. Hudson DA, Kriege JE, Stover RM, King HS. Malignant melanoma of the external ear. *Br J Plast Surg.* 1990; 43:608.
23. Batsakis JG. *Tumors of Head and Neck: Clinical and Pathological Considerations.* Baltimore: Williams & Wilkins; 1979.
24. Wanebo HJ, Cooper PH, Young DV, et al. Prognostic factors in head and neck melanoma. *Cancer.* 1988; 62:831.
25. Fitzpatrick PJ, Brown TC, Reid J. Malignant melanoma of the head and neck: A clinicopathological study. *Can J Surg.* 1972; 15:90.
26. Hyams VJ. Pathology of tumors of the ear. In: Thawley SE, Panje WR, eds. *Comprehensive Management of Tumors of the Head and Neck.* Philadelphia: WB Saunders; 1988:168.
27. Conley J, Schuller DE. Malignancies of the ear. *Laryngoscope.* 1976; 86:1147.
28. Rosenberg SI. Endoscopic otologic surgery. *Otolaryngol Clin North Am.* 1996; 29(2):291.
29. Fisch U. Infratemporal fossa approach to tumors of the temporal bone and base of the skull. *J Laryngol Otol.* 1978; 92:949.

30. Jackler RK, Pitts LH. Selection of surgical approach to acoustic neuroma. *Otolaryngol Clin North Am.* 1992; 25(2):361.

31. Brackmann DE, House JR, Hitselberger WE. Technical modifications to the middle fossa craniotomy approach in removal of acoustic neuromas. *Am J Otol.* 1994; 15:1.

32. Guild SR. A hitherto unrecognized structure: The glomus jugularis in man, abstracted. *Anat Rec.* 1941; 79(suppl 2):28.

33. Rosenwasser H. Carotid body tumor of the middle ear and mastoid. *Arch Otolaryngol.* 1945; 41:64.

34. Alford BR, Guilford FR. A comprehensive study of tumors of the glomus jugulare. *Laryngoscope.* 1962; 72:765.

35. House WF, Glasscock ME. Glomus tympanicum tumors. *Arch Otolaryngol.* 1968; 87:550.

36. Jackson G, Glasscock ME, Harris PF. Glomus tumors: Diagnosis, classification, and management of large lesions. *Arch Otolaryngol.* 1982; 108:401.

37. Salvivelli F, De la Cruz A. Glomus tumors. In: *Otoneurosurgery and Lateral Skull Base Surgery.* Philadelphia: WB Saunders; 1996:179.

38. Jackson CG, Welling DB, Chironis P. Glomus tympanicum tumors: Contemporary concepts in conservation surgery. *Laryngoscope.* 1989; 99:875.

39. Parisier SC, Edelstein DR, Levenson MJ. Tumors of the middle ear and mastoids. In: Paparilla MM, ed. *Otolaryngology.* Philadelphia: WB Saunders; 1991:1457.

40. Zak FG, Lawson W. *The Paraganglionic Chemoreceptor System: Pathology and Clinical Medicine.* New York: Springer Verlag; 1982.

41. Robinson PJ, Grant HR, Brown SG: NdYAG laser treatment of a glomus tympanicum tumor. *J Laryngol Otol.* 1993; 107:236.

42. Green JD Jr, Brackmann DE, Nguyen CD, et al. Surgical management of previously untreated glomus jugular tumors. *Laryngoscope.* 1994; 104:917.

43. Jackson CG, Woods CI, Chironis PN. Glomus jugulare tumors. In: Sekhar LN, Janecka IP, eds. *Surgery of Cranial Base Tumors.* New York: Raven Press; 1993:747.

44. Jackson CG, Haynes DS, Walker PA, et al. Hearing conservation in surgery for glomus jugulare tumors. *Am J Otol.* 1996; 17:425.

45. Cole JM, Beiler D. Long-term results of treatment for glomus jugulare and glomus vagale tumors with radiotherapy. *Laryngoscope.* 1994; 104:1461.

46. deJong AL, Coker NJ, Jenkins HA, et al. Radiation therapy in the management of paragangliomas. *J Otology (Am).* 1995; 16:283.

47. Brackmann DE, House WF, Terry R, et al. Glomus jugulare tumors: Effective radiation. *Trans Am Acad Ophthalmol.* 1972; 76:1423.

48. Bottrill ID, Chawla OP, Ramsay AD. Salivary gland choristoma of the middle ear. *J Laryngol Otol.* 1992; 106:630.

49. Kartush JM, Graham MD. Salivary gland choristoma of the middle ear: A case report and review of the literature. *Laryngoscope.* 1984; 94:228.

50. Mischke RE, Brackmann DE, Gruskin P. Salivary gland choristoma of the middle ear. *Arch Otolaryngol.* 1977; 103:432.

51. Derlacki EL, Barney PL. Adenomatous tumors of the middle ear and mastoid. 78th Annual Meeting of the American Laryngological, Rhinological and Otological Society, Inc., Atlanta, GA, April 10, 1975.

52. Jahrsdoerfer RA, Fechner RE, Moon CN, et al. Adenoma of the middle ear. *Laryngoscope.* 1983; 93:1041.

53. Eby TL, Makek MS, Fisch U. Adenomas of the temporal bone. *Ann Otol Rhinol Laryngol.* 1988; 97:605.

54. Li JC, Brackmann DE, Lo WM, et al. Reclassification of aggressive adenomatous mastoid neoplasms as endolymphatic sac tumors. *Laryngoscope.* 1993; 103:1342.

55. Mills SE, Wick MR, Weiland LH, Fu YS. *Neoplasms and Related Lesions of the Head and Neck.* Chicago: American Society of Clinical Pathologists Press; 1993:120.

56. Heffner DK. Low-grade adenocarcinoma of probable endolymphatic sac origin. *Cancer.* 1989; 64:2292.

57. Minatogawa T, Node MN, Fukuda I, et al. Dermoid cyst in the middle ear. *J Laryngol Otol.* 1993; 107:335.

58. Parnes LS, Sun AH. Teratoma of the middle ear. *J Otolaryngol.* 1995; 24:165.

59. Franklin DJ, Moore GF, Fisch U. Jugular foramen peripheral nerve sheath tumors. *Laryngoscope.* 1989; 99:1081.

60. Brackmann DE, Gherini SG. Differential diagnosis of skull base neoplasms involving the posterior fossa. In: Cummings C, ed. *Textbook of Otolaryngology.* St Louis: Mosby; 1986: 3421.

61. McElveen JT, Saunders JE. Tumors of the cerebellopontine angle: Neuro-otologic aspects of diagnosis. In: Wilkins RH, Rengachary SS, eds. *Neurosurgery.* 2nd ed. New York: McGraw-Hill; 1996:1039.

62. Selesnick SH, Jackler RK. Clinical manifestations and audiologic diagnosis of acoustic neuromas. *Otolaryngol Clin North Am.* 1992; 25:521.

63. Saunders JE, Luxford WM, Degan KK, Fetterman BL. Sudden hearing loss in acoustic neuroma patients. *Otolaryngol Head Neck Surg.* 1995; 113:23.

64. Moffat DA, Hardy DG, Baguley DM. Strategy and benefits of acoustic neuroma searching. *J Laryngol Otol.* 1989; 103:51.

65. Glass WV, Haid CT, Cidlinsky K, Stenglein C. False-positive MR imaging in the diagnosis of acoustic neurinomas. *Otolaryngol Head Neck Surg.* 1991; 104:863.

66. Wilson DF, Hodgson RS, Gustafson MF, et al. The sensitivity of auditory brainstem response testing in small acoustic neuromas. *Laryngoscope.* 1992; 102:961.

67. Chandresekhar SS, Brackmann DE, Devgan KK. Utility of auditory brainstem response audiometry in diagnosis of acoustic neuromas. *Am J Otolaryngol.* 1995; 16(1):63.

68. Kotlarz JP, Eby TL, Borton TE. Analysis of efficiency of retrocochlear screening. *Laryngoscope.* 1992; 102:1108.

69. Nedzelski JM, Schessel DA, Pfeiderer A, Kassel EE, Roweed DW. Conservative management of acoustic neuromas. *Otolaryngol Clin North Am.* 1992; 25(3):691.

70. Nadol JB Jr, Chiong CM, Ojemann RG, et al. Preservation of hearing and facial nerve function in resection of acoustic neuroma. *Laryngoscope.* 1992; 102:1153.

71. Lalwani AK, Yuan-Shin F, Jackler RK, et al. Facial nerve outcome after acoustic neuroma surgery: A study from the era of cranial nerve monitoring. *Otolaryngol Head Neck Surg.* 1994; 111:561.

72. Nedzelski JM, Chiong CM, Cashman MZ. Hearing preservation in acoustic neuroma surgery: Value of monitoring cochlear nerve action potentials. *Otolaryngol Head Neck Surg.* 1994; 111:703.

73. Hirsch JW, Noren G. Audiological findings after stereotactic radiosurgery in acoustic neurinomas. *Acta Otolaryngol (Stockh).* 1988; 106:244.

74. Lunsford LD, Linskey ME. Stereotactic radiosurgery in the treatment of patients with acoustic tumors. *Otolaryngol Clin North Am.* 1992; 25(2):471.

75. Slattery WH III, Brackmann DE. Results of surgery following stereotactic irradiation for acoustic neuromas. *Am J Otol.* 1994; 16:315.

76. Doyle KJ, Shelton C. Hearing preservation in bilateral acoustic neuroma surgery. *J Otology (Am).* 1993; 14:562.

77. Briggs RJ, Brackmann DE, Baser ME, et al. Comprehensive management of bilateral acoustic neuromas. *Arch Otolaryngol Head Neck Surg.* 1994; 120:1307.

78. Gadre AK, Kwartler JA, Brackmann DE, et al. Middle fossa decompression of the internal auditory canal in acoustic neuroma surgery: A therapeutic alternative. *Laryngoscope.* 1990; 100:948.

79. Igarashi M, Alford BR, Herndon JW, Saito R. Cerebellopontine meningiomas and the temporal bone. *Arch Otolaryngol.* 1971; 94:224.

80. Kumar A, Mafee M, Vassalli L, Applebaum E. Intracranial and intratemporal meningiomas with primary otologic symptoms. *Otolaryngol Head Neck Surg.* 1988; 99:444.

81. Gentry LR, Jacoby CG, Turski PA, Houston LW, Strother CM, Sackett JF. Cerebellopontine angle-petromastoid mass lesions: comparative study of diagnosis with MR imaging and CT. *Radiology.* 1987; 162:513.

82. Press GA, Hesselink JR. MR imaging of cerebellopontine an-

gle and internal auditory canal lesions at 1.5T. *AJR.* 1988; 150:1371.

83. Neely JG, Alford BR. Facial nerve neuromas. *Arch Otolaryngol.* 1974; 100:298.

84. Pillsbury HC, Price HC, Gardiner LJ. Primary tumors of the facial nerve: Diagnosis and management. *Laryngoscope.* 1983; 93:1045.

85. O'Donoghue GM, Brackmann DE, House JW, et al. Neuromas of the facial nerve. *J Otology (Am).* 1989; 10:49.

86. Lateck JT, Gabrielsen TO, Knake JL, et al. Facial nerve neuromas: Radiologic evaluation. *Radiology.* 1983; 149:731.

87. Inoue Y, Tabuchi T, Hakuba A, et al. Facial nerve neuromas: CT findings. *J Comp Asst Tomog.* 1987; 2:942.

88. Daniels DL, Czervionke LF, Pojunas KW. Facial nerve enhancement in MR imaging. *NJNR.* 1987; 8:605.

89. Shelton C, Brackmann DE, Lo WW, et al. Infratemporal facial nerve hemangiomas. *Otolaryngol Head Neck Surg.* 1991; 104:116.

90. Curtin HD, Jensen JE, Barnes L Jr, et al. "Ossifying" hemangiomas of the temporal bone: Evaluation with CT. *Radiology.* 1987; 164:831.

91. Lo WW, Shelton C, Waluch V, et al. Infratemporal vascular tumors: Detection with CT and MR imaging. *Radiology.* 1989; 171:445.

92. Mair IW, Roald B, Lilleas F, et al. Cavernous hemangioma of the middle ear. *J Otology (Am).* 1994; 15:254.

93. Sutbeyaz Y, Selimoglu E, Karasen M, et al. Hemangiopericytoma of the middle ear: Case report and literature review. *J Laryngol Otol.* 1995; 109:977.

94. Horn KL, Shea JJ, Brackmann DE. Congenital cholesteatoma of the petrous pyramid. *Arch Otolaryngol.* 1985; 111: 621.

95. Saunders JE, Kwartler JA, Wolf HK, et al. Lipomas of the internal auditory canal. *Laryngoscope.* 1991; 101:1031.

96. Thedinger BA, Nadol JB, Montgomery WW, Thedinger BS, Greenberg JJ. Radiographic diagnosis, surgical treatment and long term follow up of cholesterol granulomas of the petrous apex. *Laryngoscope.* 1989; 99:896.

97. Michael L, Wells M. Squamous cell carcinoma of the middle ear. *Clin Otolaryngol.* 1980; 5:235.

98. Maurer HM, Bettangady M, Gehan EA, et al. The Intergroup Rhabdomyosarcoma Study-I, a final report. *Cancer.* 1988; 61: 209.

99. Wiatrak BJ, Pensak ML. Rhabdomyosarcoma of the ear and temporal bone. *Laryngoscope.* 1989; 99:1188.

100. Glasscock ME III, McKennan KX, Levine SC, et al. Primary adenocarcinoma of the middle ear and temporal bone. *Arch Otolaryngol Head Neck Surg.* 1987; 113:822.

101. Hill BA, Kohut RI. Metastatic adenocarcinoma of the temporal bone. *Arch Otolaryngol.* 1976; 102:568.

102. Seidman MD, Nichols RD, Raju UB. Extracranial skull base chondrosarcoma. *Ear Nose Throat J.* 1989; 68:626.

III. PATHOLOGY OF THE EAR
AND TEMPORAL BONE

■ C A R O L   F .   A D A I R

■ B R U C E   M .   W E N I G

EMBRYOLOGY, ANATOMY, AND HISTOLOGY

EXTERNAL EAR

The ear can be considered as three distinct regions or compartments: the external ear, the middle ear and temporal bone, and the inner ear. The external ear develops from the first branchial groove. The external auricle (pinna) forms from the fusion of the auricular hillocks or tubercles, a group of mesenchymal tissue swellings from the first and second branchial arches that lie around the external portion of the first branchial groove.[1] The external auditory canal is considered a normal remnant of the first bran-

chial groove. The tympanic membrane forms from the first and second branchial pouches and the first branchial groove.[1] The ectoderm of the first branchial groove gives rise to the epithelium on the external side, the endoderm from the first branchial pouch gives rise to the epithelium on the internal side, and the mesoderm of the first and second branchial pouches gives rise to the connective tissue lying between the external and internal epithelia.[1] The middle ear space develops from invagination of the first branchial pouch (pharyngotympanic tube) from the primitive pharynx. The eustachian tube and tympanic cavity develop from the endoderm of the first branchial pouch; the malleus and incus develop from the mesoderm of the first branchial arch (Meckel's cartilage), while the incus develops from

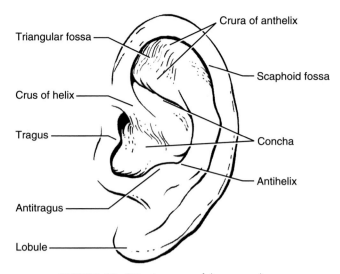

FIGURE 12-20 Anatomy of the external ear.

Labels on figure:
Triangular fossa
Crus of helix
Tragus
Antitragus
Lobule
Crura of anthelix
Scaphoid fossa
Concha
Antihelix

The anatomy of the external ear is seen in Figure 12–20. The outer portion of the external ear includes the auricle or pinna leading into the external auditory canal with its medial limit being the external aspect of the tympanic membrane. Histologically, the auricle is essentially a cutaneous structure composed of keratinizing, stratified squamous epithelium with associated dermal adnexal structures that include hair follicles, sebaceous glands, and eccrine sweat glands. The subcutaneous tissue is composed of fibroconnective tissue, fat, and elastic-type fibrocartilage that gives the auricle its structural support. In addition to the dermal adnexal structures, the outer third of the external canal is noteworthy for the presence of modified apocrine glands called ceruminal glands that replace the eccrine glands seen in the auricular dermis. Ceruminal glands produce cerumen and are arranged in clusters composed of cuboidal cells with eosinophilic cytoplasm often containing a granular, golden-yellow pigment. These cells have secretory droplets along their luminal border. In the inner portion of the external auditory canal, ceruminal glands, as well as the other adnexal structures, are absent. Similar to the auricle, the external auditory canal is lined by keratinizing squamous epithelium that extends to include the entire canal and covers the external aspect of the tympanic membrane. The inner two thirds of the external auditory canal contains bone rather than cartilage.

The anatomy of the external, middle, and inner ear is seen in Figure 12–21. The middle ear or tympanic cavity contents include the ossicles (malleus, incus, and stapes), eustachian tube, tympanic cavity proper, epitympanic recess, mastoid cavity, and the chorda tympani of the facial (VII) nerve. The middle ear and the external ear function as conduits for sound conduction for the auditory part of the

the mesoderm of the second branchial arch (Reichert's cartilage).[1] The first division of the ear to develop is the inner ear that appears toward the end of the first month of gestation.[1,2] The membranous labyrinth, including the utricle, saccule, semicircular ducts, and cochlear duct arises from the otic vesicle (otocyst). The otic vesicle forms from the invagination of the surface ectoderm, located on either side of the neural plate, into the mesenchyme. This invagination eventually loses its connection with the surface ectoderm. The bony labyrinth—including the vestibule, semicircular canals, and cochlea—arises from the mesenchyme around the otic vesicle.[1,2]

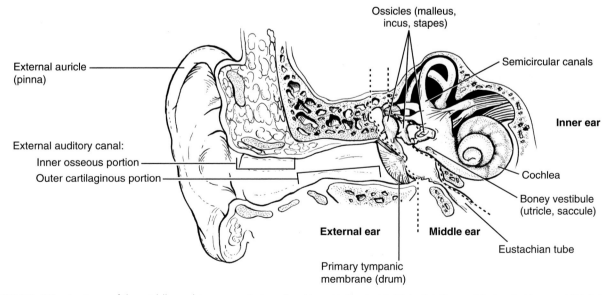

Labels on figure:
External auricle (pinna)
External auditory canal:
Inner osseous portion
Outer cartilaginous portion
Ossicles (malleus, incus, stapes)
Semicircular canals
Inner ear
Cochlea
Boney vestibule (utricle, saccule)
Eustachian tube
External ear
Middle ear
Primary tympanic membrane (drum)

FIGURE 12-21 Anatomy of the middle and inner ear. Redrawn from Hyams V, Batsakis JG, Michaels L. Tumors of the ear. In: Hartmann WH, Sobin LH, eds. *Tumors of the Upper Respiratory Tract and Ear.* 2nd series. Fascicle 25. Washington DC: Armed Forces Institute of Pathology; 1988:258, with permission.

internal ear. The anatomic limits of the middle ear include:

1. Lateral or internal aspect made up by the tympanic membrane and squamous portion of the temporal bone
2. Medial aspect bordered by the petrous portion of the temporal bone
3. Superior (roof) delimited by the tegmen tympani, a thin plate of bone separating the middle ear space from the cranial cavity
4. Inferior (floor) aspect bordered by a thin plate of bone separating the tympanic cavity from the superior bulb of the internal jugular vein
5. Anterior aspect delimited by a thin plate of bone separating the tympanic cavity from the carotid canal housing the internal carotid artery
6. Posterior aspect delimited by the petrous portion of the temporal bone containing the mastoid antrum and mastoid air cells.

Histologically, the lining of the middle ear is a respiratory epithelium varying from ciliated epithelium in the eustachian tube to a flat, single, cuboidal epithelium in the tympanic cavity and mastoid. The epithelial lining of the eustachian tube becomes pseudostratified as it approaches the pharyngeal end. Under normal conditions, there are no glandular elements within the middle ear. The eustachian tubes contain a lymphoid component, particularly in children, that is referred to as Gerlach's tubal tonsil. The ossicular articulations are typical synovial joints.

The internal ear is embedded within the petrous portion of the temporal bone and consists of the structures of the membranous and osseous labyrinth and the internal auditory canal in which the vestibulocochlear (VIII) nerve runs. The internal ear is the sense organ for hearing and balance. The anatomy and histology of this region are complex and beyond the scope of this chapter. The reader is referred to specific texts detailing the inner ear anatomy and histology.

Among the different neoplasms of the ear encountered by the surgical pathologist are those of cutaneous origin. This is true regarding biopsy material as well as frozen sections. The important issue relative to frozen section of cutaneous lesions is adequacy of tumor excision, that is, whether the margins of resection are clear of tumor. Figure 12–22 shows the handling and sectioning of external ear tumors.

Frozen sections of tumors of the external canal, middle ear, and mastoid aid in determining whether tumor is present and, if possible, the specific tumor type. The resection margins from larger resection specimens of this region are best handled at the surgical pathology bench rather than at frozen section. The gross dissection of temporal bone resections, whether total or subtotal, is problematic given the predominance of the osseous component of the specimen. Orientation of the specimen with the identification of the surgical margins of resection is

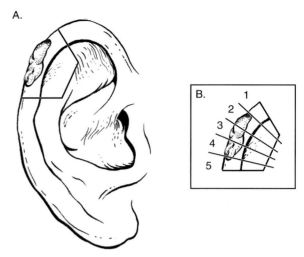

FIGURE 12–22 *A and B. Sectioning of cutaneous tumors of the external ear. Sequential sectioning of the lesion to include the entire tumor as well as the surgical margins of resection (i.e., lateral and deep).*

essential for the proper sectioning of the specimen. This requires a close interaction with the surgeon and radiologist in determining the site of origin of the tumor (e.g., external auditory canal, middle ear, mastoid, inner ear) and the extent of invasion. The surgical pathologist is responsible for determining the tumor type, site of origin and extent, and predominant direction of tumor invasion. Important questions that must be addressed include the relationship of the tumor with surrounding structures, whether there is involvement of the parotid gland, whether the tympanic membrane is intact or violated by the tumor, and whether the surgical margins of resection are free of tumor.

Non-Neoplastic Lesions

The classification of non-neoplastic lesions of the ear and temporal bone can be found in Table 12–7.

KELOID

Gross Pathology

Keloids are characterized grossly by a homogeneous rubbery white nodule, often polypoid, covered by thin glistening hairless skin. The size is variable, usually less than 2 cm in the case of keloids associated with ear piercing; however, they may attain a diameter of several centimeters, with rare gigantic examples.[3,4]

Microscopic Pathology

The histologic appearance is quite characteristic and includes haphazardly arranged fascicles of hyalinized collagenous fibers with scattered fibroblasts and myofibroblasts. The proliferation is not encapsulated, but blends subtly with the surrounding der-

TABLE 12-7	CLASSIFICATION OF NON-NEOPLASTIC LESIONS OF THE EAR, AND TEMPORAL BONE

EXTERNAL EAR

Developmental (accessory tragi, first branchial cleft anomalies, others)
Infectious
Keloid
Epidermal and sebaceous cysts
Idiopathic cystic chondromalacia
Chondrodermatitis nodularis helicis chronicus
Angiolymphoid hyperplasia with eosinophilia/Kimura's disease
Systemic disease (relapsing polychondritis, gout)
Exostosis

MIDDLE AND INNER EAR, INCLUDING TEMPORAL BONE

Developmental and congenital anomalies
Infectious (otitis media)
Otic or aural polyp
Cholesteatoma
Otosclerosis
Langerhans' cell histiocytosis (eosinophilic granuloma)
Heterotopias (central nervous system tissue, salivary gland)
Teratoma
Others

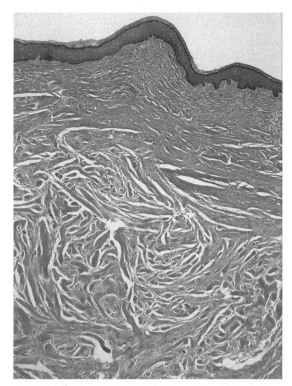

FIGURE 12-23 The haphazard fascicles of hyalinized collagen blend with the surrounding dermal fibers in this keloid. The overlying skin is thinned and hairless.

mal fibrous tissue (Fig. 12–23). The collagen bundles are often separated by dermal mucosubstances, which lend an "edematous" appearance to the nodule. The lesion is poorly vascularized, with widely scattered dilated blood vessels, and the overlying epidermis is thin and atrophic, without dermal adnexal structures. Keloids treated with corticosteroid injection may contain pools of amorphous mucin-like material, sometimes associated with a mild foreign-body type reaction (Fig. 12–24). The material is histochemically distinct from epithelial mucins and from the connective tissue mucin seen in cutaneous mucinosis.[5]

Differential Diagnosis

The clinical setting usually makes the differential diagnosis quite simple. To be considered in the gross and histologic differential are hypertrophic scar, dermatofibroma, and dermatofibrosarcoma protuberans. The distinction from hypertrophic scar is of minimal clinical importance; however, several histologic features are helpful in addition to the clinical appearance. Hypertrophic scars lack the dense hyalinized collagenous fibers seen in keloids, having more delicate fibrillar collagen. The collagen and fibroblastic cells in hypertrophic scars demonstrate a more orderly arrangement parallel to the skin surface. Mature hypertrophic scars generally do not have an abundance of mucosubstances and therefore

have a more compact microscopic appearance.[6] The extremely low cellularity of keloids distinguishes them from dermatofibromas. The latter also usually have associated hyperplasia of the overlying epidermis. Kuo et al[7] described an unusual variant of dermatofibroma characterized by keloidal type changes and referred to as keloidal dermatofibroma. Although dermatofibrosarcoma protuberans is often polypoid, it is also an intensely cellular fibrous neoplasm that is collagen-poor.

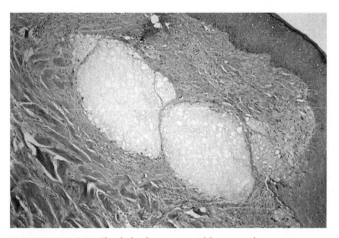

FIGURE 12-24 This keloid was treated by steroid injection, which has resulted in small steroid lakes.

Clinicopathologic Correlation

Keloids are not true neoplasms, but rather represent an exaggerated reaction to trauma. They are similar morphologically to a hypertrophic scar, and in fact represent one extreme of the spectrum of reparative reactions of the skin.

Differences in fibrin degradation between normal skin fibroblasts and keloidal fibroblasts have recently been described. These differences may be related to the exaggerated scarring seen in patients who manifest a propensity for keloid development.[8]

IDIOPATHIC CYSTIC CHONDROMALACIA OF THE AURICULAR CARTILAGE

Gross Pathology

The excised tissue may include only a fragment of the cyst wall or, less often, a full-thickness excision of the ear. An intact cyst usually contains fluid, which has been described as "olive-oil-like."[9] The cyst wall consists of a 1 to 2 mm rim of cartilage; the lining may have a smooth and glistening cartilaginous surface or may include roughened rust-colored patches. The cyst is usually an elongated cleft, but multifocal cystic degeneration may be seen.

Microscopic Pathology

The cystic cleft is centrally placed in the cartilaginous plate (Fig. 12–25). No epithelial lining is present, rather the cyst is the result of loss of cartilage, hence the term "pseudocyst." There may be a rim of fibrous tissue along the inner rim of the cyst, or granulation tissue with plump fibroblasts and a delicate vascular proliferation may form part of the pseudocyst lining, corresponding to rust-colored areas grossly (Fig. 12–26). In long-standing cases fibrous tissue may essentially obliterate the cystic space.[9–11]

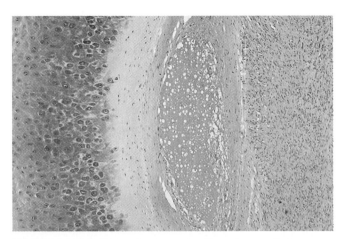

FIGURE 12–26 Idiopathic cystic chondromalacia with remaining viable cartilage seen on the left and fibroblastic tissue on the right of the cystic lesion. Note the absence of an epithelial lining; mucoid material fills the cystic space.

Differential Diagnosis

Some lesions of cystic chondromalacia are characterized by a distinctly proliferative cartilaginous response, developing a thickened cartilaginous wall. There may be slight cytologic atypia in such instances, suggesting the differential diagnostic possibility of chondrosarcoma. However, the orderly nature of the proliferation and the associated central cystic degeneration facilitate the exclusion of a malignant neoplasm.[12]

Clinicopathologic Correlation

Idiopathic cystic chondromalacia (ICC) is a cystic degenerative process of the auricular cartilage, of unknown etiology, that typically occurs in young and middle-aged men. It is uncommon in women. ICC most often occurs adjacent to the helix. Although trauma has been implicated in the development of these lesions, there is no definitive connection to prior trauma.

CHONDRODERMATITIS NODULARIS CHRONICUS HELICIS

Gross Pathology

The lesion of chondrodermatitis nodularis chronicus helicis (CNCH) usually ranges in diameter from 3 to 18 mm, with an average of 7 mm. Rare lesions achieve diameters of 2 to 3 cm. The dome-shaped nodule is usually light grey, somewhat translucent, and often has a scale crust covering the central area of ulceration.[13]

Microscopic Pathology

The lesion of CNCH is characterized by alterations in the epidermis, dermis, and, more variably, in the

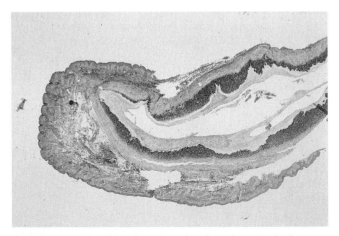

FIGURE 12–25 Idiopathic cystic chondromalacia, with elastic stain demonstrating the cystic degeneration of the central portion of the cartilaginous plate. The cyst is partially lined by connective tissue.

auricular cartilage. Some degree of acanthosis is present in the epidermis immediately surrounding a depressed ulcer in most cases. Hyperkeratosis and parakeratosis frequently accompany the epidermal hyperplasia. The ulcerated area varies in depth, from a shallow ulcer bed with exuberant granulation tissue at its base to a deep crater extending as far as the auricular cartilage (Figs. 12–27 and 12–28). The dermis lacks cutaneous adnexal structures in the area of the lesion, and the vasculature appears telangiectatic. The dermis underneath the ulcer contains chronic, and sometimes acute, inflammatory cells along with a pronounced capillary proliferation. The dermis may show areas of fibrinoid eosinophilic material or, in some cases, frank necrobiosis of the collagen may be present. Occasionally palisading histiocytes are seen in association with the necrobiotic collagen. The changes in the auricular cartilage deep to the ulcer range from mild perichondritis through variable degrees of degenerative changes characterized by edema, loss of chondrocytes, and smudging and hyalinization of the chondroid matrix. The necrotic material from the dermis, and occasionally even fragments of degenerated cartilage, may protrude into the ulcer crater.[14,15]

The uncommon lesions arising on the antihelix have been noted to differ histologically as well as

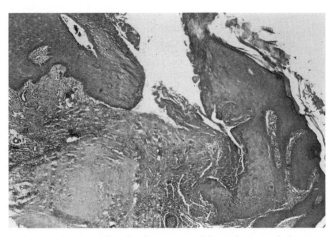

FIGURE 12–28 Chondrodermatitis nodularis chronicus helicis showing damaged dermal collagen fibers protruding into the central ulcerated area, demonstrating the concept of transepidermal elimination of collagen.

clinically from the typical helical lesions. They lack the epidermal hyperplasia of helical CNCH, and the cartilaginous changes rarely exceed mild perichondritis. The predominant alterations involve the dermal vasculature, which is dilated and thickened.[16]

Differential Diagnosis

CNCH is frequently misdiagnosed as a cutaneous malignancy, particularly as basal cell carcinoma or squamous cell carcinoma. Metzger and Goodman[17] noted a clinical diagnosis of either a malignant or premalignant lesion in 80% of the cases they reviewed. Unfortunately, the same mistake may be perpetuated by microscopic examination, particularly if the epidermal hyperplastic changes are misinterpreted as representing either squamous cell carcinoma or a hypertrophic actinic keratosis. Observation of the extensive dermal changes and usually some degree of cartilaginous alterations, along with the well-demarcated nature of the epidermal proliferation and lack of cytologic atypia in the adjacent epidermis, should help in differentiating CNCH from a squamous cell neoplasm.

Clinicopathologic Correlation

CNCH is a non-neoplastic ulcerative lesion of the ear. The etiology of CNCH is not known, but several theories have been suggested. Because the skin of the auricle is quite thin, with little subcutaneous fat, the area may be unusually sensitive to trauma. In addition, vascular supply to the area is somewhat tenuous, with the avascular cartilage depending on the dermal circulation for sustenance. These anatomic features of the auricle may predispose it to the development of CNCH. Winkler,[18] in his original description, attributed the lesions to primary cartilaginous changes; however, the cutaneous alterations, which seem to have greater significance and

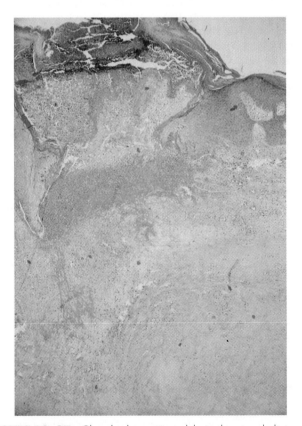

FIGURE 12–27 Chondrodermatitis nodularis chronicus helicis showing a central crust covering the area of ulceration through which dermal collagen fibers protrude through the epidermis. There is degenerative change of the dermis down to and including the cartilage.

constancy, are more likely linked to etiology. In fact, the mild changes present in the cartilage of most patients with CNCH do not differ significantly from age-related alterations normally seen in the population most at risk.[19] Carol and Van Haren[20] favored hyperkeratosis and epidermal hyperplasia as causative of the ulceration. It is more likely that the development of CNCH is multifactorial. Santa Cruz[14] postulated that CNCH is related to the perforating dermatoses, which are characterized by the transepidermal elimination of material such as elastic fibers or degenerated collagen through a disruption in the epidermis. Trauma is thought to be an initiating factor in many of the perforating dermatoses.[15]

RELAPSING POLYCHONDRITIS

Gross Pathology

The auricular cartilage is involved, usually bilaterally, in nearly 90% of patients with relapsing polychondritis (RP).[21,22] The affected ear is erythematous, swollen, and very tender. In advanced cases there may be distortion of the pinna due to destruction of the cartilage. The overlying skin is not ulcerated.

Microscopic Pathology

The primary finding in RP is perichondrial inflammation with a mixed infiltrate of lymphocytes, plasma cells, polymorphonuclear leukocytes, and occasional eosinophils that blurs the interface between the perichondrium and the auricular cartilage (Figs. 12–29 and 12–30). By hematoxylin and eosin staining, there is loss of the usual basophilia in the cartilage, which appears more eosinophilic. At the advancing edge of the inflammation there is loss of chondrocytes and destruction of lacunar architecture. As cartilage is destroyed, it is replaced by granulation tissue and eventually by fibrous tissue. Immunomicroscopic findings have been described,

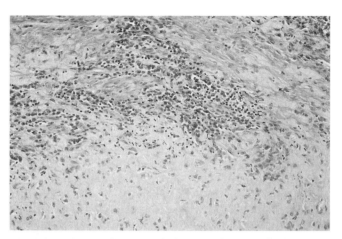

FIGURE 12–30 Relapsing polychondritis showing inflammatory cells concentrated along the irregular border of the damaged cartilaginous plate of the auricle.

in some cases showing diffuse granular deposition of IgG and C3 in the perichondrial fibrous tissue.[23]

Differential Diagnosis

The localization of the inflammatory infiltrate to the perichondrial-cartilaginous interface without significant cellulitis is helpful in excluding an infectious process such as external otitis or acute infectious perichondritis in patients with RP. Other differential diagnostic considerations are primarily clinical and include gout and a variety of rheumatologic diseases. Gout is characterized by deposition of polarizable crystalline urate that usually elicits a granulomatous inflammatory reaction. A variety of rheumatologic diseases may be associated with RP, including rheumatoid arthritis, Sjögren's syndrome, systemic lupus erythematosis, scleroderma, Reiter's syndrome, and Raynaud's syndrome.[21,24] These diseases may have manifestations in other organs, which overlap those seen in RP as well. Other associated "autoimmune" diseases have been described in patients with RP, including autoimmune thyroid disease, ulcerative colitis, glomerulonephritis, and pernicious anemia.[24] Relapsing polychondritis has also been linked to a paraneoplastic syndrome in patients with hematopoietic disorders, including leukemias and myelodysplastic syndromes.[25–27] In these diseases, RP should be considered as a possible coexistent disorder; biopsy confirmation is more often necessary for confirmation of RP in the presence of these "overlap" diseases.

Clinicopathologic Correlation

Relapsing polychondritis is an uncommon systemic relapsing disease characterized by progressive degeneration of cartilaginous structures throughout the body. Although the etiology of RP has not been clearly elucidated, there is accumulating evidence

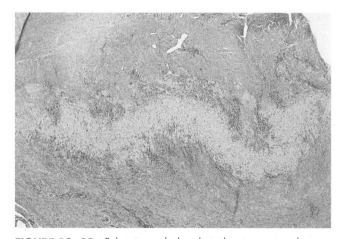

FIGURE 12–29 Relapsing polychondritis showing a mixed inflammatory infiltrate blurring the interface between the cartilaginous plate and the dermal collagen. The cartilage has a ragged border.

for an autoimmune process. Patients with RP have been known to have factors in their serum that react with cartilage.[28] Circulating antibodies to type II collagen,[29] found only in cartilage with titers reflecting the severity of disease, as well as the documentation of immunofluorescent localization of immune complex components at the perichondrial-cartilaginous interface, have been reported in patients with RP.[30–32] These findings, plus the association of RP with an array of known autoimmune systemic diseases, lend additional support to an autoimmune etiology.

GOUT

Gout is a disorder of purine metabolism or renal excretion of uric acid. In gout, there is a precipitation of monosodium urate as deposits or "tophi" throughout the body. The helix of the ear represents one of the more common sites for gouty tophi. Histologically, gouty tophi are composed of needle-shaped aggregates of urate crystals with a surrounding foreign-body giant cell reaction (Fig. 12–31). Urate crystals are water soluble; therefore, if a diagnosis of gout is suspected, the resected tissue should be fixed in absolute alcohol.

ANGIOLYMPHOID HYPERPLASIA WITH EOSINOPHILIA

Gross Pathology

Angiolymphoid hyperplasia with eosinophilia (ALHE) is characterized by either single or multiple clustered pink to red-brown indurated cutaneous papules or subcutaneous nodules, a few millimeters to 1 cm in diameter, involving the ear or periauricular skin, though they may be seen elsewhere on the face and, infrequently, on the trunk and extremities. Clusters of papules may coalesce to form a plaque

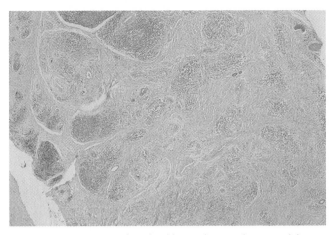

FIGURE 12–32 Angiolymphoid hyperplasia with eosinophilia showing a patchy lymphoid infiltrate accompanying a vascular proliferation.

that may be up to 8 cm in diameter.[33–35] The surface of the papule of ALHE is usually unremarkable, though some are eroded, with adherent scale crust.

Microscopic Pathology

Angiolymphoid hyperplasia with eosinophilia is characterized by a nodular vascular proliferation accompanied by a variably dense lymphoid infiltrate rich in eosinophils (Fig. 12–32). The process is circumscribed but not encapsulated and may involve the subcutis or dermis, or both. The vascular proliferation involves small vessels, ranging from capillaries to small and medium-sized arteries and veins. The vessels are increased in number and are lined by plump appearing (epithelioid) endothelial cells (Figs. 12–33 and 12–34). A lobular arrangement of the proliferating vessels may be evident, as is seen in hemangiomas, but the distribution of vessels is

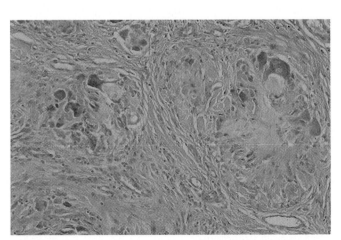

FIGURE 12–31 Gouty tophi are composed of needle-shaped aggregates of urate crystals with a surrounding foreign-body giant cell reaction.

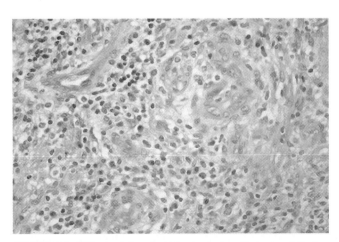

FIGURE 12–33 Angiolymphoid hyperplasia with eosinophilia in which scattered eosinophils are admixed with the lymphoplasmacytic infiltrate. Neutrophils may also be present. The vessels are thickened, with plump epithelioid endothelial cells.

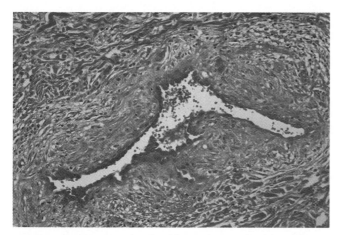

FIGURE 12–34 Angiolymphoid hyperplasia with eosinophilia. Larger vessels demonstrate the prominence of the epithelioid endothelial lining.

more haphazard. The endothelial cell nuclei are variably enlarged and display mild pleomorphism and hyperchromasia.[33,35,36] These nuclei may protrude conspicuously into the vessel lumen or may form a cobblestone-like pavement lining the vessel.[37] The vessels vary from irregular, poorly canalized, thinwalled spaces to rounded well-formed vessels with thickened walls. In some cases there is evidence of disruption or damage to some of the involved vessels.[33,34,38,39] The inflammatory infiltrate varies in density, from patchy to heavy and diffuse. The inflammatory cells are predominantly composed of lymphocytes, histiocytes, and eosinophils and surround aggregates of proliferating vessels and infiltrate between them. The proportion of eosinophils is quite variable. On occasion, eosinophils may be few in number or absent. Lymphoid follicles may be seen, but they are not a major component of ALHE. The overlying epidermis is usually acanthotic, with or without parakeratosis. Surface erosion is present in some cases.

Differential Diagnosis

The most important histologic differential diagnoses are lobular capillary hemangioma and angiosarcoma. ALHE is distinguished from hemangioma by the prominence of epithelioid endothelial features and by the associated lymphoplasmacytic and eosinophilic infiltrate. Although angiosarcoma may be suggested by the enlargement and nuclear atypia of the endothelial cells, the clinical pattern and the presence of the characteristic inflammatory infiltrate are helpful features in identifying ALHE. Further, the interconnecting or ramifying vascular pattern seen in angiosarcoma is not found in ALHE.

Clinicopathologic Correlation

Angiolymphoid hyperplasia with eosinophilia has been a controversial lesion with regard to its classification as a reactive or neoplastic process, as well as to its relationship to Kimura's disease. A history of trauma elicited in a number of cases, as well as the microscopic impression of vascular damage and the demonstration of immunoglobulin deposits in the vessels have led several observers to favor a reactive or reparative etiology.[33,35,38] Hormonal influences may play a role in some cases, as suggested by the association with pregnancy in some patients.

Kimura's disease shares many histologic features with ALHE. The two lesions have been considered a single entity; however, prominent clinical differences and more subtle histologic differences have caused reconsideration of this issue.[40] Recent studies support separation of the two as distinct clinicopathologic entities.[37,39,41–43] Kimura's disease occurs in Asians. In contrast to ALHE, Kimura's disease tends to affect males, is often associated with regional lymphadenopathy and peripheral eosinophilia, is a larger lesion than the one seen in ALHE, and tends to occur in sites other than the head and neck. The histologic features are also different in Kimura's disease. In Kimura's disease the lymphoid proliferation predominates, eclipsing the vascular proliferation, which is usually sparse and exhibits minimal epithelioid endothelial changes. Kimura's disease is usually located deeper than ALHE, often extending to the fascia and even to skeletal muscle, and the subcutaneous fat is usually fibrotic. Eosinophils are always numerous in Kimura's disease, but may be sparse or even absent in ALHE.

It has been suggested that ALHE be categorized with a group of neoplastic lesions that include epithelioid hemangioepithelioma.[43] However, the behavior of ALHE and the evidence for a reactive etiology mitigate against this approach.

NECROTIZING (MALIGNANT) EXTERNAL OTITIS

Gross Pathology

The changes of necrotizing external otitis (NEO) are most pronounced in the osseous portion of the external canal, where the destructive infection usually begins.[44–46] In this area the skin becomes ulcerated, leaving a layer of thick granulation tissue covering the underlying exposed and irregularly eroded bone, usually along the anterior and inferior surfaces of the external auditory canal.[44–47] Necrotic tissue is abundant in fully developed NEO and may, along with purulent exudate, obstruct the canal. The adjacent skin of the cartilaginous portion of the canal is erythematous and swollen and, as the disease progresses, may be covered with a yellow-grey layer of necrotic skin and exudate.

Microscopic Pathology

The histologic appearance of NEO is dominated by necrotic material and exuberant granulation tissue. If epithelium remains, it is ulcerated with pseudoepitheliomatous hyperplasia adjacent to denuded areas. Diffuse, heavy, acute, and chronic inflammation is seen in the subcutis, and a necrotizing vasculitis is commonly present. The bone and cartilage are necrotic, with acute and chronic inflammatory cells massively infiltrating adjacent viable bone. Sequestra of nonviable bone or cartilage may be seen.[48] The dermis is eventually replaced by acellular collagen.

Special Techniques

Gram-negative bacilli are easily demonstrated by tissue gram stain.

Differential Diagnosis

The infectious nature of NEO is usually evident from the clinical course and the histologic findings; however, the presence of pseudoepitheliomatous hyperplasia of the squamous epithelium along with sometimes striking reactive atypia may suggest squamous cell carcinoma. Conversely, squamous cell carcinoma, if associated with extensive necrosis, may elude diagnosis by biopsy, yielding only necroinflammatory material such as one encounters in NEO. Occasionally the clinical presentation of squamous cell carcinoma of the external auditory canal may closely mimic NEO,[49,50] or the two diseases may occur concurrently.[46]

Clinicopathologic Correlation

Whereas otitis externa (swimmer's ear), a chronic limited infection of the external auditory canal, is most often caused by *Pseudomonas aeruginosa,* the same organism responsible for NEO, the clinical course is dramatically different. Swimmer's ear involves the cartilaginous portion of the external canal and, though painful, rarely becomes life-threatening. Host alterations appear to be responsible for the aggressive course of Pseudomonas infection in NEO.

The key elements in the development of NEO are traumatic interruption, usually minor, in the integrity of the skin lining the external auditory canal and immune impairment of the host. These two factors are essential in allowing the causative organism, *Pseudomonas aeruginosa,* access to the tissue. The organism, by virtue of its endo- and exotoxins, neurotoxins, collagenases, and elastases, is capable of causing rapid extensive tissue necrosis and necrotizing vasculitis that compounds the destruction.[48] The typical clinical setting is that of a chronically debilitated or immunologically deficient patient.[51,52] The host, most often an older diabetic, usually has microangiopathy and a migratory defect of polymorphonuclear leukocytes related to systemic disease. These host factors that impede the inflammatory response to infection, combined with the destructive devices of *P. aeruginosa,* are thought to be responsible for the lethal potential of NEO.[48,53] Early fibrotic

changes in the dermis and perichondrium of the canal, suggesting a predisposing injury secondary to diabetic microangiopathy, have been also described.[54,55]

KERATOSIS OBTURANS

Gross Pathology

The plug-like mass removed from the ear canal in keratosis obturans is pearly white and densely lamellated, similar to the contents of a middle ear cholesteatoma.

Microscopic Pathology

The lesion consists of a dense plug of concentrically lamellated keratin. If canal lining epithelium is present it may be inflamed.

Differential Diagnosis

The chief differential diagnostic consideration is cholesteatoma of the external auditory canal, a rare lesion associated with unilateral pain and otorrhea.[56] It usually occurs in an older population and, in contrast to keratosis obturans, is a localized process causing bone destruction. Histologically the keratin in keratosis obturans is densely packed, whereas in cholesteatoma it is loosely layered.

EXOSTOSES

Gross Pathology

The gross appearance of exostosis is usually better appreciated by the surgeon, as only fragments are available to the pathologist in most cases. The intact exostosis is a broad-based, mound-like bony proliferation similar in color and texture to normal cortical bone. It is covered by a layer of periosteum with overlying thin meatal skin.

Microscopic Pathology

Exostoses are classically described as a compact proliferation of layers of bone in a mound. The layers are like the skin of an onion and usually lack trabecular architecture or marrow spaces (Fig. 12–35).

Differential Diagnosis

The chief differential diagnosis is osteoma, which is much less common. The distinction between exostosis and osteoma is usually readily made based on the clinical presentation. There has been some controversy regarding the ability to distinguish between the two lesions histologically. Many observers consider the lesions to be histologically different;[57–60] however, others do not find the microscopic features sufficiently distinctive to be separated.[61,62]

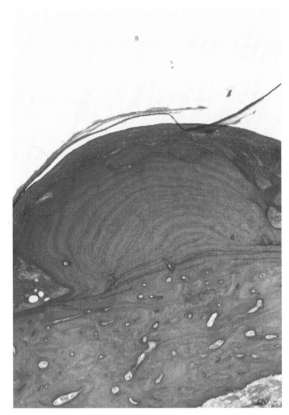

FIGURE 12–35 This exostosis is composed of laminated compact bone, giving it an "onion-skin" appearance in cross-section.

SYNOVIAL CHONDROMATOSIS

Synovial chondromatosis is a reactive process of unknown pathogenesis characterized by the formation of cartilaginous nodules in the synovium. Synovial chondromatosis of the temporomandibular joint may present as an asymptomatic mass within the external auditory canal. The histology includes nodules of mature cartilage of varying cellularity. The nodules may calcify or ossify. In some examples, there is increased cellularity with atypia, including binucleated chondrocytes. These features may suggest a chondrosarcoma. Radiographic correlation should allow for differentiating this benign proliferation from a chondrosarcoma.

Benign Neoplasms

The classification of neoplastic lesions of the external ear is listed in Table 12–8. This chapter discusses the more common and unique lesions that the pathologist can expect to confront when dealing with the surgical pathology of the ear. The most common lesions of the external ear are of cutaneous origin.

TABLE 12–8	CLASSIFICATION OF NEOPLASMS OF THE EAR AND TEMPORAL BONE

EXTERNAL EAR

Benign

Keratoacanthoma
Squamous papilloma
Seborrheic keratosis
Ceruminal gland neoplasms
Melanocytic nevi
Dermal adnexal neoplasms
Neurilemmoma/Neurofibroma
Osteoma
Chondroma
Others

Malignant

Basal cell carcinoma
Squamous cell carcinoma
Verrucous carcinoma
Ceruminal gland adenocarcinoma
Malignant melanoma
Merkel cell carcinoma
Atypical fibroxanthoma
Others

MIDDLE AND INNER EAR

Benign

Middle ear adenoma
Epithelial papilloma
Jugulotympanic paraganglioma
Meningioma
Acoustic neuroma

Indeterminant Biologic Behavior

Endolymphatic sac papillary tumor

Malignant

Middle ear adenocarcinoma
Primary squamous cell carcinoma
Rhabdomyosarcoma
Others
Secondary Tumors

KERATOACANTHOMA

Gross Pathology

Keratoacanthomas (KA) are characterized grossly by their elevated crater-like appearance, with a central depression filled with a plug-like aggregate of keratin. The mature lesion usually measures between 1.0 and 2.5 cm in diameter and is elevated 0.5 to 1.0 cm above the skin surface.[63,64] The surface, though usually not ulcerated, is irregular due to the heavy keratinization. The borders of the lesion are rolled over the central depression.

Microscopic Pathology

The cross-section of a keratoacanthoma shows an irregular proliferation of pale-staining keratinocytes with abundant cytoplasm, often with a rather "glassy" quality. Proliferating broad bulbous columns of keratinocytes extend downward into the dermis with a "pushing" border and form a cup-shaped depression filled with layers of keratin (Figs. 12–36 and 12–37). As the lesion progresses, lymphocytes and—to a lesser degree—plasma cells accumulate in the adjacent dermis. Histiocytes, some multinucleated, may be numerous. A zone of granulation tissue surrounds the keratoacanthoma. As the inflammation increases, it may infiltrate the periphery of the keratinocytic columns, causing irregularity of the deep border of the lesion. Intraepithelial microabscesses are common. Small nests of degenerated epithelium may be seen within the dermal inflammatory and fibroblastic reaction; these are not considered convincing evidence of infiltrating malignancy. The presence of nuclear atypia or thin infiltrating tongues of epithelium extending from the base of the lesion are, however, cause for concern and should preclude a simple diagnosis of keratoacanthoma.[65] A worrisome and somewhat controversial finding that has been accepted in the literature as a feature of benign keratoacanthomas is perineural invasion by the proliferating keratinocytes.[66–68] Such a finding deserves documentation and probably makes a simple benign diagnosis unwise.

Differential Diagnosis

The differential diagnosis of KA is primarily with squamous cell carcinoma. The distinction between keratoacanthoma and well-differentiated squamous cell carcinoma may be extremely difficult; it has

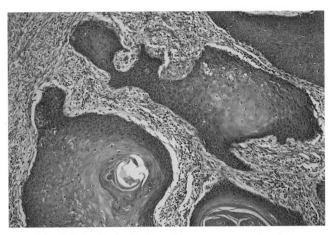

FIGURE 12–37 This keratoacanthoma is composed of anastomosing cords and islands of keratinocytes with abundant pale cytoplasm, lacking atypia.

plagued pathologists and fueled controversy for many years. The controversy is based not only on the difficulty of histologic distinction between squamous cell carcinoma and keratoacanthoma, but also on the question of the biologic potential of the lesion termed keratoacanthoma.

Clinicopathologic Correlation

Keratoacanthoma has long been a mystery for clinicians and pathologists. Its resemblance to squamous cell carcinoma contrasts with its peculiar habit of spontaneous regression or "healing." Viral and actinic influences have been suggested as etiologic factors. It has been variously considered a benign neoplasm, a tumor of uncertain malignant potential, and a variant of squamous cell carcinoma.[69,70] Much of the controversy stems from the rare, but significant, reported cases in which a lesion clinically and histologically consistent with keratoacanthoma displayed locally aggressive behavior or metastasized.[69–75] While variations in criteria for malignancy may explain many cases of "metastasizing keratoacanthoma," Hodak et al[69] have concluded that keratoacanthomas cannot reliably be distinguished from squamous cell carcinoma and should be considered one of its variants. Reed[76] proposes an indeterminant category—"carcinoma-like keratoacanthoma"—for lesions with atypical features that fall short of the criteria for carcinoma. While the controversy is by no means settled, it seems prudent when making a diagnosis of keratoacanthoma to include an annotation that these lesions cannot always be distinguished from a well-differentiated squamous cell carcinoma. Certainly, lesions with significant cytologic atypia or worrisome irregularities of the base of the lesion should not be diagnosed simply as keratoacanthoma.

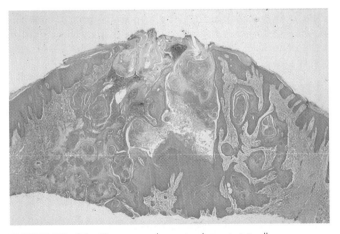

FIGURE 12–36 Keratoacanthoma is characteristically cup-shaped, with a central keratin plug. Controversy involves the distinction between keratoacanthoma and well-differentiated squamous cell carcinoma. (See Figs. 12–55 and 12–56.)

SQUAMOUS CELL PAPILLOMA AND SEBORRHEIC KERATOSIS

Squamous cell papillomas are benign epithelial neoplasms that may occur on the external ear or in the external auditory canal. Squamous cell papillomas are exophytic, tan-white lesions. Histologically, papillomas are composed of a proliferation of benign squamous cells with a central fibrovascular core. Hyperkeratosis and parakeratosis may be present.

Seborrheic keratosis (inverted follicular keratosis) may occur in the external auditory canal where differentiation from squamous cell carcinoma and basal cell carcinoma may prove difficult. The absence of cytologic atypia or invasive growth in seborrheic keratosis assists in the differential diagnosis.

CERUMINAL GLAND ADENOMA

Gross Pathology

Ceruminal gland adenomas usually range from 0.5 to 4 cm in diameter; they are slightly raised and are almost always covered by intact skin of the external auditory canal.[77,78] The cut surface may be cystic or multicystic.[78] The tumor is not encapsulated.

Microscopic Pathology

The tumor is composed of an unencapsulated, but usually well-demarcated, proliferation of variably sized, sometimes cystic glandular structures (Fig. 12–38). The glandular spaces may be scattered throughout a collagenized fibrous stroma or may be closely packed together. The apocrine-type cells that line the glands have granular eosinophilic cytoplasm with apical intraluminal projections ("snouts") and round, basally oriented nuclei with homogeneous dense chromatin (Fig. 12–39). An outer layer of flattened to cuboidal myoepithelial cells with a smaller

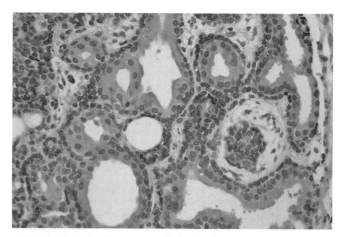

FIGURE 12–39 This ceruminal gland adenoma is characterized by well-formed glandular spaces lined by an inner layer of cuboidal to columnar cells and an outer layer of small compressed cells.

amount of clear cytoplasm and round vesicular nuclei can usually be seen in at least some of the glandular spaces.[79] The glandular lumina may contain blebs of apocrine cytoplasm and amorphous eosinophilic debris. Mitotic activity and nuclear pleomorphism are not seen.

Special Techniques

Mucin may be demonstrated in some glandular lumina and in occasional tumor cells by periodic acid-Schiff reaction with diastase digestion or with mucicarmine. Hemosiderin granules may be evident on hematoxylin-eosin stain, as well as with Prussian blue.

Clinicopathologic Correlation

The literature has been confusing with regard to glandular neoplasms of the external auditory canal, initially lumping a diverse group of lesions of variable histogenesis under the umbrella term "ceruminoma." The classification scheme utilized by Hyams and others[77,80–83] is summarized in Table 12–9 and

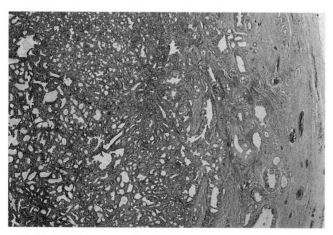

FIGURE 12–38 In ceruminal gland adenoma, the glandular proliferation is orderly and circumscribed, but not encapsulated.

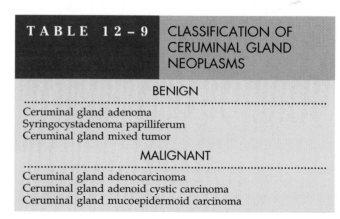

TABLE 12–9	CLASSIFICATION OF CERUMINAL GLAND NEOPLASMS
BENIGN	
Ceruminal gland adenoma	
Syringocystadenoma papilliferum	
Ceruminal gland mixed tumor	
MALIGNANT	
Ceruminal gland adenocarcinoma	
Ceruminal gland adenoid cystic carcinoma	
Ceruminal gland mucoepidermoid carcinoma	

presents these lesions in a logical manner, with consideration given to both histogenesis and biologic potential. Each entity will be discussed separately.

The ceruminal or "wax-forming" glands of the external auditory canal are apocrine-type glands, found in the lower two thirds of the dermis of the cartilaginous portion of the external auditory canal. Neoplasms of these glands are rare, but may be classified as benign ceruminal gland adenomas or as frankly malignant ceruminal gland adenocarcinomas, both of which retain the cytologic features that distinguish them as apocrine in origin. Ceruminal gland adenomas account for between 25% and 30% of glandular neoplasms of the external auditory canal.[80,84]

CERUMINAL GLAND BENIGN MIXED TUMOR

Gross Pathology

Mixed tumors arising in the external auditory canal are pathologically indistinguishable from those of salivary gland origin. The tumors reported have ranged in size from 0.5 to 3.5 cm.[85–87] They are covered by meatal skin and are circumscribed and firm. The cut surface is grey to white, often with a cartilaginous appearance.

Microscopic Pathology

Mixed tumors of the external auditory canal are well circumscribed but lack a true capsule. There may be dumbbell-shaped protrusions from the periphery of the lesion, but infiltration of surrounding tissue is not seen. Similar to salivary gland mixed tumors, ceruminal gland mixed tumors show a biphasic proliferation of epithelial cellular component and a chondromyxoid stroma. The epithelial cellular component includes tubular or ductular structures and myoepithelial cells. The latter may have an appearance ranging from spindle-shaped cells scattered through the stroma to loose aggregates of plasmacytoid-appearing cells (Fig. 12–40). The tubules often display two cell types: an inner lining cell that may bear apocrine features and an outer cuboidal to flattened myopeithelial-type cell.

Differential Diagnosis

Differential diagnostic considerations include a primary cartilaginous tumor such as chondroma or chondrosarcoma, which are both distinguished from mixed tumor by their lack of an epithelial component. A small biopsy, however, may not reflect the biphasic nature of the neoplasm and is a potential source of diagnostic error. Similarly, a cellular epithelial area of a mixed tumor may mimic a ceruminal gland adenoma if chondromyxoid stroma is not seen.

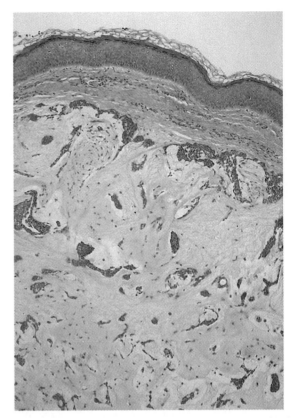

FIGURE 12–40 Like mixed tumors of the major salivary glands, ceruminal mixed tumors contain chondromyxoid stroma and an epithelial cellular component.

Clinicopathologic Correlation

Ceruminal gland mixed tumors are rare, with 26 cases reported.[85,88] Opinions vary on the histogenesis of mixed tumors of the external auditory canal; some authors postulate origin from ectopic salivary gland tissue in the canal or extension from the tail of the parotid.[88] The extreme rarity of salivary gland choristomas in the external auditory canal mitigates against this theory.[89] An origin from the ceruminal glands is favored.[84] Mixed tumors arise rarely in the auricle; these are probably cutaneous neoplasms of eccrine origin (chondroid syringoma).[84]

SYRINGOCYSTADENOMA PAPILLIFERUM

Gross Pathology

Syringocystadenoma papilliferum usually presents as a nodule or plaque, often with some degree of surface papillation, particularly in the center of the lesion. A central umbilication may be evident. The cross-sectioned specimen reveals a cyst partially filled with spongy tissue.[90] The cyst often opens to the surface through a narrow channel at its apex.

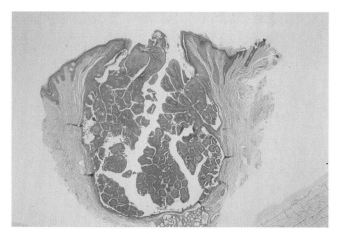

FIGURE 12–41 This cup-shaped cystic lesion, syringocystadenoma papilliferum, is filled with a papillary proliferation and communicates with the skin surface.

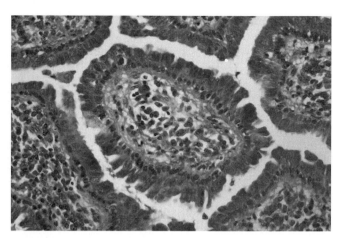

FIGURE 12–42 The papillary fronds of syringocystadenoma papilliferum are covered by two types of cells. The luminal columnar cells with eosinophilic cytoplasm demonstrating apocrine snouting, and less conspicuous flattened cuboidal inner layer.

Microscopic Pathology

Epidermal papillomatosis is common. One or several invaginations extend from the surface to form the cystic cavity, into which protrude papillary fronds that may be lined in different areas by keratinizing squamous, cuboidal, or columnar epithelium (Fig. 12–41). The glandular epithelium has granular eosinophilic cytoplasm and round, basally oriented nuclei. In many areas, particularly deeper in the lesion, two cell types are seen lining the papillae: a luminal layer of columnar cells with apocrine secretory features (snout-like blebs of cytoplasm pinching off the apical surface) and an inner layer of smaller flattened or cuboidal cells (Fig. 12–42). A fibrous stroma, with a variable lymphoplasmacytic infiltrate, forms the cores of the papillae.

Differential Diagnosis

Cystic lesions that may be mistaken clinically for syringocystadenoma papilliferum include the uncommon cholesteatoma of the external auditory canal and cysts related to the first branchial cleft. The cystic and papillary architecture of syringocytadenoma papilliferum distinguishes it from ceruminal gland adenoma, which has similar cytologic features.

OSTEOMA

Gross Pathology

An intact osteoma is a rounded, often pedunculated, protruding bony tumor 0.2 to 2.0 cm in diameter. The lesion is covered by the lining of the auditory canal.

Microscopic Pathology

The osteoma is usually composed of lamellar bone and may have distinctive outer cortical and inner medullary structure. Some osteomas, however, are predominantly of compact bone (Figs. 12–43 and 12–44). If trabecular architecture is present, the intervening marrow spaces contain adipose tissue, hematopoietic elements, or fibrous tissue. The lesion is covered by keratinizing squamous epithelium and underlying periosteum.

Differential Diagnosis

The chief differential concern is exostosis, which has been described earlier. Although exostoses are generally lamellated mounds of bone without trabecular architecture or marrow components, some controversy remains as to whether osteomas and exostoses

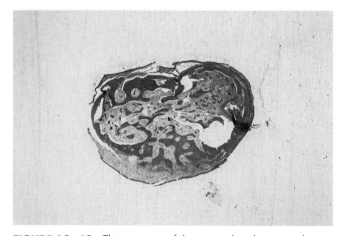

FIGURE 12–43 This osteoma of the external auditory canal shows a rounded bony proliferation composed of lamellar bone.

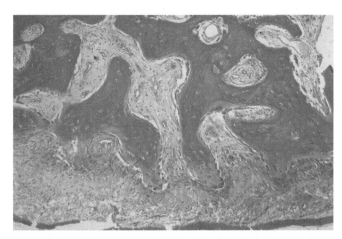

FIGURE 12–44 Distinct outer cortical and inner medullary structure is present in this osteoma of the external auditory canal.

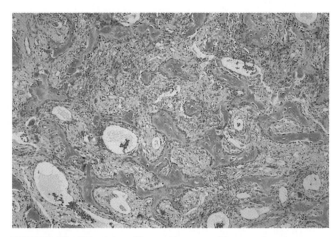

FIGURE 12–45 A lace-like proliferation of bony trabeculae is seen in a loose fibrovascular stroma in this osteoblastoma of the external auditory canal. Plump osteoblasts line the trabeculae.

are reliably distinguishable on histologic grounds alone.[58,59]

OSTEOBLASTOMA

Gross Pathology

Intact lesions are rarely seen by the pathologist, since curettage is the usual means of surgical treatment. The tumor is usually well circumscribed, with a hemorrhagic appearance and granular to somewhat gritty texture, depending on the degree of calcification in the tumor's osteoid.[91] Older lesions may be more heavily calcified, resembling cancellous bone.[91] In all skeletal locations, osteoblastomas range from 1.5 cm to 10 cm in diameter.[91] Osteoblastomas often lack the sclerotic rim so prominent in osteoid osteomas.

Microscopic Features

The well-circumscribed lesion is composed of an intricate complex of bony trabeculae that may lack mineralization or may be rather heavily calcified (Fig. 12–45). The trabeculae merge with those of the host bone at the periphery of the lesion. The bony trabeculae are lined by a single layer of plump osteoblasts that may have small bland nuclei or may have enlarged nuclei with prominent nucleoli. Scattered typical mitotic figures may be identified in the osteoblastic cells. The intertrabecular spaces contain a richly vascularized loose fibroblastic stroma (Fig. 12–46). Chondroid areas are uncommon but may be seen focally. Large, atypical, but degenerated-appearing hyperchromatic nuclei may rarely be seen.[92,93]

Differential Diagnosis

Distinction from osteoid osteoma may be difficult, as there is significant histologic similarity between the two entities. Osteoid osteoma usually is associated with a peripheral sclerotic rim and limited size (less than 1.5 cm) as well as a central nidus by microscopic examination. Osteoblastomas may contain areas that mimic aneurysmal bone cyst, giant cell tumor, and even osteosarcoma.[94] The critical distinction between osteoblastoma and osteosarcoma may be extemely difficult with a small biopsy. Unni[91] notes that the most useful features assisting in the diagnosis of osteoblastoma while excluding osteosarcoma include sharp circumscription with no permeation or entrapment of surrounding host bone, bony trabeculae embedded in loose connective tissue, and lining of trabeculae by a single layer of osteoblasts. Unni also considers the presence of sheets of osteoblasts without osteoid production to be a feature that is strongly suggestive of osteosarcoma.

Clinicopathologic Correlation

The frequent difficulty in distinguishing between osteoblastoma and osteosarcoma has led to the intro-

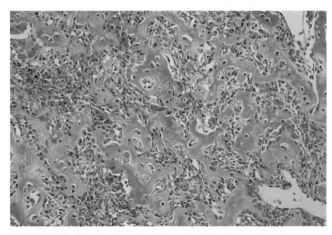

FIGURE 12–46 In this osteoblastoma of the external auditory canal, we see an area with more brisk osteoblastic proliferation.

duction of a variety of modifying terms such as "aggressive osteoblastoma" to describe cases in which atypical features such as epithelioid-appearing osteoblasts, sheet-like or trabecular areas of osteoid, and osteoclastic activity are present.[95] Metastatic disease has not been seen in the lesions categorized as histologically aggressive or malignant; the separation of an aggressive group of osteoblastomas has not been reproducible.[96]

CHONDROMA

Gross Pathology

Chondromas involving the ear are rare but may occur in the auricle and external auditory canal, as well as in the middle ear and temporal bone. In osseous locations, they may occur as endosteal lesions or as exophytic subperiosteal masses. Extraosseous chondromas are rare.[97] Seldom exceeding 1 cm in diameter, these lesions have the gross appearance of white to grey firm hyaline cartilage.

Microscopic Pathology

Chondromas are composed of mature-appearing hyaline cartilage with absent or minimal chondrocyte atypia. There may be a tendency for clustering lacunae, and multiple mononucleated chondrocytes may be seen in a single lacuna.[98] The border between the tumor and surrounding host tissue is usually distinct; however, intraosseous lesions may be lobulated and appear multifocal due to intervening areas of host bone.[98] Periosteal lesions are covered by a layer of periosteum.

Differential Diagnosis

The lack of chondrocyte atypia and the clinical and radiographic appearance distinguish chondromas from chondrosarcomas. Exophytic osseous lesions should be distinguished from osteochondromas, which have—in addition to the cartilaginous component—benign bone.

Clinicopathologic Correlation

Solitary intraosseous chondromas are benign lesions. The presence of multiple chondromas ("Ollier's disease") is associated with a significant risk (approximately 25% by age 40) of a patient developing chondrosarcoma.

MYXOMA

Gross Pathology

These tumors are usually semitranslucent, grey to white, and gelatinous. Although myxomas may appear grossly circumscribed, it is not uncommon for them to permeate surrounding tissues. Size varies greatly. Soft-tissue lesions of the head and neck are usually much smaller than intramuscular myxomas of the extremities, which may be as large as 21 cm.[99] Myxomas of the external ear and external auditory canal described in the complex of myxomas, spotty pigmentation, endocrine tumors, and schwannomas by Ferreiro and Carney[100] ranged in size from 3 mm to 2 cm in diameter. Lesions in the auditory canal are usually pedunculated.

Microscopic Pathology

Myxomas are characterized by sparse cellularity and paucity of vessels. The lesion consists chiefly of mucoid material in which are suspended a loose framework of reticulin fibers. Mature collagen is scanty. The cellular component consists of a population of spindled to stellate cells with tiny pyknotic nuclei and delicate cytoplasmic process. Cellular pleomorphism is not seen. Lipid-containing histiocytes may be seen in some cases.[99] The periphery of the tumor is surrounded by a pseudocapsule of condensed reticulin fibers and compressed host tissue, particularly skeletal muscle. The lesions seen in the complex of myxomas, spotty pigmentation, endocrine neoplasms, and schwannomas had the unusual feature of epithelial inclusions in many of the tumors.[100]

Special Techniques

The myxoid matrix in myxoma stains with alcian blue and is hyaluronidase sensitive. Mucicarmine and colloidal iron also stain the material.[99]

The cellular component of myxomas is vimentin positive but does not express skeletal muscle antigens or S-100 protein. A potential pitfall in interpretation of immunostains in these lesions is the entrapment of atrophic skeletal muscle fibers at the periphery of the lesion, which will be positive for muscle-specific actin, desmin, and myoglobin and may be misinterpreted as rhabdomyoblasts, leading to a misdiagnosis of embryonal rhabdomyosarcoma.

Differential Diagnosis

Myxoid change in a variety of benign neoplasms, including neurofibroma, neurilemmoma, and lipoma, may mimic myxoma, especially in limited biopsy material. Of more concern, however, are several myxoid malignant neoplasms overlapping myxoma in distribution and clinical appearance. These include myxoid malignant fibrous histiocytoma, myxoid liposarcoma, myxoid chondrosarcoma, and sarcoma botryoides (embryonal rhabdomyosarcoma). These malignant neoplasms display much greater cellularity and a richer vascular pattern than myxomas. The cytologic features also differ. Cellular pleomorphism, often including multinucleated giant cells, typifies myxoid malignant fibrous histiocytoma. Lipoblasts in liposarcoma, rhabdomyoblasts in rhabdomyosarcoma, and atypical chondroblastic cells in chondrosarcoma are distinctive features. The hyaluronidase-sensitive feature of alcian blue staining in myxomas differs from the alcian blue staining in chondrosarcoma, which is resistant to hyaluronidase.[99]

Clinicopathologic Correlation

Although myxomas of the head and neck are most often intraosseous lesions of the jaws, it is important to recognize the rare intramuscular or soft-tissue myxomas. The histologic pattern in these lesions may mimic myxoid soft-tissue malignancies that are much more common in this location, particularly rhabdomyosarcoma. Although soft-tissue myxomas lack a discrete capsule, they rarely recur after excision.

Of particular interest is the association of myxomas of the external ear and external auditory canal with myxomas in other locations (most notably cardiac), endocrine tumors, and schwannomas. The finding of a myxoma of the ear should alert one to the possibility of this autosomal dominant syndrome.[100]

FIBROMA

Gross Pathology

Usually firm and white, due to the high content of mature collagen, these lesions may be circumscribed or may have irregular borders. Dermatofibromas and fibrous histiocytomas may have a yellowish or brownish color due to the present of lipidized or hemosiderin-containing histiocytic cells.

Microscopic Pathology

Collagen fibers are abundant, while cellularity is relatively low in these lesions. The tumor cells are spindled, with small elongated nuclei with evenly distributed fine chromatin. Nuclear pleomorphism, hyperchromasia, and mitotic activity are not seen.

Dermatofibroma, a fibrohistiocytic tumor found in the dermis, and its soft-tissue correlate, the fibrous histiocytoma, are composed of a storiform proliferation of compact spindle cells with variable amounts of intervening collagen (Fig. 12–47). Hemosiderin deposits, either extracellular or within histiocytes, are common. Foamy histiocytes, multinucleated giant cells, or Touton giant cells with peripheral lipid accumulation are frequent findings (Fig. 12–48). Variable numbers of chronic inflammatory cells are scattered throughout the lesion. Mitotic figures are usually infrequent.

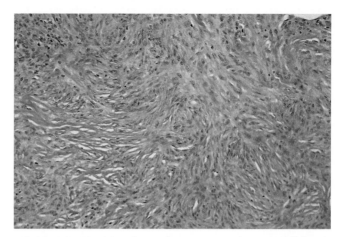

FIGURE 12–47 Note the storiform pattern in this more cellular area of a fibrous histiocytoma of the external auditory canal.

FIBROUS DYSPLASIA OF BONE

Gross Pathology

The lesion of fibrous dysplasia is usually a discrete area of dense white fibrous tissue, with a slightly gritty texture due to the presence of osseous trabeculae.

Microscopic Pathology

The dominant component of the classic lesion of fibrous dysplasia is a population of plump, bland fibroblastic cells that lack mitotic activity and cellular pleomorphism. Variable amounts of collagen fibers are present between the fibroblasts. Embedded within the fibroblastic background are haphazardly arranged, irregularly shaped trabeculae of woven bone, some of which are small, rounded "psammomatoid" structures. The trabeculae are not rimmed by osteoblasts. Aggregates of foamy histiocytes are

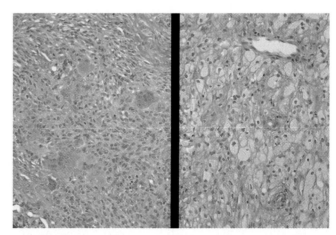

FIGURE 12–48 Other areas of the lesion seen in Figure 12–47 contain multinucleated giant cells and lipid-rich histiocytes.

common, as are small groups of giant cells. Cartilaginous foci are occasionally seen and may be prominent in some cases.[101]

Differential Diagnosis

The chief histologic differential diagnosis is ossifying fibroma, to be discussed next. In lesions with larger aggregates of giant cells, a true giant cell tumor of bone may be considered.

Clinicopathologic Correlation

Fibrous dysplasia of the temporal bone is rare, with only one case identified by Adair and Hyams[102] in the AFIP Otolaryngic Tumor Registry. Fibrous dysplasia is thought to represent a developmental anomaly of bone rather than a neoplastic process. There is controversy regarding the distinction of a separate group of lesions based on the presence of osteoblastic activity.[103,104]

OSSIFYING FIBROMA

Gross Pathology

Ossifying fibromas are virtually identical to the lesions of fibrous dysplasia on gross examination.

Microscopic Pathology

The fibroblastic background seen in ossifying fibroma is virtually identical to that of fibrous dysplasia. The bony trabeculae tend to be composed of mature (lamellar) bone without odd geometric patterns. The significant histologic difference that has been cited as distinguishing ossifying fibroma as an entity separate from fibrous dysplasia is the presence of prominent osteoblastic rimming of the bony trabeculae.

Differential Diagnosis

The histologic similarity between ossifying fibroma and fibrous dysplasia makes the two lesions of differential diagnostic interest, as well as the basis of considerable controversy regarding their classification as two distinctive entities.

Clinicopathologic Correlation

Twelve ossifying fibromas of the temporal bone were identified in the AFIP Otolaryngic Tumor Registry.[102] There has been controversy in the distinction between monostotic fibrous dysplasia and ossifying fibroma since the latter term was introduced by Kempson[103] in 1966 to describe lesions of the long bones that resembled fibrous dysplasia but with prominent osteoblastic activity. While some accept no osteoblastic activity in "fibrous dysplasia,"[105,106] others conclude that the presence of osteoblastic

rimming and some lamellar bone do not exclude a diagnosis of fibrous dysplasia in the setting of compatible radiographic and clinical features.[107,108] Polyostotic fibrous dysplasia is readily distinguished by its clinical characteristics.

GIANT CELL TUMOR OF BONE

Gross Pathology

Usually appearing before the pathologist as curetted material, the tumor is dark red-brown and friable, sometimes with firm areas related to fibrosis or osteoid production; necrotic areas or foci of cystic degeneration may be filled with blood.[109]

Microscopic Pathology

The primary cellular component is a mononuclear cell with poorly defined cell borders. The nucleus may be round or ovoid or sometimes spindle shaped. Nuclear hyperchromasia and pleomorphism are not seen. Mitotic figures are usually present and may be numerous; atypical mitoses are not seen. Giant cells, which seem to form from the coalescence of mononuclear cells, are scattered rather evenly throughout the tumor (Fig. 12–49). The giant cells contain between 40 and 60 nuclei. Other, more variable, findings include the presence of foamy histiocytic cells, prominent spindle cell proliferation in areas, reactive bone formation, and areas resembling aneurysmal bone cyst. The presence of intravascular tumor at the advancing edge of the lesion does not indicate malignancy.[109]

Differential Diagnosis

Chondroblastoma, though rich in both mononuclear and giant cells, is distinguished by the more irregular distribution of giant cells as well as by the presence of at least focal chondroid. Giant cell tumors

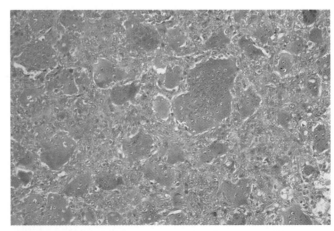

FIGURE 12–49 In this giant cell tumor of the temporal bone, plump mononucleated stromal cells are evenly admixed with multinucleated giant cells containing between 40 and 60 nuclei.

may be confused with osteosarcoma if there are areas of reactive bone formation; infiltration of soft tissue by giant cell tumor is often accompanied by some degree of osteoid production. Giant cell tumors, however, lack the cytologic atypia of osteosarcoma. In giant cell tumors with a predominance of spindle cells, fibrosarcoma or malignant fibrous histiocytoma may be considered, but the absence of cytologic atypia does not support these diagnoses.

Clinicopathologic Correlation

True giant cell tumors of bone, when they occur in the skull, usually involve the sphenoid bone.[110,111] Adair and Hyams[112] identified only three cases arising in the temporal bone. The biologic behavior of giant cell tumor of bone is quite unpredictable and is difficult to correlate with the histologic features of the tumor. Cases of histologically "benign" giant cell tumors that metastasized have been reported.[113,114] Features such as mitotic rate and local vascular invasion, which might suggest aggressive behavior, do not correlate with clinical course. Frank malignant change has been described in a small subset of giant cell tumors in extracranial locations.[115]

Malignant Neoplasms

BASAL CELL CARCINOMA

Gross Pathology

Several gross patterns may be seen in basal cell carcinoma. The typical noduloulcerative lesion is characterized by a firm pearly-white to grey papule with subtle telangiectasia, which ulcerates as it enlarges. The enlarging "rodent" ulcer is rimmed by a rolled border. Though usually limited in size, neglected lesions may be extremely disfiguring. A variant of the noduloulcerative form is pigmented basal cell carcinoma, distinguished by dark brown pigmentation imparted by melanin in the tumor cells. Morphea-like or sclerosing basal cell carcinoma presents as an ill-defined yellow-white shiny plaque, which may be slightly raised or depressed and scar-like. Superficial basal cell carcinoma is the most subtle, with one or several slightly erythematous scaly patches; the periphery may be slightly raised and pearly, while the center may appear depressed and shiny, suggesting an atrophic area of scarring.[116]

Microscopic Pathology

The tumor cells of basal cell carcinoma are small, with a high nuclear-to-cytoplasmic ratio and an ovoid nucleus with fine evenly distributed chromatin. The cytoplasm is scanty and poorly defined, giving the cells a syncytial appearance. Except in areas of keratinization, which are usually localized, intercellular bridges are not frequently seen. Mitotic figures vary in number but are not atypical. Cells at

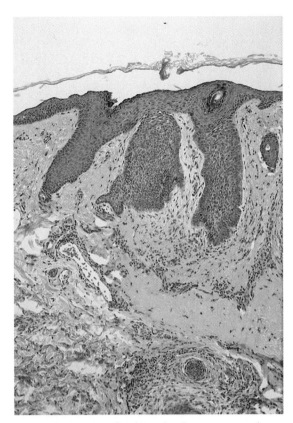

FIGURE 12–50 A superficial basal cell carcinoma is characterized by small nests arising from the basal epidermis; they may resemble follicular strucures at first glance.

the periphery of the nests exhibit palisading. In the typical basal cell carcinoma, the tumor nests are sharply circumscribed and distinct from the surrounding proliferating fibroblastic stroma (Figs. 12–50 through 12–52). There may be cleft-like areas in which the tumor appears to retract from the stroma. Collections of blue mucinous material and, less frequently, amyloid may be seen in the stroma

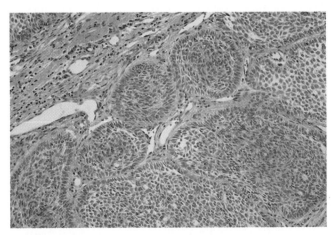

FIGURE 12–51 Rounded or rosette-shaped nests of basaloid tumor cells exhibit peripheral palisading of nuclei.

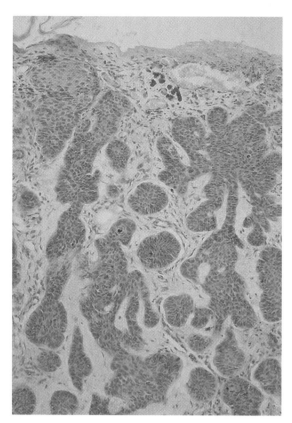

FIGURE 12–52 Melanin present in the tumor cells gives this lesion a brown-to-black apperance, possibly causing confusion with melanoma.

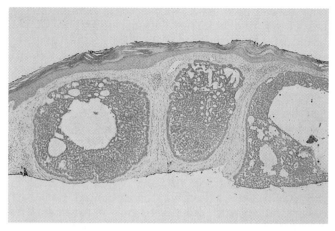

FIGURE 12–53 A glandular appearance is seen in the tumor nests in this adenoid basal cell carcinoma. Note the bluish mucoid material often seen in basal cell carcinomas of any pattern.

cell carcinoma merge with areas typical of squamous cell carcinoma. This lesion is distinct from the keratotic basal cell carcinoma previously described and may be more prone to metastasize than the usual basal cell carcinoma.[117]

as well as within the tumor nests. The tumor cells may exhibit histologic evidence of "differentiation" toward follicular structures (keratotic basal cell carcinoma), sebaceous structures, or tubuloglandular structures (adenoid basal cell carcinoma). The keratotic basal cell carcinoma forms horn cysts surrounded by parakeratotic cells. Sebaceous differentiation is expressed as the presence of groups of vacuolated lipid-rich sebaceous cells scattered through an otherwise typical basal cell carcinoma. Adenoid basal cell carcinoma has an intricate lacelike histologic pattern that gives the impression of attempted formation of tubuloglandular structures; however, secretory activity is not demonstrable (Figs. 12–53 and 12–54).[116]

The microscopic appearance of morphea-like basal cell carcinoma is distinctive: the tumor cells form elongated strands in a background of dense fibrous tissue and may extend deep into the dermis or subcutis. Superficial basal cell carcinoma is characterized by multiple elongated or rounded nests of tumor emanating from the basal layer of the epidermis with little or no infiltration of the dermis. The nests may be rather widely separated, making close attention to margins important.

Metatypical basal cell carcinoma represents a "hybrid" tumor, in which areas with features of basal

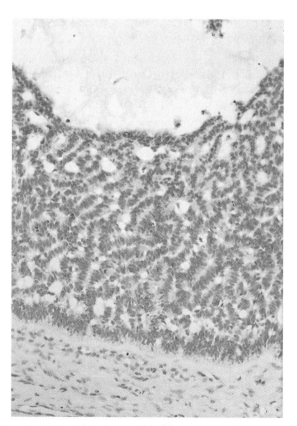

FIGURE 12–54 The intricate glandular pattern seen in adenoid basal cell carcinoma may cause confusion with other adenexal tumors. Look for architectural and histologic clues throughout the lesion.

Differential Diagnosis

The differential diagnosis chiefly concerns squamous cell carcinoma, particularly in the case of keratotic basal cell carcinoma. In keratotic basal cell carcinoma, the horn cysts show abrupt keratinization and general lack of atypia, while the squamous pearls of squamous cell carcinoma form from whorls of dyskeratotic cells showing more variable irregular keratinization and usually more cytologic atypia.

Of special concern is the distinction of morphea-form basal cell carcinoma from desmoplastic tricho-epithelioma, which also contains compressed elongated strands of tumor and an abundant dense fibroblastic stroma. The key distinguishing feature is the prominence of horn cysts in desmoplastic tricho-epithelioma. Horn cysts are not usually seen in the morphea-like type of basal cell carcinoma.

Clinicopathologic Correlation

Although basal cell carcinoma may be clinically extemely destructive, and even life-threatening when neglected, metastatic disease is very rare, with estimated incidence of 0.1% or less.[118-120] Although there may be some evidence that metatypical basal cell carcinomas are more likely to metastasize, no specific pattern of usual basal cell carcinoma has been linked to likelihood of metastasis.[120] While metastatic disease is more likely to occur in patients with a very large ulcerated, long-standing, and locally aggressive tumor, most tumors that fulfill this description never metastasize. Metastatic spread is both lymphatic and hematogenous, commomly involving the lungs, bone, and—less often—the liver and other intra-abdominal organs.[120]

SQUAMOUS CELL CARCINOMA

Gross Pathology

Squamous cell carcinoma of the pinna forms a raised indurated nodule, frequently with central ulceration, which may yield a crater-like appearance. Sectioning through the lesion reveals a firm white tumor that may be partially necrotic or may contain foci of yellow-white granular keratinous material. Lesions in the external auditory canal may be obscured by exudate or necrotic debris on the surface and may be difficult to sample. Superficial biopsies may suggest necrotizing external otitis.

Microscopic Pathology

Typical squamous cell carcinoma of the ear is frequently well differentiated, with abundant keratinization exemplified by formation of keratin pearls (whorled aggregates of anucleated squames) in addition to individual cell keratinization (Figs. 12–55 and 12–56). The well-differentiated tumor consists of anastomosing cords and irregular islands of squamous epithelium, usually with intercellular bridges

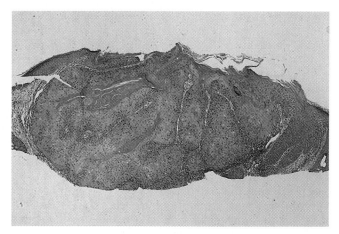

FIGURE 12–55 Note the architectural similarity of this squamous cell carcinoma of the pinna to the keratoacanthoma seen in Figure 12–36.

visible in areas. There is usually some disturbance of cellular polarity, giving the tumor cells a slightly disheveled appearance when compared to normal epidermis. Nuclear atypia is present but is quite variable; it is characterized by nuclear enlargement, anisonucleosis, hyperchromasia with irregularities of chromatin distribution within an individual nucleus, and variations in nucleolar size and shape. Mitoses

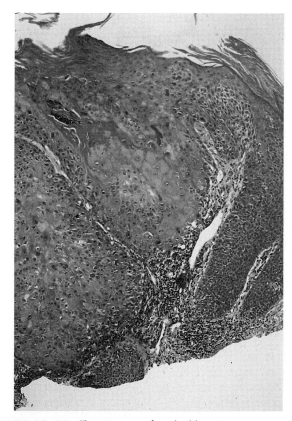

FIGURE 12–56 The presence of marked keratinocytic atypia helps distinguish this lesion (a squamous cell carcinoma of the pinna) from keratoacanthoma.

may be few or numerous, and some may be atypical. Frequently there is irregular budding of the basal epithelium from the skin surface in earlier lesions, which—when pronounced and associated with a stromal reaction—may reflect superficial invasion. More obvious invasion is characterized by irregular tongues of tumor projecting downward from the surface epithelium and by disconnected irregular strands of atypical epithelial cells extending between dermal collagen fibers. Moderately differentiated squamous cell carcinoma lacks keratin pearls but has scattered individual keratinized cells. In poorly differentiated squamous cell carcinoma, keratinization is very difficult to identify, and classification as squamous cell carcinoma is based on features such as associated squamous epithelial dysplasia, a pavement-like squamoid cellular pattern, or foci in which intercellular bridges or some evidence of keratinization is seen.

Spindle squamous cell carcinoma, or sarcomatoid carcinoma, of the external ear is a pattern of particular interest for differential diagnostic reasons. In spindle squamous cell carcinoma the predominant, and often exclusive, cell pattern is one of elongated tumor cells with elongated and variably pleomorphic hyperchromatic nuclei (Fig. 12–57). While some of the nuclei are long and thin, others may be lobulated and quite bizarre, mimicking the cells typically seen in malignant fibrous histiocytoma. Mitotic activity is usually high and often atypical. The amount of cytoplasm is variable; some cells with little cytoplasm suggest a mesenchymal neoplasm, while some cells with abundant eosinophilic cytoplasm may appear more epithelioid and even show evidence of keratinization. The surface of spindle squamous cell carcinoma is often ulcerated; however, areas of intact surface epithelium may offer evidence of the epithelial nature of the lesion by the presence of surface dysplasia or by areas in which the spindle cells appear to arise from the squamous epithelium. Some spindle squamous cell carcinomas may exhibit evidence of divergent differentiation, with production of atypical chondroid or osteoid matrix.[121]

Adenoid squamous cell carcinoma is an unusual variant of squamous cell carcinoma with a propensity to occur on the face and scalp and especially the periauricular area.[122] The "adenoid" appearance refers to a pseudoglandular appearance that results from tumor cell acantholysis (Fig. 12–58). Islands of tumor cells show central acantholysis, in which cohesiveness is lost and the tumor cells crumble apart, leaving a relatively intact peripheral rim of more cohesive tumor cells. This results in the illusion of a glandular lumen. The acantholytic cells in the false "lumen" often show the deeply eosinophilic cytoplasm common in exfoliated dyskeratotic cells. The glandlike spaces often contain some amorphous basophilic material; however, there is no evidence of glandular epithelial differentiation histochemically: the material is periodic acid–Schiff negative and positive for alcian blue (pH 2.5) with hyaluronidase lability. The tumor can usually be seen emanating from dysplastic surface epithelium, further supporting its squamous origins.

Special Techniques

Immunohistochemistry is not usually required in the diagnosis of squamous cell carcinomas of the pinna and external auditory canal, except in the case of

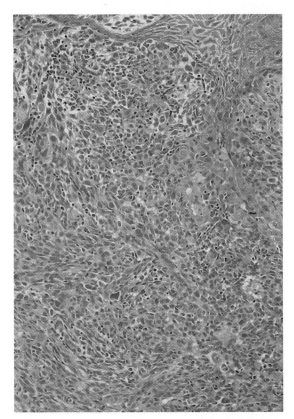

FIGURE 12–57 This squamous cell carcinoma (spindle cell type) of the pinna demonstrates a transition from dysplastic surface epithelium to infiltrating spindle cells, making the diagnosis easy.

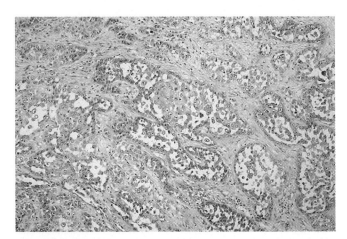

FIGURE 12–58 The large islands of invasive tumor in this squamous cell carcinoma have developed a pseudoglandular appearance as a result of tumor cell acantholysis.

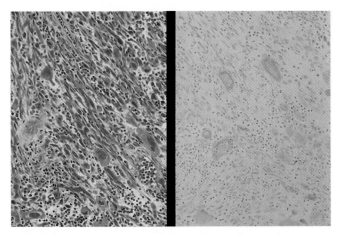

FIGURE 12-59 Immunohistochemistry for cytokeratin shows tumor cell staining in the right frame (spindle squamous cell carcinoma, pinna).

spindle squamous cell carcinoma. Spindle squamous cell carcinoma is almost always reactive for cytokeratin (Fig. 12–59) and/or epithelial membrane antigen (cell membrane staining pattern), though staining may be focal. Vimentin, though not specific, is almost always reactive as well. Tumor cells do not mark with S-100 protein or HMB-45.[121]

Differential Diagnosis

The differential diagnosis includes hypertrophic actinic keratosis, which is distinguished from squamous cell carcinoma by its lack of invasive features. Adenoid squamous cell carcinoma may be distinguished from adenocarcinoma, either primary or metastatic, by the association with surface squamous epithelial dysplasia, the acantholytic origin of the pseudoglandular spaces, and the absence of epithelial mucin by histochemistry. Adenoid squamous cell carcinoma may also be mistaken for angiosarcoma in some instances. In such instances, immunohistochemical studies for cytokeratin and epithelial membrane antigen are positive in carcinoma, whereas angiosarcoma expresses endothelial antigens such as Factor VIII–related antigen, CD31, and CD34.[123] Spindle squamous cell carcinoma must be differentiated from atypical fibroxanthoma and spindle cell malignant melanoma. Immunohistochemistry is extremely helpful in the differential diagnosis of these malignant spindle cell neoplasms (Table 12–10).

Clinicopathologic Correlation

Squamous cell carcinoma of the ear has unusually high recurrence (18.7%) and metastatic (11%) rates, more than twice the rates observed in squamous cell carcinomas of other cutaneous sites.[124] Factors identified in a large study of squamous cell carcinomas of the skin by Rowe et al[124] linked several pathologic factors to propensity for local recurrence and metastasis, including diameter greater than 2 cm, depth greater than 4 mm, poor differentiation, perineural invasion, development within a scar, previously treated squamous carcinoma in the site, and host immunosuppression.[124–127]

VERRUCOUS CARCINOMA

Verrucous carcinoma of the external ear and temporal bone is extremely rare.[128–130] The gross appearance of a warty papillated surface with abundant keratosis and the verruciform proliferation of cytologically bland squamous epithelium with subtle pushing infiltration of the underlying dermis is characteristic of verrucous carcinoma in other more common locations. Diagnosis of these lesions is impossible based on superficial biopsy material, because examination of the tumor-dermal interface is essential for establishing the diagnosis of verrucous carcinoma. There is a spectrum of very well-differentiated squamous cell carcinomas arising in the external auditory canal, some of which may lack the exophytic architecture defining verrucous carcinoma. The illustrated case (Figs. 12–60 and 12–61) demonstrates an infiltrative squamous neoplasm with a desmoplastic stromal response; although the exophytic features of typical verrucous carcinoma are lacking, the bland cytologic appearance is quite similar to that of verrucous carcinoma. Perhaps "verrucoid squamous cell carcinoma" would describe many of these intermediate cases between classical verrucous carcinoma and the more common forms

TABLE 12-10	IMMUNOHISTOCHEMISTRY IN PLEOMORPHIC AND SPINDLE CELL NEOPLASMS OF THE SKIN				
TUMOR	CYTOKERATIN	S-100 PROTEIN	HMB-45	VIMENTIN	MUSCLE-SPECIFIC ACTIN
Spindle cell squamous carcinoma	+/–	–	–	+/–	–
Malignant melanoma	–	+	+	+	–
Atypical fibroxanthoma[a]	–	–	–	+	+/–
Dermatofibrosarcoma protuberans	–	–	–	+	–

[a] Atypical fibroxanthoma may be positive for alpha-1-antitrypsin, chymotrypsin, or alpha-1-antichymotrypsin, but these are rather nonspecific and may yield equivocal positive results in other neoplasms in this category.

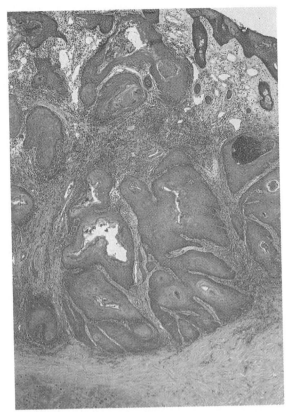

FIGURE 12-60 This well-differentiated lesion (a squamous cell carcinoma of the external auditory canal) might be termed "verrucoid" because of its resemblance to the bland tumor islands of verrucous carcinoma. The growth pattern is not so exophytic as verrucous carcinoma. This lesion was biopsied several times and was thought to represent a reactive process in external otitis.

of squamous cell carcinoma with significant cytologic atypia.

Distinction from reactive processes associated with otitis externa may be extremely difficult. In the middle ear, verrucous carcinoma is differentiated from the more common cholesteatoma on the basis of papillary growth and thickened epithelium—neither of which occur in cholesteatoma.

CERUMINAL GLAND ADENOCARCINOMA

Gross Pathology

Ceruminal gland adenocarcinomas are rounded to polypoid fleshy or indurated lesions, often ulcerated. The size ranges from 1 to 4 cm.[77,78,131–134]

Microscopic Pathology

Like ceruminal gland adenomas, ceruminal gland adenocarcinomas are unencapsulated lesions composed of glandular spaces lined by cuboidal to columnar cells with granular eosinophilic cytoplasm (Fig. 12–62). Some degree of apocrine "snouting" may be seen, but this feature is less common than in adenomas and is not seen in less differentiated carcinomas. Unlike ceruminal adenoma, the glandular spaces are lined by a single type of epithelial cells, lacking the outer myoepithelial layer. Nuclear pleomorphism in carcinoma is obvious, and mitotic activity is usually evident (Fig. 12–63). A deeply infiltrative pattern is present, with destruction of underlying structures, including cartilage and bone in more advanced lesions. Although hemosiderin granules may be focally present in tumor cells, they are much less common than in adenomas. Poorly differentiated ceruminal gland adenocarcinomas occur and are recognized based on their localization to the external auditory canal. Extramammary Paget's disease has been described in the skin of the external auditory canal in association with ceruminal gland adenocarcinoma.[134]

Differential Diagnosis

The chief differential diagnostic consideration is ceruminal gland adenoma, which has been detailed

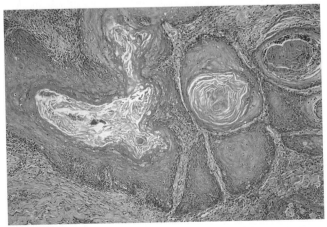

FIGURE 12-61 A closer view of the cytology of the tumor seen in Figure 12–60 demonstrates the bland cytologic features. The lesion was deeply infiltrative.

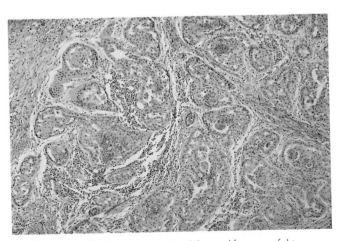

FIGURE 12-62 The irregular glandular proliferation of this ceruminal gland adenocarcinoma contains foci of necrosis.

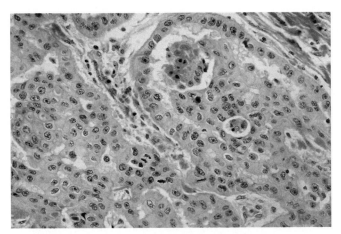

FIGURE 12–63 Unlike ceruminal gland adenoma, these glands are not lined by two cell types. Marked cytologic atypia indicated malignancy in this ceruminal gland adenocarcinoma.

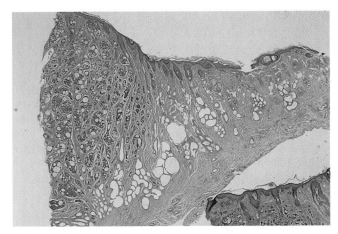

FIGURE 12–64 A low-power view of a ceruminal gland adenoid cystic carcinoma demonstrates the relationship of this neoplasm to the neighboring benign ceruminal glands, supporting an origin from them.

previously. In the setting of a poorly differentiated adenocarcinoma of the external auditory canal, the possibility of metastatic carcinoma from another site, such as the breast, should be considered.

Clinicopathologic Correlation

Ceruminal gland adenocarcinoma is a rare lesion that should be separated from two other carcinomas of ceruminal gland origin: adenoid cystic carcinoma and mucoepidermoid carcinoma (soon to be discussed). The distinction between adenoid cystic carcinoma and ceruminal gland adenocarcinoma is of prognostic importance. Ceruminal gland adenocarcinoma may be locally aggressive with recurrences if incompletely excised, but metastasis has not been documented. Adenoid cystic carcinoma of ceruminal origin, however, is extremely aggressive, with a high incidence of metastasis and a high mortality rate.

CERUMINAL GLAND ADENOID CYSTIC CARCINOMA

Gross Pathology

Adenoid cystic carcinomas of the external auditory canal are similar to those of primary salivary gland origin. The tumors are often described as yellow, firm, and translucent, sometimes giving the impression of a cyst. The size ranges from 0.6 to 1.5 cm by clinical observation, but more extensive infiltration is common at microscopic examination.[135,136]

Microscopic Pathology

The microscopic features are identical to those of adenoid cystic carcinoma of the salivary gland. The predominant pattern is the classic cribriform type in which islands of small cells with dark monotonous nuclei and scanty, slightly eosinophilic cytoplasm

contain cylindrical aggregates of loose basophilic material or more condensed eosinophilic reduplicated basement membrane–like material. The tumor cells lack pleomorphism, and mitoses are uncommon. The tumor islands are surrounded by a dense fibrous stroma in which strands of tumor cells or comma-shaped tubular structures are seen (Figs. 12–64 and 12–65). Some areas may exhibit a more solid pattern. Perineural invasion is common.

Differential Diagnosis

Adenoid cystic carcinoma of ceruminal glands should be distinguished from ceruminal gland adenocarcinoma, which has a much more favorable prognosis. While ceruminal gland adenocarcinoma does not metastasize, adenoid cystic carcinoma metastasizes to regional lymph nodes and to distant sites in many cases. Multiple recurrences are com-

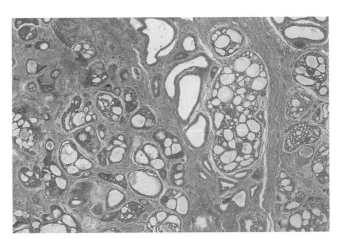

FIGURE 12–65 The histologic features of this ceruminal gland adenoid cystic carcinoma are identical to those of adenoid cystic carcinomas of major salivary glands and other sites.

mon, with extensive, locally destructive disease and a high mortality rate.[135–137] Extension from a primary parotid adenoid cystic carcinoma must also be considered. Rare examples of cutaneous eccrine cylindroma involving the external ear and external auditory canal may resemble adenoid cystic carcinoma.[138] These are two distinct entities that were confused in the older literature by the use of the term "cylindroma" in reference to both lesions. The pathologist must make the diagnosis very clear, preferably by avoiding the term cylindroma except in describing the benign eccrine tumor. ("Benign eccrine cylindroma" is a useful diagnostic phrase that helps to avoid confusion of these two lesions.)

Clinicopathologic Correlation

Adenoid cystic carcinoma has a marked propensity for recurrence, which may be explained by its extremely infiltrative nature and by the common finding of extensive perineural invasion. Not surprisingly, Perzin et al[135] found the following factors associated with recurrence to portend a dire outcome: tumor at or near the margin of resection, extension into the parotid gland, bone involvement, and histologically identified perineural invasion.

CERUMINAL GLAND MUCOEPIDERMOID CARCINOMA

Few cases of the rare ceruminal gland mucoepidermoid carcinoma have been reported in the literature, and those appear to have been low-grade tumors.[139] Histologically, these tumors are characterized by cystic areas with abundant mucin and a predominance of intermediate type cells and mucocytes (Figs. 12–66 and 12–67). A single case has been reported of mucinous carcinoma of the external auditory canal postulated to be of primary cutaneous origin.[140] This lesion contained small clusters of neoplastic cells with associated large pools of mucin. Subsequent parotid metastases developed.

MALIGNANT MELANOMA

Gross Pathology

Melanomas of the skin of the pinna and external auditory canal vary greatly in morphology, as they do elsewhere in the body, ranging from circumscribed, small, flat, hyperpigmented lesions resembling melanocytic nevi to large polypoid ulcerated masses. Pigment may be grossly obvious or inconspicuous.

Microscopic Pathology

In situ melanoma consists of a proliferation of atypical melanocytes limited to the epidermis. It is characterized by an irregular proliferation of cytologically atypical melanocytes with varying degrees of

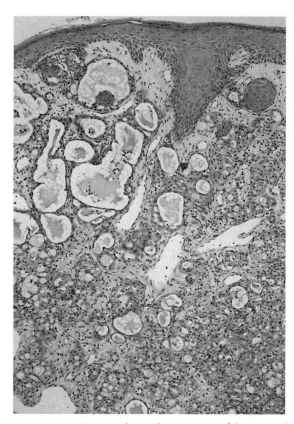

FIGURE 12–66 Mucoepidermoid carcinomas of the external auditory canal are exceedingly rare lesions, thought to arise from ceruminal glands. The cystic spaces and abundance of mucin are typical of low-grade mucoepidermoid carcinomas of any site.

nuclear enlargement and pleomorphism, often with prominent nucleoli, and arranged either in nests of variable size or as increased numbers of single melanocytes replacing extensive areas of basal keratinocytes. A common finding indicative of neoplasia that will be helpful in the diagnosis is the presence of

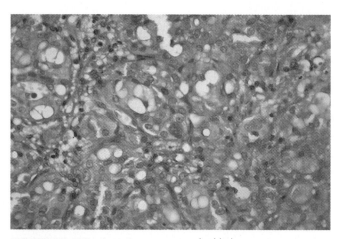

FIGURE 12–67 A mucicarmine stain highlights rare mucocytes in this mucoepidermoid carcinoma of the external auditory canal, which contains predominantly intermediate-type cells.

pagetoid spread of melanocytes into the upper epidermis, often in a haphazard "buckshot scatter" fashion.

Invasive melanoma adds to the above in situ component an intradermal melanocytic cell infiltration consisting of epithelioid and/or spindle-shaped melanocytes consisting of pleomorphic and hyperchromatic nuclei, prominent nucleoli, and variable amounts of eosinophilic cytoplasm (Figs. 12–68 and 12–69). Mitotic figures with atypical forms are commonly identified in the intradermal component and may also be seen in the intraepidermal component. Neurotropism is occasionally present and should be documented. The intradermal component may be arranged in nests, cords, or as single infiltrating cells. By light microscopy, intracytoplasmic brown-to-black melanin pigment with a fine, granular appearance may be readily apparent or may be completely absent (amelanotic melanoma).

Depth or thickness of malignant melanomas is an important part of evaluation with prognostic significance. As described by Breslow,[141] depth is measured perpendicularly from the granular layer of the epidermis to the deepest dermal extent of the neoplasm.

Special Techniques

Histochemical staining for melanin pigment includes the Fontana stain in which the melanin apppears black. This stain may be quite helpful in the identification of melanin in those cases where little pigment is identifiable through conventional light microscopic staining.

The immunohistochemical staining profile of malignant melanoma includes S-100 protein, HMB-45, and vimentin. S-100 protein, though not specific, is a sensitive marker identified in virtually all cases of malignant melanoma. HMB-45 is more specific; it is usually present in cases of epithelioid or pleomor-

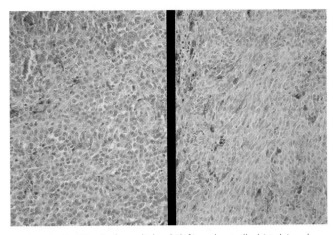

FIGURE 12–69 Both epithelioid (*left*) and spindled (*right*) melanocytic cells are seen infiltrating the dermis in this melanoma of the external ear. Pigment is readily identified.

phic malignant melanoma but often absent in spindle cell melanoma.[121] The lack of HMB-45 staining in spindle cell malignant melanomas is thought to reflect the paucity of premelanosomes in those tumors.[121]

Electron Microscopy

The development of effective and readily available immunohistochemical procedures has reduced the number of cases requiring electron microscopy, although it may occasionally be necessary for diagnostic confirmation. In such cases the organelle of interest is the premelanosome, which is specific evidence of melanocytic differentiation. More mature melanosomes contain heavy deposits of melanin that obscure the ultrastructural features of the organelles, making it difficult to distinguish them from secondary lysosomes and other structures. The premelanosome is a membrane-bound structure with an internal lamellar lattice-like framework.[142]

Differential Diagnosis

The differential diagnosis includes benign melanocytic nevi, which may be seen on and around the pinna and, less commonly, in the external auditory canal. Findings of melanocytic atypia, architectural asymmetry, and pagetoid migration of melanocytes into the upper epidermis distinguish melanoma from benign nevi. Malignant neoplasms that may resemble epithelioid melanoma include metastatic poorly differentiated carcinoma and lymphoma. The presence of an in situ component in melanoma is a helpful discriminator. The differential diagnosis of spindle cell melanoma includes atypical fibroxanthoma, spindle cell carcinoma, and occasionally dermatofibrosarcoma protuberans. Ulceration may obscure an intraepidermal component in some melanomas, making exclusion of metastatic melanoma difficult.

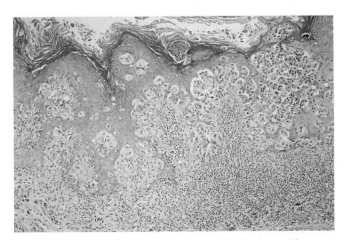

FIGURE 12–68 The epidermis is remarkable for the proliferation of variable-sized nests and single melanocytes, with pagetoid spread into the epithelium. An atypical melanocytic proliferation replaces the underlying dermis in this melanoma of the external ear.

Clinicopathologic Correlation

Primary melanoma of the external ear accounts for between 7% and 16% of melanomas of the head and neck region with 60% of these occuring on the helix and antihelix.[143–145] Melanoma of the external auditory canal is rare, with only six cases identified in a review by Langman et al.[146] Melanomas of the head and neck are generally found in an older population than those of the trunk and extremities; they involve a larger percentage of males, have a greater mean thickness, and have shorter survival time. Primary melanomas of the ear have shorter survivals than facial or scalp lesions, a fact partially explained by the frequency of thicker lesions on the ear.[144] Melanomas involving the central portion of the external ear or external auditory canal have been found to have a less favorable prognosis than those of the peripheral portion of the external ear, probably related to delay in diagnosis and difficulty of surgical resection.[147,148] The histologic feature of most prognostic significance is tumor thickness as defined by Breslow.[141]

MERKEL CELL CARCINOMA

Merkel cell carcinoma, or neuroendocrine carcinoma of the skin, is a slow-growing tumor with a predilection for cutaneous sites of the head and neck. Merkel cell carcinoma may involve the region of the external ear.[149–151] Histologically, Merkel cell carcinomas are characterized by a diffuse cellular infiltrate, often in a trabecular growth pattern, but also growing in cords and cell nests. Usually, the epidermis is not involved; the neoplastic infiltrate is confined to the dermis and subcutaneous tissues. Intraepithelial involvement can occur. The neoplastic cells have round nuclei with dispersed or stippled chromatin, small nucleoli, and scant cytoplasm. Increased mitotic activity and necrosis are often present. Immunohistochemical staining will show cytokeratin reactivity with a characteristic paranuclear punctate or dotlike pattern. In addition, staining will be seen with chromogranin, synaptophysin, and neuron-specific enolase. Chan et al[152] reported Merkel cell carcinomas to be CK20 positive. In contrast, small cell neuroendocrine carcinomas often will not express CK20.

ATYPICAL FIBROXANTHOMA

Gross Pathology

Atypical fibroxanthomas (AFX) usually measure between 1 and 2 cm. They are flesh-colored rubbery nodules and are frequently ulcerated.[153]

Microscopic Pathology

Atypical fibroxanthoma is an unencapsulated, but generally circumscribed, spindle cell neoplasm aris-

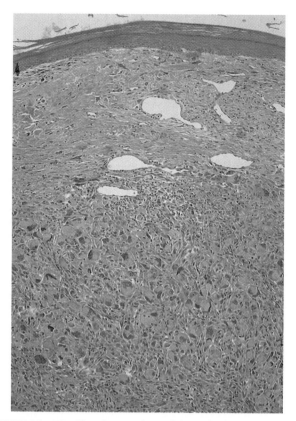

FIGURE 12–70 The pleomorphic cellular proliferation is localized to the dermis in this atypical fibroxanthoma of the pinna. The epidermis is thinned.

ing in the dermis (Fig. 12–70). The cellular component is varied, including a spectrum of elongated to plump spindle cells, pleomorphic spindle cells with hyperchromatic nuclei, and bizarre multinucleated cells (Fig. 12–71). The larger cells may have foamy cytoplasm reminiscent of lipid-rich histiocytic cells. In some cases a pleomorphic component may be

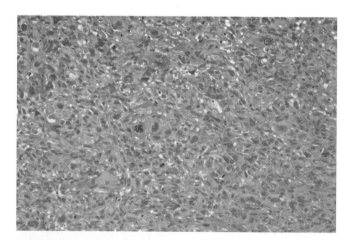

FIGURE 12–71 The pleomorphic tumor cells of this atypical fibroxanthoma of the pinna resemble those of malignant fibrous histiocytoma of deeper tissues. Mitotic figures, some atypical, are present.

absent.[154] Atypical mitoses are common. Some areas may exhibit a storiform pattern, but this is not usually prominent. A chronic inflammatory infiltrate may accompany the tumor. Vascular invasion may be seen, but necrosis is uncommon.

Special Techniques

Tumor cells may demonstrate intracytoplasmic diastase-resistant, PAS-positive granular material.[153] Immunohistochemistry is extremely valuable in the differential diagnosis of AFX by virtue of its lack of staining for cytokeratin, S-100 protein (except for scattered non-neoplastic dendritic cells) and HMB-45.[121,155] The presence of S-100 protein–positive dendritic cells scattered singly through the neoplasm should not be misinterpreted as tumor positivity for that antigen (Fig. 12–72). Variable staining for other antigens—including Factor VIII–related antigen (uncommon), vimentin, muscle-specific actin, smooth muscle actin, and KP1 (a monocyte-macrophage marker)—has been described, suggesting both fibrohistiocytic and myofibroblastic features (Fig. 12–73).[156] Alpha-1-antitrypsin and alpha-1-antichymotrypsin may also be demonstrated but are considered as relatively nonspecific staining.

Electron Microscopy

Electron microscopy is not particularly helpful in confirming a diagnosis of AFX, as the findings are nonspecific and overlap with other fibroblastic and myofibroblastic lesions. The presence of desmosomes in spindle squamous cell carcinoma or premelanosomes in spindle cell malignant melanoma is helpful in excluding AFX.

Differential Diagnosis

The key differential diagnostic considerations are spindle squamous cell carcinoma and malignant

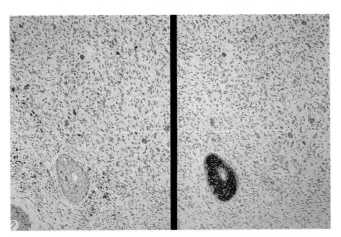

FIGURE 12–72 S-100 stains scattered non-neoplastic dendritic cells at left; cytokeratin stains only benign cutaneous adnexal structures, at right, in this atypical fibroxanthoma.

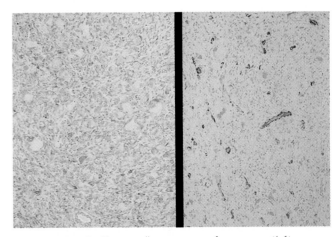

FIGURE 12–73 Tumor cells are positive for vimentin (*left*); muscle-specific actin stains only vascular structures. This is an atypical fibroxanthoma.

melanoma, which have been previously discussed. AFX is distinguished from malignant fibrous histiocytoma (MFH). If a tumor has the histologic features of AFX but is large (greater than 2.0 cm in diameter), has extensive infiltrative growth, necrosis, and vascular invasion then it should be considered to be MFH. Deeply occurring MFH has a propensity for recurrence and metastasis. The treatment for this tumor includes surgery and supplemental irradiation. Superficial malignant fibrous histiocytoma is considered a fully malignant lesion but is associated with a better prognosis than its deep, soft-tissue counterparts because its superficial location leads to earlier diagnosis. Immunohistochemical staining for desmin will allow for differentiating AFX from leiomyosarcoma.

Clinicopathologic Correlation

The relationship of AFX to malignant fibrous histiocytoma has been a source of controversy. AFX occurs in two clinical settings: elderly patients (75%), usually involving the skin of the head and neck, and younger patients (most of the remaining cases), involving the superficial soft tissues of the extremities and trunk. MFH, on the other hand, is typically a deep-seated tumor of the soft tissues or bone, though superficial lesions localized to the subcutis are recognized. The behavior of AFX, which is usually cured by complete excision, contrasts dramatically with that of deep MFH, a sarcoma with a propensity for recurrences and metastases, and a poor prognosis. The behavior of superficial MFH is closer to that of AFX, but these lesions should be considered definite malignancies, as well.

Atypical fibroxanthoma has been considered a mesenchymal tumor of "uncertain" or "borderline" malignant potential, since there are instances of recurrence and rare reports of metastasis. Attempts to explain the behavioral differences between the two entities using DNA content have produced conflicting results.[157,158] The apparent association of AFX with cutaneous sun damage is interesting as a possible correlate with the radiation-induced cases of MFH. Large, deep, recurrent cases of AFX should be approached clinically as MFH.

DERMATOFIBROSARCOMA PROTUBERANS

Gross Pathology

Dermatofibrosarcoma protuberans (DFSP) is a protuberant nodular cutaneous neoplasm averaging 5 cm in diameter.[159] The tumor is covered by thinned shiny skin, which may be ulcerated in larger examples. The circumscribed grey-white firm mass involves the dermis and subcutis but rarely extends deeper except in neglected or recurrent cases. Hemorrhage, cystic degeneration, or myxoid alterations may be evident.[159]

Microscopic Pathology

Although DFSP appears circumscribed, it is not encapsulated, but rather is very infiltrative. It may abut the epidermis, or a narrow uninvolved zone of dermis may be present. Deep infiltration involves the dermis and subcutis, with tumor entrapping adipocytes and even adnexal structures; extension of tumor cells from the main mass along connective tissue septa is common and is responsible for the high recurrence rate in these lesions. The tumor is composed of plump spindle cells with scanty, poorly delineated cytoplasm arranged in a prominent storiform pattern (Fig. 12–74). The cellularity is relatively high in the center of the tumor, less conspicuous at the periphery. Nuclear pleomorphism is minimal, and the mitotic rate is usually low. Multinucleated giant cells and foamy histiocytes are uncommon.[159]

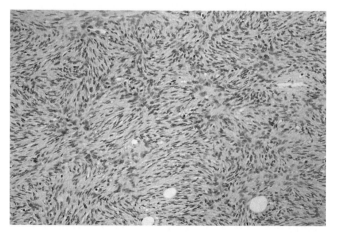

FIGURE 12–74 This preauricular dermatofibrosarcoma is characterized by a highly cellular, but rather uniform, spindle-cell proliferation.

Special Techniques

Immunohistochemical staining is not specific in DFSP. Vimentin is diffusely positive, muscle-specific actin (HHF-35) is positive in some examples, and there is no reactivity with cytokeratin, S-100 protein, and HMB-45.[155]

Electron Microscopy

Ultrastructural studies are nonspecific with evidence suggesting fibroblastic (fusiform cells with orderly lamellae of rough endoplasmic reticulum) or histiocytic (some cells with cell processes, intracytoplasmic lipid, and phagolysosomes) differentiation.[159]

Differential Diagnosis

The chief differential diagnostic considerations are dermatofibroma ("fibrous histiocytoma") and malignant fibrous histiocytoma. Dermatofibroma is usually more variable in its appearance than the monotonous proliferation of DFSP; multinucleated giant cells and lipidized histiocytes are common in dermatofibroma. Dermatofibroma, though unencapsulated, is not so deeply infiltrative as DFSP. In addition, CD34 is negative in dermatofibroma and positive in most DFSPs. Malignant fibrous histiocytoma also contains more pleomorphic cellular components, with more dramatic nuclear variability and hyperchromasia, high mitotic rate, and necrosis.[159] Neurofibroma and neurilemmoma are readily distinguished by their S-100 protein positivity. Rare examples of DFSP contain areas of high-grade sarcoma resembling MFH or fibrosarcoma; these behave aggressively.[159]

Clinicopathologic Correlation

DFSP is a neoplasm of either fibroblastic or fibrohistiocytic derivation with an intermediate malignant potential. The infiltrative nature of the lesion, which spreads along connective tissue planes, sometimes forming "satellite nodules," makes local recurrence a serious problem in patient management. Multiple recurrences may result in deformity and loss of function; however, metastasis is very rare.

ANGIOSARCOMA

Gross Pathology

Angiosarcomas appear first as macular blue-to-purple areas, later becoming multinodular, sometimes with ulceration or spontaneous hemorrhage.[160–162] Exact size is often difficult to determine from the gross appearance because of the tumor's tendency for irregular infiltration and formation of satellite nodules; tumors larger than 5 cm are not rare.[160]

Microscopic Pathology

Angiosarcomas exhibit a range of vasoformative patterns, often within a single tumor. Well-formed vascular spaces, with irregular shapes and sizes, may dissect through the dermis (Fig. 12–75). The spaces are lined by endothelial cells with enlarged, spindled to plump, hyperchromatic nuclei. The endothelial cells may line papillae that protrude into the lumen of the vascular space (Fig. 12–76). Well-formed vascular spaces may infiltrate the dermis singly or may form an anastomosing meshwork.[160] In some areas, the endothelial cells may form several layers, with tufts projecting into the vascular lumen. Vascular lumina usually contain only a few red blood cells but may appear empty or may contain eosinophilic coagulum and degenerating endothelial cells.[160] Other areas of angiosarcoma may contain predominantly spindle cells or elongated epithelioid cells in fascicles dissecting the dermis; the vasoformative nature of the proliferation is less obvious, with formation of cleft-like spaces containing scattered erythrocytes. In less "differentiated" areas of angiosarcoma, the tumor cells are found in nodular aggregates and sheets in which vasoformative features are difficult to recognize. Usually some slit-like or irregular spaces representing abortive vascular lumina contain rare red blood cells. Mitotic figures may be rare in areas with well-formed vascular spaces but are usually more readily identified in areas with less distinct vasoformative patterns.[160]

Special Techniques

Reticulin stains are sometimes helpful in defining the vascular network in angiosarcomas, but the reticulin network may be sparse in the less vasoformative patterns. Immunohistochemical stains include Factor VIII–related antigen, *Ulex europaeus* lectin, CD31, and CD34—useful markers of endothelial

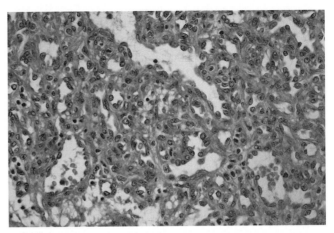

FIGURE 12–76 The endothelial cells in the tumor illustrated in Figure 12–75 are large, hyperchromatic, and protrude into the vessel lumen.

cells that are positive in most angiosarcomas. It has been noted that Factor VIII–related antigen stains poorly differentiated areas less intensely than does *Ulex* lectin.[160] The endothelial cells generally do not stain for cytokeratin.

Electron Microscopy

Tumor cells display some of the features of normal endothelial cells, depending on the degree of differentiation of the tumor. These features include pinocytotic vesicles, intercellular connections, formation of either well-developed lumina or intracytoplasmic lumina, presence of basal lamina that may be continuous or discontinuous, intermediate filaments, cytoplasmic protrusions, and Weibel-Palade bodies.[160]

Differential Diagnosis

The differential diagnosis includes Kaposi's sarcoma, particularly in areas of predominant spindle cells without obvious vasoformative features. A poorly differentiated carcinoma, either primary or metastatic, is considered in those angiosarcomas with prominent epithelioid cytologic features. Malignant melanoma is also a frequent consideration because of the biphasic spindle and epithelioid patterns in some tumors. Other spindle cell neoplasms also may be included in the differential diagnosis.

Clinicopathologic Correlation

Cutaneous angiosarcomas occur almost exclusively in three clinical settings. They are associated with chronic lymphedema of the extremities (most commonly postmastectomy), in an area of previous irradiation, and involving the face and scalp of elderly individuals. Angiosarcomas of the head and neck usually involve the scalp or soft tissue of the face

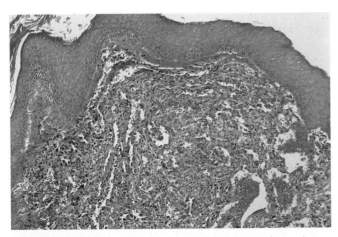

FIGURE 12–75 A cutaneous vascular proliferation of irregular anastomosing vascular spaces in a periaural angiosarcoma occurred in an elderly man.

but are confined only rarely to the ear. In the ear, angiosarcomas typically occur in elderly men. The propensity for cutaneous angiosarcomas not associated with lymphedema or radiation to occur almost exclusively in the head and neck region suggests some etiologic factor specific for that region. A logical explanation would be actinic damage, since the head and neck are high-risk areas for other sun-related cutaneous malignancies, such as squamous cell carcinoma and malignant melanoma. There are problems with this explanation, however, since angiosarcomas often arise in areas of scalp well protected by the hair and may occur in black individuals.[160] No other predisposing factors have been recognized in head and neck angiosarcomas.

The poor outcome in patients with angiosarcoma may be linked to several pathologic features of the neoplasm. Local recurrences are very common and appear to be related, first, to the rather insidious infiltrative pattern of angiosarcoma that makes complete resection challenging and, second, to the frequency of multiple foci of tumor developing as satellite nodules in the region of the initial primary lesion. Tumor grade does not appear to be closely linked with prognosis in angiosarcoma.

KAPOSI'S SARCOMA

Gross Pathology

The gross appearance of Kaposi's sarcoma (KS) varies with duration of the disease. Early cutaneous lesions appear as a pink-to-blue patch resembling a bruise, while more advanced lesions may present as purple plaques or nodules, sometimes with ulceration. A brownish color may result from the deposition of hemosiderin. Tumor size is quite variable, from a few millimeters to several centimeters.[163–165]

Microscopic Pathology

The histologic features of KS are essentially the same whether the lesions occur in patients with classical disease, in transplant patients, or in patients with acquired immunodeficiency syndrome (AIDS). The early lesions, referred to as the "patch stage," may be very subtle and consist of a proliferation of tiny blood vessels surrounding larger ectatic vessels. As the lesion progresses, more irregular small vessels produce a more obvious network infiltrating the dermal collagen fibers. A few extravasated erythrocytes may be present, along with a scanty lymphoplasmacytic infiltrate.

More advanced lesions of the "plaque stage" feature an extensive vascular proliferation involving the dermis and usually subcutis as well. A progressive accumulation of uniform spindle cells builds around the proliferating vessels, gradually coalescing into the typical nodules of KS. The vascular component in this stage becomes increasingly slit-like as the spindle cells begin to predominate. Eryth-

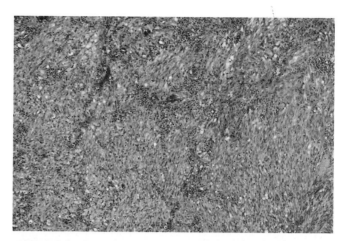

FIGURE 12–77 Kaposi's sarcoma, ear. The spindle cell neoplasm contains a patchy chronic inflammatory infiltrate composed of plasma cells and lymphocytes.

rocytes are seen coursing through these very narrow channels (Figs. 12–77 and 12–78). More distinctly angiomatous vascular channels are retained in areas, usually at the periphery of nodules, and these call attention to the vascular nature of the tumor. Inflammatory cells and hemosiderin deposits are also more prominent at the periphery. A nonspecific feature found in KS but which may be seen in other vascular proliferations is the presence of periodic acid Schiff–positive, diastase-resistant hyaline globules. These globules measure 1 to 7 microns in diameter and are seen intra- and extracellularly.[165] Mitotic activity is usually low in KS, except in occasional cases with more aggressive behavior.

Special Techniques

The spindle cells of KS do not usually react with Factor VIII–related antigen, though the endothelial lining of the ectatic vessels do. Several other "endothelial markers" have been demonstrated in many

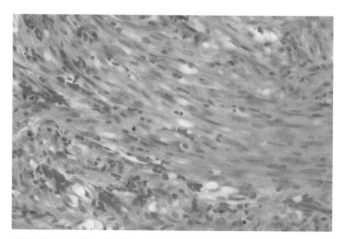

FIGURE 12–78 Slit-like spaces containing red blood cells are interspersed between bundles of uniform spindle cells in this Kaposi's sarcoma of the ear.

cases of KS, even in the spindle cells, suggesting that they may be a modified form of endothelial cell. The variable reports of staining of KS with endothelial markers is thought to reflect the spectrum of antigen expression seen in vascular malignancies in general.[165] The presence or absence of staining with endothelial markers does not define the diagnosis of KS.

Electron Microscopy

The EM findings are not specific but support the idea of endothelial differentiation of KS. The slit-like lumina of KS are lined by cells with endothelial features, with interruptions in the continuity of the lining and a discontinuous basal lamina. Pericyte-like cells with phagocytic properties are seen in more advanced lesions with a significant spindle cell component.

Differential Diagnosis

The early patch stage of KS may be very difficult to distinguish from vascular ectasia related to a chronic inflammatory process. As the vascular component becomes more prominent, hemangioma enters the differential diagnosis. Fully developed lesions with the biphasic spindle cell and vascular proliferation are usually easily recognized, though some areas closely mimic the pattern of angiosarcoma. The clinical setting is usually helpful in separating KS from angiosarcoma. Advanced lesions with a cellular spindle cell component may be confused with fibrosarcoma; however, the vascular proliferation is usually evident at least focally, and the presence of red blood cells between the spindle cells and the inflammatory infiltrate at the periphery are features that favor KS.

Clinicopathologic Correlation

The behavior of Kaposi's sarcoma is very closely related to the clinical situation in which it occurs. Although classical KS is associated with a very low mortality rate of 10% to 20%, patients with AIDS-related KS have a far more aggressive course. Even among the AIDS-related cases, the outcome is greatly influenced by the presence or absence of concomitant opportunistic infections. The etiology of KS is far from clear. There is substantial evidence for the role of viruses in the development of the neoplasm, including the association with human immunodeficiency virus, as well as possible links to other viral agents.[166-168]

MIDDLE EAR AND TEMPORAL BONE

The classification of non-neoplastic lesions of the middle ear and temporal bone is listed in Table 12–7.

Non-Neoplastic Lesions

OTITIS MEDIA

Gross Pathology

There are no specific macroscopic features. The tissue specimens are usually received as multiple small fragments of soft to rubbery granulated tissue. If tympanosclerosis is present, the tissues may be firm to hard, consisting of calcific debris. In general, all the tissue fragments should be processed for histologic examination.

Microscopic Pathology

The histology of otitis media varies and depends on the disease state.[169] Acute otitis media is virtually never a surgical disease. The inflammatory infiltrate in acute otitis media is composed of acute inflammatory cells (i.e., polymorphonuclear leukocytes). Acute inflammatory cells may be superimposed in a case of chronic otitis media (COM). The histologic changes in COM include a variable amount of chronic inflammatory cells, including lymphocytes, histiocytes, plasma cells, and eosinophils. Multinucleated giant cells and foamy histiocytes may be present. The middle ear low cuboidal epithelium may or may not be seen. However, glandular metaplasia (Fig. 12–79), a response of the middle ear epithelium to the inflammatory process, may be present, simulating the appearance of a glandular neoplasm (e.g., middle ear adenoma). The glands tend to be more common in nonsuppuratve otitis media than in suppurative otitis media. The metaplastic glands are unevenly distributed in the tissue specimens, variable in shape, and separated by abundant stromal tissue. The glands are lined by a columnar to cuboidal epithelium with or without

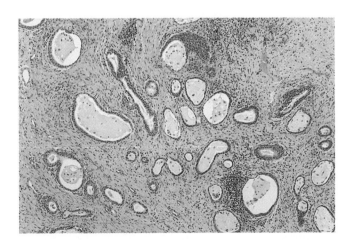

FIGURE 12–79 Chronic otitis media with associated glandular metaplastic proliferation. The metaplastic glands are unevenly distributed, and proliferate in the setting of fibrosis and chronic inflammation.

cilia or goblet cell metaplasia (Fig. 12–80). Glandular secretions may or may not be present, so the glands may appear empty or may contain varying secretions, including thin (serous) or thick (mucoid) fluid content. The identification of cilia is confirmatory of middle ear glandular metaplasia and is a feature that is not found in association with middle ear adenomas.[170]

In addition to the inflammatory cell infiltrate and glandular metaplasia, other histopathologic findings usually seen in association with COM include fibrosis, granulation tissue, tympanosclerosis, cholesterol granulomas, and reactive bone formation.

Tympanosclerosis represents dystrophic mineralization (calcification or ossification) of the tympanic membrane or middle ear that is associated with recurrent episodes of otitis media.[171] Tympanosclerotic foci may be localized or diffuse and appear as white nodules or plaques. Histologically, dense clumps of mineralized, calcified, or ossified material or debris can be seen within the stromal tissues or in the middle (connective tissue) aspect of the tympanic membrane (Fig. 12–81). Tympanosclerosis may cause scarring and ossicular fixation.

Cholesterol granulomas represent a foreign-body granulomatous response to cholesterol crystals derived from the rupture of red blood cells with breakdown of the lipid layer of the erythrocyte cell membrane. Cholesterol granulomas arise in the middle ear in any condition in which there is hemorrhage combined with interference in drainage and ventilation of the middle ear space.[172,173] The histology of cholesterol granulomas includes the presence of irregular-shaped clear-appearing spaces surrounded by histiocytes and/or multinucleated giant cells (foreign-body granuloma) (Fig. 12–82). Cholesterol granulomas are not related to cholesteatomas but may occur in association with or independent of a cholesteatoma. Tympanosclerosis and cholesterol

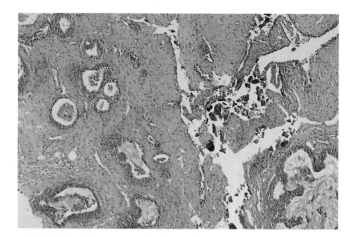

FIGURE 12–81 Tympanosclerotic foci appearing as mineralized debris is seen in association with other tissue alterations of chronic otitis media.

granulomas may occur independent of otitis media; cholesteatomas may or may not be associated with otitis media.

Differential Diagnosis

The inflammatory cell infiltrate seen in cases of otitis media may be extremely dense and can obscure cells that are diagnostic for another condition. This is especially true in diseases that favor the pediatric-aged population, including rhabdomyosarcoma and Langerhans' cell histiocytosis (i.e., eosinophilic granuloma). The glandular metaplasia may be mistaken for middle ear adenoma. In contrast to adenomas, glandular metaplasia is limited in extent, with the glands haphazardly arrayed rather than the diffuse glandular proliferation seen in adenomas.

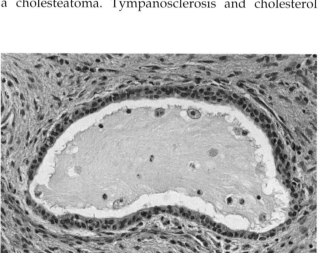

FIGURE 12–80 Metaplastic glands are lined by a cuboidal epithelium and contain serous-appearing fluid with scattered inflammatory cells.

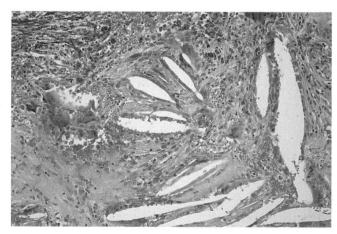

FIGURE 12–82 Cholesterol granuloma appears as empty, irregularly shaped clefts or as spaces surrounded by histiocytes and multinucleated giant cells. Fresh hemorrhage and hemosiderin pigment are apparent.

Clinicopathologic Correlation

In general, otitis media is managed medically, but sometimes tissue is removed for histopathologic examination. In the antibiotic era, complications associated with otitis media are not generally seen; however, if left unchecked, complications of otitis media include acute mastoiditis, suppurative labyrinthitis (inflammation of the inner ear), meningitis, and brain abscess. As will be discussed later in this chapter, primary squamous cell carcinoma of the middle ear is rare but typically occurs in patients suffering from long-standing (decades) chronic otitis media.

Miscellaneous Infections

Uncommonly, otitis media may be caused by tuberculosis, syphilis, fungi (including *Candida, Mucor, Cryptococcus,* and *Aspergillus*), and actinomycosis.[174–177] The setting for some of these infections, particularly mycoses, is in patients who are diabetic or debilitated.[176] In patients infected with human immunodeficiency virus (HIV) or who suffer from acquired immunodeficiency syndrome (AIDS), *Pneumocystis carinii* may seed from pulmonary lesions to the middle ear and temporal bone.[178] In this setting, the initial clinical presentation may occur as an aural polyp that by histologic examination shows characteristic foamy exudate containing the causative organisms. Viruses—including herpes, cytomegalovirus, rubella, rubeola, and mumps—can infect this region and may result in labyrinthitis and sensorineural hearing loss.[179,180]

OTIC OR AURAL POLYP

Gross Pathology

The gross appearance of otic polyps is that of a polypoid, soft to rubbery, tan-white to pink-red appearing lesion.

Microscopic Pathology

The polypoid mass is composed of a cellular infiltrate primarily consisting of a chronic inflammatory cell infiltrate, including mature lymphocytes, plasma cells, histiocytes, and eosinophils (Fig. 12–83). Russell bodies or Mott cells containing large eosinophilic immunoglobules can be seen and are indicative of a benign plasma cell proliferation. Polymorphonuclear leukocytes may be present. The stroma includes granulation tissue varying in appearance from edematous and richly vascularized to fibrous with a decreased vascular component. Multinucleated giant cells, cholesterol granulomas, and calcific debris (tympanosclerosis) may be present. An overlying epithelium may not be seen, but when present it appears as pseudostratified columnar or

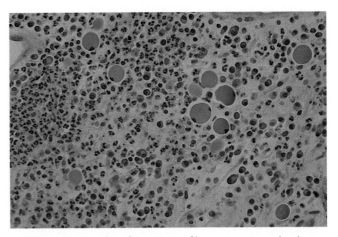

FIGURE 12–83 The inflammatory infiltrate seen in aural polyps is heterogenous, including an admixture of mature plasma cells, polymorphonuclear leucocytes, and scattered lymphocytes. Russell bodies or Mott cells containing large eosinophilic immunoglobules are present.

cuboidal cells with or without cilia. Foci of squamous metaplasia and a glandular metaplastic proliferation may also be seen.

Special Techniques

Special stains for microorganisms are indicated in order to rule out an infectious etiology.

Differential Diagnosis

In general, the presence of a mixed cell population of chronic inflammatory cells is benign, and a diagnosis of a malignant lymphoproliferative process is not an issue. Rarely, lymphomatous or leukemic involvement of the middle ear and temporal bone occur secondary to systemic disease. The dense plasma cell component may lead to consideration of a plasmacytoma. While plasma cell dyscrasia may rarely occur in this site, the presence of mature plasma cells, Russell bodies, and polyclonality by immunohistochemistry should preclude a diagnosis of plasmacytoma.[181] The cellular component in otic polyps may be very dense and may obscure an underlying neoplastic process (e.g., rhabdomyosarcoma, Langerhans' cell histiocytosis, carcinoma).

Clinicopathologic Correlation

Otic (aural) polyp is an inflammatory polypoid proliferation that originates from the middle ear mucosa and may result secondary to chronic otitis media. Despite origin from the middle ear, otic polyps may cause perforation of the tympanic membrane with extension into the external auditory canal. In this situation, the polyp may appear to be originating from the external auditory canal.

CHOLESTEATOMA (KERATOMA)

Gross Pathology

Cholesteatomas appear as a cystic, white to pearly-appearing mass of varying size containing creamy or waxy granular material.

Microscopic Pathology

The histologic diagnosis of cholesteatoma is made in the presence of a stratified keratinizing squamous epithelium, subepithelial fibroconnective or granulation tissue, and keratin debris. The essential diagnostic feature is the keratinizing squamous epithelium; the presence of keratin debris alone is not diagnostic of a cholesteatoma. The keratinizing squamous epithelium is cytologically bland and shows cellular maturation without evidence of dysplasia (Fig. 12–84). In spite of its benign histology, cholesteatomas are invasive and have widespread destructive capabilities. The destructive properties of cholesteatomas result from a combination of interrelated reasons, including mass effect with pressure erosion of surrounding structures from the cholesteatoma, the production of collagenase (which has osteodestructive capabilities by its resorption of bony structures), and bone resorption.[182,183] Collagenase is produced by both the squamous epithelial and the fibrous tissue components of the cholesteatoma.

Special Techniques

The histologic diagnosis of cholesteatomas is relatively straightforward in the presence of keratinizing squamous epithelium. In the differentiation of congenital from acquired cholesteatomas, Frankel et al[184] found an absolute increase in the number of S-100 protein–reactive dendritic cells within the squamous epithelium as compared to the number of S-100 protein–reactive dendritic cells in congenital cholesteatomas.

Differential Diagnosis

In contrast to cholesteatomas, squamous cell carcinoma shows dysplastic or overt malignant cytologic features with a prominent desmoplastic stromal response to its infiltrative growth. Cholesteatomas do not transform into squamous cell carcinomas.

Clinicopathologic Correlation

Cholesteatoma is a pseudoneoplastic middle ear disease characterized by invasive growth and the presence of stratified squamous epithelium that forms a sac-like accumulaton of keratin within the middle ear space.[185,186] Despite their invasive growth, cholesteatomas are not considered to be true neoplasms. In an attempt to determine whether cholesteatomas were low-grade squamous carcinomas, Desloge et al[187] performed DNA analysis on human cholesteatomas to determine whether genetic (ploidy) abnormalities were present. In ten cases with interpretable data, nine had euploid DNA and one was aneuploid. These authors concluded that, due to a lack of overt genetic instability, cholesteatomas could not be considered malignant neoplasms.

The term cholesteatoma is a misnomer in that it is not a neoplasm nor does it contain cholesterol.[186] Perhaps the designation of keratoma would be more accurate, but the term cholesteatoma is entrenched in the literature. Cholesterol granuloma is not synonymous with cholesteatoma. These entities are distinctly different pathologic entities and should not be confused with each other.[188]

LANGERHANS' CELL HISTIOCYTOSIS, LANGERHANS' CELL (EOSINOPHILIC) GRANULOMATOSIS, EOSINOPHILIC GRANULOMA

Microscopic Pathology

Histologically, Langerhans' cell histiocytosis (LCH) is characterized by a proliferation of Langerhans' cells (LC), which are members of the dendritic cell system.[189] The Langerhans' cells in LCH are arranged in sheets, nests, or clusters composed of reniform nuclei characterized by nuclear membrane lobations or indentations. The nuclei have a vesicular chromatin with inconspicuous to small, centrally located basophilic nucleoli and a moderate amount of eosinophilic cytoplasm (Figs. 12–85 and 12–86). The LC may show mild pleomorphism, and mitotic figures are uncommonly seen. LC may display emperipolesis. An inflammatory cell infiltrate accompanies the LC and primarily consists of eosinophils. Other inflammatory cells are present, including polymorphonuclear leukocytes, plasma cells, and lymphocytes. Foamy histiocytes and multinucleated giant

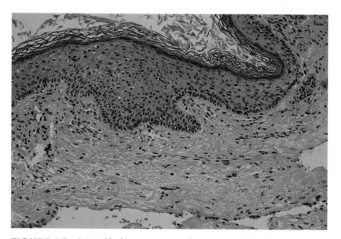

FIGURE 12–84 Cholesteatoma is characterized by the presence in the middle ear of a keratinizing squamous epithelium lacking cytologic atypia.

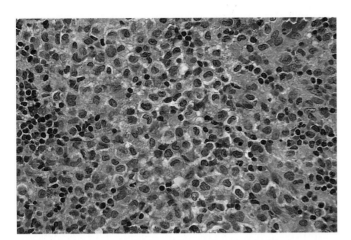

FIGURE 12–85 Langerhans' cell granulomatosis. The characteristic Langerhans' cells have reniform nuclei characterized by nuclear membrane lobations or indentations. Typically, an associated inflammatory infiltrate rich in eosinophils is seen in association with the Langerhans' cells.

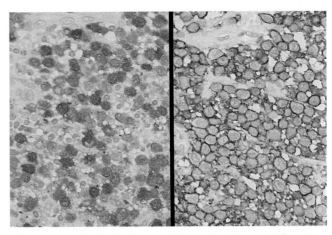

FIGURE 12–87 Immunoreactivity with S-100 protein (*left*) and CD1a (*right*) assists in the diagnosis of Langerhans' cell granulomatosis.

cells may be present. The histiocytes may show phagocytosis of mononuclear cells.

Special Techniques

The diagnosis of LCH is facilitated by immunohistochemical evaluation. LC are diffusely immunoreactive with S-100 protein and CD1a (Fig. 12–87).[190]

Electron Microscopy

By ultrastructural evaluation, elongated granules referred to as Langerhans' or Birbeck granules can be seen within the cytoplasm of the LC.[191]

Differential Diagnosis

The histologic differential diagnosis of LCH includes extranodal sinus histiocytosis with massive lym-

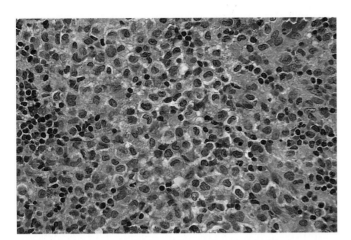

FIGURE 12–86 In this example of Langerhans' cell granulomatosis, there is almost no accompanying inflammatory cell infiltrate.

phadenopathy (Rosai-Dorfman disease), and non-Hodgkin's malignant lymphoma. Like LC, the cells of Rosai-Dorfman disease are S-100 protein–reactive, but they differ in that these cells are nonreactive with CD1a.[190]

Clinicopathologic Correlation

Lieberman et al[189] proposed the designation of Langerhans' cell granulomatosis (LCG) to replace the previous nomenclature of histiocytosis X, including eosinophilic granuloma, to indicate that the Langerhans' cell represents a cellular component of the dendritic cell system rather than a tissue macrophage (histiocyte). LCH is characterized by single or multiple bone lesions. Previous designations have fallen under the rubric of "Histiocytosis X," which include eosinophilic granuloma, Letterer-Siwe disease, and Hand-Schüller-Christian disease.

EXTRANODAL SINUS HISTIOCYTOSIS WITH MASSIVE LYMPHADENOPATHY OR ROSAI-DORFMAN DISEASE

Gross Pathology

Descriptions of the gross appearance of extranodal sinus histiocytosis with massive lymphadenopathy (SHML) lesions vary and include polypoid, nodular, or exophytic growths with a tan-white to yellow appearance.[192–195] Dimensions of the resected specimens were difficult to determine, as many of the specimens were removed in pieces.

Microscopic Pathology

At low power, the histopathologic features include the presence of lymphoid aggregates alternating with pale-appearing areas that are composed of a polymorphous cellular infiltrate consisting of mature lymphocytes, plasma cells, and histiocytes. The histiocytes, or so-called SHML cells, appear in clusters or cell nests but may be obscured by the nonhistiocytic cell population (particularly the plasma cells).[195] The SHML cells are characterized by round to oval, vesicular to hyperchromatic nuclei, with an abundant amphophilic to eosinophilic, granular to foamy to clear appearing cytoplasm (Fig. 12–88). Cell borders are poorly defined but occasionally are delineated by deposition of delicate fibrillar material. Nucleoli vary from prominent and eosinophilic to inconspicuous. Mild cellular pleomorphism and scattered mitoses can be seen. A characteristic finding is the presence of phagocytized cells (emperipolesis) within the SHML cell cytoplasm. The engulfed cells are most often lymphocytes but may also include plasma cells, erythrocytes, and polymorphonuclear leukocytes (see Fig. 12–88). In lymph nodes, emperipolesis is usually readily identifiable, but in extranodal sites emperipolesis has been considered a less frequently identified feature.[194]

The lymphocytic and plasma cell infiltrates are mature (benign) cells. True germinal centers are not seen. The lymphoid aggregates are composed of mature lymphocytes and occasionally contain histiocytic cells imparting a mottled appearance. An indication of benignancy relative to the plasma cells is the presence of intracytoplasmic eosinophilic globules (Russell bodies). In addition to the lymphocytes and plasma cells, scattered eosinophils may be present and may rarely represent the dominant nonhistiocytic cell type.[195] Well-formed granulomas or multinucleated giant cells are not seen. Fibrosis may be present and occasionally may take the form of prominent fibrotic bands, giving the appearance of a nodular proliferation. In mucosal sites, the surface epithelium is usually intact and not involved. Rather, the SHML proliferation diffusely involves the submucosal tissues. In the temporal bone region, the cellular proliferation may diffusely involve bone and other soft-tissue components.[195]

Special Techniques

Histochemical stains for microorganisms, including gram, periodic acid-Schiff (PAS), Gomori methenamine silver (GMS), acid-fast bacilli (AFB), and Warthin-Starry are indicated in order to exclude an infectious etiology. These stains are invariably negative.[195]

The SHML cells demonstrate diffuse and intense S-100 protein reactivity (Fig. 12–89). The SHML cells also demonstrate consistent immunoreactivity with alpha-1-antichymotrypsin (ACT), KP1, lysozyme, and MAC-387. SHML cells are not immunoreactive with Leu-M1 or CD1a.[190] The immunophenotypic antigenic profile of SHML supports the concept that the SHML cells are part of the mononuclear phagocyte and immunoregulatory effector (M-PIRE) system belonging to the macrophage/histiocytic family.[196-198] The plasma cells demonstrate a polyclonal pattern of proliferation as seen by the cytoplasmic positivity for both kappa and lambda light chains.[195]

Differential Diagnosis

Among the lesions included in the differential diagnosis of SHML are infectious (granulomatous) diseases, Wegener's granulomatosis, Langerhans' cell histiocytosis, and Hodgkin's disease. Microbiologic evaluation (cultures and special stains for microorganisms) fail to identify a known pathogen in SHML. Wegener's granulomatosis is characterized by a combination of a benign polymorphous inflammatory cell infiltrate composed of lymphocytes, plasma cells, and histiocytes—and occasionally with eosinophils, vasculitis, "ischemic"-type necrosis, and scattered giant cells. S-100 protein immunoreactivity

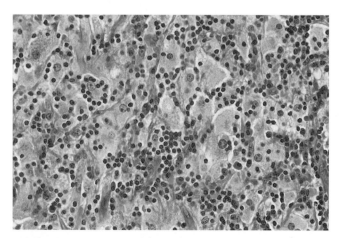

FIGURE 12–88 Extranodal sinus histiocytosis with massive lymphadenopathy involving the temporal bone. The SHML cells have abundant foamy-appearing eosinophilic cytoplasm with ill-defined borders. Phagocytized mononuclear cells are seen within the cytoplasm of some of the SHML cells.

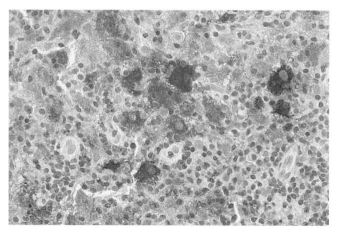

FIGURE 12–89 SHML cells are S-100 protein positive.

is not seen in Wegener's granulomatosis. Of importance in the diagnosis of Wegener's granulomatosis is the identification of increased serologic titers of (cytoplasmic) antineutrophil cytoplasmic autoantibodies (ANCA).[199,200] ANCA levels are not elevated in SHML.

In contrast to SHML cells, the cells in Langerhans' cell histiocytosis are characterized by the presence of nuclear lobation, indentation, or longitudinal grooving. Both SHML cells and Langerhans' cells will be S-100 protein–reactive. However, Langerhans' cells react with CD1a, a marker not identified in SHML cells. Further, Langerhans' cells have characteristic intracytoplasmic rod-shaped granules (Birbeck granules), a feature not seen in association with SHML cells. Azumi et al[201] demonstrated an antigenic phenotype of the proliferating cells in Langerhans' cells that, in addition to S-100 protein, included reactivity with LN-2 and LN-3, representing HLA-DR antigens. SHML cells do not demonstrate the presence of these HLA-DR antigens.

Clinicopathologic Correlation

Sinus histiocytosis with massive lymphadenopathy is an idiopathic, nodal-based histiocytic proliferative disorder that usually resolves spontaneously.[192–194] Extranodal sinus histiocytosis with massive lymphadenopathy may occur as part of a generalized process involving lymph nodes or may involve extranodal sites independent of the lymph node status.[194] The head and neck region represents one of the more common extranodal areas affected by SHML.[195] In addition to lymph nodes, SHML may affect a variety of extranodal sites. A review of registry SHML reported 43% of patients with SHML having at least one site of extranodal involvement.[194] Within the head and neck, there is predilection for the nasal cavity and paranasal sinuses; however, virtually all head and neck sites may be affected, including the temporal bone.[194,195]

Rosai-Dorfman disease is considered an indolent, self-limiting disease. Increased morbidity and mortality have been attributed to complications of SHML.[202] There is no ideal treatment for SHML.[203] The etiology for SHML remains obscure. Rosai and Dorfman[192,193] theorized an infectious etiology as a possible cause of SHML. However, an infectious agent has never been isolated. Other etiologic considerations implicated but never substantiated include immunodeficiency, autoimmune disease, or a neoplastic process.[194]

HETEROTOPIAS (CHORISTOMAS) OF THE MIDDLE EAR AND MASTOID

Microscopic Pathology

Microscopically, heterotopic salivary tissues are composed of an admixture of seromucous glands (Fig. 12–90) and adipose tissue. Rarely, these sali-

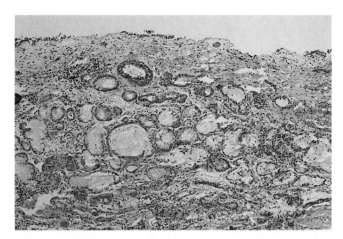

FIGURE 12-90 Salivary gland heterotopic tissue lying beneath the the cuboidal epithelial-lined middle ear mucosa.

vary gland heterotopias may produce a neoplastic proliferation (mixed tumor).[204,205]

Neuroglial heterotopia includes a heterogenous population of cells, including glial cells, histiocytes, and mature lymphocytes (Fig. 12–91). Reactive alterations of the neuroglial tissue (gliosis) may be present. In addition, granulation tissue and keratinizing squamous epithelium (cholesteatoma) may be seen.

Special Techniques

Immunohistochemical confirmation of neuroglial tissues includes reactivity with glial filament acidic protein (GFAP).

Differential Diagnosis

In chronic otitis media, a fibrillary stroma is often present that may simulate the appearance of neuro-

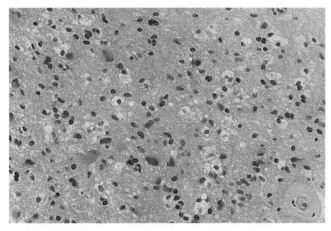

FIGURE 12-91 Neuroglial tissue within the middle ear cavity. This is an example of acquired encephalocele in which the brain tissue herniated through a compromised tegmen.

fibrillary matrix. GFAP will assist in confirming or excluding neuroglial tissues.

Clinicopathologic Correlation

Heterotopias, also referred to as choristomas and ectopias, include the presence of normal-appearing tissue(s) in an anatomic location in which they normally are not found. Heterotopias that occur in the middle ear include salivary gland tissue and neuroglial tissue. Salivary gland choristomas may present with unilateral conductive hearing loss, tend to occur more often in women, and occur over a wide age range.[206–208]

Neuroglial tissues in the middle ear and mastoid generally represent an acquired encephalocele with herniation of the brain into the middle ear and mastoid via compromise of the tegmen, a thin bony shell that separates the middle ear and mastoid cavity from the temporal lobe. The tegmen may be compromised or destroyed secondary to trauma, prior surgery, complication of otitis media, or congenital defect.[209] Potential complications include brain abscess. True neuronal heterotopias, in which isolated neuroglial tissue is located in the middle ear and temporal bone without continuity with the central nervous system is rare, but has been reported.[210,211]

CONGENITAL ANOMALIES

The ear—including the external, middle, and internal ear—often is a target organ for congenital anomalies. These congenital abnormalities occur as isolated defects or in combination with other aural and extra-aural abnormalities; they vary from cosmetic defects to complete hearing loss. A complete discussion of the developmental defects of the ear is beyond the scope of this chapter. The interested reader is referred to other texts.[212] This section includes the more common developmental abnormalities with which the surgical pathologist is likely to be confronted in daily practice.

Accessory Tragi (Accessory or Supernumerary Ears)

Gross Pathology

Accessory tragi may be solitary or multiple, unilateral or bilateral, sessile or pedunculated, soft or cartilaginous skin-covered nodules or papules.

Microscopic Pathology

Histologically, accessory tragi recapitulate the normal external auricle and include skin, cutaneous adnexal structures, and a central core of cartilage (Fig. 12–92). Squamous papillomas lack cutaneous adnexal structures and cartilage.[213]

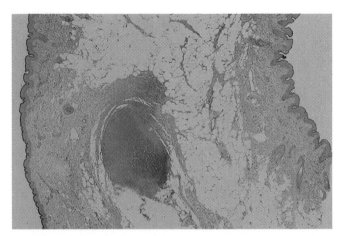

FIGURE 12–92 Accessory tragus resembles the normal external ear as seen by the presence of skin, cutaneous adnexa, and a central core of cartilage.

Clinicopathologic Correlation

Accessory tragi appear at birth. They are located on the skin surface often anterior to the auricle and may clinically be mistaken for a papilloma. Accessory tragi are thought to be related to second branchial arch anomalies. Accessory tragi may occur independent of other congenital anomalies but may occur in association with cleft palate or lip, mandibular hypoplasia, or with other anomalies such as Goldenhar's syndrome (oculoauriculovertebral dysplasia).[213]

First Branchial Cleft Anomalies

Gross Pathology

First branchial cleft anomalies typically occur in the area of the external ear and may include cysts, sinuses, and fistulas.[214]

Microscopic Pathology

Some authors feel that first branchial cleft lesions can be divided into two types.[215,216] Type I contains only ectodermal elements (keratinizing squamous epithelium without adnexal structures or cartilage), thereby duplicating the membranous external auditory canal (Fig. 12–93). Type II shows both ectodermal and mesodermal elements, including keratinized squamous epithelium, cutaneous adnexa and cartilage, thereby duplicating the external auditory canal and pinna (see Fig. 12–93). Olsen et al[214] proposed overlapping histology between Types I and II and therefore recommended classifying these anomalies into cyst, sinus, or fistula.

Differential Diagnosis

The differential diagnosis for Type I and Type II defects include epidermoid cyst and dermoid, re-

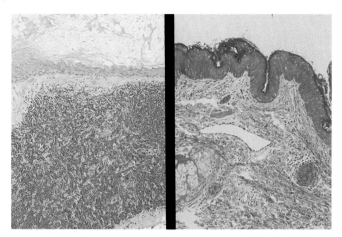

FIGURE 12–93 Type I first branchial cleft lesion contains only ectodermal elements (keratinizing squamous epithelium) without adnexal structures or cartilage (*left*). Type II first branchial cleft lesion shows both ectodermal and mesodermal elements, including keratinized squamous epithelium and cutaneous adnexa (*right*).

spectively. Clinical correlation will help in the differentiation of these histologically similar lesions.

Clinicopathologic Correlation

In comparison to second branchial cleft anomalies, first branchial cleft anomalies are uncommon, representing from 1% to 8% of all branchial apparatus defects. First branchial cleft anomalies may be identified in a variety of locations, including pre-, post-, or infra-auricular; at the angle of the jaw; associated with the ear lobe; and in the external auditory canal or involving the parotid gland. Involvement of the external auditory canal may result in otalgia or otorrhea. Parotid involvement may result in an intra- or periparotid mass. The majority of first branchial cleft anomalies are cysts representing over two thirds (68%) of these anomalies.[214,217] Sinuses and fistulas, equally, make up the remainder of these lesions. The fistula tract in first branchial cleft anomalies may extend from the skin over or through the parotid and open in the external auditory canal.

OTOSCLEROSIS

Microscopic Pathology

Histologically, the initial alterations include resorption of bone around blood vessels. The cellular fibrovascular tissue replaces the resorbed bone resulting in softening of the bone (otospongiosis). Immature bone is laid down with continuous active resorption and remodeling. The new bone is rich in ground substance and deficient in collagen, but over time more mature bone with increased collagen and less ground substance is produced, resulting in densely sclerotic bone. This process most often begins anterior to the oval window, eventually involving the footplate of the stapes. Stapedial involve-

ment causes fixation of the stapes and the inability to transmit sound waves, resulting in conductive hearing loss. Similar pathologic involvement of the inner ear may produce sensorineural hearing loss.

Clinicopathologic Correlation

Otosclerosis is a disorder of the bony labyrinth and stapedial footplate that occurs exclusively in humans and is of unknown etiology. Otosclerosis more often affects women than men, and a family history occurs in over 50% of cases. Otosclerosis primarily causes conductive hearing loss that usually begins in the second and third decades of life and is slowly progressive. The extent of the hearing loss directly correlates with the degree of stapedial footplate fixation. It is not uncommon for patients with otosclerosis to have vestibular disturbances also.[218,219] Otosclerosis usually involves both ears; however, unilateral disease can occur in up to 15% of cases.[220]

WEGENER'S GRANULOMATOSIS

Microscopic Pathology

The histologic features are similar to those described in the upper aerodigestive tract, lower aerodigestive tract, or kidney (see Chapter 6).

Special Techniques

Special stains for microorganisms are indicated to exclude an infectious etiology. Elevation of serum levels of antineutrophil cytoplasmic autoantibodies (ANCA) are of great assistance in those cases where the diagnosis is suspected but where the histology may not be definitively diagnostic of Wegener's granulomatosis (WG).

Clinicopathologic Correlation

Wegener's granulomatosis is a systemic necrotizing vasculitis that typically involves the kidneys, lung, and upper aerodigestive tract. Otologic involvement by WG occurs in 20% to 60% of patients with disease in these more usual sites.[221,222] The most common otologic manifestations include unilateral or bilateral otitis media (serous or suppurative), perforation of the tympanic membrane, sensorineural hearing loss, cutaneous involvement of the external ear with perforation of the ear lobes, and external otitis.[221–224] Facial palsy may occur as the intial manifestation of disease.[225] Involvement of the middle ear may occur secondary to nasopharyngeal and sinonasal disease via the eustachian tube or may be due to direct involvement by disease. Combined corticosteroid and immunosuppressive therapy may result in long-term remissions and is capable of reversing the hearing loss and facial palsy if the diagnosis can be established and treatment initiated early in the disease course.[226]

Other autoimmune or systemic diseases that may involve the middle or inner ear include polyarteritis nodosa and rheumatoid arthritis. Polyarteritis nodosa is a necrotizing vasculitis of small and medium-sized muscular arteries. Aural-related symptoms include otitis media with effusion.[227] Sensorineural hearing loss may be the initial presentation or may occur after the diagnosis has already been established.[227] The histologic diagnosis is dependent on the presence of necrotizing vasculitis. The manifestations of rheumatoid arthritis of the audiovestibular system include conductive hearing loss due to involvement of the incudomalleal and incudostapedial articulations.[228]

PAGET'S DISEASE (OSTEITIS DEFORMANS)

Microscopic Pathology

Paget's disease is characterized by three histologic phases. In the first, or osteolytic, phase, there is excessive osteoclastic activity resulting in bone resorption. In the second, or mixed or combined, phase, new bone formation (osteoblastic activity) predominates over bone resorption (osteoclastic activity) with deposition of new bone next to areas of bone resorption. In the third, or osteoblastic, phase, there is increased new bone characterized by dense irregular masses showing a mosaic pattern referred to as cement lines. Sarcomatous transformation occurs in approximately 1% of cases and usually transforms to an osteosarcoma. Osteosarcomas arising in Paget's disease are highly malignant with less than 10% 5-year survival rates.[229,230]

Clinicopathologic Correlation

Paget's disease is a disorder of unknown etiology. The skull and temporal bone are involved in approximately 70% of cases of Paget's disease.[231] Other sites of involvement include the external auditory canal, tympanic membrane, eustachian tube, ossicles, oval window, round window, internal auditory canal, cochlea, and endolymphatic sac.[231] Symptoms include hearing loss and vertigo. The hearing loss is mixed sensorineural and conductive.

Benign Neoplasms of the Middle Ear

The classification of middle ear and temporal bone neoplasms are listed in Table 12–8.

MIDDLE EAR ADENOMA

Gross Pathology

The gross appearance of middle ear adenoma (MEA) includes a grey-white to red-brown, rubbery to firm mass free of significant bleeding on manipulation.

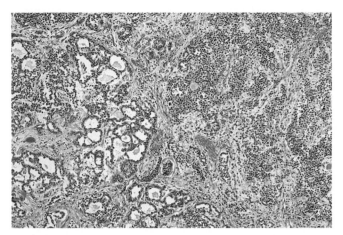

FIGURE 12–94 Diffuse proliferation of neoplastic cells in this middle ear adenoma forms glands with back-to-back growth (*left*) adjacent to an area with a more solid pattern of growth (*right*).

Microscopic Pathology

Histologically, MEA are unencapsulated glandular lesions with gland or tubule formation, as well as solid, sheet-like, trabecular, cystic, and cribriform growth patterns (Fig. 12–94). Rarely, papillary growth may predominate (Fig. 12–95). The usual appearance is that of a densely cellular gland-forming neoplasm. The neoplastic glands occur individually or have back-to-back growth. Often adjacent to or intimately admixed with the glands is a more solid or sheet-like growth of similar appearing neoplastic cells. The glands are composed of a single layer of cuboidal to columnar cells with a varying amount of eosinophilic cytoplasm and a round to oval hyperchromatic nucleus. Nucleoli may be seen and are generally eccentrically located. The cells may have a prominent plasmacytoid appearance, particularly evident in the more solid areas of growth but also in the cells forming the glandular

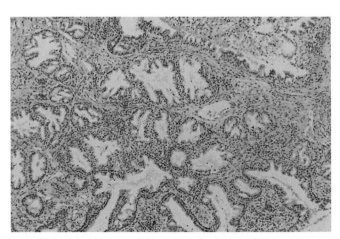

FIGURE 12–95 This middle ear adenoma with a dominant papillary pattern of growth was not associated with aggressive growth or aggressive biologic behavior.

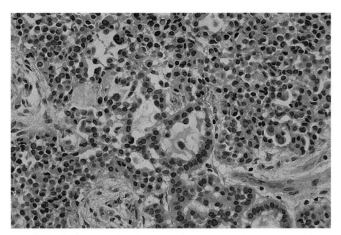

FIGURE 12–96 Both the glands and solid areas of this middle ear adenoma are composed of the same cells showing plasmacytoid features.

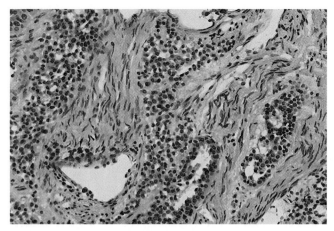

FIGURE 12–98 An otherwise typical middle ear adenoma with neurotropism. This feature by itself is not indicative of malignancy in these tumors. This patient is alive and well, free of tumor two decades after removal of his neoplasm. The patient never experienced any recurrences or metastases from his tumor.

structures (Fig. 12–96). A paranuclear clear zone is not present. Less often, the cells have a more dispersed or stippled nuclear chromatin with the "salt and pepper" pattern suggestive of neuroendocrine differentiation (Fig. 12–97). Cellular pleomorphism may be prominent, but mitoses are uncommon. Perineural invasion is rare but may occur (Fig. 12–98). Neurotropism in the absence of cytologic features of malignancy (see middle ear adenocarcinoma) is not indicative of malignant behavior. The stromal component is sparse and may appear fibrous or myxoid.

Middle ear adenoma may perforate the tympanic membrane and appear to represent a neoplasm of the external auditory canal. In this situation, the MEA lies subjacent to the keratinizing squamous epithelium of the tympanic membrane or external canal. These tumors should not be mistaken for ceruminal gland neoplasms that are histologically different.

Special Techniques

Histochemical stains show the presence of intraluminal but not intracytoplasmic mucin-positive material. PAS-positive material is not present. The neoplastic cells may be argentaffin and argyrophilic positive. By immunohistochemical evaluation, the neoplastic cells are cytokeratin positive. Some MEA may show immunoreactivity with neuroendocrine markers such as chromogranin and synaptophysin (Fig. 12–99). Neuron-specific enolase and Leu-7 reactivity may also be seen. S-100 protein and bombesin have been reported to be negative.[232] Desmin and actin are not found.

Differential Diagnosis

The differential diagnosis of MEA includes metaplastic glandular proliferation secondary to otitis media, ceruminal gland adenoma, jugulotympanic

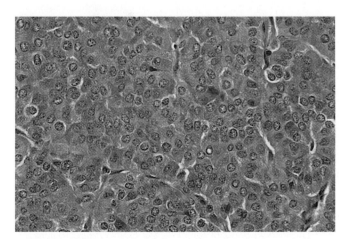

FIGURE 12–97 Middle ear adenoma with a stippled chromatin pattern suggestive of neuroendocrine differentiation.

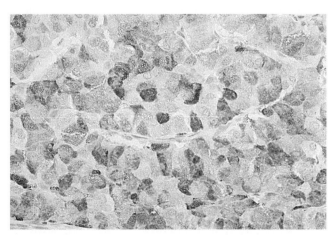

FIGURE 12–99 Chromogranin reactivity is confirmatory of neuroendocrine differentiation in the tumor illustrated in Figure 12–97.

paraganglioma, acoustic neuroma, meningioma, middle ear adenocarcinoma, rhabdomyosarcoma, plasmacytoma, and endolymphatic sac papillary tumor. In general, the clinical, radiologic, and pathologic findings indicate that the tumor is benign (absence of associated neural deficits, invasion or destruction of adjacent structures or pleomorphism, and increased mitotic activity). Nevertheless, the histologic appearance is not always predictive of the clinical behavior.

Clinicopathologic Correlation

MEA are benign glandular neoplasms originating from the middle ear mucosa.[233] MEA are not related to a prior history of chronic otitis media. Concomitant cholesteatomas may occur and may be the cause of bone destruction and/or facial nerve abnormalities.

Middle ear adenomas with neuroendocrine differentiation have been termed carcinoid tumors of the middle ear.[234–237] Rather than representing a separate, distinct neoplasm of the middle ear, we agree with Batsakis[238] and El-Naggar et al[232] that these "carcinoid tumors" are better viewed as part of the histologic spectrum of MEA, albeit one with neuroendocrine differentiation. This concept is supported by the findings of El-Naggar and colleagues[232] who showed the presence of chromogranin positive cells within hyperplastic but non-neoplastic middle ear epithelium overlying an MEA.

Another histologic type of MEA is one with papillary growth. The papillary MEA is one that is confined to the middle ear, is not related to the endolymphatic sac papillary tumor, and has a similar indolent behavior as other MEA (personal observation).

JUGULOTYMPANIC PARAGANGLIOMA

Gross Pathology

The gross appearance of jugulotympanic paragangliomas (JTP) include a polypoid, red, friable mass identified behind an intact tympanic membrane or within the external auditory canal, measuring from a few millimeters to a large mass completely filling the middle ear space.

Microscopic Pathology

Irrespective of the site of origin, the histologic appearance of all extra-adrenal paragangliomas is the same. The hallmark histologic feature is the presence of a cell nest or "zellballen" pattern (Fig. 12–100). The stroma surrounding and separating the nests is composed of a prominent fibrovascular tissue. While this pattern is characteristic of paragangliomas, it is not unique to paragangliomas. It can be seen in other tumors, such as all types of other neuroendocrine tumors, including carcinoid and atypical carci-

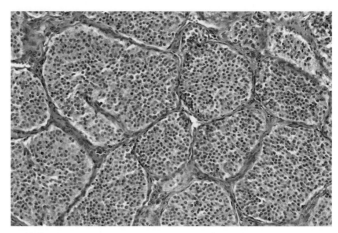

FIGURE 12–100 Jugulotympanic paraganglioma showing the classic cell nest ("zellballen") or organoid growth.

noid tumors, as well as in melanomas and carcinomas. Paragangliomas are predominantly composed of chief cells, which are round or oval with uniform nuclei, dispersed chromatin pattern, and abundant eosinophilic, granular, or vacuolated cytoplasm (Fig. 12–101). The sustentacular cells, representing modified Schwann cells, are located at the periphery of the cell nests as spindle-shaped, basophilic-appearing cells but are difficult to identify by light microscopy. Cellular and nuclear pleomorphism can be seen, but these features are not indicative of malignancy. Mitoses and necrosis are infrequently identified. Paragangliomas lack glandular or alveolar differentiation.

Special Techniques

Paragangliomas are often readily identified by light microscopic evaluation. However, in certain in-

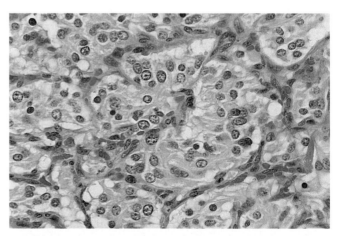

FIGURE 12–101 Paragangliomas are predominantly composed of chief cells characterized by uniform nuclei with stippled chromatin and abundant eosinophilic cytoplasm. Sustentacular cells are spindle-shaped, basophilic appearing cells situated at the periphery of the cell nests but are virtually undetectable by light microscopy.

stances paragangliomas may be difficult to differentiate from other tumors that have similar histomorphologic features. Frequently, middle ear and temporal paragangliomas do not show the characteristic cell nest appearance as occurs in other sites (Figs. 12–102 and 12–103). This "loss" of the organoid growth may be artifactually induced by surgical manipulation ("squeezing") of the tissue during removal. The absence of the typical growth pattern may result in diagnostic confusion with other middle ear tumors. In such instances, histochemical stains may be of assistance in the diagnosis. Reticulin staining may better delineate the cell nest growth pattern with staining of the fibrovascular cores surrounding the neoplastic nests. In addition, the tumor cells are argyrophilic (Churukian-Schenk or Grimelius stains). Argentaffin (Fontana), mucicarmine, and periodic acid-Schiff stains are negative.

The diagnosis of paragangliomas is facilitated by immunohistochemical stains. The immunohistochemical antigenic profile of paragangliomas includes chromogranin, synaptophysin, neuron-specific enolase positivity in the chief cells, and S-100 protein staining localized to the peripherally located sustentacular cells (Fig. 12–104). In general, epithelial markers, including cytokeratin as well as HMB-45 and mesenchymal markers (desmin and other markers of myogenic differentiation), are negative. Rare examples of cytokeratin reactive paragangliomas have been reported.[239] Vimentin is variably reactive in both the chief cells and sustentacular cells.

Electron Microscopy

Ultrastructural evaluation of paragangliomas shows the presence of neurosecretory granules.[240]

Differential Diagnosis

The histologic differential diagnosis of paragangliomas include middle ear adenoma (with or without

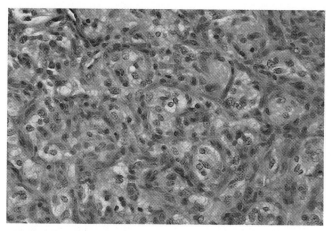

FIGURE 12–103 Although a vague cell nest pattern is seen in this jugulotympanic paraganglioma, the characteristic cell nests were absent for most of the tumor. The pattern of growth in this neoplasm was suggestive of a meningioma, but the nuclear features were more those of a tumor of neuroendocrine origin.

neuroendocrine differentiation), acoustic neuroma, and meningioma.

Clinicopathologic Correlation

The histologic appearance of paragangliomas does not correlate to the biologic behavior of the tumor. JTP are slow-growing tumors but may be locally invasive with extension into and destruction of adjacent structures, including the temporal bone and mastoid.[241,242] Intracranial extension may occur in up to 15% of cases.[243] Neurologic abnormalities—including cranial nerve palsies, cerebellar dysfunction, dysphagia, and hoarseness—may be seen and correlate to the invasive capabilities of this neoplasm. DNA ploidy studies by image analysis are not predictive of the behavior of paragangliomas, in general. Barnes and Taylor[244] reported that in the (be-

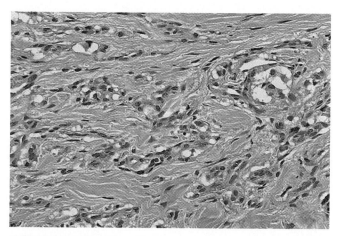

FIGURE 12–102 This infiltrative jugulotympanic paraganglioma lacks the characteristic cell nest pattern of growth.

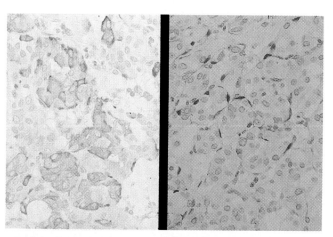

FIGURE 12–104 Chromogranin reactivity in the chief cells (*left*) and S-100 protein reactivity in the peripherally situated sustentacular cells (*right*) confirm the diagnosis of paraganglioma.

nign) carotid body tumors they evaluated, 31% were DNA diploid while 69% showed ploidy anomalies (diploid-tetraploid, tetraploid, aneuploid, or polyploid). Malignant jugulotympanic paragangliomas are rare. These tumors are associated with histologic criteria of malignancy, including increased mitotic activity, necrosis usually seen within the center of the cell nests, and vascular invasion. Metastasis to cervical lymph nodes, lungs, and liver may occur.[245,246]

ACOUSTIC NEUROMA

Gross Pathology

The gross appearance of acoustic neuroma includes a circumscribed, tan-white, rubbery to firm mass that may appear yellow and have cystic change. Tumor sizes range from a few millimeters up to 4 to 5 cm in greatest diameter.

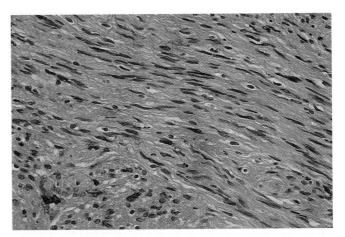

FIGURE 12–106 The nuclei in acoustic neuroma are elongated and twisted with hyperchromatic nuclei and indistinct cytoplasmic borders.

Microscopic Pathology

Histologically, the tumors are unencapsulated and composed of alternating regions of compact spindle cells (called Antoni A areas) and loose, hypocellular zones (called Antoni B areas) (Fig. 12–105). For any given tumor, the proportion of these components varies. Antoni B areas display a disorderly cellular arrangement, myxoid stroma, and a chronic inflammatory cell infiltrate. The nuclei are vesicular to hyperchromatic, elongated, and twisted, with indistinct cytoplasmic borders (Fig. 12–106). The cells are arranged in short interlacing fascicles, and whorling or palisading of nuclei may be seen. Nuclear palisading with nuclear alignment in rows is called Verocay bodies (Fig. 12–107). The cellularity may vary, and some benign schwannomas can be very cellular (so-called cellular schwannoma). Mitoses are usually sparse in number, and cellular pleomorphism with hyperchromasia can be identified, but these are

not features of malignancy. Retrogressive changes—including cystic degeneration, necrosis, hyalinization, calcification, and hemorrhage—may be seen. Schwannomas have prominent vascularity composed of large vessels with thickened (hyalinized) walls.

Special Techniques

Immunohistochemical staining shows the presence of diffuse and intense S-100 protein reactivity. There is no immunoreactivity with cytokeratin or the neuroendocrine markers chromogranin and synaptophysin.

Differential Diagnosis

The histologic differential diagnosis of acoustic neuromas include middle ear adenoma (with or without

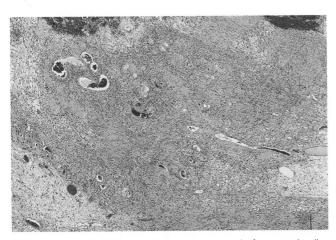

FIGURE 12–105 Acoustic neuroma composed of a central cellular zone of spindle cells (Antoni A areas) and loose, hypocellular zones (Antoni B areas) at the outer aspects of the illustration.

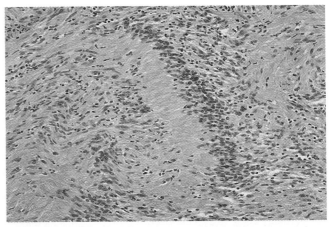

FIGURE 12–107 When present, a characteristic feature of acoustic neuromas is the presence of Verocay bodies characterized by a nuclear palisading with an orderly alignment of the nuclei in rows.

neuroendocrine differentiation), paraganglioma, and meningioma.

Clinicopathologic Correlation

Acoustic neuromas are benign neoplasms arising from Schwann cells specifically originating from the eighth cranial nerve. The histologic appearance is similar to benign peripheral nerve sheath tumors (schwannomas) of all other sites. Acoustic neuromas are the most common tumor of the cerebellopontine angle. Up to 8% may be bilateral, a potential indicator of neurofibromatosis type 2.[247–251] Malignant acoustic neuromas are exceedingly rare and, if present, neurofibromatosis should be suspected.

MENINGIOMA

Gross Pathology

The gross appearance of meningioma includes a lobular appearing, tan-white to grey, rubbery to firm, mass with a gritty consistency. In contrast to their intracranial counterparts, which are well-delineated and circumscribed lesions, meningiomas of the middle ear tend to be infiltrative with extension and invasion of adjacent structures.

Microscopic Pathology

Four histologic variants have been described and include syncytial or meningothelial, fibroblastic, transitional (combination of syncytial and fibroblastic), and angioblastic. In the middle ear, the most common histologic subtype is the meningothelial meningioma. The histologic features include a lobular growth with tumor nests separated by a variable amount of fibrous tissue. The cells have a whorled appearance and are composed of round to oval or spindle-shaped nuclei with pale staining cytoplasm and indistinct cell borders (Fig. 12–108). Characteristically, the nuclei have a punched-out or empty appearance resulting from intranuclear cytoplasmic inclusions. Psammoma bodies, typical and numerous in intracranial meningothelial meningiomas, may be seen but are not as common in meningiomas of the middle ear region (Fig. 12–109).

Special Techniques

The immunohistochemical antigenic profile of meningiomas include reactivity with epithelial membrane antigen (EMA) and vimentin. In contrast with middle ear adenomas, meningiomas are generally nonreactive with cytokeratin and—in contrast to jugulotympanic paragangliomas—meningiomas are nonreactive with neuroendocrine markers (i.e., chromogranin and synaptophysin).

Differential Diagnosis

The histologic differential diagnosis of meningioma includes middle ear adenoma (with or without neu-

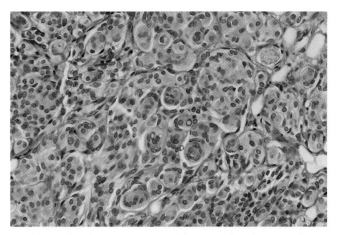

FIGURE 12–108 Meningioma of the internal auditory canal showing a cell nest or lobular growth separated by fibrovascular tissue. The cells have a whorled appearance and are composed of round to oval or spindle-shaped nuclei with pale staining cytoplasm and indistinct cell borders. The nuclei have a characteristic punched-out or empty appearance due to intranuclear cytoplasmic inclusions.

roendocrine differentiation), acoustic neuroma, and paraganglioma.

Clinicopathologic Correlation

Meningiomas are benign neoplasms arising from arachnoid cells forming the arachnoid villi seen in relation to the dural sinuses. Meningiomas occurring outside the central nervous system (CNS) are considered ectopic and can be divided into those meningiomas with no identifiable CNS connection (primary meningioma) and those with CNS connection (secondary meningioma). The development of primary meningiomas in the middle ear and temporal bone results from either direct extension or from the presence of ectopically located arachnoid cells. A diagnosis of middle ear meningioma should be made

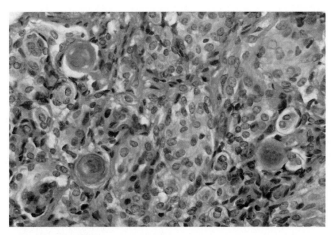

FIGURE 12–109 Psammoma bodies are a helpful diagnostic feature in this internal auditory canal meningioma.

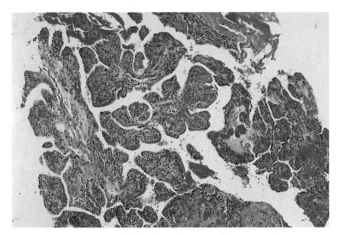

FIGURE 12–110 Endolymphatic sac papillary tumor showing a papillary growth pattern. A richly vascular stroma is present below the epithelial lining of the tumor.

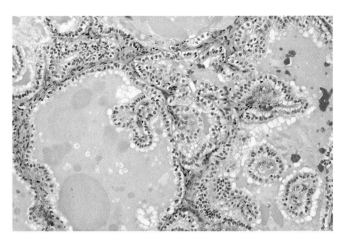

FIGURE 12–112 This endolymphatic sac papillary tumor has the morphologic appearance of thyroid papillary carcinoma.

only after clinical evaluation to exclude secondary extension from an intracranial neoplasm.[252]

ENDOLYMPHATIC SAC (PAPILLARY) TUMOR

Microscopic Pathology

The histopathologic appearance of endolymphatic sac (papillary) tumor (ELST) is quite variable. ELST are papillary and focally cystic tumors. The papillary structures are generally not complex in their growth and are perhaps not as well developed as in other papillary neoplasms (Fig. 12–110). The neoplastic cells vary in appearance from flattened or attenuated to columnar (Fig. 12–111). Most often there is only a single row of cells. Occasionally, the surface epithelial cells may have an appearance suggesting a double layer of cells (epithelial and myoepithelial). However, the "outer" row of cells, in all probability, represent a stromal element, as they

have not been shown to be immunoreactive with epithelial markers.[253] The epithelial cells have uniform nuclei (usually situated either in the center of the cells or toward the luminal aspect) and a pale eosinophilic to clear appearing cytoplasm. The latter may predominate in any given tumor. Cell borders may be seen but, not infrequently, the neoplastic cells lack a distinct cell membrane. In some cases, there are hypercellular areas with crowded, variably sized cystic glandular spaces that contain eosinophilic (colloid-like) material (Figs. 12–112 and 12–113). The latter appear remarkably similar to thyroid tissue. In all cases, pleomorphism is minimal, and mitotic activity and necrosis are rarely present.

A granulation tissue reaction is seen in association with the neoplastic cells and includes small vascular spaces lying in close proximity to the surface epithelium and/or within the stroma of the papillary fronds. Due to the absence of a distinct cell mem-

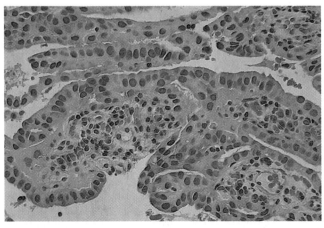

FIGURE 12–111 Higher magnification of Figure 12–110 showing distinct columnar-appearing cells aligned in a single row.

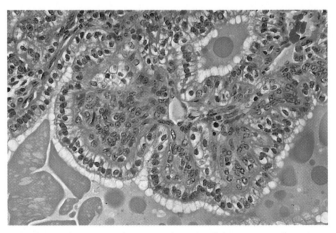

FIGURE 12–113 Higher magnification of the previous illustration shows the cytomorphologic similarities of this endolymphatic sac papillary tumor with thyroid papillary carcinoma, but thyroglobulin staining is not present.

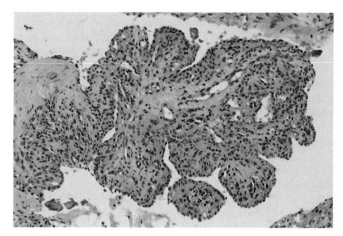

FIGURE 12–114 Another endolymphatic sac papillary tumor showing papillary growth pattern and vascular stroma but with a less discernible surface epithelial component.

brane around the neoplastic cells, a sharp demarcation separating the neoplastic cells from the subjacent granulation tissue may not be present. This appearance may create diagnostic confusion—the neoplastic proliferation may not be appreciated, and the neoplastic proliferation may be misdiagnosed as a reactive process (Figs. 12–114 and 12–115). This misinterpretation is further enhanced by the presence in the stroma of a mixed inflammatory cell infiltrate, fibrosis, vascular proliferation, fresh hemorrhage and/or hemosiderin (within the neoplastic cells or within macrophages), cholesterol granulomas, and dystrophic calcification. The latter does not include laminated calcific concretions (psammomatoid bodies).

Special Techniques

Intracytoplasmic diastase-sensitive, PAS positive material can be seen. The colloid-like luminal material

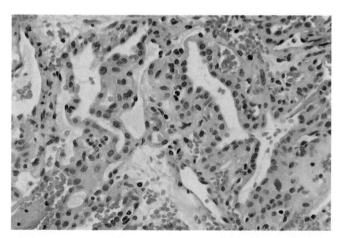

FIGURE 12–115 Higher magnification of the previous illustration showing the absence of a distinct cell membrane around the neoplastic epithelial cells. In this situation, the epithelial component of the tumor may be overlooked and considered as part of a reactive granulation tissue process.

stains strongly with PAS with and without diastase digestion. Intracytoplasmic and intraluminal mucin staining are rarely positive. Iron stains are positive.

ELST are diffusely cytokeratin positive and also show variable reactivity with epithelial membrane antigen (EMA), S-100 protein, vimentin, neuron-specific enolase (NSE), glial fibrillary acidic protein (GFAP), Ber-EP4, synaptophysin, and Leu-7.[254] Thyroglobulin immunoreactivity is not seen.

Electron Microscopy

Ultrastructurally, ELST show the presence of intercellular junctional complexes, microvilli, basement membrane material, rough endoplasmic reticulum, and intracytoplasmic glycogen and secretory granules.[253]

Differential Diagnosis

The differential diagnosis includes choroid plexus papilloma and metastatic papillary carcinoma of thyroid gland origin. These are differentiated on the basis of anatomic location and histologic and immunohistochemical findings.[254]

Clinicopathologic Correlation

The ELST—also referred to as adenoma of endolymphatic sac, adenoma/adenocarcinoma of temporal bone or mastoid, low-grade adenocarcinoma of probable endolymphatic sac origin, papillary adenoma of temporal bone, aggressive papillary tumor of temporal bone, aggressive papillary middle ear tumor, and more recently as the Heffner tumor—is an uncommon neoplasm representing a distinct clinicopathologic entity and possibly representing a manifestation of von Hippel-Lindau (VHL) syndrome.[232,238–240,243–245,255–266] An endolymphatic sac origin is supported by:

1. Early clinical manifestations of vestibular disease including sensorineural hearing loss, tinnitus, and episodic vertigo
2. Radiographic features showing the tumor to grow in the region of the posterior-medial petrous ridge, a site where the endolymphatic sac is located
3. Intraoperative identification of an in situ tumor (originating from within the endolymphatic sac)
4. Morphologic similarities and shared immunohistochemical and ultrastructural features of the tumor with the normal endolymphatic sac epithelium.[254]

The diagnosis of this tumor is one of clinical, radiographic, and pathologic correlation. In this way, diagnostic confusion may be minimized. A diagnosis of ELST should prompt the clinician to exclude the possibility that the patient has von Hippel-Lindau syndrome.

EPITHELIAL (SCHNEIDERIAN-TYPE) PAPILLOMAS

Gross Pathology

The intraoperative gross description of the tumor varies and includes a cauliflower-appearing mass to numerous grape-like or polypoid lesions filling the middle ear.[267] These lesions are described as yellow-tan to tan-white, soft to rubbery, and measuring from 0.2 cm to 0.7 cm in greatest diameter.[267]

Microscopic Pathology

The histologic appearance is that of a polypoid epithelial cell neoplasm. The predominant growth pattern is exophytic, composed of papillary fronds with a fibrovascular core. An endophytic or inverted growth pattern can also be seen. These tumors are histologically identical to the inverted or cylindrical cell types of sinonasal (Schneiderian) papilloma (Fig. 12–116). The epithelial component includes multilayered epidermoid and ciliated columnar cells with cellular uniformity, cell maturation, and retention of cell polarity. These different cell types may represent the sole component of a given tumor, or they may be admixed within the same case. Intercellular bridges can be seen in the epidermoid-appearing cells, and cilia can be seen along the surface of the columnar cells. In addition, mucocytes and acute and chronic inflammatory cells, as well as intraepithelial cysts are identified in the epithelial layer. Surface keratinization is not present.

Special Techniques

Intracytoplasmic and extracellular mucicarminophilic and diastase-resistant, PAS positive material is present within the cytoplasm of the mucocytes as well as within the intraepithelial cystic structures.[267]

The epithelial neoplastic cells are cytokeratin reactive but not reactive with chromogranin.[267] Immunohistochemical evaluation for human papillomavirus particles (6/11 and 16/18) failed to demonstrate reactivity in the five cases reported by Wenig.[267]

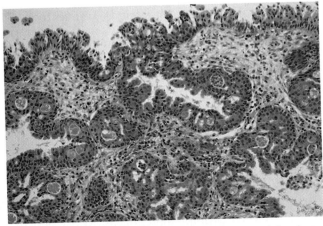

FIGURE 12–116 Middle ear epithelial papilloma with histologic features of a cylindrical cell papilloma of the sinonasal tract.

Differential Diagnosis

The differential diagnosis primarily is with a middle ear adenoma. In contrast to middle ear adenomas, the Schneiderian papillomas are not gland-forming tumors, nor do they demonstrate the cytomorphologic features seen in middle ear adenomas and described previously. Other tumors occurring in the middle ear—such as jugulotympanic paraganglioma, acoustic neuroma, and meningioma—should not present diagnostic difficulties with middle ear Schneiderian papillomas, and should be readily distinguished on the basis of light microscopic evaluation. Differentiation from the endolymphatic sac papillary tumor can be made on the basis of histologic differences between these two tumors, as well as the localization of ESPT to the temporal bone petrous ridge and/or endolymphatic sac.

Clinicopathologic Correlation

Stone and colleagues[268] invoke the notion that the Schneiderian type of middle ear papilloma may occur via transmission of a prior sinonasal-tract Schneiderian papilloma through the eustachian tube to the middle ear space. However, this would appear to be a remote possibility, especially in the absence of identifying nasopharyngeal papillomas colonizing the eustachian tube. Stone and colleagues[268] did not identify a nasopharyngeal neoplasm, nor were any nasopharyngeal tumors seen in the cases reported in the study by Wenig.[267] Kaddour and Woodhead[269] also reject the notion of transmission via the eustachian tube, suggesting a multicentric primary origin of the Schneiderian papillomas. As indicated by Kaddour and Woodhead[269] and Wenig,[267] a more plausible explanation for the occurrence of Schneiderian papillomas in the middle ear possibly relates to extensive embryologic migration of the Schneiderian mucosa to include ectopic distribution in the middle ear. A diagnosis of middle ear Schneiderian-type papilloma should be made only following clinical exclusion of a primary paranasal sinus or nasopharyngeal papilloma secondarily involving the middle ear via extension through the eustachian tube.

OTHER BENIGN TUMORS

While uncommon, a number of other primary benign tumors can be found in the middle ear or temporal bone. These tumors are primarily mesenchymal, including hemangiomas, lipoma, osteoma, chondroblastoma, and teratomas.[270–280]

Malignant Neoplasms of the Middle Ear

The classification of malignant neoplasms of the middle ear and temporal bone are listed in Table 12–8.

SQUAMOUS CELL CARCINOMA

Microscopic Pathology

The histology is similar to squamous carcinomas of other sites and includes infiltrative malignant cells with associated keratinization and/or intercellular bridges (Fig. 12–117). The neoplasms may vary from well to poorly differentiated and may or may not be seen arising from the middle ear mucosa. Often there is evidence of chronic otitis media seen in association with the infiltrating carcinoma as demonstrated by the presence of a chronic inflammatory cell infiltrate, calcifications (tympanosclerosis), and glandular proliferation (Fig. 12–118). A concomitant cholesteatoma may be present, but these tumors do not develop from cholesteatomas.

Differential Diagnosis

The differential diagnosis includes a cholesteatoma and metastatic squamous cell carcinoma. Cholesteatomas do not have the dysplastic cytologic changes seen in squamous carcinoma. Secondary involvement of this area by squamous cell carcinoma may originate from a distant site and metastasize to the middle ear and temporal bone. Alternatively, a cutaneous squamous cell carcinoma from an adjacent site (external ear, nasopharynx, parotid gland, or skin) can directly invade into the middle ear or temporal bone. Detailed clinical history or physical examination would assist in identifying a squamous carcinoma that is metastatic to this site or extends to the middle ear from an adjacent primary tumor.

Clinicopathologic Correlation

Primary malignant neoplasms with squamous differentiation originating from the middle ear mucosal epithelium are rare.[281–283] The majority of patients have a history of chronic otitis media usually longer

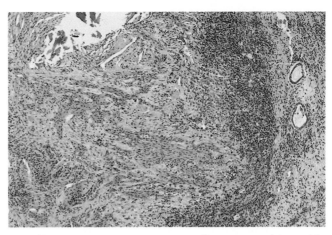

FIGURE 12–118 Primary squamous cell carcinoma of the middle ear occurring in the setting of chronic otitis media. Histologic features of the latter include chronic inflammation, glandular metaplasia, and mineralized debris (tympanosclerosis).

than 20 years in duration.[281] The development of a middle ear squamous cell carcinoma should be suspected in patients with a long history of chronic otitis media who present with sudden onset of pain out of proportion to the clinical extent of disease, onset or increase of otorrhea that is often hemorrhagic, and a lack of clinical resolution following therapeutic doses of antibiotics. The development of middle ear squamous cell carcinoma is also linked to radiation treatment for intracranial neoplasms and, although no longer used, radiotherapy for middle ear inflammatory conditions.

MIDDLE EAR ADENOCARCINOMA

Gross Pathology

Middle ear adenocarcinomas may attain large sizes, filling the middle ear space and encasing the ossicles.[284]

Microscopic Pathology

The histology includes an unencapsulated and infiltrative glandular proliferation that in many respects is similar to adenomas but includes the presence of pleomorphism, increased mitotic activity, and extensive infiltration of surrounding soft tissue structures involving nerves, lymph-vascular spaces, and bone (Fig. 12–119).

Special Techniques

Histochemical stains may show intraluminal mucin positive material. Immunohistochemical reactivity with epithelial markers such as cytokeratin will be reactive. Immunoreactivity is not seen with prostate specific antigen, prostatic acid phosphatase, estrogen or progesterone receptors, BRST-2, or thyroglobulin.

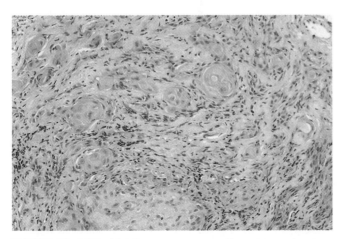

FIGURE 12–117 Middle ear squamous cell carcinoma showing an infiltrative cancer with the conventional features of well-differentiated squamous cell carcinoma.

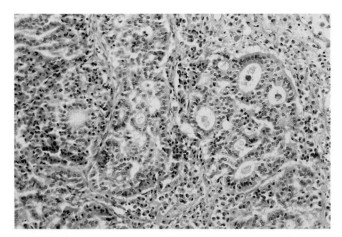

FIGURE 12–119 *Primary middle ear adenocarcinoma characterized by its complex cribriform growth, cytologic atypia, mitotic activity, and focal necrosis. This tumor was widely invasive within the temporal bone.*

Differential Diagnosis

The histologic differential diagnosis includes a middle ear adenoma. While adenomas may be locally infiltrative, including neurotropism, they lack the complexity of growth and cytologic anaplastic alterations seen in adenocarcinomas. Given the rarity of primary middle ear adenocarcinomas, a metastasis from a distant primary site should be clinically excluded. The absence of immunoreactivity with a potentially organ-specific immunohistochemical marker (e.g., prostate, breast, or thyroid) assists in the diagnosis. Further, confinement of the tumor to the middle ear and the association with the middle ear mucosa support origin from the middle ear and temporal bone.

Clinicopathologic Correlation

Middle ear adenocarcinoma is a malignant glandular neoplasm arising from the middle ear mucosa. Middle ear adenocarcinomas are rare.[284–288] In the presence of a malignant glandular neoplasm of the middle ear and temporal bone secondary metastasis to this region should be excluded.

RHABDOMYOSARCOMA

Gross Pathology

The gross appearance of aural rhabdomyosarcoma (RMS) most commonly presents as an otic (external or middle ear) polyp. Sarcoma botryoides (botryoid RMS) is a variant of embryonal RMS characterized by its gross appearance that includes a polypoid and myxoid mass.

Microscopic Pathology

According to the WHO classification, RMS is divided into six histologic subtypes, including embry-

onal, botryoid, spindle cell, alveolar, pleomorphic, and RMS with ganglionic differentiation (so-called ectomesenchymoma).[289] The Intergroup classification of RMS proposed four groups based on prognosis, including (I) Superior prognosis (botryoid RMS and spindle cell RMS), (II) Intermediate prognosis (embryonal RMS), (III) Poor prognosis (alveolar RMS and undifferentiated RMS), and (IV) Subtypes whose prognosis is not presently evaluable (RMS with rhabdoid features).[290]

The majority of RMS of the head and neck are of the embryonal type that includes botryoid type, representing 80% to 85% of cases. This is followed by alveolar RMS, representing 10% to 15% of cases. The other histologic types may occur in the head and neck but are considered uncommon.

Embryonal RMS represents the most common histologic variant seen in head and neck RMS. Typically, there is a variation in the cellularity of these tumors with alternating hyper- and hypocellular areas; the latter often is associated with a myxoid stroma (Fig. 12–120). The cellular components consist of both round and spindle cells. The round cells resemble lymphocytes and are round to oval with hyperchromatic nuclei and an acidophilic to amphophilic, distinct to indistinct cytoplasm (Fig. 12–121). The spindle cells are elongated with central hyperchromatic nuclei and eosinophilic cytoplasm. The nuclei tend to have pointed ends. Mitoses and necrosis are commonly seen. The stroma may be myxoid, fibrillar, or edematous. The histologic appearance of sarcoma botryoides (botryoid RMS) includes the presence of a cambium layer in which a subepithelial condensation of the neoplastic cells are seen.

Alveolar RMS is characterized by the presence of ill-defined collections of noncohesive tumor cells, the central portions of which appear empty or markedly hypocellular, giving the appearance of forming spaces or alveoli (Fig. 12–122). Portions of the tumor do not take on the alveolar appearance but are

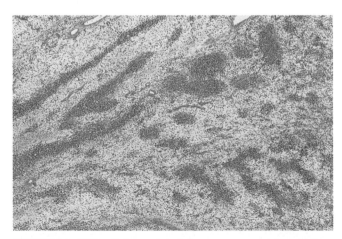

FIGURE 12–120 *Embryonal rhabdomyosarcoma of the middle ear showing variable cellularity including hyper- and hypocellular (myxoid) areas.*

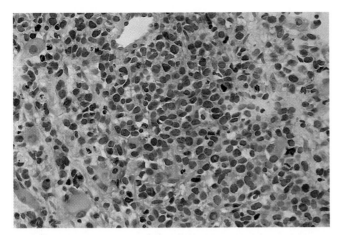

FIGURE 12–121 Rhabdomyosarcoma composed of small round cells with hyperchromatic nuclei and acidophilic to amphophilic to indistinct cytoplasm. Mitotic figures are present.

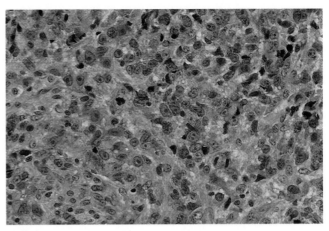

FIGURE 12–123 Malignant undifferentiated cellular infiltrate. This neoplasm was poorly differentiated, lacking evidence of cross striations, and was confirmed as a rhabdomyosarcoma only after special stains were performed.

rather composed of solid aggregates of tumor cells arranged in a trabecular pattern. The cellular portions of the tumor are separated by dense fibrous connective tissue forming septa and associated with prominent vascular spaces. The tumor cells are round to oval to spindle-shaped with hyperchromatic nuclei, inconspicuous nucleoli, and an acidophilic to amphophilic cytoplasm. Increased mitotic activity, including atypical mitoses, may be present, and necrosis can be seen. Multinucleated giant cells with peripherally placed nuclei are a prominent feature.

Irrespective of the histologic variant, general histologic considerations of RMS include the presence of rhabdomyoblasts, the cell of origin for this sarcoma, which may take on numerous appearances, including small round cells to ribbon- or strap-shaped to large and pleomorphic. Rhabdomyoblasts with cross-striations are not always identified, and their

absence does not exclude the diagnosis of rhabdomyosarcoma. An associated benign inflammatory infiltrate may predominate, overrunning and masking the presence of the neoplastic cells. In the presence of a poorly differentiated neoplasm lacking evidence of cross-striations, special stains are invaluable in confirming the diagnosis of rhabdomyosarcoma (Fig. 12–123).

Special Techniques

Histochemical stains may be of assistance in the diagnosis. The neoplastic cells demonstrate the presence of intracytoplasmic glycogen (diastase-sensitive, PAS-positive) (Fig. 12–124). Stains for epithelial mucin are negative. Intracellular myofibrils can be seen by Masson's trichrome and phosphotungstic acid–hematoxylin stains.

Immunohistochemistry is an important adjunct in

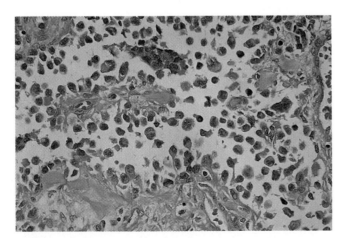

FIGURE 12–122 Alveolar rhabdomyosarcoma is characterized by the presence of noncohesive tumor cells, the central portions of which appear empty or markedly hypocellular, seeming to form spaces or alveoli.

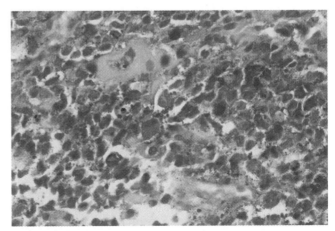

FIGURE 12–124 Rhabdomyosarcomas typically show intracytoplasmic PAS-positive material that is cleared following diastase digestion. This diastase-sensitive, PAS-positive material is glycogen, present in the neoplastic cells of rhabdomyosarcoma.

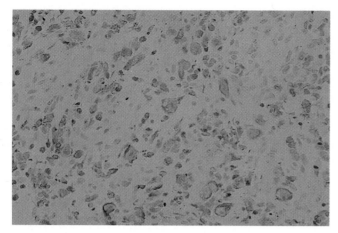

FIGURE 12-125 The neoplastic cells of rhabdomyosarcoma are immunoreactive with desmin.

the diagnosis of RMS and includes immunoreactivity with desmin (Fig. 12–125), myoglobin, actin (muscle-specific), and vimentin. In general, there is no immunoreactivity seen with epithelial markers (cytokeratin, EMA, CEA, others), LCA, neuroendocrine markers (chromogranin, synaptophysin, NSE, Leu-7, GFAP, NFP), S-100 protein, HMB-45, or Ewing's marker.

Differential Diagnosis

The histologic diagnosis of RMS may be overlooked in the presence of obscuring inflammatory cells as may occur in an aural polyp. The differential diagnosis of middle ear RMS includes other round cell malignancies, including malignant melanoma, malignant lymphoma, and poorly differentiated epithelial and mesenchymal tumors. Generally, differentiation can be established on the basis of the combined light microscopic, histochemical, and immunohistochemical findings.

Clinicopathologic Correlation

RMS is a malignant tumor of skeletal muscle cells (rhabdomyoblasts). In the head and neck, RMS is primarily, but not exclusively, a disease of the pediatric population.[291–295] If all ages are considered, RMS comprises up to half of all soft-tissue sarcomas of the head and neck. RMS restricted to pediatric ages represents up to 75% of all soft-tissue sarcomas of the head and neck.[291,292] In the pediatric age group, RMS represents the most common aural malignant neoplasm.[293] There is no gender predilection. In the head and neck, the most common sites of occurrence of RMS (in descending order of occurrence) include the orbit, nasopharynx, middle ear/temporal bone, and the sinonasal tract.[293] If only adults are considered, the most frequent site of occurrence is the sinonasal tract.[296–298] RMS is associated with chromosomal abnormalities, includ-

ing chromosomal translocations [t(2;13)(q35;q14) and t(1;13)(p36q14)] in alveolar RMS, but other changes occur, including structural abnormalities, translocations, and nonrandom chromosome alterations.[299–301]

OTHER MALIGNANT TUMORS

While uncommon, a number of other malignant tumors can originate in the middle ear or temporal bone. These tumors are primarily mesenchymal, including matrix-forming neoplasms such as osteosarcoma and chondrosarcoma. Osteosarcomas of the skull are uncommon, with approximately 1% to 2% of all osteosarcomas occurring in this location.[302,303] Osteosarcomas of the skull often arise in the setting of Paget's disease of bone, fibrous dysplasia, or secondary to radiotherapy.[302,303] Chondrosarcomas of the temporal bone are rare. The petrous apex and posteromedial aspect of the temporal bone are perhaps the most common sites of occurrence.[304] Osteosarcomas of the skull are aggressive tumors with a tendency for metastasis to the lungs and brain and with less than 15% 5-year survivals.[302,303,305] As reported by Coltera and colleagues,[304] chondrosarcomas of the temporal bone are not necessarily lethal tumors, as 13 of their 17 cases with follow-up survived their tumors over periods ranging up to 8 years.

Other malignancies of the middle ear and temporal bones include hematolymphoid neoplasms, including malignant lymphomas (non-Hodgkin's and Hodgkin's), leukemia, and plasma cell dyscrasias.[306–308] Middle ear and temporal bone involvement by a malignant hematolymphoid neoplasm is often secondary to primary disease elsewhere.

SECONDARY TUMORS

Metastatic tumors secondarily involving the middle ear and temporal bone originate from virtually

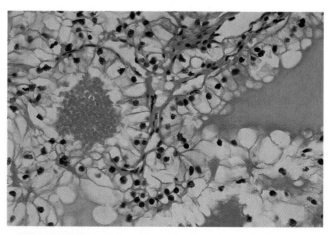

FIGURE 12-126 Metastatic renal cell carcinoma to the temporal bone showing characteristic cells with clear cytoplasm, distinct cell borders, intraluminal red blood cells, and fibrovascular stroma separating neoplastic nests.

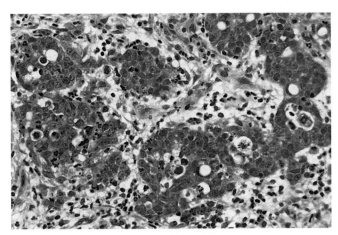

FIGURE 12-127 Metastatic prostate adenocarcinoma with gland formation and neoplastic cells showing prominent nucleoli. These histologic features are not diagnostic of prostatic adenocarcinoma; immunohistochemical stains showed reactivity with both prostatic acid phosphatase (PAP) and prostate specific antigen (PSA), confirming the diagnosis.

every site. The more common malignant tumors to metastasize to this region include breast adenocarcinoma, pulmonary adenocarcinoma, renal cell carcinoma (Fig. 12–126), malignant melanoma, and prostatic adenocarcinoma (Fig. 12–127).[309–312] While metastases to the temporal bone often occur late in the disease course, metastatic involvement of the temporal bone may represent the initial presentation of a distant malignant disease.[313–315] Metastatic disease to the temporal bone occurs via hematogenous spread but may also occur by direct extension from a nearby primary tumor (e.g., squamous cell carcinoma), meningeal carcinomatosis, or leptomeningeal extension from an intracranial primary neoplasm.[316]

REFERENCES

1. Moore KL. The ear. In: Moore KL, ed. *The Developing Human: Clinically Oriented Embryology.* 4th ed. Philadelphia: WB Saunders; 1988:412.
2. Dayal VS, Farkashidy J, Kokshanian A. Embryology of the ear. *Can J Otolaryngol.* 1973; 2:136.
3. Cheng LH. Keloid of the ear lobe. *Laryngoscope.* 1972; 82:673.
4. Murray JC, Pollack SV, Pinnel SR. Keloids: A review. *J Am Acad Dermatol.* 1981; 4:461.
5. Santa Cruz DJ, Ulbright TM. Mucin-like changes in keloids. *Am J Clin Pathol.* 1981; 75:18.
6. Blackburn WR, Cosman B. Histologic basis of keloid and hypertrophic scar differentiation. *Arch Pathol.* 1966; 82:65.
7. Kuo TT, Hu S, Chan HL. Keloidal dermatofibroma. Report of 10 cases of a new variant. *Am J Surg Pathol.* 1998; 22:564.
8. Tuan T-L, Zhu JY, Sun B, et al. Elevated levels of plasminogen activator inhibitor-1 may account for altered fibrinolysis by keloid fibroblasts. *J Dermatol.* 1996; 106:1007.
9. Engel D. Pseudocysts of the auricle in Chinese. *Arch Otolaryngol.* 1966; 83:29.
10. Glamb R, Kim R. Pseudocyst of the auricle. *J Am Acad Dermatol.* 1984; 11:58.
11. Heffner DK, Hyams VJ. Cystic chondromalacia (endochondral pseudocyst) of the auricle. *Arch Pathol Lab Med.* 1986; 110:740.
12. Choi S, Lam K, Chan K, et al. Endochondral pseudocyst of the auricle in Chinese. *Arch Otolaryngol.* 1984; 110:792.
13. Shuman R, Helwig EB. Chondrodermatitis helicis. *Am J Clin Pathol.* 1954; 24:126.
14. Santa Cruz DJ. Chondrodermatitis nodularis helicis: A transepidermal perforating disorder. *J Cutan Pathol.* 1980; 7:70.
15. Mehregan AH. Perforating dermatosis: A clinicopathologic review. *Int J Dermatol.* 1977; 16:19.
16. Barker LP, Young AW, Sachs W. Chondrodermatitis of the ears. *Arch Dermatol.* 1960; 81:15.
17. Metzger SA, Goodman ML. Chondrodermatitis helicis: A clinical re-evaluation and pathological review. *Laryngoscope.* 1976; 86:1402.
18. Winkler M. Knotchenformige erkrankung am helix. Chondrodermatitis nodularis chronica helicis. *Arch Dermatol Syphilol.* 1915; 212:278.
19. Newcomer VD, Steffan CG, Sternberg TH, Lichtenstein L. Chondrodermatitis nodularis chronica helicis. *Arch Dermatol Syphilol.* 1953; 68:241.
20. Carol ELL, Van Haren HB. Chondrodermatitis nodularis chronica helicis. *Dermatologica.* 1941; 83:353.
21. McAdam LP, O'Hanlan MA, Bluestone R, Pearson CM. Relapsing polychondritis: Prospective study of 23 patients and a review of the literature. *Medicine.* 1976; 55:193.
22. Damiani JM, Levine HL. Relapsing polychondritis—report of ten cases. *Laryngoscope.* 1979; 89:929.
23. Irani BS, Martin-Hirsch DP, Clark D, et al. Relapsing polychondritis—a study of four cases. *J Laryngol Otol.* 1992; 106: 911.
24. Harisdangkul V, Johnson WW. Association between relapsing polychondritis and systemic lupus erythematosus. *South Med J.* 1994; 87:753.
25. Diebold L, Rauh G, Jager K, Lohrs U. Bone marrow pathology in relapsing polychondritis: High frequency of myelodysplastic syndromes. *Br J Haematol.* 1995; 89:820.
26. Hebbar M, Brouillard M, Wattel E, et al. Association of myelodysplastic syndrome and relapsing polychondritis: Further evidence. *Leukemia.* 1995; 9:731.
27. Shirota T, Hayashi O, Uchida H, et al. Myelodysplastic syndrome associated with relapsing polychondritis: Unusual transformation from refractory anemia to chronic myelomonocytic leukemia. *Ann Hematol.* 1993; 67:45.
28. Dolan DL, Lemmon GB Jr, Teitelbaum SL. Relapsing polychondritis: Analytical literature review and studies on pathogenesis. *Am J Med.* 1966; 41:285.
29. Froidart J-M, Abe S, Martin GR, et al. Antibodies to type II collagen in relapsing polychondritis. *N Engl J Med.* 1978; 299: 1203.
30. Valenzuela R, Cooperrider PA, Gogate P, et al. Relapsing polychondritis immunomicroscopic findings in cartilage of ear biopsy specimens. *Hum Pathol.* 1980; 11:19.
31. Helm TN, Valenzuela R, Glanz S, et al. Relapsing polychondritis: A case diagnosed by direct immunofluorescence and coexistng with pseudocyst of the auricle. *J Am Acad Dermatol.* 1992; 26:315.
32. Lang B, Rothenfusser A, Lanchbury JS, et al. Susceptibility to relapsing polychondritis is associated with HLA-DR4. *Arthritis Rheum.* 1993; 36:660.
33. Olsen TG, Helwig EB. Angiolymphoid hyperplasia with eosinophilia. A clinicopathologic study of 116 patients. *J Am Acad Dermatol.* 1985; 12:781.
34. Mehregan AH, Shapiro L. Angiolymphoid hyperplasia with eosinophilia. *Arch Dermatol.* 1971; 103:50.
35. Barnes L, Koss W, Nieland ML. Angiolymphoid hyperplasia with eosinophilia: A disease that may be confused with malignancy. *Head Neck Surg.* 1980; 2:425.
36. Rosai J, Gold J, Landy R. The histiocytoid hemangiomas. A unifying concept embracing several previously described entities of skin, soft tissue, large vessels, bone, and heart. *Hum Pathol.* 1979; 10:707.
37. Chun SI, Goo H. Kimura's disease and angiolymphoid hyperplasia with eosinophilia: Clinical and histopathologic differences. *J Am Acad Dermatol.* 1992; 27:954.

38. Fetsch JF, Weiss SW. Observations concerning the pathogenesis of epithelioid hemangioma (angiolymphoid hyperplasia). *Mod Pathol.* 1991; 4:449.

39. Urabe A, Tsuneyoshi M, Enjoji M. Epithelioid hemangioma versus Kimura's disease: A comparative clinicopathologic study. *Am J Surg Pathol.* 1987; 11:758.

40. Wells GC, Whimster IW. Subcutaneous angiolymphoid hyperplasia with eosinophilia. *Br J Dermatol.* 1969; 81:1.

41. Googe PB, Harris NL, Mihm MC Jr. Kimura's disease and angiolymphoid hyperplasia with eosinophilia: Two distinct histopathological entities. *J Cutan Pathol.* 1987; 14:263.

42. Kuo TT, Shih LY, Chan HL. Kimura's disease: Involvement of regional lymph nodes and distinction from angiolymphoid hyperplasia with eosinophilia. *Am J Surg Pathol.* 1988; 12:843.

43. Allen PW, Ramakrishna B, MacCormac LB. The histiocytoid hemangiomas and other controversies. *Pathol Ann.* 1992; 27(2):51.

44. Chandler JR. Malignant otitis externa. *Laryngoscope.* 1968; 78:1257.

45. Chandler JR. Malignant external otitis: Further considerations. *Ann Otol Rhinol Laryngol.* 1986; 84:417.

46. Chandler JR. Pathogenesis and treatment of facial paralysis due to malignant otitis externa. *Ann Otol Rhinol Laryngol.* 1987; 101:211.

47. Bernheim J, Sade J. Histopathology of the soft parts in 50 patients with malignant external otitis. *J Laryngol Otol.* 1989; 103:366.

48. Nager GT. Necrotizing ("malignant") granulomatous external otitis and osteomyelitis. In: Nager GT, ed. *Pathology of the Ear and Temporal Bone.* Baltimore: Williams & Wilkins; 1993:192.

49. Al-Shihabi BA. Carcinoma of the temporal bone presenting as malignant otitis externa. *J Laryngol Otol.* 1992; 106:908.

50. Grandis JR, Hirsch BE, Yu VL. Simultaneous presentation of malignant external otitis and temporal bone cancer. *Arch Otolaryngol Head Neck Surg.* 1993; 119:687.

51. Weinroth SE, Schessel D, Tuazon CU. Malignant otitis externa in AIDS patients: Case report and review of the literature. *Ear Nose Throat J.* 1994; 73:772.

52. Shpitzer T, Stern Y, Cohen O, et al. Malignant external otitis in nondiabetic patients. *Ann Otol Rhinol Laryngol.* 1993; 102:870.

53. Corberand J, Nguyen F, Fraysse B, Enjalbert L. Malignant external otitis and polymorphonuclear leukocyte migration impairment. *Arch Otolaryngol.* 1982; 108:122.

54. Kohut RI, Lindsay JR. Necrotizing external otitis: Histopathologic processes. *Ann Otol Rhinol Laryngol.* 1979; 88:714.

55. Ostfeld E, Segal M, Czernobilsky B. Malignant external otitis: Early histopathologic changes and pathogenetic mechanism. *Laryngoscope.* 1981; 91:965.

56. Piepergerdes JC, Kramer BM, Behnke EE. Keratosis obturans and external auditory canal cholesteatoma. *Laryngoscope.* 1980; 90:383.

57. Adair CF, Hyams VJ. Pathology of the ear and temporal bone. In: English GM, ed. *Otolaryngology.* Vol 1. Philadelphia: Lippincott-Raven; 1996:1.

58. Nager GT. Osteomas and exostoses. In: Nager GT, ed. *Pathology of the Ear and Temporal Bone.* Baltimore: Williams & Wilkins; 1993:483.

59. Graham MD. Osteomas and exostoses of the external auditory canal. A clinical, histopathological, and scanning electron microscopic study. *Ann Otol.* 1979; 88:566.

60. Schuknecht H. Exostoses of the external auditory canal. In: Schuknect H, ed. *Pathology of the Ear.* Philadelphia: Lea & Febiger; 1993:398.

61. Friedmann I, Arnold W. Cartilaginous and osteogenic neoplasms. In: Friedmann I, ed. *Pathology of the Ear.* Edinburgh: Churchill Livingston; 1993:307.

62. Fenton JE, Turner J, Fagan PA. A histopathologic review of temporal bone exostoses and osteomata. *Laryngoscope.* 1996; 106:624.

63. Goodwin RE, Fisher GH. Keratoacanthoma of the head and neck. *Ann Otol.* 1980; 89:72.

64. Patterson HC. Facial keratoacanthoma. *Otolaryngol Head Neck Surg.* 1983; 91:263.

65. Reed RJ. Actinic keratoacanthoma. *Arch Dermatol.* 1972; 106:858.

66. Janecka IP, Wolff M, Crikelair GF, Cosman B. Aggressive histological features of keratoacanthoma. *J Cutan Pathol.* 1978; 4:342.

67. Wade TR, Ackerman AB. The many faces of keratoacanthoma. *J Dermatol Surg Oncol* 1978; 4:498.

68. Lapins NA, Helwig EB. Perineural invasion by keratoacanthoma. *Arch Dermatol.* 1980; 116:791.

69. Hodak E, Jones RE, Ackerman AB. Solitary keratoacanthoma is a squamous-cell carcinoma: Three examples with metastases. *Am J Dermatopathol.* 1993; 15:332.

70. Grant-Kels JM. Response. *Am J Dermatopathol.* 1993; 15:343.

71. Davies DG. Keratoacanthoma or squamous carcinoma? *J Laryngol Otol.* 1969; 83:333.

72. Iverson RE, Vistnes LM. Keratoacanthoma is frequently a dangerous diagnosis. *Am J Surg.* 1973; 126:359.

73. Schnur PL, Bozzo P. Metastasizing keratoacanthomas? *Plast Reconst Surg.* 1978; 62:258.

74. Sullivan JJ, Colditz GA. Keratoacanthoma in a subtropical climate. *Aust J Dermatol.* 1979; 20:34.

75. Piscioli F, Boi S, Zumiani G, Cristofolini M. A gigantic metastasizing keratoacanthoma. *Am J Dermatopathol.* 1984; 6:123.

76. Reed RJ. Response. *Am J Dermatopathol.* 1993; 15:347.

77. Hyams VJ, Batsakis JG, Michaels L. Neoplasms of the external ear. In: Hartmann WH, Sobin LH, eds. *Tumors of the Upper Respiratory Tract.* 2nd series. Fascicle 25. Washington, DC: Armed Forces Institute of Pathology; 1988:281.

78. Batsakis JG, Hardy GC, Hishiyama RH. Ceruminous gland tumors. *Arch Otolaryngol.* 1967; 86:92.

79. Leitner MJ. Adenoma of the ceruminous glands. *Am J Clin Pathol.* 1952; 22:466.

80. Hicks GW. Tumors arising from the glandular structures of the external auditory canal. *Laryngoscope.* 1983; 93:326.

81. Wetli CV, Pardo V, Millard M, Gerston K. Tumours of the ceruminous glands. *Cancer.* 1972; 29:1169.

82. Moss R, Labay G, Mehta N. Ceruminoma revisited. *Am J Otol.* 1987; 8:485.

83. Mansour P, George MK, Pahor AL. Ceruminous gland tumors: A reappraisal. *J Laryngol Otol.* 1992; 106:727.

84. Nager GT. Neoplasms and other lesions of the external ear. In: Nager GT, ed. *Pathology of the Ear and Temporal Bone.* Baltimore: Williams & Wilkins; 1993:387.

85. Haraguchi H, Hentona H, Tanaka H, Komatuzaki A. Pleomorphic adenoma of the external auditory canal: A case report and review of the literature. *J Laryngol Otol.* 1996; 110:52.

86. Fink H. External auditory canal: Mixed tumor of salivary gland type. *Brooklyn Hospital Journal.* 1953; 11:104.

87. Smith HW, Duarte I. Mixed tumors of the external auditory canal. *Arch Otolaryngol.* 1962; 75:108.

88. Goldenberg RA, Block BL. Pleomorphic adenoma manifesting as aural polyp. *Arch Otolaryngol.* 1980; 106:440.

89. Braun GA, Lowry LD, Meyers A. Bilateral choristomas of the external auditory canals. *Arch Otolaryngol.* 1978; 104:467.

90. Nissim F, Czernobilsky B, Ostfeld E. Hidradenoma papilliferum of the external auditory canal. *J Laryngol Otol.* 1981; 95:843.

91. Unni KK. Benign osteoblastoma. In: Unni KK, ed. *Dahlin's Bone Tumors.* 5th ed. Philadelphia: Lippincott-Raven; 1996:131.

92. Mirra JM, Kendrick RA, Kendrick RE. Pseudomalignant osteoblastoma versus arrested osteosarcoma: A case report. *Cancer.* 1976; 37:2005.

93. Lucas DR, Unni KK, McLeod RA, et al. Osteoblastoma: Clinicopathologic study of 306 cases. *Hum Pathol.* 1994; 25:117.

94. Bertoni F, Unni KK, McLeod RA, Dahlin DC. Osteosarcoma resembling osteoblastoma. *Cancer.* 1985; 55:416.

95. Dorfman HD, Weiss SW. Borderline osteoblastic tumors:

Problems in the differential diagnosis of aggressive osteoblastoma and low-grade osteosarcoma. *Semin Diagn Pathol.* 1984; 1:215.

96. Della Roca C, Huvos AG. Osteoblastoma: Do histologic features predict clinical behavior? A study of 55 patients (abstract). *Mod Pathol.* 1994; 7:6A.

97. Quercetani R, Gelli R, Pimpinelli N, Reali U. Bilateral chondroma of the auricle. *J Dermatol Surg Oncol.* 1988; 14:436.

98. Unni KK. Chondroma. In: Unni KK, ed. *Dahlin's Bone Tumors.* 5th ed. Philadelphia: Lippincott-Raven; 1996:25.

99. Enzinger FM, Weiss SW. Intramuscular myxoma. In: Enzinger FM, Weiss SW, eds. *Soft Tissue Tumors.* 3rd ed. St. Louis: Mosby; 1995:1045.

100. Ferreiro JA, Carney JA. Myxomas of the external ear and their significance. *Am J Surg Pathol.* 1994; 18:274.

101. Unni KK. Fibrous dysplasia. In: Unni KK, ed. *Dahlin's Bone Tumors.* 5th ed. Philadelphia: Lippincott-Raven; 1996: 367.

102. Adair CF, Hyams VJ. Pathology of the ear and temporal bone. In: English GM, ed. *Otolaryngology.* Vol 1. Philadelphia: Lippincott-Raven; 1996:53.

103. Kempson RL. Ossifying fibroma of the long bones. *Arch Pathol.* 1966; 82:218.

104. Waldron CA. Fibro-osseous lesions of the jaws. *J Oral Maxillofac Surg.* 1985; 63:249.

105. Pindborg JJ, Kramer IRH. Histologic typing of odontogenic tumors, jaw cysts and allied lesions. Geneva: World Health Organization, 1971.

106. Schajowicz F, Ackerman LV, Sissons HA. Histologic typing of bone tumors. Geneva: World Health Organization, 1972.

107. Waldron CA, Giansanti JS. Benign fibro-osseous lesions of the jaws. Part I: Fibrous dysplasia of the jaws. *Oral Surg.* 1973; 35:190.

108. Eversole LR, Sabes WR, Rovin S. Fibrous dysplasia: A nosologic problem in the diagnosis of fibro-osseous lesions of the jaws. *J Oral Pathol.* 1972; 1:189.

109. Unni KK. Giant cell tumor. In: *Dahlin's Bone Tumors.* 5th ed. Philadelphia: Lippincott-Raven; 1996:263.

110. Wolfe JY, Scheitauer BW, Dahlin DC. Giant cell tumor of the sphenoid bone: Review of 10 cases. *J Neurosurg.* 1983; 59:322.

111. Bertoni F, Unni KK, Beabout JW, Ebersold MJ. Giant cell tumor of the skull. *Cancer.* 1992; 70:1124.

112. Adair CF, Hyams VJ. Pathology of the ear and temporal bone. In: English GM, ed. *Otolaryngology.* Vol 1. Philadelphia: Lippincott-Raven; 1996:54.

113. Bertoni F, Present D, Sudanese A, Baldini N, Bacchini P, Campanacci M. Giant cell tumor of bone with pulmonary metastases. Six case reports and a review of the literature. *Clin Orthop.* 1988; 237:275.

114. Kay RM, Eckardt JJ, Seeger LL, Mirra JM, Hak DJ. Pulmonary metastasis of benign giant cell tumor of bone. Six histologically confirmed cases, including one of spontaneous regression. *Clin Orthop.* 1994; 302:219.

115. Rock MG, Sim FH, Unni KK, et al. Secondary malignant giant-cell tumor of bone. Clinicopathologic assessment of nineteen patients. *J Bone Joint Surg.* 1986; 68A:1073.

116. Kirkham N. Tumors and cysts of the epidermis. In: Elder D, ed. *Lever's Histopathology of the Skin.* 8th ed. Philadelphia: Lippincott-Raven; 1997:685.

117. Borel DM. Cutaneous basosquamous carcinoma. Review of the literature and report of 35 cases. *Arch Pathol.* 1973; 95: 293.

118. Farmer ER, Helwig EB. Metastatic basal cell carcinoma. A clinicopathologic study of 17 cases. *Cancer.* 1980; 46:748.

119. Von Domarus H, Stevens PJ. Metastatic basal cell carcinoma. Report of five cases and review of 170 cases in the literature. *J Am Acad Dermatol.* 1984; 10:1043.

120. Cotran RS. Metastasizing basal cell carcinomas. *Cancer.* 1961; 14:1036.

121. Wick MR, Fitzgibbon J, Swanson PE. Cutaneous sarcomas and sarcomatoid neoplasms of the skin. *Sem Diagn Pathol.* 1993; 10:148.

122. Johnson WC, Helwig EB. Adenoid squamous cell carcinoma: Adenoacanthoma. *Cancer.* 1966; 19:1639.

123. Nappi O, Wick MR, Pettinato G, et al. Pseudovascular adenoid squamous cell carcinoma of the skin. *Am J Surg Pathol.* 1992; 16:429.

124. Rowe DE, Carroll RJ, Day CL. Prognostic factors for local recurrence, metastasis, and survival rates in squamous cell carcinoma of the skin, ear, and lip. *J Am Acad Dermatol.* 1992; 26:976.

125. Goepfert H, Dichtel WJ, Medina JE, et al. Perineural invasion in squamous cell skin carcinoma of the head and neck. *Am J Surg.* 1984; 148:542.

126. Marshall V. Premalignant and malignant skin tumors in immunosuppressed patients. *Transplantation.* 1984; 17:272.

127. Dinehart SM, Chu DZL, Maners AW, et al. Immunosuppression in patients with metastatic squamous cell carcinoma from the skin. *J Dermatol Surg Oncol.* 1990; 16:271.

128. Stafford ND, Frootko NJ. Verrucous carcinoma in the external auditory canal. *Am J Otol.* 1986; 7:443.

129. Edelstein DR, Smouha E, Sacks SH, Biller HF, Kaneko M, Parisier SC. Verrucous carcinoma of the temporal bone. *Ann Otol Rhinol Laryngol.* 1986; 95:447.

130. Proops DW, Hawke WM, van Nostrand AWP, Harwood AR, Lunan M. Verrucous carcinoma of the ear. *Ann Otol Rhinol Laryngol.* 1984; 93:385.

131. Peel RL: Ceruminous gland tumors. In: Barnes L, ed. *Surgical Pathology of the Head and Neck.* Vol 1. New York: Dekker; 1985:473.

132. Dehner LP, Chen KTK. Primary tumors of the external and middle ear—benign and malignant glandular neoplasms. *Arch Otolaryngol.* 1980; 106:13.

133. Warren S, Gates O. Carcinoma of the ceruminous gland. *Am J Pathol.* 1941; 22:821.

134. Fliegel Z, Kaneko M. Extramammary Paget's disease of the external auditory canal in association with ceruminous gland adenocarcinoma. *Cancer.* 1975; 36:1072.

135. Perzin KH, Gullane P, Conley J. Adenoid cystic carcinoma involving the external auditory canal. A clinicopathologic study of 16 cases. *Cancer.* 1982; 50:2873.

136. Pulec JL, Parkhill EM, Devine KD. Adenoid cystic carcinoma (cylindroma) of the external auditory canal. *Am Acad Opthalmol Otolaryngol.* 1963; 67:673.

137. DalMaso M, Lippi L. Adenoid cystic carcinoma of the head and neck: A clinical study of 37 cases. *Laryngoscope.* 1985; 95: 177.

138. Wilson RS, Johnson JT. Benign eccrine cylindroma of the external auditory canal. *Laryngoscope.* 1980; 90:379.

139. Pulec JL. Glandular tumors of the external auditory canal. *Laryngoscope.* 1977; 87:1601.

140. Kitamura K, Asai M, Kubo T, Harii K, Hasagawa A. Mucinous carcinoma of the external auditory canal: Case report. *Head Neck.* 1990; 12:417.

141. Breslow A: Thickness, cross-sectional areas and depth of invasion in the prognosis of cutaneous melanoma. *Ann Surg.* 1970; 172:902.

142. Dickersin GR. *Diagnostic Electron Microscopy: A Text/Atlas.* New York: Igaku-Shoin; 1988.

143. Pack G, Conley J, Oropeza R. Melanoma of the external ear. *Arch Otolaryngol.* 1970; 92:106.

144. Byers RM, Smith JL, Russell N, Rosenberg V. Malignant melanoma of the external ear. Review of 102 cases. *Am J Surg.* 1980; 140:518.

145. Conley J. *Melanoma of the Head and Neck.* New York: Thieme Medical Publishers; 1990.

146. Langman AW, Yarington CT Jr, Patterson SD. Malignant melanoma of the external auditory canal. *Otolaryngol Head Neck Surg.* 1996; 114:645.

147. Gussack GS, Reintgen D, Cox E, Fisher SR, Cole B, Seigler HF. Cutaneous melanomas of the head and neck. A review of 399 cases. *Arch Otolaryngol.* 1983; 109:803.

148. Ward NO, Acquarelli MJ. Malignant melanoma of the external ear. *Cancer.* 1968; 21:226.

149. al-Dousary S, Maqbool S, Zaid MA, et al. Merkel cell carcinoma of the auricle. *J Otolaryngol.* 1996; 25:408.

150. Skia B, Bibas A, Hickey SA, et al. Merkel cell carcinoma of the pinna. *J Laryngol Otol.* 1997; 111:1195.
151. Yanguas I, Goday JJ, Gonzalz-Guemes M, et al. Spontaneous regression of Merkel cell carcinoma of the skin. *Br J Dermatol.* 1997; 137:296.
152. Chan JKC, Suster S, Wenig BM, et al. Cytokeratin 20 immunoreactivity distinguishes Merkel cell (primary cutaneous neuroendocrine) carcinomas from salivary gland small cell carcinomas and small cell carcinomas of various sites. *Am J Surg Pathol.* 1997; 21:226.
153. Enzinger FM, Weiss SW. Malignant fibrohistiocytic tumors. In: Enzinger FM, Weiss SW, eds. *Soft Tissue Tumors.* 3rd ed. St. Louis: Mosby; 1995:351.
154. Calonje E, Wadden C, Wilson-Jones E, Fletcher CDM. Spindle-cell non-pleomorphic atypical fibroxanthoma: Analysis of a series and delineation of a distinctive variant. *Histopathol.* 1993; 22:247.
155. Ma CK, Zarbo RJ, Gown AM. Immunohistochemical characterization of atypical fibroxanthoma and dermatofibrosarcoma protuberans. *Am J Clin Pathol.* 1992; 97:478.
156. Longacre TA, Smoller BR, Rouse RV. Atypical fibroxanthoma. Multiple immunohistologic profiles. *Am J Surg Pathol.* 1993; 17:1199.
157. Worrell JT, Ansari MQ, Ansari SJ, Cockerell CJ. Atypical fibroxanthoma: DNA ploidy analysis of 14 cases with possible histogenetic implications. *J Cutan Pathol.* 1993; 20:215.
158. Michie BA, Reid RP, Fallowfield ME. Aneuploidy in atypical fibroxanthoma: DNA content quantification of 10 cases by image analysis. *J Cutan Pathol.* 1994; 21:404.
159. Enzinger FM, Weiss SW. Fibrohistiocytic tumors of intermediate malignancy. In: Enzinger FM, Weiss SW, eds. *Soft Tissue Tumors.* 3rd ed. St. Louis: Mosby; 1995:325.
160. Cooper PH. Angiosarcoma of the skin. *Sem Diagn Pathol.* 1987; 4:2.
161. Mark RJ, Tran LM, Sercarz J, et al. Angiosarcoma of the head and neck. The UCLA experience 1955 through 1990. *Arch Otolaryngol Head Neck Surg.* 1993; 119:973.
162. Lydiatt WM, Shaha AR, Shah JP. Angiosarcoma of the head and neck. *Am J Surg.* 1994; 168:451.
163. Stearns MP, Hibbard AA, Patterson HC. Kaposi's sarcoma of the ear: A case study. *J Laryngol Otol.* 1983; 97:641.
164. Gnepp DR, Chandler W, Hyams V. Primary Kaposi's sarcoma of the head and neck. *Ann Intern Med.* 1984; 100:107.
165. Enzinger FM, Weiss SW. Kaposi's sarcoma. In: Enzinger FM, Weiss SW, eds. *Soft Tissue Tumors.* 3rd ed. St. Louis: Mosby; 1995:658.
166. Lothe F. Kaposi's sarcoma. *Acta Pathol Microbiol Scand.* 1963; 161:1.
167. Jones RR, Jones EW. The histogenesis of Kaposi's sarcoma. *Am J Dermatopathol.* 1986; 8:369.
168. Jones RR, Spaull J, Spry C, et al. The histogenesis of Kaposi's sarcoma in patients with and without AIDS. *J Clin Pathol.* 1986; 39:742.
169. Friedmann I. The pathology of acute and chronic infections of the middle ear cleft. *Ann Otol Rhinol Laryngol.* 1971; 80:390.
170. Wenig BM. *Atlas of Head and Neck Pathology.* Philadelphia: WB Saunders; 1994.
171. Ferlito A. Histopathogenesis of tympanosclerosis. *J Laryngol Otol.* 1979; 93:25.
172. Godolfsky E, Hoffman RA, Holliday RA, Cohen NL. Cholesterol cysts of the temporal bone: Diagnosis and treatment. *Ann Otol Rhinol Laryngol.* 1991; 100:181.
173. Nager GT, Vanderveen TS. Cholesterol granuloma involving the temporal bone. *Ann Otol Rhinol Laryngol.* 1985; 85:204.
174. Windle-Taylor PC, Bailey CM. Tuberculous otitis media: A series of 22 patients. *Laryngoscope.* 1980; 90:1039.
175. McNulty JS, Fassett RL. Syphilis: An otolaryngolic perspective. *Laryngoscope.* 1981; 91:889.
176. McGill TJI. Mycotic infections of the temporal bone. *Arch Otolaryngol.* 1978; 104:140.
177. Leek JH. Actinomycosis of the tympanomastoid. *Laryngoscope.* 1974; 84:290.
178. Sandler ED, Sandler JM, Leboit P, et al. Pneumocystis carinii otitis media in AIDS: A case report and review of the literature regarding extrapulmonary pneumocystosis. *Otolaryngol Head Neck Surg.* 1990; 103:817.
179. Schuknecht HF. Infection. In: Schuknecht HF, ed. *Pathology of the Ear.* 2nd ed. Philadelphia: Lea & Febiger; 1993:191.
180. Wilson WR. The relationship of herpesvirus family to sudden hearing loss: A prospective clinical study and literature review. *Laryngoscope.* 1986; 96:870.
181. Marks PV, Brookes GB. Myelomatosis presenting as an isolated lesion in the mastoid. *Laryngoscope.* 1985; 99:903.
182. Abramson M, Moriyama H, Huang CC. Histology, pathogenesis, and treatment of cholesteatoma. *Otol Rhinol Laryngol.* 1984; 112:125.
183. Schecter G. A review of cholesteatoma pathology. *Laryngoscope.* 1969; 79:1907.
184. Frankel S, Berson S, Godwin T, et al. Differences in dendritic cells in congenital and acquired cholesteatomas. *Laryngoscope.* 1993; 103:1214.
185. Michaels L. Pathology of cholesteatomas: A review. *J R Soc Med.* 1979; 72:366.
186. Schuknecht HF. Cholesteatoma. In: Schuknecht HF, ed. *Pathology of the Ear.* 2nd ed. Philadelphia: Lea & Febiger; 1993: 31.
187. Desloge RB, Carew JF, Finstad CL, et al. DNA analysis of human cholesteatomas. *Am J Otol.* 1997; 18:155.
188. Ferlito A, Devaney KO, Rinaldo A, et al. Ear cholesteatoma versus cholesterol granuloma. *Ann Otol Rhinol Laryngol.* 1997; 106:79.
189. Lieberman PH, Jones CR, Steinman RM, et al. Langerhans cell (eosinophilic) granulomatosis: A clinicopathologic study encompassing 50 years *Am J Surg Pathol.* 1997; 20:519.
190. Emile JF, Wechsler J, Brousse N, et al. Langerhans' cell histiocytosis. Definitive diagnosis with the use of monoclonal antibody O10 on routinely paraffin-embedded samples. *Am J Surg Pathol.* 1995; 19:636.
191. Ide F, Iwase T, Saito I, et al. Immunohistochemical and ultrastructural analysis of the proliferating cells in histiocytosis X. *Cancer.* 1984; 53:917.
192. Rosai J, Dorfman RF. Sinus histiocytosis with massive lymphadenopathy: A newly recognized benign clinicopathologic entity. *Arch Pathol.* 1969; 87:63.
193. Rosai J, Dorfman RF. Sinus histiocytosis with massive lymphadenopathy: A pseudolymphomatous benign disorder. *Cancer.* 1972; 30:1174.
194. Foucar E, Rosai J, Dorfman R. Sinus histiocytosis with massive lymphadenopathy (Rosai-Dorfman disease): Review of the entity. *Semin Diagn Pathol.* 1990; 7:19.
195. Wenig BM, Abbondanzo SL, Childers E, et al. Extranodal sinus histiocytosis with massive lymphadenopathy (Rosai-Dorfman disease) of the head and neck. *Hum Pathol.* 1993; 24:483.
196. Foucar K, Foucar E. The mononuclear phagocyte and immunoregulatory effector (M-PIRE) system: Evolving concepts. *Semin Diagn Pathol.* 1990; 7:4.
197. Eisen RN, Buckley PJ, Rosai J. Immunophenotypic characterization of sinus histiocytosis with massive lymphadenopathy (Rosai-Dorfman disease). *Semin Diagn Pathol.* 1990; 7:74.
198. Paulli M, Rosso R, Kindl S, et al. Immunophenotypic characterization of the cell infiltrate in five cases of sinus histiocytosis with massive lymphadenopathy (Rosai-Dorfman disease). *Hum Pathol.* 1992; 23:647.
199. Nolle B, Specks U, Ludemann J, et al. Anticytoplasmic autoantibodies: Their immunodiagnostic value in Wegener's granulomatosis. *Ann Int Med.* 1989; 111:28.
200. Specks U, Wheatley CL, McDonald TJ, et al. Anticytoplasmic autoantibodies in the diagnosis and follow-up of Wegener's granulomatosis. *Mayo Clin Proc.* 1989; 64:28.
201. Azumi N, Sheibani K, Swartz WG, et al. Antigenic phenotype of Langerhans cell histiocytosis: An immunohistochemical study demonstrating the value of LN-2, LN-3, and vimentin. *Hum Pathol.* 1988; 19:1376.
202. Foucar E, Rosai J, Dorfman RF. Sinus histiocytosis with massive lymphadenopathy. Ear, nose, and throat manifestations. *Arch Otolaryngol.* 1978; 104:687.

203. Comp DM. The treatment of sinus histiocytosis with massive lymphadenopathy (Rosai-Dorfman disease). *Semin Diagn Pathol.* 1990; 7:83.

204. Saeed YM, Bassis ML. Mixed tumor of the middle ear. A case report. *Arch Otolaryngol.* 1971; 93:433.

205. Moore PJ, Benjamin BNP, Kan AE. Salivary gland choristoma of the middle ear. *Int J Pediatr Otorhinolaryngol.* 1984; 8:91.

206. Cannon CR. Salivary gland choristoma of the middle ear. *Am J Otol.* 1980; 1:250.

207. Kenneth KL, Gruskin P, Carberry JN. Salivary gland choristoma of the middle ear. *Arch Pathol Lab Med.* 1982; 106:39.

208. Bottrill ID, Chawla OP, Ramsay AD. Salivary gland choristoma of the middle ear. *J Laryngol Otol.* 1992; 106:630.

209. Glassock ME III, Dickins JRE, Jackson CR, et al. Surgical management of brain tissue herniation into the middle ear and mastoid. *Laryngoscope.* 1979; 89:1743.

210. Gulya AJ, Gassock ME III, Pensak ML. Neural choristoma of the middle ear. *Otolaryngol Head Neck Surg.* 1987; 97:52.

211. Wazen J, Silverstein H, McDaniel A, Hays A. Brain tissue heterotopia in the eighth cranial nerve. *Otolaryngol Head Neck Surg.* 1987; 96:373.

212. Schuknecht HF. Developmental defects. In: Schuknecht HF, ed. *Pathology of the Ear.* 2nd ed. Philadelphia: Lea & Febiger; 1993:115.

213. Brownstein MH, Wanger N, Helwig EB. Accessory tragi. *Arch Dermatol.* 1971; 104:625.

214. Olsen KD, Maragos NE, Weiland LH. First branchial cleft anomalies. *Laryngoscope.* 1980; 90:423.

215. Work WP. Newer concepts of first branchial cleft defects. *Laryngoscope.* 1972; 81:1581.

216. Aronsonn RS, Bataskis JG, Rice DH, et al. Anomalies of the first branchial cleft. *Arch Otolaryngol.* 1976; 102:737.

217. Greenway RE, Hurst L, Fenton NA. An unusual first branchial cleft cyst. *J Laryngol.* 1981; 10:219.

218. Morales-Garcia C. Cochleo-vestibular involvement in otosclerosis. *Acta Otolaryngol (Stockh).* 1972; 73:484.

219. Cody DTR, Baker HL Jr. Otosclerosis: vestibular symptoms and sensorineural hearing loss. *Ann Otol Rhinol Laryngol.* 1978; 87:778.

220. Schuknecht HF: Otosclerosis. In: *Pathology of the Ear.* 2nd ed. Philadelphia: Lea & Febiger; 1993:365.

221. McCaffrey TV, McDonald TJ, Facer GW, et al. Otologic manifestations of Wegener's granulomatosis. *Otolaryngol Head Neck Surg.* 1980; 88:586.

222. Fauci AS, Haynes BF, Katz P, et al. Wegener's granulomatosis: Prospective clinical and therapeutic experience with 85 patients for 21 years. *Ann Intern Med.* 1983; 98:76.

223. Okamura H, Ohtani I, Anzai T. The hearing loss in Wegener's granulomatosis: Relationship between hearing loss and serum ANCA. *Auris Nasus Larynx.* 1992; 19:1.

224. Illum P, Thorling K. Otologic manifestations of Wegener's granulomatosis. *Laryngoscope.* 1982; 92:801.

225. Kornblut AD, Wolff SM, Fauci AS. Ear disease in patients with Wegener's granulomatosis. *Laryngoscope.* 1982; 92:713.

226. McDonald TJ, Remee RA. Wegener's granulomatosis. *Laryngoscope.* 1983; 93:220.

227. Wolf M, Kronenberg J, Engelberg S, et al. Rapidly progressive hearing loss as a symptom of polyarteritis nodosa. *Am J Otolaryngol.* 1987; 8:105.

228. Gussen R. Atypical ossicle joint lesions in rheumatoid arthritis with sicca syndrome (Sjögren's syndrome). *Arch Otolaryngol.* 1977; 103:284.

229. Wick MR, McLeod RA, Siegel GP, et al. Sarcomas of bone arising complicating osteitis deformans (Paget's disease). Fifty years' experience. *Am J Surg Pathol.* 1981; 5:47.

230. Haibach H, Farrell C, Dittrich FJ. Neoplasms arising in Paget's disease of bone: A study of 82 cases. *Am J Clin Pathol.* 1985; 83:594.

231. Schuknecht HF. Paget's disease. In: Schuknecht HF, ed. *Pathology of the Ear.* 2nd ed. Philadelphia: Lea & Febiger; 1993: 379.

232. El-Naggar AK, Pflatz M, Ordóñez NG, Batsakis JG. Tumors of the middle ear and endolymphatic sac. *Pathol Annual.* 1994; Part 29(2):199.

233. Hyams VJ, Michaels L. Benign adenomatous neoplasm (adenoma) of the middle ear. *Clin Otolaryngol.* 1976; 1:17.

234. Stanley MW, Horwitz CA, Levinson RM, Sibley RK. Carcinoid tumors of the middle ear. *Am J Clin Pathol.* 1987; 87:592.

235. Latif MA, Madders DJ, Shaw PAV. Carcinoid tumour of the middle ear associated with systemic symptoms. *J Laryngol Otol.* 1987; 101:480.

236. Manni J, Faverly DRGS, van Haelst UJGM. Primary carcinoid tumor of the middle ear: Report of four cases and a review of the literature. *Arch Otolaryngol Head Neck Surg.* 1992; 118:1341.

237. Faverly DRGS, Manni J, Smedts F, et al. Adenocarcinoid or amphicrine tumors of the middle ear. *Pathol Res Pract.* 1992; 188:162.

238. Batsakis JG. Adenomatous tumors of the middle ear. *Ann Otol Rhinol Laryngol.* 1989; 98:749.

239. Johnson TL, Zarbo RJ, Lloyd RV, Crissman JD. Paragangliomas of the head and neck: Immunohistochemical neuroendocrine and intermediate filament typing. *Modern Pathol.* 1988; 1:216.

240. Kliewer KE, Wen DR, Cancilla PA, Cochran AJ. Paragangliomas: Assessment of prognosis by histologic, immunohistochemical, and ultrastructural techniques. *Hum Pathol.* 1989; 20:29.

241. Hyams VJ, Batsakis JG, Michaels L. Jugulotympanic paraganglioma. In: Hartmann WH, Sobin LH, eds. *Tumors of the Upper Respiratory Tract and Ear.* Atlas of tumor pathology, Fascicle 25, second series. Washington, DC: Armed Forces Institute of Pathology; 1988:306.

242. Larson TC, Reese DF, Baker HL, McDonald TJ. Glomus tympanicum chemodectomas: Radiographic and clinical characteristics. *Radiology.* 1987; 163:801.

243. Spector GJ, Ciralsky RH, Ogura JH. Glomus tumors in the head and neck. III. Analysis of clinical manifestaions. *Ann Rhinol Otol Laryngol.* 1975; 84:73.

244. Barnes L, Taylor SR. Carotid body paragangliomas: A clinicopathologic and DNA analysis of 13 cases. *Arch Otolaryngol Head Neck Surg.* 1990; 116:447.

245. Taylor DM, Alford BR, Greenberg SD. Metastases of glomus jugulare tumors. *Arch Otolaryngol.* 1965; 82:5.

246. Johnstone PAS, Foss RD, Desilets DJ. Malignant jugulotympanic paraganglioma. *Arch Pathol Lab Med.* 1990; 114:976.

247. Erickson LS, Sorenson GD, McGavran MH. A review of 140 acoustic neurinomas (neurilemmoma). *Laryngoscope.* 1965; 75: 601.

248. Kasantikul V, Netsky MG, Glassock ME III, et al. Acoustic neurilemmoma. Clinicoanatomical study of 103 patients. *J Neurosurg.* 1980; 52:28.

249. Martuza RL, Ojemann RG. Bilateral acoustic neuromas: Clinical aspects, pathogenesis and treatment. *Neurosurgery.* 1982; 10:1.

250. Anand T, Byrnes DP, Walby AP, Kerr AG. Bilateral acoustic neuromas. *Clin Otolaryngol.* 1993; 18:365.

251. Moffat DA, Irving RM. The molecular genetics of vestibular schwannomas. *J Laryngol Otol.* 1995; 109:381.

252. Rietz DR, Ford CN, Kurtycz DF, et al. Significance of apparent intratympanic meningiomas. *Laryngoscope.* 1983; 93:1397.

253. Heffner DK. Low-grade adenocarcinoma of probable endolymphatic sac origin. A clinicopathologic study of 20 cases. *Cancer.* 1989; 64:2292.

254. Wenig BM, Heffner DK. Endolymphatic sac tumors: Fact or fiction? *Adv Anat Pathol.* 1996; 3:378.

255. Megerian CA, McKenna MJ, Nuss RC, et al. Endolymphatic sac tumors: Histopathologic confirmation, clinical characterization, and implication in von Hippel-Lindau disease. *Laryngoscope.* 1995; 105:801.

256. Manski TJ, Heffner DK, Glenn GM, et al. Endolymphatic sac tumors: The basis of morbid hearing loss in von Hippel-Lindau disease. *JAMA.* 1997; 277:1461.

257. Hassard AD, Boudreau SF, Cron CC. Adenoma of the endolymphatic sac. *J Otolaryngol.* 1984; 13:213.

258. Eby TL, Makek MS, Fisch U. Adenomas of the temporal bone. *Ann Otol Rhinol Laryngol.* 1988; 97:605.

259. Benecke JE, Noel FL, Carberry JN, et al. Adenomatous tumors of the middle ear and mastoid. *Am J Otol.* 1990; 11:20.

260. Goebel JA, Smith PG, Kemink JL, Graham MD. Primary adenocarcinomas of the temporal bone mimicking paragangliomas: Radiographic and clinical recognition. *Otolaryngol Head Neck Surg.* 1987; 96:231.

261. Palmer JM, Coker NJ, Harper RL. Papillary adenoma of the temporal bone in von Hippel-Lindau disease. *Otolaryngol Head Neck Surg.* 1989; 100:64.

262. Poe DS, Tarlov EC, Thomas CB, Kveton JF. Aggressive papillary tumors of temporal bone. *Otolaryngol Head Neck Surg.* 1993; 108:86.

263. Thomas CB, Kveton JF, Poe DS, et al. Aggressive papillary tumor of temporal bone in von Hippel-Lindau disease. *Surg Pathology.* 1993; 5:63.

264. Gaffey MJ, Mills SE, Fechner RE, et al. Aggressive papillary middle-ear tumors: A clinicopathologic entity distinct from middle-ear adenoma. *Am J Surg Pathol.* 1988; 12:790.

265. Gaffey MJ, Mills SE, Boyd JC. Aggressive papillary tumor of middle ear/temporal bone and adnexal papillary cystadenoma. Manifestations of von Hippel-Lindau disease. *Am J Surg Pathol.* 1994; 18:1254.

266. Batsakis JG, El-Naggar AK. Papillary neoplasms (Heffner's tumors) of the endolymphatic sac. *Ann Otol Rhinol Laryngol.* 1993; 102:648.

267. Wenig BM. Schneiderian papillomas of the middle ear. *Ann Otol Rhinol Laryngol.* 1996; 105:226.

268. Stone DM, Berktold RE, Ranganathan C, Wiet RJ. Inverted papilloma of the middle ear and mastoid. *Otolaryngol Head Neck Surg.* 1987; 97:416.

269. Kaddour HS, Woodhead CJ. Transitional papilloma of the middle ear. *J Laryngol Otol.* 1992; 106:628.

270. Andrade JM, Gehris CW Jr, Breitnecker R. Cavernous hemangioma of the tympanic membrane. A case report. *Am J Otol.* 1983; 4:198.

271. Jackson CG, Levine SC, McKennan KX. Hemangioma of the middle ear. *Am J Otol.* 1987; 8:131.

272. Eby TL, Fisch U, Malek MS. Facial nerve management in temporal bone hemangiomas. *Am J Otol.* 1992; 13:223.

273. Olson JE, Glassock ME III, Britton BH. Lipomas of the internal auditory canal. *Arch Otolaryngol.* 1978; 104:431.

274. Huang TS. Primary intravestibular lipoma. *Ann Otol Rhinol Laryngol.* 1989; 98:393.

275. Ishikawa T, Saito H, Takahashi K. Osteoma of the mastoid. *Arch Otorhinolaryngol.* 1977; 217:93.

276. Denia A, Perez F, Canalis RR, et al. Extracanalicular osteomas of the temporal bone. *Arch Otolaryngol.* 1975; 105:706.

277. Marlowe FI, Dave U, Wolfson RJ. Giant osteoma of the mastoid. *M J Otolaryngol.* 1980; 1:191.

278. Bertoni F, Unni KK, Beabout JW, et al. Chondroblastoma of the skull and facial bones. *Am J Clin Pathol.* 1987; 88:1.

279. Navrátil J. Teratome der paukenhöhle und der tuba eustachii. *Acta Otolaryngol (Stockh).* 1965; 60:36.

280. Silverstein H, Griffin WL Jr, Balough K Jr. Teratoma of the middle ear and mastoid process. A case with aberrant innervation of the facial musculature. *Arch Otolaryngol.* 1967; 85: 243.

281. Hyams VJ, Batsakis JG, Michaels L. Squamous cell carcinoma of the middle ear. In: *Tumors of the Upper Respiratory Tract and Ear.* Atlas of tumor pathology, Fascicle 25, second series. Washington, DC: Armed Forces Institute of Pathology; 1988: 326.

282. Michaels L, Wells M. Squamous cell carcinoma of the middle ear. *Clin Otolaryngol.* 1980; 5:235.

283. Kenyon GS, Marks PV, Scholtz CL, Dhillon R. Squamous cell carcinoma of the middle ear; a 25-year retrospective study. *Ann Otol Rhinol Laryngol.* 1985; 94:273.

284. Hyams VJ, Batsakis JG, Michaels L. Adenocarcinoma of the middle ear. In: *Tumors of the Upper Respiratory Tract and Ear.* Atlas of tumor pathology, Fascicle 25, second series. Washington, DC: Armed Forces Institute of Pathology; 1988:320.

285. Pallanch JF, McDonald TJ, Weiland LH, et al. Adenocarcinoma and adenoma of the middle ear. *Laryngoscope.* 1982; 92: 47.

286. Schuller DE, Conley JJ, Goodman JH, et al. Primary adenocarcinoma of the middle ear. *Otolaryngol Head Neck Surg.* 1983; 91:280.

287. Gulya AJ, Glassock ME, Pensack ML. Primary adenocarcinoma of the temporal bone with middle cranial fossa extension: Case report. *Laryngoscope.* 1986; 96:675.

288. Glassock ME, McKennan KX, Levine SC, Jackson CG. Primary adenocarcinoma of the middle ear and temporal bone. *Arch Otolaryngol Head Neck Surg.* 1987; 113:822.

289. Weiss SW. *World Health Organization International Histological Classification of Tumours.* Histological typing of soft tissue tumours. 2nd ed. Berlin: Springer-Verlag; 1995.

290. Newton WA, Gehan EA, Webber BL, et al. Classification of rhabdomyosarcomas and related sarcomas: Pathologic aspects and proposal for a new classification—an Intergroup rhabdomyosarcoma study. *Cancer.* 1995; 76:1073.

291. Mauer HM, Beltangady M, Gehan EA, et al. The Intergroup rhabdomyosarcoma study-I. a final report. *Cancer.* 1988; 61: 209.

292. Enzinger FW, Weiss SW. Rhabdomyosarcoma. In: *Soft Tissue Tumors.* 2nd ed. St. Louis: Mosby; 1995:539.

293. Barnes L. Tumors and tumor-like lesions of the soft tissues. In: Barnes L, ed. *Surgical Pathology of the Head and Neck.* New York: Marcel Dekker Inc.; 1985:725.

294. Anderson GJ, Tom LWC, Womer RB, et al. Rhabdomyosarcoma of the head and neck in children. *Arch Otolaryngol Head Neck Surg.* 1990; 116:428.

295. Callender TA, Weber RS, Janjan N, et al. Rhabdomyosarcoma of the nose and paranasal sinuses in adults and children. *Head Neck Surg.* 1995; 112:252.

296. El-Naggar AK, Batsakis JG, Ordóñez NG, et al. Rhabdomyosarcoma of the adult head and neck: A clinicopathological study and DNA ploidy study. *J Laryngol Otol.* 1993; 107:716.

297. Nakhleh RE, Swanson PE, Dehner LP. Juvenile (embryonal and alveolar) rhabdomyosarcoma of the head and neck in adults. A clinical, pathologic, and immunohistochemical study of 12 cases. *Cancer.* 1991; 67:1019.

298. Nayar RC, Prudhomme F, Parise O Jr, et al. Rhabdomyosarcoma of the head and neck in adults. A study of 26 patients. *Laryngoscope.* 1993; 103:1362.

299. Ladanyi M. The emerging molecular genetics of sarcoma translocations. *Diagn Mol Pathol.* 1995; 4:162.

300. Parham DM, Shapiro DN, Downing X Jr, et al. Solid alveolar rhabdomyosarcoma with the t(2;13). Report of two cases with diagnostic implications. *Am J Surg Pathol.* 1994; 18:474.

301. Coffin CM. The new international rhabdomyosarcoma classification, its progenitors, and considerations beyond morphology. *Adv Anat Pathol.* 1997; 4:1.

302. Nora FE, Unni KK, Pritchard DJ. Osteosarcoma of extragnathic craniofacial bones. *Mayo Clin Proc.* 1983; 58:268.

303. Huvos AG, Sandaresan N, Bretsky SS. Osteogenic sarcoma of the skull. A clinicopathologic study of 19 patients. *Cancer.* 1985; 56:1214.

304. Coltera MC, Googe PB, Harrist TJ, et al. Chondrosarcoma of the temporal bone. Diagnosis and treatment in 13 cases and review of the literature. *Cancer.* 1986; 58:2689.

305. Caron AS, Hajdu SI, Strong EW. Osteogenic sarcoma of the facial and cranial bones. A review of forty-three cases. *Am J Surg.* 1971; 122:719.

306. Schuknecht HF: Neoplastic growths. In: Schuknecht HF, ed. *Pathology of the Ear.* Philadelphia: Lea & Febiger; 1993:447.

307. Malik MK, Gupta RK, Samuel KC. Primary lymphoma of the middle ear—a case report. *Indian J Cancer.* 1976; 13:188.

308. Peperella MM, el-Finky FM. Ear involvement in malignant lymphoma. *Ann Otol Rhinol Laryngol.* 1972; 81:352.

309. Hill BA, Kohut RI. Metastatic adenocarcinoma of the temporal bone. *Arch Otolaryngol.* 1976; 102:568.

310. Jahn AF, Farkashidy J, Berman JM. Metastatic tumours in the temporal bone—a physiologic study. *J Otolaryngol.* 1979; 8:85.

311. Morton AL, Butler SA, Khan A, et al. Temporal bone metastases—pathophysiology and imaging. *Otolaryngol Head Neck Surg.* 1987; 97:583.

312. Sahin AA, Ro JY, Ordóñez NG, et al. Temporal bone involvement by prostatic adenocarcinoma: Report of two cases and review of the literature. *Head Neck.* 1991; 13:349.

313. Bergstrom LV, Baker BB, Sando I. Sudden deafness and facial palsy from metastatic bronchogenic carcinoma. *J Laryngol Otol.* 1977; 91:787.

314. Alberts MC, Terrence CF. Hearing loss in carcinomatous meningitis. *J Laryngol Otol.* 1978; 92:233.

315. Igarashi M, Card GG, Johnson PE, Alford BR. Bilateral hearing loss and metastatic pancreatic adenocarcinoma. *Arch Otolaryngol.* 1979; 105:196.

316. Berlinger NT, Koutroupas S, Adams G, et al. Patterns of involvement of the temporal bone in metastastic and systemic malignancy. *Laryngoscope.* 1980; 90:619.

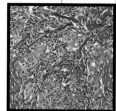

CHAPTER 13

Neck

I. CLINICAL CONSIDERATIONS FOR NON-NEOPLASTIC LESIONS OF THE NECK

■ ROBERT M. KELLMAN

■ JAMES E. FREIJE

ANATOMY

Thorough knowledge of neck anatomy is essential for a proper understanding of disorders of the head and neck. There are a number of methods to separate the anatomy into subdivisions, making the structures more easily classified. These include:

1. Triangles of the neck
2. Fascial compartments
3. Visceral compartments
4. Neurovascular structures
5. Extensive lymphatic system

Triangles

The neck can be divided into anterior and posterior triangles. The *anterior triangle* is bordered by the anterior border of the sternocleidomastoid muscle (SCM) laterally, the midline medially, and the body of the mandible superiorly. The *posterior triangle* is contained between the posterior border of the sternocleidomastoid muscle anteriorly, the anterior border of the trapezius muscle posteriorly, and the clavicle inferiorly. It is divided by the inferior belly of the omohyoid into the *occipital triangle* above and the *subclavian triangle* below. Subdivisions of the anterior triangle are also described. The *submental triangle* lies between the two anterior bellies of the digastric muscles bilaterally, with the hyoid forming the inferior border. The *submandibular* (or *digastric*) *triangle* lies above and between the anterior and posterior bellies of the digastric below and the mandible above on each side. The *carotid triangle* is bounded by the anterior border of the sternocleidomastoid muscle posteriorly, the posterior belly of the digastric muscle superiorly, and the anterior belly of the omohyoid muscle anteroinferiorly. These subdivisions of the neck are also important clinically since lymph node metastases to various zones in the neck are predictive of the site of primary tumors of the head and neck (Fig. 13–1).

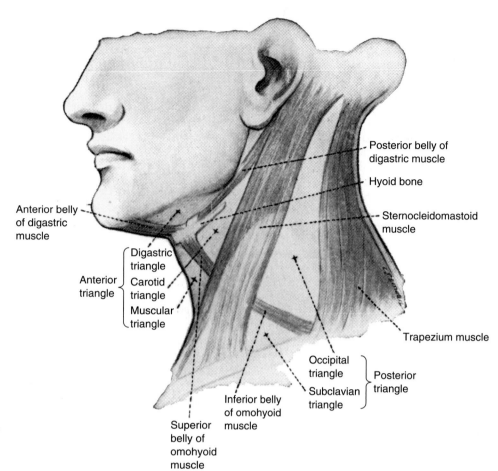

FIGURE 13-1 The triangles of the neck. From Thorek P., *Anatomy in Surgery.* 2nd ed. Philadelphia: JB Lippincott; 1985: 124, with permission.

Fascial Planes

The fascia of the neck consists of both superficial and deep layers. The superficial fascia consists of the subcutaneous tissue and surrounds the platysma muscle. The deep cervical fascia is further divided into superficial, middle, and deep layers.

The superficial layer of the deep cervical fascia encompasses the submandibular gland and splits superiorly to surround the trapezius muscle, the sternocleidomastoid muscle, and the omohyoid muscles. It is attached to the base of the skull, mandible, and hyoid bones superiorly and the clavicle and manubrium inferiorly. The space created by its attachment inferiorly between the clavicular heads is known as the suprasternal space of Burns and contains the anterior jugular veins. The deep portion of the superficial layer contributes to the formation of the carotid sheath, as do all three layers of the deep cervical fascia. The middle layer of the deep cervical fascia, also known as the pretracheal fascia, again forms a portion of the anterior aspect of the carotid sheath and overlies the thyrohyoid muscle, thyroid gland, and trachea. Finally, the deepest layer of the cervical fascia of the neck, also referred to as the fascial carpet, covers the prevertebral musculature as

well as the splenius capitis, levator scapula, and scalene muscles.

Musculature

In addition to their functions, the muscles of the neck are important as surgical landmarks. The platysma muscle is innervated by the cervical branch of the facial nerve. It attaches over the inferior border of the mandible, blending with the inferior facial muscles, and extends over the clavicle below. The platysma is an important landmark since, when raising most skin flaps for neck surgery, the plane of dissection is usually directly under this muscle, allowing for elevation of the flaps in a relatively avascular plane. The muscle is well developed in young patients but may be more difficult to identify in the older population as it becomes relatively thin and atrophic. The muscle is absent in the midline over the strap muscles.

The digastric, stylohyoid, and mylohyoid muscles are found in the submental and submandibular triangles. The digastric muscle has two bellies. The posterior belly, innervated by cranial nerve VII, passes from the mastoid tip to the lesser cornu of the hyoid bone. The anterior belly, innervated by cranial nerve V, attaches to the deep surface of the mentum. The digastric muscle is an important surgical landmark since vital structures in this region (i.e., the internal jugular vein, carotid artery, and hypoglossal nerve) all run deep to this structure. The thin stylohyoid muscle passes from the styloid process to the hyoid bone and splits to surround the outer belly of the digastric. The mylohyoid muscle forms a portion of the floor of the mouth and is also innervated by cranial nerve V. The muscle extends from the mylohyoid line on the undersurface of the mandible to the hyoid bone. When this muscle is retracted anteriorly the lingual nerve, submandibular duct, and hypoglossal nerve can all be identified easily during a submental dissection or a submandibular gland excision. The sternocleidomastoid muscle passes from the mastoid tip to the clavicle and sternum, where it splits into two heads, one of which inserts on the sternum and the other on the anterosuperior clavicle. The external jugular vein and greater auricular nerve can easily be identified on the lateral surface of the muscle. At approximately the midpoint of the posterior margin of the sternocleidomastoid muscle, the greater auricular nerve crosses over its outer surface, in an area known as Erb's point. This is an important surgical landmark for identifying the spinal accessory nerve that exits the posterior portion of the SCM at or below this point and enters the posterior triangle. It provides innervation for the sternocleidomastoid muscle as well as the trapezius muscle. The spinal accessory nerve can, in most instances, be easily identified just inferolateral and deep to Erb's point. The nerve can then be traced inferoposteriorly to the anterior border of the trapezius muscle, which forms the posterior limit of a standard neck dissection.

The infrahyoid strap muscles pass from the hyoid or thyroid ala to attachments on the sternum or scapula. The most lateral strap muscle is the omohyoid, which consists of two bellies. Its anterior attachment is to the hyoid bone while the posterior attachment is to the scapula. The junction of the anterior and posterior bellies of the omohyoid lies directly underneath the clavicular and sternal heads of the sternocleidomastoid muscle, where it provides a good landmark for the internal jugular vein that lies deep to the muscle in this area. The other strap muscles include the sternohyoid and thyrohyoid muscles that overlie the larynx. These muscles are supplied by the ansa cervicalis that separates from the hypoglossal nerve high in the neck and then passes over the internal jugular vein and carotid sheath as it travels inferoanteriorly. The muscles underlying the deep cervical fascia include the splenius capitis and levator scapulae muscles laterally and the anterior, middle, and posterior scalene muscles more medially. The muscles under the fascial carpet are very important as surgical landmarks. More specifically, the phrenic nerve is easily identified as it passes from a lateral to medial direction over the anterior scalene muscle. Likewise, the brachial plexus can be found passing laterally between the anterior and middle scalene muscles. Passing through the musculature of the fascial carpet, the cutaneous branches of the cervical plexus that supply sensation to the skin are encountered. These are derived from the second through fourth cervical nerves.

Neurovascular Structures

Many vital neural structures occur in the head and neck, some of which have been previously mentioned. Branches of cranial nerve VII as well as cranial nerves IX, X, XI, and XII are readily identified and protected during head and neck surgery whenever possible. The cervical branch of cranial nerve VII passes from the lower division of the facial nerve along the angle of the mandible into the submandibular triangle to the orbicularis oris. The nerve can be identified and protected by reflecting the fascia of the submandibular gland superiorly during standard dissection of the neck. Cranial nerves IX, X, and XI pass through the jugular foramen to enter the neck. Although the glossopharyngeal nerve (cranial nerve IX) is not routinely identified in the neck, it can be found deep to the styloid muscles innervating the stylopharyngeus muscle. The vagus nerve (cranial nerve X) lies within the carotid sheath in close proximity to the carotid artery and jugular vein. Important branches include the superior laryngeal nerve that exits high from the vagus, passing under the carotid artery to form external and internal divisions. The external branch innervates the cricothyroid muscle, while the internal branch supplies sensation to the endolarynx and pharynx. The recurrent laryngeal nerve supplies the remaining innervation to the intrinsic muscles of the larynx. The recurrent nerve passes around the ligamentum arteriosum on the left and subclavian artery on the right. A nonrecurrent laryngeal nerve on the right may be associated with an aberrant right subclavian artery. As previously noted, cranial nerve XI (the spinal accessory nerve) also exits from the jugular foramen and passes over the jugular vein to supply the sternocleidomastoid muscle and trapezius muscle. It is most easily identified in the posterior triangle of the neck and can be traced through the sternocleidomastoid muscle to the skull base. Finally, the hypoglossal nerve (cranial nerve XII), which exits the skull base through a separate foramen, is found in the neck passing over the carotid artery approximately 1 to 2 cm above the bifurcation in the carotid. It then passes under the digastric muscle to supply motor innervation to the tongue. The hypoglossal nerve also contributes to the strap muscle innervation via the ansa hypoglossi.

The arterial and venous structures are, for the

most part, branches of the jugular and carotid artery systems. Superficial veins include the external and anterior jugular veins. The external jugular vein passes from the area of the parotid gland over the anterior aspect of the sternocleidomastoid muscle and most commonly drains directly into the subclavian vein. The anterior jugular vein begins in the suprahyoid region of the neck and drains into the subclavian or jugular veins in the superior mediastinum. The internal jugular vein passing from the jugular foramen to the subclavian vein receives numerous branches in the neck, the most prominent of which is commonly the middle thyroid vein. The internal jugular vein is not only important for its venous drainage, but also because it is intimately related with the major lymphatic drainage of the neck, making this structure extremely important in oncologic neck procedures.

Most arterial supply to the neck originates from the carotid artery. The common carotid artery divides into internal and external branches at the level of the hyoid bone. The internal branch usually remains lateral and has no branches external to the skull base. The external carotid has several named branches in the neck including the superior thyroid, ascending pharyngeal, lingual, and facial arteries anteriorly with the occipital, posterior auricular, superficial temporal, and maxillary arteries more posteriorly. Tributaries from the thyrocervical trunk may also be found in the neck and include the inferior thyroid and transverse cervical arteries.

Lymphatic Drainage

An in-depth understanding of the cervical lymphatic system is vital when treating various disorders of the head and neck. There are approximately 600 lymph nodes in the body, 200 of which are located in the neck. A standard classification of neck nodes most recently described by Robbins et al[1] divides the nodal group into six levels. For oncological consideration, the level of nodal disease becomes significant, not only in predicting the location of the primary tumor, but also for prognostic treatment purposes.

Level I includes the submental and submandibular nodes. This area receives drainage from the lips, anterior oral cavity, and skin of the midface. *Level II,* the upper jugular nodal group, drains the soft palate, tonsillar fossa, posterior tongue and tongue base, pyriform sinus, and the supraglottic larynx. *Level III* includes the midjugular nodes, which primarily drain the supraglottic larynx and hypopharynx. *Level IV,* the lower jugular chain, receives primary drainage from the thyroid, trachea, and cervical esophagus. *Level V,* the posterior triangle nodes, primarily drain the posterior scalp and nasopharynx. *Level VI* refers to the anterior nodal compartment and includes the pretracheal (Delphian)

nodes and paratracheal nodes. Drainage to level VI is primarily from the larynx, trachea, and thyroid gland.

Other nodal groups that may not be specifically categorized in the six levels just described include the retropharyngeal, anterior scalene (Virchow's), and supraclavicular nodes. Retropharyngeal nodes, which are commonly overlooked, drain the nasopharynx, posterior nasal cavity, hypopharynx, and paranasal sinuses. Disease in the anterior scalene and supraclavicular nodes is most commonly an indication of infraclavicular disease.

EMBRYOLOGY

The embryologic development of the head and neck structures can be classified through the development of branchial arches, clefts, and pharyngeal pouches in the embryo. By the age of 5 weeks, the head and neck structures become recognizable as five or six pairs of branchial arches. Between the arches are clefts externally and pouches or outpouchings of the foregut internally. The arches and pharyngeal pouches are lined by ectoderm.

Branchial Arches and Clefts

Each branchial arch contains a cartilage bar, nerve, and artery from which skeletal, muscular, and neurovascular structures of the neck develop (Table 13–1). (Note the absence of a "fifth branchial arch.")

Pharyngeal Pouches

As previously mentioned, the pharyngeal pouches are endodermal-lined outpouchings of the foregut. The endodermal lining of each pouch lies adjacent to the ectodermal lining of its associated cleft externally (Table 13–2).

CONGENITAL NECK MASSES

Branchial Cleft Abnormalities

Branchial cleft cysts are congenital cysts believed to result from persistence of the cervical sinus, which is the ectodermally lined sinus tract that develops as the branchial arches are submerged within the endodermally lined branchial pouches. When separated from the skin, a branchial cyst develops. A tract may open either into the pharynx or out through the skin. When the tract is continuous from the skin to the pharynx, it is designated as a branchial fistula.

TABLE 13-1　BRANCHIAL ARCHES

First Branchial Arch

Cartilage bar (Meckel's cartilage)
  Ramus and body of the mandible
  Spheno-mandibular ligament
  Anterior malleolar ligament
  Malleus except manubrium
  Incus
Musculature
  Temporalis muscle
  Masseter muscle
  Medial and lateral pterygoid muscles
  Tensor tympani
  Tensor veli palatini
  Anterior belly of digastric
  Mylohyoid
Innervation
  Trigeminal nerve
Vascular structures degenerate

Second Branchial Arch

Cartilage bar of Reichert's cartilage
  Styloid process
  Stylohyoid ligament
  Manubrium of malleus
  Long process of incus and stapes
  Body and lesser cornu of the hyoid bone
Musculature
  Facial muscles
  Platysma
  Posterior belly digastric
  Stylohyoid muscle
  Stapedius
Innervation
  Facial nerve
Vascular structures (stapedial artery) degenerates

Third Branchial Arch

Cartilage bar
  Remaining portions of hyoid bone
Musculature
  Stylopharyngeus muscle
  Superior pharyngeal constrictor
  Middle pharyngeal constrictor
Innervation
  Glossopharyngeal nerve
Vascular structures: Internal carotid artery

Fourth Branchial Arch

Cartilage bar
  Thyroid cartilage
Musculature
  Cricothyroid muscle
Innervation
  Vagus nerve: Superior laryngeal branch
Vascular structures
  Aorta
  Proximal subclavian artery

Sixth Branchial Arch

Cartilage bar
  Cricoid cartilage
  Arytenoid cartilages
Musculature
  Intrinsic muscles of the larynx
  Upper esophageal musculature
Innervation
  Vagus nerve: Recurrent laryngeal branch
Vascular structures
  Pulmonary arteries
  Ductus arteriosus

TABLE 13-2　PHARYNGEAL POUCHES

First Pharyngeal Pouch (Along with Part of Second)

Endodermal derivatives
  Epithelium of middle ear
  Tympanic membrane
Ectodermal derivatives
  External auditory canal

Second Pharyngeal Pouch

Epithelial lining of the palatine tonsil

Third Pharyngeal Pouch

Inferior parathyroids
Thymus gland

Fourth Pharyngeal Pouch

Superior parathyroids
Some thymus gland (occasionally)

Sixth Pharyngeal Pouch

Ultimobranchial body, which gives rise to parafollicular C
  cells of the thyroid gland

Branchial cysts and sinuses associated with the development of the first, second, third, and fourth arches are well-described, with the second being the most common, followed by the first and third, and the fourth being extremely rare. While sixth-arch anomalies are theoretically possible, they have not been described.

Since these anomalies are developmental structural abnormalities, they do not resolve spontaneously. Careful and complete surgical excision is the treatment of choice.

FIRST BRANCHIAL CLEFT CYSTS

According to Batsakis,[2] true anomalies of the first branchial groove probably represent less than 1% of all anomalies of the developing branchial system. This relative rarity may lead to misdiagnosis. Failure to recognize these anomalies and, therefore, the relationship of such preauricular lesions to the facial nerve, can lead to surgical misadventure and avoidable facial paralyses.

First branchial groove anomalies are distinctly divided into type I and type II. Type I anomalies are derived only from the first cleft and are therefore of ectodermal origin; they represent a reduplication of the external auditory canal and typically drain into or around the area of the external auditory canal. They are generally above the facial nerve but may be very close to it. The more common type II anomalies are of both ectodermal and mesodermal origin and are duplications of the membranous and cartilaginous portions of the ear canal. They typically present beneath the angle of the mandible along the anterior edge of the sternocleidomastoid muscle, though they may be found in the parotid gland overlying the horizontal ramus (body) of the mandi-

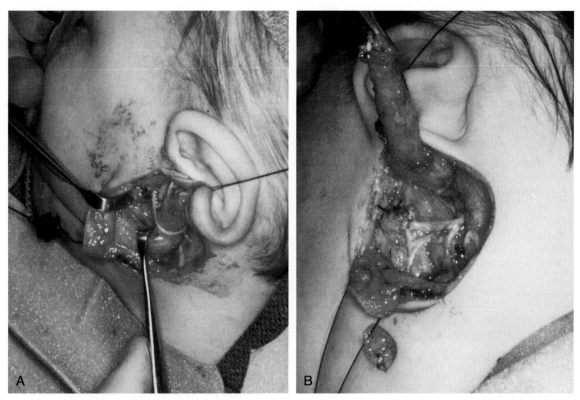

FIGURE 13–2 *A,* Child with a type II first branchial cleft cyst showing the cyst separating branches of the facial nerve. *B,* The nerve in position after the cyst has been lifted from between the nerve fibers. Note the cyst tracking toward the ear canal.

ble. They are intimately related to the facial nerve and may pass lateral to, medial to, or even between fibers of the facial nerve (Fig. 13–2 *A* and *B*). To avoid complications, excision of these lesions generally requires a superficial parotidectomy with facial nerve dissection. First branchial cleft cysts should not be confused with pretragal cysts or sinuses, which are associated with developmental abnormalities of the pinna and are not true branchial cleft anomalies.

SECOND BRANCHIAL CLEFT CYSTS

Second branchial cleft cysts are the most common type of branchial cleft abnormalities, representing approximately 95% of all branchial cleft cysts.[3] The cyst is found along the midportion of the anterior border of the sternocleidomastoid muscle, and its tract passes over the internal carotid artery (which is of third arch origin, and thus between the internal and external carotid arteries). It passes over other third arch structures (cranial nerve IX, hyoid bone), over the hypoglossal nerve, and under second arch structures (posterior belly of digastric and stylohyoid), opening into the tonsillar fossa. These cysts are generally lined with stratified squamous epithelium, though respiratory (columnar) epithelium may be seen as well.

THIRD BRANCHIAL CLEFT CYSTS

Third branchial cleft cysts are relatively rare. The cyst is found along the anterior border of the inferior portion of the sternocleidomastoid muscle. The tract passes behind the internal carotid artery, but over cranial nerve X, over cranial nerve XII, and under cranial nerve IX. It opens into the pyriform sinus.

FOURTH BRANCHIAL CLEFT CYSTS

Fourth branchial cleft cysts are extremely rare.[3-6] The cyst appears low in the neck along the anterior border of the sternocleidomastoid muscle. A sinus opens either to the skin or into the apex of the pyriform sinus. A complete fistula would have a tract that passes under either the aortic arch on the left or the subclavian artery on the right, and it would ascend from the mediastinum over cranial nerve XII and open into the esophagus. A complete fistula of the fourth cleft has never been described.

Thyroglossal Duct Cysts

Thyroglossal duct cysts develop along the path of the embryologic development of the thyroid gland.

The thyroglossal duct, which begins as the foramen caecum at the base of the tongue, descends into the neck, eventually developing into the thyroid gland proper. As it descends into the neck, it passes very close to or through the developing hyoid bone. The duct normally undergoes obliteration by 6 weeks; failure of the thyroglossal duct obliteration results in the potential for cysts to develop.

Thyroglossal duct cysts are characterized by being midline cystic structures usually found between the hyoid bone and the thyorid cartilage, though one third occur either at or above the level of the hyoid bone. They typically enlarge and may become infected following an upper respiratory infection. The lesions are epithelial-lined and often contain thick mucoid material. Treatment of thyroglossal duct cysts requires complete removal of the cyst and tract. Because of its embryologic relationship to the hyoid bone, the central portion of the hyoid bone must be removed with the tract (Sistrunk procedure), to avoid an otherwise unacceptably high recurrence rate.[7] The tract should be followed as proximally as possible to the area of the foramen caecum.

Thymic Cysts

The thymus gland develops from the third and fourth pharyngeal pouches descending into the superior mediastinum via the thyropharyngeal duct. Much like the thyroglossal duct cysts, failure of the thyropharyngeal duct to undergo complete obliteration may lead to the formation of a thymic cyst. While solid thymic rests occur either laterally or in the midline, thymic cysts present laterally and are clinically very much like second branchial cleft cysts. They are distinguished from the latter histologically. The treatment of choice is complete excision of the cyst and epithelial tract, which may open into the pharynx through the thyrohyoid membrane or may remain attached to the thymus gland itself. There has been no association with myasthenia gravis.

Laryngoceles

Laryngoceles are congenital cysts of the larynx that arise in the laryngeal ventricle and saccule. The saccule consists of an epithelial-lined sac that extends from the anterior ventricle superiorly along the inner aspect of the thyroid cartilage. The saccule contains mucous glands that produce secretions in the endolarynx. A distinction between a laryngocele and a saccular cyst should be made. Laryngoceles represent abnormal dilatation of the saccule and ventricle. They are air-filled and communicate with the laryngeal lumen. In contrast, saccular cysts are fluid-filled lesions that do not communicate with the endolarynx.

Laryngoceles may have an external component, an internal component, or an external and internal component simultaneously. The external portion of the laryngocele exits the larynx through the thyrohyoid membrane along the superior laryngeal neurovascular structures. The internal component usually extends posteriorly into the false vocal cord. Infection of these lesions may result in the formation of a laryngopyocele, which is potentially life-threatening due to airway obstruction or aspiration of the cyst contents. Treatment of laryngoceles involves complete excision via an external approach or an endoscopic laser excision. The superior portion of the thyroid cartilage on the ipsilateral side can be removed for improved exposure. A prophylactic tracheotomy may be considered at the time of excision.

Teratomas and Dermoid Cysts

Teratomas represent a group of lesions of embryonic origin arising from pluripotential cells; they show varying degrees of differentiation. Unlike hamartomas, the tissue of origin is not local tissue. Teratomas can be classified into four groups. For all of these, the treatment of choice is surgical excision when the lesions are symptomatic.

1. Dermoid cysts are the most common teratomas of the head and neck. These are midline structures consisting of ectodermal and mesodermal tissue and often present as a small pit containing hair and sebaceous elements.
2. Teratoid cysts are derived from all three germ layers. However, these lesions remain poorly differentiated.
3. True teratomas are also derived from ectoderm, mesoderm, and endoderm—but in contrast to teratoid cysts, teratomas are well differentiated to the level of specific tissues and organs. The most common site of teratomas in the head and neck is the nasopharynx. They are found at birth (or before) and cause symptoms arising from compression of surrounding structures.
4. Epignathic lesions have the highest degree of differentiation representing reduplicated fetal organs and limbs. The presence of epignathi is rarely compatible with life.

Hamartomas

Unlike teratomas, hamartomas represent a benign overgrowth of the tissue (cells) native to the area. Although a hamartoma may present as an enlarging mass, it is not a true neoplasm. According to Batsakis,[2] it may be more accurately described as a malformation. Examples of hamartomas of the head and neck include, among others, hemangiomas and lymphangiomas (see following sections) and congenital lipomas.

Hemangiomas

Hemangiomas (and lymphangiomas, next section) are believed to result from arrested development of mesenchymal vascular primordia and are thus true congenital malformations rather than neoplastic processes.[8] However, there is endothelial proliferation during the growing phase, typically during the first year, followed by slow involution. Still, this may be more a response to pressure and flow, rather than cellular neoplasia. (True neoplasia is seen in angiofibromas and angiosarcomas.) Hemangiomas are the most common congenital lesions, occurring in almost 3% of newborns and, with a larger number developing during the first month of life, nearly 12% of 1-year-olds have hemangiomas.

Hemangiomas have been divided into capillary, cavernous, and mixed. While it has been suggested that the type of hemangioma depends upon the embryologic stage of vascular development at which the hemangioma begins,[8] Batsakis[2] has suggested that the cavernous form is actually the result of dilatation of the vessels in a capillary hemangioma.

The head and neck are the most common sites for the development of hemangiomas. They commonly occur in the skin (subdermal or subcutaneous), though visceral lesions occur in the head and neck as well. Subglottic hemangiomas often lead to upper-airway dysfunction varying from mild croup to severe airway obstruction. Therapy ranges from watchful waiting (since many begin to involute by the end of the first year of life, and the majority do so by age 7), to aggressive surgical excision (with or without preoperative embolization) for deforming and/or obstructing lesions. Pharmacotherapy with systemic and/or intralesional steroids and interferon as well as various laser treatments, are also used. Cryotherapy and the injection of sclerosing agents, no longer considered useful, have been abandoned. Ionizing radiation may lead to malignant transformation as well as inhibition of normal growth and, therefore, more severe deformities.

Lymphangiomas (Cystic Hygromas)

Like hemangiomas, lymphangiomas are the result of abnormal development of vascular (lymphatic) channels. The lymphatic system develops as endothelial sacs within the venous capillary system.[8] Endothelial sprouting leads to the development of the mature lymphatic system. When development is aberrant, lymphangiomas may result. Like hemangiomas, lymphangiomas are thus technically malformations; unlike hemangiomas, however, lymphangiomas have a single layer of endothelial lining, and a lower rate of cell turnover.[9]

Like hemangiomas, lymphangiomas are divided into capillary (vascular channels only) and cavernous (composed of large cystic lymphatic compo-

nents). When the cavernous type degenerates into larger cystic structures (it is unclear whether this represents a distinct form of lymphangioma or merely an obstruction of lymphatic channels followed by dilatation into larger cystic structures) it is called a cystic lymphangioma or cystic hygroma. When there is a vascular component as well, the lesion is classified as a lymphangiohemangioma. Lymphangiomas are far less common than hemangiomas, and lymphangiohemangiomas are considered rare.

More than half of lymphangiomas are noted at birth, and almost 90% are found by age 2, though they can be diagnosed initially in adults as well. They can enlarge in response to a regional infection, which may result in diagnosis or in complications in a previously diagnosed lesion. The vast majority of lymphangiomas occur in the head and neck region.

Lymphangiomas present as soft, compressible masses and can present due to their deforming cosmetic appearance and/or symptoms caused by encroachment on regional structures generally affecting the upper aerodigestive tract (Fig. 13–3). Though completely benign and noninvasive, cystic hygromas develop without respect for tissue planes and thus insinuate themselves between and around vital structures. This pattern of growth and the fact that their walls are often very thin make complete surgical excision extremely difficult, leading to high recurrence rates. Therefore, excision of asymptomatic lesions is ill-advised. Surgery should be considered

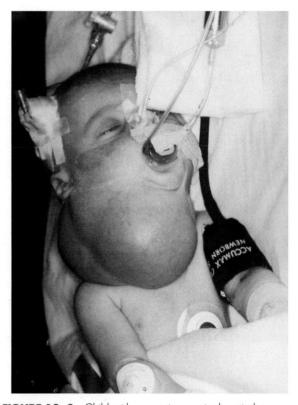

FIGURE 13–3 Child with a massive cervical cystic hygroma.

early only for visceral compromise to preserve the function of the airway and alimentary tract. Parents of infants often want surgery performed quickly because of the dramatic deformity that large hygromas create. These cases should be delayed as long as is reasonable to allow the infant to grow; the parents must be counseled carefully regarding the surgical risks to neurovascular structures, as well as the risk of recurrence. While the use of sclerosing agents has historically been unsuccessful, the risks and challenges of surgery for these lesions has led to a recent resurgence of interest in the newer experimental sclerosing agents.[10]

Lingual Thyroid

Lingual thyroid is represented by ectopic thyroid tissue that may or may not be associated with functioning thyroid tissue in the neck. In most instances, it is the only functioning thryoid tissue in the body. Incidence of lingual thyroid is significantly higher in females.

These lesions usually present as midline masses in the posterior tongue in the area of the foramen caecum (Fig. 13–4), with the most common presenting symptom being dysphagia. When the diagnosis of lingual thyroid is being considered, radionuclide studies should be performed to determine the level of thyroid activity in the tongue base as well as any normal-appearing thyroid tissue in the neck. Treatment includes thyroid suppression, radioactive io-

dine ablation, and surgical excision with thyroid replacement, depending upon the status of the patient's symptoms and thyroid function.

Congenital Torticollis (Fibromatosis Colli, Pseudotumor of Infancy)

Congenital torticollis represents varying degrees of sternocleidomastoid fibrosis. It presents at birth or soon after, and it has been associated with birth trauma, though there is no clear evidence of a cause-and-effect relationship. It presents as a slowly enlarging mass in the inferior third of the sternocleidomastoid muscle, and it must be differentiated from a true neoplasm such as a fibrosarcoma or rhabdomyosarcoma. Recently, fine-needle aspiration has been found helpful.[11] Most of these masses disappear spontaneously before age 1, and surgery is indicated only for those few infants with progressive torticollis (wry neck). Physical therapy may help maintain mobility and prevent foreshortening of the growing sternocleidomastoid muscle.

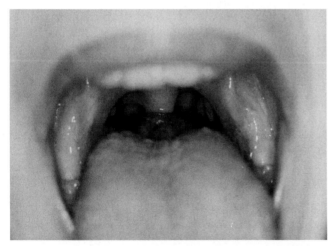

FIGURE 13–4 A lingual thyroid mass at the base of the tongue of a child.

REFERENCES

1. Robbins KT, Medina JE, Wolfe GT, Levine PA, Sessions RB, Pruet CW. Standardizing neck dissection terminology. Official report of the academy's committee for head and neck surgery and oncology. *Arch Otolaryngol Head Neck Surg.* 1991; 117:601–605.
2. Batsakis JG. *Tumors of the Head and Neck. Clinical and Pathological Considerations.* 2nd ed. Baltimore; Williams & Wilkins; 1979.
3. Cote DN, Gianoli GJ. Fourth branchial cleft cysts. *Otolaryngol Head Neck Surg.* 1996; 114(1):95–97.
4. Sanborn WD. A branchial cleft cyst of fourth pouch origin. *J Pediatr Surg.* 1972; 7:82.
5. Rosenfeld RM, Biller HF. Fourth branchial pouch sinus: Diagnosis and treatment. *Otolaryngol Head Neck Surg.* 1991; 105:44–50.
6. Tucker HM, Skolnick ML. Fourth branchial cleft (pharyngeal pouch) remnant. *Trans Am Acad Ophthalmol Otolaryngol.* 1973; 77:368–371.
7. Sistrunk WE. The surgical treatment of cysts of the thyroglossal tract. *Annals Surg.* 1920; 71:120.
8. Stal S, Hamilton S, Spira M. Hemangiomas, lymphangiomas, and vascular malformations of the head and neck. *Otolaryngol Clin North Am.* 1986; 19(4):769–796.
9. Mulliken JB, Glowacki J. Hemangiomas and vascular malformations in infants and children: A classification based on endothelial characteristics. *Plastic Recon Surg.* 1982; 69(3):412–422.
10. Smith RJ, Burke DK, Sato Y, et al. OK-432 therapy for lymphangiomas. *Arch Otolaryngol Head Neck Surg.* 1996; 122(11):1195–1199.
11. Schwartz RA, Powers CN, Wakely PE Jr, Kellman RM. Fibromatosis colli. The utility of fine needle aspiration in diagnosis. *Arch Otolaryngol Head Neck Surg.* 1997; 123(3):301–304.

II. CLINICAL CONSIDERATIONS FOR NEOPLASMS OF THE NECK

■ JOHN F. CAREW

■ DENNIS H. KRAUS

GENERAL CONSIDERATIONS

Neoplasms of the neck represent a vast array of benign and malignant tumors that can develop in a variety of sites throughout the cervical region. To treat these neoplasms surgically depends on a complete understanding of the regional anatomy of the neck. For this reason, a general overview of the surgical anatomy of the neck is presented here. Special anatomical considerations for the various neoplasms will then be addressed.

Most descriptions of the anatomy of the neck divide its contents into the fascial compartments or the various triangles. Obviously, an understanding of these compartments and divisions is fundamental. For the purpose of avoiding redundancy and to emphasize the surgical anatomy, it seems worthwhile to divide the neck into the various levels encompased in a neck dissection (levels I through V). Certainly, in the absence of regional lymph node metastasis, few of the lesions described in this chapter would require a standard comprehensive neck dissection. By understanding the anatomical relationships of the structures encountered in each level, however, the surgeon is able to design a surgical procedure allowing an en bloc resection of these tumors.

Many of the aggressive neoplasms developing in the neck do not respect the anatomic boundaries. Additionally, tumors of various histologies tend to occur at sites outside those routinely encompassed in a standard neck dissection. With this consideration, the anatomy of several other regions of the neck, such as the skull base and cervicothoracic junction, are discussed.

Levels I through IV are found in the anterior triangle of the neck. The significant structures in level I include the submandibular gland, marginal mandibular branch of the facial nerve, lingual nerve, hypoglossal nerve, facial artery and vein, digastric muscle, mylohyoid muscle, and hyoglossus muscle. The marginal mandibular branch of the facial nerve exits the parotid gland and sweeps down inferior to the lower border of the mandible, beneath the platysma on the fascia overlying the submandibular gland. It usually does not sweep lower than 2 cm below the border of the mandible; therefore, incisions are often designed 2 cm beneath the angle of the mandible to protect this branch of the facial nerve.

Whenever surgery is performed in level I of the neck (Fig. 13–5), every effort should be made to identify and preserve the marginal mandibular nerve, as its sacrifice leads to deformity of the lower lip. The facial artery, looping around the border of the posterior belly of the digastric and passing through the submandibular gland and over the mandible to enter the face, is a key anatomic relationship within level I. The anterior belly of the digastric and mylohyoid muscles are seen anteriorly. The submental triangle is bound laterally on either side by the anterior bellies of the digastric muscles. The lingual nerve, Wharton's duct, and the hypoglossal nerve are located deep to the digastric and mylohyoid muscles and superficial to the hyoglossus muscle. The lingual artery can sometimes be seen at the depths of level I, passing deep to the hyoglossus muscle. The submandibular ganglion, carrying the postganglionic parasympathetic fibers to the submandibular gland, can be identified emerging from the lingual nerve.

The sternocleidomastoid muscle (SCM) overlies levels II to IV (Fig. 13–6). Levels II and III are arbi-

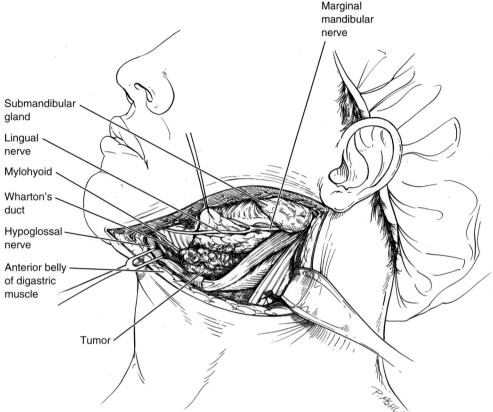

Marginal
mandibular
nerve

Submandibular
gland

Lingual
nerve

Mylohyoid

Wharton's
duct

Hypoglossal
nerve

Anterior belly
of digastric
muscle

Tumor

FIGURE 13-5 Schematic diagram of anatomy and tumor resection of a lesion found at level I of the neck.

trarily divided by the upper and middle third of the SCM, while levels III and IV are divided by the omohyoid muscle. Beneath the upper SCM, at level II, the posterior belly of the digastric muscle, stylohyoid muscle, spinal accessory nerve, hypoglossal nerve, glossopharyngeal nerve, internal jugular vein (IJV), and internal and external carotid arteries can be seen. The key landmark in the upper limits of level II is the posterior belly of the digastric muscle. This muscle lies superficial to the spinal accessory nerve, IJV, and carotid artery and protects them. The spinal accessory nerve passes posteriorly from beneath the inferior border of the digastric toward the posterior triangle. If oncologically feasible, this nerve should be identified and preserved during any resection, including level II. The hypoglossal nerve, passing over the carotid bifurcation and deep to the digastric muscle as it enters level I, should also be preserved. The vagus nerve lies deep to the IJV on the lateral aspect of the carotid artery and should always be identified and preserved when working in the region of the IJV. The glossopharyngeal nerve lies more anterior and superior in level II and seldom requires sacrifice. The main structures included in level III are those in the carotid sheath—the IJV, carotid artery, and vagus nerve. The ansa cervicalis can also be seen coursing from the hypoglossal nerve to the strap muscles inferiorly. The omohyoid muscle divides level III from level IV. Again, the contents of the carotid sheath

are found passing through level IV. The thoracic duct also can be found at the inferior aspect of level IV, being more prominent on the left side. There are many anatomical variants of the thoracic duct, and care should be taken to ligate these lymphatics with nonabsorbable sutures to prevent chyle leaks. The transverse cervical artery and inferior thyroid artery pass transversely through the lower aspect of level IV. The cervical sympathetic chain lies posterior to the carotid sheath in levels II to IV.

The posterior triangle, or level V, is located between the SCM, trapezius muscle, and the clavicle (Fig. 13–7). The spinal accessory nerve passes from the posterior border of the SCM to the trapezius, sending branches to both these muscles. Often it can be identified at the posterior border of the SCM just above the point where the great auricular nerve wraps around the SCM known as Erb's point. It runs through the muscle in most instances (82%) but can also lie deep to the muscle.[1] The spinal accessory nerve courses in a relatively superficial plane in the posterior triangle. The cervical trunks may contribute motor fibers to the spinal nerve and occasionally may be the only source of motor innervation to the trapezius. When oncologically feasible, the spinal accessory nerve should be preserved to avoid significant shoulder morbidity. In the lower region of the posterior triangle, the omohyoid muscle is seen, with the transverse cervical artery traveling transversely deep to it. The floor of the posterior

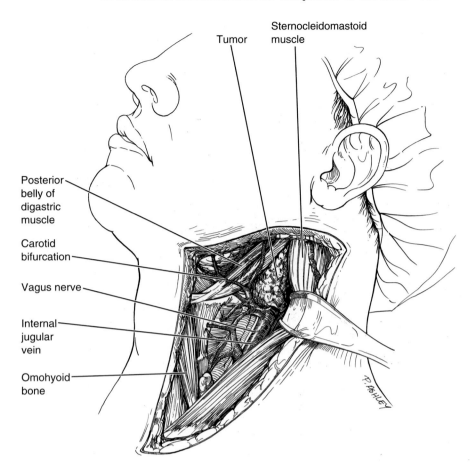

FIGURE 13-6 Schematic diagram of anatomy and tumor resection of a lesion found at level II of the neck.

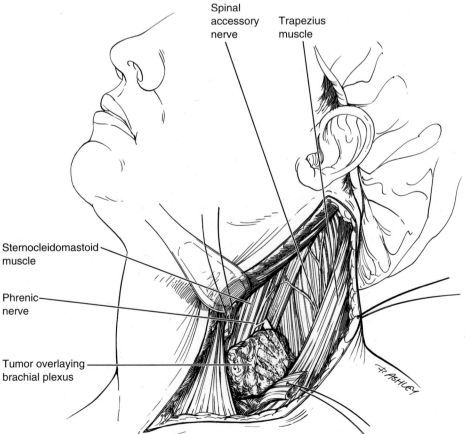

FIGURE 13-7 Schematic diagram of tumor overlying the brachial plexus in the posterior triangle of the neck.

triangle is formed by several muscles (from posterior to anterior): the splenius capitus, levator scapulae, scalenus posterior, medius, and anterior. The nerves to the splenius capitus and levator scapulae pass below the prevertebral fascia. Dissection in this region should be superficial to this fascia to preserve innervation. Proceeding along the floor of the posterior triangle from posterior to anterior, the brachial plexus is seen between the scalenus medius and anterior; the phrenic nerve is seen traveling on the surface of the scalenus anterior.

The central compartment, or level VI, contains the strap muscles (sternohyoid, sternothyroid, and thyrohyoid), thyroid gland, parathyroid glands, recurrent laryngeal nerve, superior laryngeal nerve, laryngotracheal complex, and thymus inferiorly.

Last we consider lesions in the supraclavicular region, or root of the neck, which straddle the cervicothoracic junction.[2] Lesions at this site may encroach upon or invade central visceral structures—the laryngotracheal complex and esophagus, neural structures (the brachial plexus, phrenic nerve, cervical sympathetics, and vagus-recurrent laryngeal nerve) major vessels (including the carotid, innominate, subclavian arteries, and corresponding venous anatomy), as well as the lungs and upper mediastinum. The deepest soft tissue structures of the root of the neck include the longus capitus and longus colli anteriorly and the semispinalis capitus and semispinalis cervicis posteriorly. In the center of the neck is the vertebral column. The vertebral artery enters the transverse foramen of the vertebral column at the level of C6.

BENIGN NEOPLASMS

Teratomas

Clinical Presentation

Teratomas occur in about one in 4000 births, with approximately 2% to 4% occurring in the cervical region.[3,4] They arise in both sexes with equal frequency.[5,6] Unlike teratomas of the nasopharynx, which are associated with palatal and craniofacial abnormalities, cervical teratomas are not associated with any other congenital anomalies.[7] Cervical teratomas usually present as a semicystic mass in a para-axial or midline region of the neck. This is observed at birth or soon thereafter. They are often diagnosed prenatally by ultrasound, in which case, securing the neonatal airway can be accomplished at the time of planned cesarean section.[8] Cervical teratomas have been classified by Jordan and Gauderer[3] based on age, birth status, and symptoms (Table 13–3). Although the vast majority of teratomas present during the first year, cases of adult teratomas have been reported.[9] In an adult, however, most of these lesions are malignant and are discussed later in this chapter.

T A B L E 1 3 – 3	CLASSIFICATION OF CERVICAL TERATOMAS		
		NUMBER	MORTALITY
I	Stillborn and moribund newborns	27	100%
II	Newborns with respiratory distress	29	43.4%
III	Newborns without respiratory distress	37	2.7%
IV	Children (1 month–18 years)	31	3.2%
V	Adults	23	43.5%

Symptoms and Signs

Teratomas in the neonate are associated with polyhydraminos in 18% to 53% of cases.[7,10] This is due to the mass effect of the teratoma on the pharynx or esophagus, preventing the fetus from swallowing amniotic fluid. On physical examination, a firm multilobular mass is seen, which shows rapid growth and does not transilluminate. Teratomas usually are located in the midline, but may be more prominent on one side.[11] Cervical teratomas in the neonate usually cause symptoms related to the midline structures of the aerodigestive tract, which they compress. Patients with cervical teratomas can experience dyspnea, stridor, airway obstruction, and dysphagia. The magnitude of these symptoms depends primarily on the size and location of the tumor.

Radiology

On CT scan (Fig. 13–8), mature teratomas usually demonstrate cystic regions with the density of water or fat. Radiographic evidence of calcification in the mass has been reported in 16% of cases, reflecting the variety of tissue types found in teratomas.[3] Sometimes a fat-fluid level can be visualized, which

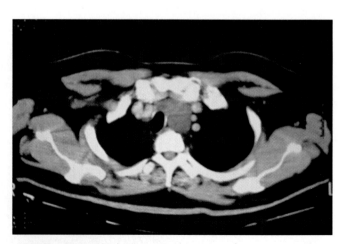

FIGURE 13–8 Axial CT scan with contrast of a teratoma in the left superior mediastinum that required a cervicothoracic approach.

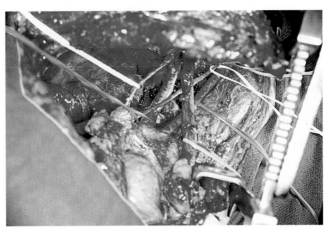

FIGURE 13-11 Operative photo postresection of the teratoma of the superior mediastinum. The arch of the aorta, vagus nerve (white vessel loop to the right), and phrenic nerve (white vessel loop to the left) are preserved.

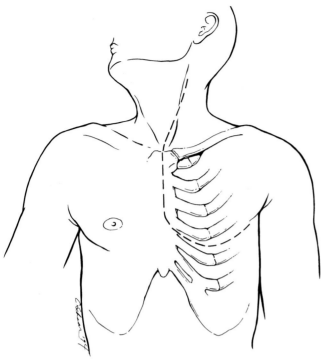

FIGURE 13-9 The surgical incision is designed along the anterior sternocleidomastoid muscle, through the midline sternotomy, and laterally to the fourth interspace. From Kraus DH, Huo J, Burt M. Surgical access to tumors of the cervicothoracic junction. *Head & Neck.* 1995; 17:134. Copyright 1995 John Wiley & Sons, with permission.

is virtually pathognomonic of a teratoma.[9] Ultrasound shows a heterogeneous echogenicity, which can help differentiate it from the multiocular pattern of a cystic hygroma.

Treatment

The treatment of cervical teratomas involves securing the airway along with prompt and complete surgical excision (Figs. 13-9 through 13-16). They can grow rapidly and compress the airway, so early surgical removal is recommended. An 80% mortality rate has been reported for patients who did not undergo expeditious surgical management during the neonatal period.[12] Operative mortalities ranging from 9% to 15% have been reported for patients undergoing prompt surgical excision.[8,12] These lesions are often encapsulated, enabling complete removal. Although cervical metastasis has been reported, it is rare.[13]

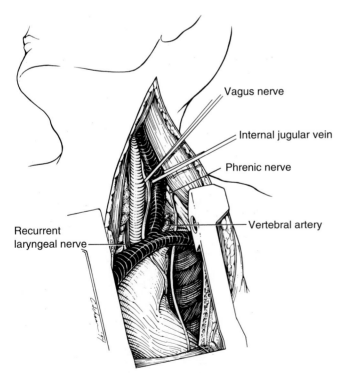

Vagus nerve

Internal jugular vein

Phrenic nerve

Recurrent laryngeal nerve

Vertebral artery

FIGURE 13-10 Dissection of mobilization of the paravertebral neurovascular structures with isolation of the mediastinal chordoma. From Kraus DH, Huo J, Burt M. Surgical access to tumors of the cervicothoracic junction. *Head & Neck.* 1995;17:134. Copyright 1995 John Wiley & Sons, with permission.

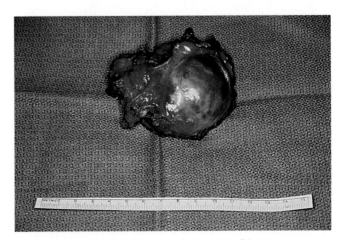

FIGURE 13-12 The surgical specimen of the teratoma.

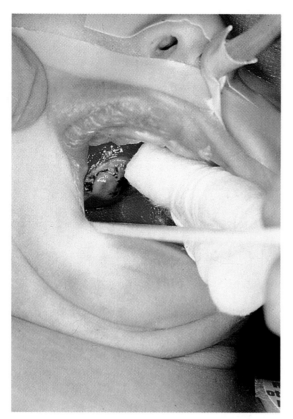

FIGURE 13-13   Teratoma in the right oropharynx of an infant.

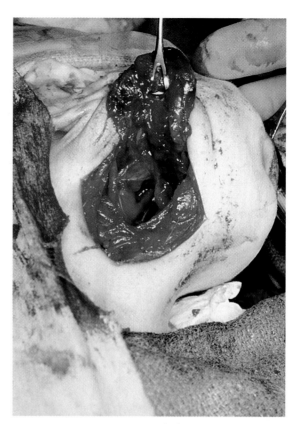

FIGURE 13-15   Operative removal of teratoma through a cervical approach. A portion of the lateral pharyngeal wall was resected and closed primarily.

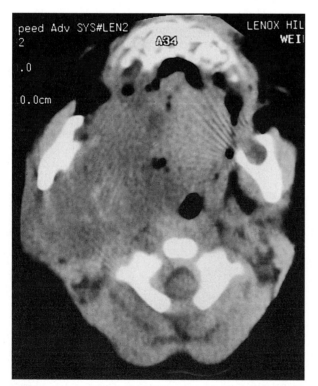

FIGURE 13-14   Axial CT scan of teratoma showing characteristic radiographic appearance. The CT reveals significant impingement on the oropharyngeal airway.

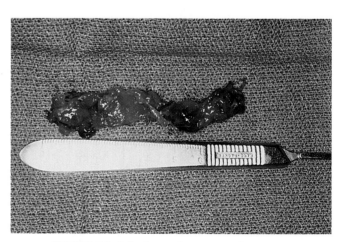

FIGURE 13-16   Surgical specimen of teratoma.

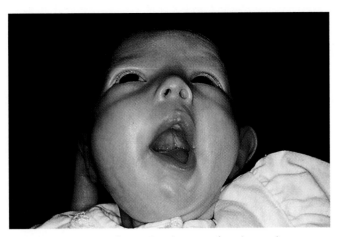

FIGURE 13-17 Infant with right cervicofacial cystic hygroma.

Prognosis

With early treatment and complete excision, prognosis is very good. When mortality occurs, it is usually due to delayed treatment or failure to secure the airway. The most significant factors affecting clinical course are the size and location of the teratoma.

Controversies

Classification of teratomas has been attempted based on their relationship to the thyroid gland.[14] This is probably unnecessary, as most teratomas are intimately related to the thyroid gland, and classification has little clinical importance.

Cystic Hygroma (Lymphangioma)

Clinical Presentation

Lymphangiomas occur in as many as 12 of every 1000 fetuses, as examined on maternal ultrasound. Approximately 50% to 60% are clinically apparent at birth, and 80% to 90% present before 2 years (Fig. 13–17).[4,15] In the 10% that present in adults, the question arises whether they are congenital or posttraumatic. Males and females are equally affected.[16] Lymphangiomas occur throughout the body, but most are found in the neck (up to 90% of cases).[17] There they are found most commonly in the posterior triangle, but they can extend anterior to the sternocleidomastoid muscle and cross the midline. Lymphangiomas have been associated with Turner's syndrome and various trisomies.[4] They have also been associated with congenital anomalies including thyroglossal duct cysts, congenital heart anomalies, and hand and foot deformities.[5]

Lymphangiomas have been classified into three groups:[18]

1. Lymphangioma simplex (capillary-like lymphatic vessels)
2. Cavernous lymphangioma (dilated lymphatic chan-

nels with one or several endothelial layers with or without an adventitial layer)
3. Cystic hygroma or cystic lymphangiomas (large multiloculated cysts)

Cystic hygroma is the most common type, and 75% occur in the neck.[19]

Symptoms and Signs

Lymphangiomas present as soft, cystic, sometimes multilocular painless masses that can be transilluminated. They are found most commonly in the posterior triangle.[4] Compression of nearby structures can lead to symptoms of stridor, dyspnea, dysphagia, and pain. Cervical lesions may extend into the axilla, mediastinum, or thorax.[4] When lesions extend into the mediastinum, they are associated with venous aneurysms.[20] Although growth rates vary, the majority of lymphangiomas grow in proportion with the infant or show slow progressive enlargement.[4,7] Occasionally, hemorrhage into the lymphangioma or infection can result in rapid enlargement and potentially life-threatening airway compression.[4,7]

Radiology

On CT (Fig. 13–18), lymphangiomas are low-density, nonenhancing cystic lesions that may be unilocular or multilocular. The cyst wall is thin and not usually seen radiographically unless previous infection or hemorrhage has caused it to thicken.[15] Lymphangioma can displace or surround neurovascular structures and muscles, but rarely is found to infiltrate on radiographic examination.[15] On MR, the lesions have low intensity on T1W and high intensity on T2W. On T1W images they may, however, have foci of high-intensity signal representing fat or methemoglobin within the lesion.[19] If previous hemorrhage has occurred, fluid-fluid levels may be visualized and are best seen on T2W images.[15]

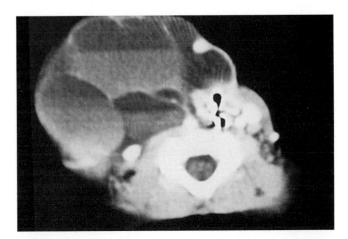

FIGURE 13-18 Axial CT scan with intravenous contrast showing multilocular cystic hygroma with fluid-fluid levels.

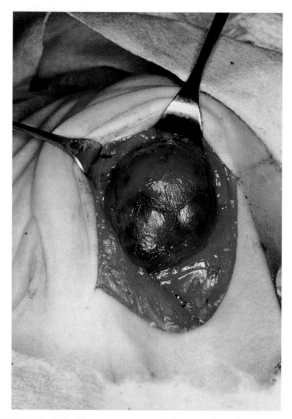

FIGURE 13–19   Operative removal of cervicofacial cystic hygroma.

Treatment

Surgical excision is the mainstay of treatment (Figs. 13–19 and 13–20). Lymphangiomas can extend locally to surround neurovascular structures, making complete surgical removal a challenge. Most surgeons advocate delayed removal, suggesting surgery at the age of 2 to 4 years, unless there are symptoms of compression or an uncertainty of diagnosis in the infant.[5,7,16] Others advocate early surgical excision for infants born with cystic hygromas to avoid the problems of airway obstruction when hemorrhage or

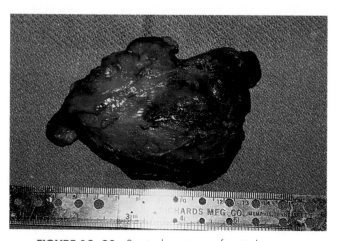

FIGURE 13–20   Surgical specimen of cystic hygroma.

infection cause rapid enlargement.[4] Regardless of timing, every attempt should be made to avoid rupturing the cyst during surgery to allow complete removal. Lymphangiomas can adhere to adjacent structures, making dissection tedious.

Prognosis

Recurrence rates ranging from 5% to 10% have been reported.[16] As expected, larger lymphangiomas and the cavernous type have a higher recurrence rate.[4,7] The location also affects recurrence rates, with 81% of extraparotid suprahyoid lesions recurring compared to only 15% of infrahyoid lesions.[21]

Controversies

Nonsurgical treatment modalities such as sclerotherapy, aspiration, radiation therapy, and diathermy have been reported in treating lymphangiomas. Most of these techniques are associated with high complication rates and inconsistent or unsatisfactory results.[4] The use of these nonsurgical methods, specifically sclerotherapy, may assist in treating large, extensively invasive, unresectable lymphangiomas. The mainstay of therapy, however, remains surgical excision. As stated earlier, there is not a consensus in the literature on the ideal timing of surgery for lesions that do not compromise the airway.

Hemangiomas

Clinical Presentation

Hemangiomas represent the most common lesion of the head and neck found in infants and children, and occur in one to three of every 100 live births (Fig. 13–21).[4] The term hemangioma has been used to describe a variety of lesions that differ vastly in clinical behavior, including strawberry hemangioma, cavernous hemangioma, and capillary hemangioma. A recent classification system of vascular lesions proposes defining them as either hemangiomas or vascular malformations based on clinical behavior and cell kinetics.[22] The defining characteristic of a hemangioma is rapid neonatal growth and endothelial proliferation, followed by involution beginning at age 1 to 2 years and lasting up to 12 years.[22,23] Vascular malformations, in contrast, are true structural anomalies that grow in proportion with the child and show a normal rate of endothelial turnover.[22]

Symptoms and Signs

Hemangiomas can appear as either cutaneous skin lesions or subcutaneous masses. Hemangiomas that are both cutaneous and subcutaneous are called compound lesions. Cutaneous lesions appear as erythematous vascular macules. Subcutaneous hemangiomas appear as soft, cystic, compressible lesions with a bluish discoloration of the overlying skin as well as audible bruits that change in size on crying or straining. They are often associated with heman-

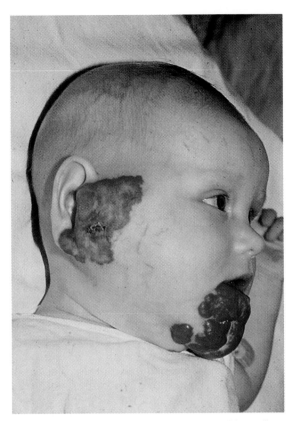

FIGURE 13-21 Infant with right preauricular and lower lip and chin hemangioma.

giomas elsewhere in the body. When they are large, hemangiomas can cause severe systemic complications, including a consumptive coagulopathy (Kasabach-Merritt syndrome) and even high-output cardiac failure.

Radiology

On CT and MR, intravenous contrast results in intense enhancement of hemangiomas.[15] On CT, phleboliths may be visualized within the lesion.[15] On MR, these lesions have variable intensity on T1W and high intensity on T2W images. Vascular flow voids are usually present on MR, resulting in a heterogeneous appearance.[15]

Treatment

With the clinical course of hemangiomas being ultimately involution, a conservative approach to treatment is often warranted unless they threaten function, grow at unacceptable rates, or cause complications. Approximately 10% to 20% of hemangiomas require some form of treatment.[23] Steroids have become the first line of therapy in controlling hemangiomas that require treatment. In one series, 30% of patients had dramatic responses to steroids, with most receiving doses of 2 to 3 mg/kg/day.[24] It should be noted, however, that steroids are useful

only during the proliferative phase.[23] Note, too, that in approximately 40% of cases, the lesions begin to grow after cessation of steroid therapy, necessitating a prolonged course of steroid therapy at a reduced dose (0.75 to 1 mg/kg/day).[23] For patients requiring treatment of hemangiomas who fail to respond to steroids, interferon alpha-2a has been used. In a series of 20 patients who failed steroid therapy, interferon alpha-2a caused a 50% or more regression of the hemangioma after an average of 7.8 months.[25] Long-term toxicity of interferon alpha-2a was not seen in any of these patients. Surgical intervention is reserved for cases threatening function or causing significant complications in patients who fail nonsurgical therapies. Blood loss can be significant, and preoperative embolization should be considered to minimize intraoperative blood loss.[16] Many of the deep-seated lesions can be infiltrative, making complete surgical excision difficult. Sacrifice of vital structures should be avoided in treating these benign lesions. Some authors have begun to advocate early surgical treatment of select patients with the copper vapor laser of flash lamp pumped-dye laser. These pulsed lasers emit yellow light that is readily absorbed by hemoglobin and melanin. The parameters of the pulsed light are manipulated to maximize absorption by hemoglobin within the hemangioma and to minimize absorption by melanin in the adjacent skin. The rationale for treating lesions that will spontaneously involute is to halt or inhibit visible changes of the skin and subcutaneous tissue that often persist after complete involution.[23] This group suggests treating early cutaneous hemangiomas, late proliferative lesions failing medical therapy, and the early involutional phase of cutaneous and compound hemangiomas.[23]

Prognosis

As the natural history of hemangiomas is ultimate involution, most patients do not require treatment. As mentioned, however, visible changes persist even after complete involution. Lesions that grow rapidly or impinge on vital structures continue to challenge clinicians despite the growing options of clinical tools used to treat these lesions.

Controversies

The unresolved issues in the treatment of hemangiomas involve minimizing the long-term sequelae and treating rapidly growing, aggressive lesions that impair function and cause complications. The use, sequence, and timing of steroid therapy, interferon alpha-2a, and laser therapy continue to evolve.

Lipoma (Hibernoma)

Clinical Presentation

Lipomas occur infrequently in the head and neck region, accounting for less than 15% of all lipomas.

Those few are found throughout the head and neck region, most frequently in the cervical region.[5,15] There is no gender predilection, and they most commonly occur in the fifth and sixth decades. Lipomas usually grow with age; malignant degeneration is extremely rare. Lipomas enlarge with weight gain but generally do not shrink with weight loss, making them more apparent after a patient loses weight. Benign fatty tumors arising from the brown fat are called hibernomas.

Other clinical entities involving the deposition of lipomatous tissue in the neck include benign symmetric lipomatosis, or Madelung's disease, a disorder characterized by an abnormal accumulation of lipomatosis tissue around the entire cervical region.

Symptoms and Signs

A lipoma usually presents as a slowly enlarging painless mass in the neck. On physical examination, a soft fatty mass is usually found in the subcutaneous tissues. It can also occur deeper in the neck and have a more infiltrative nature.[26] Lipomas can also occur within the upper aerodigestive tract, causing symptoms related to the function of these structures, such as dysphagia or change in voice.

Radiology

On CT scan, lipomas are isointense with the low-intensity subcutaneous fat. On MR, lipomas are again isointense with fat showing a high signal on T1W images and low intensity on T2W images.[15] Soft-tissue densities found within a lipoma may represent previous hemorrhage or suggest liposarcoma.[15]

Treatment

The treatment of lipomas is complete surgical excision. Although asymptomatic lipomas may be observed, surgical excision allows histologic confirmation of these benign tumors.

Prognosis

Lipomas rarely recur after excision, and even after enucleation, the reported recurrence rate is less than 5%.[5,27] A variant classified as infiltrating lipoma can occur deep in the neck; these are nonencapsulated, making complete excision difficult and recurrence more common.

Controversies

Another variant is spindle cell lipoma. This lesion most commonly occurs in the posterior triangle and supraclavicular region of older males. Histologically, these can be confused with liposarcoma but are composed of uniform spindle cells without lipoblasts.[27]

Fibrous Histiocytoma

Clinical Presentation

Fibrous histiocytoma refers to a wide variety of benign lesions containing fibroblasts and histiocytes. Until recently, these lesions were classified separately as dermatofibroma, atypical fibroxanthoma, pigmented villonodular synovitis, nodular tenosynovitis, juvenile xanthogranuloma, xanthoma, and xanthofribroma. In the mid-1970s, however, these related lesions were grouped and classified as fibrous histiocytomas.[28] These lesions can occur either cutaneously or in the subcutaneous soft tissues (noncutaneous). The noncutaneous lesions show a male predilection, a male:female ratio of 2.5:1, and an average age of patients with noncutaneous lesions of 37 years.[29]

The cutaneous form of fibrous histiocytoma occurs most frequently in patients with sun-exposed skin, the majority of them under 50 years old.[30]

Symptoms and Signs

Fibrous histiocytoma usually presents as a slow-growing painless mass and can cause symptoms related to structures within the upper aerodigestive tract, as it compresses or invades that area. Symptoms of nasal obstruction, epistaxis, dysphagia, and dyspnea have been reported.[29]

Radiology

The cutaneous forms of fibrous histiocytomas are readily accessible to clinical examination and rarely require radiologic imaging. When imaging studies are obtained, lesions are seen to have a well-defined homogeneous appearance. On MRI, the intensity of the fibrous histiocytomas on T2W image depends on the cellularity of the tumor. Hypercellular tumors have an increased signal, and hypocellular tumors have a decreased signal.[31] Some of the specific types of noncutaneous fibrous histiocytomas have a characteristic appearance. Pigmented villonodular synovitis, for example, on T2W MRI, displays areas of marked signal loss due to the presence of hemosiderin-laden tissue.[31]

Treatment

The standard treatment for fibrous histiocytomas is local excision. Because these tumors are benign, major neurovascular structures should not be sacrificed in resecting these lesions.

Prognosis

Recurrence rates of 11% have been reported after local excision.[29] If positive margins are seen, recurrence is more frequent.

Controversies

Past controversy existed regarding the histologic criteria for the diagnosis of fibrous histiocytoma and for defining the malignant potential of these lesions. Additionally, prior to the advent of immunohistochemical analysis, other pathologic entities were included with fibrous histiocytoma.

Rhabdomyoma

Clinical Presentation

Adult rhabdomyomas are rare benign tumors arising in striated muscle that occur most commonly in the myocardium.[32] The second most common location of rhabdomyomas is the head and neck region, with close to 90% of extracardiac rhabdomyomas occurring in the head and neck.[7,32] The most common sites in the head and neck include the larynx, submandibular region, pharynx, mouth, and nasopharynx.[32] The male:female ratio is 2:1, and the mean age of patients with rhabdomyomas is 40 years.[33] The majority of adult rhabdomyomas are solitary lesions, although 18% of extracardiac lesions are multifocal.[32]

Based on gross and histopathologic examination, two types of rhabdomyomas are recognized: adult and fetal. Fetal rhabdomyomas show the presence of myoblasts in early stages of development and suggest that this lesion may be a hamartoma rather than a true neoplasm.[7] Fetal rhabdomyomas usually present before the age of 3 years and arise more commonly in males. As with adult rhabdomyomas, fetal rhabdomyomas show a predilection for the head and neck, specifically for the postauricular region.

Symptoms and Signs

Clinically, adult rhabdomyomas present as a slow-growing painless mass. On physical examination, a well-demarcated soft mass is seen. As with other benign tumors, they usually cause symptoms related to their location in the head and neck region. Fetal rhabdomyomas usually present early in life as well-defined, rubbery, mobile masses.

Radiology

On CT, rhabdomyomas are well-circumscribed lesions that are isointense with muscle. On MRI, rhabdomyomas are slightly hyperintense to muscle on T1W images and even more hyperintense to muscle on T2W images. They enhance mildly with intravenous contrast.[15]

Treatment

Surgical excision is the treatment of choice for rhabdomyomas. They are often well demarcated, facili-

tating complete excision. Definitive resection establishes the diagnosis and relieves symptoms caused by these slow-growing lesions.

Prognosis

If completely excised, the prognosis is good. If not completely excised, recurrence is common.

Peripheral Nerve Sheath Tumors

It is now widely accepted that Schwann cells are the cells of origin of the peripheral nerve sheath tumors, including schwannomas and neurofibromas. Although they are rare tumors, approximately 45% of peripheral nerve sheath tumors occur in the head and neck region. Neurogenic tumors account for 17% to 25% of lesions in the parapharyngeal space, second only to salivary gland tumors.[15] Although schwannomas and neurofibromas share the same progenitor cell, these neoplasms display different clinical behavior and are considered separately.

SCHWANNOMA

Clinical Presentation

Schwannomas can arise anywhere in the body but have a predilection for the head and neck region. They affect females more commonly than males and occur most commonly in the 40-to-70-year age group. Within the head and neck, the most common site is the lateral cervical region, although they can occur in other areas such as the internal auditory canal, where they are commonly referred to as acoustic neuromas or vestibular nerve schwannomas. Within the neck, they can arise from the cranial nerves, cervical sensory nerves, cervical sympathetic chain, and brachial plexus. Malignant degeneration is extremely rare.

Symptoms and Signs

Schwannomas usually present as a solitary, slow-growing neck mass that may cause symptoms related to compression of neighboring structures. Occasionally pain occurs, which is located distal to the lesion and can be exacerbated by pressure on the lesion. Neurologic deficits from schwannomas are rare.

Radiology

On CT, benign nerve sheath tumors are isointense to soft tissue. Both schwannomas and neurofibromas may appear cystic. In schwannomas, this appearance is indeed due to cysts, while in neurofibroma it is due to fatty regions within the lesion. Although these lesions are hypovascular, they tend to enhance with intravenous contrast.[15] On MRI these lesions have intermediate intensity on T1W images and high intensity on T2W images.[34] If they extend through foramina, nerve sheath tumors can form a dumbbell-shaped tumor.

In the specific cases where schwannomas arise from neural structures within the parapharyngeal space or from the cervical sympathetic chain, they tend to occur in the post-styloid compartment and displace the carotid artery anteriorly.[35]

Treatment

Schwannomas arise from the perineural elements and histologically appear to push axons aside rather than incorporating the axons in the tumor.[5,7] Surgery remains the treatment of choice. These encapsulated lesions can, on rare occasions, be dissected off the nerve of origin with preservation of neural function.

Prognosis

Once again, with complete excision, prognosis is good and local recurrence is rare. The ability to completely excise schwannomas depends primarily on the size, location, and proximity of the tumor to vital structures.

NEUROFIBROMA

Clinical Presentation

Neurofibromas can occur as an isolated lesion, as part of the syndrome of neurofibromatosis (von Recklinghausen's disease), or—rarely—as multiple neurofibromas not associated with a syndrome. Mucosal neuromas can occur in association with medullary thyroid carcinoma and pheochromocytoma (multiple endocrine neoplasia [MEN] 2B).

Solitary neurofibromas occur equally in both sexes and most commonly in the 20-to-30-year age group. They can be located anywhere in the head and neck region and are seen most commonly in the skin and subcutaneous tissues. Occasionally they can be found in the upper aerodigestive tract. Malignant transformation in isolated neurofibromas is rare.

Neurofibromatosis, or von Recklinghausen's disease, is transmitted by autosomal dominant inheritance with variable but high penetrance. It can also occur through spontaneous mutation; positive family histories are found in only one half of patients.[27]

Neurofibromatosis is classified as type I or type II; the following discussion applies primarily to type I. A plexiform neurofibroma, which involves a major nerve trunk with the characteristic fusiform multilobular enlargement, is virtually pathognomonic of neurofibromatosis. The diagnosis of neurofibromatosis (type I) is made by the presence of two or more of the following:[5]

1. Six café au lait spots (light brown macules) greater than 5 mm in diameter

2. Two or more neurofibromas or one plexiform neurofibroma
3. Axillary or inguinal freckling
4. Optic gliomas
5. Two or more Lisch nodules (optic harmartomas)
6. Distinctive osseous lesions (sphenoid dysplasia or thinning of long bone cortex)
7. First-degree relative with neurofibromatosis (type I)

Two thirds of patients manifest symptoms of neurofibromatosis by the age of 1 year, and onset after age 25 is rare.[5,27] The genetic abnormality resulting in neurofibromatosis has been localized to chromosome 17.[36] A second form of neurofibromatosis (type II) is associated with multiple cranial nerve neurofibromas. Sarcomatous changes have been reported in 10% of plexiform neurofibromas and 6% to 16% of all patients with neurofibromatosis.[27,37]

Symptoms and Signs

Neurofibromas, whether solitary or in neurofibromatosis, present as slow-growing painless masses that are otherwise asymptomatic.

Radiology

Although schwannomas and neurofibromas differ histologically, their radiographic appearance on CT and MRI is similar; the reader is referred to the radiology section on schwannomas.

Treatment

Neurofibromas are intimately associated with the axons of the nerve, often requiring nerve sacrifice, in contrast to schwannomas, which may be dissected off the nerve.[15] Complete surgical excision is the standard treatment of solitary neurofibromas. In neurofibromatosis, surgical treatment is indicated for lesions that are large, painful, rapidly growing, or suspected of being malignant.[5] These lesions are not encapsulated but are infiltrative, making complete excision a challenge.

Prognosis

Neurofibromatosis presents a challenge to the clinician. The majority of cases are benign. When sarcomatous changes occur, however, a 5-year survival rate of 20% has been reported.[5]

Carotid Body Tumors

Clinical Presentation

The carotid body is the second most common site for paragangliomas of the head and neck (Fig. 13–22). Approximately equal numbers of females

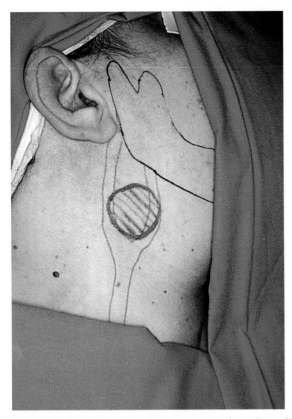

FIGURE 13-22 Carotid body tumor seen in the right neck.

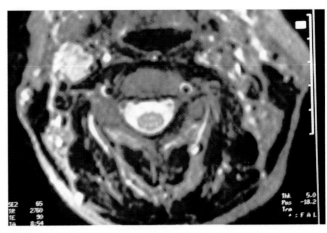

FIGURE 13-23 Axial MRI (T2W) of the left carotid body tumor. The tumor is seen to splay the carotid bifurcation.

and males develop carotid body tumors, and the mean age of patients is 42 years.[38]

Carotid body tumors can arise in a familial autosomal dominant form or sporadically. In one series, approximately one half of patients demonstrated a familial pattern.[38] Approximately 10% of all patients with paragangliomas of the head and neck have a family history of paragangliomas.[39] In patients with a familial pattern, other family members should be screened with MRI. Multiple paragangliomas are seen in over 80% of patients with the familial form and 31% to 43% of patients with the sporadic form.[38,39] The most common second site for patients with multiple paragangliomas is a contralateral carotid body tumor.

Symptoms and Signs

Patients with carotid body tumors present with a slow-growing painless neck mass. Larger tumors can cause symptoms related to compression of the upper aerodigestive tract. On physical examination, a pulsatile mass is seen at the level of the carotid bifurcation, which has decreased vertical mobility. On auscultation, a bruit is commonly appreciated. Fewer than one in five patients present with cranial nerve deficits.[38] The most common cranial nerves involved are the hypoglossal and vagus nerves.[39] It is rare for these tumors to produce catecholamines and uncom-

mon (10% to 15%) for the tumors to spread to regional lymph nodes or to distant sites.[39–41]

Radiology

On MRI, carotid body tumors can be seen splaying the carotid bifurcation. They are isointense or slightly hyperintense to muscle on T1W images and hyperintense to muscle on T2W images (Fig. 13–23).[42] Signal voids from the vascularity of these tumors give them a characteristic "salt and pepper" appearance on MRI.[42] They enhance with intravenous contrast. MRI and MR angiography can usually confirm the diagnosis; invasive angiography is rarely required but it is necessary when preoperative embolization is planned (Fig. 13–24).[42] Studies of contralateral cerebral blood flow and the conse-

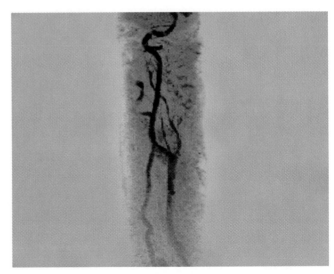

FIGURE 13-24 MR angiography of the left carotid body tumor. Again, the carotid vessels are splayed apart at the carotid bifurcation.

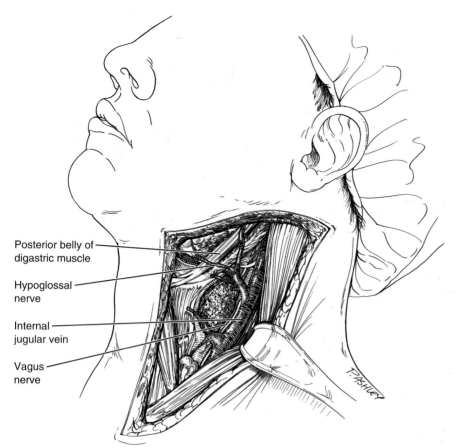

Posterior belly of
digastric muscle

Hypoglossal
nerve

Internal
jugular vein

Vagus
nerve

FIGURE 13–25   A schematic diagram of the operative exposure of a carotid body tumor.

quence of carotid sacrifice should be considered for patients with recurrent or massive tumors.

Treatment

Surgical excision is the primary treatment of carotid body tumors (Figs. 13–25 through 13–27). In cases of bilateral tumors, the contralateral side can be treated with external beam radiation therapy or observation. When bilateral carotid body tumors are resected, patients can experience baroreceptor failure manifested postoperatively by wide variations in blood pressure and heart rate. The hyperintense and tachycardiac episodes seen with bilateral barorecep-

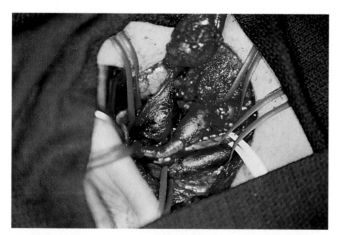

FIGURE 13–26   Operative photo of dissection of the carotid body tumor. The carotid artery is isolated in red vessel loops, the internal jugular vein in blue vessel loops, and the vagus nerve in the white vessel loop. The tumor has been meticulously dissected off the bifurcation with liberal use of bipolar cautery.

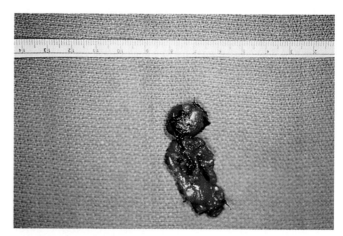

FIGURE 13–27   Surgical specimen of the carotid body tumor. Note that hyperplastic level II lymph nodes have been removed to facilitate tumor removal and remain attached to the specimen.

tor failure may be controlled with the alpha-2 adrenergic agonist chonidine.[38] Patients with significant medical co-morbidities may choose external beam radiation therapy or observation.

Surgical Anatomy

Carotid body tumors are approached through a horizontal cervical incision in a natural skin crease at the level of the carotid bifurcation. Subplatysmal flaps are elevated to give wide exposure of the operative field. Care should be taken to preserve the great auricular nerve when possible. The anterior border of the SCM is skeletonized. Hyperplastic lymph nodes are commonly seen at levels II to III and are removed to allow an unhindered view of the carotid body tumor. The landmarks at this level—the spinal accessory nerve, posterior belly of the digastric muscle, hypoglossal nerve, and internal jugular vein (IJV)—are identifed and preserved. Inferiorly, below the tumor, the carotid sheath is identified and opened; the common carotid artery, IJV, and vagus nerve are isolated. At this point, the tumor is meticulously dissected off the carotid artery with liberal use of bipolar cautery to minimize blood loss and maximize visualization. Usually, this dissection is done in a subadventitial plane, but occasionally it can be done without violating the adventitia. Dissection proceeds superiorly until the tumor is freed from the carotid bifurcation. The ascending pharyngeal artery often can be seen supplying the tumor from the medial surface of the carotid bifurcation and must be controlled. The sympathetic chain and superior laryngeal nerve can often be seen deep to the tumor and should be preserved. Throughout the dissection, care is taken to preserve critical neurovascular structures. Rarely does tumor removal require carotid resection or sacrifice of cranial nerves. When large or adherent tumors require resection of the carotid artery wall, reconstruction is performed with a vein or synthetic patch graft or interposition graft.

Prognosis

Carotid body tumors rarely recur after surgical excision. Permanent nerve injuries occur in 17% to 57% of patients.[39,43] These tumors rarely metastasize, and disease-related mortality is low. In a series of seven carotid body tumors treated with radiation therapy (4000 to 4850 cGy) with 5- to 8.5-year follow-up, two had complete regression, two had partial regression, two remained stable, and one progressed, resulting in a disease-related mortality at 5 years.[4]

Controversies

Preoperative embolization of carotid body tumors remains controversial. Some authors advise against preoperative embolization, citing the difficulty of embolizing the multitude of vascular connections, the high risk of intracranial embolization and the inflammatory response resulting from embolization that obliterates normal planes and makes subsequent dissection difficult.[27] Others, however, have used preoperative embolization to minimize blood loss in larger tumors.[38,39] The authors of this chapter have not performed preoperative embolization of carotid body tumors.

The role of radiation therapy or observation in the treatment of carotid body tumors remains controversial. At this time, the standard treatment of most carotid body tumors remains surgical. The role of radiation therapy or observation for patients with significant co-morbidities, elderly patients, or those with advanced or recurrent tumors continues to evolve.

Glomus Vagale

Clinical Presentation

Approximately 3% to 5% of all paragangliomas originate from the vagus nerve (Fig. 13–28).[27,44] The female:male ratio is approximately 2.7:1, and the mean age of patients is 48 years.[44]

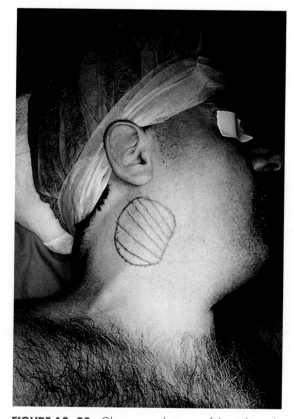

FIGURE 13-28 Glomus vagale tumor of the right neck.

Glomus vagale tumors can arise in a familial autosomal dominant form or sporadically. In one series, approximately one half of patients demonstrated a familial pattern.[44] Approximately 10% of all patients with paragangliomas of the head and neck have a family history of paragangliomas.[27,39] Other family members of these patients should be screened with MRI. Multiple paragangliomas are seen in approximately 35% to 89% of patients with the familial form and 10% of patients with the sporadic form.[44,45] The most common second site in patients with multiple paragangliomas is a carotid body tumor.

Symptoms and Signs

Patients with glomus vagale tumors present with a slow-growing painless neck mass. Hoarseness and aspiration of liquids can result from vagal nerve paralysis, seen in 47% of patients.[44] On physical examination, a mass is seen behind the angle of the mandible. If there is large and significant parapharyngeal space involvement, a mass can be seen in the oropharynx, displacing the tonsil medially. Nearly one half of patients present with vocal cord paralysis.[44] Other cranial nerve deficits can occur, such as glossopharyngeal nerve paralysis, jugular foramen syndrome, and Horner's syndrome. Although only four cases of metabolically active tumors secreting catecholamines have been reported, 24-hour urine metanephrine and vanillylmandelic acid tests should be done in patients with symptoms of increased sympathetic activity.[44] Spread to regional lymph nodes or distant spread is uncommon (10%).[41]

Radiology

On MRI, glomus vagale tumors can be at or above the carotid bifurcation (Fig. 13–29). The mass dis-

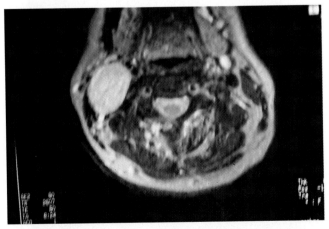

FIGURE 13–29 Axial MRI (T2W) of the left glomus vagale tumor. The tumor is seen to displace the carotid system anteriorly and medially.

places the carotid vessels anteriorly and medially without widening the carotid bifurcation, in contrast to the carotid body tumor, which splays and displaces the carotid vessels posteriorly. They are isointense or slightly hyperintense to muscle on T1W images, and hyperintense to muscle on T2W images. Signal voids from the vascularity of these tumors give them a characteristic "salt and pepper" appearance on MRI. They enhance with intravenous contrast.

Treatment

Surgical excision is the primary treatment of glomus vagale tumors. In cases of bilateral tumors, the contralateral or nonparalyzed side can be treated with external beam radiation therapy or observation to avoid the consequences of bilateral vocal cord paralysis. Patients with significant medical co-morbidities may decide upon external beam radiation therapy or observation.

Surgical Anatomy

Glomus vagale tumors are accessed by a lateral cervical approach (Figs. 13–30 through 13–32). On rare occasion, a mandibulotomy is required for exposure of the superior parapharyngeal space. When intracranial extension occurs, a posterior fossa craniotomy allows removal of the intracranial component. In the cervical approach, a transverse incision is made and subplatysmal flaps are elevated, giving wide exposure of the operative field. Care is taken to preserve the great auricular nerve when possible. The anterior border of the SCM is skeletonized to the carotid sheath, which is opened below the tumor. This exposes the common carotid artery, IJV, and carotid artery from inferiorly to superiorly, until the tumor is freed from the carotid and IJV at the skull base. Again, if the tumor has extended intracranially, a posterior fossa craniotomy allows complete tumor removal. The sympathetic chain can often be seen deep to the tumor and should be preserved. Throughout the dissection, care is taken to preserve critical neurovascular structures. The vagus nerve must be sacrificed in order to remove an en bloc tumor, and vocal cord medialization techniques should be used for voice rehabilitation and to prevent aspiration.

Prognosis

Glomus vagale tumors rarely recur after surgical excision. Vagal paralysis is an accepted result of surgery, and permanent injuries to the ninth and twelfth cranial nerves occur in 31% of patients.[44] These tumors rarely metastasize, and disease-related mortality is low. In a series of 32 glomus jugulare

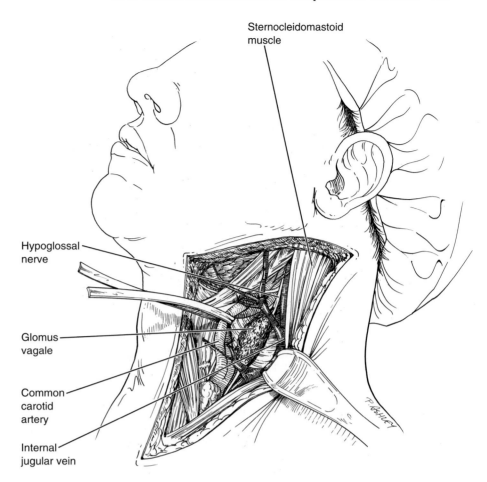

Sternocleidomastoid
muscle

Hypoglossal
nerve

Glomus
vagale

Common
carotid
artery

Internal
jugular vein

FIGURE 13–30 A schematic diagram of the operative exposure of a glomus vagale tumor.

and vagale tumors treated with megavoltage radiation therapy with 5- to 27-year follow-up, only one had disease progression, while the remainder had stabilization or regression.[46] It should be noted, however, that the vast majority of tumors in this series were glomus jugulares.

Controversies

The role of radiation therapy in the treatment of glomus vagale tumors remains controversial. At this time, the standard treatment of glomus vagale tumors is surgical. Radiation therapy remains an op-

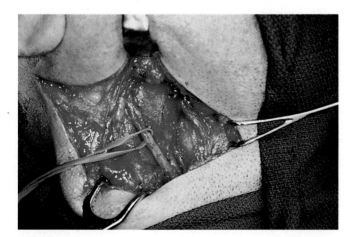

FIGURE 13–31 Operative photo of surgical resection of the glomus vagale tumor.

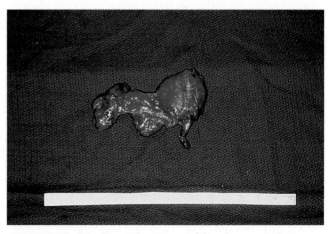

FIGURE 13–32 Surgical specimen of the glomus vagale tumor.

tion, however, in the elderly, medically unstable, or patients with bilateral tumors in whom bilateral vagus sacrifice would cause significant sequelae.

MALIGNANT NEOPLASMS

Soft-tissue sarcomas of the head and neck are a rare group of heterogeneous tumors. Their clinical behavior varies considerably from locally aggressive lesions to locally destructive neoplasms with a potential for regional and distant metastasis. Sarcomas of the head and neck account for less than 1% of all neoplasms of the head and neck; in a prospective database of patients admitted to Memorial Sloan-Kettering Cancer Center, only 60 of 1400 (4.3%) had lesions arising in the head and neck region.[47] Unlike squamous cell carcinomas, which arise from the mucosal lining of the upper aerodigestive tract, sarcomas can arise from soft tissues located anywhere in the head and neck region. The plethora of histologies, clinical behaviors, and primary locations in these uncommon tumors makes it difficult to determine the optimal treatment.

Despite the diversity of histologies, the grade of a sarcoma determines its behavior more often than its histologic tissue type. In this section, rather than considering each tumor separately, sarcomas will be considered as a whole. This allows the most meaningful interpretation of the limited data available for these rare tumors. Unique characteristics of clinical presentation, behavior, and treatment results for each histologic type of sarcoma are then presented.

Clinical Presentation

The clinical presentation and distribution of sarcomas is strongly dependent upon the histologic type; these will be addressed in each subheading. One issue related to all sarcomas is the small but well-defined propensity of radiation-induced sarcomas. Post-irradiation sarcoma has been defined as microscopic or radiographic evidence of nonmalignant tissue prior to irradiation, tumor occurring in the radiation portal, a minimum latent period of 3 years, and histologically proven sarcoma.[48] Radiation for other cancers, such as mantle radiation for lymphoma, is associated with the development of sarcoma. In one series, 9 of 164 patients (5.5%) with head and neck sarcomas had previous irradiation with a latent period ranging from 4 to 18 years.[49]

Symptoms and Signs

In the neck, a sarcoma usually presents as a painless, rapidly enlarging subcutaneous mass.[50] In one series, approximately 80% of sarcomas presented as a painless lesion.[47] Pain may be present in 25% of patients.[51] Besides the appearance of a mass and oc-

casional pain, the other symptoms caused by a sarcoma are usually determined by the location of the tumor and the adjacent structures that may be compressed or invaded. As sarcomas grow, they may compress or invade cervical sensory roots, resulting in pain, paresthesia, or a pressure sensation. Invasion of cranial nerves is responsible for paresis or paralysis of the vagus, spinal accessory, hypoglossal, or sympathetic chain (Horner's syndrome). Impingement on the central visceral structures can create dysphagia, stridor, dyspnea, and airway obstruction. Neurosarcomas arising from the brachial plexus can present with weakness in the corresponding motor innervation of the upper extremity. Phrenic paralysis is extremely rare, usually being asymptomatic, but may be incidentally noted on a preoperative chest x-ray.

Radiology

Radiographic imaging of suspected sarcomas should be obtained prior to biopsy or surgical manipulation. MRI offers excellent soft-tissue definition, while CT gives better bone imaging. The characteristic radiographic appearance of each type of sarcoma is presented in each subheading.

Treatment

Representative tissue for histologic diagnosis should be obtained in a site-specific manner that does not impair subsequent treatment. Tumors in the neck are most commonly approached by the technique of fine-needle aspiration biopsy. For sarcomas, however, a tissue core technique may be used if the mass is not in proximity to major neurovascular structures. Caution in interpretation of these results should be used; both fine-needle aspiration biopsy and core biopsy techniques for extremity and trunk soft-tissue sarcomas are considered unreliable by some authors.[52,53] Care must be taken in evaluating these patients to exclude the more common entities of metastatic squamous cell carcinoma from an upper aerodigestive tract primary metastatic thyroid carcinoma and other, less common, entities. In lesions raising suspicion for soft-tissue sarcoma of the neck, the optimal approach is preoperative counseling with the patient that allows for diagnostic biopsy and definitive resection through a single incision and under a single anesthetic. This requires the pathologist to identify a sarcoma, independent of grade, on frozen section analysis without the aid of immunohistochemical staining. When the biopsy is performed as an isolated procedure, every attempt should be made to design incisions in the same location and axis as would be employed for definitive resection. Dissection should be limited in order to prevent local dissemination of tumor during biopsy. Suspected lesions arising in the skin should be biopsied by incisional biopsy, as excisional biopsy obscures the margins and may result in a larger definitive resection due to the indeterminate nature of the extent of the lesion. Vascular lesions, such as angiosarcomas, may be quite vascular and present difficulties in obtaining hemostasis at time of biopsy.

Pretreatment assessment should consist of a directed metastatic work-up including chest x-ray, screening blood tests including liver function tests, bone profile, and hematologic evaluation. Any abnormality in these studies may prompt further laboratory and radiographic evaluation.

Multimodality therapy is the cornerstone of therapy for most soft-tissue sarcomas of the head and neck. Obtaining wide negative surgical margins in the head and neck is more difficult than in the extremities and trunk. The adjacent major neurovascular structures in the head and neck, and the functional and cosmetic morbidity related to their sacrifice, limits the application of a wide resection in many cases. Radiation is employed in a large percentage of high-risk patients, particularly in those with high-grade or large lesions. Chemotherapy, as will be discussed, remains under investigation for reducing the risk of distant metastasis.

As sarcomas enlarge, a pseudocapsule is formed by the compression of adjacent tissue. This pseudocapsule contains neoplastic cells. Adjacent to the pseudocapsule is a reactive tissue component of inflammatory and malignant cells. Tumor subsequently extends along the adjacent fascial planes and muscle fibers. It is this mechanism of tumor extension that necessitates the wide en bloc resection technique required in sarcomas that include normal tissue well beyond identifiable margins of the tumor.[50] It cannot be overemphasized that this capsule is not an accurate indicator of the margin of the lesion.

Surgery followed by postoperative radiation therapy is the mainstay of treatment of sarcomas. Most sarcomas have a low risk of regional lymph node metastasis; therefore, a comprehensive neck dissection is rarely required. Resections should be performed to achieve an en bloc resection of the tumor. This may entail nothing more than a wide local excision for a level I or level V mass. Cases of larger or more aggressive lesions invading adjacent structures may require extended procedures encompassing structures not ordinarily included in a comprehensive neck dissection. No attempt should be made to preserve structures that are circumferentially involved with the tumor or invaded by the capsule of the tumor. Resection of cranial nerves can be performed with limited but acceptable morbidity and, in some instances, rehabilitative strategies (e.g., vocal cord medialization after vagal sacrifice) can be employed.[54]

The decision to resect lesions involving vital structures such as the carotid artery, brachial plexus, central visceral structures, and mediastinum is more difficult. Occasionally, low-grade sarcomas may involve these vital structures and can be resected with a reasonable outlook for long-term survival and acceptable morbidity. More commonly, however, high-grade lesions require extensive resections with significant morbidity. In the face of the poor prognosis of these extensive lesions, each decision to resect must be considered individually. When central visceral structures are involved, they often can be reconstructed with a jejunal free tissue transfer or gastric pull-up. The morbidity from these procedures must be weighed against the patient's long-term prognosis. Resection of the carotid artery should be performed only under special circumstances—lesions involving the carotid artery commonly require resection of cranial nerves and paravertebral musculature, resulting in significant functional impairment and the risk of a major cerebrovascular event or death.[55] The patency of the circle of Willis should be assessed preoperatively by angiography in these patients. Temporary carotid occlusion with intra-arterial balloons and xenon cerebral imaging detect with reasonable reliability those patients who can tolerate carotid sacrifice and those who will require reconstruction.[56] Major involvement of the cervical vertebral body or intraspinal extension with extradural or intradural invasion are general contraindications to resection.[55] The ability to widely resect the prevertebral muscles, whether in the anterior neck or posterior neck, is limited, making radiation a requirement. Tumors that involve both the supraclavicular region and the superior mediastinum often require the assistance of a thoracic surgeon. Low-grade lesions such as desmoid tumors can be resected with a hemi–clam shell thoracotomy with excellent exposure and preservation of uninvolved structures.[2]

As mentioned previously, multimodality therapy including surgery and postoperative radiation therapy is the mainstay of treatment for resectable lesions. The majority of the data supporting postoperative radiation therapy is extrapolated from the treatment of patients with sarcomas of the extremities. Significantly improved local control has been demonstrated with adjuvant radiation therapy for sarcomas greater than 5 cm. In a prospective, randomized trial for high-grade sarcomas of the extremities and superficial trunk, brachytherapy was shown to improve local control (90% versus 60%) but did not improve rates of distant metastasis and survival.[57] Current strategy is to use adjuvant external beam radiation therapy in all but the smallest lesions that have been resected with negative margins. When external beam is used, the dose is usually 60 to 65 Gy for low-grade lesions and 65 to 70 Gy for high-grade lesions.[57] Treatment plans for the neck usually deliver postoperative radiation therapy to the involved neck. This can sometimes be done with opposed AP/PA portals, but often requires a CT-based treatment plan. The technical problems relate to the need to deliver 60 to 70 Gy to the bed without exceeding spinal cord tolerance, and to minimize the dose to the contralateral neck to decrease acute toxicity (mucositis) and late effects (xerostomia). If the low neck is involved, concerns about the brachial plexus must also be addressed. In this situation, we often advocate an interstitial implant at the time of surgery, followed by limited external beam radiation (45 Gy) in an effort to maximize tumor dose and minimize neurologic toxicity.

To date, there is limited experience with chemotherapy for soft-tissue sarcomas of the head and neck. Although some studies have shown a trend toward improved survival, none has shown a statistically significant improvement in outcome.[58-62] The use of chemotherapy in the treatment of sarcomas, therefore, should continue to be studied in the setting of a randomized, controlled trial.

In the management of local-regional recurrence, initial efforts should be directed toward detection of distant disease, most commonly found in the lungs, bones, central nervous system, or liver. If the metastatic work-up is negative, patient factors must then be considered. Patients with massive recurrence, extensive high-grade lesions, or poor functional status are poor candidates for definitive surgical salvage and are best served by palliative care. In the majority of instances, surgery plays a central role in local and/or regional recurrence. The ability to resect locally recurrent disease is determined by clinical assessment and radiographic imaging. In patients who have undergone surgery only as the initial management, postoperative radiation therapy should be employed. In some instances, radiation alone may serve as definitive treatment for local recurrence. In patients previously irradiated, an interstitial implant may remain an option to boost the tumor bed after re-resection, to minimize local complications occuring with external beam radiation therapy.[63] For the rare patient with local disease but isolated regional lymph node metastasis, therapeutic lymphadenectomy (neck dissection and/or parotidectomy) with postoperative radiation therapy, depending upon prior radiation therapy portals, offers good potential for regional control, although virtually all patients develop systemic disease.[49]

The ability to salvage isolated systemic metastasis is limited. The optimal setting for resection of a metastasis is an isolated pulmonary nodule. In patients with extremity sarcomas presenting with distant disease, approximately 19% have isolate pulmonary metastasis.[64] Survival was statistically improved with complete resection with a 3-year survival of 23% for patients undergoing complete resection.[64] The role of chemotherapy in this cohort also remains undetermined.

Prognosis

Tumor grade has a significant impact on the natural history of sarcomas. Low-grade well-differentiated sarcomas (i.e., low-grade fibrosarcoma, dermatofibrosarcoma protuberans) are less locally invasive due to pushing margins rather than destructive permeation. These lesions are more indolent and have a low metastatic potential. Conversely, high-grade poorly differentiated sarcomas (i.e., malignant fibrous histiocytoma, angiosarcoma) are locally invasive, tracking along major nerves, bones, and blood vessels. Consistent with their highly aggressive local behavior is the increased risk of developing distant metastasis. It is important to note, however, that low-grade lesions still require aggressive local treatment as their propensity for local recurrence is significant.

Tumor size as a predictor of outcome of head and neck sarcomas is somewhat controversial. In several studies, size was a predictor of survival but was not evaluated with respect to local control.[49-51] In another series, size was not identified as a predictor of either local recurrence or survival.[47] The patient who is referred after unplanned surgical excision exemplifies another factor that is important in the local control of a sarcoma. In one study, nearly one half of patients with an unplanned total surgical resection of an extremity sarcoma had residual tumor on wide re-excision.[65]

Regional lymph node mestastases are rare and occur almost exclusively in high-grade sarcomas. Reported incidence of lymph node metastasis ranged from 3% to 36%, although the higher rate occurred in a series including rhabdomyosarcomas.[66-71] Other series have reported a 3% to 9% incidence of nodal metastasis at presentation.[47,49] The most common pathology to develop nodal metastasis (excluding rhabdomyosarcomas and angiosarcomas) includes epithelioid sarcoma, myogenic sarcoma, malignant fibrous histiocytomas (MFH), and synovial cell sarcoma.[71]

The development of distant metastasis appears to be primarily a function of tumor grade. In one series, distant metastasis occurred in 6% of patients with low-grade lesions and 44% of patients with high-grade lesions.[49] Another study identified direct local tumor extension to vital structures, placing patients at increased risk for distant metastasis.[72] The most common site of distant metastasis is the lungs, followed by bone, central nervous system, and liver.[50] Size does not appear to be a major risk factor for the development of distant metastasis, with a reported rate of 33% in lesions less than 5 cm and 45% in those greater than 5 cm.[50]

Interpretation of outcomes for sarcoma of the head and neck must be cautious because of the inherent heterogeneity regarding pathologic subtypes, location, grade, treatment plans, and method of reporting results. Despite these shortcomings, meaningful information may still be acquired by comparing large reports from tertiary referral centers.[47,49-51,71-73] With the exception of Willers' series, patients were treated with surgical resection; of those, a large percentage received postoperative radiation therapy. Due to the low incidence of lymph node metastasis, survival is defined primarily by lo-

TABLE 13 – 4	LOCAL CONTROL AND SURVIVAL IN PATIENTS WITH HEAD AND NECK SARCOMAS			
	NUMBER	5-YEAR LOCAL CONTROL	5-YEAR CAUSE-SPECIFIC SURVIVAL	5-YEAR OVERALL SURVIVAL
LeVay	52	59%	62%	—
Kraus	60	70%	—	71%
Willers	57	60%	—	66%
Greager	53	81%	54%	—
Weber	188	77%	—	—
Tran	164	41%	—	57%
Farhood	176	—	—	55%

From Kraus DH, Harrison LB. Soft tissue sarcomas of the head and neck. In: Harrison LB, Sessions RS, Hong KW, eds. *Head and Neck Cancer—A Multidisciplinary Approach.* Philadelphia: Lippincott; 1996:884, with permission.

cal and distant disease. Table 13–4 summarizes the reported 5-year local control rates and survival rates for the preceding studies.[55] The 5-year local control rate ranges from 41% to 81%. Table 13–5 shows the factors affecting local control.[55] Although grade, size, and extent of tumor have all been reported to affect local control, status of the margins is the factor most consistently seen to predict local recurrence (see Table 13–5).[47,49–51,71–73] It should be noted that grade was a prognostic factor for local recurrence in one of the three studies examining this issue.[47,72,73] In the other two studies, however, a trend was noted toward increased local recurrence with high-grade lesions; it might have reached statistical significance with a larger sample size.[72,73] Reported survival rates (disease-specific or overall) range from 54% to 71% at 5 years. Primary tumor grade, size, and margins were the most significant and most commonly studied factors predicting survival.[47,49–51,71–73] Two studies examined the effect of direct extension on sur-

vival, but only one found a statistically significant effect.[72,73] Many of these prognostic factors are probably related, but the limited sample sizes preclude meaningful multivariate analysis. With low-grade trunk and extremity lesions, multimodality therapy has improved local control rates.[57] This increase in local control, however, has not translated into an increase in survival. Similar patterns can be extrapolated to head and neck sarcomas, although this has not been established in the form of a prospective, randomized trial.

Malignant Teratoma

Clinical Presentation

While benign teratomas are relatively common, malignant teratomas are rare tumors. Of adult teratomas, reported rates of malignancy exceed 90%.[74]

TABLE 13 – 5	IMPACT OF GRADE, MARGIN STATUS, SIZE, AND DIRECT EXTENSION ON LOCAL RECURRENCE AND SURVIVAL							
		LOCAL RECURRENCE PROGNOSTIC FACTORS				SURVIVAL			
	Number	Grade	Margin	Size	Extent	Grade	Margin	Size	Extent
LeVay	52	–	+	–	+	+	–	+	+
Kraus	60	+	+	–	NS	+	+	–	NS
Willers	57	–	NS	+	–	+	NS	–	–
Greager	53	NS	NS	NS	NS	+	NS	+	NS
Weber	188	NS	NS	NS	NS	+	+	+	NS
Tran	164	NS	+	NS	NS	+	+	+	NS
Farhood	176	NS	NS	NS	NS	+	+	+	NS

NS, not stated; +, statistically significant; –, not statistically significant.
From Kraus DH, Harrison LB. Soft tissue sarcomas of the head and neck. In: Harrison LB, Sessions RS, Hong KW, eds. *Head and Neck Cancer—A Multidisciplinary Approach.* Philadelphia: Lippincott; 1996:884, with permission.

They occur more commonly in females.[75] Malignant teratomas rarely occur in the neonatal or infantile form, and the clinical significance of lymph node metastasis is unclear.[75]

Symptoms and Signs

Malignant teratomas usually present as a rapidly growing neck mass in an adult. Other symptoms may be related to nearby structures that they invade or compress.

Radiology

CT scans of malignant teratomas often show a low-attenuation locally destructive process that can cause bone erosion. When imaged with the contrast, malignant teratomas can appear as a nonenhancing necrotic process with a zone of peripheral enhancement.[76] If a dynamic CT is performed, it may reveal a vascular outer rim due to the vascularity of the capsule of this lesion.[76]

Treatment

With less than 20 cases of malignant teratomas reported in the literature, it is difficult to determine the optimal treatment of this rare neoplasm.[74] From these reports, however, it is apparent that malignant teratomas carry a dismal prognosis and that combined surgery and radiation therapy should be considered.

Prognosis

Despite multimodality therapy (surgery, radiation therapy, and chemotherapy), survival in patients with malignant teratomas remains anecdotal. Local-regional recurrence and pulmonary metastasis are common. Pulmonary metastases have been reported to occur via local invasion of the mediastinum and neck veins.[74]

Angiosarcoma

Clinical Presentation

Angiosarcomas account for 2% to 3% of soft-tissue sarcomas.[15] Approximately one half of all angiosarcomas occur in the head and neck, but they account for less than 0.1% of malignancies in that area.[77] Most common sites within the head and neck are the scalp and soft tissues of the neck.[78] Several factors that have been associated with angiosarcoma include prior irradiation, chronic lymphedema, thoridium dioxide, vinyl chloride, insecticides, anabolic steroids, and synthetic estrogens.[78]

Symptoms and Signs

The angiosarcomas in the head and neck region commonly present as a vascular, purple, macular scalp or neck lesion with poorly defined margins.[78] The margins often extend laterally throughout the dermis beyond where they are clinically apparent, making wide excision with negative margins difficult.[79] They are often mistaken for a bruise or hemangioma, resulting in a delay in diagnosis and treatment. Often the lesion is ulcerated, and the patient reports a history of bleeding.[72] Angiosarcomas are also often multifocal.[79] Relative to other sarcomas, angiosarcomas display a high incidence (10% to 15%) of regional lymph node metastasis.[78,80] Although this rate is relatively high, most authors agree that elective treatment of the neck is not warranted.

Radiology

On CT and MRI, the vascularity of angiosarcomas results in significant enhancement with intravenous contrast.[15] Their radiographic appearance reflects their aggressive clinical behavior and bone destruction is often shown.

Treatment and Prognosis

Angiosarcomas require multimodality treatment with wide excision followed by postoperative radiation treatment. They have a poor prognosis, with 5-year survival ranging from 12% to 33%, with a propensity for local recurrence and distant dissemination.[78–80] (See also Treatment and Prognosis, Malignant Neoplasms, pages 788–791).

Liposarcoma

Clinical Presentation

Liposarcomas of the head and neck are relatively rare, with only 76 cases reported in the world literature over the last 80 years.[81] Liposarcomas represent 1% of all head and neck sarcomas.[82] They occur more commonly in males (65%) and in the fifth to seventh decades of life.[81] The neck is the most common site (38% of occurrences) in the head and neck region.[82]

Symptoms and Signs

As with other sarcomas, liposarcomas most commonly present as a painless, rapidly enlarging subcutaneous or submucosal mass.

Radiology

While lipomas are significantly more common than liposarcomas, several radiographic features may allow the head and neck surgeon to predict when a malignant lesion may be encountered. When a fatty mass demonstrates a nonhomogeneous dense matrix or soft-tissue densities within the lesion, the possibility of a liposarcoma must be entertained.[83] On T1W MRIs, a lesion with high signal intensity and ill-defined margins invading surrounding tissue is seen.[15]

Treatment and Prognosis

As with other sarcomas, the mainstay of treatment is surgery and postoperative radiation. Aside from the other factors predicting survival in sarcomas the histologic type is a determinant of survival in patients with liposarcomas.[5] Patients with the well-differentiated and myxoid types have 5-year survival rates of 71% to 100%, while patients with the round cell and pleomorphic varieties have 5-year survival rates ranging from 0% to 55%.[5] (See also Treatment and Prognosis, Malignant Neoplasms, pages 788–791.)

Fibrosarcoma

Clinical Presentation

Fibrosarcomas account for 12% to 19% of all soft-tissue sarcomas. Fifteen percent of fibrosarcomas occur in the head and neck region.[15] Fibrosarcomas show a male predilection and occur most commonly in the fourth to sixth decades of life.[7] Within the head and neck region, they occur most commonly in the neck. Fibrosarcomas can occur in the pediatric age group, and are associated with a better prognosis.

Symptoms and Signs

As with other sarcomas, fibrosarcomas most commonly present as a painless, rapidly enlarging subcutaneous or submucosal mass.

Radiology

On CT, fibrosarcomas are homogeneous and non-enhancing.[15] They tend to remodel bone. On MRI they have a low to intermediate sequence on T1W and T2W images.

Treatment and Prognosis

As with other sarcomas, the mainstay of treatment is surgery and postoperative radiation. Compared to other sarcomas, fibrosarcomas are associated with a favorable prognosis. (See also Treatment and Prognosis, Malignant Neoplasms, pages 788–791.)

Malignant Fibrous Histiocytoma

Clinical Presentation

Malignant fibrous histiocytomas (MFH) are relatively rare in the head and neck region, accounting for less than 5% of all cases of MFH.[84,85] They occur most commonly between the ages of 50 and 70 years and have a slight male predominance.[84] Within the head and neck they occur most commonly in the sononasal tract (30%), with the neck accounting for 10% to 15% of cases.[85]

Symptoms and Signs

As with other sarcomas, MFH most commonly present as a painless, rapidly enlarging, subcutaneous mass. (See also Symptoms and Signs, Malignant Neoplasms, page 788.) Relative to other sarcomas, high-grade MFH displays one of the higher incidences of regional lymph node metastases.

Radiology

These lesions have a nonspecific appearance, with low to moderate enhancement on CT and intermediate signal on T1W and T2W MRIs.[15] Both bone destruction and remodeling can be seen in these lesions, making the radiographic differentiation difficult.

Treatment and Prognosis

The mainstay of treatment is surgery and postoperative radiation. (See also Treatment and Prognosis, Malignant Neoplasms, page 788.)

Malignant Peripheral Nerve Sheath Tumors

Clinical Presentation

Malignant peripheral nerve sheath tumors (MPNST) are also called neurofibrosarcomas, malignant schwannomas, neurogenic sarcomas, and malignant neurilemmomas. They can occur sporadically or be associated with neurofibromatosis or von Recklinghausen's disease. Approximately one quarter to one half of cases occur in patients with neurofibromatosis.[15,86] Of all cases of MPNST, 9% to 14% arise in the head and neck, and the most common site in this region (44% of cases) is the neck.[86] A male:female ratio of 3.5:1 has been reported. These tumors occur most commonly between the third and sixth decades.[86] Cranial nerves (except for optic and olfactory), large cervical nerves, the sympathetic chain, inferior alveolar, and brachial plexus are the nerves most commonly involved.[15,86]

Symptoms and Signs

As with other sarcomas, MPNSTs most commonly present as a painless, rapidly enlarging subcutaneous or submucosal mass. (See Symptoms and Signs, Malignant Neoplasms, page 788.) Pain and paresthesia or dysfunction of the involved nerve have been noted to occur in over one third of cases.[86]

Radiology

MPNSTs have been reported to have a low T1W signal and intermediate T2W weighted signal on MRI.[15] They can show bony erosion on CT scan, which has been reported in 30% of cases.[86]

Treatment and Prognosis

As with other sarcomas, the mainstay of treatment is surgery and postoperative radiation. Reported 5-year survival rates are higher for the sporadic type (50%) compared to 15% to 30% for the tumors associated with neurofibromatosis. (See also Treatment and Prognosis, Malignant Neoplasms, page 788.)

Synovial Sarcoma

Clinical Presentation

Synovial sarcomas are rare tumors of the head and neck, with fewer than 75 cases reported in the literature.[87] It is estimated that between 3% and 10% of synovial sarcomas arise in the head and neck region.[79] It is important to note that few synovial-type sarcomas arise in close proximity to articulating joints, the most common source of synovial tissue. Synovial sarcomas of the head and neck tend to occur in the second and third decades, and more commonly in males.[87] In the head and neck region, they occur most commonly in the parapharyngeal space and occasionally in proximity to articulations such as the cricoarytenoid, temporomandibular, and sternoclavicular joints.[79]

Symptoms and Signs

As with other sarcomas, synovial sarcomas most commonly present as a painless, rapidly enlarging subcutaneous mass. (See Symptoms and Signs, Malignant Neoplasms, page 788.)

Radiology

CT imaging shows an invasive soft-tissue mass which often has areas of calcification.[15]

Treatment and Prognosis

The mainstay of treatment is surgery and postoperative radiation. Reported 5-year survival rates range from 36% to 55%.[87,88] Late distant metastasis, specifically pulmonary metastasis, is common; reported 10-year survival rates range from 18% to 38%.[88] (See also Treatment and Prognosis, Malignant Neoplasms, pages 788–791.)

Alveolar Soft Part Sarcoma

Clinical Presentation

Alveolar soft part sarcoma (ASPS) is a rare tumor, accounting for less than 1% of all soft-tissue sarcomas.[89] It shows a slight female predominance and occurs most frequently in the second and third decades of life. It usually arises in skeletal muscle.[89] When it occurs in children, ASPS is located most commonly in the head and neck region.[90]

Symptoms and Signs

Alveolar soft part sarcomas most commonly present as a painless, rapidly enlarging, subcutaneous mass. (See Symptoms and Signs, Malignant Neoplasms, page 788.)

Radiology

On unenhanced CT images, the lesion usually demonstrates a lower attenuation than muscle.[91] In CT images with contrast, the lesion typically shows peripheral enhancement with a low attenuation center consistent with central necrosis. If central necrosis is not present, the entire lesion may enhance. On MRI, the lesion usually has high signal intensity on T1W and T2W.[91] Flow voids are often seen both at the core and margins of the lesions.[91]

Treatment and Prognosis

With ASPS also, the mainstay of treatment is surgery and postoperative radiation. Late distant metastases are the rule, and survival decreases from 87% at 2 years to 18% at 20 years.[92] Patients in the younger age groups tend to have a better prognosis.[92]

METASTATIC TUMORS FROM AN OCCULT PRIMARY

The cervical region, with its rich lymphatic network, is a site for metastatic disease most commonly from squamous cell carcinomas of the upper aerodigestive tract. It can, however, develop metastasis from primaries below the clavicles, or cutaneous lesions of the head and neck such as melanomas and squamous cell carcinoma. Thyroid neoplasms can also occasionally present as an unknown primary. Finally, lymphomas can often present with cervical lymph node involvement. As the vast majority of metastatic lesions from occult primaries are squamous cell carcinomas, the bulk of this section focuses on regional lymph node metastasis from an occult supraclavicular squamous cell carcinoma primary. Occult primaries from other sites are also reviewed.

Clinical Presentation

Occult primary squamous cell carcinomas show a patient distribution similar to that of patients who have squamous cell carcinomas of the upper aerodigestive tract. This includes a male preponderance, with the most common ages being the fifth to seventh decades. Some of these tumors may have been associated with Epstein-Barr virus. Alcohol and tobacco use are significant risk factors. Certain sites of occult primary tumors have characteristic epidemiologic distributions; occult primaries located in the nasopharynx, for instance, most commonly affect Chinese people.

Patients with occult non–squamous cell carcinoma primaries have epidemiologic characteristics determined by their primary tumor. For example, a patient with a regional metastasis from an occult thyroid cancer may have a history of radiation exposure to the neck or a family history of thyroid cancer. Likewise, a patient with metastasis from an occult melanoma may have a history of significant solar radiation exposure. It should be noted that the lung is the most common site of an occult primary lesion below the clavicles metastasizing to the neck.[5]

Symptoms and Signs

Nearly all patients with metastatic tumors of an occult primary present with a painless neck mass.[93] The location of the metastatic disease often can be a clue to the location of the primary. For example, level I disease would most commonly arise from a primary in the oral cavity while bulky disease at level II extending into the posterior triangle is often found with a nasopharyngeal primary. Patients commonly present with level II disease (34%), a catch-all nodal basin for primary sites of many locations.[94] The majority of patients with regional cervical lymph node metastasis from an unknown squamous cell carcinoma primary present with advanced neck disease—between 75% and 88% with N2/N3 disease.[93,94]

In non–squamous cell carcinomas, the location of the neck metastasis often can give a clue as to the site of the primary. Occult thyroid primaries most commonly metastasize to the central compartment as well as levels II through V. Metastasis from occult primaries below the clavicles typically develops low in the neck in the supraclavicular region, including level IV and level V. Lymphomas often present with diffuse and sometimes bulky disease. The location of regional metastasis from occult cutaneous lesions, such as melanomas, is related to the location of the primary. Lesions of the posterior neck and scalp often result in metastasis in the suboccipital region and levels II through V and rarely in level I. Lesions of the ear, face, and anterior scalp usually result in parotid and level I through IV metastasis.[95]

Radiology

Metastatic squamous cell carcinomas of an occult primary have the same radiologic appearance as regional lymph node metastasis from a known primary. The characteristic CT appearance of regional lymph node metastasis is defined by three criteria:

1. Size greater than 1 cm
2. Central necrosis
3. Peripheral enhancement

In cases of non–squamous cell carcinoma occult primaries, the radiographic appearance of the neck metastasis can give the physician additional insight as to the site of the primary. For example, papillary thyroid cancers often have cystic lymph node metastasis. Radiographically, however, it is difficult to differentiate between a cystic lymph node metastasis and a metastatic lymph node with central necrosis. Lymphomas often show diffuse and bulky lymph node disease.

While advances in imaging techniques offer improved detection of regional metastasis, progress in identifying the location of an occult primary through head and neck examination has been disappointing. With advances in upper aerodigestive tract examination with flexible fiberoptic endoscopes and rigid telescopes, the failure of radiographic tests to determine the location of an unknown primary has become even more apparent. This, however, may change in the future with the application of advanced radiologic techniques that allow the functional assessment of tissues. Single photon emission computed tomography (SPECT) using 2-[F-18] fluoro-2-deoxy-D-glucose was able to detect nine of eleven histologically proven occult primary neoplasms of the upper aerodigestive tract.[96]

Treatment

The fundamental aspect in treating patients with cervical lymph node metastasis from an occult primary is the initial evaluation, including the history and physical examination. The first goal is to detect the location of the primary. The patient should be evaluated for symptoms referable to the upper aero-digestive tract, risk factors for squamous cell carcinomas (such as alcohol and tobacco use), and risk factors for squamous cell carcinomas of skin origin. A complete head and neck examination should be performed, giving special attention to the scalp and skin, region of Waldeyer's ring (nasopharynx, tonsils, and the base of tongue), and pyriform sinuses. Attention should also be directed to regions outside the head and neck, such as the chest, abdomen, breasts, and other nodal regions (axilla).

A central component of the work-up for these patients, if a primary cannot be located, involves obtaining tissue for diagnosis from the involved lymph node. A fine-needle aspiration biopsy is usually adequate to differentiate a squamous cell carcinoma metastasis from other histologic types. If the pathologist has difficulty in determining the cell of origin with hematoxylin and eosin stains, immunohistochemical stains may be helpful. In non–squamous cell carcinomas, the fine-needle aspiration biopsy often can determine the general histologic class, such as adenocarcinoma. It may even be able to suggest the exact histologic type, such as with differentiated thyroid carcinomas. Again, immunohistochemical staining can be helpful in determining the histologic type of tumor. Examples include thyroglobulin for thyroid carcinomas, calcitonin and CEA for medullary thyroid carcinomas, and S-100 and HMB-45 for melanomas. With current cytopathological and immunohistochemical techniques, an open biopsy is required less frequently to determine the histologic nature of a lesion. When possible, open biopsy should be avoided because of complications in later surgical management. In poorly differentiated or difficult-to-access lesions, an open biopsy occasionally may be required. If so, the surgical incision should be designed to be easily encompassed in a standard neck dissection incision. Once the histologic type of tumor is determined the work-up can proceed in a directed manner.

If the head and neck examination for squamous cell carcinomas of occult origin does not detect the location of the primary lesion, radiographic imaging studies can be considered. As mentioned earlier, in the setting of a negative head and neck examination, radiographic imaging is often fruitless in the search for the primary. This may change, however, with advances in functional radiographic techniques.[96] Serologic markers such as antibody titers to the early antigen and viral capsid antigen of the Epstein-Barr virus in nasopharyngeal carcinoma occasionally aid in locating the primary.[97] If the preoperative search for the primary is unsuccessful, endoscopic examination of the upper aerodigestive tract under general anesthesia should be performed, with special attention to the region of Waldeyer's ring (nasopharynx, tonsils, base of tongue), and pyriform sinuses. This endoscopic evaluation can be performed immediately prior to definitive surgical management of the neck.

When all means for locating the occult primary lesion of squamous cell carcinoma are exhausted, the focus turns toward treatment. A comprehensive neck dissection should be performed in this population. Over 70% of these patients have N2/N3 neck disease.[93,94] Postoperative radiation therapy is recommended for patients with ominous histologic features such as multiple histologically positive lymph nodes, extracapsular spread, vascular invasion, or perineural invasion.[94] In a single lymph node metastasis without these adverse histologic features, the use of radiation therapy is less well defined, but is often employed. Postoperative radiation therapy to potential mucosal sites of the primary lesions is often incorporated, and is discussed in a later section. These patients require close postoperative follow-up to detect the possible appearance of a primary lesion as well as second primaries, assessment of neck disease, and risk of developing distant metastasis. The occult primary is eventually identified in 12% to 18% of patients receiving multimodality therapy.[94,98]

Prognosis

Reported overall 5-year survival rates are in the 46% to 63% range.[93,94,98] The addition of postoperative radiation therapy in patients with indications mentioned previously has led to improved regional control rates (74%), but has not translated into improved survival.[94] The addition of radiation therapy has led to fewer patients whose primary lesion subsequently becomes apparent.[94,98] The clinical stage of the neck is the most consistent factor in predicting survival as well as control of the neck.[93,94] Other prognostic factors include complete resection of the neck disease, failure of the treated neck, and development of a primary lesion.[94]

Controversies

The diagnosis and management of patients with neck metastasis from an occult primary is surrounded by controversy. Again, this discussion will be limited to occult squamous cell carcinomas of the head and neck. The results of radiotherapy alone after excisional biopsy of only the involved lymph nodes are limited.[99] After excisional biopsy of a solitary cervical lymph node in which all gross tumor is removed, radiation therapy resulted in a 90% control rate above the clavicles and a 77% 5-year survival rate.[99] It should be noted in this study, however, that only one patient had N3 neck disease.[99] The indication for and extent of postoperative radiation therapy in patients with regional metastasis from occult squamous cell carcinomas tends to be the most controversial aspect of this disease. Postoperative radiation therapy has been shown to increase regional control rates as well as control of the occult primary lesions. This, however, has not translated into improved survival, and there is significant morbidity in wide-field radiation of all potential mucosal sites of primary lesions. The use of multimodality therapy (surgery and RT) in patients with N2/N3 disease, or N1 disease with multiple nodes or extracapsular spread, has been shown to improve regional control rates to greater than 70% and is thus indicated.[93,94] The next question is whether all potential primary sites need to be irradiated. More specifically, does the nasopharynx need to be irradiated? The morbidity of irradiating the nasopharynx is substantial, and patients experience significantly more xerostomia, trismus, and other related symptoms. Exclusion of the nasopharynx obviates these symptoms. The radiation dose to the oropharynx and hypopharynx approaches the therapeutic when radiation portals are limited to the neck. It may be reasonable, then, to limit the radiation to the neck unless a high index of suspicion is raised for a potential nasopharyngeal primary, such as high level V metastasis, Asian descent, or positive serologic testing for Epstein-Barr virus. This controversy, however, remains unresolved.

REFERENCES

1. Hollinshead WH. The head and neck. In: Hollinshead WH, ed. *Anatomy for Surgeons*. Vol. 1. 3rd ed. Philadelphia: Harper & Row; 1982:497.
2. Kraus DH, Huo J, Burt M. Surgical access to tumors of the cervico-thoracic junction. *Head Neck Surg*. 1995; 17:131.
3. Jordan RB, Gauderer MWL. Cervical teratomas: An analysis, literature review and proposed classification. *J Pediatric Surg*. 1988; 23:583.
4. Filston HC. Hemangiomas, cystic hygromas and teratomas of the head and neck. *Semin Pediatr Surg*. 1994; 3(3):147.
5. Wenig BM. *Atlas of Head and Neck Pathology*. Philadelphia: W.B. Saunders; 1993.
6. El-Sayed Y. Teratoma of the head and neck. *J Laryngol Otol*. 1992; 106:836.
7. Batsakis JG. *Tumors of the Head and Neck*. 2nd Ed. Baltimore: Williams & Wilkins; 1979.
8. Zerella JT, Finberg FJ. Obstruction of the neonatal airway from teratomas. *Surg Gynecol Obstet*. 1990; 170:126.
9. Kuhel WI, Yagoda M, Peterson P. Benign cervical teratomas in the adult: Report of a case with dense fibrosis involving adjacent vital structures. *Otolaryngol Head Neck Surg*. 1996; 115(1):152.
10. Rothschild MA, Catalano P, Urken M, et al. Evaluation and management of congenital cervical teratoma. *Arch Otolaryngol Head Neck Surg*. 1994; 120:444.
11. Ward RF, April M. Teratomas of the head and neck. *Otolaryngol Clin North Amer*. 1989; 22:621.
12. Gundry SR, Wesley JR, Klein MD, Barr M, Covan AG. Cervical teratomas in the newborn. *J Pediatr Surg*. 1983; 18:382.
13. Batsakis JG, Littler ER, Oberman HA. Teratomas of the neck: A clinicopathological assessment. *Arch Otolaryngol*. 1964; 79:619.
14. Bale GF. Teratoma of the neck in the region of the thyroid gland: Review of the literature and report of four cases. *Am J Pathol*. 1950; 26:565.
15. Som PM. Head and neck imaging. In: Som PM, Curtin HD, eds. *Head and Neck Imaging*. Vol. 1. 3rd ed. New York: Mosby; 1996:533.
16. Donegan JO. Congenital neck masses. In: Cummings CW, Fredrickson JF, Harker LA, Krause CJ, Schuller DE, eds. *Otolaryngology–Head and Neck Surgery*. Vol. 2. 2nd ed. St. Louis: Mosby; 1993.
17. Hancok BJ, St-Vil D, Luks FI, et al. Complications of lymphangioma in children. *J Pediatr Surg*. 1992; 27:220.
18. Landing BH, Farber S. Tumors of the cardiovascular system. In: Landing BH, Farber S, eds. *Atlas of Tumor Pathology*. Washington DC: Armed Forces Institute of Pathology; 1956: 124.
19. Siegel MJ, Glazer HS, St. Amour TE, et al. Lymphangiomas in children: MR imaging. *Radiology*. 1989; 170:467.
20. Joseph AE, Donaldson JS, Reynolds M. Neck and thorax venous aneurysms: Association with cystic hygromas. *Radiology*. 1989; 170:109.
21. Ricciardelli EJ, Richardson MA. Cervicofacial cystic hygromas. Patterns of recurrence and management of the difficult case. *Arch Otolaryngol Head Neck Surg*. 1991; 117:546.
22. Mulliken JB, Glowacki J. Hemangiomas and vascular malformations in infants and children: A classification based on endothelial characteristics. *Plast Reconstr Surg*. 1982; 69:412.
23. Waner M, Suen JY, Dinehart S. Treatment of hemangiomas of the head and neck. *Laryngoscope*. 1992; 102:1123.
24. Enjolras O, Riche MC, Merland JJ, et al. Management of alarming hemangiomas in infancy: A review of 25 cases. *Pediatrics*. 1990; 85:491.
25. Ezekowitz RAB, Mulliken JB, Folkman J. Interferon alpha-2a therapy for life threatening hemangiomas of infancy. *N Engl J Med*. 1992; 326:1456.
26. Dionne CP, Seemayer TA. Infiltrating lipomas and angiolipomas revisited. *Cancer*. 1974; 33:732.
27. Myers EN, Johnson JT. Neoplasms. In: Cummings CW, Fredrickson JF, Harker LA, Krause CJ, Schuller DE, eds. *Otolaryngology—Head and Neck Surgery*. Vol. 2. 2nd ed. St. Louis: Mosby; 1993:1601.
28. Kempson R, Kyriakos M. Fibroxanthosarcoma of the soft tissue. *Cancer*. 1972; 29:961.
29. Bielamowicz S, Dauer MS, Chang B, Zimmerman MC. Noncutaneous benign fibrous histiocytoma of the head and neck. *Arch Otolaryngol Head Neck Surg*. 1995; 113(1):140.
30. Gonzalez S, Duarte I. Benign fibrous histiocytoma of the skin: A morphologic study of 290 cases. *Pathol Res Pract*. 1982; 174:379.
31. Kransdorf MJ, Jelinek JS, Moser RP. Imaging of soft tissue tumors. *Rad Clin North America*. 1993; 31(2):359.
32. Shemen L, Spiro R, Tuazon R. Multifocal adult rhabdomyomas of the head and neck. *Head Neck*. 1992; 14:395.
33. Van der Waal I, Snoe GB. Benign tumors and tumorlike lesions of oral cavity and oropharynx. In: Cummings CW, Fredrickson JF, Harker LA, Krause CJ, Schuller DE, eds. *Otolaryngology–Head and Neck Surgery*. Vol. 2. 2nd ed. St. Louis: Mosby; 1993:1246.
34. Suh IS, Abenoza P, Galloway HR, et al. Peripheral nerve tumors: Correlation of MR imaging and histologic findings. *Radiology*. 1992; 183:341.
35. Carrau RL, Myers EN, Johnson JT. Management of tumors arising in the parapharyngeal space. *Laryngoscope*. 1990; 100:583.
36. Brackman DE, Arriaga MA. Differential diagnosis of neoplasms of the posterior fossa. In: Cummings CW, Fredrickson JF, Harker LA, Krause CJ, Schuller DE, eds. *Otolaryngology—Head and Neck Surgery*. Vol. 2. 2nd ed. St. Louis: Mosby; 1993: 272.
37. Malis LI. Neurofibromatosis (von Recklinghausen's disease). In: Cummings CW, Fredrickson JF, Harker LA, Krause CJ, Schuller DE, eds. *Otolaryngology—Head and Neck Surgery*. Vol. 2. St. Louis: Mosby; 1986.
38. Netterville JL, Reilly KM, Robertson D, Reiber ME, Armstrong WB, Childs P. Carotid body tumors: A review of 30 patients with 46 tumors. *Laryngoscope*. 1995; 105:115.

39. Wax MK, Briant DR. Carotid body tumors: A review. *J Otolaryngol.* 1992; 21(4):277.

40. Gudea F, Mendenhall WM, Parsons JT, Millon RR. Radiotherapy for chemodectoma of the carotid body and ganglion nodosum. *Head Neck.* 1991; 13:509.

41. Lawson W. Glomus bodies and tumors. *NY State J Med.* 1980; 80:1567.

42. Win T, Lewin JS. Imaging characteristics of carotic body tumors. *Am J Otolaryngology.* 1995; 16(5):325.

43. McPherson GA, Halliday AW, Mansfield AO. Carotid body tumors and other cervical paragangliomas: Diagnosis and management in 25 patients. *Br J Surg.* 1989; 76:33.

44. Uruquhart AC, Johnson JT, Myers EN, Schecter GL. Glomus vagale: Paraganlioma of the vagus nerve. *Laryngoscope.* 1994; 104:440.

45. Parkin J. Familial multiple glomus tumors and pheochromocytomas. *Ann Otolaryngol.* 1981; 90:60.

46. Cole JM, Beiler D. Long-term results of treatment for glomus jugulare and glomus vagale tumors with radiotherapy. *Laryngoscope.* 1994; 104:1461.

47. Kraus DH, Dubner S, Harrison LB, et al. Prognostic factors for recurrence and survival in head and neck soft tissue sarcomas. *Cancer.* 1994; 74:697.

48. Cahan WG. Sarcomas arising in irradiated bone. *Cancer.* 1948; 1:3.

49. Tran LM, Rufus M, Meier R, Calcaterra TC, Parker RG. Sarcomas of the head and neck. Prognostic factors and treatment strategies. *Cancer.* 1992; 169:70.

50. Weber RS, Benjamin RS, Peters LJ, Ro JY, Anchon O, Goepfert H. Soft tissue sarcomas of the head and neck in adolescents and adults. *Am J Surg.* 1986; 386:152.

51. Farhood AI, Hadju SI, Shiu MH, Strong EW. Soft tissue sarcomas of the head and neck. *Am J Surg.* 1990; 365:160.

52. Hadju SI, Shiu MH, Brennan MF. The role of the pathologist in the management of soft tissue sarcomas. *World J Surg.* 1988; 12:326.

53. Hadju SI. *Differential Diagnosis of Soft Tissue and Bone Tumors.* Philadelphia: Lea and Feiberger; 1985.

54. Kraus DH, Ali MK, Ginsberg RJ, et al. Vocal cord medialization for unilateral paralysis associated with intrathoracic malignancies. *J Thoracic Cardiovascular Surg.* 1996; 111:334.

55. Kraus DH, Harrison LB. Soft tissue sarcomas of the head and neck In: Harrison LB, Sessions RS, Hong KW, eds. *Head and Neck Cancer—A Multidisciplinary Approach.* Philadelphia: Lippincott; 1996.

56. Lawson MT, Spetzler RF. Internal carotid artery sacrifice for radical resection of skull base tumors. *Skull Base Surgery.* 1996; 6:119.

57. Harrison LB, Franzese F, Gaynor JJ, Brennan MF. Long-term results of a prospective randomized trial of adjuvant brachytherapy in the management of completely resected soft tissue sarcomas of the extremity and superficial trunk. *Int J Rad Oncol Biol Phys.* 1993; 27:259.

58. Glenn J, Kinsella T, Glatstein E, et al. A randomized prospective trial of adjuvant chemotherapy in adults with soft tissue sarcomas of the head and neck, breast and trunk. *Cancer.* 1985; 55:1206.

59. Elias AD, Antman KH. Adjuvant chemotherapy for soft tissue sarcomas: An approach in search of an effective regimen. *Semin Oncol.* 1989; 16:305.

60. Pezzi CM, Pollock RE, Evans HL, et al. Preoperative chemotherapy for soft tissue sarcomas of the extremity. *Ann Surg.* 1990; 211:476.

61. Rouesse JG, Friedman S, Sevin DM, et al. Preoperative induction chemotherapy in the management of locally advanced soft tissue sarcomas. *Cancer.* 1987; 60:296.

62. Chang EA, Kinsella T, Glatstein E, et al. Adjuvant chemotherapy for patients with high grade soft tissue sarcomas of the extremity. *J Clin Oncol.* 1988; 6:1491.

63. Nori D, Schupak K, Shiu M, et al. Role of brachytherapy in recurrent extremity sarcoma in patients treated with prior surgery and radiation therapy. *Int J Rad Oncol Biol Phys.* 1991; 20:1229.

64. Gadd MA, Casper ES, Woodruff JM, McCormack PM, Brennan MF. Development and treatment of pulmonary metastasis in adult patients with soft tissue sarcomas. *Ann Surg.* 1993; 218:705.

65. Giuliano AE, Eilber FR. The rationale for planned reoperation after unplanned total excision of soft tissue sarcomas. *J Clin Oncol.* 1985; 3:1344.

66. Goepfert H, Lindberg RD, Sinkovics JG, Ayala AG. Soft tissue sarcoma of the head and neck after puberty. *Arch Otolaryngol.* 1977; 103:365.

67. Blitzer A, Lawson W, Zak FG, Biller HF, Som ML. Clinical-pathological determinance in prognosis of fibrous histiocytomas of the head and neck. *Laryngoscope.* 1981; 91:2053.

68. Daou RA, Attia EL, Viloria JB. Malignant fibrous histiocytoma of the head and neck. *J Otolaryngol.* 1983; 12:383.

69. Newman AN, Rice DH. Rhabdomyosarcoma of the head and neck. *Laryngoscope.* 1984; 94:234.

70. Farr HW. Soft part sarcomas of the head and neck. *Seminars in Oncology.* 1981; 8:185.

71. Greager JA, Patel MK, Briele HA, Walker MJ, DasGupta TK. Soft tissue sarcomas of the adult head and neck. *Cancer.* 1985; 56:820.

72. Willers H, Hug EB, Spiro IJ, Efrid JT, Rosenberg AE, Wang CC. Adult soft tissue sarcomas of the head and neck treated by radiation and surgery or irradiation alone: Patterns of failure and prognostic factors. *Int J Radiat Oncol Biol Phys.* 1995; 33:585.

73. Levay J, O'Sullivan B, Catton C, et al. An assessment of prognostic factors in soft tissue sarcoma of the head and neck. *Arch Otolaryngol Head Neck Surg.* 1994; 129:981.

74. Buckley NJ, Burch WM, Leight GS. Malignant teratoma of the thyroid gland of an adult. A case report and review of the literature. *Surgery.* 1986; 100:932.

75. Batsakis JG, El-Naggar AK, Luna MA. Pathology consultation: Teratomas of the head and neck with emphasis on malignancy. *Ann Otol Rhinol Laryngol.* 1995; 104:496.

76. Sacher M, Som PM, Lanzieri CF, Solodnik P, Rotham A, Biller HF. Malignant teratoma of the parapharyngeal space in an adult presenting as cervical cord compression. *J Comp Asst Tomog.* 1986; 10:37.

77. Maddox JC, Evans HL. Angiosarcoma of skin and soft tissue: A study of forty-four cases. *Cancer.* 1981; 48:1907.

78. Mark RJ, Tran LM, Secarz J, Fu YS, Calcaterra TC, Jullard GF. Angiosarcoma of the head and neck: The UCLA experience 1955 through 1990. *Arch Otolaryngol Head Neck Surg.* 1993; 119:973.

79. Lydiatt WM, Shaha AR, Shah J. Angiosarcoma of the head and neck. *Am J Surg.* 1994; 168:451.

80. Hoolden CA, Spittle MF, Wilson-Jones E. Angiosarcoma for the face and scalp, prognosis and treatment. *Cancer.* 1987; 59:1046.

81. McCulloch TM, Makielski KH, McNutt MA. Head and neck liposarcoma: A histopathologic revaluation of reported cases. *Arch Otolaryngol Head Neck Surg.* 1992; 118:1045.

82. Golledge J, Fisher C, Rhys-Evans PH. Head and neck liposarcoma. *Cancer.* 1995; 76:1051.

83. Som PM, Scherl MP, Rao VM, et al. Rare presentations of ordinary lipomas of the head and neck: A review. *AJNR.* 1986; 7:657.

84. Singh B, Shaha A, Har-El G. Malignant fibrous histiocytoma of the head and neck. *J Craniomaxillofac Surg.* 1993; 21:262.

85. Barnes L, Verbin RS, Gnepp DR. Diseases of the ear, nose, paranasal sinuses and nasopharynx. In: Barnes L, ed. *Surgical Pathology of the Head and Neck.* Vol. 1. New York: Marcel Dekker; 1985:725.

86. Vege DS, Chinoy RF, Ganesh B, Parikh DM. Malignant peripheral nerve sheath tumors of the head and neck: A clinicopathological study. *J Surg Oncol.* 1994; 55:100.

87. Bukachevsky RP, Pincus RL, Schectman FG, Sarti E, Chodosh P. Synovial sarcoma of the head and neck. *Head Neck.* 1992; 14:44.

88. Carrillo R, Rodriguez-Peralto JL, Batsakis JG. Pathology consultation: Synovial sarcomas of the head and neck. *Ann Otol Rhinol Laryngol.* 1992; 101:367.

89. Foschini MP, Eusebi V. Alveolar soft-part sarcoma: A new type of rhabdomyosarcoma? *Semin Diag Pathol.* 1994; 11(1):58.

90. Spector RA, Travis LW, Smith J. Alveolar soft part sarcoma of the head and neck. *Laryngoscope.* 1979; 89:1301.
91. Iwamoto Y, Morimoto N, Chuman H, Shinohara N, Sugioka Y. The role of MR imaging in the diagnosis of alveolar soft part sarcoma: A report of 10 cases. *Skeletal Radiol.* 1995; 24:267.
92. Lieberman PH, Brennan MF, Kimmel M, et al. Alveolar soft part sarcoma. A clinicopathological study of half a century. *Cancer.* 1989; 63:1.
93. Nguyen C, Shenouda G, Black MJ, Vuong T, Donath D, Yassa M. Metastatic squamous cell carcinoma to cervical lymph nodes from unknown primary mucosal sites. *Head Neck.* 1994; 16(1):58.
94. Davidson BJ, Spiro RH, Patel S, Patel K, Shah J. Cervical metastasis of occult origin: The impact of combined modality therapy. *Am J Surg.* 1994; 168:395.
95. Shah J, Kraus DH, Dubner S, Sarkar S. Patterns of regional lymph node metastases from cutaneous melanomas of the head and neck. *Am J Surg.* 1991; 162:320.
96. Mukherji SK, Drane WE, Mancuso AA, Parsons JT, Mendenhall WM, Stringer S. Occult primary tumors of the head and neck: Detection with 2-[F-18] fluoro-2-deoxy-d-glucose SPECT. *Radiology.* 1996; 199(3):761.
97. Neel HB, Pearson GR, Weiland LH, et al. Application of Epstein-Barr virus serology to the diagnosis and staging of North American patients with nasopharyngeal carcinoma. *Otolaryngol Head Neck Surg.* 1983; 91:255.
98. Wang RC, Goepfert H, Barber AE, Wolf P. Unknown primary squamous cell carcinoma metastatic to the neck. *Arch Otolaryngol Head Neck Surg.* 1990; 116:1388.
99. Mack YM, Parsons JT, Mendenhall WM, Stringer SP, Cassisi NJ, Million RR. Squamous cell carcinoma of the head and neck: Management after excisional biopsy of a solitary node. *Int J Radiat Oncol Biol Phys.* 1993; 25:619.

III. PATHOLOGY OF LESIONS OF THE NECK

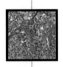

■ KENNETH DEVANEY

GENERAL CONSIDERATIONS

The discovery of a neck mass usually invites consideration of a wide range of potential causes—including infectious lesions, cervical nodal metastases from a known primary squamous carcinoma of the head and neck region, and malignant lymphoma. While these are indeed common causes of masses in this area, an occasional patient develops either a developmental lesion or a true soft-tissue tumor. This chapter covers lesions from either end of the spectrum of neck masses—the rather more common non-neoplastic congenital (developmental) lesions and the much less frequently encountered true soft-tissue neoplasms. Cervical metastases from an occult primary source are considered here as well. Soft-tissue tumors of the neck are uncommon lesions; when they do occur, they are more often benign than malignant.[1-3] The cervical region may give rise to the same range of benign and malignant tumors as other regions of the body, although true malignant soft-tissue tumors are encountered much more frequently elsewhere. (The extremities and the retroperitoneum are common sites of origin for soft-tissue sarcomas in adults.)

In children, the upper aerodigestive tract is one of the principal sites of development of rhabdomyosarcomas. The neck proper—the region of interest for this chapter—is not, however, a particularly common site of origin of soft-tissue sarcomas. The soft-tissue lesions seen in clinical practice are usually found in adults, and these may include both benign and malignant tumors. By some estimates, the benign soft-tissue tumors outnumber the malignant ones by a ratio of 30:1 in the head and neck.[1] It should be acknowledged that, especially with larger bulkier lesions, it may be difficult to determine whether the tumor (which at the time of biopsy may span several discrete anatomic territories) originally arose in the soft tissues of the neck, the larynx, or the adjacent skin or subcutis. In such situations, the pathologist usually defers to the clinician's best judgment of the most likely primary site and then tempers this judgment by an evaluation of the pathologic findings.

Benign developmental lesions of the neck are more frequently encountered in general practice in children, and so it is here that the consideration of these cervical-based entities begins.[4-9]

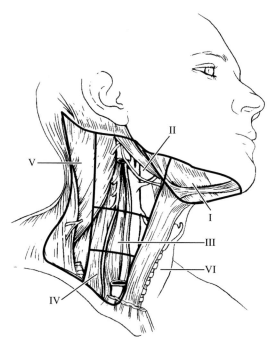

FIGURE 13–33 Lymph node regions of the neck. From Robinson KT, Medina JE, Wolfe GT, et al. Standardizing neck dissection terminology: Official report of the Academy's Committee for Head and Neck Surgery and Oncology. *Arch Otolaryngol Head Neck Surg.* 1991; 117:602. Copyright American Medical Association, with permission.

SPECIMEN HANDLING AND NECK DISSECTION

Figure 13–33 illustrates the lymph node regions of the neck. The neck is divided into the anterior and posterior triangles by the sternocleidomastoid muscle. Region I includes the submental and submandibular triangle. Regions II, III, and IV include the lymph nodes found along the internal jugular vein and the lymph nodes identified in the fibroadipose tissue medial to the sternocleidomastoid muscle. From superior to inferior, regions II, III, and IV are divided into thirds. Region II is the upper third and includes the upper jugular, jugular digastric, and upper posterior cervical lymph nodes, identified in close proximity to the spinal accessory nerve. Region II is separated from region III by the hyoid bone. Region III is the middle third and is separated from region IV at the point that the omohyoid muscle crosses the internal jugular vein or by the cricothyroid membrane. Region IV is the lower third and includes the lower jugular, the scalene, and the supraclavicular lymph nodes lying deep to the lower third of the sternocleidomastoid muscle. Region V includes the contents of the posterior triangle.

The classification of neck dissections is dependent on the divisions of the lymph node groups in the neck (Table 13–6). Neck dissections are classified as comprehensive, selective, and extended. Unless otherwise stated, this discussion is limited to one side of the neck.

A comprehensive neck dissection includes the removal of all lymph node regions (I–V), and these are divided into radical and modified radical neck dissections. Modifications of the radical neck dissec-

tion are based on preservation of one or more of the following structures: the spinal accessory nerve, the internal jugular vein, or the sternocleidomastoid muscle. Modified radical neck dissection (type I) includes preservation of only the spinal accessory nerve; type II includes the preservation of two structures, the spinal accessory nerve and the internal jugular vein. Type III, also referred to as the "functional neck dissection," includes the preservation of all three structures.

The selective neck dissection includes the removal of the lymph node groups that are at the highest risk of harboring metastatic disease based on the location of the primary tumor. It preserves the spinal accessory nerve, the internal jugular vein, and the sternocleidomastoid muscle. Selective neck dis-

TABLE 13–6	CLASSIFICATION OF NECK DISSECTIONS

Comprehensive
  Radical
  Modified radical
    Type I
    Type II
    Type III
Selective
  Lateral
  Anterolateral
  Expanded supraomohyoid
Posterolateral
Extended

section is subdivided into three different neck dissections, including:

1. Lateral neck dissection—en bloc resection of the lymph nodes in regions II to IV
2. Supraomohyoid neck dissection—en bloc removal of the lymph nodes in regions I to III—and expanded supraomohyoid neck dissection that consists of en bloc removal of the lymph nodes in regions I to IV
3. Posterolateral neck dissection—removal of the suboccipital and retroauricular lymph nodes as well as removal of the lymph nodes in regions II to V.

The extended neck dissection includes any of the above-described neck dissections that have been "extended" to include lymph nodes (e.g., paratracheal, retropharyngeal) or anatomic structures (e.g., carotid artery) that are not routinely removed. Once resected, the neck dissection falls under the purview of the surgical pathologist, who must describe the gross findings and properly section the resected specimen. The orientation of the neck dissection is critical to the proper sectioning of the specimen. To this end, the surgeon may delineate the anatomic regions or boundaries of the neck by one or more black sutures. If necessary the surgeon should assist the pathologist in properly orienting the specimen. Proper orientation and sectioning of the neck dissection will allow the pathologist to issue a report with clinical and prognostic value. For head and neck metastatic carcinoma to lymph nodes, factors that may have prognostic significance and that should be mentioned in the pathology report include the presence of extracapsular extension by the tumor, site of nodal metastasis, number of lymph nodes with metastatic disease, node fixation, tissue response to metastatic tumor, and presence of vascular or perineural invasion.

NON-NEOPLASTIC LESIONS

Branchial Cleft Anomalies

Gross Pathology

Branchial cleft fistulas, sinuses, and cysts share a common feature: when intact, they consist of a unilocular central cavity with a relatively thin, smooth inner wall.[10-18] The cyst contents may be serous, mucinous, or purulent (in those lesions where secondary infection has supervened). Most branchial cleft anomalies are cysts and so may not be accompanied by skin or mucosa; they may consist of a soft-tissue mass. The remainder of the branchial cleft anomalies are divided between sinus tracts and fistulous connections linking pharyngeal mucosa with the skin surface.

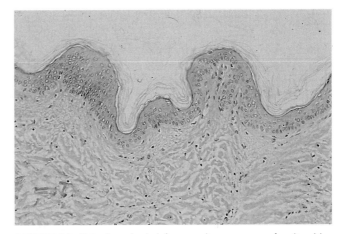

FIGURE 13–34 Branchial cleft anomalies are most often lined by a keratinizing squamous epithelium (H&E, × 100).

As the cycle of inflammation and repair evolves in some of the branchial cleft anomalies, the lining epithelium may be obliterated, leaving in its wake only a dense fibrosis with a mixed acute and chronic inflammatory reaction. Such a change may result in the gross appearance of a solid rather than a cystic mass.[19,20]

Microscopic Pathology

The lining epithelium of a branchial cleft anomaly is, in most instances, a simple keratinizing squamous epithelium—not surprising, in view of the fact that it develops from ectodermally derived tissues (Fig. 13–34). Variations on this basic theme include the occasional ciliated pseudostratified respiratory epithelium (lining a portion or even the entirety of the lesion), adnexal structures (including sebaceous glands and hair shafts), and even islands of cartilage (Fig. 13–35).[10-16]

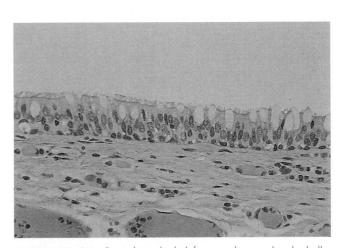

FIGURE 13–35 Some branchial cleft anomalies are lined wholly or in part by ciliated pseudostratified columnar respiratory-type epithelium (H&E, × 260).

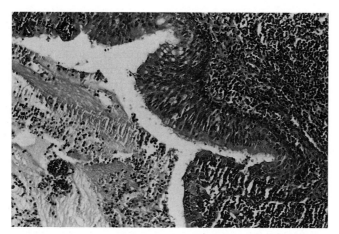

FIGURE 13-36 In addition to the epithelial lining, the second common feature of a branchial cleft anomaly is the presence within the wall of a dense lymphoid infiltrate that may include germinal centers; here, the left portion of the figure shows the amorphous debris accumulated within the central cystic space, while the right portion of the figure shows the dense lymphoid infiltrate underlying a ciliated pseudostratified epithelial cyst lining (H&E, ×260).

In addition to an epithelial lining, branchial cleft anomalies are often identified by a second feature: the presence of a benign lymphoid infiltrate within the wall of the lesion (Fig. 13–36). This infiltrate is typically rather dense (and is so commonly encountered in these lesions that some observers have suggested that branchial cleft anomalies are actually the result of epithelial inclusions within true cervical lymph nodal tissues).

The cyst contents are typically fluid, and may include shed epithelial cells, amorphous material, and cholesterol crystals; when secondary infection has developed, an acute inflammatory exudate may appear in both the cyst contents and the wall of the lesion. This inflammatory infiltrate, when present, may be quite florid and may obscure or replace the underlying epithelial lining (Fig. 13–37).

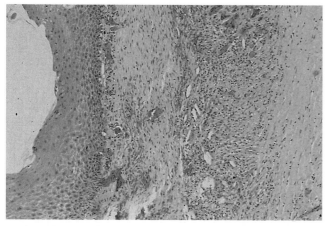

FIGURE 13-37 Some branchial cleft anomalies are modified by secondary infection and inflammation; here, the right portion of the figure is occupied by a pattern of dense fibrosis with inflammatory cells, hemorrhage, and scattered cholesterol clefts (H&E, ×100).

Differential Diagnosis

On a clinical plane, the finding of a soft compressible lesion within the soft tissues of the neck is likely to evoke a differential that includes a branchial cleft anomaly, an epidermoid cyst, a thyroglossal duct cyst, a salivary gland lesion (either inflammatory or neoplastic), cystic hygroma (particularly in a child), hemangioma, lymph node based disease (including inflammatory lymphadenitis, primary malignant lymphoma, or metastatic carcinoma), carotid body tumor, a lipoma, or even a laryngocele. The classic anatomic distribution of branchial cleft anomalies falls within a territory defined by a line drawn from just anterior to the tragus at one end and, proceeding inferiorly, paralleling the anterior of the sternocleidomastoid muscle. Such a topographic restriction excludes from consideration, in most instances, such potential histologic "look-alikes" as an epidermoid cyst of the posterior neck, or a midline thyroglossal duct cyst.

Special Techniques

The branchial cleft anomalies are sometimes approached initially by means of fine-needle aspiration cytology. In older adults, the finding of well-differentiated squamous epithelium on cytologic study should be reaffirmed by surgical excision of the mass (to avoid confusing a well-differentiated squamous carcinoma metastatic to a regional lymph node from a benign developmental lesion). Other special techniques, such as electron microscopy or immunohistochemistry, have not proven significantly useful in the diagnosis of these lesions.[21]

Clinicopathologic Correlations

Some debate has centered about the distinction between branchial cleft anomalies and lymphoepithelial cysts (the latter being diagnosed most often in lesions of the oral cavity). In general, the diagnosis of a lymphoepithelial cyst is probably best reserved for those lesions developing in the oral cavities of older adults (as contrasted with the usually younger patients with true branchial cleft anomalies). It must be conceded, however, that the histologic overlap between these two lesions is great, and distinction is not reliably made on histologic grounds alone.

The definitive therapy for a branchial cleft anomaly is complete excision of the lesion. Save for the potential for secondary infection, they are not a significant cause of morbidity in most patients and have no significant premalignant potential. A very few individuals, suffering from a secondary infection of a branchial cleft anomaly, may present with signs and symptoms deriving from pressure of the mass upon adjacent structures and producing dysphagia or dyspnea.

The branchial cleft anomalies, taken together, are wholly benign and lack any significant premalignant potential; while older reports made occasional reference to squamous carcinomas arising in pre-existing branchial cleft remnants, many of these reports probably described cervical nodal metastases from occult primary squamous carcinomas elsewhere in the head and neck region. A convincing proof of a true carcinoma arising within a branchial cleft cyst would require, among other findings, a follow-up period of several years duration so as to exclude the possibility of an occult primary elsewhere—a requirement that most putative "branchial cleft carcinomas" cannot satisfy.[22-29]

Thyroglossal Cyst

Gross Pathology

On surgical exploration or at the time of pathologic dissection, thyroglossal cysts may resemble branchial cleft cysts in their gross appearance, as they usually consist of a central cystic space lined by a thin smooth cyst wall.[30-40] As with the branchial cleft anomalies, the thyroglossal-derived anomalies may also sometimes take the form of a sinus tract or a fistulous connection (although the great majority are cystic lesions).

Microscopic Pathology

The thyroglossal cyst, as the name suggests, may contain recognizable thyroidal epithelial tissue; unfortunately for the surgical pathologist, however, not all thyroglossal cysts will show foci of thyroid tissue (which may in some instances be related to the vagaries of sampling). The cyst lining may be either a keratinizing squamous epithelium or a pseudostratified ciliated columnar epithelium. Such a nondescript squamous epithelium, of course, will differ little microscopically from the lining of a branchial cleft anomaly or an epidermal inclusion cyst (Figs. 13–38 through 13–40).[41,42]

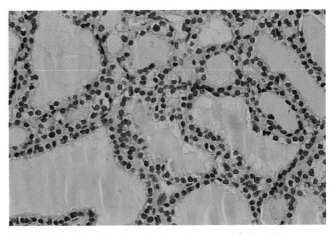

FIGURE 13-39 On close scrutiny, the areas of thyroid tissue within a thyroglossal cyst consist of epithelial-lined spaces filled with a dense eosinophilic acellular material (colloid) (H&E, ×260).

Differential Diagnosis

The usual midline location within the neck of thyroglossal cysts (and their tendency to cluster about the hyoid bone) aids greatly in their clinical recognition. Branchial cleft anomalies and the wide range of lymph node based lesions are located in the lateral neck, while epidermoid cysts (discussed later) are most often found in the posterior neck.

With regard to the interpretation of the histologic evidence alone, in those samplings including only a squamous epithelial lined cyst and no thyroid tissue, confusion with a branchial cleft cyst or epidermoid cyst would be understandable. In this instance, knowledge of the cervical region from which the specimen was obtained (often posterior neck for epidermoid cyst, virtually always lateral neck for branchial cleft anomaly, anterior midline of the neck for thyroglossal cyst) is of immeasurable aid to the diagnostic pathologist.

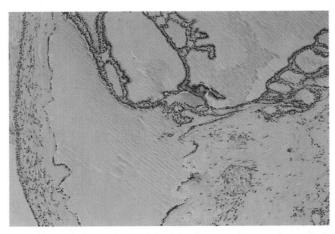

FIGURE 13-38 At the far left of this figure is the pseudostratified columnar epithelial lining of this midline anterior neck mass; the remainder of the figure is occupied by thyroid tissue, which identifies this lesion as a thyroglossal duct cyst (H&E, ×80).

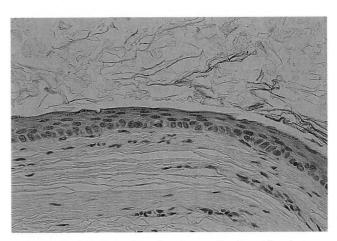

FIGURE 13-40 Some thyroglossal cysts, like this midline lesion which was attached to the hyoid bone, reveal a squamous (or respiratory-type) epithelial-lined cyst but no recognizable thyroid tissue (H&E, ×260).

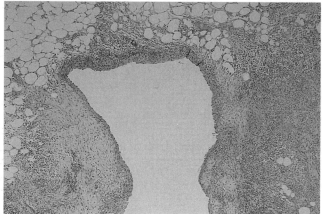

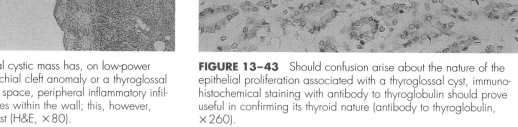

FIGURE 13-41 This cervical cystic mass has, on low-power view, many features of a branchial cleft anomaly or a thyroglossal cyst—a central epithelial-lined space, peripheral inflammatory infiltrates, and epithelial aggregates within the wall; this, however, proved to be a parathyroid cyst (H&E, ×80).

FIGURE 13-43 Should confusion arise about the nature of the epithelial proliferation associated with a thyroglossal cyst, immunohistochemical staining with antibody to thyroglobulin should prove useful in confirming its thyroid nature (antibody to thyroglobulin, ×260).

The occasional differential diagnostic problem may be introduced by the uncommon parathyroid cyst, in which another type of epithelial proliferation may appear in the setting of a cystic neck mass; in parathyroid cysts, however, the epithelial elements are thyroglobulin negative and parathyroid hormone positive on immunohistochemical study (Figs. 13–41 and 13–42).

Special Techniques

The recognition of a thyroglossal cyst as a benign epithelial lined lesion with thyroid tissue embedded in its wall in most instances will be a straightforward matter for the light microscopist. In the event that the thyroid tissue is present and is not immedi-

ately recognized as thyroid, then positive immunohistochemical staining with antibody to thyroglobulin suggests the correct diagnosis (Fig. 13–43).

Clinicopathologic Correlations

The thyroglossal duct cysts are usually not apparent at birth, although the majority of cases are diagnosed in the first two decades of life. Only a very occasional thyroglossal cyst will be found lateral to the midline (usually attributed to prior surgery); in such an instance, the microscopic identification of thyroid tissue will clinch the diagnosis.

When a Sistrunk-type procedure (that is, removal of the midportion of the hyoid bone and the residuum of the tract extending to the foramen caecum, in addition to the lesion identified on physical examination itself) is not performed, thyroglossal duct cysts may recur in a minority of patients. These lesions lack a significant capacity for malignant change, however, and so the rare recurrences are a fairly straightforward problem in local control.

While occasional reports of the development of thyroid carcinoma (particularly papillary thyroid carcinoma) within thyroglossal duct cysts have appeared, at least some of these lesions have represented metastatic deposits from primary thyroid carcinoma, while others have represented direct extension from an adjacent thyroid lesion.[43–49] Rare reports of squamous carcinoma arising in a thyroglossal duct cyst have appeared as well. As with putative carcinomas arising in branchial cleft cysts, the suspicion should always be that such lesions are more likely to represent metastases from occult primaries. Reports of primary tumors arising in such circumstances (while not unheard of) should therefore be viewed with a healthy dose of skepticism.[50–52]

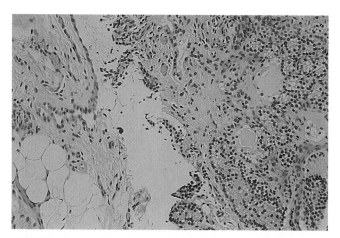

FIGURE 13-42 This cystic neck mass contains glandular epithelial islands within its walls—however, in contrast to the glands of true thyroid tissue, the glands filling the right portion of this figure are not filled with colloid. These are islands of parathyroid epithelium, and so this lesion is a parathyroid cyst (H&E, ×180).

Thymic Cyst

Gross Pathology

The cervical thymic cyst may be unilocular or multilocular; cyst contents may be a colorless, yellow-brown, or (in those cysts in which secondary infection has supervened) purulent fluid. The associated solid areas are soft to rubbery septa with a tan-white color.[53–61]

Microscopic Pathology

The low-power microscopic appearance of a thymic cyst most often suggests a lymphoid lesion of some sort—a lymph node, perhaps, or the wall of a branchial cleft anomaly (Fig. 13–44). One key light microscopic difference between a thymic cyst and a branchial cleft anomaly or lymph node relates to the presence of identifiable thymic tissue in the former lesion and its absence in the latter two entities. This thymic tissue is distinctive in that it includes both lymphoid follicles and the pathognomonic epithelial islands known as the Hassall's corpuscles (Fig. 13–45).[56]

The accompanying cystic spaces may be lined by squamous epithelium, a simple cuboidal epithelium, or both. As with the branchial cleft anomalies, when infection supervenes, the lining epithelium may be focally or wholly denuded and replaced by fibrous tissue. Other reactive changes, such as foreign body giant cell formation or cholesterol cleft formation, are common accompaniments of thymic cysts (Fig. 13–46).

Differential Diagnosis

Thymic cysts may arise in either the lateral neck or in the midline, so physical examination may suggest a variety of possibilities including a branchial cleft

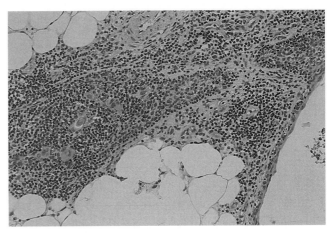

FIGURE 13–45 The Hassall's corpuscles of a thymic cyst, as seen here, consist of insular aggregates of squamous cells (often with central keratinization), which are in turn associated with lymphoid tissue (H&E, × 120).

anomaly, a thyroglossal cyst, a teratoma, or a lymphangioma.

When a cervical mass has been correctly identified as thymic in nature, consideration may turn to the possibility of a thymoma. Neoplastic thymomas, however, differ from thymic cysts in their greater volume of solid thymic tissue. Most of the bulk of a thymic cyst is provided by the cystic spaces, with a lesser contribution by the thymic tissue proper.

Special Techniques

The aid of special techniques is not often sought in the recognition of thymic cysts, although two instances might arise in which immunohistochemical studies might be employed: (1) a lymphoid lesion in which consideration is being given to the possibility of a malignant lymphoma (polyclonality by immu-

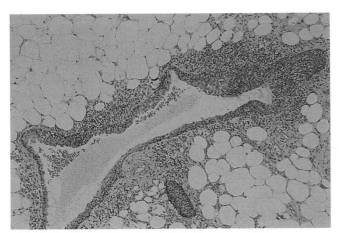

FIGURE 13–44 This cervical thymic cyst superficially resembles a branchial cleft anomaly; however, on close scrutiny, the lymphoid tissue is seen to contain the epithelial islands (Hassall's corpuscles), which are not a feature of branchial cleft anomalies (H&E, × 100).

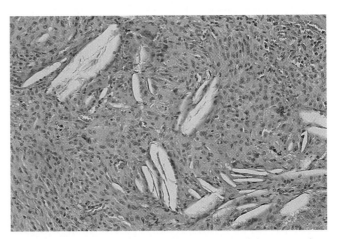

FIGURE 13–46 A common finding within the solid portions of a thymic cyst is an accumulation of histiocytes, chronic inflammatory cells, and cholesterol clefts (H&E, × 200).

nohistochemistry will support a diagnosis of a thymic cyst over one of lymphoma), and (2) thymic cysts in which the epithelial component is difficult to appreciate by light microscopy (the subtle epithelial component may be highlighted by immunohistochemical staining with antibody to cytokeratin).

Clinicopathologic Correlations

As with branchial cleft anomalies, most thymic cysts of the neck will be identified in the first two decades of life. They are most uncommon cervical lesions, and a tentative diagnosis should be accepted only after considering the differential diagnoses previously discussed and following histologic confirmation. While hyperplasia of mediastinal thymic tissue has been associated in some patients with myasthenia gravis, no such association has been drawn with cervical thymic tissue and myasthenia.

The thymic cyst is a benign lesion, and so complete excision will be curative. It is not a premalignant lesion, so failure to perform a complete excision will not place the patient at risk for the subsequent development of a thymoma, lymphoma, or carcinoma.

Dermoid Cyst

Gross Pathology

The gross appearance of a dermoid cyst does not diverge appreciably from that of an epidermoid cyst (epidermal cyst, discussed later). It typically takes the form of a thin-walled cystic lesion that contains a grey-white friable material. When the cyst contents have been evacuated, the internal aspect of the cyst wall has a smooth, featureless appearance.[62–69]

Microscopic Pathology

There are many microscopic similarities between a dermoid cyst and an epidermoid cyst. Both are lined by stratified squamous epithelium that produces a central accumulation of material. The dermoid cyst differs in one key way, however; its wall contains adnexal structures (such as hair shafts and sebaceous, eccrine, or apocrine glands) (Fig. 13–47).[62] As with epidermoid cysts, dermoid cysts may rupture, releasing their contents into the adjacent soft tissues, inciting a florid foreign-body giant cell reaction that can obscure the underlying cyst wall.

Differential Diagnosis

As noted above, the critical distinction between a dermoid cyst and an epidermoid cyst lies in its microscopic appearance. The dermoid cyst includes, within its wall, cutaneous-type adnexal structures (including sebaceous glands and/or hair shafts)

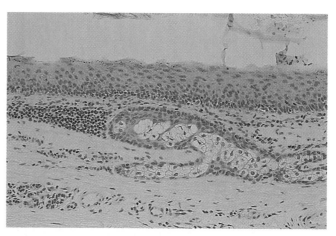

FIGURE 13–47 The squamous epithelial lining of a dermoid cyst differs from that of an epidermoid cyst in that it includes adnexal structures, including sebaceous glands (shown here), hair shafts, eccrine glands, and/or apocrine glands (H&E, × 260).

which are not part of the wall of an epidermoid cyst. Each of these tissues is cytologically benign.

Special Techniques

As with its cousin, the epidermoid cyst, recognition of a dermoid cyst lies in the province of the light microscopist, and special techniques are not called for here.

Clinicopathologic Correlations

In view of their status as developmental lesions, it is not surprising that dermoid cysts are pediatric lesions. It is uncommon indeed to diagnose dermoid cysts of the neck in adults. Dermoid cysts are wholly benign developmental anomalies, and have no premalignant potential. When completely excised, these lesions do not recur.

Epidermoid Cyst

Gross Pathology

Epidermoid cysts often rupture in the course of their excision and so may appear as an admixture of friable grey-white material and the soft tissue which at one time made up the wall of the lesion. When intact, epidermoid cysts consist of a thin (usually no more than a few millimeters) smooth wall surrounding a single space, wherein the friable contents are contained.[70–72]

Microscopic Pathology

The lining of an epidermoid cyst is a stratified squamous epithelium that includes a defined granular cell layer; the central contents are masses of anu-

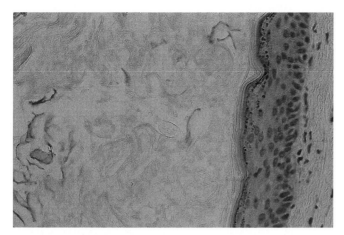

FIGURE 13–48 An epidermoid cyst is lined by a keratinizing squamous epithelium without cutaneous adnexal structures—and so may resemble the lining of some branchial cleft anomalies, thyroglossal duct cysts, and thymic cysts (H&E, ×260).

cleate keratin material (Fig. 13–48). When these lesions rupture in situ and spill their contents into the adjacent soft tissues, a florid inflammatory reaction (marked by numerous multinucleated giant cells and acute and chronic inflammatory cells) may develop. When such an inflammatory reaction is particularly pronounced, the only sign of the pre-existing epidermoid cyst may be scattered keratin flakes caught up in an overwhelming foreign-body giant cell reaction.[71,72]

Differential Diagnosis

The absence of associated adnexal structures (such as hair follicles or sebaceous glands) serves to distinguish an epidermoid cyst from a dermoid cyst; otherwise, the rather undistinguished squamous lining of an epidermoid cyst may invite comparison with a branchial cleft or thyroglossal cyst (when thyroid tissue is not found)—and in these instances the location of the lesion will aid in making the distinction.

The rupture of an epidermoid cyst may spill keratin material into the adjacent soft tissues, which will incite an inflammatory reaction. Should this finding be the only change noted on biopsy, the patient's age and the depth of the biopsy must be considered when interpreting these findings. In a superficial lesion from a child, keratin debris alone may indeed represent the residua of a ruptured benign cyst; in a deep lesion from an older adult, however, that keratin material may represent the residua of a well-differentiated metastatic squamous carcinoma which has spread to a cervical lymph node and incited so florid an inflammatory reaction that both the host lymph node and the cytologically malignant metastatic carcinoma cells are obscured.

Special Techniques

The diagnosis of an epidermoid cyst is sufficiently straightforward to preclude special diagnostic techniques. Light microscopy serves admirably to aid in its recognition.

Clinicopathologic Correlations

The vast majority of these relatively common lesions are believed to derive from the infundibulum of the hair shaft. As a point of nomenclature, they are properly designated as epidermoid or infundibular cysts. By contrast, a true epidermal inclusion cyst—resulting from traumatic implantation of a portion of epidermis into the underlying dermis—is a decidedly uncommon lesion. It must be conceded, however, that many pathologists use these terms interchangeably. These subcutaneous lesions may be solitary or multiple; when multiple, they are occasionally associated with Gardner's syndrome (occurrence of intestinal polyps, multiple epidermoid cysts, and skeletal lesions—usually an autosomal dominant inheritance pattern).

Epidermoid cysts are benign lesions without a significant capacity for undergoing malignant degeneration. Only rare accounts exist of malignant degeneration—usually in the form of a basal cell carcinoma or a squamous carcinoma. Total excision is curative.

Nodular Fasciitis

Gross Pathology

A focus of nodular fasciitis may reach a maximum dimension of a few centimeters, but it is uncommon for these masses to exceed 5 cm in diameter. These lesions are almost always solitary masses, well circumscribed but unencapsulated. The cut surface of nodular fasciitis varies from firm and rubbery to soft and frankly myxoid; scattered small cysts are occasionally seen.[73–76]

Microscopic Pathology

In its early phase of development, nodular fasciitis consists of a loosely arranged grouping of spindle cells that are set in a myxoid to collagenous stroma. The spindle cells are gathered into short fascicles that may intersect one another at varying angles but do not reach the high degree of storiform organization which has been likened to a "tissue culture" appearance. The latter arrangement is seen in fibrous histiocytoma, which is discussed later. The myxoid stroma often contains a scattering of extravasated erythrocytes and chronic inflammatory cells (principally small mature lymphocytes). One particularly deceptive finding may be the presence of readily identifiable mitotic figures in some lesions. The nuclei are uniform, vesicular, and often

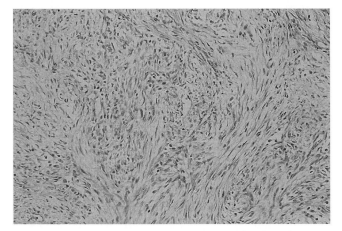

FIGURE 13-49 The low-power appearance of nodular fasciitis is characterized by rather cellular proliferation of spindle cells gathered together into short loose fascicles (H&E, ×120).

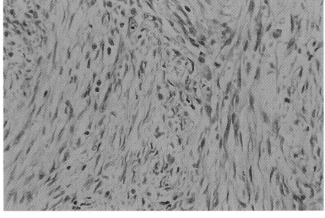

FIGURE 13-51 The individual cells of nodular fasciitis are spindled, with monomorphous nuclei that are neither pleomorphic nor hyperchromatic. While mitoses may be present, they are not atypical division figures and so do not make this a malignant lesion (H&E, ×260).

possess small distinct nucleoli (Figs. 13–49 through 13–51).[73-75]

As lesions of nodular fasciitis mature, they often become increasingly collagenized and fibrotic, losing some of their stromal myxoid character. While the masses appear to be rather well circumscribed on gross examination, microscopic study may reveal tongues of spindle cells projecting for a short distance into the adjacent soft tissues; such a finding should not be mistaken for evidence of malignancy.

Clearly delineated light microscopic subtypes of nodular fasciitis exist: lesions associated with a vessel wall (intravascular fasciitis), lesions with areas of bone formation (ossifying fasciitis), and variants marked by a dominant population of large ganglion-like cells with prominent nucleoli (proliferative fasciitis or proliferative myositis, depending upon the location of the lesion) (Fig. 13–52).[77]

Differential Diagnosis

Its self-limited clinical nature notwithstanding, nodular fasciitis has been an unrelenting source of confusion for the diagnostic pathologist. Neural lesions, the occasional metastatic sarcomatoid carcinoma, and fibromatoses have all been mistaken for nodular fasciitis at one time or another. Fibromatoses are typically larger lesions, with a more aggressive pattern of infiltration of the adjacent tissues. With regard to a malignant differential, nodular fasciitis

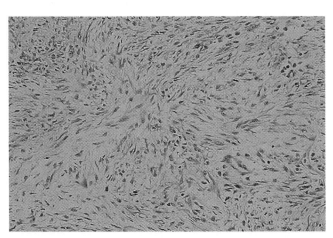

FIGURE 13-50 Architecturally, the hallmark of nodular fasciitis is a loosely fascicular arrangement of spindle cells set in a myxoid background (H&E, ×200).

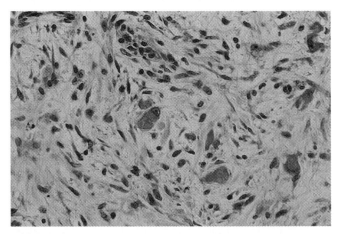

FIGURE 13-52 One variant of nodular fasciitis, seen here, is proliferative fasciitis. The central portion of proliferative fasciitis contains a mass of large cells with basophilic cytoplasm and prominent nucleoli (ganglion-like cells), which are each separated from their neighboring cells. The periphery of these lesions is more reminiscent of conventional nodular fasciitis (H&E, ×320).

does not manifest the degree of nuclear atypia or pleomorphism seen in most sarcomas; while mitotic activity may be found in nodular fasciitis, these mitotic figures are not atypical (that is, they are not bizarre, multipolar structures). Fibrosarcomas, monophasic synovial sarcomas, and malignant peripheral nerve sheath tumors are larger, more cellular lesions than are foci of nodular fasciitis. Perhaps the greatest overlap in light microscopic pattern is between nodular fasciitis and fibrous histiocytoma; in general, a somewhat greater variation in cellular appearance is the hallmark of the fibrous histiocytoma, while the cells of nodular fasciitis are a more homogeneous population. In addition, the storiform pattern quite prominent in fibrous histiocytoma is less well developed in nodular fasciitis.

Special Techniques

The spindle cell character of nodular fasciitis will, as noted above, sometimes invite consideration of other lesions, both benign and malignant, in the differential diagnosis. As a consequence, immunohistochemical studies may be used to refine a tentative diagnosis; nodular fasciitis will be vimentin positive, and often actin (both smooth muscle actin and muscle-specific actin, or HHF-35) positive as well. Importantly, nodular fasciitis should not be S-100 protein, desmin, or cytokeratin positive.

In the uncommon variants of proliferative fasciitis and proliferative myositis, the large centrally placed polygonal cells have been confused both with ganglionic elements (sparking consideration of a ganglioneuromatous lesion) and with rhabdomyoblasts (prompting consideration of malignant and benign skeletal muscle lesions). The periphery of the lesion usually retains its nodular fasciitis–like appearance, however, and so confusion should be minimized. Moreover, proliferative fasciitis/myositis will be S-100 protein and desmin negative on immunohistochemical study, which should aid in the resolution of these differential diagnostic problems.

Clinicopathologic Correlations

Clinically, nodular fasciitis is a paradoxical lesion. Its rapid development (typically described as a subcutaneous mass developing over a brief period of weeks to a few months) is often a cause for concern, raising the specter of a malignant process. However, a parallel may be drawn here between nodular fasciitis and a cutaneous keratoacanthoma: in both instances the rapid growth of these benign lesions actually outstrips the typical growth of their malignant counterparts, helping to support clinical diagnosis of a benign lesion.

The prognosis for nodular fasciitis is excellent, as these lesions may spontaneously regress after only an incisional biopsy; as a consequence, there is no pressing reason to aggressively re-excise them when

a previous biopsy is reported to have microscopic positive margins of excision. The local recurrence rate is quite low.

Hamartomatous Lesions

Gross Pathology

Depending upon the precise tissue type(s) involved, a hamartoma may be solid, cystic, or a combination thereof. Its contours may be either sharply demarcated or ill-defined; the latter gross appearance does not indicate an invasive aggressive neoplasm, but rather reflects its nature as a developmental defect. The mass-like proliferation of benign structures native to the area in question simply blends inextricably into the adjacent (more normally arranged) host tissues.[78–82]

Microscopic Pathology

By definition, a hamartoma is a mass lesion that, on microscopic examination, proves to consist of a proliferation of tissues normally found in the region in question; they are wholly benign, but typically are arranged in an abnormal architecture (often characterized as an "overgrown" appearance). For example, Figure 13–53 shows a lateral neck mass adjacent to the trachea (from which it presumably derived). On surgical exploration, the mass was well circumscribed. Microscopically, it consisted of an intimate admixture of chondroid islands and epithelial structures (and so resembled the more commonly encountered pulmonary hamartomas). No matter the tissue type involved, the key to recognizing a hamartoma microscopically is identification of its component parts as benign, architecturally abnormal (over-

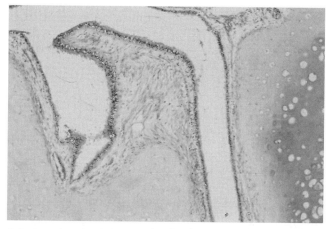

FIGURE 13–53 One example of a hamartoma, shown here, arose in association with the trachea and consisted of an intimate admixture of cartilaginous islands and benign columnar ciliated epithelium (an appearance reminiscent of the pulmonary hamartomas) (H&E, ×80).

grown), and indigenous to the area from which the biopsy was obtained.

Differential Diagnosis

In view of the fact that hamartomas are uncommon lesions, the clinical differential diagnosis will usually center around other slowly growing lesions, such as branchial cleft cysts, epidermoid cysts, and lymphangiomas. The microscopic differential will usually rest between a hamartoma, a choristoma, and a teratoma. Choristomas (or heterotopias) are perfectly normal-appearing tissues (that is, architecturally normal on light microscopic study) found in an abnormal location (in other words, they are not indigenous to the area in which they appear). The teratomas (considered next) are classically defined as masses derived from all three germ layers (both hamartomas and choristomas are usually composed of derivatives of one, or rarely two, germ layers) that are both foreign to the area in which they develop, and possessed of a capacity for continued growth. Thus, they are true neoplasms.

Special Techniques

The recognition of a hamartoma is within the province of the light microscopist, so special techniques do not play a significant role here.

Clinicopathologic Correlations

While no age is exempt from a diagnosis of a hamartoma, most of the cervical lesions are recognized in the first two decades of life. They are slow growing and painless and so present problems that are either cosmetic in nature or the product of their compression of adjacent structures. The hamartoma, by virtue of its status as a non-neoplastic mass lesion, lacks a capacity for unrestrained growth, and so its prognosis is excellent following surgical excision.

BENIGN NEOPLASMS

Teratomas

Gross Pathology

Benign teratomas, whatever their site of origin, usually consist of a predominance of cystic spaces, with a lesser component of solid tissue. These cystic spaces may be filled with colorless to yellow-green liquid, sebaceous material, or even hair. The solid areas are soft to rubbery and grey-tan to brown; on rare occasion, a grossly recognizable tooth will be formed within the wall of one of the cystic spaces. The masses overall may be quite large, rivaling the size of the head itself in some exceptional instances.

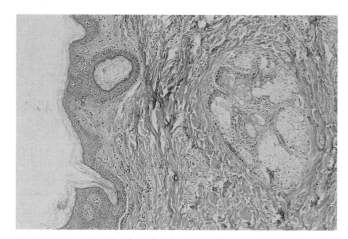

FIGURE 13–54 This field from a cervical teratoma contains a proliferation of keratinizing squamous epithelium with associated adnexal structures—and so resembles a dermoid cyst; elsewhere, however, this lesion contained areas of brain tissue, vascular tissue, cartilaginous islands, and both respiratory and gastrointestinal epithelium (H&E, ×100).

Benign teratomas are either circumscribed or frankly encapsulated masses.[83–95]

Microscopic Pathology

In its best defined form, a teratoma consists of contributions from all three germ layers—the ectoderm (including skin), the mesoderm (including cartilage, bone, and muscle), and the endoderm (including respiratory and gastrointestinal epithelium). These tissues are blended inextricably together, so that a given low-power microscopic field may include islands of cartilage, spaces lined by ciliated respiratory epithelium, brain tissue, and keratinizing squamous epithelium (Figs. 13–54 and 13–55).[83,88,91,92] The proportions of the relative components may vary widely, so a given benign teratoma may consist

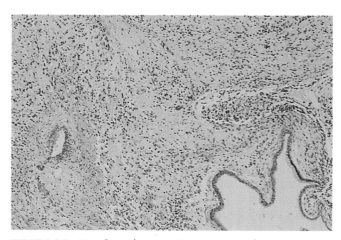

FIGURE 13–55 Central nervous tissue (*upper right*), gastrointestinal epithelium (*lower right*) and vascular tissue (*left of figure*) of the cervical teratoma from Figure 13–54. (H&E, ×100).

primarily of hair-forming epithelium, or of neural tissues, or any other tissue type. Clearly, in such cases thorough sampling may be important in uncovering the other (less well-represented) components.

Differential Diagnosis

The finding of all three lines of differentiation—ectodermal, mesodermal, and endodermal derivatives—serves to distinguish a teratoma from a branchial cleft anomaly, epidermoid cyst, hamartoma, or choristoma. Thorough sampling is mandated, however, to exclude the possibility of a potentially aggressive component such as immature neural elements or yolk sac tumor (considered later under the heading of malignant teratoma).

Special Techniques

The distinction of a benign teratoma from a choristoma from a hamartoma is a light microscopic exercise, and so special techniques will not add a great deal to the evaluation.

Clinicopathologic Correlations

The vast majority of benign teratomas will appear in the first year of life—many, in fact, are congenital lesions. The behavior of benign teratomas of childhood is well established, and they seem to lack capacity for undergoing malignant degeneration. When large, however, they may compress vital structures within the neck and may present some technical difficulties in complete surgical excision. As congenital lesions, they may be associated with maternal polyhydramnios and result in acute respiratory distress at the time of delivery.

Surgical excision of a benign cervical teratoma may be an easy matter (for smaller encapsulated lesions) or more challenging (for larger lesions impinging upon vital structures). When the lesions have been removed in their entirety with surgical margins free of disease, this procedure will prove curative. Benign teratomas are not metastasizing tumors.

Cystic Hygroma (Lymphangioma)

Gross Pathology

Incision of a cystic hygroma (either intraoperatively or at the time of initial pathologic examination) typically exposes a multilocular cystic lesion that contains clear fluid. Indeed, in light of the fact that lymphangiomas and hemangiomas may show some similarities on microscopic examination, pathologists are often anxious to learn from the attending surgeons the character of the fluid expressed at the time of surgery—clear, colorless, lymphatic fluid or bloody fluid. This interest is motivated by the obser-

vations that blood may be drained from what was initially a blood-filled specimen (and so mimic a lymphangioma from the microscopist's perspective) and that intraoperative trauma may cause bleeding into what was initially a lymph-filled lesion (and so deceive the microscopist into thinking that the lesion is best diagnosed as an hemangioma). These lesions are not particularly well circumscribed, and so a clear-cut plane of dissection may not be apparent at the time of intraoperative exploration.[96–113]

Microscopic Pathology

Taken as a group, lymphangiomas differ from one another by the size of the lymphatic channels formed, ranging from tiny capillary structures to large, gaping cavernous spaces (Fig. 13–56). The predominant pattern of cervical lymphangiomas is that of a cavernous lesion—that is, a profusion of large spaces that are either empty or filled with a colorless, finely granular material (lymphatic fluid) in which small numbers of lymphocytes may be found. These spaces are lined by flattened to attenuated endothelial cells with small opaque nuclei. The surrounding solid areas of a lymphangioma consist of loose fibrous connective tissue that may contain scattered aggregates of small mature lymphocytes and/or thin bundles of smooth muscle cells.[111–113]

One potential complication of a cervical lymphangioma is the development of secondary infection within it. As a consequence, the stroma may take on an increasingly sclerotic character, with patches of acute and chronic inflammatory cell infiltrate. When particularly pronounced, these secondary changes may obscure the underlying vascular nature of the process.

Differential Diagnosis

The clinical impression may take into account the possibilities of a branchial cleft anomaly, a thyro-

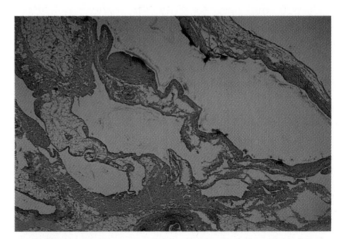

FIGURE 13–56 The typical cystic hygroma is composed of large spaces filled with colorless fluid and lined by flattened endothelial cells (H&E, × 100).

glossal duct cyst, or a teratoma in the differential diagnosis of a cystic hygroma. Microscopically, the differential will usually lie between a lymphangioma (filled with clear lymphatic fluid) and a hemangioma (filled with blood). As noted previously, the intraoperative characteristics of the lesion in question will aid greatly in making such a distinction. One point should be made here: lymphangiomas are not well circumscribed, and as a consequence their microscopic borders exhibit an infiltrative character that should not be confused with an invasive (malignant) growth pattern. The endothelial cells lining the individual spaces are small and nondescript, lacking the nuclear atypia, mitotic activity, and other attributes of a malignant tumor.

Special Techniques

Light microscopy is the key to confirming an intraoperative diagnosis of lymphangioma, leaving only a slight role for application of special techniques. Immunohistochemistry has not proven particularly helpful in distinguishing lymphatic from hemangiomatous tissues.

Clinicopathologic Correlations

The spectrum of lesions encompassed by the clinical term "cystic hygroma" ranges from small localized lesions, easily cured by simple excision, to extensive lesions extending from the base of the skull to the mediastinum. The latter lesions are not generally amenable to surgical cure. In view of the extensive nature of some of these lesions, they are probably best considered a form of angiomatosis (specifically, lymphangiomatosis)—and when particularly extensive should prompt clinical evaluation to exclude the possibility of lesions elsewhere (the skeleton, for example, or the viscera).[111]

As with benign hemangiomas (considered next), patients of any age may develop a lymphangioma, although the vast majority of cervical lymphangiomas are diagnosed between the time of birth and the child's second birthday. One well-recognized association of cervical lymphangiomas is with Turner's syndrome (a chromosomal abnormality with a 45 XO karyotype, short stature, and absent or rudimentary gonads, among other signs). Indeed, in stillborn infants, a finding of bilateral cervical lymphangiomas may be the only external clue to the presence of Turner's syndrome.

Small localized lesions are of only limited clinical import; the more extensive lesions, however, may pose significant problems. They can be difficult to control surgically and so may serve as foci for development of (potentially life-threatening) infections as they grow and ulcerate. When large, lymphangiomas may, by their very bulk, compress adjacent vital structures. Some regression in the size of con-genital lymphangiomas may be anticipated over the first few years of life.

The premalignant potential for extensive lesions of lymphangiomatosis is slight. It does exist, however, for chronically edematous lesions in the extremities. Chronic lymphedema can function as a precursor to angiosarcoma in patients with longstanding lymphedema, both congenital and postsurgical. In the neck, however, cervical lymphangiomas show no predisposition to herald angiosarcoma. These site-specific lesions appear to possess no significant premalignant character.

Hemangioma

Gross Pathology

Hemangiomas may be large or small, superficial or deep; despite these variables, all hemangiomas appear grossly as blood-filled cystic structures. Smaller lesions may appear somewhat circumscribed, but hemangiomas are not encapsulated.[111–120]

Microscopic Pathology

The microscopic patterns of hemangiomas include capillary-sized proliferations, larger (cavernous) proliferations, venous proliferations, mixed arteriovenous proliferations, or any combination of these types (Figs. 13–57 through 13–59). The vascular spaces are filled with erythrocytes and lined by nondescript flattened endothelial cells. As with the just-discussed lymphangiomas, hemangiomas are not well-circumscribed lesions, and so their borders often blend inextricably with the surrounding host tissues. Rather than indicate malignancy, this feature merely reflects the developmental nature of most of

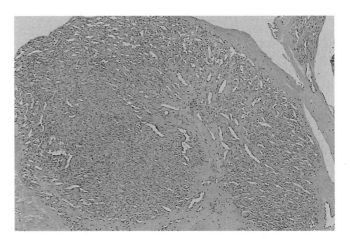

FIGURE 13–57　Among the patterns that may be adopted by a hemangioma is the lobular capillary arrangement shown here, in which larger caliber vessels supply alveolar groupings of smaller capillaries (H&E, ×80).

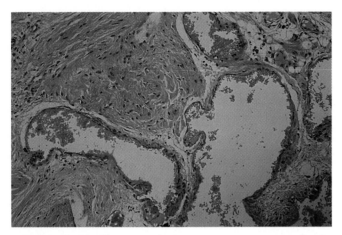

FIGURE 13-58 This venous hemangioma consists principally of large blood-filled spaces with thin muscular walls but no elastic lamellae (H&E, ×100).

these lesions and their formation in concert with the formation of the surrounding tissues.[111-113]

Differential Diagnosis

The practical differential problems presented by hemangiomas are few. Once grossly identified as blood-filled (not conduits for clear lymphatic fluid), it remains only for the light microscopist to confirm that they are cytologically benign. As with lymphangiomas, the microscopist must not confuse an infiltrative pattern of growth with unequivocal evidence of malignancy. Angiosarcomas exhibit nuclear atypia and mitotic activity, classical definitions of malignant tumors of other tissue types. The absence of these features should support a diagnosis of a benign vascular tumor.

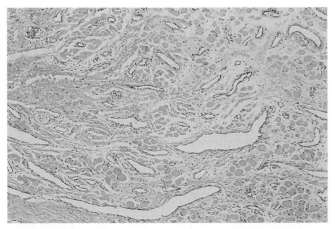

FIGURE 13-59 In angiomatosis, the proliferation of vascular spaces differs little, in a given microscopic field, from that seen in a hemangioma; the angiomatoses are defined rather by their extensive involvement of either a large surface area or multiple tissues (H&E, ×80).

Special Techniques

Immunohistochemical methods exist for endothelial tissue identification (see page 824). Hemangiomas, however, are well differentiated and render the use of these special techniques unnecessary. Light microscopy will serve quite well for diagnostic purposes.

Clinicopathologic Correlations

After the lipoma, the hemangioma is the most frequently diagnosed benign tumor arising within the soft tissues of the neck proper. A wide age range is covered by these tumors, from newborn to elderly. No age group is immune to a diagnosis of hemangioma, although most patients are in the first two decades of life at initial diagnosis.

One vexing feature of the larger hemangiomas is their poor circumscription, which can lead to great difficulties in achieving a complete surgical excision, resulting in an annoying incidence of local recurrence. The larger lesions are usually referred to as angiomatosis and, when particularly extensive, may suggest the possibility of a greater involvement of the body than is immediately apparent on physical examination.

The smaller hemangiomas represent simple cosmetic problems and are usually cured by simple surgical excision. In view of their poor circumscription, however, the larger lesions are more difficult to control surgically and so may recur when incompletely excised. Despite the application of other modalities—including sclerotherapy and radiation therapy—these larger lesions have proven in many instances to be stubbornly recurring processes.

Lipoma (Including Hibernoma and Lipoblastoma)

Gross Pathology

The archetype of a benign lipoma, on gross examination, is a soft, yellow, spherical to oval mass of adipose tissue that appears to be encapsulated. As these lesions are sometimes removed in portions, the capsule may be disrupted, hence, inapparent. A lobular pattern is often appreciable on cut section. The light microscopic variants of lipoma discussed here share this basic appearance (save for the hibernomas, which have more of a tan to red-brown cut surface).[121-125]

Microscopic Pathology

Lipomas of the type most often encountered in general practice are virtually identical to normal adult adipose tissue; that is, most lipomas consist of a proliferation of adipocytes with rather undistinguished peripheral nuclei surrounding a single large

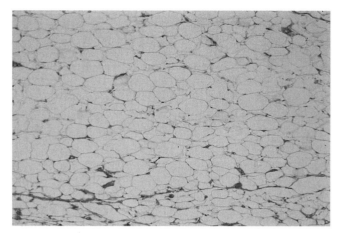

FIGURE 13–60 The usual lipoma consists largely of cytoplasmic aggregates of lipid material, with few nuclei apparent at this magnification (H&E, ×80).

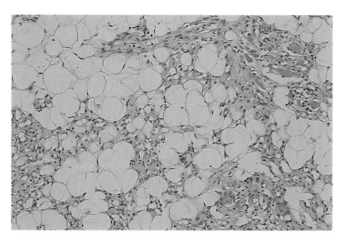

FIGURE 13–62 Among the variants of lipoma is the angiolipoma, in which capillary vessels may be quite prominent, overshadowing in some instances the adipose tissue component (H&E, ×120).

vacuole of lipid and small quantities of associated fibrous tissue and/or vasculature (Figs. 13–60 and 13–61). Variations upon this basic theme include lipomas with a more prominent fibrous stroma than that usually seen (fibrolipomas), with prominent blood vessels (angiolipomas; see Fig. 13–62), with admixed smooth muscle fascicles (myolipomas), and even with metaplastic islands of bone or cartilage (chondrolipoma or osteolipoma).[125]

When a lipoma is traumatized (not an uncommon event, in light of its superficial location), its stroma may become hemorrhagic or even necrotic; these secondary changes (particularly fat necrosis) may include a prominence of endothelial cells and the accumulation of foamy histiocytes—all of which may be mistaken for evidence of a sarcoma.

Two histologic (light microscopic) variants of lipoma are particularly pertinent here, as they are peculiarly associated with the cervical region. These variants are spindle cell lipoma (Figs. 13–63 and 13–64) and pleomorphic lipoma (Figs. 13–65 and 13–66). Neither of these lesions is particularly remarkable grossly; they are superficial, circumscribed yellowish masses presumed by the surgeon to be lipomas. On microscopic examination, the potential for a great deal of confusion arises, for the spindle cell lipomas consist of variable amounts of a cytologically benign spindle cell proliferation,[126,127] while the pleomorphic lipomas include scattered, profoundly atypical, large cells that may be mistaken for malignant cells.[128] In neither variant, however— spindle cell or pleomorphic—will mitotic activity or areas of necrosis be found. These light microscopic features, coupled with the superficial location of the mass, should aid greatly in recognizing these lesions as variants of benign lipoma.

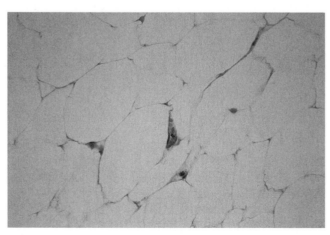

FIGURE 13–61 Nuclei are widely scattered in a lipoma and have an opaque chromatin pattern (H&E, ×260).

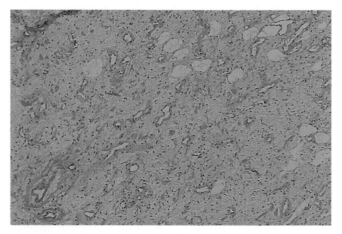

FIGURE 13–63 In a spindle cell lipoma, recognizable vacuolated adipocytes may be a minor component of the lesion, overshadowed by myxoid zones containing spindle cells (H&E, ×120).

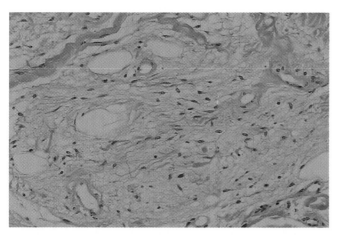

FIGURE 13-64 The spindle cell component of a spindle cell lipoma is a proliferation of dark monomorphous oval cells set in a myxoid background; occasional adipocytes are present, as here—a finding that sometimes invites confusion with a spindle cell tumor invading fat (H&E, ×200).

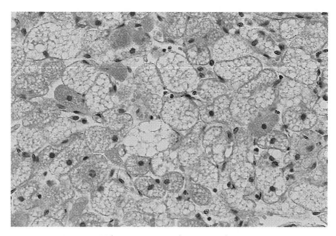

FIGURE 13-67 Hibernomas are benign adipose tissue tumors that consist of a sheet-like proliferation of coarsely granular to finely vacuolated cells, reminiscent of fetal fat (H&E, ×180).

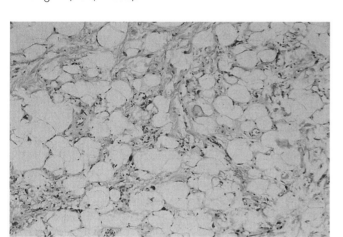

FIGURE 13-65 Pleomorphic lipomas, at scanning power, are marked by the presence of scattered hyperchromatic cells set against an adipose tissue background (H&E, ×80).

Another variant of lipoma that may appear in the head and neck region is the hibernoma. A hibernoma, as a pure lesion, consists of a lobular proliferation of granular to multivacuolated adipocytes resembling nothing more than fetal (brown) fat (Fig. 13-67). In many cases, the proliferation of hibernomatous tissue will not be pure, but will rather be admixed with mature adipose tissue, leading to diagnosis as a mixed hibernomalipoma.[129-133] As with other lipoma variants, hibernomas are well-circumscribed masses.

The last benign tumor of adipose tissue for consideration here is the lipoblastoma. This is a tumor restricted to the pediatric age group. By light microscopic criteria, it has much in common with liposarcoma (including the presence of multivacuolated lipoblasts and a myxoid stroma) (Figs. 13-68 and

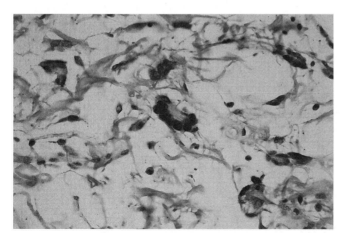

FIGURE 13-66 The nuclei of a pleomorphic lipoma are often characterized as floret-like—that is, they have multiple lobes arrayed about the periphery of the nucleus, are enlarged, and hyperchromatic. In contrast to a sarcoma, however, these are superficial masses lacking mitotic activity or necrosis (H&E, ×260).

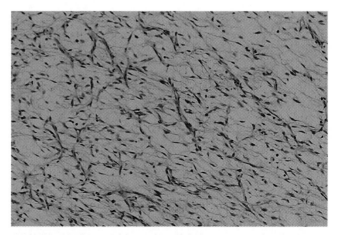

FIGURE 13-68 Lipoblastomas, while benign, may be misinterpreted as sarcomas. Here, for example, is a lipoblastoma with a prominent stromal vasculature and myxoid change, findings which, in an adult, would suggest the possibility of a myxoid sarcoma (H&E, ×120).

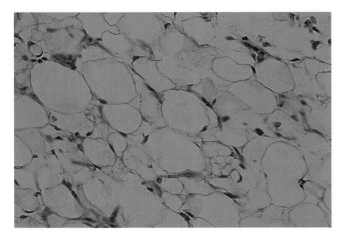

FIGURE 13–69 On closer scrutiny, it is possible to find multivacuolated lipoblast-like cells within most lipoblastomas—a finding that heightens the resemblance to a liposarcoma. These, however, are entirely benign tumors of childhood (H&E, ×200).

13–69). The behavior of a lipoblastoma is very different indeed from that of a liposarcoma. Lipoblastomas are benign tumors with no capacity for metastasis and only a limited capacity for local recurrence. When lipoblastomas are particularly extensive, the lesion is known as lipoblastomatosis.[134–137]

Differential Diagnosis

For differential diagnostic purposes, one critical characteristic of the majority of benign lipomas is their superficial location, in the vicinity of the subcutis. This serves to separate them from the liposarcomas, which are usually more deeply seated and with which they might otherwise be confused.

On microscopic grounds, the resemblance between a lipoma of the usual type and host adipose tissue is sufficiently close to make it one of the most commonly encountered differential diagnostic pairings.

Spindle cell lipoma may resemble a low-grade liposarcoma (in view of its apparent infiltration of mature adipose tissue), but its superficial location and lack of either pleomorphism or lipoblast formation will aid in its recognition.

Pleomorphic lipoma, like spindle cell lipoma, may suggest the possibility of a liposarcoma; again, its superficial location and lack of lipoblasts will serve to point the pathologist in the correct direction.

Hibernomas may superficially resemble granular cell tumors; however, the frank vacuolation of some of the hibernoma's tumor cells serves to differentiate them from granular cell tumors.

Lipoblastoma is best thought of as a histologically immature form of lipoma, one in which occasional multivacuolated cells are found. Here, it is the patient's age in particular that leads the pathologist towards the correct diagnosis.

Special Techniques

The lipomas of the usual type are handily managed by light microscopy alone, without the aid of ancillary diagnostic testing.

Clinicopathologic Correlations

The lipoma is probably the most common benign soft-tissue lesion excised from the cervical region (hemangiomas increase in incidence as attention shifts from the neck proper to the cutaneous regions of the head and neck). Both the lipomas of the usual type and the light microscopic variants thereof are seen more often in adulthood than in childhood. The only exception to this generalization is the lipoblastoma, which is an exclusively pediatric tumor. The spindle cell and the pleomorphic variants of lipoma are peculiarly common in the vicinity of the posterior neck and usually develop in older male patients; the other lipoma variants show no sex predilection.

A rare clinical condition pertinent here is Madelung's disease (benign symmetrical lipomatosis). This is a disease of older men, in which a soft tissue mass enlarges the neck symmetrically. This mass proves, on light microscopic study, to be mature adipose tissue, and the pathologist will usually diagnose it as consistent with a lipoma.[138–141]

Lipomas are benign tumors, which do not appear to undergo "malignant degeneration." We have seen, however, that it can be difficult to distinguish lipoma from host adipose tissue on both gross and microscopic grounds, so in some patients it may be difficult to delineate a clear plane of surgical dissection. In those patients, an incomplete excision may result in a local recurrence of the lipoma some years later. This uncommon event should provoke skepticism; that is, sections of the original lesion as well as a thorough sampling of the recurrent mass should be reviewed to exclude the possibility of well-differentiated liposarcoma. An occasional recurrent lipoma will be encountered, however, and in such an instance, complete surgical excision will be curative.

Fibrous Histiocytoma

Gross Pathology

The cutaneous fibrous histiocytomas (often called dermatofibromas) are rather small lesions with an appreciable degree of circumscription and yellow-grey cut surfaces.[142–148]

The more deeply seated fibrous histiocytomas may arise in the cervical region, albeit much less often than the cutaneous ones. These deeper lesions are often larger than their cutaneous counterparts, but they possess similar circumscribed contours and a yellow-grey cut surface.

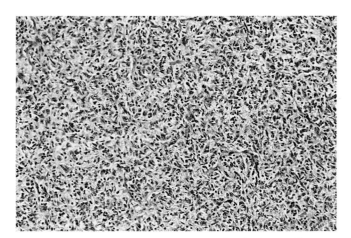

FIGURE 13–70 The polygonal to oval cells of a benign fibrous histiocytoma are arranged in a well-developed storiform pattern (H&E, ×160).

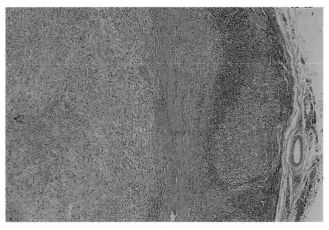

FIGURE 13–72 Angiomatoid fibrous histiocytomas are arranged in a distinct way. A dense fibrous capsule surrounds an internal lymphoid infiltrate at right and an interior proliferation of relatively monomorphous histiocytic cells at left (H&E, ×80).

Microscopic Pathology

The principal cell type comprising the fibrous histiocytoma is the spindle cell; these spindle cells are arranged in short bundles, or fascicles, which meet in a crisscrossing pattern described as "woven" or "storiform." These are, in turn, associated with a collagenous matrix. Interspersed among these fascicles of spindle cells are chronic inflammatory cells, usually small mature lymphocytes, with lesser numbers of plasma cells (Figs. 13–70 and 13–71). Scattered polygonal cells (particularly at the periphery) often occur; these may contain lipid material or hemosiderin pigment.[147,148]

The angiomatoid fibrous histiocytoma is a fibrohistiocytic lesion that has been reclassified in only the past few years—taken out of the malignant category. It consists of a peripheral fibrous capsule surrounding lymphoid infiltrate and a central prolifera-

tion of rather bland monomorphous histiocytic elements (Figs. 13–72 and 13–73).[149–152]

Differential Diagnosis

The spindled character of a benign fibrous histiocytoma may invite consideration of nodular fasciitis (a more myxoid, less collagenous lesion); a neural tumor (S-100 protein positive); a smooth muscle tumor (desmin positive); or dermatofibrosarcoma protuberans (paradoxically, a more monomorphous, repetitively storiform lesion than a fibrous histiocytoma).

Special Techniques

In general, recognition of a fibrous histiocytoma is a light microscopic exercise. The immunoprofile of a fibrous histiocytoma may be helpful in some cases,

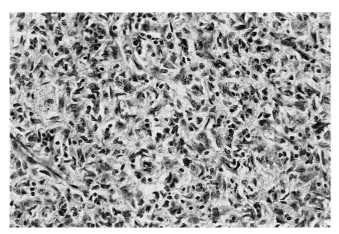

FIGURE 13–71 On close scrutiny, the cells of a benign fibrous histiocytoma manifest a slight variation in size and staining features (paradoxically, a greater variation than that seen in dermatofibrosarcoma protuberans, a low-grade malignancy) (H&E, ×200).

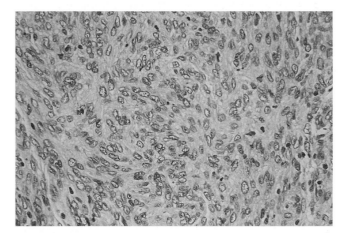

FIGURE 13–73 The central histiocytic cells of an angiomatoid fibrous histiocytoma are monomorphous, with scattered mitotic figures and an arrangement less firmly grounded in a rigid storiform pattern than that seen in conventional fibrous histiocytomas (H&E, ×200).

however. Fibrous histiocytomas are factor XIIIa–positive, but are negative for desmin, cytokeratin, S-100 protein, and CD34.

Clinicopathologic Correlations

No associations are recognized between the development of fibrous histiocytomas and recognized syndromes or other tumor types. While these were at one time thought of as reactive processes, they are now believed to be true neoplasms. When incompletely excised, fibrous histiocytomas may recur locally; they are not, however, premalignant and so local excision is usually curative.

The particular pediatric subset of angiomatoid fibrous histiocytomas was initially thought to be a subset of malignant fibrous histiocytoma. Further experience with this lesion has shown that, while it may recur locally if incompletely excised, it almost never metastasizes and for this reason has been reclassified as a nonmalignant lesion.

Rhabdomyoma (Adult and Fetal)

Gross Pathology

The gross appearance of an adult rhabdomyoma usually suggests a benign tumor, in that the mass appears to be encapsulated or at least well circumscribed. The same is true of fetal rhabdomyomas; their cut sections are grey to red-brown.[153–162]

Microscopic Pathology

Rhabdomyomas are divided on both clinical (age) and light microscopic grounds into two subtypes—adult and fetal. The adult rhabdomyoma consists of a sheet-like proliferation of large polygonal cells with capacious, finely granular, eosinophilic cytoplasm; in a very few tumor cells, intracytoplasmic cross-striations may be identified. The tumor cell nuclei are centrally located and usually possess prominent nucleoli. Peripheral cytoplasmic vacuolation is prominent, the result of glycogen accumulation (Fig. 13–74).[159,162]

While the cells of an adult rhabdomyoma are usually readily identified as benign skeletal muscle elements, the same cannot be said for the fetal counterpart. The tumor cells of a fetal rhabdomyoma are spindled, a finding suggesting to the unwary the possibility of a malignant tumor. (Remember that the age group in which the fetal rhabdomyoma is found is identical to that in which the majority of true rhabdomyosarcomas are diagnosed.) (Figs. 13–75 and 13–76). The fetal rhabdomyoma, however, does not manifest the same degree of cytologic atypia/pleomorphism or mitotic activity seen in rhabdomyosarcomas; this fact, coupled with its gross circumscription (which would be unusual in a

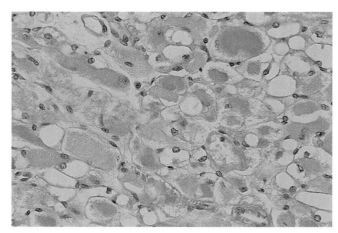

FIGURE 13–74 Adult-type rhabdomyomas are distinctive lesions, in that their component cells are large polygonal cells with abundant brightly eosinophilic cytoplasm and numerous large areas of cytoplasmic clearing (H&E, ×200).

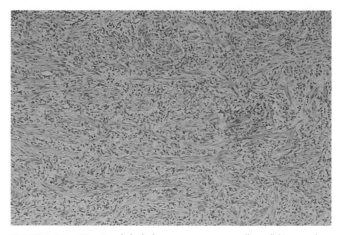

FIGURE 13–75 Fetal rhabdomyomas are spindle cell lesions that lack both a striking degree of nuclear atypia and mitotic activity (and so differ from another more common pediatric tumor, the rhabdomyosarcoma) (H&E, ×80).

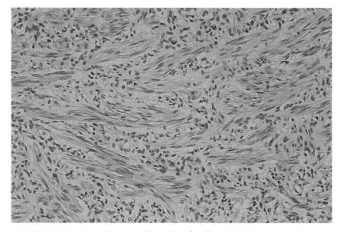

FIGURE 13–76 The spindle cells of a fetal rhabdomyoma have eosinophilic cytoplasm and are arranged in short fascicles (H&E, ×160).

rhabdomyosarcoma), should aid in correctly identifying these tumors.[158,162]

Differential Diagnosis

The critical differential diagnostic consideration here lies between the rhabdomyoma and the rhabdomyosarcoma. In general, rhabdomyosarcomas are more pleomorphic, mitotically active, and infiltrative lesions than are rhabdomyomas.

Special Techniques

The adult-type rhabdomyomas may contain cytoplasmic granules (corresponding ultrastructurally to myoid type Z-band material). This feature is well shown (when present) by histochemical staining with phosphotungstic acid–hematoxylin. As the fetal type of rhabdomyoma is a more primitive sort of proliferation, the cytoplasm does not usually contain such structures. While adult rhabdomyomas are usually readily recognized as muscular in origin, fetal rhabdomyomas occasionally are confused with other spindle cell proliferations. Immunohistochemical staining with antibody to desmin will serve to confirm the myoid nature of the lesion (Fig. 13–77).

Clinicopathologic Correlations

While cardiac rhabdomyomas have been associated with tuberous sclerosis, no such association has been reported with extracardiac rhabdomyomas. Rhabdomyomas of the adult type are more common than fetal rhabdomyomas. Both types are usually solitary masses, but on occasion are multifocal, not to be confused with metastasizing malignant lesions. While benign, rhabdomyomas may recur locally if incompletely excised; they are not, however, premalignant lesions.

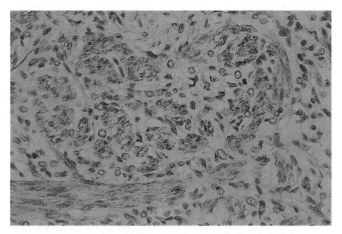

FIGURE 13–77 Should the myoid nature of a fetal rhabdomyoma be in question, the positive desmin staining of rhabdomyomas as shown here should help to resolve any confusion in that regard (antibody to desmin, ×160).

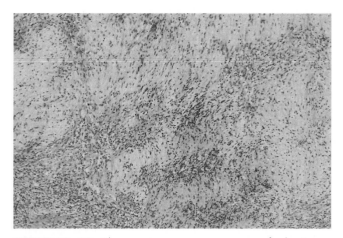

FIGURE 13–78 The scanning power appearance of a benign schwannoma is dominated by a pattern of alternating light (less cellular Antoni B) and dark (more cellular Antoni A) areas (H&E, ×80).

Schwannoma

Gross Pathology

The schwannoma, or neurilemmoma, is usually received by the pathologist as an intact encapsulated mass with a firm rubbery texture; in some instances, an attached nerve of origin is identified as well. The cut section is grey-tan and glistening; small cysts may be noted.[163–172]

Microscopic Pathology

Schwannomas are spindle cell lesions. The classic microscopic pattern of a schwannoma is made up of two zones: the Antoni A areas (marked by a rather dense proliferation of short fascicles of spindle cells) and the Antoni B areas (less densely populated, more myxoid regions) (Figs. 13–78 and 13–79). The

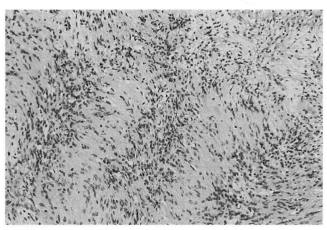

FIGURE 13–79 The nuclei of a benign schwannoma align themselves in areas in parallel arrays of palisading nuclei (Verocay bodies) (H&E, ×120).

individual tumor cells are small, with pointed nuclei and occasional wavy or buckled contours. In addition to these mixed Antoni A and B areas are thick-walled vessels, areas of nuclei aligning themselves into parallel arrays (Verocay bodies), and scattered inflammatory cells.[171,172]

One peculiar degenerative change may occur in schwannomas—the microscopic appearance often designated as "ancient change." This pattern encompasses a modicum of nuclear atypia among the tumor cell nuclei, areas of necrosis or cyst formation, and even scattered mitotic figures. Lacking, however, are the infiltrative (invasive) borders and atypical mitoses of a sarcoma, and so distinction from a malignant process remains possible, albeit difficult in some cases.

Another variant of schwannoma is the cellular schwannoma, marked by a greater degree of cellularity than usually seen in schwannomas. These variants are still well circumscribed, however, and follow a benign course.[172]

On rare occasion a schwannoma will grossly adopt a plexiform pattern (and so resemble the plexiform neurofibromas of von Recklinghausen's disease). Plexiform schwannomas, however, are not associated with neurofibromatosis.

Differential Diagnosis

Confusion with other spindle cell lesions is possible; however, positive immunohistochemical staining with antibody to S-100 protein should serve to distinguish these lesions from myoid and fibrous proliferations. When present, "ancient change" may cause some confusion with a malignancy; however, the circumscription and small size of a schwannoma aid in its recognition. It is not always comfortable to assign a given tumor to either the schwannoma or neurofibroma category, owing to overlapping features of both lesions; when this occurs, a simple designation of "benign peripheral nerve sheath tumor" will suffice.

Special Techniques

When faced with a tiny biopsy sampling containing a nondescript proliferation of benign spindle cells, the pathologist may find support for a diagnosis of benign peripheral nerve sheath tumor in a strong diffuse nuclear positivity of the tumor cells with antibody to S-100 protein.

Clinicopathologic Correlations

While it is not impossible to find schwannomas in patients with von Recklinghausen's (neurofibromato-sis), it is uncommon. The vast majority of benign peripheral nerve sheath tumors that develop in these patients prove to be neurofibromas (considered next).

Classically, schwannomas were thought of as solitary lesions. Of late, however, it has become apparent that multiple lesions—known as schwannomatosis—may affect some rare individuals just as multiple neurofibromas may be found in patients with neurofibromatosis. In contrast to neurofibromatosis (NF1), however, the lesions of schwannomatosis do not appear to be premalignant and do not seem to be a manifestation of neurofibromatosis.[173-175]

The schwannoma is a benign lesion, with little or no propensity for undergoing malignant degeneration. Complete surgical excision may be difficult in some instances, however, and incompletely excised lesions may recur locally.

Neurofibroma

Gross Pathology

Unlike schwannomas, neurofibromas are unencapsulated but remain well circumscribed nevertheless. They are firm masses with grey-tan myxoid cut surfaces. An associated nerve may be excised at the same time as the neurofibroma.[176-181]

Microscopic Pathology

Like schwannomas, neurofibromas are derivatives of Schwann cells and so consist microscopically of a proliferation of benign spindle cells. Neurofibromas differ from schwannomas in their lack of division into relatively more cellular and relatively less cellular Antoni A and B areas. The pattern of a neurofibroma is marked instead by a homogeneity from one area to another, a profusion of monomorphous spindle cells (some showing "wavy" or "buckled" nuclear contours) (Fig. 13–80). The intervening stroma is myxoid, with small numbers of chronic inflammatory cells interspersed throughout.[171,172]

Two variants of neurofibroma have been delineated: plexiform and diffuse. Plexiform neurofibromas are defined by their gross characteristics. Let us say that they are multinodular (contrast with usual presentation of solitary neurofibroma as single dominant mass) and have been likened, on physical examination, to a "bag of worms" (Fig. 13–81). Diffuse neurofibromas are not as well circumscribed as the usual solitary lesions, and so are more difficult to excise surgically (and thus, more likely to recur locally).

Differential Diagnosis

Should the neural origin of a neurofibroma be suspect, positive immunohistochemical staining with

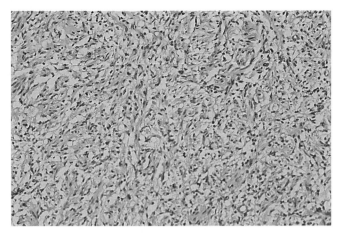

FIGURE 13-80 Neurofibromas lack the variable cellularity of the schwannomas; wavy pointed nuclei are distributed throughout a loosely collagenized stroma (H&E, ×160).

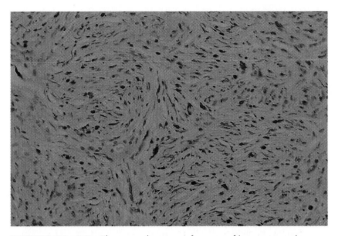

FIGURE 13-82 The neural nature of a neurofibroma may be confirmed by finding positive immunostaining of the tumor cells with antibody to S-100 protein (antibody to S-100 protein, ×160).

antibody to S-100 protein should distinguish neurofibroma from similar spindle cell lesions of fibrous or myoid origin.

Special Techniques

As with schwannoma, a tentative diagnosis of neurofibroma may be buttressed by a finding of strong diffuse nuclear S-100 protein positivity among the tumor cells (Fig. 13–82). In contrast to the usual case with the schwannomas (strongly positive in the majority of cells), however, neurofibromas exhibit a more variable pattern of S-100 protein positivity.

Clinicopathologic Correlations

A neurofibroma may be a solitary lesion, with no other underlying condition. But when multiple neurofibromas are identified in a given patient, a strong

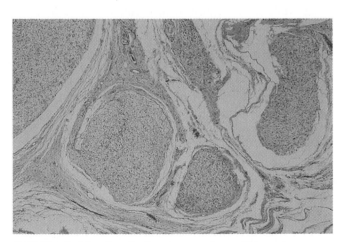

FIGURE 13-81 The plexiform variant of neurofibroma (associated with von Recklinghausen's disease) is recognized as a multinodular proliferation as seen here; the individual nodules have the appearance of neurofibromas of the usual sort (H&E, ×80).

suspicion of autosomal dominant neurofibromatosis (von Recklinghausen's disease) will be raised. Other supporting signs and symptoms of neurofibromatosis (including pigmented cutaneous lesions or café au lait spots; ocular abnormalities, including hamartomas and gliomas; skeletal lesions; and relatives with a previous diagnosis of neurofibromatosis) should be sought. Still, about half the cases are sporadic (new mutations).

Plexiform neurofibromas (defined strictly by their gross or physical examination characteristics) arise, for all practical purposes, only in von Recklinghausen's disease patients; diffuse neurofibromas may be seen sporadically or consistently in von Recklinghausen's patients.

In contrast to their benign nerve sheath cousins, the schwannomas, neurofibromas may undergo malignant degeneration, usually to a high-grade malignant peripheral nerve sheath tumor—rarely, to angiosarcoma and other exotic malignancies. Patients with neurofibromatosis (von Recklinghausen's disease, or NF1) are likely to see one of their neurofibromas undergo malignant degeneration: an estimated 10% of neurofibromatosis patients may develop such a sarcoma.

By contrast, it is decidedly uncommon for a solitary neurofibroma to undergo malignant change. When this does take place, the malignant peripheral nerve sheath tumor usually proves to be an aggressive high-grade sarcoma with a poor prognosis.

MALIGNANT NEOPLASMS

Malignant Teratoma

Gross Pathology

A malignant teratoma may be deceptively circumscribed grossly, raising the possibility of a benign lesion. However, on cut section, the mass reveals a variety of worrisome patterns including myxoid, hemorrhagic, and necrotic areas.[182–190]

Microscopic Pathology

In order to recognize a given malignancy as teratomatous in nature, it might seem reasonable to expect that areas of benign teratoma will be present, as well as the malignant component(s). Indeed, that is usually the case. This rule will be violated only in the setting of a pure proliferation of a form of tumor (such as a yolk sac tumor) associated exclusively with teratomas—in such a setting, the associated teratoma is presumed to have been overgrown and thus replaced by the malignant component.

The aggressive components of a malignant teratoma in a pediatric patient will most often consist of yolk sac tumor, a lesion marked by an arrangement of medium-sized polygonal cells in a variety of patterns, including cords, perivascular arcades (Schiller-Duval bodies), and solid regions perforated by numerous glandular spaces (Fig. 13–83). The individual tumor cells are rather similar to one another with regard to size and staining characteristics; in some lesions, scattered globular cytoplasmic aggregates of eosinophilic material are found.[191–196]

Immature elements in a cervical teratoma are controversial. Immature teratomas (recognized as a proliferation of primitive neural tissue, reminiscent to some extent of a neuroblastoma, as seen in Fig. 13–84) may be aggressive lesions when arising in the ovary. In the head and neck, however, opinions diverge over the import of such a finding. Immature teratomas may be less ominous in the head and neck because of the volume of immature neural tissue present. On the other hand, the greater the vol-

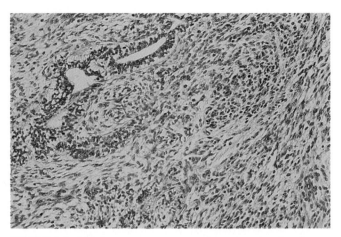

FIGURE 13–84 Immaturity in a cervical teratoma usually takes the form of an expanse of primitive neural tissue with neural tubules and closely packed small hyperchromatic cells (which differs from the less cellular cerebral-type tissue often seen in benign teratomas) (H&E, ×120).

ume of immature neural elements, the greater the likelihood of distant spread. For this reason, immature teratomas are considered here rather than with the benign lesions.[184–186]

In adults, the malignant elements are more likely to take the form of a poorly differentiated carcinoma. Yolk sac tumor is not a common finding in the adult lesion.[187–190]

Differential Diagnosis

The principal differential problem is in part theoretical, related to a malignant cervical tumor, apparently composed of several different tissues, arising in an adult. While such a finding in a child usually prompts a diagnosis of malignant teratoma, a similar finding in an adult is difficult for some to think of as a teratoma and so an alternative diagnosis such as carcinosarcoma may be offered. In general, the principal differential problem posed by the finding of immature neural tissue in a cervical lesion in a child is one of distinguishing an immature teratoma from a true neuroblastoma (primary or metastatic); here, thorough sampling so as to reveal the other teratomatous elements of an immature teratoma will be most helpful.

Special Techniques

Should a yolk sac tumor be under consideration, immunohistochemical staining with antibody to alpha fetoprotein may be of some aid; however, both true yolk sac tumors and their eosinophilic inclusions may fail to stain for alpha fetoprotein, and so a negative result does not exclude this diagnosis.

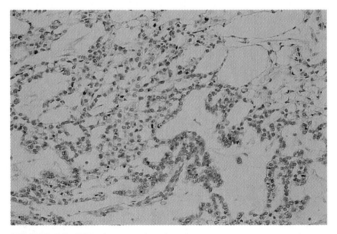

FIGURE 13–83 A cervical malignant teratoma may contain a variety of malignant tissues; in children, the aggressive component is most often a yolk sac tumor as seen here—a proliferation of epithelial cells arranged in cords, trabeculae, forming large spaces, and surrounding blood vessels (Schiller-Duval bodies) (H&E, ×120).

Clinicopathologic Correlations

Malignant teratomas in newborns or pediatric patients are well-established entities; difficulties arise, however, with regard to adult patients.[197-201] Distinguishing between an adult carcinosarcoma and a malignant teratoma will, in some instances, be more a matter of opinion than one of right or wrong. The prognosis of malignant teratoma depends, in part, upon the definitions applied for recognizing these tumors in the first place. In children, teratomas with immature elements seem to have a less-aggressive course than do histologically similar lesions arising in the ovary. The same cannot be said for yolk sac tumors, however—these are fully malignant tumors, with capacity for local recurrence as well as metastasis. The same is true of other germ cell-derived malignancies (including embryonal carcinoma and seminoma) arising in the setting of a teratoma.

Setting aside for the moment the issue of distinguishing between malignant teratomas and carcinosarcomas, malignant teratomas in adults seem to have a uniformly poor prognosis, with the majority of these tumors causing the death of the patients involved within a few years of diagnosis.

Angiosarcoma

Gross Pathology

The most striking feature of most angiosarcomas on initial surgical incision is their highly vascular nature, and hence a propensity to bleed at a terrific rate both spontaneously and when incised. The hemorrhagic areas may form a single dominant mass (particularly in the deep-seated lesions) or may appear to be a multifocal process (especially in the more superficial lesions).[202-211]

Microscopic Pathology

The patterns an angiosarcoma may adopt will range across a broad area, from subtle proliferations of individual vascular channels separated by a loose fibrous stroma (more often found in cutaneous angiosarcomas) to more densely cellular proliferations of highly anaplastic cells immediately recognizable as some form of malignancy (more often seen in the deeper-seated angiosarcomas) (Figs. 13–85 and 13–86).[113,210,211]

While modern soft-tissue pathology usually separates the hemangiopericytomas (benign and malignant) from the true angiosarcomas as a form of perivascular tumor, older classifications have considered these two tumor types together. A word about the pattern of the pericytic tumors is therefore appropriate here. The essence of a pericytic tumor is a distinctive arrangement of tumor cells about the prominent vascular spaces of the stroma, with closely packed tumor cells closely applied to the periphery of the thin-walled (often gaping) vessels (Fig. 13–87).[212-214]

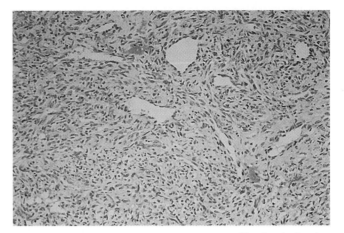

FIGURE 13-85 Angiosarcomas are most readily identified with the finding of true vascular spaces containing red cells lined by pleomorphic sarcoma cells, as seen here. (H&E, × 80).

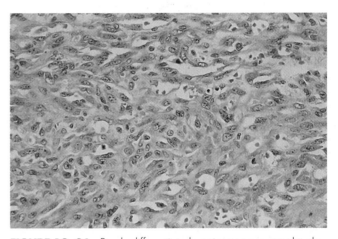

FIGURE 13-86 Poorly differentiated angiosarcomas may be deceptive lesions, particularly when the sarcoma cells adopt a polygonal shape and so mimic an epithelial lesion (H&E, × 200).

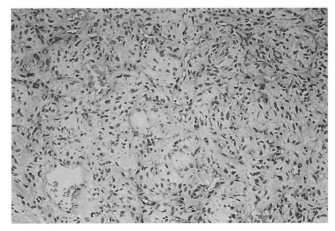

FIGURE 13-87 The architecture of a hemangiopericytoma is distinctive—the tumor cells show a greater density about the (abundant) stromal vessels than at a distance from them (H&E, × 200).

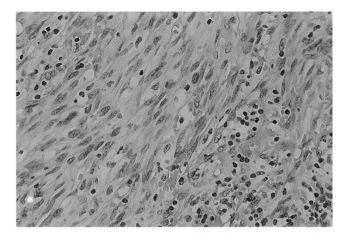

FIGURE 13-88 Kaposi's sarcoma differs from a conventional angiosarcoma in that it is often a less pleomorphic and less mitotically active lesion (H&E, ×120).

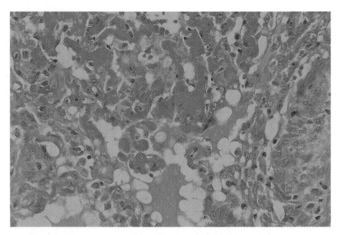

FIGURE 13-89 Benign papillary endothelial hyperplasia may, on high power study, raise a suspicion of malignancy, in view of the high cellularity and scattered mitotic figures (H&E, ×200).

Kaposi's sarcoma has been discussed of late as an entity separate and discrete from the conventional angiosarcomas, in light of its association with AIDS and speculation about its neoplastic versus non-neoplastic nature. A brief description of its appearance is appropriate here, however. While the earliest cutaneous manifestations of Kaposi's sarcoma (patch stage) are subtle, well-established lesions are spindle cell proliferations marked in most instances by a lesser degree of pleomorphism and mitotic activity than is seen in conventional angiosarcomas (Fig. 13–88).[210]

Differential Diagnosis

The presence of vascular channels lined by cytologically atypical tumor cells usually suggests to the light microscopist the possibility of a vascular malignancy. In the poorly differentiated angiosarcomas, the tumor cells may take on an epithelioid appearance (and so mimic a carcinoma) or a spindled appearance (and so resemble a fibrosarcoma). In both instances, it will be necessary to search for the true vascular spaces lined by sarcoma cells that will reveal the vascular nature of such a tumor.

Pericytoma-like patterns may be found in fibrous histiocytomas, synovial sarcomas, and mesenchymal chondrosarcomas; the diagnosis of hemangiopericytoma rests on the distribution of this peculiar arrangement of tumor cells throughout the entire tumor, not just as a focal phenomenon.

One particularly deceptive vascular lesion is papillary endothelial hyperplasia, a wholly benign process marked by an intensely cellular organization of blood clot; lacking here, however, is the cytologic atypia that is the hallmark of a conventional angiosarcoma (Figs. 13–89 and 13–90).[215,216]

Special Techniques

Immunohistochemistry may be used to aid in the recognition of some angiosarcomas—particularly the poorly differentiated ones. While Factor VIII is less successful at marking poorly differentiated tumors than benign vascular lesions, both CD34 and CD31 have proven to be useful in supporting a tentative diagnosis of a vascular tumor. Hemangiopericytomas and Kaposi's sarcoma also have proven to be CD34 positive in many instances.

Clinicopathologic Correlations

It is usually held that either malignant fibrous histiocytoma or liposarcoma is the most frequently encountered sarcoma in adults, while angiosarcomas are generally regarded as quite uncommon. However, angiosarcomas are rather more frequently seen in the head and neck region than are these other sarcoma types.[1] The head and neck angiosarcomas are usually cutaneous lesions centered about the face and scalp, but occasional angiosarcomas involving the soft tissues of the neck (either directly or by extension from adjacent cutaneous or laryngeal sites) have been diagnosed.[1]

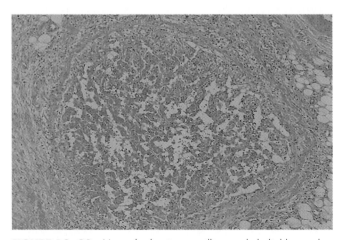

FIGURE 13-90 Here, the benign papillary endothelial hyperplasia shown in Figure 13–89 clearly resolves into an intravascular process—in essence, an organizing blood clot (H&E, ×80).

An association between tobacco or alcohol use and angiosarcoma development has not been drawn. A very few angiosarcomas have developed in the setting of neurofibromatosis, but this is an extraordinary association. A previous course of radiation therapy will, in a minority of patients, be associated with the subsequent development of an angiosarcoma. Angiosarcomas are extremely aggressive tumors, and so the likelihood is great that patients with angiosarcomas, no matter what the precise histologic subtype, will ultimately succumb to their disease. The 5-year survival for conventional angiosarcomas is no more than approximately 15%.

Liposarcoma

Gross Pathology

A liposarcoma is usually a large mass that may appear deceptively circumscribed; on cut section, the mass may have a yellow or shiny grey myxoid appearance (lower-grade tumors) or an extensively necrotic, hemorrhagic appearance (high-grade liposarcomas).[217-224]

Microscopic Pathology

Well-differentiated (low-grade) lipoma-like liposarcoma has many areas resembling mature adipose tissue; among them, however, are scattered large hyperchromatic cells and occasional lipoblasts (defined in the following paragraph) (Fig. 13–91). A variation on this basic theme is the sclerosing liposarcoma, another low-grade liposarcoma distinguished by its abundance of fibrous stroma with scattered tumor cells (Fig. 13–92). Myxoid liposarcomas are another type of low-grade liposarcoma, defined by their prominent plexiform vasculature (described by some

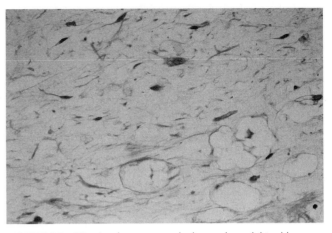

FIGURE 13–92 Another pattern which may be exhibited by a low-grade (well-differentiated) liposarcoma is the sclerosing pattern, in which scattered hyperchromatic tumor cells and multivacuolated lipoblasts are distributed throughout a relatively acellular stroma (H&E, ×200).

as a "chicken wire" pattern of vessels), stromal myxoid change, and scattered lipoblasts (Figs. 13–93 and 13–94). The round cell liposarcoma is a high-grade tumor with a profusion of closely packed, poorly differentiated small round cells and scattered lipoblasts (Fig. 13–95). Finally, the pleomorphic liposarcoma is a highly anaplastic tumor with scattered lipoblasts but many other areas suggestive only of a high-grade sarcoma (not further subclassified) (Fig. 13–96).[217,223,224]

Irrespective of histologic subtype or grade, the hallmark of a liposarcoma is the presence of lipoblasts, which are defined as tumor cells containing one or more lipid vacuoles that indent and displace the nuclei to the cell's periphery.

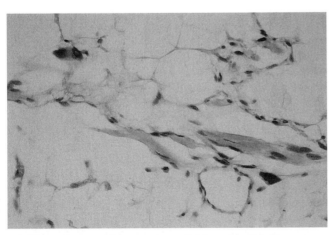

FIGURE 13–91 The low-grade (well-differentiated) liposarcomas may adopt a variety of patterns; here, a lipoma-like liposarcoma is seen—a tumor marked by numerous benign-appearing adipocytes, with only scattered enlarged hyperchromatic cells recognizable as malignant (H&E, ×200).

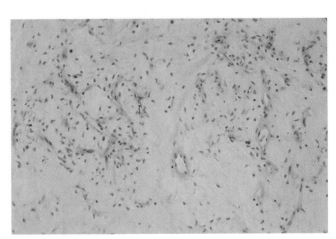

FIGURE 13–93 A myxoid liposarcoma is first recognized on low power by its combination of a myxoid stroma with a prominent vascular pattern (described as a "chicken wire" vascular pattern) (H&E, ×100).

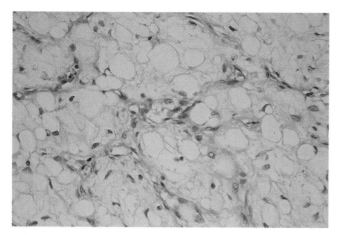

FIGURE 13-94 On close scrutiny, the prominent vasculature of a myxoid liposarcoma is joined by occasional lipoblasts (usually univacuolate lipoblasts) (H&E, ×200).

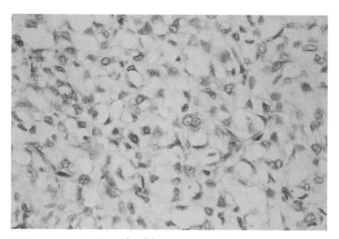

FIGURE 13-95 Round cell liposarcomas, like the example seen here, are much more cellular than are the lipoma-like or the myxoid liposarcomas (H&E, ×260).

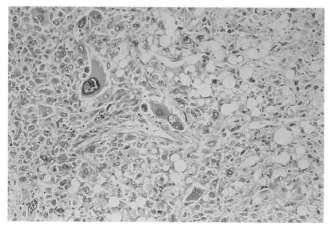

FIGURE 13-96 A pleomorphic liposarcoma combines high cellularity and a pronounced degree of cellular pleomorphism to yield a tumor which, absent the occasional multivacuolated lipoblast, may in some microscopic fields be difficult to recognize as being of adipose tissue origin (H&E, ×120).

Differential Diagnosis

The finding of cytoplasmic vacuolation is not exclusively within the province of the liposarcomas. Virtually any sarcoma (or, for that matter, many carcinomas) may exhibit vacuolar change, as may degenerative changes in a host of other lesions and tissues. The keys to recognizing vacuolar change in nonadipose tissue tumors include maintenance of a central location within the cells for the nuclei and a failure of the vacuoles to indent the nuclei in the "faux lipoblasts."

Lipoblastomas are quite reminiscent of low-grade liposarcomas; attention to the patient's age will aid in reminding the pathologist of the existence of these benign lesions of childhood.

Special Techniques

As with the benign tumors of adipose tissue origin, the liposarcomas are best diagnosed by light microscopy. Special techniques add little to their recognition.

Clinicopathologic Correlations

A link between tobacco or alcohol use and the development of liposarcoma has not been suggested. While the development of other sarcoma types has been associated with prior courses of therapeutic radiation, a similar association with the development of liposarcomas has not been drawn.

The prognosis of a liposarcoma is linked directly to the grade of the lesion. Low-grade tumors (lipoma-like, sclerosing, or myxoid liposarcomas) have a high likelihood of recurring locally but usually do not metastasize, while high-grade liposarcomas (round cell and pleomorphic liposarcomas) are more aggressive lesions, with a high incidence both of local recurrence and distant metastasis.

Fibrosarcoma

Gross Pathology

The usual fibrosarcoma is a large lesion with a firm to rubbery consistency; its cut surface usually ranges from grey to tan, with foci of hemorrhage or necrosis in some cases. A deceptive suggestion of circumscription is often noted, but these lesions are microscopically invasive.[225-231]

Microscopic Pathology

Fibrosarcomas are often described as "herringbone." That is, the tumor cells (which are close-packed hyperchromatic spindle cells with little in the way of intervening stroma) are gathered together into tight fascicles that intersect one another at acute angles, an arrangement reminiscent of the fabric pattern of

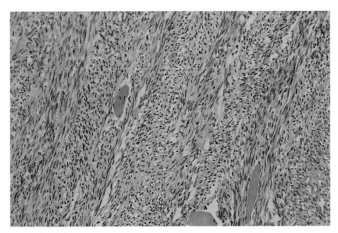

FIGURE 13-97 The long fascicles of hyperchromatic spindle cells in a fibrosarcoma are often described as a "herringbone" pattern (H&E, ×100).

the same name. Mitotic figures are numerous and readily identified (Figs. 13–97 and 13–98).[231]

Differential Diagnosis

A spindle cell malignancy may be a fibrosarcoma, a monophasic synovial sarcoma, a malignant peripheral nerve sheath tumor, or even a sarcomatoid carcinoma. Immunohistochemistry aids in distinguishing between these possibilities. Fibrosarcomas are rather inert lesions by immunohistochemistry, showing only vimentin positivity but no desmin, S-100 protein, or keratin positivity.

Special Techniques

The recognition of a fibrosarcoma is regarded by many observers as a process of exclusion: when faced with a spindle cell malignancy in which competing diagnoses such as sarcomatoid carcinoma,

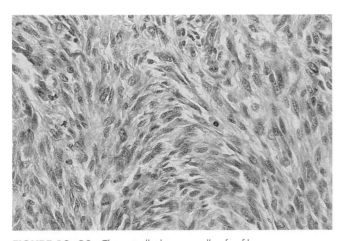

FIGURE 13-98 The spindled tumor cells of a fibrosarcoma are hyperchromatic with minimal cytoplasm; mitotic figures are abundant (H&E, ×260).

malignant peripheral nerve sheath tumor, and monophasic synovial sarcoma can be excluded, most pathologists will make a confident diagnosis of fibrosarcoma. To that end, immunohistochemistry is a valuable aid to differential diagnosis.

As the typical fibrosarcoma patient is an older adult, a tentative diagnosis of fibrosarcoma in a young adult should prompt consideration of a lesion such as the synovial sarcoma (discussed later), which is a form of spindle cell malignancy more often found in the young adult population.

Clinicopathologic Correlations

No association between alcohol or tobacco use and the subsequent development of fibrosarcomas has been drawn. Both therapeutic radiation and the presence of a pre-existing burn scar have been associated with the subsequent development of both soft-tissue and skeletal sarcomas (including fibrosarcomas) in some patients. Most fibrosarcomas are high-grade lesions, fully capable of recurring locally and of metastasizing. The 5-year survival is on the order of 50%.

Malignant Fibrous Histiocytoma

Gross Pathology

The typical malignant fibrous histiocytoma (MFH) is a bulky grey-tan mass that may be punctuated by foci of hemorrhage and/or necrosis. The myxoid subtype differs from this general description in that its gross appearance is dominated by a myxoid character.[232–238]

Microscopic Pathology

The patterns MFH may adopt are varied. They include the storiform-pleomorphic MFH, with an admixture of spindled and polygonal tumor cells arranged in a pattern reminiscent of that seen in the benign fibrous histiocytomas (Figs. 13–99 and 13–100); the myxoid MFH, in which half or more of the tumor sampled has a predominantly myxoid stroma with scattered tumor cells and a lesser volume of tumor resembling the usual storiform-pleomorphic MFH (Fig. 13–101); and the giant cell MFH, marked by a storiform-pleomorphic pattern with a superimposed infiltrate of numerous osteoclast-like giant cells. What each of these subtypes has in common is a profound degree of cytologic atypia among the individual tumor cells.[238]

Differential Diagnosis

The rarity of malignant fibrous histiocytomas in the cervical region makes such a diagnosis in this region suspect; to this end, efforts should be made to exclude other competing possibilities such as a sarco-

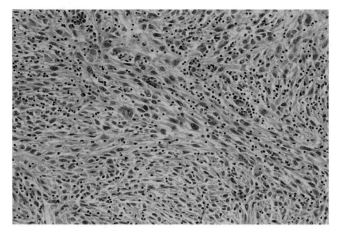

FIGURE 13-99 Malignant fibrous histiocytomas are most often arranged in a storiform-pleomorphic pattern, with both polygonal and spindled tumor cells (H&E, ×100).

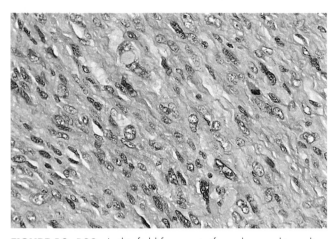

FIGURE 13-100 In this field from a storiform-pleomorphic malignant fibrous histiocytoma, the highly pleomorphic, mitotically active, spindled tumor cells are grouped in a fascicular arrangement (H&E, ×260).

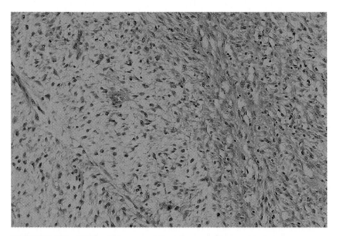

FIGURE 13-101 This myxoid malignant fibrous histiocytoma combines less cellular myxoid areas with more cellular areas typical of the usual storiform-pleomorphic malignant fibrous histiocytoma (H&E, ×100).

matoid carcinoma. MFH will diverge from other spindle cell sarcomas (such as fibrosarcoma or monophasic synovial sarcoma) in its heterogeneity; that is, while areas of MFH may show a focal fascicular arrangement of oval to spindle tumor cells, elsewhere these tumor cells will adopt different architectural patterns and often become polygonal in shape. These other spindle cell lesions, by contrast, maintain a fascicular arrangement of tumor cells throughout their extent.

Special Techniques

Immunohistochemical studies may be carried out to confirm that a given tumor is not actually an epithelial tumor masquerading as a sarcoma. MFH is, in general, negative for cytokeratin, S-100 protein, and desmin. However, there are occasional mesenchymal lesions showing focal cytokeratin positivity among scattered tumor cells, but this degree of positivity falls far short of the intensity seen in most true carcinomas.

Clinicopathologic Correlations

The typical MFH patient is an older adult, and so diagnosis of this lesion in children and young adults should be met with some skepticism. MFH does not appear to be linked to smoking, alcohol consumption, or any other occupational exposure. There is, however, an association between radiation therapy and the subsequent development of soft-tissue sarcomas, including MFH. As a consequence, when MFH is diagnosed in this unusual locale, it is of interest to know if the tumor is a therapy-associated sarcoma. MFH is usually a high-grade lesion, likely to recur locally and metastasize widely. Accordingly, surgical therapy is directed toward aggressive attempts at removal of the mass, while both chemotherapy and radiation therapy are directed towards achieving local and systemic control.

Malignant Peripheral Nerve Sheath Tumor

Gross Pathology

Grossly, a malignant peripheral nerve sheath tumor (MPNST) may resemble a benign neural tumor in its rubbery consistency and grey-tan cut surface but tends to be much larger than its benign counterparts. There may also be foci of hemorrhage and/or necrosis.[239-245]

Microscopic Pathology

The cellularity of an MPNST is high—higher, in fact, than that of the typical neurofibroma or schwannoma. In addition to this increase in cellularity, MPNSTs are further distinguished from benign

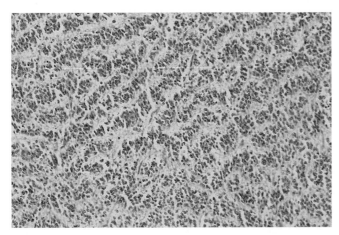

FIGURE 13–102 Malignant peripheral nerve sheath tumors are sometimes arranged in a palisading pattern; however, in contrast to a benign schwannoma, the palisading here is done by appreciably more pleomorphic and mitotic sarcoma cells (H&E, × 100).

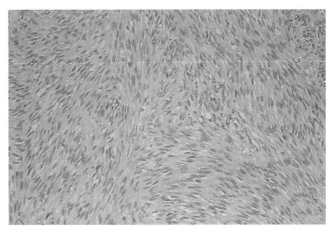

FIGURE 13–104 Spindle cell lesions often evoke a lengthy differential diagnosis; in the head and neck region in particular, attention should be paid to the possibility of site-specific tumors, like this pleomorphic adenoma (benign mixed tumor) (H&E, × 100).

lesions by the presence of pronounced cytologic atypia, numerous mitotic figures, and patches of necrosis; however, the tumor cells still, in areas, adopt the same wavy or buckled contours seen in benign nerve sheath tumors (Figs. 13–102 and 13–103). The hypercellular areas are interwoven with less cellular, more myxoid regions. Other secondary (not pathognomonic) features seen in neural tumor include hyalinization of the stroma and perivascular aggregation of tumor cells.[244,245]

Differential Diagnosis

The differential diagnosis of MPNST—typically, a high-grade spindle cell sarcoma—includes fibrosarcoma, monophasic synovial sarcoma, sarcomatoid carcinoma, and some malignant melanomas. Unless the MPNST is S-100 protein positive (which would

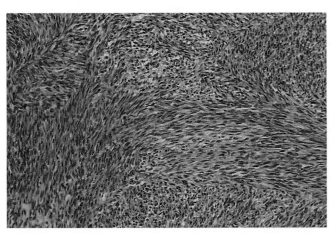

FIGURE 13–103 This malignant peripheral nerve sheath tumor possesses a fascicular arrangement of tumor cells, with alternately more and less cellular zones; again, the individual tumor cells are cytologically malignant and mitotically active (H&E, × 100).

not be characteristic of a fibrosarcoma), light microscopy is necessary to distinguish between a fibrosarcoma and MPNST. Melanomas present an even greater problem, and a clinical history of a previous cutaneous lesion is indispensable. Both sarcomatoid carcinoma and monophasic synovial sarcoma will show, at least focally, cytokeratin and/or epithelial membrane antigen–positive tumor cells by immunohistochemistry.

The less cellular areas of a MPNST may be mistaken for cellular benign lesions marked by some hyperchromasia of their cellular elements. See, for example, the spindle cell–rich area from a pleomorphic adenoma (benign mixed tumor) in Figure 13–104.

Special Techniques

In view of the distinctive differential diagnostic considerations just noted, it is often the case that immunohistochemical support is drawn upon to buttress an impression of MPNST; these investigations must, however, be interpreted with some caution. Approximately half of MPNSTs will exhibit nuclear S-100 protein positive on immunohistochemical study; thus, S-100 protein negativity does not by itself exclude a neural sarcoma. Moreover, while S-100 protein positivity is relatively specific for neural lesions, recall that malignant melanoma—another malignant tumor that may adopt a spindled configuration—is typically strongly S-100 protein positive. Finally, focal S-100 protein positivity may appear in other lesions such as synovial sarcomas; this fact must be borne in mind when interpreting a weak focal positivity for this antibody.

Clinicopathologic Correlations

While MPNSTs are not associated with prior smoking or alcohol consumption, there is a well-established link between von Recklinghausen's disease and MPNST development; thus, head and neck MPNSTs may be divided into two clinical groups—those in patients with von Recklinghausen's disease and those whose MPNSTs are sporadic tumors. Whether sporadic or associated with von Recklinghausen's disease (NF1), most MPNSTs are high-grade sarcomas and hence have a poor overall prognosis. The sporadic MPNSTs are more favorable (5-year survival on the order of 50% or so), while the neurofibromatosis-associated MPNSTs often prove fatal within 3 to 4 years after diagnosis.

Synovial Sarcoma

Gross Pathology

Synovial sarcomas, like many other types of sarcoma, may be deceptively circumscribed masses; their cut sections are yellow-tan to grey and may be cystic. Some lesions, particularly those with a high-grade light microscopic appearance, may be hemorrhagic and necrotic.[246-258]

Microscopic Pathology

The classic synovial sarcoma is a biphasic tumor, with malignant epithelial areas (usually gland-forming zones) intimately admixed with spindle cell sarcomatous regions (Figs. 13–105 and 13–106). A variant on this basic theme is the monophasic synovial sarcoma, in which the spindle cell component is the dominant or exclusive component of the tumor, with little in the way of recognizable glandular areas. The existence of monophasic epithelial predominant synovial sarcomas has been proposed, but these are such exotic tumors as to warrant no further consideration here.[258]

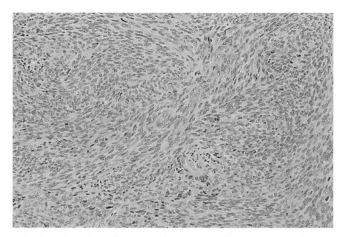

FIGURE 13-106 The monophasic synovial sarcomas are deceptive lesions, insofar as their epithelial natures are submerged beneath a sea of spindle cells (H&E, ×100).

Differential Diagnosis

The biphasic synovial sarcoma is sufficiently distinctive, when deeply seated, to be difficult to confuse with another tumor type. When only the most superficial extent of a synovial sarcoma is biopsied, there is some potential for confusion with a form of cutaneous malignancy derived from adnexal structures (which may also give rise to biphasic tumors). In such a setting, knowledge that the tumor has its epicenter in the deep soft tissues will aid in its classification as a synovial sarcoma.

The monophasic synovial sarcoma, on the other hand, may be confused with a fibrosarcoma, a malignant peripheral nerve sheath tumor, or malignant melanoma; in this regard, immunohistochemical findings will aid in the exclusion of these other differential diagnostic considerations. Cytokeratin (and/or epithelial membrane antigen) positivity is typical of a synovial sarcoma (Fig. 13–107), and so

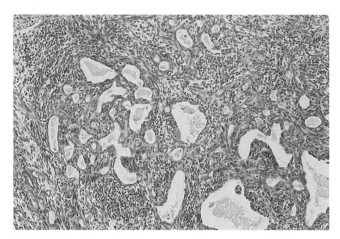

FIGURE 13-105 The classic synovial sarcoma is a biphasic lesion, with an intimate admixture of epithelial and spindle cell components (H&E, ×80).

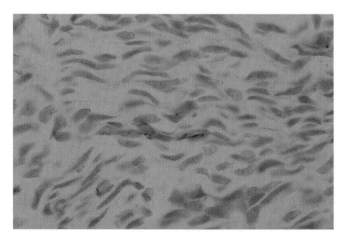

FIGURE 13-107 Immunohistochemistry will confirm a diagnosis of monophasic synovial sarcoma—as here, scattered tumor cells will prove to be keratin positive (antibody to cytokeratin, ×380).

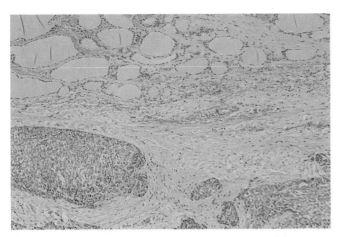

FIGURE 13-108 While rare, one very close mimic of the monophasic synovial sarcoma is the spindle epithelial tumor with thymus-like differentiation (SETTLE); this spindle cell proliferation, which arises in children, is associated with thyroid tissue (*top*) (H&E, ×80).

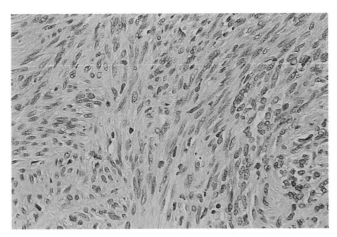

FIGURE 13-109 The tumor cells of a SETTLE are similar to those of a monophasic synovial sarcoma—including their positive immunohistochemical reaction with antibody to cytokeratin (H&E, ×260).

differs from the keratin negative fibrosarcomas, malignant peripheral nerve sheath tumors, and melanomas. Sarcomatoid carcinomas—which may also show immunohistochemical evidence of cytokeratin positivity among tumor cells—are usually more pleomorphic proliferations than are the monophasic synovial sarcomas.

The spindle epithelial tumor with thymus-like differentiation (SETTLE) is a rare, distinctive, lesion of childhood, similar to a monophasic synovial sarcoma. SETTLEs develop in association with thyroid tissue; they are a proliferation of spindle cells with admixed benign epithelial-lined cystic spaces. These spindle cells are keratin positive, as are the monophasic synovial sarcomas, which heightens the resemblance between the two lesions (although the intensity of keratin staining in a SETTLE exceeds that seen in monophasic synovial sarcomas) (Figs. 13-108 and 13-109).[259]

Special Techniques

The classic biphasic synovial sarcoma, with its intimate admixture of spindled and gland-forming areas, is usually readily recognized by light microscopy. More difficulties are presented by the monophasic synovial sarcomas, tumors that may prompt consideration of other possibilities, such as fibrosarcoma or malignant peripheral nerve sheath tumor. In this setting, a finding of at least focal cytokeratin and/or epithelial membrane antigen positivity among the tumor cells on immunohistochemical study may be employed to support a diagnosis of synovial sarcoma.

A distinctive chromosomal translocation—t(X;18)—has been found in the majority of synovial sarcomas. This translocation may be identified either by culture of tumor cells (which requires the harvesting and utilization of living tissue) or by means of polymerase chain reaction when only paraffin-embedded tissue is available. As neither of these techniques has as yet become universally available, most synovial sarcomas are diagnosed by light microscopy with or without the aid of immunohistochemistry.

Clinicopathologic Correlations

In contrast to most other soft-tissue sarcomas, which shun the regional draining lymph nodes in their metastatic pathways, the synovial sarcoma has a well-recognized propensity for involving nodes. This fact will be useful in planning definitive therapy. Affected patients are also younger than the usual sarcoma patients; often they are young adults. Synovial sarcomas do not seem to develop any more often in those who smoke or drink alcohol than in those who do not. Synovial sarcomas are relatively aggressive tumors; they have achieved some notoriety for their tendency to develop metastases several years after initial diagnosis. The 10-year survival is on the order of some 30%.

Alveolar Soft Part Sarcoma

Gross Pathology

Alveolar soft part sarcomas (ASPS) usually do not manifest the deceptive pseudoencapsulation seen in many other pseudosarcomas; instead, they are poorly circumscribed soft masses with a red to grey-white cut surface. Foci of hemorrhage and/or necrosis are usually prominent.[260-266]

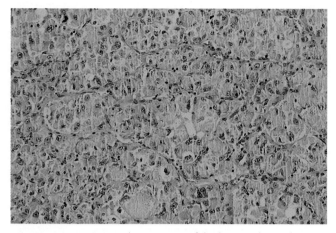

FIGURE 13-110 It is the grouping of the large polygonal tumor cells together into rounded aggregates that gives the alveolar soft part sarcoma its name (H&E, × 160).

Microscopic Pathology

The most striking feature of the ASPS is its low-power architecture. Large polygonal cells are grouped together into distinctive aggregates of a dozen or so cells (often characterized as an organoid arrangement, reminiscent of the pattern of some neuroendocrine tumors) separated by thin, richly vascularized, septa. These alveolar groupings of tumor cells typically show a loss of cohesion of individual cells centrally, and hence the alveolar groupings. Nuclei are central, with prominent nucleoli; mitotic figures are found only occasionally (Fig. 13–110).[265,266]

Differential Diagnosis

In view of the fact that ASPS are rare tumors in their own right and particularly uncommon in the head and neck region, it is perhaps not surprising that they may be misdiagnosed on initial viewing. Their alveolar arrangement may be reminiscent of a neuroendocrine tumor (including the extra-adrenal paragangliomas) or a metastasis from a primary renal carcinoma; immunohistochemistry (discussed next) will aid in making some of these distinctions.

Special Techniques

The architectural arrangement of the tumor cells in an ASPS will often suggest the correct diagnosis. In light of the likelihood of confusion of this tumor with other similarly arranged tumors, however, ancillary techniques are often relied upon. Histochemical staining has traditionally been employed to reveal the presence of periodic acid-Schiff–positive, diastase-resistant, intracytoplasmic crystalline material within tumor cells; however, only some 50% or so of ASPS show this histochemical attribute. An absence of cytokeratin and epithelial membrane anti-

gen staining by immunohistochemistry may be relied upon to support a diagnosis of ASPS over one of renal carcinoma, while the finding of S-100 protein positivity among the sustentacular cells of a neuroendocrine tumor differs from the usual S-100 negativity of an ASPS.

Clinicopathologic Correlations

Those ASPS that do arise in the head and neck are most often situated in the periorbital soft tissues or the tongue. As with synovial sarcomas, ASPS have a predilection for developing in young adults. The behavior ASPS is capricious. While they are clearly malignant tumors, those which do metastasize can do so either in the immediate postdiagnosis period, or many years after initial evaluation. No technique presently available can distinguish nonmetastasizing from early-metastasizing from late-metastasizing tumors.

METASTATIC TUMORS FROM AN OCCULT PRIMARY

Gross Pathology

A metastatic deposit may adopt any of a multitude of appearances—from the solid white-grey deposits of a metastatic carcinoma to a soft hemorrhagic deposit of metastatic renal carcinoma to a deeply pigmented focus of metastatic malignant melanoma.[267–275]

By definition, an occult metastasis includes the presence of an overt neck mass harboring a histologically proven metastatic neoplasm in the absence of a clinically detectable primary neoplasm. The most common clinical manifestation of a metastatic tumor to the neck from an occult primary neoplasm is that of a unilateral, fixed mass.

Microscopic Pathology

The light microscopic appearances of a metastatic deposit may range over the entirety of lesions considered in this volume and beyond, and so a unifying description is impossible here. Suffice it to say that the pathologist will be obliged to consider both architecture and cytology in the diagnostic process. Distinction must be made between a sheet-like proliferation of polygonal cells (possible epithelial tumor), a pattern of discrete round tumor cells (possible hematopoietic process), or a proliferation of spindled tumor cells (possible mesenchymal tumor or sarcomatoid carcinoma). Clearly, this is a process that is aided immeasurably by advance knowledge of the patient's previous medical history and status of present evaluation. Providing this information at the time of pathology consultation is vital. Failure to do so may result in an incorrect diagnosis, adversely

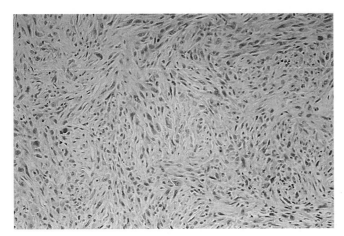

FIGURE 13–111 This cervical lesion has a storiform arrangement of pleomorphic spindle cells and so resembles a storiform-pleomorphic malignant fibrous histiocytoma; each tumor cell proved to be cytokeratin positive, however. This is a sarcomatoid carcinoma, a metastasis from this patient's renal carcinoma (diagnosed 5 years earlier) (H&E, ×120).

affecting the course of the patient's future care (Figs. 13–111 and 13–112).

The majority of metastatic tumors to the cervical lymph nodes originate from a head and neck primary tumor; therefore, the most common histologic appearance is that of a squamous cell carcinoma. Except for the metastatic thyroid papillary carcinoma, the histologic appearance of metastatic cystic (squamous cell) carcinoma to cervical lymph nodes does not allow confirmation of a specific site of origin. This is especially true for keratinizing squamous cell carcinomas, which could originate from any head and neck mucosal site. However, metastatic tumors with a morphologic appearance that includes nonkeratinizing or undifferentiated carcinoma are

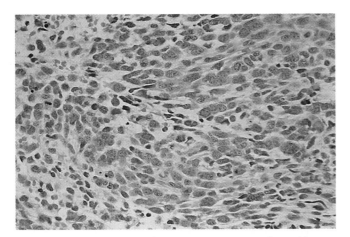

FIGURE 13–112 This neck mass raises a variety of possible primary tumors on light microscopy, including epithelial and neural lesions; it actually represents a metastasis from a previously diagnosed cutaneous malignant melanoma (H&E, ×260).

likely to have originated from Waldeyer's tonsillar ring.[276]

Differential Diagnosis

The differential diagnosis of a metastatic deposit often taxes the capabilities of the diagnostic pathologist, as the patient's clinicians not only want to identify the mass as a metastasis, but also to know from whence it derived—and this may be a difficult question to answer. Often, the best that can be offered will be an educated guess so as to direct further investigations.

Controversy exists between the diagnosis of metastatic cystic squamous cell carcinoma versus a carcinoma arising in a branchial cleft cyst (branchiogenic carcinoma). The criteria, established by Martin et al,[27] for diagnosing a brachiogenic carcinoma include the following:

1. The metastatic tumor occurs along the line extending from a point anterior to the tragus along the anterior border of the sternocleidomastoid muscle to the clavicle.
2. Histology supports origin from a branchial cleft–derived structure
3. Histology supports carcinoma arising in the wall of an epithelial-lined cyst.
4. A minimum of 5-year follow-up demonstrates no evidence of a primary source for this neoplasm.

Despite the fulfillment of these criteria, it is highly unlikely that carcinoma arises in a branchial cleft cyst.[278,279] Rather, all these cystic nodal lesions represent metastatic cystic squamous cell carcinoma most often originating from a primary tumor in Waldeyer's tonsillar ring. The primary Waldeyer's ring neoplasm may be so small as to defy clinical detection, but nevertheless it is capable of metastasizing.

Special Techniques

The full range of immunohistochemistry is brought to bear on the problem of the metastatic deposit derived from an occult primary when it is necessary to distinguish epithelial from hematopoietic from mesenchymal tumors. Unfortunately, in most instances cervical metastases will prove to be carcinomas.

Recently, Paccioni et al[280] evaluated 25 cases of occult metastasis to cervical lymph nodes for the presence of EBV by in situ hybridization following fine-needle aspiration biopsies of the neck mass and correlated with the histology of the surgical specimens (after locating the primary site of origin). These authors report that EBV was expressed in all seven metastases ultimately proving origin from the nasopharynx, while the remaining 18 cases (not of Waldeyer's ring origin) were negative for EBV.[280] The authors indicate that detection of EBV in cervical metastatic foci may assist in localization of the occult primary to Waldeyer's ring.[280]

Clinicopathologic Correlations

The nasopharynx, tonsils, and base of tongue, collectively referred to as Waldeyer's tonsillar ring, are the areas harboring the occult primary tumor in the great majority of squamous carcinomas metastatic to the neck.[281] Other common but less frequent sites of the occult tumor include the thyroid gland (papillary carcinoma), hypopharynx, and larynx (supraglottic region). Metastatic tumors to the neck originate not only from head and neck neoplasms but also may represent primary occult neoplasms from organ systems in the thorax, abdomen, and pelvis.[281] The most common primary site for a metastatic tumor originating from below the clavicle is the lungs. Virtually every organ may be the primary focus of a metastasis to the head and neck. A malignant neoplasm of the head and neck with an unsual histologic appearance or presenting difficulty in its histologic classification should alert the pathologist that the neoplasm may represent a metastasis from a distant site. The pathologist should not be lulled into a false sense of security by "playing the odds," as the possibility exists that an entirely unexpected primary site—such as the kidney or a cutaneous malignant melanoma—will prove to be responsible for the cervical deposit.

Treatment methods for the occult metastatic tumor are not fixed and are dependent on the clinical stage, location of the lymph node(s) involved, and histologic appearance of the tumor. A combination of surgery (neck dissection) and radiotherapy is the preferred therapeutic approach.[281–283] The single most important factor in prognosis is the clinical stage.[281,284] Other factors that correlate with prognosis include the location of the lymph node (e.g., supraclavicular nodal involvement has a poor prognosis) and the histologic appearance (e.g., metastatic adenocarcinomas have worse survival rates).

Common sense would suggest that the prognosis of a metastasizing lesion is likely to be rather unfavorable. While in most instances experience has borne out this supposition, there are occasional anecdotal reports of occult primary tumors that present with a solitary cervical metastasis and nevertheless remain compatible with a subsequent long survival. The presence of nodal metastasis with extension of the tumor outside the capsular confines of the lymph node and into perithyroidal soft tissues (extracapsular spread or ECS) is generally associated with increased risk of recurrent disease, increased risk of distant metastasis, and a reduction in long-term survival by as much as 50%.[285–296]

REFERENCES

1. Makino Y. A clinicopathological study on soft tissue tumors of the head and neck. *Acta Pathol Jpn.* 1979; 29:389.
2. Batsakis JG, Manning JT. Soft tissue tumors: Unusual forms. *Otolaryngol Clin N Am.* 1986; 19:659.
3. Setzen M, Sobol S, Toomey JM. Clinical course of unusual malignant sarcomas of head and neck. *Ann Otol.* 1979; 88:486.
4. Knight PJ, Reiner CB. Superficial lumps in children: What, when, and why? *Pediatrics.* 1983; 72:147.
5. Friedberg J. Pharyngeal cleft sinuses and cysts, and other benign neck lesions. *Pediatr Clin N Am* 1989; 36:1451.
6. Schewitsch I, Stalsberg H, Schroder KE, Mair IWS. Cysts and sinuses of the lateral head and neck. *J Otolaryngol.* 1980; 9:1.
7. Todd NW. Common congenital anomalies of the neck—embryology and surgical anatomy. *Surg Clin N Am.* 1993; 73:599.
8. Telander RL, Filston HC. Review of head and neck lesions in infancy and childhood. *Surg Clin N Am.* 1992; 72:1429.
9. Telander RL, Deane SA. Thyroglossal and branchial cleft cysts and sinuses. *Surg Clin N Am.* 1977; 57:779.
10. Gaisford JC, Anderson VS. First branchial cleft cysts and sinuses. *Plast Reconstr Surg.* 1975; 55:299.
11. Howie AJ, Proops DW. The definition of branchial cysts, sinuses and fistulae. *Clin Otolaryngol.* 1982; 7:51.
12. Chandler JR, Mitchell B. Branchial cleft cysts, sinuses, and fistulas. *Otolaryngol Clin N Am.* 1981; 14:175.
13. Golledge J, Ellis H. The aetiology of lateral cervical (branchial) cysts: Past and present theories. *J Laryngol Otol.* 1994; 108:653.
14. Doi O, Hutson JM, Myers NA, McKelvie PA. Branchial remnants: A review of 58 cases. *J Pediatr Surg.* 1988; 23:789.
15. Friedberg J. Pharyngeal cleft sinuses and cysts, and other benign neck lesions. *Pediatr Clin N Am.* 1989; 36:1451.
16. Little JW, Rickles NH. The histogenesis of the branchial cyst. *Am J Pathol.* 1967; 50:533.
17. Rickles NH, Little JW. The histogenesis of the branchial cyst II. A study of the lining epithelium. *Am J Pathol.* 1967; 50:765.
18. Choi SS, Zalzal GH. Branchial anomalies: A review of 52 cases. *Laryngoscope.* 1995; 105:909.
19. Fleming WB. Infection in branchial cysts. *Aust NZ J Surg.* 1988; 58:481.
20. Myers EN, Cunningham MJ. Inflammatory presentations of congenital head and neck masses. *Pediatr Infect Dis J.* 1988; 7 (suppl 11):S162.
21. Crocker J, Jenkins R. An immunohistochemical study of branchial cysts. *J Clin Pathol.* 1985; 38:784.
22. Jablokow VR, Kathuria S, Wang T. Squamous cell carcinoma arising in branchiogenic cyst-branchial cleft carcinoma. *J Surg Oncol.* 1982; 20:201.
23. Cinberg JZ, Silver CE, Molnar JJ, Vogl SE. Cervical cysts: Cancer until proven otherwise? *Laryngoscope.* 1982; 92:27.
24. Khafif RA, Prichep R, Minkowith S. Primary branchiogenic carcinoma. *Head Neck.* 1989; 11:153.
25. Foss RD, Warnock GR, Clark WB, et al. Malignant cyst of the lateral aspect of the neck: Branchial cleft carcinoma or metastasis. *Oral Surg Oral Med Oral Pathol.* 1991; 71:214.
26. Burgess KL, Hartwick RWJ, Bedard YC. Metastatic squamous carcinoma presenting as a neck cyst—differential diagnosis from inflamed branchial cleft cyst in fine needle aspirates. *Acta Cytol.* 1993; 37:494.
27. Hall SF, Dexter DF. Cystic cervical metastases are not branchiogenic carcinomas. *J Otolaryngol.* 1993; 22:184.
28. Carroll WR, Zappia JJ, McClatchey KD. Branchiogenic carcinoma. *J Otolaryngol.* 1993; 22:26.
29. Flanagan PM, Roland NJ, Jones AS. Cervical node metastases presenting with features of branchial cysts. *J Laryngol Otol.* 1994; 108:1068.
30. Ward GE, Hendrick JW, Chambers RG. Thyroglossal tract abnormalities—cysts and fistulas. *Surg Gynecol Obstet.* 1949; 89:727.
31. Judd ES. Thyroglossal-duct cyst and sinuses. *Surg Clin N Am.* 1963; 43:1023.
32. Pollack WF, Stevenson EO. Cysts and sinuses of the thyroglossal duct. *Am J Surg.* 1966; 112:225.

33. Allard RHB. The thyroglossal duct cyst. *Head Neck Surg.* 1982; 5:134.

34. Ellis PDM, van Nostrand AWP. The applied anatomy of thyroglossal duct remnants. *Laryngoscope.* 1977; 87:765.

35. Howard DJ, Lund VJ. Thyroglossal ducts, cysts and sinuses: A recurrent problem. *Ann R Coll Surg.* 1986; 68:137.

36. deMello DE, Lima JA, Liapis H. Midline cervical cysts in children—thyroglossal anomalies. *Arch Otolaryngol Head Neck Surg.* 1987; 113:418.

37. van der Wal N, Weiner JD, Allard RH, et al. Thyroglossal cysts in patients over 30 years of age. *Int J Oral Maxillofac Surg.* 1987; 16:416.

38. Shanmugham MS, Todd GB. Thyroglossal cyst in the elderly patient. *Ear Nose Throat J.* 1983; 62:215.

39. Katz AD, Hachigian M. Thyroglossal duct cysts—a thirty year experience with emphasis on occurrence in older patients. *Am J Surg.* 1988; 155:741.

40. Topf P, Fried MP, Strome M. Vagaries of thyroglossal duct cysts. *Laryngoscope.* 1988; 98:740.

41. Soucy P, Penning J. The clinical relevance of certain observations on the histology of the thyroglossal tract. *J Pediatr Surg.* 1984; 19:506.

42. Hoffman MA, Schuster SR. Thyroglossal duct remnants in infants and children: Reevaluation of histopathology and methods for resection. *Ann Otol Rhinol Laryngol.* 1988; 97:483.

43. LiVolsi VA, Perzin KH, Savetsky L. Carcinoma arising in median ectopic thyroid (including thyroglossal duct tissue). *Cancer.* 1974; 34:1303.

44. Joseph TJ, Komorowski RA. Thyroglossal duct carcinoma. *Hum Pathol.* 1975; 6:717.

45. Trail ML, Zeringue GP, Chicola JP. Carcinoma in thyroglossal duct remnants. *Laryngoscope.* 1977; 87:1685.

46. Fernandez JF, Ordonez NG, Schultz PN, et al. Thyroglossal duct carcinoma. *Surgery.* 1991; 110:928.

47. Van Vuuren PA, Balm AJ, Gregor RT, et al. Carcinoma arising in thyroglossal remnants. *Clin Otolaryngol.* 1994; 19:509.

48. Tew S, Reeve TS, Poole AG, Delbridge L. Papillary thyroid carcinoma arising in thyroglossal duct cysts: Incidence and management. *Aust NZ J Surg.* 1995; 65:717.

49. Hilger AW, Thompson SD, Smallman LA, Watkinson JC. Papillary carcinoma arising in a thyroglossal duct cyst: A case report and literature review. *J Laryngol Otol.* 1995; 109: 1124.

50. White IL, Talbert WM. Squamous cell carcinoma arising in thyroglossal duct remnant cyst epithelium. *Otolaryngol Head Neck Surg.* 1982; 90:25.

51. Yanagisawa K, Eisen RN, Sasaki CT. Squamous cell carcinoma arising in a thyroglossal duct cyst. *Arch Otolaryngol Head Neck Surg.* 1992; 118:538.

52. Deshpande A, Bobhate SK. Squamous cell carcinoma in thyroglossal duct cyst. *J Laryngol Otol.* 1995; 109:1001.

53. Mikal S. Cervical thymic cyst. *Arch Surg.* 1974; 109:558.

54. Fielding JF, Farmer AW, Lindsay WK, Cohen PE. Cystic degeneration in persistent cervical thymus. *Can J Surg.* 1963; 6:178.

55. Lewis MR. Persistence of the thymus in the cervical area. *J Pediatr.* 1962; 61:887.

56. Behring C, Bergman F. Thymic cyst of the neck. *Acta Pathol Microbiol Scand.* 1963; 59:45.

57. Sanusi ID, Carrington PR, Adams DN. Cervical thymic cyst. *Arch Dermatol.* 1982; 118:122.

58. Carpenter RJ. Thymic cyst of the neck with prolongation to the thymus gland. *Otolaryngol Head Neck Surg.* 1982; 90:494.

59. Yamashita H, Murakami N, Noguchi S, et al: Cervical thymoma and incidence of cervical thymus. *Acta Pathol Jpn.* 1983; 33:189.

60. Barat M, Sciubba JJ, Abramson AL. Cervical thymic cyst: Case report and review of the literature. *Laryngoscope.* 1985; 95:89.

61. Cure JK, Tagge EP, Richardson MS, Mulvihill DM. MR of cystic aberrant cervical thymus. *Am J Neuroradiol.* 1995; 16: 1124.

62. Brownstein MH, Helwig EB. Subcutaneous dermoid cysts. *Arch Dermatol.* 1973; 107:237.

63. Katz AD. Midline dermoid tumors of the neck. *Arch Surg.* 1974; 109:822.

64. McAvoy JM, Zuckerbraun L. Dermoid cysts of the head and neck in children. *Arch Otolaryngol.* 1976; 102:529.

65. Holt GR, Holt JE, Weaver RG. Dermoids and teratomas of the head and neck. *Ear Nose Throat J.* 1979; 58:520.

66. Leveque H, Saraceno CA, Tang CK, Blanchard CL. Dermoid cysts of the floor of the mouth and lateral neck. *Laryngoscope.* 1979; 89:296.

67. Tuffin JR, Theaker E. True lateral dermoid cyst of the neck. *Int J Oral Maxillofac Surg.* 1991; 20:275.

68. Young BK, Davies AS. A large dermoid cyst of the neck—case report. *Aust Dent J.* 1991; 36:206.

69. Smirniotopoulos JG, Chiechi MV. Teratomas, dermoids, and epidermoids of the head and neck. *Radiographics.* 1995; 15: 1437.

70. Wein MD, Caro MR. Traumatic epithelial cysts of the skin. *JAMA.* 1934; 102:197.

71. Love WR, Montgomery H. Epithelial cysts. *Arch Dermatol Syphilol.* 1943; 47:185.

72. McGavran MH, Binnington B. Keratinous cysts of the skin: Identification and differentiation of pilar cysts from epidermal cysts. *Arch Dermatol.* 1966; 94:499.

73. Konwaler BE, Keasbey L, Kaplan L. Subcutaneous pseudosarcomatous fibromatosis (fasciitis). *Am J Clin Pathol.* 1955; 25:241.

74. Dahl I, Jarlstedt J. Nodular fasciitis of the head and neck: A clinicopathological study of 18 cases. *Acta Otolaryngol.* 1980; 90:152.

75. Montgomery EA, Meis JM. Nodular fasciitis: Its morphologic spectrum and immunohistochemical profile. *Am J Surg Pathol.* 1991; 15:942.

76. DiNardo LJ, Wetmore RF, Potsic WP. Nodular fasciitis of the head and neck in children: A deceptive lesion. *Arch Otolaryngol Head Neck Surg.* 1991; 117:1001.

77. Enzinger FM, Weiss SW. Benign fibrous lesions. In: *Soft Tissue Tumors.* 3rd ed. St. Louis: Mosby; 1995:165.

78. Newmark H, Chantaratherakitti C, Sims CA. An osteocartilaginous hamartoma of the neck seen on computerized tomography. *Comput Tomogr.* 1981; 5:283.

79. Samuel J, Fernandes CC. Hamartomas of the head and neck—a report of 4 cases. *S Afr Med J.* 1985; 68:265.

80. Iyer RS, Shanthalaxmi MN. Cervical hamartoma. *Indian Pediatr.* 1990; 27:1310.

81. Rosai J, Limas C, Husband EM. Ectopic hamartomatous thymoma—a distinctive benign lesion of lower neck. *Am J Surg Pathol.* 1984; 8:501.

82. Armour A, Williamson JM. Ectopic cervical hamartomatous thymoma showing extensive myoid differentiation. *J Laryngol Otol.* 1993; 107:155.

83. Ferlito A, Devaney KO. Developmental lesions of the head and neck: Terminology and biologic behavior. *Ann Otol Rhinol Laryngol.* 1995; 104:913.

84. Jordan RB, Gauderer MWL. Cervical teratomas: An analysis, literature review and proposed classification. *J Pediatr Surg.* 1988; 23:583.

85. Abamayor E, Newman A, Bergstrom L, et al. Teratomas of the head and neck in childhood. *Laryngoscope.* 1984; 94: 1489.

86. Ward RF, April M. Teratomas of the head and neck. *Otolaryngol Clin North Am.* 1989; 22:621.

87. Colton JJ, Batsakis JG, Work WP. Teratomas of the neck in adults. *Arch Otolaryngol.* 1978; 104:271.

88. Batsakis JG, Littler ER, Oberman HA. Teratomas of the neck—a clinicopathologic appraisal. *Arch Otolaryngol.* 1964; 79:619.

89. Ward RF, April M. Teratomas of the head and neck. *Otolaryngol Clin North Am.* 1989; 22:621.

90. Kountakis SE, Minorri AM, Maillard A, Stierberg CM. Teratomas of the head and neck. *Am J Otolaryngol.* 1994; 15:292.

91. Carney JA, Thompson DP, Johnson CL, Lynn HB. Teratomas in children: Clinical and pathologic aspects. *J Pediatr Surg.* 1972; 7:271.

92. Tapper D, Lack EE. Teratomas in infancy and childhood: A

54-year experience at the Children's Hospital Medical Center. *Am J Clin Pathol.* 1983; 198:398.

93. Jordan RB, Gauderer MW. Cervical teratomas: An analysis. Literature review and proposed classification. *J Pediatr Surg.* 1988; 23:583.

94. Rothschild MA, Catalano P, Urken M, et al. Evaluation and management of congenital cervical teratoma—case report and review. *Arch Otolaryngol Head Neck Surg.* 1994; 120:444.

95. Azizkhan RG, Haase GM, Applebaum H, et al. Diagnosis, management, and outcome of cervicofacial teratomas in neonates: A Children's Cancer Group study. *J Pediatr Surg.* 1995; 30:312.

96. Bill AH, Sumner DS. A unified concept of lymphangioma and cystic hygroma. *Surg Gynecol Obstet.* 1965; 120:79.

97. Saijo M, Munro IR, Mancer K. Lymphangioma—a long-term follow-up study. *Plast Reconstr Surg.* 1975; 56:642.

98. Emery PJ, Bailey CM, Evans JNG. Cystic hygroma of the head and neck: A review of 37 cases. *J Laryngol Otol.* 1984; 98:613.

99. Bowman CA, Witte MH, Witte CL, et al. Cystic hygroma reconsidered: Hamartoma or neoplasm? Primary culture of an endothelial cell line from a massive cervicomediastinal hygroma with bony lymphangiomatosis. *Lymphology.* 1984; 17:15.

100. Carr RF, Ochs RH, Ritter DA, et al. Fetal cystic hygroma and Turner's syndrome. *Am J Dis Child.* 1986; 140:580.

101. Langer JC, Fitzgerald PG, Desa D, et al. Cervical cystic hygroma in the fetus: Clinical spectrum and outcome. *J Pediatr Surg.* 1990; 25:58.

102. Glasson MJ, Taylor SF. Cervical, cervicomediastinal and intrathoracic lymphangioma. *Prog Pediatr Surg.* 1991; 27:62.

103. Ricciardelli E, Richardson MA. Cervicofacial cystic hygroma: Patterns of recurrence and management of difficult cases. *Arch Otolaryngol Head Neck Surg.* 1991; 117:546.

104. Hellman JR, Prenger EC, Myer CM. Therapeutic alternatives in the treatment of life-threatening vasoformative tumors. *Am J Otolaryngol.* 1992; 13:48.

105. Heether J, Whalen T, Doolin E. Follow-up of complex unresectable lymphangiomas. *Am Surg.* 1994; 60:840.

106. Ikarashi T, Inamura K, Kinmra Y. Cystic lymphangioma and plunging ranula treated by OK-423 therapy: A report of two cases. *Acta Otolaryngol Suppl.* 1994; 511:196.

107. Nussbaum M, Buchwald RP. Adult cystic hygroma. *Am J Otolaryngol.* 1981; 2:159.

108. Karmody CS, Fortson JK, Calcaterra VE. Lymphangiomas of the head and neck in adults. *Otolaryngol Head Neck Surg.* 1982; 90:283.

109. Baer S, Davis J. Cystic hygroma presenting in adulthood. *J Laryngol Otol.* 1989; 103:976.

110. Scally CM, Black JH. Cystic hygroma: Massive recurrence in adult life. *J Laryngol Otol.* 1990; 104:908.

111. Devaney K, Vinh TN, Sweet DE. Skeletal-extraskeletal angiomatosis—a clinicopathologic study of 14 cases; nosologic considerations. *J Bone Joint Surg.* 1994; 76A:878.

112. Enzinger FM, Weiss SW. Benign tumors and tumorlike lesions of blood vessels. In: *Soft Tissue Tumors.* 3rd ed. St. Louis: Mosby; 1995:579.

113. Devaney KO. Vascular neoplasms. In: Ferlito A, ed. *Surgical Pathology of Laryngeal Neoplasms.* London: Chapman & Hall Medical; 1966:341.

114. Garfinkle TJ, Handler SD. Hemangiomas of the head and neck in children—a guide to management. *J Otolaryngol.* 1980; 9:439.

115. Persky MS. Congenital vascular lesions of the head and neck. *Laryngoscope.* 1986; 96:1002.

116. Morgan RF, Horowitz JH, Wanebo HJ, Edgerton MT. Surgical management of vascular malformations of the head and neck. *Am J Surg.* 1986; 152:424.

117. Rossiter JL, Handrix RA, Tom LW, Potsic WP. Intramuscular hemangioma of the head and neck. *Otolaryngol Head Neck Surg.* 1993; 108:18.

118. Jackson IT, Carraeno R, Potparic Z, Hussain K. Hemangiomas, vascular malformations, and lymphovenous malfor-

119. Kane WJ, Morris S, Jackson IT, Woods JE. Significant hemangiomas and vascular malformations of the head and neck: Clinical management and treatment outcomes. *Ann Plast Surg.* 1995; 35:133.

120. Soumekh B, Adams GL, Shapiro RS. Treatment of head and neck hemangiomas with recombinant interferon alpha 2B. *Ann Otol Rhinol Laryngol.* 1996; 105:201.

121. Som PM, Scherl MP, Rao VM, Biller HF. Rare presentations of ordinary lipomas of the head and neck: A review. *Am J Neuroradiol.* 1986; 7:657.

122. Mattel SF, Persky MS. Infiltrating lipoma of the sternocleidomastoid muscle. *Laryngoscope.* 1983; 93:205.

123. Scherl MP, Som PM, Biller HF, Shah K. Recurrent infiltrating lipoma of the head and neck; case report and literature review. *Arch Otolaryngol Head Neck Surg.* 1986; 112:1210.

124. Johnson JT, Curtin HD. Deep neck lipoma. *Ann Otol Rhinol Laryngol.* 1987; 96:472.

125. Enzinger FM, Weiss SW. Benign lipomatous tumors. In: *Soft Tissue Tumors.* 3rd ed. St. Louis: Mosby; 1995:381.

126. Enzinger FM, Harvey DA. Spindle cell lipoma. *Cancer.* 1975; 36:1852.

127. Fletcher CDM, Martin-Bates E. Spindle cell lipoma: A clinicopathological study with some original observations. *Histopathology.* 1987; 11:803.

128. Shmookler BM, Enzinger FM. Pleomorphic lipoma: Benign tumor simulating liposarcoma. *Cancer.* 1979; 47:574.

129. Lawson W, Biller HF. Cervical hibernoma. *Laryngoscope.* 1976; 86:1258.

130. Kristensen S. Cervical hibernoma—review of the literature and a new case. *J Laryngol Otol.* 1985; 99:1055.

131. Abamayor E, McClean PH, Cobb CJ, et al. Hibernomas of the head and neck. *Head Neck Surg.* 1987; 9:362.

132. Hall RE, Kooning J, Hartman L, Del Balso A. Hibernoma—an unusual tumor of adipose tissue. *Oral Surg Oral Med Oral Pathol.* 1988; 66:706.

133. Worsey J, McGuirt W, Carrau RL, Peitzman AB. Hibernoma of the neck: A rare cause of neck mass. *Am J Otolaryngol.* 1994; 15:152.

134. Vellios F, Baez JM, Shumacker HB. Lipoblastomatosis: A tumor of fetal fat different from hibernoma: Report of a case, with observations on the embryogenesis of human adipose tissue. *Am J Pathol.* 1958; 34:1149.

135. Chung EB, Enzinger FM. Benign lipoblastomatosis: An analysis of 35 cases. *Cancer.* 1973; 32:482.

136. Solem BS, Eide TJ, Elverland HH, Mair IW. Benign lipoblastomatosis: A cervical tumor of children. *Int J Pediatr Otorhinolaryngol.* 1981; 3:163.

137. Gammaelgaard N, Jorgensen K, Lund C. Benign lipoblastoma in the neck causing respiratory insufficiency. *Laryngoscope.* 1983; 93:935.

138. Luscher NJ, Prein J, Spiessl B. Lipomatosis of the neck (Madelung's neck). *Ann Plastic Surg.* 1986; 16:502.

139. Plotnicov NA, Babayev TA, Lamberg MA, et al. Madelung's disease (benign symmetrical lipomatosis). *Oral Surg Oral Med Oral Pathol.* 1988; 66:171.

140. John DG, Fung HK, van Hasselt CA, King WW. Multiple symmetrical lipomatosis in the neck. *Eur Arch Otorhinolaryngol.* 1992; 249:277.

141. Kitano H, Nakanishi Y, Takeuchi E, Nagahara K. Multiple symmetrical lipomatosis: No longer just a Mediterranean disease? *J Otorhinolaryngol Relat Spec.* 1994; 56:177.

142. Gross RE, Wolbach SB. Sclerosing hemangiomas—their relationship to dermatofibroma, histiocytoma, xanthoma and to certain pigmented lesions of the skin. *Am J Pathol.* 1943; 19:533.

143. Meister P, Hohne N, Konrad E, Eder M. Fibrous histiocytoma: An analysis of the storiform pattern. *Virch Arch [A].* 1979; 383:31.

144. Li D-F, Iwasaki H, Kikuchi M, et al. Dermatofibroma: superficial fibrous proliferation with reactive histiocytes. *Cancer.* 1994; 74:66.

145. Bielamowicz S, Dauer MS, Chang B, Zimmerman MC. Non-cutaneous benign fibrous histiocytoma of the head and neck. *Otolaryngol Head Neck Surg.* 1995; 113:140.

146. Calonje E, Fletcher CDM. Aneurysmal benign fibrous histio-cytoma: Clinicopathological analysis of 40 cases of a tumour frequently misdiagnosed as a vascular neoplasm. *Histopathology.* 1995; 26:323.

147. Enzinger FM, Weiss SW. Benign fibrohistiocytic tumors. In: *Soft Tissue Tumors.* 3rd ed. St. Louis: Mosby; 1995:293.

148. Devaney KO. Fibrous and histiocytic neoplasms. In: Ferlito A, ed. *Surgical Pathology of Laryngeal Neoplasms.* London: Chapman & Hall Medical; 1966: 295.

149. Enzinger FM. Angiomatoid malignant fibrous histiocytoma—a distinct fibrohistiocytic tumor of children and young adults simulating a vascular neoplasm. *Cancer.* 1979; 44:2147.

150. Costa MJ, Weiss SW. Angiomatoid malignant fibrous histio-cytoma—a follow-up study of 108 cases with evaluation of possible histologic predictors of outcome. *Am J Surg Pathol.* 1990; 14:1126.

151. Smith MEF, Costa MJ, Weiss SW. Evaluation of CD68 and other histiocytic antigens in angiomatoid malignant fibrous histiocytoma. *Am J Surg Pathol.* 1991; 15:757.

152. Fletcher CDM. Angiomatoid "malignant fibrous histiocy-toma": An immunohistochemical study indicative of myoid differentiation. *Hum Pathol.* 1991; 22:563.

153. Di Sant'Agnese PA, Knowles DM. Extracardiac rhabdomyo-ma: A clinicopathologic study and review of the literature. *Cancer.* 1980; 46:780.

154. Gardner DG, Corio RL. Multifocal adult rhabdomyoma. *Oral Surg Oral Med Oral Pathol.* 1983; 56:76.

155. Helliwell TR, Sissons MC, Stoney PJ, Ashworth MT. Immu-nohistochemistry and electron microscopy of head and neck rhabdomyoma. *J Clin Pathol.* 1988; 41:1058.

156. Blaauwgeers JL, Troost D, Dingemans KP, et al. Multifocal rhabdomyoma of the neck—report of a case studied by fine-needle aspiration, light and electron microscopy, histochem-istry, and immunohistochemistry. *Am J Surg Pathol.* 1989; 13: 791.

157. Shemen L, Spiro R, Tuazon R. Multifocal adult rhabdomyo-mas of the head and neck. *Head Neck.* 1992; 14:395.

158. Kapadia SB, Meis JM, Frisman DM, et al. Fetal rhabdomyo-ma of the head and neck: A clinicopathologic and immuno-phenotypic study of 24 cases. *Hum Pathol.* 1993; 24:754.

159. Kapadia SB. Adult rhabdomyoma of the head and neck: A clinicopathologic and immunophenotypic study. *Hum Pathol.* 1993; 24:608.

160. Cleveland DB, Chen SY, Allen CM, et al. Adult rhabdomy-oma—a light microscopic, ultrastructural, virologic, and im-munohistochemical analysis. *Oral Surg Oral Med Oral Pathol.* 1994; 77:147.

161. Box JC, Newman CL, Anastasiades KD, et al. Adult rhabdo-myoma: Presentation as a cervicomediastinal mass (case re-port and review of the literature). *Am Surg.* 1995; 61:271.

162. Enzinger FM, Weiss SW. Rhabdomyoma. In: *Soft Tissue Tu-mors.* 3rd ed. St. Louis: Mosby, 1995:523.

163. Gooder P, Farrington T. Extracranial neurilemmomata of the head and neck. *J Laryngol Otol.* 1980; 94:243.

164. Hawkins DB, Luxford WM. Schwannomas of the head and neck in children. *Laryngoscope.* 1980; 90:1921.

165. Sharaki MM, Talaat M, Hamam SM. Schwannoma of the neck. *Clin Otolaryngol.* 1982; 7:245.

166. Kun Z, Qi DDY, Zhang KH. A comparison between the clinical behavior of neurilemomas in the neck and oral and maxillofacial region. *J Oral Maxillofac Surg.* 1993; 51:769.

167. Oberman HA, Sullenger G. Neurogenous tumors of the head and neck. *Cancer.* 1967; 20:1992.

168. Rosenfeld L, Graves H, Lawrence R. Primary neurogenic tu-mors of the lateral neck. *Ann Surg.* 1968; 167:847.

169. Rice DH, Coulthard SW. Neurogenic tumors of the head and neck in children. *Ann Plast Surg.* 1979; 2:441.

170. Wilson JA, McLaren K, McIntyre MA, et al. Nerve-sheath tumors of the head and neck. *Ear Nose Throat J.* 1988; 67:103.

171. Bruner JM. Peripheral nerve sheath tumors of the head and neck. *Semin Diagn Pathol.* 1987; 4:136.

172. Enzinger FM, Weiss SW. Benign tumors of peripheral nerves. In: *Soft Tissue Tumors.* 3rd ed. St. Louis: Mosby; 1995: 821.

173. Shishibo T, Niimura M, Ohtsuka F, et al. Multiple cutaneous neurilemomas as a skin manifestation of neurilemomatosis. *J Am Acad Dermatol.* 1984; 10:744.

174. Purcell SM, Dixon SL. Schwannomatosis: An unusual variant of neurofibromatosis or a distinct clinical entity? *Arch Derma-tol.* 1989; 125:390.

175. Buenger KM, Porter NC, Dozier SE, et al. Localized multiple neurilemomas of the lower extremity. *Cutis.* 1993; 51:36.

176. Mukherji MM. Giant neurofibroma of the head and neck. *Plast Reconstr Surg.* 1974; 53:184.

177. Griffith BH, Lewis VL, McKinney P. Neurofibromas of the head and neck. *Surg Gynecol Obstet.* 1985; 160:534.

178. Peetermans JF, Van de Heyning PH, Parizel PM, et al. Neu-rofibroma of the vagus nerve in the head and neck: A case report. *Head Neck.* 1991; 13:56.

179. Raffensperger J, Cohen R. Plexiform neurofibromas in child-hood. *J Pediatr Surg.* 1972; 7:144.

180. Holt GR. E.N.T. manifestations of von Recklinghausen's dis-ease. *Laryngoscope.* 1978; 88:1617.

181. Krueger W, Weisberger E, Ballantyne AJ, Goepfert H. Plexi-form neurofibroma of the head and neck. *Am J Surg.* 1979; 138:517.

182. Shoenfeld A, Ovadia J, Edelstein T, Liban E. Malignant cer-vical teratoma of the fetus. *Acta Obstet Gynecol Scand.* 1982; 61:7.

183. Touran T, Applebaum H, Frost DP, et al. Congenital meta-static cervical teratoma: Diagnostic and management consid-erations. *J Pediatr Surg.* 1989; 24:21.

184. Baumann FR, Nerlich A. Metastasizing cervical teratoma of the fetus. *Pediatr Pathol.* 1993; 13:21.

185. Rostad S, Kleinschmidt-DeMasters BK, Manchester DK. Two massive congenital intracranial immature teratomas with neck extension. *Teratology.* 1985; 32:163.

186. Uchiyama M, Iwafuchi M, Naitoh S, et al. A huge immature cervical teratoma in a newborn: Report of a case. *Surg Today.* 1995; 25:737.

187. Colton JJ, Batsakis JG, Work WP. Teratomas of the neck in adults. *Arch Otolaryngol.* 1978; 104:271.

188. Kimler SC, Muth WF. Primary malignant teratoma of the thyroid: Case report and literature review of cervical terato-mas in adults. *Cancer.* 1978; 42:311.

189. Tobey DN, Mangham C. Malignant cervical teratomas. *Oto-laryngol Head Neck Surg.* 1980; 88:215.

190. Batsakis JG, el-Naggar AK, Luna MA. Teratomas of the head and neck with emphasis on malignancy. *Ann Otol Rhinol Laryngol.* 1995; 81:848.

191. Lack EE. Extragonadal germ cell tumors of the head and neck region: Review of 16 cases. *Hum Pathol.* 1985; 16:56.

192. Dehner LP. Gonadal and extragonadal germ cell neoplasia of childhood. *Hum Pathol.* 1983; 14:493.

193. Dehner LP, Mills A, Talerman A, et al. Germ cell neoplasms of head and neck soft tissues: A pathologic spectrum of teratomatous and endodermal sinus tumors. *Hum Pathol.* 1990; 21:309.

194. Devaney KO, Ferlito A. Yolk sac tumors (endodermal sinus tumors) of the head and neck. *Ann Otol Rhinol Laryngol.* 1997; 106:254.

195. Lanza J, Wooh K, Goldberg S, Har-El G. Malignant head and neck germ cell tumours. *J Laryngol Otol.* 1992; 106:268.

196. Nogales FF. Embryologic clues to human yolk sac tumors: A review. *Int J Gynecol Pathol.* 1993; 12:101.

197. O'Sullivan P, Daneman A, Chan HSL, et al. Extragonadal endodermal sinus tumors in children: A review of 24 cases. *Pediatr Radiol.* 1983; 13:249.

198. Stephenson JA, Mayland DM, Kun LE, et al. Malignant germ cell tumors of the head and neck in childhood. *Laryngoscope.* 1989; 99:732.

199. Ulbright TM, Roth LM, Brodhecker CA. Yolk sac differentia-

tion in germ cell tumors—a morphologic study of 50 cases with emphasis on hepatic, enteric, and parietal yolk sac features. *Am J Surg Pathol.* 1986; 10:151.

200. Teilum G. Endodermal sinus tumors of the ovary and testis: Comparative morphogenesis of the so-called mesonephroma ovarii (Schiller) and extraembryonic (yolk sac-allantoic) structures of the rat's placenta. *Cancer.* 1959; 12:1092.

201. Kurman RJ, Norris HJ. Endodermal sinus tumor of the ovary: A clinical and pathologic analysis of 71 cases. *Cancer.* 1976; 38:2404.

202. Bardwil JM, Mocega EE, Butler JJ, Russin DJ. Angiosarcomas of the head and neck region. *Am J Surg.* 1968; 116:548.

203. Hodgkinson DJ, Soule EH, Woods JE. Cutaneous angiosarcoma of the head and neck. *Cancer.* 1979; 44:1106.

204. Cochran JH, Fee WE. Angiosarcoma of the head and neck. *Otolaryngol Head Neck Surg.* 1979; 87:409.

205. Panje WR, Moran WJ, Bostwick DG, Kitt VV. Angiosarcoma of the head and neck: Review of 11 cases. *Laryngoscope.* 1986; 96:1381.

206. Holden CA, Spittle MF, Wilson Jones E. Angiosarcoma of the face and scalp: Prognosis and treatment. *Cancer.* 1987; 59:1046.

207. Mark RJ, Tran LM, Sercarz J, et al. Angiosarcoma of the head and neck—the UCLA experience 1955 through 1990. *Arch Otolaryngol Head Neck Surg.* 1993; 119:973.

208. Lydiatt WM, Shaha AR, Shah JP. Angiosarcoma of the head and neck. *Am J Surg.* 1994; 168:451.

209. Morrison WH, Byers RM, Garden AS, et al. Cutaneous angiosarcoma of the head and neck—a therapeutic dilemma. *Cancer.* 1995; 76:319.

210. Enzinger FM, Weiss SW. Malignant vascular tumors. In: *Soft Tissue Tumors.* 3rd ed. St. Louis: Mosby; 1995:641.

211. Weiss SW. Vascular tumors: A deductive approach to diagnosis. *Surg Pathol.* 1989; 2:185.

212. Delsupehe KG, Jorissen M, Sciot R, et al. Hemangiopericytoma of the head and neck: A report of four cases and a literature review. *Acta Otorhinolaryngol Belg.* 1992; 46:421.

213. Jones DC, Vaughan ED. Haemangiopericytomas of the head and neck: A report of two cases. *Br J Maxillofac Surg.* 1988; 26:107.

214. Volpe AG, Sullivan JG, Chong FK: Aggressive malignant hemangiopericytoma in the neck. *J Surg Oncol.* 1991; 47:136.

215. Kuo T, Sayers CP, Rosai J. Masson's "vegetant intravascular hemangioendothelioma": A lesion often mistaken for angiosarcoma: Study of seventeen cases located in the skin and soft tissues. *Cancer.* 1976; 38:1227.

216. Devaney K. Papillary endothelial hyperplasia of the synovium. *Hum Pathol.* 1993; 24:1264.

217. Kindblom LG, Angervall L, Jarlstedt J. Liposarcoma of the neck: A clinicopathologic study of 4 cases. *Cancer.* 1978; 42:774.

218. Saunders JR, Jacques DA, Casterline PF, et al. Liposarcoma of the head and neck: A review of the literature and addition of four cases. *Cancer.* 1979; 43:162.

219. Otte T, Kleinsasser O. Liposarcoma of the head and neck. *Arch Otorhinolaryngol.* 1981; 232:285.

220. McCulloch TM, Makielski KH, McNutt MA. Head and neck liposarcoma—a histopathologic reevaluation of reported cases. *Arch Otolaryngol Head Neck Surg.* 1992; 118:1045.

221. Stewart MG, Schwartz MR, Alford BR. Atypical and malignant lipomatous lesions of the head and neck. *Arch Otolaryngol Head Neck Surg.* 1994; 120:1151.

222. Golledge J, Fisher C, Rhys-Evans PH. Head and neck liposarcoma. *Cancer.* 1995; 76:1051.

223. Enzinger FM, Weiss SW. Liposarcoma. In: *Soft Tissue Tumors.* 3rd ed. St. Louis: Mosby; 1995:431.

224. Evans HL. Liposarcoma: A study of 55 cases with a reassessment of its classification. *Am J Surg Pathol.* 1979; 3:507.

225. Conley J, Stout AP, Healey MV. Clinicopathologic analysis of eighty-four patients with an original diagnosis of fibrosarcoma of the head and neck. *Am J Surg.* 1967; 114:564.

226. Swain RE, Sessions DG, Ogura JH. Fibrosarcoma of the head and neck: A clinical analysis of forty cases. *Ann Otol.* 1974; 83:439.

227. Frankenthaler R, Ayala AG, Hartwick RW, Goepfert H. Fibrosarcoma of the head and neck. *Laryngoscope.* 1990; 100:799.

228. Mark RJ, Sercarz JA, Tran L, et al. Fibrosarcoma of the head and neck—the UCLA experience. *Arch Otolaryngol Head Neck Surg.* 1991; 117:396.

229. Gartlan MG, Haller JR, Hoffman HT, Dolan KD. Fibrosarcoma of the posterior neck. *Ann Otol Rhinol Laryngol.* 1993; 102:820.

230. Greager JA, Reichard K, Campana JP, Das Gupta TK. Fibrosarcoma of the head and neck. *Am J Surg.* 1994; 167:437.

231. Enzinger FM, Weiss SW. Fibrosarcoma. In: *Soft Tissue Tumors.* 3rd ed. St. Louis: Mosby; 1995:269.

232. Blitzer A, Lawson W, Biller HF. Malignant fibrous histiocytoma of the head and neck. *Laryngoscope.* 1977; 87:1479.

234. Ogura JH, Toomey JM, Setzen M, Sobol S. Malignant fibrous histiocytoma of the head and neck. *Laryngoscope.* 1980; 90:1429.

235. Barnes L, Kanbour A. Malignant fibrous histiocytoma of the head and neck—a report of 12 cases. *Arch Otolaryngol Head Neck Surg.* 1988; 114:1149.

236. Singh B, Santos V, Guffin TN, et al. Giant cell variant of malignant fibrous histiocytoma of the head and neck. *J Laryngol Otol.* 1991; 105:1079.

237. Singh B, Shaha A, Har-El G. Malignant fibrous histiocytoma of the head and neck. *J Craniomaxillofac Surg.* 1993; 21:262.

238. Enzinger FM, Weiss SW. Malignant fibrohistiocytic tumors. In: *Soft Tissue Tumors.* 3rd ed. St. Louis: Mosby; 1995: 351.

239. Hutcherson RW, Jenkins HA, Canalis RF, et al. Neurogenic sarcoma of the head and neck. *Arch Otolaryngol.* 1979; 105:267.

240. Martin G, Kleinsasser O. Neurogenic sarcomas of the neck in neurofibromatosis. *Arch Otorhinolaryngol.* 1981; 232:273.

241. Gullane PJ, Gilbert RW, van Nostrand AW, Slinger RP. Malignant schwannoma in the head and neck. *J Otolaryngol.* 1985; 14:171.

242. Chaudhuri B, Ronan SG, Manaligod JR. Angiosarcoma arising in a plexiform neurofibroma: A case report. *Cancer.* 1980; 46:605.

243. Bailet JW, Abemayor E, Andrews JC, et al. Malignant nerve sheath tumors of the head and neck: A combined experience from two university hospitals. *Laryngoscope.* 1991; 101:1044.

244. Enzinger FM, Weiss SW. Malignant tumors of the peripheral nerves. In: *Soft Tissue Tumors.* 3rd ed. St. Louis: Mosby; 1995: 889.

245. Ducatman BS, Scheithauer BW, Piepgras DG, et al. Malignant peripheral nerve sheath tumors: A clinicopathologic study of 120 cases. *Cancer.* 1986; 57:2006.

246. Harrison E, Black BM, Devine KD. Synovial sarcoma primary in the neck. *Arch Pathol.* 1961; 71:137–141.

247. Jacobs LA, Weaver AW. Synovial sarcoma of the head and neck. *Am J Surg.* 1974; 128:527.

248. Liebman EP, Harwick RD, Ronis ML, et al. Synovial sarcoma of the cervical area. *Laryngoscope.* 1984; 84:889.

249. Mitcherling JJ, Collins EM, Tomich CE, et al. Synovial sarcoma of the neck: Report of a case. *J Oral Surg.* 1976; 34:64.

250. Roth JA, Enzinger FM, Tannenbaum M. Synovial sarcoma of the neck: Follow-up study of 24 cases. *Cancer.* 1975; 35:1243.

251. Mamelle G, Richard J, Luboiski B, et al. Synovial sarcoma of the head and neck: An account of four cases and review of the literature. *Eur J Surg Oncol.* 1986; 12:347.

252. Bukachevsky RP, Pincus RL, Shechtman FG, et al. Synovial sarcoma of the head and neck. *Head Neck.* 1992; 14:44.

253. Carillo R, Rodriguez-Peralto JL, Batsakis JG. Synovial sarcomas of the head and neck. *Ann Otol Rhinol Laryngol.* 1992; 101:367.

254. Amble FR, Olsen KD, Nascimento AG, Foote RL. Head and neck synovial sarcoma. *Otolaryngol Head Neck Surg.* 1992; 107:631.

255. Miloro M, Quinn PD, Stewart JC. Monophasic spindle cell synovial sarcoma of the head and neck: Report of two cases and review of the literature. *J Oral Maxillofac Surg.* 1994; 52:309.

256. Robinson DL, Destain S, Hinton DR. Synovial sarcoma of the

neck: Radiographic findings with a review of the literature. *Am J Otolaryngol.* 1994; 15:46.

257. Lombardi LJ, Cleri DJ, Horten BC, et al. Synovial sarcoma of the occipital region of the neck. *Am J Orthop.* 1995; 24:553.

258. Enzinger FM, Weiss SW. Synovial sarcoma. In: *Soft Tissue Tumors.* 3rd ed. St. Louis: Mosby; 1995:757.

259. Chan JKC, Rosai J. Tumors of the neck showing thymic or related branchial pouch differentiation: A unifying concept. *Hum Pathol.* 1991; 22:349.

260. Spector RA, Travis LW, Smith J. Alveolar soft part sarcoma of the head and neck. *Laryngoscope.* 1979; 89:1301.

261. Simmons WB, Haggerty HS, Ngan B, Anonsen CK. Alveolar soft part sarcoma of the head and neck—a disease of children and young adults. *Int J Pediatr Otorhinolaryngol.* 1989; 17:139.

262. Auerbach HE, Brooks JJ. Alveolar soft part sarcoma: A clinicopathologic and immunohistochemical study. *Cancer.* 1987; 60:66.

263. Lieberman PH, Brennan MF, Kimmel M, et al. Alveolar soft part sarcoma: A clinicopathologic study of half a century. *Cancer.* 1989; 63:1.

264. Matsuno Y, Mukai K, Itabashi M, et al. Alveolar soft part sarcoma—a clinicopathologic and immunohistochemical study of 12 cases. *Acta Pathol. Jpn.* 1990; 40:199.

265. Rosai J, Dias P, Parham DM, et al. MyoD1 protein expression in alveolar soft part sarcoma as confirmatory evidence of its skeletal muscle nature. *Am J Surg Pathol.* 1991; 15:974.

266. Foschini MP, Eusebi V. Alveolar soft-part sarcoma: A new type of rhabdomyosarcoma? *Semin Diagn Pathol.* 1994; 11:58.

267. France CJ, Lucas R. The management and prognosis of metastatic neoplasms of the neck with an unknown primary. *Am J Surg.* 1963; 106:835.

268. Barrie JR, Knapper WH, Strong EW. Cervical nodal metastases of unknown origin. *Am J Surg.* 1970; 120:466.

269. Butler JJ, Howe CD, Johnson DE. Enlargement of the supraclavicular lymph nodes as the initial sign of prostatic carcinoma. *Cancer.* 1971; 27:1055.

270. Batsakis JG, McBurney TA. Metastatic neoplasms to the head and neck. *Surgery Gynecol Obstet.* 1971; 133:673.

271. MacComb WS. Diagnosis and treatment of metastatic cervical cancerous nodes from an unknown primary site. *Am J Surg.* 1972; 124:441.

272. Miyamoto R, Helmus C. Hypernephroma metastatic to the head and neck. *Laryngoscope.* 1973; 83:898.

273. Jesse RH, Perez CA, Fletcher GH. Cervical lymph node metastasis: Unknown primary cancer. *Cancer.* 1973; 31:854.

274. Frieo MP, Deihl WH, Brownson RJ, et al. Cervical metastasis from an unknown primary. *Ann Otol.* 1975; 84:152.

275. Davis RS, Flynn MB, Moore C. An unusual presentation of carcinoma of the lungs: 26 patients with cervical node metastases. *J Surg Oncol.* 1977; 9:503.

276. Thompson LDR, Heffner DK. The clinical importance of cystic squamous cell carcinomas in the neck. A study of 136 cases. *Cancer.* 1998; 82:944.

277. Martin H, Morfit MH, Ehrilich G. The case for branchiogenic cancer (malignant branchioma). *Ann Surg.* 1950; 132:867.

278. Batsakis JG, McBurney TA. Metastatic neoplasms to the head and neck. *Surg Gynecol Obstet.* 1971; 133:673.

279. Compagno J, Hyamns VJ, Safavian M. Does branchiogenic carcinoma really exist? *Arch Pathol Lab Med.* 1976; 100: 311.

280. Paccioni D, Negro F, Valente G, Bussolati G. Epstein-Barr virus by in situ hybridization in fine-needle aspiration biopsies. *Diagn Mol Pathol.* 1994; 3:100.

281. Luna MA. The occult primary and metastatic tumors to and from the head and neck. In: Barnes L, ed. *Surgical Pathology of the Head and Neck.* New York: Marcel Dekker; 1985: 1211.

282. Schwarz D, Hamberger AD, Jesse RH. The managment of squamous cell carcinoma in cervical lymph nodes in the clinical absence of a primary lesion by combined surgery and radiotherapy. *Cancer.* 1981; 48:1746.

283. Shenoy AM, Hasan S, Nayak U, et al. Neck metastasis from an occult primary—the Kiwai experience. *Indian J Cancer.* 1992; 29:203.

284. Shah JP, Lydiatt W. Treatment of cancer of the head and neck. *Ca Cancer J Clin.* 1995; 45:352.

285. Cerezo L, Millan I, Torre A, Aragon G, Otero J. Prognostic factors for survival and tumor control in cervical lymph node metastases from head and neck cancers. A multivariate analysis. *Cancer.* 1992; 69:1224.

286. Olsen KD, Caruso M, Foote RL, et al. Primary head and neck cancer. Histopathologic predictors of recurrence after neck dissection in patients with lymph node involvement. *Arch Otolaryngol Head Neck Surg.* 1994; 120:1370.

287. Snow GB, Annyas AA, Van Slooten EA, Bartelink H, Hart AA. Prognostic factors of neck node metastasis. *Clin Otolaryngol.* 1982; 7:185.

288. Kalnins IK, Leonard AG, Sako K, Razack MS, Shedd DP. Correlation between prognosis and degree of lymph node involvement in carcinoma of the oral cavity. *Am J Surg.* 1977; 134:450.

289. Johnson JT, Myers EN, Bedetti CD, Barnes L, Schramm VL, Thearle PB. Cervical lymph node metastasis: Incidence and implications of extracapsular carcinoma. *Arch Otolaryngol.* 1985; 111:534.

290. Snyderman NL, Johnson JT, Schramm VL, Myers EN, Bedetti CD, Thearle PB. Extracapsular spread of carcinomas in cervical lymph nodes: Impact upon survival in patients with carcinomas of the supraglottic larynx. *Cancer.* 1985; 56:1597.

291. Richard JM, Sancho-Garnier H, Michaeu C, Saravane D, Cachin Y. Prognostic factors in cervical lymph node metastasis in upper respiratory and digestive tract carcinomas: Study of 1713 cases during a 15-year period. *Laryngoscope.* 1987; 97:97.

292. Leemans CR, Tiwari R, van der Waal I, Karim ABMF, Nauta JJP, Snow GB. The efficacy of comprehensive neck dissection with or without postoperative radiotherapy in nodal metastases of squamous cell carcinoma of the upper respiratory and digestive tracts. *Laryngoscope.* 1990; 100:1194.

293. Hirabayashi H, Koshii K, Kohei U, et al. Extracapsular spread of squamous cell carcinoma in neck lymph nodes: Prognostic factor of laryngeal cancer. *Laryngoscope.* 1991; 101: 502.

294. Esclamado RM, Carroll WR. Extracapsular spread and the perineural extension of squamous cell cancer in the cervical plexus. *Arch Otolaryngol Head Neck Surg.* 1992; 118:1157.

295. Leemans CR, Tiwari R, Nauta JJP, van der Waal I, Snow GB. Regional lymph node involvement and its significance in the development of distant metastases in head and neck carcinoma. *Cancer.* 1993; 71:452.

296. Leemans CR, Tiwari R, Nauta JJP, van der Waal I, Snow GB. Recurrence at the primary site in head and neck cancer and the significance of neck lymph node metastases as a prognostic factor. *Cancer.* 1994; 73:187.

Lip and Oral Cavity

STAGE GROUPING

0	Tis	N0	M0
I	T1	N0	M0
II	T2	N0	M0
III	T3	N0	M0
	T1	N1	M0
	T2	N1	M0
	T3	N1	M0
IVA	T4	N0	M0
	T4	N1	M0
	Any T	N2	M0
IVB	Any T	N3	M0
IVC	Any T	Any N	M1

DEFINITIONS

Primary Tumor (T)

TX   Primary tumor cannot be assessed

T0   No evidence of primary tumor

Tis   Carcinoma in situ

T1   Tumor 2 cm or less in greatest dimension

T2   Tumor more than 2 cm but not more than 4 cm in greatest dimension

T3   Tumor more than 4 cm in greatest dimension

T4   Lip: Tumor invades adjacent structures (e.g., through cortical bone, inferior alveolar nerve, floor of mouth, skin of face)

T4   Oral cavity: Tumor invades adjacent structures (e.g., through cortical bone, into deep [extrinsic] muscle of tongue, maxillary sinus, skin. Superficial erosion alone of bone/tooth socket by gingival primary is not sufficient to classify as T4.)

Regional Lymph Nodes (N)

NX   Regional lymph nodes cannot be assessed

N0   No regional lymph node metastasis

N1   Metastasis in a single ipsilateral lymph node, 3 cm or less in greatest dimension

N2   Metastasis in a single ipsilateral lymph node, more than 3 cm but not more than 6 cm in greatest dimension; or in multiple ipsilateral lymph nodes, none more than 6 cm in greatest dimension; or in bilateral or contralateral lymph nodes, none more than 6 cm in greatest dimension

N2a   Metastasis in a single ipsilateral lymph node more than 3 cm but not more than 6 cm in greatest dimension

N2b   Metastasis in multiple ipsilateral lymph nodes, none more than 6 cm in greatest dimension

N2c   Metastasis in bilateral or contralateral lymph nodes, none more than 6 cm in greatest dimension

N3   Metastasis in a lymph node more than 6 cm in greatest dimension

Distant Metastasis (M)

MX   Distant metastasis cannot be assessed

M0   No distant metastasis

M1   Distant metastasis

* From *AJCC Cancer Staging Manual*. 5th ed. Philadelphia: Lippincott-Williams & Wilkins; 1995:29, 37–39, 45, 46, 51, 52, 57, 58, 63, 64, with permission of the American Joint Committee on Cancer.

Pharynx (Including Base of Tongue, Soft Palate, and Uvula)

STAGE GROUPING: NASOPHARYNX

0	Tis	N0	M0
I	T1	N0	M0
IIA	T2a	N0	M0
IIB	T1	N1	M0
	T2	N1	M0
	T2a	N1	M0
	T2b	N0, N1	M0
III	T1	N2	M0
	T2a, T2b	N2	M0
	T3	N0, N1, N2	M0
IVA	T4	N0, N1, N2	M0
IVB	Any T	N3	M0
IVC	Any T	Any N	M1

STAGE GROUPING: OROPHARYNX, HYPOPHARYNX

0	Tis	N0	M0
I	T1	N0	M0
II	T2	N0	M0
III	T3	N0	M0
	T1	N1	M0
	T2	N1	M0
	T3	N1	M0
IVA	T4	N0	M0
	T4	N1	M0
	Any T	N2	M0
IVB	Any T	N3	M0
IVC	Any T	Any N	M1

DEFINITIONS

Primary Tumor (T)

TX   Primary tumor cannot be assessed
T0   No evidence of primary tumor
Tis   Carcinoma in situ

Nasopharynx

T1   Tumor confined to the nasopharynx
T2   Tumor extends to soft tissues of oropharynx and/or nasal fossa
    T2a   without parapharyngeal extension
    T2b   with parapharyngeal extension
T3   Tumor invades bony structures and/or paranasal sinuses
T4   Tumor with intracranial extension and/or involvement of cranial nerves, infratemporal fossa, hypopharynx, or orbit

Oropharynx

T1   Tumor 2 cm or less in greatest dimension
T2   Tumor more than 2 cm but not more than 4 cm in greatest dimension
T3   Tumor more than 4 cm in greatest dimension
T4   Tumor invades adjacent structures (e.g., pterygoid muscle[s], mandible, hard palate, deep muscle of tongue, larynx)

Hypopharynx

T1   Tumor limited to one subsite of hypopharynx and 2 cm or less in greatest dimension
T2   Tumor involves more than one subsite of hypopharynx or an adjacent site, or measures more than 2 cm but not more than 4 cm in greatest diameter without fixation of hemilarynx
T3   Tumor measures more than 4 cm in greatest dimension or with fixation of hemilarynx
T4   Tumor invades adjacent structures (e.g., thyroid/cricoid cartilage, carotid artery, soft tissues of neck, prevertebral fascia/muscles, thyroid and/or esophagus)

Regional Lymph Nodes (N): Nasopharynx

The distribution and the prognostic impact of regional lymph nodes spread from nasopharynx cancer, particularly of the undifferentiated type, is different from that of other head and neck mucosal cancers and justifies use of a different N classification scheme.

NX   Regional lymph nodes cannot be assessed
N0   No regional lymph node metastasis
N1   Unilateral metastasis in lymph node(s), 6 cm or less in greatest dimension, above the supraclavicular fossa
N2   Bilateral metastasis in lymph node(s), 6 cm or less in greatest dimension, above the supraclavicular fossa
N3   Metastasis in a lymph node(s)
    N3a   greater than 6 cm in dimension
    N3b   in the supraclavicular fossa

Regional Lymph Nodes (N): Oropharynx and Hypopharynx

NX   Regional lymph nodes cannot be assessed
N0   No regional lymph node metastasis
N1   Metastasis in a single ipsilateral lymph node, 3 cm or less in greatest dimension
N2   Metastasis in a single ipsilateral lymph node, more than 3 cm but not more than 6 cm in greatest dimension, or in multiple ipsilateral lymph nodes, none more than 6 cm in greatest dimension, or in bilateral or contralateral lymph nodes, none more than 6 cm in greatest dimension

   N2a   Metastasis in a single ipsilateral lymph node more than 3 cm but not more than 6 cm in greatest dimension
   N2b   Metastasis in multiple ipsilateral lymph nodes, none more than 6 cm in greatest dimension
   N2c   Metastasis in bilateral or contralateral lymph nodes, none more than 6 cm in greatest dimension
N3   Metastasis in a lymph node more than 6 cm in greatest dimension

Distant Metastasis (M)

MX   Distant metastasis cannot be assessed
M0   No distant metastasis
M1   Distant metastasis

Histopathologic Type

The predominant cancer type is squamous cell carcinoma for all pharyngeal sites. Nonepithelial tumors such as those of lymphoid tissue, soft tissue, bone, and cartilage are not included in this system.

Histopathologic Grade (G): Oropharynx, Hypopharynx

GX   Grade cannot be assessed
G1   Well differentiated
G2   Moderately differentiated
G3   Poorly differentiated

Larynx

STAGE GROUPING

0	Tis	N0	M0
I	T1	N0	M0
II	T2	N0	M0
III	T3	N0	M0
	T1	N1	M0
	T2	N1	M0
	T3	N1	M0
IVA	T4	N0	M0
	T4	N1	M0
	Any T	N2	M0
IVB	Any T	N3	M0
IVC	Any T	Any N	M1

DEFINITIONS

Primary Tumor (T)

TX   Primary tumor cannot be assessed
T0   No evidence of primary tumor
Tis   Carcinoma in situ

Supraglottis

T1   Tumor limited to one subsite of supraglottis with normal vocal cord mobility
T2   Tumor invades mucosa of more than one adjacent subsite of supraglottis or glottis or region outside the supraglottis (e.g., mucosa of base of tongue, vallecula, medial wall of pyriform sinus) without fixation of the larynx
T3   Tumor limited to larynx with vocal cord fixation and/or invades any of the following: postcricoid area, pre-epiglottic tissues
T4   Tumor extends through the thyroid cartilage, and/or extends into soft tissues of the neck, thyroid, and/or esophagus

Glottis

T1   Tumor limited to vocal cord(s) (may involve anterior or posterior commissures) with normal mobility
   T1a   Tumor limited to one vocal cord
   T1b   Tumor involves both vocal cords
T2   Tumor extends to supraglottis and/or subglottis, and/or with impaired vocal cord mobility

T3   Tumor limited to the larynx with vocal cord fixation
T4   Tumor invades through thyroid cartilage and/or to other tissues beyond the larynx, e.g., trachea, soft tissues of neck, including thyroid, pharynx

Subglottis

T1   Tumor limited to the subglottis
T2   Tumor extends to vocal cord(s) with normal or impaired mobility
T3   Tumor limited to larynx with vocal cord fixation
T4   Tumor invades through cricoid or thyroid cartilage and/or extends to other tissues beyond the larynx (e.g., trachea, soft tissues of neck, including thyroid, esophagus)

Regional Lymph Nodes (N)

NX   Regional lymph nodes cannot be assessed
N0   No regional lymph node metastasis
N1   Metastasis in a single ipsilateral lymph node, 3 cm or less in greatest dimension
N2   Metastasis in a single ipsilateral lymph node, more than 3 cm but not more than 6 cm in greatest dimension, or multiple ipsilateral lymph nodes, none more than 6 cm in greatest dimension, or bilateral or contralateral lymph nodes, none more than 6 cm in greatest dimension
   N2a   Metastasis in a single ipsilateral lymph node more than 3 cm but not more than 6 cm in greatest dimension
   N2b   Metastasis in multiple ipsilateral lymph nodes, none more than 6 cm in greatest dimension
   N2c   Metastasis in bilateral or contralateral lymph nodes, none more than 6 cm in greatest dimension
N3   Metastasis in a lymph node more than 6 cm in greatest dimension

Distant Metastasis (M)

MX   Distant metastasis cannot be assessed
M0   No distant metastasis
M1   Distant metastasis

Histopathologic Type

The predominant cancer type is squamous cell carcinoma. Nonepithelial tumors such as those of lymphoid tissue, soft tissue, bone and cartilage are not included in this system.

Histopathologic Grade (G)

GX   Grade cannot be assessed
G1   Well differentiated
G2   Moderately differentiated
G3   Poorly differentiated

Paranasal Sinuses

STAGE GROUPING

0	Tis	N0	M0
I	T1	N0	M0
II	T2	N0	M0
III	T3	N0	M0
	T1	N1	M0
	T2	N1	M0
	T3	N1	M0
IVA	T4	N0	M0
	T4	N1	M0
IVB	Any T	N2	M0
	Any T	N3	M0
IVC	Any T	Any N	M1

DEFINITIONS

Primary Tumor (T)

TX   Primary tumor cannot be assessed
T0   No evidence of primary tumor
Tis   Carcinoma in situ

Maxillary Sinus

T1   Tumor limited to the antral mucosa with no erosion or destruction of bone
T2   Tumor causing bone erosion or destruction, except for the posterior antral wall, including extension into the hard palate and/or the middle nasal meatus
T3   Tumor invades any of the following: bone of the posterior wall of maxillary sinus, subcutaneous tissues, skin of cheek, floor or medial wall of orbit, infratemporal fossa, pterygoid plates, ethmoid sinuses
T4   Tumor invades orbital contents beyond the floor or medial wall including any of the following: the orbital apex, cribiform plate, base of skull, nasopharynx, sphenoid, frontal sinuses

Ethmoid Sinus

T1   Tumor confined to the ethmoid with or without bone erosion
T2   Tumor extends into the nasal cavity
T3   Tumor extends to the anterior orbit and/or maxillary sinus

T4   Tumor with intracranial extension, orbital extension including apex, involving sphenoid and/or frontal sinus and/or skin of external nose

Regional Lymph Nodes (N)

NX   Regional lymph nodes cannot be assessed
N0   No regional lymph node metastasis
N1   Metastasis in a single ipsilateral lymph node, 3 cm or less in greatest dimension
N2   Metastasis in a single ipsilateral lymph node, more than 3 but not more than 6 cm in greatest dimension, or in multiple ipsilateral lymph nodes, none more than 6 cm in greatest dimension, or in bilateral or contralateral lymph nodes, none more than 6 cm in greatest dimension
N2a   Metastasis in a single ipsilateral lymph node more than 3 cm but not more than 6 cm in greatest dimension
N2b   Metastasis in multiple ipsilateral lymph nodes, none more than 6 cm in greatest dimension
N2c   Metastasis in bilateral or contralateral lymph nodes, none more than 6 cm in greatest dimension
N3   Metastasis in a lymph node more than 6 cm in greatest dimension

Distant Metastasis (M)

MX   Distant metastasis cannot be assessed
M0   No distant metastasis
M1   Distant metastasis

Histopathologic Type

The predominant cancer is squamous cell carcinoma. Nonepithelial tumors such as those of lymphoid tissue, soft tissue, bone and cartilage are not included in this system.

Histopathologic Grade (G)

GX   Grade cannot be assessed
G1   Well differentiated
G2   Moderately differentiated
G3   Poorly differentiated

Major Salivary Glands (Parotid, Submandibular, and Sublingual)

STAGE GROUPING

I	T1	N0	M0
	T2	N0	M0
II	T3	N0	M0
III	T1	N1	M0
	T2	N1	M0
IV	T4	N0	M0
	T3	N1	M0
	T4	N1	M0
	Any T	N2	M0
	Any T	N3	M0
	Any T	Any N	M1

DEFINITIONS

Primary Tumor (T)

TX   Primary tumor cannot be assessed
T0   No evidence of primary tumor
T1   Tumor 2 cm or less in greatest dimension without extraparenchymal extension
T2   Tumor more than 2 cm but not more than 4 cm in greatest dimension without extraparenchymal extension
T3   Tumor having extraparenchymal extension without seventh nerve involvement and/ or more than 4 cm but not more than 6 cm in greatest dimension
T4   Tumor invades base of skull, seventh nerve, and/or exceeds 6 cm in greatest dimension

Regional Lymph Nodes (N)

NX   Regional lymph nodes cannot be assessed
N0   No regional lymph node metastasis
N1   Metastasis in a single ispilateral lymph node, 3 cm or less in greatest dimension
N2   Metastasis in a single ipsilateral lymph node, more than 3 cm but not more than 6 cm in greatest dimension, or in multiple ipsilateral lymph nodes, none more than 6 cm in greatest dimension or in bilateral or in contralateral lymph nodes, none more than 6 cm in greatest dimension

N2a   Metastasis in a single ipsilateral lymph node more than 3 cm but not more than 6 cm in greatest dimension
N2b   Metastasis in multiple ipsilateral lymph nodes, none more than 6 cm in greatest dimension
N2c   Metastasis in bilateral or contralateral lymph nodes, none more than 6 cm in greatest dimension
N3   Metastasis in a lymph node more than 6 cm in greatest dimension

Distant Metastasis (M)

MX   Distant metastasis cannot be assessed
M0   No distant metastasis
M1   Distant metastasis

Histopathologic Type

The suggested histopathologic typing is that proposed by the World Health Organization. Other more rare entities also exist and are classified in the WHO fascicle.

Acinic cell carcinoma
Adenoid cystic carcinoma
Salivary duct carcinoma
Carcinoma ex pleomorphic adenoma
Adenocarcinoma
Mucoepidermoid carcinoma
Polymorphous low-grade adenocarcinoma (terminal duct adenocarcinoma).

Histopathologic Grade (G)

Histologic grading is applicable only to some types of salivary gland cancer: mucoepidermoid, adenoid cystic, and acinic cell carcinomas. In other instances the histologic type defines the grade.

Thyroid Gland

STAGE GROUPING

Separate stage groupings are recommended for papillary, follicular, medullary, or undifferentiated (anaplastic)

PAPILLARY OR FOLLICULAR
Under 45 years

Stage I	Any T, Any N, M0
Stage II	Any T, Any N, M1

45 Years and Over

Stage I	T1, N0, M0
Stage II	T2, N0, M0
	T3, N0, M0
Stage III	T4, N0, M0
	Any T, N1, M0
Stage IV	Any T, Any N, M1

MEDULLARY

Stage I	T1	N0	M0
Stage II	T2	N0	M0
	T3	N0	M0
	T4	N0	M0
Stage III	Any T	N1	M0
Stage IV	Any T	Any N	M1

UNDIFFERENTIATED (ANAPLASTIC)

All cases are Stage IV

Stage IV	Any T	Any N	Any M

DEFINITIONS

Primary Tumor (T)

All categories may be subdivided: (a) solitary tumor; (b) multifocal tumor (the largest determines the classification)

TX	Primary tumor cannot be assessed
T0	No evidence of primary tumor
T1	Tumor 1 cm or less in greatest dimension limited to the thyroid
T2	Tumor more than 1 cm but not more than 4 cm in greatest dimension limited to the thyroid
T3	Tumor more than 4 cm in greatest dimension limited to the thyroid
T4	Tumor of any size extending beyond the thyroid capsule

Regional Lymph Nodes (N)

Regional nodes are the cervical and upper mediastinal lymph nodes

NX	Regional lymph nodes cannot be assessed
N0	No regional lymph node metastasis
N1	Regional lymph node metastasis
N1a	Metastasis in ipsilateral cervical lymph node(s)
N1b	Metastasis in bilateral, midline, or contralateral cervical or mediastinal lymph node(s)

Distant Metastasis (M)

MX	Distant metastasis cannot be assessed
M0	No distant metastasis
M1	Distant metastasis

Histopathologic Type

There are four major histopathologic types:

Papillary carcinoma (including those with follicular foci)
Follicular carcinoma
Medullary carcinoma
Undifferentiated (anaplastic) carcinoma

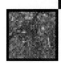

Index

Note: Page numbers in *italics* refer to illustrations; page numbers followed by t refer to tables.

ISBN 0-443-07558-1

90071

9 780443 075582